Advances in Geology of the Porphyry Copper Deposits

Southwestern North America

Contributing Authors

Daniel M. Aiken
James A. Anderson
Kent D. Aveson
Norman G. Banks
Charles F. Barter
Richard E. Beane
David W. Blake
Maurice A. Chaffee
David S. Cook
Henry R. Cornwall
Robert B. Cummings
Peter G. Dunn
Marco T. Einaudi
Paul Gilmour
Frederick T. Graybeal
Tom L. Heidrick
Louis J. Jansen
James L. Kelly
John R. King
Joseph Kolessar
Randolph A. Koski
Edward L. Kretschmer
Jackson M. Langton
Philip W. Nason
Denis L. Norton
Allen V. Shaw
Ted G. Theodore
Spencer R. Titley
Luis A. Vega
Richard J. West
William H. Wilkinson, Jr.
Sidney A. Williams

Advances in Geology of the Porphyry Copper Deposits

Southwestern North America

Spencer R. Titley, *Editor*

THE UNIVERSITY OF ARIZONA PRESS / TUCSON, ARIZONA

About the Editor . . .

Spencer R. Titley, professor of geology and geosciences, has taught at the University of Arizona since 1960. He has worked for industry as employee and consultant and has carried out research and taught in the field of mineral deposits and economic geology. In 1975 he was awarded the Medal for Distinguished Achievement in Mineral Engineering by the Colorado School of Mines. He has served on the Editorial Board of *Economic Geology* and has published numerous articles based on research conducted on ore deposits in the Pacific Basin region. He was senior editor of the University of Arizona Press book *Geology of the Porphyry Copper Deposits, Southwestern North America* (1966).

Second printing 1983

THE UNIVERSITY OF ARIZONA PRESS

This book was set in 10/12 Videocomp Times Roman.
Manufactured in the U.S.A.

Government funds have not been involved in this publication.

Library of Congress Cataloging in Publication Data

Advances in geology of the porphyry copper deposits.

Includes bibliographical references and index.
1. Copper ores—North America. 2. Porphyry—North America. I. Titley, Spencer Rowe, 1928-
TN443.A1A38 553.4'3'0979 81-16461

ISBN 0-8165-0730-9 AACR2

In memory of

Enfield Benton Bell

1926–1979

Geologist and Friend

Contents

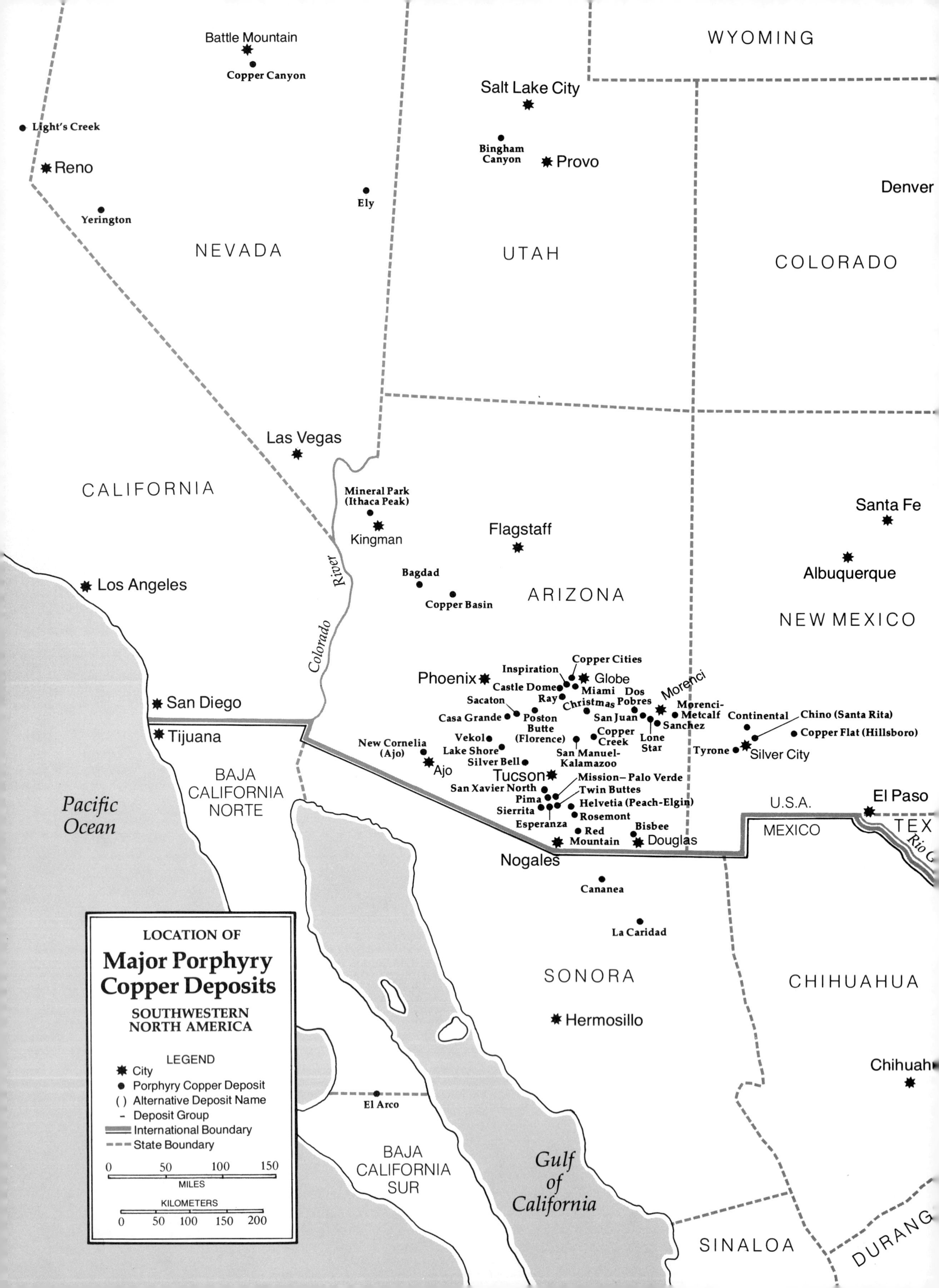
LOCATION OF
Major Porphyry Copper Deposits
SOUTHWESTERN NORTH AMERICA
LEGEND
City
Porphyry Copper Deposit
( ) Alternative Deposit Name
- Deposit Group
International Boundary
State Boundary
0 50 100 150
MILES
KILOMETERS
0 50 100 150 200
Battle Mountain
Copper Canyon
Light's Creek
Reno
Yerington
Ely
NEVADA
WYOMING
Salt Lake City
Bingham Canyon
Provo
UTAH
Denver
COLORADO
Las Vegas
CALIFORNIA
Mineral Park (Ithaca Peak)
Kingman
Flagstaff
Santa Fe
Albuquerque
Los Angeles
Colorado River
Bagdad
Copper Basin
ARIZONA
NEW MEXICO
Copper Cities
Inspiration
Phoenix
Globe
Castle Dome
Miami
Dos Pobres
Morenci
Ray
Sacaton
Christmas
Morenci-Metcalf
Continental
Chino (Santa Rita)
Casa Grande
Poston Butte (Florence)
San Juan
Sanchez
Copper Flat (Hillsboro)
Vekol
Copper Creek
Lone Star
Tyrone
Silver City
New Cornelia (Ajo)
Lake Shore
San Manuel-Kalamazoo
Silver Bell
Ajo
San Diego
Tijuana
Tucson
Mission–Palo Verde
San Xavier North
Twin Buttes
Pima
Helvetia (Peach-Elgin)
Sierrita
Rosemont
Esperanza
Bisbee
Red Mountain
Douglas
Nogales
U.S.A.
MEXICO
El Paso
TEX
Rio G
BAJA CALIFORNIA NORTE
Pacific Ocean
Cananea
La Caridad
SONORA
CHIHUAHUA
Hermosillo
Chihuah
El Arco
BAJA CALIFORNIA SUR
Gulf of California
SINALOA
DURANG

Preface

Porphyry copper deposits of southwestern North America compose one of the richest and most densely clustered groups of such deposits on earth. In this region, which includes Utah, Nevada, and most importantly, Arizona and contiguous New Mexico and Mexico, 50 named, explored, or actively mined deposits occur, most of which are in southeastern Arizona. The economic importance of the region is significant and is revealed by production statistics through 1976 reported by Greeley (1978). Copper produced from Arizona, New Mexico, Nevada, and Utah—almost entirely from porphyry copper deposits or their weathered products—was over 89 percent of total U.S. output. Arizona alone accounted for over 63 percent of the U.S. total.

In addition to their economic importance, the porphyry copper systems of the American Southwest have also served as an important base of geologic information to which deposits in other parts of the world may be compared, and as a basis from which many scientific investigations in ore genesis have been carried out over many decades. Geologic investigations of these large hydrothermal systems by many individuals and groups, including industry, government, and academia, have contributed significantly to the understanding of many aspects of ore-forming processes. Results of these studies have been widely reported in a variety of geological and geochemical publications, and a great number of such reports have been generated since publication of the first volume on porphyry copper deposits in this region (Titley and Hicks, 1966). The great interest in these deposits has been revealed in the many symposia that have been convened to discuss porphyry copper deposit geology in numerous local and national meetings; further, porphyry copper deposits were the subject of discussion at the First Penrose Conference of the Geological Society of America in 1969 (Skinner, 1969).

Geologic study and detailing of phenomena in the porphyry systems have continued unabated since 1966 and have resulted in an immense body of information in the 1980s. Works that have collated information for deposits in other parts of the world have been published (Sutherland Brown, 1976; Gustafson and Titley, 1978; Hollister, 1978), as have detailed and exhaustive studies of specific deposits, such as El Salvador (Gustafson and Hunt, 1975). In the American Southwest the task of broadening and refining the geologic data base has been carried out by members of corporate geologic staffs who work with the rocks on a day-to-day basis. Without this basic information concerning geology of the ores, other meaningful studies are not possible.

In addition to new geologic information about deposits discovered in the 1960s and 1970s and deposits that have been mined and studied for many decades, many types of new data have been derived from laboratory studies and modeling. This information has been utilized to re-examine older concepts and, if necessary, to advance new hypotheses. The hypotheses have been and continue to be tested against the reality of the rocks; well-defined ore deposit geology continues to be the standard against which exciting new hypotheses must be tested.

Because of the discovery of many porphyry copper deposits in the American Southwest since 1960 and the development of basic geologic information about some of them, and because of the evolution of many concepts in ore genesis since publication of the first volume, it is appropriate to draw information together once again. This volume presents the information in two parts: the first treats topical subjects that generally have wide application; the second describes geology in specific deposits of the region. The topics in Part I are arranged in order of generally small to large scale, and the deposit descriptions in Part II are presented in geographical order, from east to west. The deposits discussed and described are both those for which no previous reports have been published, and those for which the information presented reflects a substantial augmentation to earlier studies.

The encouragement of many colleagues brought about the compilation of this second volume on the deposits. The path has been somewhat tortuous in pulling the information together. For many different reasons, hoped-for reports on some deposits in Mexico were not available. Another problem existed in attempts to bring metrication into engineering systems based upon existing English grids and bench levels. It was possible in only a few instances, but metric scales have been provided in most cases where appropriate.

It is my hope that the new information presented here will continue to stimulate the studies of these deposits. As more is learned about the nature and genesis of porphyry copper deposits, the potential becomes broader for increasing our ability to discover and exploit the important resource that these deposits represent.

ACKNOWLEDGMENTS

A book such as this necessarily involves the contributions of a great number of people, foremost among whom are the authors themselves. The chapters in this book, with few exceptions, are the results of study and writing for the express purpose of presenting data and ideas for the volume. I am indebted to the authors who contributed to this undertaking. Cooperation was positive and always constructive, notwithstanding the fact that many authors had to work initial preparation and revisions into already heavy professional schedules.

I thank James H. Courtright and Frederick T. Graybeal of ASARCO, who coordinated contributions on the geology at Mission, North San Xavier, Sacaton, and Silver Bell; I also acknowledge with thanks the assistance of Robert A. Metz and John I. Sharpe of the Duval Corporation, who coordinated preparation of the chapters on Mineral Park and Sierrita-Esperanza, and Arthur H. Kinneberg and John A. Lentz of the Phelps Dodge Corporation, who made possible the contributions on geology at Tyrone and Dos Pobres.

Joyce A. Lekawa, Merlene P. Lopez, and Linda F. Smith of the Department of Geosciences at the University of Arizona assisted in preparation of parts of the manuscript. Deborah C. Church assisted by drafting and redrafting many figures, and by producing some fine art work. Throughout the development of the volume, at many times and in many different ways, colleagues at the University of Arizona provided assistance and advice. I particularly acknowledge editorial advice and encouragement from Richard E. Beane, John M. Guilbert, and Denis L. Norton.

The detailed editing of the manuscript for publication was facilitated by Clare C. Spera, the assigned editor from the University of Arizona Press, whose sharp eyes, concern for detail, and careful work has helped bring this volume into being. I thank Elizabeth Y. Anthony for her assistance and Gulf Mineral Resources for financial support in preparation of the index. Lastly, I wish to acknowledge the continuing encouragement and patience of my wife, Helen, who kept the paths clear for this effort during the busy two years that it took to put the manuscripts between hard covers.

SPENCER R. TITLEY

REFERENCES CITED

Greeley, M. N., 1978, The primary copper industry of Arizona: Ariz. Dept. of Mineral Res., Spec. Rept. 2, 87 p.

Gustafson, L. B., and Hunt, J. P., 1975, The porphyry copper deposits at El Salvador, Chile: Econ. Geol., v. 70, p. 857–912.

Gustafson, L. B., and Titley, S. R., eds., 1978, Porphyry copper deposits of the southwestern Pacific islands and Australia: Econ. Geol., Spec. Issue v. 73, no. 5, p. 597–986.

Hollister, V. F., 1978, Geology of the Porphyry Copper Deposits of the Western Hemisphere: New York, AIME, 219 p.

Skinner, B. J., 1969, First Penrose Conference: Geotimes, v. 14, p. 15–16.

Sutherland Brown, A., ed., 1976, Porphyry Deposits of the Canadian Cordillera: CIM Spec. Vol. 15, 510 p.

Titley, S. R., and Hicks, C. L., eds., 1966, Geology of the Porphyry Copper Deposits, Southwestern North America: Tucson, Univ. Ariz. Press, 287 p.

PART I

Topics In Porphyry Copper Geology

Introduction

The chapters in Part I, arranged in order of generally small to large scale, discuss and review some important topics related to geology of porphyry copper deposits. These topics and their treatment here reflect the accumulation, evaluation, and interpretation of basic field and laboratory data and interpretations of many aspects of ore genesis based upon such studies. The scope of the subject matter in Part I is broad and ranges from information concerning grades and tonnage, through reviews of genesis and alteration, petrology, and field data, to research in exploration techniques. The content of these chapters reflects advances made in the decades between 1960 and 1980. The focus is upon geology of porphyry copper systems, although many of the concepts outlined and suggested have much broader application in the science of ore genesis at a wide range of scales. Although comparative examples are often drawn from other areas, the topical subject matter is related to porphyry copper deposits in southwestern North America. While the decades of the 1960s and 1970s were witness to an extraordinary number of discoveries of porphyry copper systems in the Pacific Basin rim environment, and while scientific studies have been reported for deposits in many other regions, the basis for elucidation of many fundamentals of occurrence, genesis, and processes was developed in studies of deposits of the American Southwest.

The decade of the 1970s was a period during which many concepts of porphyry copper genesis, in both localized and global settings, were outlined. Continued elaboration of these concepts progressed simultaneously with tests of the ideas against the reality of nature. The orderly arrangement of sulfide minerals and alteration products—zoning—was detailed (Lowell and Guilbert, 1970; Rose, 1970; James, 1971; Hollister, 1975). The typical zoning patterns or models that were proposed have widespread application in interpretive studies and exploration, and they have provided an important basis for comparison of porphyry copper deposits in many regions of the world. The reader will note the influence of these concepts on the discussions of zoning in many deposits described in this volume. As zoning hypotheses have grown, many attempts have been made to explain processes in such a context; however, the details of mineralization and alteration have also been subjects of continuing scrutiny in some deposits of the region. As a result, an enhanced recognition of the fourth dimension of geology—time—has emerged and is now considered important in the context of zoning and of hydrothermal genesis. Some aspects of the nature and process of metallization and zoning in porphyry copper deposits are discussed in Part I in reports on tonnages and grades of porphyry copper systems (Chapter 1, by Paul Gilmour); on elemental zoning in the Kalamazoo orebody (Chapter 9, by M. A. Chaffee); in a review of the features of skarn-related porphyry ores (Chapter 7, by M. T. Einaudi); and in a review of the progress of alteration and mineralization in porphyry systems as interpreted from field data (Chapter 5, by S. R. Titley).

The development of important chemical and modelling tools by H. L. Helgeson (1970, and in many subsequent publications) has provided a basis for study of the high-temperature chemistry of hydrothermal reactions. The principles and techniques developed by Helgeson continue to have wide application in studies of porphyry copper hydrothermal genesis. Many publications by H. P. Taylor, Jr. (particularly the summary in 1974) outline the results of many studies of oxygen and hydrogen isotopes in minerals of porphyry systems; these studies, initiated in deposits of the American Southwest, have resulted in a more advanced

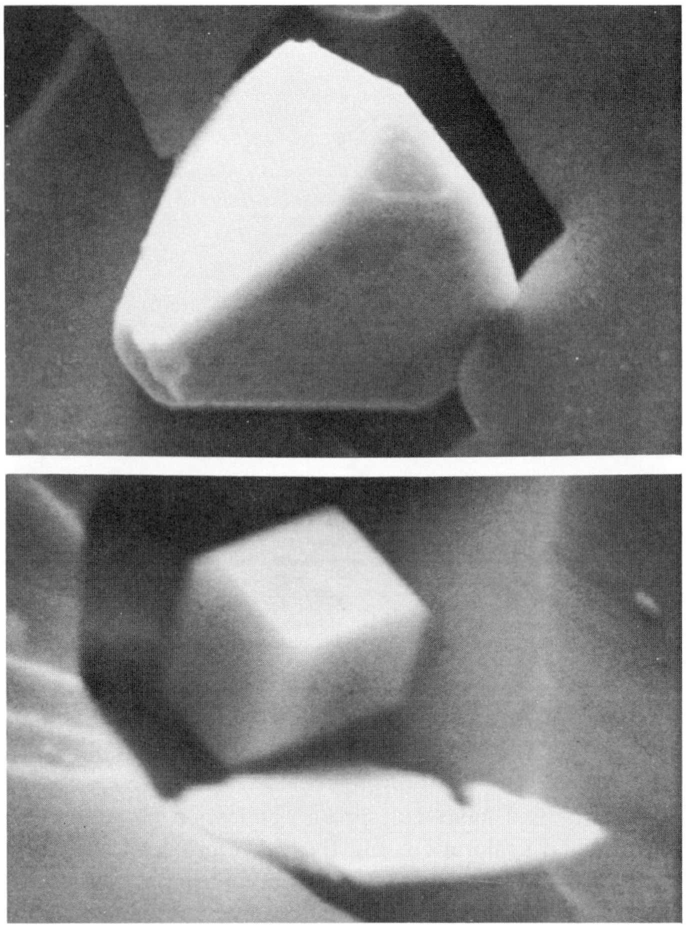

SEM photographs of minerals in fluid inclusions from porphyry at Chino, New Mexico: *above,* a crystal of chalcopyrite; *below,* a cubic crystal of pyrite and a plate of mica. Edges on the chalcopyrite crystal are about 4 microns in length; scale is the same for both photographs. These illustrations show the detail and scales at which much work has been carried out in studies of porphyry copper systems between the mid-1960s and 1980. Photographs courtesy of R. E. Beane.

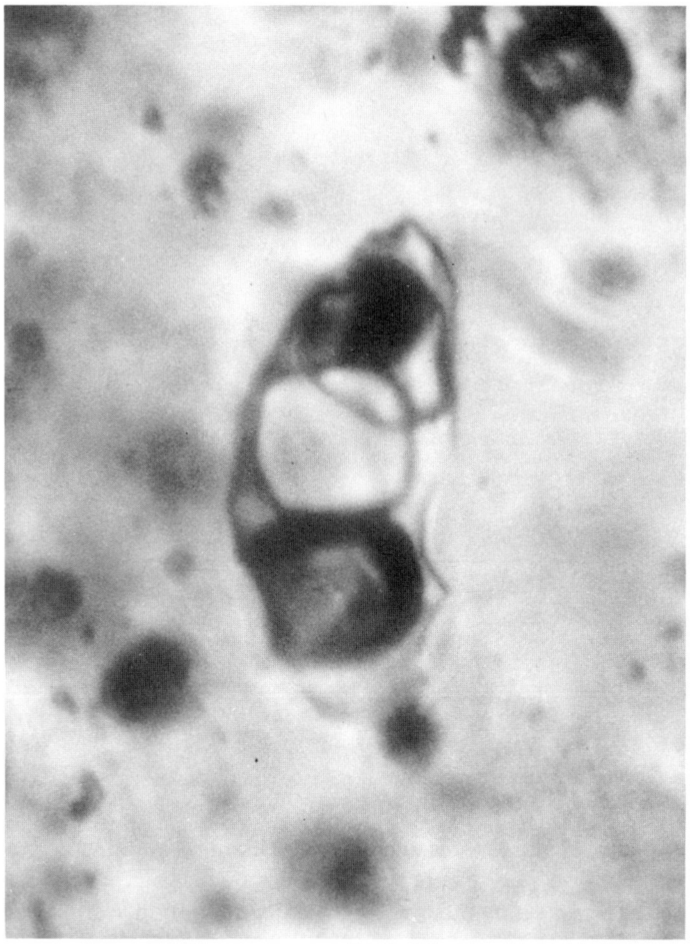

Photograph of a fluid inclusion from porphyry at Chino, New Mexico. This inclusion, for which filling temperatures in excess of 800°C have been measured, contains, in addition to its probable magmatic water, a vapor bubble (at the bottom), a crystal of sylvite (center), and a plate of mica above an opaque crystal of hematite. Photograph courtesy of R. E. Beane.

understanding of the sources and roles of different waters at different stages of the hydrothermal process. Chemical and isotopic tools have been augmented by the techniques of measurement, analysis, and interpretation of fluid inclusions advanced by Edwin Roedder (1971, and many other publications). The study of these inclusions in detailing hydrothermal genesis and some physical conditions extant at the time of ore formation had become commonplace by 1980. The importance of these three areas of research is emphasized in several chapters in Part I. Modelling of hydrothermal flow, with particular reference to rocks of southeastern Arizona, is discussed in Chapter 3, by D. L. Norton; alteration in potassium-silicate rocks is detailed in Chapter 6, by R. E. Beane; and alteration in skarns is reported in Chapter 8, by M. T. Einaudi, while Chapter 10, by N. G. Banks, reviews the evidence for metal and sulfur sources, with particular reference to Ray, Arizona.

Re-establishment of the ideas of continental drift on a firm scientific basis since the mid-1960s has resulted in different bases for interpretation of the geologic history of the earth. Since porphyry copper deposits are integral parts of this history, explanations of their genesis and copper metallogeny have been sought in the cause and effect of continental and oceanic plate interactions. Although the concept has been applied in a geometrical sense to continental and arc edges in many parts of the Pacific Basin (Sillitoe, 1972), the complex geologic history that both preceded and followed porphyry copper evolution in southwestern North America has resulted in unanswered questions about many aspects of the process in this area. Because the concept relates evolution of the porphyries to effects of plate interactions, a knowledge of rock compositions is essential to evaluate application of the theory. However, the relatively older ages of deposits in this region (ca. 55–75 m.y. old), the existence of alteration aureoles many kilometers in diameter around porphyry systems, and the presence of widespread, deeply penetrating supergene effects makes the task difficult for the petrologist; thus, little of the necessary, high-quality petrochemical information has been developed for deposits of this region. However, careful petrologic work has been carried out in the deposit at Ray, Arizona, and the results are reported in Chapter 11, by H. R. Cornwall.

Some aspects of the nature of rock failure in porphyry systems and its geologic and tectonic implications are discussed in the study on Laramide fracturing (Chapter 4, by T. L. Heidrick and S. R. Titley). Regional geology, a necessary

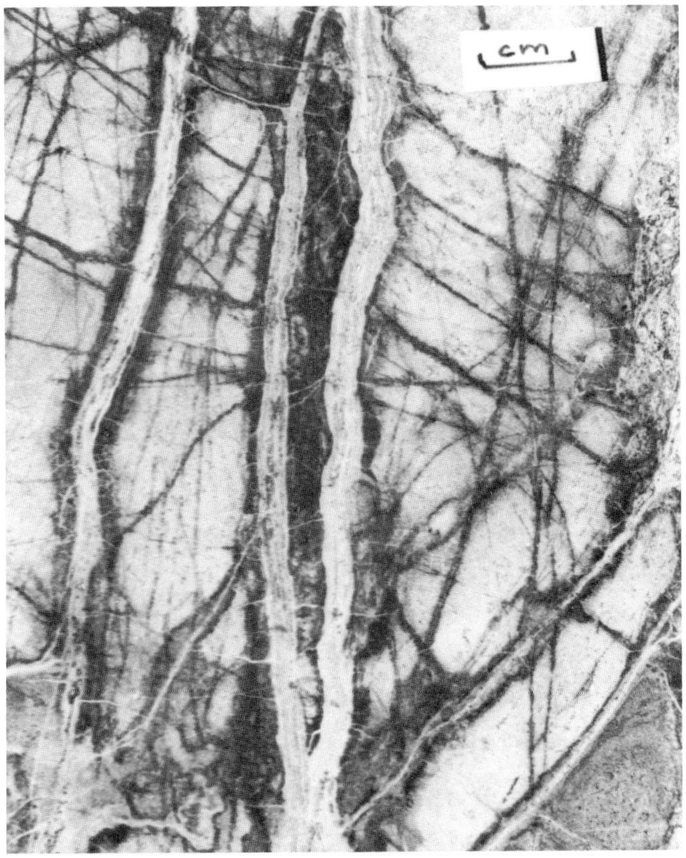

Mineralization and fracture patterns in skarn from porphyry copper deposits in the Rosemont area, Arizona. Early development of pervasive calc-silicate minerals took place, followed by rock failure and a second stage of alteration along cracks. Copper ore in the skarn-altered wall rocks of porphyry intrusions has become an increasingly major source of the metal since the mid-1960s. Photograph by S. R. Titley.

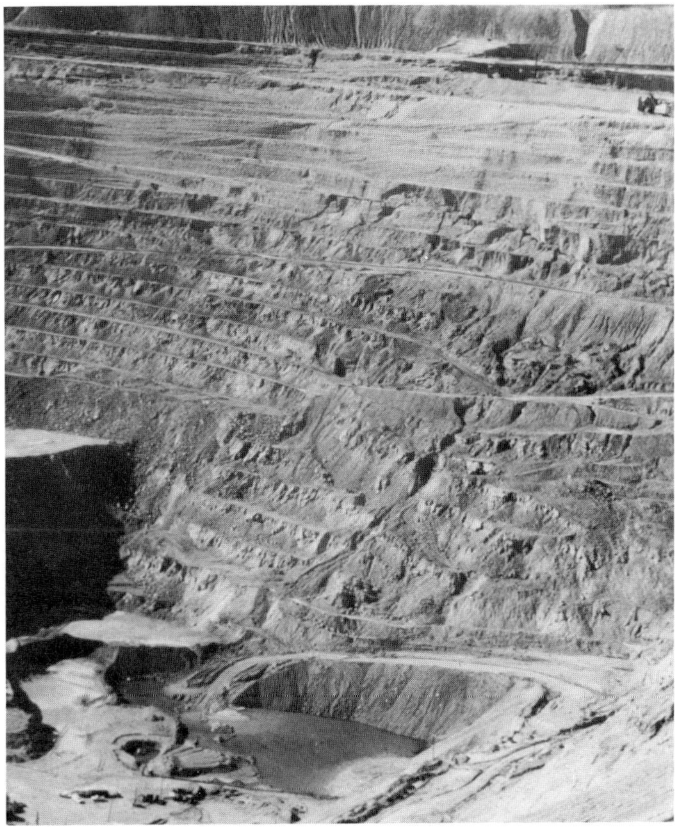

A view southward across the open pit at Twin Buttes, Arizona. This orebody has stimulated the evolution of concepts of many aspects of ore genesis and ore search in southwestern North America. Dominated by skarn mineralization, it is centered on a porphyry stock, exposures of which are in a bench at the left center of the picture. The orebody was completely covered by geologically youthful alluvium, exposures of which may be seen high on the pit wall near the top of the photograph. Photograph by S. R. Titley.

basis to the interpretation of geotectonic phenomena, is also outlined in Part I (Chapter 2, by S. R. Titley); however, as is the case with studies in petrology, the complex geologic history of weathering and alteration, coupled with the superposition of many episodes of tectonism in this region, has left many features of geology poorly understood and probably even unrecognized.

Information presented in Chapter 1 on grade and tonnage reveals many discoveries of porphyry systems in southwestern North America during the 1960s and 1970s. The search for more deposits continues, and the exploration geologist continues to be faced with problems of interpretation of the surface. It is hoped that the scientific advances summarized above, together with the related topical chapters in Part I will aid that search. In spite of knowledge gained about hydrothermal processes, manifestations of alteration, and regional geology, the exploration geologist is still faced with working outcrop. The interpretation of leached capping remains an honorable art and science that, together with application of geochemical prospecting techniques, will continue to be widely applied. Techniques of appraising leached capping, based upon experimental and field studies, are discussed in Chapter 12, by J. A. Anderson. Application of geochemical prospecting techniques in the semi-arid areas of the region is reviewed in Chapter 13, by M. A. Chaffee.

The chapters in Part I, thus, contain a broad sampling of different phenomena of porphyry copper genesis, and the advances made in knowledge about the genesis and discovery of ore are constructively considered and reviewed in the chapters that follow.

S.R.T.

References Cited

Helgeson, H. C., 1970, A chemical and thermodynamic model of ore deposition in hydrothermal systems: Mineral. Soc. America, Spec. Paper 3, p. 155–186.

James, A. H., 1971, Hypothetical diagrams of several porphyry copper deposits: Econ. Geol., v. 66, p. 43–47.

Lowell, J. D., and Guilbert, J. M., 1970, Lateral and vertical alteration-mineralization zoning in porphyry ore deposits: Econ. Geol., v. 65, p. 373–408.

Roedder, Edwin, 1971, Fluid inclusion studies on the porphyry-type ore deposits at Bingham, Utah; Butte, Montana; and Climax, Colorado: Econ. Geol., v. 66, p. 98–120.

Rose, A. W., 1970, Zonal relations of wallrock alteration and sulfide distribution at porphyry copper deposits: Econ. Geol., v. 63, p. 920–936.

Sillitoe, R. H., 1972, A plate tectonic model for the origin of porphyry copper deposits: Econ. Geol., v. 67, p. 184–197.

Taylor, H. P. Jr., 1974, The application of oxygen and hydrogen isotope studies to problems of hydrothermal alteration and ore deposition: Econ. Geol., v. 69, p. 843–883.

1

Grades and Tonnages of Porphyry Copper Deposits

Paul Gilmour

If it is true that "pure science" avoids lines of research which could by any possibility have a practical application, such a course would seem a near-absurdity in studies such as these. . . .

(Perret, 1937, p. 8)

Consideration of metallic mineral deposits as natural phenomena requires reconciliation of two conflicting geological points of view: on the one hand, economics must be de-emphasized—or even temporarily abandoned; on the other hand, publications on the geology of ore deposits are inevitably influenced to varying degrees by financial considerations. Economics must be temporarily de-emphasized because it would, for example, be inconvenient if the statistics for various classes of mineral deposits rose or fell in sympathy with demand and metal prices. As for the fact that reports are at least colored by economics, it might be noted that the failure of some published descriptions of deposits to record the presence of any given mineral or metal does not necessarily mean that it is not present. The omission may simply mean that the amount present is insignificant compared to other economically more important metals or minerals, or even that deliberate attempts were made to conceal its presence. A large, high-grade, lead-zinc deposit with which I am familiar contains an appreciable amount of copper—perhaps 0.25 percent overall, with large volumes containing up to 1.0 percent—yet, to my knowledge, in no published account is the presence of copper even mentioned. Presumably this is because 0.25 percent copper seems insignificant alongside 20 to 25 percent combined lead and zinc. In another example, involving a massive sulfide, information on the presence of lead was actually suppressed, lest the miners emulate the employees in another camp and demand a lead bonus. Pity the poor geologist who—dependent on published reports alone—devises an elegant theory to account for the absence of lead in that deposit!

With few, if any, other groups of metallic mineral deposits is this distinction more important or easier to bear in mind than with porphyry copper deposits—more important because grade is so critical, and easier because no other important group of deposits contains a reference to grade (economics) in its title, "porphyry" being synonymous in the minds of most mining people with "large-tonnage, low-grade." Thus, in one of the earliest comprehensive reviews of operations exploiting this group of copper deposits, Parsons (1933, p. 2) wrote that representatives of the class are characterized by "their huge size, particularly with respect to their horizontal dimensions; the relative uniformity with which the copper minerals are disseminated through the mass; *and the low average per-ton copper content of the exploitable ore*" (italics added). In the sequel to Parsons' volume the reference to amenability to exploitation by "large-scale, low-per-ton-cost methods"—with its corollary of large tonnage as well as low grade—was promoted to first place in the list of characteristics cited (Parsons, 1957, p. 8). Titley and Hicks (1966, p. ix) stated the case quite explicitly when they wrote:

> Originally applied in a genetic sense to disseminated copper mineralization in acid igneous porphyritic rocks, its [the term "porphyry copper"] definition has now come to be more closely allied to economic considerations and engineering characteristics. The present sense of meaning is broad and general but is essentially applicable to large, low-grade, epigenetic, hypogene copper deposits that can be mined by mass-mining methods.

The geologic problem posed by definitions phrased too narrowly in engineering terms is that they can be applied to almost any large deposit amenable to surface or underground bulk (low-cost) mining methods—including some which most geologists would prefer to class otherwise, e.g., Palabora (World Mining, 1963). In a study which has been very widely cited Lowell and Guilbert (1970) obviate this problem by employing mainly geologic terms in a comprehensive definition of porphyry copper deposits, but they also emphasize the importance of economic considerations, noting that such deposits are "generally large" with dimensions on a "scale of several thousands of feet" and of low grade, the tenor of "primary mineralization in a typical porphyry copper deposit ranging up to 0.8% Cu and 0.02% Mo." The authors continue, "All porphyry copper deposits contain at least traces of molybdenite, and all porphyry molybdenite deposits contain some chalcopyrite. Many deposits contain recoverable amounts of both minerals. . . . " These and other figures cited by Lowell and Guilbert (1970, Table 1) provide valuable guides for tonnage and grade, but they do not attempt to tell the whole story.

Since a characteristic of porphyry copper deposits is their low grade, an obvious question which arises is: How low is "low"? The answer depends on the place and time to which reference is made; for the present, at least, place refers to southwestern North America and attention is focussed on the factor of time. In order to place the temporal (and, to a lesser degree, spatial) factors in perspective it is useful to separate porphyry copper deposit grades into three classes, which arise from the mode of occurrence of the copper minerals and reflect the evolution of mined grades or mill-heads for the group as a whole. Individual deposits may or may not recapitulate this evolution, since many of the discoveries of recent years have short-circuited the process by starting on primary sulfides.

GRADE CLASSES

The three principal grade classes into which the mined grade of porphyry copper deposits or systems can be divided are as follows:

High—grades over 2.5 percent copper. This group includes the veins and tactite, or skarn, deposits (which may be locally enriched) commonly associated with porphyry systems. This grade class represents a pre-porphyry stage of mining activity.

Intermediate—grades between 1.0 and 2.5 percent copper. Typically copper contents in this range result from the exploitation of a secondary or chalcocite blanket of the type associated with the classical (approximately, pre–World War II) period of porphyry copper mining. Similar values may also be found in tactite deposits and in portions of some bodies of primary mineralization.

Low—grades below 1.0 percent copper. This tenor generally results from the mining of primary mineralization in either an intrusion or a wall-rock porphyry (Titley, 1972). Ordinarily this type of mineralization and the attendant grade are associated with the modern period of porphyry development (roughly, the period which has elapsed since the end of World War II).

These grade classes correspond to geological modes of occurrence and also bear some relationship to the historical development of the group as a whole and to some individual deposits (as well as to geographical distribution). Most of the classical deposits of the southwestern U.S. have passed through each of the stages of evolution with which the grade classes are typically associated, while most (but not all) modern deposits or recent discoveries were initiated on the strength of primary sulfides with low grades (i.e., less than 1%). Other characteristics of the three grade classes are summarized below.

High-Grade Mineralization

High-grade mineralization (over 2.5% copper) is recovered from the veins and skarn deposits associated with porphyry systems. In the southwestern U.S. such mineralization was mined 80 to 100 years ago in underground workings and small open-cuts from which grades well over 2.5 percent were commonly obtained. Hammond (1961) noted, for example, that in 1896 the Highland Boy mine in the Bingham, Utah, district produced 5,000 tons which averaged 12 percent copper (plus $4 in gold and $3 in silver per ton). Lindgren (1905) recorded that in 1879 the Longfellow mine in the Morenci, Arizona, district had a daily production of 40 tons of 20 percent copper ore. In 1903 the annual output of the Morenci area as a whole was 27,000 short tons of copper which was recovered from ore containing 3 to 4 percent copper (Lindgren, 1905). At that time miners' wages were between $2.25 and $3.00 per day, while the direct cost of underground mining was between $1.50 and $3.00 per ton (Lindgren, 1905). In 1903 copper sold for 14¢ per pound—a considerably better price, in relation to wages and other costs, than those prevailing in the mid-1970s.

In the classical porphyry deposits of the U.S. Southwest, Chile, and Peru this period of high grade, pre-porphyry activity lasted from 1876 or so until mining of each deposit as a porphyry was begun (Parsons, 1933, Table 1). In some areas relatively high-grade mineralization which was being mined in 1980 may have represented the pre-porphyry stage of exploitation of as-yet unrecognized (or unexplored) porphyry systems. In still others the cessation of mining high-grade copper and the recognition of the porphyry affinities of the mineralization occurred only at the end of the 1970s (e.g., Saindak, Pakistan [Min. Mag., 1978]).

Intermediate-Grade Mineralization

It is well known that exploitation of the intermediate range of produced grade, 1.0 to 2.5 percent, is mostly coincident with the early years of production from the type deposits, which began when the first porphyry copper went on stream in 1904–1905—an event generally associated with the name of Daniel C. Jackling. (Ransome [1919] has some interesting comments on the early history of porphyry mining.) Between 1899, when Jackling first visited the Bingham district, and 1903, when Utah Copper Company was formed, at least two estimates of reserves were made on the property which was to become the nucleus of the Company's mineral-land holdings. In the first, Jackling and his colleague, Robert C. Gemmell, calculated the reserves of developed ore to be 12,385,000 tons averaging 2 percent copper, while additional probable ore was conservatively estimated at 25,000,000 tons (Hammond, 1961). Four years later, when Utah Copper Company was being formed, F. H. Minard was asked to check the earlier estimate. He described the presence of a leached zone about 50 ft. thick, succeeded downward by a copper-enriched zone which varied in thickness between 100 and 150 ft., both lying within a porphyry intrusion. The average of all available samples taken from the enriched blanket was 1.6 percent copper, and Minard concluded that it was "reasonable to suppose" that 9,000,000 tons having that average grade were available (Hammond, 1961, p. 126).

At the time when Jackling and Gemmell were evaluating what was to become the Utah Copper property, Thomas Weir, manager of the adjacent Boston Consolidated ground, estimated that his Company's holdings contained a mass of mineralized porphyry which measured 3,500 by 2,500 by 500 ft. thick (for a total of roughly 300,000,000 tons) and assayed between 0.75 and 2.5 percent copper. These, then, were the figures representing the grade (and tonnage) of the reserves in what was to be the prototype of all porphyry copper mining operations.

Large-scale mining began on the Utah property in 1904 and on the Boston Consolidated ground shortly thereafter. In those days Utah Copper treated between 4,000 and 5,000 tons per day. During the first two years of production, between start-up and 1906, the mineralized porphyry was exclusively mined underground, employing block caving. Open-pit mining was initiated in 1906, and both systems were retained until 1914, when underground mining of the porphyry orebody on the Utah property ceased. In the meantime, Utah Copper and Boston Consolidated merged in 1910. (For a more detailed account of these developments see, for example, Hammond, 1961.

From 1905 to 1912 another six porphyry copper deposits located in the U.S. Southwest and Chile were brought into production and the classical period of porphyry development (both individually for the famous deposits involved and collectively for the group as a whole) was under way (Parsons, 1933, Table 1).

The tonnage and grade of minable reserves of the major deposits during their collective classical period, when chalcocite blankets were still being exploited, were tabulated by Parsons (1933, Table 3). From the earliest days the diminution in grades and concomitant very large increases in tonnages which still characterize porphyry developments had become evident. By 1929 the 1.6 to 2.5 percent of Utah Copper had dropped to 1.07, while reported tonnage had bounded upward from 9, 12 or even 37 (Jackling and Gemmel's 12 "developed" plus 25 "probable") million tons to 640 million tons. Similarly, between 1911 and 1917, the mill heads at Miami Copper in the Globe-Miami district in Arizona declined from 1.82 to 1.44 percent copper, while annual production more than quadrupled from just under 500,000 tons to over 2,000,000: by 1929 the grade of reserves had dropped to 0.95 percent (Parsons, 1933, Table 3).

Although initially many of the operations employed underground mining either solely or in part, the amenability to open-pit mining of the tabular, sub-horizontal, chalcocite blankets was such that with a few notable exceptions this method was generally adopted during the collective classical period. According to figures quoted by Parsons (1933), the metallurgical recovery of copper in these secondary sulfides and mixed oxide-sulfide ores averaged a relatively low (compared to results obtained with primary mineralization) 77 percent in the pre-1933 period. Figures compiled by Greeley (1978) for Arizona operations in 1975 and 1976 show a spread from a low of 42 percent in oxides (Ox Hide) during 1971 to a high of 93 percent in primary sulfides (San Manuel) during 1967 and 1968, with most recoveries lying between 70 and 90 percent. The comparable figures for molybdenum recovery range from the low teens to a high of 86 percent for primary sulfides (Sierrita), with most mixed oxide-sulfide and secondary sulfide ores returning 45 to 75 percent.

Parsons (1933) reported that in 1930 the average cost of producing refined copper in the U.S. was 9.93¢ per pound. In the meantime, between 1929 and 1930 (the last years shown in Parsons' Table 2), the domestic U.S. price of copper was sliding from 18 to 15¢ per pound on its way to the low of 5¢ reached in 1932, resulting in a loss per pound of more than 4¢.

It is worth observing that in the free enterprise nations of the non-Communist world the prices of raw materials, including metals, are virtually alone in responding to the law of supply and demand, in contrast with the cost of the vast majority of goods and services which tend to climb inexorably upward, more or less in proportion to inflation. Thus, the windfall profits of, say, the farming and mining industries obtained during periods of high demand and high prices are required to offset the effects of inevitable intervening periods of low demand (relative to production) and low prices.

In the U.S. Southwest and in Chile and Peru, both for individual deposits and collectively, the classical period continued beyond the watershed years of 1929 to 1932, and numerous new mines were actually brought in between that time and the outbreak of World War II (Parsons, 1957, Table 1). The economics, geological mode of occurrence, tonnage, and grade were not qualitatively changed, although acceptable cut-offs, and, hence, average grades continued to fall in response to the interplay of changing costs, efficiencies, and metal prices. Minable reserves continued to increase, and the increase generally more than compensated for previous production, so that reserves of copper actually grew.

Low-Grade Mineralization

Mined grades significantly less than 1.0 percent or so are principally associated with the exploitation of primary sulfides. The mining of what was known as "protore" came about in two ways: (a) through the exhaustion of chalcocite blankets at the "type" porphyries which were mined through the classical period of their existence and (b) through the discovery of new primary sulfide deposits. The decline in copper grades gave added impetus to the increasing importance attached to the minor metals, notably molybdenum, gold and silver.

The changeover from mining intermediate grade, enriched ore to mining primary sulfides at the classical occurrences cannot be precisely identified. At operating mines secondary sulfides did not give way to primary mineralization either at the same time or at the same rate (although the differing demands of the necessary metallurgical treatments require that an engineering limit be drawn at individual deposits). Most of the mines opened prior to the time of World

War II are now largely or entirely dependent on exploiting primary sulfides. At least one classical deposit (Castle Dome in the Miami district of Arizona) was reopened (after a dormant period which lasted around 30 years) with a new name, Pinto Valley, as a modern low-grade operation mining primary sulfides.

Perhaps the first modern deposit developed as such was San Manuel, drilled by the U.S. Geological Survey and the U.S. Bureau of Mines during World War II. Although it possesses a leached capping and a zone of supergene mineralization, the latter is covered by Quaternary conglomerate, and the thickness of the barren material (conglomerate plus leached cap) ranges up to nearly 2,000 ft., so that it has not been possible to develop a pit and recover the enriched ore. Fortunately, the primary sulfide grade is a relatively high 0.75 percent copper (with a 0.5% cut-off), accompanied by an appreciable amount of molybdenum, so it was deemed feasible to exploit the primary mineralization underground, allowing the secondary mineralization to cave with the leached capping and conglomerate.

After the discovery and development of San Manuel another hiatus in exploration occurred until around 1950, when the Esperanza and Pima deposits were found and the modern period of exploration and development was well and truly launched. Gaspé Copper, in the Gaspé Peninsula of Eastern Quebec, was found at nearly the same time, although some 10 years were to elapse before the general affiliations of the discovery were recognized (Gilmour, 1962). Although Esperanza was classical in the sense that it possessed a leached capping and chalcocite blanket, it was modern in the sense that the decision to develop a mine was based on the unprecedentedly low estimated grade of 0.51 percent copper (and 0.028% molybdenum). Pima, on the other hand, was thoroughly modern in every sense: it was discovered by means of geophysical surveys conducted over an alluvium-covered pediment adjacent to (pre-porphyry) bedded replacement mineralization in limestone (Thurmond et al., 1958). It is a skarn or tactite deposit which exemplifies the increasingly important class of wall-rock deposits emphasized by Titley (1972). Pima also provides an instructive example of the manner in which even low-grade porphyries can be economically mined by handling larger tonnages at progressively declining grades. It was initially regarded as an orebody of 1.5 million tons, averaging 1.75 percent copper and containing 26,250 short tons of copper (the fault-localized, high-grade mineralization which evidently gave the geophysical response). Drilling was resumed when the presence of widely disseminated copper minerals was recognized, and a large, low-grade deposit was eventually outlined. Production from an open pit began in 1955 at a rate of 2,500 t.p.d. with a mill-head described as over 1 percent. In the 26 months from November, 1955, to January, 1958, 1.1 million tons of sulfide ore averaging 1.7 percent copper and 660,000 million tons of oxide material of unspecified grade were handled (Thurmond et al., 1958). This mill-head was achieved at the cost of a very high ratio of waste to ore. This stripping ratio was 7:1, and it resulted in an effective mined grade of 0.217 percent copper. By 1965 the average grade of treated ore had declined to 1.0 percent and daily capacity had grown to 8,500 t.p.d. Daily production during 1972 averaged 40,000 t.p.d., and between May, 1952, and December, 1970, 73 million tons (with an average grade of 0.72% copper) had been mined (Himes, 1972). In other words, up to 1970, over 540,000 short tons of copper in concentrates were recovered, in contrast with the 26,250 tons of copper of the original ore-reserve estimate.

Perhaps the best example in the Southwest of newly discovered, low-grade, primary mineralization (as distinct from primary mineralization associated with a classical porphyry—e.g., Pinto Valley, on the site of the former Castle Dome, or Bagdad before and after recent exploration) is provided by Sierrita. Found through geochemical surveys conducted by Bear Creek Mining Company, this deposit was placed in production by Duval Corporation in 1969. Announced reserves were 0.35 percent copper and 0.036 percent molybdenum, for a total copper equivalent (eCu) of between 0.49 and 0.53 percent (depending on whether the molybdenum assay was multiplied by a factor of 4 or 5). Sierrita is also a good illustration of the increasing importance of minor metals: the value of the molybdenum present is roughly 50 percent of that of the copper alone. In order to liberate the stated reserves, 634 million tons of waste had to be removed; this figure results in an overall stripping ratio of 1.5:1 and an effective copper equivalent grade of between 0.33 and 0.35 (Mining Magazine, 1971).

Most of the modern, low-grade deposits which have been developed lie outside of the traditional porphyry districts of the Southwest and Latin America and, accordingly, beyond the geographical scope of this volume. They are, nevertheless, highly instructive from the standpoint of grade and tonnage and, after representative examples in southwestern North America have been reviewed, some comparative statistics from other regions will be listed.

PRODUCTION AND RESERVES IN SOUTHWESTERN NORTH AMERICA

Statistics concerning production and reserves in representative porphyry copper deposits for past and present producers in Arizona are given in Table 1.1; Tables 1.2 and 1.3 show reserves in deposits in, respectively, western states exclusive of Arizona, and Mexico. Since the emphasis is on southwestern North America and on economics, the standard U.S. conventions (short tons and Troy ounces rather than metric units) were adopted. With few exceptions (e.g., Butte, Montana) the examples presented in the latter two tables belong to "southwestern North America." Since the information shown in the Tables is abbreviated, a few explanatory notes are required.

First, in many cases several sets of figures for tonnage, grade, and cut-off are presented. This was done for a number of reasons, including, but not limited to, the following: In some examples giving more than one set permits the growth of tonnage and decline of grade to be charted, as in Mineral Park (Table 1.1) and Bingham (Table 1.2). In others the distinctive features of different classes or types of ore are

TABLE 1.1
Production and Reserves in Representative Porphyry Copper Deposits in Arizona

DEPOSIT	PRODUCTION/ RESERVES	TONNAGE (s.t. × 10^6)	GRADE Cu %	Mo %	Au oz./s.t.	Ag oz./s.t.	CUT-OFF GRADE (% Cu)	RATIO W:O	SOURCES
Bagdad (Bagdad-Cyprus)	Ann. prod., 1973	2.1	0.67	0.012	—	0.0220	—	6:1(?)	E&MJ, Jun. 1974, p. 205
	Est. res., 1973	264	0.51	—	—	—	—	1.3:1	E&MJ, Jun. 1973, p. 200 & 259
		550	0.46	—				1.6:1	
	Planned ann. prod.	±14	±0.50	±0.03	—	—	—	1.5:1	E&MJ, Apr. 1978, p. 133; Min. Eng., Apr. 1978, p. 351 & 352
Bisbee (Lavender Pit)	Total reserves	±120	0.81	—	—	—	—	4.3:1	Min. Eng., Oct. 1965, p. 89 & 90, Lowell and Guilbert, 1970, p. 390 & 391
Casa Grande	Initial res., 1978	350	1.0	—	—	—	—	—	Min. Eng., June 1979, p. 626
Castle Dome	Prod., 1943–1953	41.5	0.62 (rec)	—	0.0002	0.013	—	—	Peterson, 1962, p. 88
Christmas	Reserves, 1978	100+	0.4+	—	—	—	—	±3.5:1	Lowell, 1978, p. 176
Copper Basin (Yavapai Co.)	Initial reserves	±175	0.55	0.02	—	—	—	—	E&MJ, May 1974, p. 37; E&MJ, Sept. 1975, p. 193 & 197; Greeley, 1978, p. 86
Copper Cities	Ann. prod., 1965	3.6	0.66	—	—	—	—	3.3:1	Author's estimate
Copper Creek (Pinal & Graham Co.)	Reserves, 1978	50+	0.74	—	—	—	—	UG(?)	Lowell, 1978, p. 176
Esperanza	Initial res., 1962	52.9 (mill)	0.51	0.028	—	—	—	—	Lynch, 1966, p. 267
		32.5 (leach)	—	—	—	—	—	—	
	Prod., 1959–1978	86.3	0.442	0.021	—	—	—	1.6:1	NMGS GB, 1978, p. 90
	Reserves, 1978	22.8 (mill)	0.42	0.022	—	—	—	—	NMGS GB, 1978, p. 91
		8.0 (leach)	0.23	—	—	—	—	—	
		26.0 (both)	0.38	0.027	—	—	—	—	Aiken and West, 1978, p. 119
Florence	Initial res., 1978	800	0.4	—	—	—	—	—	Min. Eng., Jun. 1979, p. 626
Inspiration	Prod., 1915–1962	180.9	1.123	0.007	—	—	—	—	Olmstead and Johnson, 1966, p. 114
	Ann. prod., 1969	±7.5	0.90	0.009	—	—	—	2.6:1	E&MJ, May 1969, p. 122 & 124
Lakeshore	Initial reserves	500 (con)	0.70	—	—	—	—	UG	Min. Mag., May 1975, p. 335
		25.0 (tac)	1.70	—	—	—	—	UG	
Miami									
"Old"	Prod., 1911–1953	135.4	0.786 (rec)	—	—	—	—	UG	Peterson, 1962, p. 86
East	Initial reserves	50	1.95	—	—	—	—	UG	Min. Eng., May 1975, p. 8

(continued)

Table 1.1 (*continued*)

DEPOSIT	PRODUCTION/ RESERVES	TONNAGE (s.t. × 10^6)	GRADE Cu %	Mo %	Au oz./s.t.	Ag oz./s.t.	CUT-OFF GRADE (% Cu)	RATIO W:O	SOURCES
Mineral Park (Ithaca Peak)	Initial reserves Production to and reserves in 1978	50 175	0.50 0.53	0.020 0.040	— —	— —	— —	1.4:1 —	Lowell and Guilbert, 1970, p. 390 & 391; Lowell, 1978, p. 176; Greeley, 1978, p. 86
Morenci	Prod. to 1972 Ann. prod., 1965 Reserves, 1970	435 18 500+	0.96 (rec) 0.90 (rec) 0.88	— 0.007 0.007	— — —	— — —	— — —	±1.8:1 2.5:1 —	Langton, 1972, p. 31 Min. Eng., Oct. 1975, p. 88 & 89 Lowell and Guilbert, 1970, p. 390 & 391
Metcalf (King Peak)	Reserves, 1978	400 419	±0.75 0.77	— —	— —	— —	— —	— —	Lowell, 1978, p. 176; Greeley, 1978, p. 86
New Cornelia (Ajo)	Prod., 1917–1962 Ann. prod., 1965	255 ±9.6	0.80 0.78	— —	0.0054 0.0052	— —	— —	1.1:1 1.7:1	Gilluly, 1946, p. 102; Min. Eng., Oct. 1965, p. 88 & 89; Dixon, 1966, p. 123
Peach-Elgin	Reserves, 1973	23	0.75	—	—	—	—	—	NMGS GB, 1978, p. 90; Greeley, 1978. p. 83
Pima	Prod., 1952–1954 Prod., 1955–1977 Reserves, 1977	0.06 199.8 146.0	5.83 0.477 (rec) 0.48 (ind)	— 0.004 0.015	— — —	— 0.060 —	— 0.3(?)	UG 2.6:1 —	
Mission	Prod., 1959–1977 Reserves, 1977	108.9 135.0	0.626 (rec) 0.73 (ind)	0.019 —	— —	0.11 —	0.3(?) —	3.4:1 —	NMGS GB, 1978, p. 89 & 90; Greeley, 1978, p. 83–87
Palo Verde	Prod., 1960–1963 Reserves, 1977	0.5 125.0	2.06 (rec) 0.61 (ind)	— —	— —	— —	— —	UG —	
ALL (Pima, Mission & Palo Verde)	Prod. & Reserves, 1952–1977	715.3	0.573 (rec & ind)	±.006	—	0.06	—	—	
Pinto Valley	Initial res., 1975	350	0.44 (ind)	0.009	—	—	—	1.4:1	Min. Eng., Jun. 1975, p. 25–31
Boston Butte (Florence)	Initial res., 1978	400(?)	0.45(?)	—	—	—	—	—	Lowell, 1978, p. 176
Ray	Production to 1966 Annual production "silicate" ore	187.5 2.5	0.80–0.85 { 1.12 (rec) ±1.75 (ind) }	— —	0.0002 (rec?) —	0.0213 (rec?) —	— —	2.5:1 —	Author's estimate Gambell, 1978, p. 35
Rosemont	Initial res., 1973	{ 320 20	0.64 (S_2) 0.55 (ox)	— —	— —	— —	— —	— —	NMGS GB, 1978, p. 67

Sacaton									
West	Initial res., 1975	33.9	0.76	—	—	0.07	0.3	±6:1	Min. Mag., Feb. 1975, p. 90–97
East	Initial res., 1975	14.0	1.37	—	—	—	—	UG	
Safford-Kennecott (Lone Star)	Initial reserves	500+	0.50+	—	—	—	—	UG	Lowell, 1978, p. 176; Greeley, 1978, p. 85
		2,000	0.41	—	—	—	—	UG	
Safford-Phelps Dodge (Dos Pobres)	Initial reserves	400 ±	0.72(?)	—	—	—	—	—	Lowell, 1978, p. 176; Greeley, 1978, p. 86
San Manuel-Kalamazoo									
San Manuel	Initial res., 1949	339.3	0.789 (S_2)	—	—	—	0.5	UG	Schwartz, 1953, p. 62
		123.5	0.767 (ox)	—	—	—	0.5	UG	
	Reserves, 1978	457	0.75	0.017	—	—	0.5	UG	Lowell, 1978, p. 176
Kalamazoo	Reserves, 1978	500	0.73	0.015	—	—	0.5(?)	UG	Lowell, 1978, p. 176
TOTAL	(including San Manuel ox)	1,080	±0.74	0.015	—	—	0.5	UG	
San Xavier North	Initial reserves	±10	1.0 (ox)	—	—	—	—	—	Author's estimate
			0.57 (S_2)	—	—	—	—	—	
	Reserves, 1978	1	0.48 (ox)	—	—	—	—	—	NMGS GB, 1978, p. 90
		167	0.52 (S_2)	—	—	—	—	—	
Sierrita	Initial res., 1967	414	0.35	0.036	—	±0.02	0.15(?)	1.5:1	Min. Mag., Mar. 1971, p. 192–199
	Prod. 1968–1978	224.7	0.27 (rec)	0.022	—	—	0.15(?)	2.2:1	NMGS GB, 1978, p. 91; Aiken and West, 1978, p. 119
	Reserves, 1978	460	0.32 (ind)	0.033	—	—	0.15(?)	0.7:1	
Silver Bell	Total reserves(?)	±100	0.75 (con)	0.017	—	0.07	—	2.5:1	Lowell and Guilbert, 1970, p. 390 & 391
			0.80 (tac)						
Twin Buttes	Prod., 1965–1977	69.3	0.702 (rec)	0.008	—	—	—	16:1(?)	NMGS GB, 1978, p. 90
	Reserves, 1978	329 (mill)	0.670 (S_2)	0.030	—	—	—	3.3:1	
		57 (leach)	1.100 (ox)	—	—	—	—	—	
Vekol	Res. during devel.	±75	0.6	—	—	—	—	OP(?)	E&MJ, Dec. 1967, p. 14
	Reserves	105	0.56	0.014	—	—	—	OP	Greeley, 1978, p. 85

NOTE: Names of the principal deposits are given in boldface; alternative names (or, where there might be confusion, counties) are shown in parentheses; and names of individual orebodies are in italics.

KEY: con = conventional or intrusion mineralization
ind = indicated, as distinct from recovered, grade
leach = reserves of oxides amenable to leaching
mill = reserves requiring conventional milling
NMGS GB = New Mexico Geological Society Guidebook
ox = oxides
OP = open pit
rec = recovered, as distinct from indicated or estimated, grade
S_2 = sulfides
tac = tactite or wall-rock mineralization
UG = underground

TABLE 1.2

Production and Reserves in Representative Porphyry Copper Deposits in the Western United States, Exclusive of Arizona

DEPOSIT	PRODUCTION/ RESERVES	TONNAGE (s.t. × 10^6)	GRADE				CUT-OFF GRADE (% Cu)	RATIO W:O	SOURCES
			Cu %	Mo %	Au oz./s.t.	Ag oz./s.t.			
MONTANA									
Butte (Berkeley Pit)	Reserves, 1971	500+	±0.8	—	Yes	Yes	—	—	Author's estimate
NEVADA									
Battle Mountain									
Copper Canyon	Reserves, 1968	25 (mill) 14 (leach)	0.79 (S_2) 0.30 (ox)	— —	} 0.025	0.47	—	0.7:1	Sayers, et al., 1968, p. 56
Copper Basin	Reserves, 1968	3 (mill) 23 (leach)	1.75 (S_2) 0.41 (ox)	— —	} 0.011	0.26	—	0.7:1	
Ely (Ruth)	Production to 1960 Production, 1960	225 —	1.14 0.80	Yes —	— —	— —	— —	— 2:1	Bauer, et al., 1960, p. 222
NEW MEXICO									
Hillsboro (Copper Flat)	Reserves, 1978	±70	0.7(?)	—	—	—	—	—	Lowell, 1978, p. 176
Santa Rita (Chino)	Prod., 1911–1962 Reserves, 1970	230 500+	0.93 (rec) 0.97	— —	— —	— —	— —	2.4:1 —	Lowell and Guilbert, 1970, p. 390–391
Tyrone	Reserves, 1978	±400	0.70	—	—	—	—	—	Lowell, 1978, p. 176
UTAH									
Bingham	Prod., 1904–1915 1904–1930 1904–1970	34.05 192.73 1,170.04	1.464 (rec) 1.191 (rec) 0.927 (rec)	— — —	— — —	— — —	— — —	0.4:1 1.1:1 1.1:1	} Natl. Acad. Sci., 1975, p. 153; James, 1978, p. 1219
	Prod., 1904–1972	1,240.19	0.912 (rec)	0.036	0.0064	0.058	—	—	James, 1978, p. 1219
	Reserves, 1972	1,773.30	0.71 (ind)	0.053	—	—	—	—	Natl. Acad. Sci., 1975, p. 173
WASHINGTON									
Brenmac (Bren Mac, Sunrise)	Initial res., 1971 Reserves, 1979	49 60	0.3 0.8 eCu (Cu, Mo, W)	0.02	—	—	— —	— —	Min. Eng., Feb, 1971; Hollister, 1979, p. 32
Glacier Peak	Initial reserves	100+	0.50	Yes	—	—	—	—	Hollister, 1979, p. 28
Mazama	Initial reserves	470	0.37	Yes	Yes	—	—	—	Hollister, 1979, p. 27
Middle Fork	Initial reserves	100	0.4	0.02	—	—	—	—	Hollister, 1979, p. 32
Mt. Tolman	Initial reserves	300	0.13	0.13	—	—	0.1 (Mo)	—	Min. Mag., Mar. 1979
North Fork	Initial reserves	44.0	0.5	—	Yes	—	—	—	Hollister, 1979, p. 32

NOTE: States are given in all capitals; names of the principal deposits are shown in boldface; alternative names or spellings are in parentheses; and names of individual orebodies are in italics.

KEY: eCu = copper equivalent
ind = indicated, as distinct from recovered, grade
leach = reserves of oxides amenable to leaching
mill = reserves requiring conventional milling
ox = oxides
rec = recovered, as distinct from indicated or estimated, grade
S_2 = sulfides

TABLE 1.3
Production and Reserves in Representative Porphyry Copper Deposits in Mexico

DEPOSIT	PRODUCTION/ RESERVES	TONNAGE (s.t. × 10^6)	GRADE Cu %	Mo %	Au oz./s.t.	Ag oz./s.t.	CUT-OFF GRADE (% Cu)	RATIO W:O	SOURCES
BAJA CALIFORNIA									
El Arco	Reserves, 1976	600	0.6	—	—	—	—	—	Sillitoe, 1976, p. B175
SINALOA									
Santo Tomás	Reserves, 1976	80+	0.55	—	—	—	—	—	Sillitoe, 1976, p. B175
SONORA									
La Caridad	Initial reserves	660	0.8 eCu		—	—	—	—	Saegart, et al., 1974, p. 1061
	Reserves, 1979	750	0.67	0.02	—	—	—	0.51:1	E&MJ, Oct. 1979, p. 72–88
La Florida-Barricón	Reserves, 1976	90	0.3	—	—	—	—	—	Sillitoe, 1976, p. B174
Nacozari									
Santa Rosa and *Pilares*	Reserves, 1974	±130	0.80	Yes	—	Yes	—	—	Min. Mag., Dec. 1974, p. 431
Los Pilares (alone)	Past production	19	2.6	—	—	—	—	—	Sillitoe, 1976, p. B174
	Reserves, 1976	44	0.8	—	—	—	—	—	
MICHOACÁN									
Inguarán	Reserves, 1976	6.6	1.2–1.5	—	—	—	—	—	Sillitoe, 1976, p. B176
La Verde	Initial reserves	81.3	0.699	—	0.0026	0.075	—	—	E&MJ, Mar. 1973, p. 207

NOTE: States are given in all capitals; names of the principal deposits are shown in boldface; and names of individual ore-bodies are in italics.

KEY: eCu = copper equivalent

shown, as between oxide and sulfide (in some examples designated as leaching and milling, respectively), or between intrusion and wall rock (skarn or tactite). In still other examples differences may exist between the figures presented in various sources, and these are cited in order to give the reader some idea of the nature of the problem or of the range of uncertainty which exists in published data. Finally, a scatter of figures may show how, if cut-off grades are raised or lowered, mill-heads may be increased or decreased (in response to changing metal prices or costs), accompanied by a concomitant reduction or expansion of tonnage.

Of necessity the data were collected from diverse sources, requiring different types of treatment. Broadly speaking, these fall into three groups: (a) conventional scientific or technical papers, cited in the usual manner (name, year), with the details in the reference list at the end of the chapter; (b) anonymous items in technical journals, which are listed by title of the journal in the tables and are complete (including pages numbers); (c) entries in guidebooks and symposia, etc., the titles of which are abbreviated in the tables and completed in the reference list.

Important differences exist among the terms "indicated" (more or less "geological") and "minable" (or "engineering") tonnage and grade, and "recovered" grade. The first two refer to the distinction between estimates derived directly from raw data (drill holes, adits, cross-cuts, etc.) and those allowing for engineering considerations (such as dilution, and mining recovery), which are dependent on the depth and configuration of the mineralization, the strength of host rocks, etc. The last refers to the grade calculated from the amount of metal actually produced; the principal difference between this figure and the other two estimates is attributable to metallurgical losses. The point of importance here is that, although the distinction between geologic and engineering estimates on the one hand, and recovered grade on the other, is nearly always clear where copper is concerned, it may not be made explicit with respect to minor metals. With recovery of molybdenum, for example, ranging from 75 down to 26 percent, it may readily be seen that the difference between estimated and recovered grade can be very significant. As a very rough guide, the grades given in the tables for molybdenum generally refer to either geological or engineering grade estimates (the difference between these two being relatively minor), whereas the assays given for gold and silver include both estimated and recovered figures (the distinction commonly being unclear in the source material). If the content of precious metals is relatively high, the published figures tend to be estimates derived from assays of the ore, whereas, if the precious metal content is low, the grades are typically based on recovered metals. The published grades therefore tend to exaggerate any real differences which may exist in the amounts of precious metals present in the orebodies.

It should not be assumed that the published statistics (notably those for tonnage) represent the total amount of ore-grade material in any given deposit. Were it not for the tax laws in Arizona, which impose a financial penalty on exploration for and/or disclosure of reserves, the state might well boast one or more porphyry deposits the size of Bingham or El Teniente.

PRODUCTION AND RESERVES IN OTHER AREAS

In order to place the statistics for southwestern North America in perspective it is necessary to examine the grades of porphyry copper deposits in other parts of the world. One of the advantages of looking outside the Southwest is that some features or trends may be better illustrated elsewhere than in this "type" area. For example, the growing importance of modern primary grade mineralization is exemplified by deposits in British Columbia, and the increasing emphasis on minor metals, notably gold and silver, is shown in southeastern Asia and in the southwestern Pacific.

Deposits in areas which lack adequate infrastructure require very large capital sums for their development and tend to have high operating costs. In order to be profitable these areas need the range of grades typically associated with secondary enrichment (e.g., Sar Chesmeh, Iran; Cerro Colorado, Panama), skarn mineralization (e.g., Gaspé, Quebec), or exceptional primary grades—especially in minor metals (e.g., Lornex, B.C.; Panguna, Papua New Guinea). In regions which have adequate infrastructure and favorable investment climates, new records for acceptably low grades have been established (e.g., parts of B.C., Europe, and the Southwest). In short, "low" can mean different things in different places.

In light of the foregoing it would be useful to briefly review recent developments in areas outside the Southwest and to summarize the reserves of a number of representative deposits in tabular form.

Gaspe Mines (Quebec) was developed in the early 1950s—i.e., about the same time as Esperanza and Pima. This event was to prove a signal step in the unfolding story of primary sulfide exploration—especially in British Columbia—and was to have a profound impact on thinking about porphyries in general, but over ten years were to elapse before the porphyry affiliations of the mineralization were recognized (Gilmour, 1962; Hollister et al., 1974; Kirkham and Soregaroli, 1975). Until the late 1960s or so conventional wisdom held that porphyry copper deposits were somehow restricted to certain segments of the Cordilleran portion of the cirum-Pacific "ring of fire"—the implications of the principle of uniformitarianism notwithstanding. Whether or not any given body of mineralization constitutes a porphyry in the economic-engineering sense depends on numerous geologic and non-geologic factors. Gaspe was instructive in that it lies in the Appalachian belt and is associated with igneous rocks of Devonian age. Initially, only tactite mineralization (wall rock porphyry), capable of providing a mill-head of around 1.5 percent copper, was mined in the underground operation at Gaspe. Low-grade material was subsequently exploited in an open-pit operation on Copper Mountain and the porphyry affiliations of the deposit became incontestable. Statistics for production and reserves in the tactite (or skarn) of the Needle Mountain orebody and the low-grade deposits of the Copper Mountain orebody are shown in Table 1.4. Interestingly enough, another deposit in eastern Canada with porphyry affinities was also mined for several years before its nature was recognized (Blecha, 1965, 1974): the Tribag deposit, near Sault St. Marie, Ontario, lies in the Superior

TABLE 1.4
Production and Reserves of Porphyry Copper Deposits in Eastern Canada

DEPOSIT	PRODUCTION/ RESERVES	TONNAGE (s.t. × 10^6)	GRADE Cu %	Mo %	Au oz./s.t.	Ag oz./s.t.	CUT-OFF GRADE (% Cu)	RATIO W:O	SOURCES
ONTARIO									
Tribag									
Breton	Estimated reserves	±40.0	0.2	—	—	—	—	UG	
	Production to 1973	0.901	1.64	—	—	—	—	UG	
East	Estimated total	{125.0	0.13	—	—	—	—	UG(?)	Blecha, 1974, p. 71 & 72
	(including)	4.27	0.27	±0.03	—	—	—	UG(?)	
West	Prod., 1967–1973	0.121	2.35	—	—	—	—	UG	
QUEBEC									
Gaspe Mines									
Needle Mtn.	Initial res., ±1955	48.32 (tac)	1.54	—	—	—	—	UG	Ford, 1959, p. 425
	Production, 1977	1.376 (tac)	1.13	—	—	—	—	UG	} Can. Mines Handbook, 1978–1979, p. 118
	Reserves, Dec. 1977 (proven & probable)	12.321 (tac)	1.15	—	—	—	—	UG	
Copper Mtn.	Prod., 1968–1977	±100.00	0.415	—	—	—	—	OP	
	Reserves, Dec. 1977	29.95 (ox)	0.435	—	—	—	—	OP	
		182.061 (S_2)	0.378	—	—	—	—	OP	

NOTE: Provinces are given in all capitals; names of the principal deposits are shown in boldface; and names of individual orebodies are in italic.

KEY: OP = open pit
ox = oxides
S_2 = sulfides
tac = tactite or wall-rock mineralization
UG = underground

province of the Canadian shield and is evidently Precambrian in age. When in 1967 Blecha visited the Copper Creek area (in Pinal and Graham counties, Arizona), accompanied by the present writer, the former remarked on the very strong similarity between some of the 100-odd Laramide intrusive breccia pipes and those at Tribag with which he was familiar. Figures for actual production and reserves estimated by Blecha are shown in Table 1.4.

The first porphyry (i.e., in the modern, loose sense, which includes wall-rock mineralization) developed in British Columbia was, not surprisingly, a tactite deposit, roughly similar to Gaspe. Craigmont was found in the late 1950s and went on stream as an open-pit operation in the early 1960s (Rennie et al., 1961; Carr, 1966). Its development was closely followed by that of the intrusive Bethlehem deposit in the Highland Valley, and the era of primary deposits—with grades substantially less than 1 percent copper—was truly inaugurated.

As at Pima, its contemporary in Arizona, Bethlehem began small, mining relatively high-grade material, and then grew up. The initial Bethlehem reserves are shown in Table 1.5. Besides emphasizing the nature of the initial reserves, the table also reveals the fact that the original cut-off grade actually exceeded the overall or average grade of subsequent mining operations (0.45–0.47%). The table also shows the effect that the stripping ratio has had on the effective mined grade (the grade which must support mining, as distinct from all other, costs). In other terms, if at a given mining operation the cost of mining a ton of rock is 50¢ and the stripping ratio (W:O) is 2:1, the actual mining cost—the cost of delivering a ton of ore to the concentrator—will be $1.50.

Numerous deposits have been found in other parts of Canada; some statistics for alkaline and calc-alkaline occurrences are shown in Tables 1.6 and 1.7 respectively. Since (like Sierrita, Pinto Valley, etc.) these are new developments, some of which have been partly financed through public participation, and since Canadian companies are freer with information than some of their counterparts elsewhere, a good deal of economic and other information on these deposits is available.

Various technical and economic developments accompanied or flowed from the exploitation of the modern, low-grade primary deposits. One of these was improved metallurgical recoveries: the performance at many B.C. operations equaled or rivaled San Manuel's 98 percent recovery of copper. Indeed, one might say that the low average grades made improved recovery—compared with the classical porphyries—imperative. A drill-indicated grade of 0.6 percent copper with only 80 percent recovery is equivalent to 0.5 percent at 95 percent recovery.

A trend already noted which was emphasized by the new developments was the increased importance of minor metals. The value of the molybdenum exceeds that of copper in a number of B.C. deposits, while the preoccupation with gold and silver is evidenced by the number of assays available (cf. Tables 1.6 and 1.7 with Tables 1.1, 1.2, and 1.3). The emphasis on precious metals in British Columbia also pointed up some of the differences between calc-alkaline and alkaline porphyries, the latter generally containing more gold and silver and very much less molybdenum than the former (see Tables 1.6 and 1.7).

The best expression of the greater emphasis placed on precious metals is to be seen in the results of exploration of porphyry mineralization in southern Asia (Table 1.8), the southwestern Pacific (Table 1.9), and the Philippines (Table 1.10). Prigogine (1975) noted, for example, that Mamut in Malaysia will produce each year, in addition to 27,000–30,000 tons of copper, some 2 tons of gold and 14 tons of silver, worth nearly (US) $50,000,000 at the prices prevailing in late 1980. The presence of these "minor" metals was to prove a boon to many mines in the middle and late 1970s, when (during a time of recession and reduced prices for most metals) the value of molybdenum, gold and silver climbed.

Statistics for examples from other parts of the world are shown in Table 1.11 (Central America), Table 1.12 (South America), and Table 1.13 (Europe). Not all of these are commercial—e.g., the mineralization believed to be of late Cambrian age from the forest of Coed-y-Brenin in Wales (Rice and Sharp, 1976), which is added for purposes of comparison. The existence of mineralization with porphyry affiliations in Paleozoic intrusions in the Scottish Highlands has been noted (Gallagher et al., 1971; Ellis, 1977; Evans, 1977; Rice and Davies, 1979), although not enough is known about it to permit its inclusion in a table.

CAPITAL COSTS OF PORPHYRY COPPER PRODUCTION

As noted at the outset, even if the economic factor has to be de-emphasized in certain circumstances, the ultimate reasons for studying metallic mineral deposits as discrete geologic phenomena are economic, and porphyry copper deposits are no exception. One of the outstanding features of very large mining projects (such as the grade and tonnage of porphyries demand) is that they are almost independent of

TABLE 1.5
Initial Reserves in the Bethlehem Porphyry Copper Deposit in the Highland Valley, British Columbia

MINE	INDIVIDUAL DEPOSIT	TONNAGE (s.t. × 10^6)	GRADE (% Cu)	CUT-OFF GRADE (% Cu)	RATIO W:O	EFFECTIVE GRADE	SOURCE
Bethlehem	*East Jersey*	3.37	1.12*	0.6	2.2:1	0.373	Metal Min. & Proc., Mar. 1964,
	Jersey	14.7	0.82	—	0.6:1	0.513	p. 31–32

*Diluted grade. The undiluted figure was 1.19% Cu.

TABLE 1.6

Production and Reserves in Representative "Alkaline" Porphyry Copper Deposits in Western Canada

DEPOSIT	PRODUCTION/ RESERVES	TONNAGE (s.t. × 10^6)	GRADE				CUT-OFF GRADE (% Cu)	RATIO W:O	SOURCES
			Cu %	Mo %	Au oz./s.t.	Ag oz./s.t.			
BRITISH COLUMBIA **Afton**	Initial res., 1975	34	1.00	—	0.0168	0.1215	0.25	4.2:1	Min. Mag., Dec. 1975, p. 416; Carr and Reed, 1976, p. 376
Caribou-Belle	Reserves in #2 and #5 Zones, 1975	28	0.49	—	0.0162	0.0325	0.3	2.4:1	Hodgson et al., 1976, p. 393
Copper Mountain & Ingerbelle	Res. in Ingerbelle & Cu Mtn, #1 & #2, 1976	61.3	0.53	—	Yes	Yes	0.2–0.3	±2:1	Fahrni et al., 1976*b*, p. 368
Galore Creek (Alice Arm)	Reserves in Central Zone, 1975	137.5	1.06	trace	0.0116	0.2233	—	—	Allen et al., 1976, p. 411
Lorraine	Reserves, 1975 { U^r Zone L^r Zone	4.95 6.05	0.75 0.60	— —	0.0099 0.0029	— —	— —	— —	Wilkinson et al., 1976, p. 397

NOTE: The province is shown in all capitals; names of principal deposits are given in boldface; and alternative names are in parentheses.

TABLE 1.7
Production and Reserves of Representative "Calc-Alkaline" Porphyry Copper Deposits in Western Canada

DEPOSIT	PRODUCTION/ RESERVES	TONNAGE (s.t. × 10^6)	GRADE Cu %	Mo %	Au oz./s.t.	Ag oz./s.t.	CUT-OFF GRADE (% Cu)	RATIO W:O	SOURCES
BRITISH COLUMBIA **Axe**	Initial res., 1976	63 (?)	0.50 (?)	—	—	—	—	—	J. Newell, 1976, pers. comm.
Bell (Babine Lake)	Geologic reserves Minable reserves	127.6 46.2	0.48 0.50	±0.005 —	0.01310 —	0.0435 —	0.3 0.3	— 0.5:1	Carson et al., 1976, p. 247
Berg	Geological reserves	±440	0.40	0.050	—	—	0.25	—	Panteleyev et al., 1976, p. 274
Bethlehem *East Jersey*	Initial res., 1964	3.37	1.19	—	—	—	0.6	2.2:1	Met. Min. & Proc., Mar. 1964, p. 31 & 32
Jersey	Initial res., 1964 Prod., 1964–1974 Reserves, 1975	14.7 31.5 34.8	0.82 — 0.46	— ±0.10 (?) —	— — —	— ±0.0435 —	— — 0.25	0.6:1 — —	Met. Min. & Proc., Mar. 1964, p. 31 & 32 (Initial res.); Briskey and Bellamy, 1976, p. 105
Heustis	Prod., 1970–1974 Reserves, 1975	18.88 8.17	— 0.45	— —	— —	— —	— 0.25	— —	Briskey and Bellamy, 1976, p. 105
Iona	Reserves, 1975	13.25	0.47	—	—	—	0.25	—	Briskey and Bellamy, 1976, p. 105
Brenda	Initial res., 1970 (including) Ann. prod., e.g., 1974 Reserves, 1975	{ 192.75 { 27.72 9.34 127.74	0.183 0.212 0.186 0.177	0.049 0.063 0.051 0.046	— — — —	— — — —	— 0.3 eCu —	— — 0.8:1 —	Min. Mag., Apr. 1971, p. 269; Min. Mag., June 1972, p. 416–423; Soregaroli and Whitford, 1976, p. 196
Cache Creek	Estimated res., 1976	100	0.40 eCu		—	—	—	—	J. Newell, 1976, pers. comm.
Copper Mountain (Granby)	Prod., 1925–1957	35	1.08	—	—	—	—	—	J. Newell, 1976, pers. comm.
Craigmont	Prod. and res., 1966 Average annual prod., 1974–1976	±29 1.81	1.77 (tac) 1.53 (head) 1.36 (rec)	— —	— —	±0.30 —	— —	UG UG	Rennie et al., 1961; Carr, 1966, p. 321; E&MJ, Feb. 1975, p. 119; E&MJ, Mar. 1977, p. 259; Canadian Mines Handbook 1977–1978, p. 93
Fish Lake	Reserves, 1975	"several tens"	±0.30	—	0.0145	—	—	—	Wolfard, 1976, p. 317
Gibraltar *Gibraltar East & West; Pollyana;* and *Granite Lake*	Initial res., 1972	358+	0.373	0.011	—	—	0.25	—	Min. Mag., Jul. 1972, p. 37–41; Min. Eng., Jul. 1972, p. 84–90
Gnat Lake	Reserves, 1972	20	0.44	—	—	—	—	—	J. Newell, 1976, pers. comm.
Granisle	Initial res., 1966 Prod., 1966–1975 Reserves, 1975	22 27.5 66.0	0.53 0.456 (rec) 0.43	— — —	— 0.0038 —	— 0.0356 —	— — —	0.15:1 — 1.1:1	West. Miner, May 1967, p. 31–38; Fahrni et al., 1976*a*, p. 239

Highmont	Res. in #1 deposit #2 #3, 4, and 6 #5 #7	121.0 26.4 — 0.13 0.20	0.287 0.273 — 1.1 1.0	0.042 0.093 — — —	— — — — —	} 0.0007 — —	— — — — —	1:1 1.8:1 — — —	Reed and Jambor, 1976, p. 163
Huckleberry	Initial reserves { Geologic Minable	96.0 85.5	0.408 0.401	0.025 0.025	— —	— —	0.30 0.25	— 1.2:1	James, 1976, p. 284
Island Copper	Initial res., 1971 Prod., 1971–1975 Prod. per day, 1975	283 28 0.035	0.52 — 0.39 (rec)	0.017 — 0.0043	— — ±0.0002	— — ±0.0008	— — —	2.4:1 2.7:1 2.5:1	Min. Mag., Oct. 1972, p. 344–349; Cargill et al., 1976, p. 206
J.A. (J–A)	Geologic reserves Minable reserves	286 126–148	0.43 0.60–0.65 eCu	0.017	— —	— —	— —	— 2.5:1	McMillan, 1976, p. 144 & 145
Krain	Initial reserves { Oxidized Sulfide Total	5.4 10.0 15.4	0.64 0.53 0.56	— — 0.010	— — —	— — —	— — —	— — —	Christie, 1976, p. 182
Lornex	Initial res., 1968 Reserves, Dec. 1974 Reserves, Dec. 1976	292.6 432 500	0.427 0.411 0.412	0.014 0.015 0.015	— — —	— — —	0.26 0.26 (?) —	1.2:1 2.1:1 —	Min. Mag., Mar. 1973, p. 154–163 } Canadian Mines Handbook, 1977–1978, p. 182 & 184
Maggie	Estimated res., 1975 {	200 199.5	0.40 eCu (?) 0.28	 0.029	— Yes	— —	— —	— —	J. Newell, 1976, pers. comm. Millar, 1976, p. 329
Morrison	Estimated res., 1973 (?)	95	0.42	0.010	0.0087	0.087	0.30	—	Carson and Jambor, 1976, p. 264
Mount Nansen	Estimated res., 1973 (?)	—	0.1–0.15	0.01–0.06	—	—	—	—	Sawyer and Dickinson, 1976, p. 342
OK	Indicated reserves Inferred reserves	54 21	0.30 0.26	0.016 0.020	— —	— —	0.20 —	— —	} Meyer et al., 1976, p. 311
Ox Lake	Estimated res., 1970	23.6	0.35 eCu		—	—	—	—	Richards, 1976, p. 289
Poison Mountain	Estimated res., 1975	±192	0.33	0.015	0.0087	—	0.25	0.7:1	Seraphim and Rainboth, 1976, p. 324
Schaft Creek	Estimated res., 1975	363	0.40	0.036	0.0093	0.0435	—	1.5:1	Fox et al., 1976, p. 219
Valley Copper	Estimated res., 1975	940	0.48	—	—	—	—	0.9:1	Osatenko and Jones, 1976, p. 130
YUKON **Casino**	Initial res., 1975	178	0.37	0.026	—	—	—	1.7:1	Godwin, 1976, p. 344

NOTE: Provinces are given in all capitals; name of principal deposits are shown in boldface; alternative names are in parentheses; and names of individual orebodies are in italics.

KEY: eCu = copper equivalent
head = mill-head (grade)
rec = recovered, as distinct from indicated or estimated, grade
tac = tactite or wall-rock mineralization

TABLE 1.8
Reserves in Representative Porphyry Copper Deposits in Southern Asia

DEPOSIT[a]	RESERVES	TONNAGE (s.t. × 10^6)	GRADE				CUT-OFF GRADE (% Cu)	RATIO W:O	SOURCES
			Cu %	Mo %	Au oz./s.t.	Ag oz./s.t.			
BURMA									
Moniwa (Monywa)	Initial reserves	66.0	0.8	—	—	—	—	—	Min. Jour., May 14, 1976, p. 389
IRAN									
Sar Cheshmeh	Initial reserves: Supergene	101.5	1.996	—	—	—	0.4	—	Waterman and Hamilton, 1975, p. 575;
	Initial reserves: Hypogene	368.7	0.896	—	—	—	0.4	—	Min. Mag., Mar. 1975, p. 182–185;
	Total	470.2	1.132	±0.03	Yes	Yes	0.4	0.6:1	E&MJ, Feb. 1978, p. 57–60
MALAYASIA									
Mamut (Sabah)	Initial reserves: Indicated	195.8	0.476	—	—	—	0.2	—	Min. Mag., Apr. 1975, p. 252–259
	Initial reserves: Minable	91.3	0.590	—	0.01841	—	0.4	1.1:1	(Min. Mag., Apr. 1975, p. 252–259)
	Minable reserves	77.0	0.61	—	0.01885	0.116	0.4	—	World Mining, Oct. 1975, p. 42–48
PAKISTAN									
Saindak									
North	Initial reserves	22.0	0.5	—	—	—	0.25	—	Min. Mag., Nov. 1978, p. 484–493
South	Initial reserves: Geologic	122.1	0.407	—	—	—	0.25	—	
	Initial reserves: Minable	83.1	0.426	0.0063	0.01479	—	0.25	3.3:1	
East	Initial reserves	300.3	0.004	—	—	—	0.25	—	

NOTE: Countries are given in all capitals; names of the principal deposits are shown in boldface; alternative names or spellings are in parentheses; and names of individual orebodies are in italics.

[a] Numerous porphyry copper deposits occur in the southern part of the Soviet Union, especially in the Asian territories (Sutulov, 1973; Laznicka, 1976), but figures for production and reserves are sketchy.

Table 1.9
Reserves in Representative Porphyry Copper Deposits in the Southwestern Pacific

DEPOSIT	RESERVES	TONNAGE (s.t. × 10^6)	GRADE Cu %	Mo %	Au oz./s.t.	Ag oz./s.t.	CUT-OFF GRADE (% Cu)	RATIO W:O	SOURCES
FIJI									
Namosi	Tot. ind. res., 1978	±440.0	0.4–0.5	—	—	—	—	—	Min. Jour., Feb. 2, 1979
	Res., 1979 *Waisoi East*	±165	0.50	—	—	—	—	±2:1	Min. Eng., Nov. 1979, p. 1550
	Res., 1979 *Waisoi West*	±330	0.48	—	—	—	—	±2:1	Min. Eng., Nov. 1979, p. 1550
INDONESIA									
Gulun Bijih (Ertzberg)	Initial reserves	33.0 (tac)	2.50	—	0.0217–0.0247	0.2305–0.2552	—	UG	Titley, 1978, p. 978
PAPUA–NEW GUINEA									
Frieda River									
Horse-Ivaal	Indicated reserves	550.0	0.50	0.003	0.010	—	—	—	Titley, 1978, p. 978
Koki Creek	Indicated reserves	286.0	0.41	0.006	0.007	—	—	—	Titley, 1978, p. 978
Manus Island	Indicated reserves	181.5	0.32	"minor" Mo, Au and Ag			—	—	Min. Jour., Jun. 17, 1975, p. 467
OK Tedi	Interim reserves	275.0	0.75	0.012	0.016	—	—	—	Min. Mag., Apr. 1975, p. 245
	Reserves, 1978	330.0 (con)	0.75	0.01	0.018	—	—	—	Titley, 1978, p. 978
	Reserves, 1978	27.5 (tac)	2.33	—	0.050	—	—	—	Titley, 1978, p. 978
Panguna	Reserves, 1972	±1,000.0	0.46–0.48	±0.0050	0.0148–0.0180	0.0603	—	0.7:1	Fountain, 1972, p. 1049; Titley, 1978, p. 978
Yandera	Indicated reserves	371.8	0.42	0.016	0.0029	0.0626	—	—	Titley, 1978, p. 978

NOTE: Countries are given in all capitals; names of the principal deposits are shown in boldface; alternative names are in parentheses; and names of individual orebodies are in italics.

KEY:
con = conventional or intrusion mineralization
tac = tactite or wall-rock mineralization
UG = underground

TABLE 1.10
Production and Reserves in Representative Porphyry Copper Deposits in the Philippines

DEPOSIT	PRODUCTION/ RESERVES	TONNAGE (s.t. × 10^6)	GRADE Cu %	Mo %	Au oz./s.t.	Ag oz./s.t.	CUT-OFF GRADE (% Cu)	RATIO W:O	SOURCES
CEBU ISLAND									
Atlas									
Lutopan	Total res. and prod.	217	0.70	Minor Au, Ag, py, and Fe_3O_4			0.5 (?)	UG	Bryner, 1969, p. 656; Min. Mag., Jan. 1974, p. 9; W. M., Dec. 1974, p. 28–33; Min. Mag., Aug. 1976, p. 107; E&MJ, Feb. 1977, p. 117–118; E&MJ, Jun. 1977, p. 43
Greater Biga and *Frank*	Initial reserves	690	0.47	—	Yes	Yes	—	—	
Carmen	Initial res. (devel)	328	0.43	—	Yes	Yes	—	—	
LUZON ISLAND									
Balatoc	Initial res. (devel)	60.0	0.5–0.6	—	0.010	—	—	—	W. M., May 1976, p. 101
Bessemer	Interim res. (expl)	17.0	0.56	—	—	—	—	—	W. M., Dec. 1974, p. 28–33
Boneng-Lobo	Reserves, 1974 (expl)	99.0	0.48	—	0.01 Au and Ag		—	—	W. M., Dec. 1974, p. 28–33
Butilao	Interim res. (expl)	30.0	0.6	—	—	—	—	—	W. M., Dec. 1974, p. 28–33
Cordon	Interim res. (expl)	50.0	0.31–1.75	—	—	—	—	—	W. M., Dec. 1974, p. 28–33
Dizon	Interim res. (devel)	{ 75.0 90.0 100.0	0.5 0.442 0.442	— — —	0.029 0.026 0.027	— — —	— — —	— — —	Min. Mag., May 1971, p. 401 W. M., Dec. 1974, p. 28–33 W. M., Nov. 1975, p. 81
Hale-Mayabo-Uban	Interim res. (expl)	46.0	0.50	—	—	—	—	—	W. M., Dec. 1974, p. 28–33
Kennon (Black Mountain)	Initial res. (expl)	— 27.0	0.63 0.47	— —	0.02 Yes	0.32 Yes	— —	UG UG	Min. Eng., Apr. 1969, p. 69; E&MJ, Jun. 1969, p. 287; W. M., Dec. 1974, p. 28–33
Lumbay	Interim res. (expl)	100.0	0.42	—	—	—	—	—	W. M., Dec. 1974, p. 28–33
Philex (San Antonio)	Reserves, 1967 Reserves, 1969 Reserves, 1974	— 56–60 28.0	0.7 0.6 0.50	— — —	0.030 0.024 —	— 0.450 —	— — —	UG UG UG	Min. Eng., Apr. 1967, p. 74 Min. Eng., Apr. 1969, p. 68 W. M., Dec. 1974, p. 28–33
Santo Niño	Reserves, 1975 (prod)	30	0.38	—	0.011	—	—	—	Min. Mag., Dec. 1975, p. 421
Santo Tomás II	Total prod. and res.	48.0	0.7	—	Yes	Yes	—	UG	Bryner, 1969, p. 657
Tawi-Tawi	Interim res. (expl)	178	0.393	—	Yes	Yes	—	—	W. M., Dec. 1974, p. 28–33
Taysan	Interim reserves (expl-devel)	60.0	0.38	—	—	—	—	—	W. M., Dec. 1974, p. 28–33
MARINDUQUE ISLAND									
Ino-Capayang-Bintakay	Interim reserves (expl-devel)	76.0	0.61	—	—	—	—	—	W. M., Dec. 1974, p. 28–33

Santa Cruz (Marcopper)	Init. res. oxide ore	4.7	0.89	Yes	Yes	Yes	—	1.8:1	Min. Eng., Apr. 1969, p. 64; Min. Mag., Jun. 1971, p. 438–455; Min. Mag., Jun. 1976, p. 547
	Init. res. high grade	85.7	0.752	—	—	—	0.4 (?)	1.8:1	
	Init. res. low grade	63.5	0.28	—	—	—	0.25	1.8:1	
	Reserves, 1974	103.0	0.58	—	0.005	0.0230	—	—	W. M., Dec. 1974, p. 28–33
	Reserves, 1978	102.3	0.58	0.011	0.0101	0.0452	—	—	Titley, 1978, p. 978
MINDANAO									
Kalamatan	Interim res. (expl)	12	0.383	—	—	—	—	—	W. M., Dec. 1974, p. 28–33
Masara	Reserves, 1974 (prod)	28	0.39–0.53	—	Yes	—	—	—	W. M., Dec. 1974, p. 28–33
Pantukan	Interim res. (expl)	45	0.45	—	—	—	—	—	W. M., Dec. 1974, p. 28–33
Sabena	Reserves, 1977	42	0.50	—	0.01 (rec)	0.017 (rec)	—	—	E&MJ, Mar. 1977, p. 271
Tagpura	Initial res., 1974	8	0.632	—	—	—	—	—	W. M., Dec. 1974, p. 28–33
NEGROS									
Aya-Aya	Interim res. (expl)	30	0.5	—	—	—	—	—	W. M., Dec. 1974, p. 28–33
Basay	Initial reserves (expl-devel)	65	0.56	—	—	—	—	—	W. M., Dec. 1974.
	Reserves, 1978	220	0.41	0.0080	0.0084	—	—	—	Titley, 1978, p. 978
Hinoban	Reserves (devel)	99	0.50	—	0.0029	0.090	—	—	W. M., Dec. 1974, p. 28–33
Sipalay (Cansibit)	Interim reserves	70	0.51	Yes	—	—	—	2.6:1 (to 800′)	Min. Eng., 1967, p. 74; Min. Eng., 1969, p. 64; Min. Eng., Aug. 1978, p. 1171; Min. Mag., Jun. 1976, p. 547
	Interim reserves	550	0.5	—	Yes	Yes	—	—	
	Reserves, 1978	884	0.50	0.015	0.0101	0.0452	—	—	Titley, 1978, p. 978

NOTE: Individual islands are given in all capitals; names of the principal deposits are shown in boldface; alternative names are in parentheses; and names of individual orebodies are in italics.

KEY: devel = during mine development
expl = during exploration
expl-devel = between exploration and development
prod = production or in production
rec = recovered, as distinct from indicated or estimated, grade
UG = underground
W. M. = World Mining

TABLE 1.11
Reserves in Representative Porphyry Copper Deposits in Central America

DEPOSIT	RESERVES	TONNAGE (s.t. × 10^6)	GRADE Cu %	GRADE Mo %	GRADE Au oz./s.t.	GRADE Ag oz./s.t.	CUT-OFF GRADE (% Cu)	RATIO W:O	SOURCES
PANAMA									
Cerro Colorado	Initial reserves	2,000 ±	0.6	0.015	0.0022	0.154	—	—	Min. Mag., Aug. 1974, p. 86 & 89
Cobre Panama	Initial reserves	300	0.65	—	—	—	—	—	Min. Mag., Mar. 1975, p. 217
Petaquilla	Reserves	500	0.4	Yes	—	—	—	—	Min. Eng., Feb. 1971, p. 131

NOTE: Country is given in all capitals, and names of the principal deposits are shown in boldface.

TABLE 1.12
Production and Reserves in Representative Porphyry Copper Deposits in South America

DEPOSIT	PRODUCTION/ RESERVES	TONNAGE (s.t. × 10^6)	GRADE Cu %	Mo %	Au oz./s.t.	Ag oz./s.t.	CUT-OFF GRADE (% Cu)	RATIO W:O	SOURCES
ARGENTINA									
Bajo Alumbrera	Reserves	?	0.38	0.04	0.0230	—	—	—	Hollister, 1973, p. 52 & 53
(Farellon Negro)	Reserves	±275	±0.5	—	—	—	—	—	Min. Jour., June 24, 1977, p. 491
El Pachón	Early reserves, 1972	80	1.0	—	—	—	—	—	E&MJ, Jun. 1972, p. 21
	Early reserves, 1972	60	0.6	—	—	—	—	—	E&MJ, Jun. 1972, p. 21
	Interim reserves 1973	270	0.7	—	—	—	—	—	E&MJ, May 1973, p. 17;
	Interim reserves 1976	600	0.59	0.016	—	—	—	—	Min. Jour., Jun. 4, 1976, p. 456;
	Interim reserves 1976	850	0.59	0.016	—	—	—	—	Min. Mag., Jul. 1976, p. 55
Paramillos Sur	Reserves	±115	0.38	0.020	—	—	—	—	Hollister, 1973, p. 52 & 53; Lowell, 1975, p. 34
CHILE									
Andacollo	Reserves, 1975	350	0.69	0.015	—	—	—	—	Lowell, 1975, p. 34; Min. Mag., Feb. 1976, p. 75 & 77
Andina (Rio Blanco)	Reserves, 1972	140	1.56	0.03	—	—	—	UG	Min. Mag., May 1972, p. 333
	Reserves Proven	120	1.29	0.02	—	—	—	UG	E&MJ, Sept. 1977, p. 36 & 41
	Reserves Probable	200	1.10	0.02	—	—	—	UG	E&MJ, Sept. 1977, p. 36 & 41
	Reserves Possible	100	0.80	0.02	—	—	—	UG	E&MJ, Sept. 1977, p. 36 & 41
Cerro Blanco	Reserves, 1973	120	1.58	0.03	—	—	—	—	Hollister, 1973, p. 52 & 53
Cerro Colorado	Reserves, 1975	?	1.0 +	—	—	—	—	—	Lowell, 1975, p. 34
Chuquicamata	Production	±2,000	0.61 (rec)	0.06	(?)	Yes	—	0.6 : 1	Min. Eng., Nov. 1969, p. 62 & 68–72
	Reserves Proven	624	1.38	—	—	—	—	—	E&MJ, Sept. 1977, p. 36 & 41
	Reserves Probable	910	0.99	—	—	—	—	—	E&MJ, Sept. 1977, p. 36 & 41
	Reserves Possible	8,853	0.46	—	—	—	—	—	E&MJ, Sept. 1977, p. 36 & 41
	Reserves Total	10,387	0.56	—	—	—	—	—	E&MJ, Sept. 1977, p. 36 & 41
Disputada	Reserves	100	1.40	—	—	—	—	—	E&MJ, Sept. 1977, p. 36 & 41
El Abra (San Jose del Abra)	Reserves Proven	60 (leach)	0.9 (ox)	—	—	—	—	—	Min. Eng., Nov. 1974, p. 22–28; Lowell, 1975, p. 34
	Reserves Proven	400 (mill)	0.9 (S_2)	—	—	—	—	—	Min. Eng., Nov. 1974, p. 22–28; Lowell, 1975, p. 34
	Reserves Possible	1,300 +	0.6	—	—	—	—	—	E&MJ, Sept. 1977, p. 36 & 41
El Salvador	Reserves Proven	150	1.28	0.033	—	—	—	—	Min. Eng., Apr. 1960, p. 339–382; Gustafson and Hunt, 1975; E&MJ, Sept. 1977, p. 36 & 41
	Reserves Probable	125	1.04	—	—	—	—	—	
	Reserves Possible	37	1.16	—	—	—	—	—	
	Reserves Total	312	1.17	—	—	—	—	—	
El Teniente (Braden)	Reserves Proven	2,850	1.16	0.03	—	—	—	UG	Howell and Molloy, 1960; E&MJ, Jun. 1969, p. 103–112; E&MJ, Sept. 1977, p. 36 & 41; E&MJ, Jun. 1978, p. 141–151
	Reserves Probable	1,200	0.90	0.05(?)	—	—	—	UG	
	Reserves Possible	4,300	0.30	—	—	—	—	UG	
	Reserves Total (or Potential)	8,350	0.68	—	—	—	—	UG	
Los Bronces	Reserves	±50	1.70	—	—	—	—	—	Hollister, 1973, p. 52 & 53

Los Pelambres	Reserves	±430	0.78	0.033	—	—	—	—	Lowell, 1975, p. 34; E&MJ, Sept. 1977, p. 36 & 41; Min. Eng., Jan. 1979, p. 17
	Reserves	±475	0.78	0.03	—	—	—	—	
Mantos Blancos	Reserves	55	0.85 (ox)	—	—	—	—	—	E&MJ, Sept. 1977, p. 36 & 41
	Reserves	50	1.50 (S_2)	—	—	—	—	—	
Pampa Norte	Reserves	242	0.70	—	—	—	—	—	E&MJ, Sept. 1977, p. 36 & 41
Potrerillos	Total, or past, prod.	±110	1.65	—	—	—	—	—	Lowell, 1975, p. 34, and author's estimate
COLOMBIA									
Pegadorcito and **Pantanos**	Reserves	625	±0.70	—	—	—	—	—	E&MJ, Jan. 1973, p. 17
	Prelim. reserves, Pegadorcito alone	275–690	0.7–1.2	—	—	—	—	—	Min. Eng., 1979, p. 1550
ECUADOR									
Chaucha	Reserves	74	0.7	0.02–0.04	—	—	—	—	Goossens and Hollister, 1973, p. 321
	Reserves	100	0.5	0.030	—	—	—	—	Min. Eng., Dec. 1972, p. 18
	Reserves	400 –	0.4	0.030	—	—	—	—	Lowell, 1975, p. 34
PERU									
Antamina	Reserves "Possible"	9.0 (tac)	2.6 (3.1 Zn)	—	—	—	—	—	Min. Mag., Oct. 1974, p. 277
		80.0	1.3 (1.4 Zn)	—	—	0.7	—	—	
Cerro Verde and **Santa Rosa**	Reserves	67.0	0.67	—	—	—	0.25	±2:1	Min. Mag., Oct. 1974, p. 273 & 275
	Reserves	250	1.10	—	—	—	—	—	Min. Eng., Sept. 1972, p. 12
	Santa Rosa reserves	1,172	0.55	—	—	—	—	—	Min. Mag., Oct. 1974, p. 273 & 275
Chalcobamba-Ferrobamba	Chalcobamba reserves, 1972	27.8 (tac)	2.1	—	—	—	—	—	Min. Eng., May 1972
	Ferrobamba reserves, 1972	±1.75 (tac)	3.4	—	—	0.7	—	—	
Cuajone	Reserves	22 (ox)	1.32	0.033	—	—	—	2.6:1	Lowell, 1975, p. 34; Min. Mag., Aug. 1976, p. 110–115
	Reserves	470 (S_2)	0.99	0.033	—	—	0.2	2.6:1	
Michiquillay	Reserves	±630	0.72	0.022	—	—	—	—	Min. Jour., Jan 9, 1970
Morococha	Reserves	360	0.76	0.02	—	—	—	—	Lowell, 1975, p. 34
Pashpa	Reserves	50	0.80	—	0.050	—	—	—	Min. Mag., Dec. 1976
Quellaveco (Quelloveco)	Reserves	200	0.98	0.03	—	—	—	—	Lowell, 1975, p. 34
	Reserves	300	0.98	—	—	—	—	—	Min. Mag., Oct. 1974, p. 275
Toquepala	Prod. 1960–1969	100	1.22	0.08	—	—	0.45 (?)	6.2:1	E&MJ, Apr. 1960, p. 81–116
	Reserves	262	0.9	0.040	—	—	0.45	±3:1	Lowell, 1975, p. 34
	Reserves	470	0.99	0.02	—	—	—	0.5:1	Min. Mag., Oct. 1974, p. 267
Toro Mocho	Reserves	±400	0.70	—	—	—	—	—	Min. Mag., Oct. 1974, p. 275
Tintaya	Reserves	50 (tac)	2.2	—	—	—	—	—	Min. Mag., Oct. 1974, p. 275 & 277

NOTE: Countries are given in all capitals; names of the principal deposits are shown in boldface; and alternative names are in parentheses.

KEY: leach = reserves of oxides amenable to leaching
mill = reserves requiring conventional milling
ox = oxides
rec = recovered, as distinct from indicated or estimated, grade
S_2 = sulfides
tac = tactite or wall-rock mineralization
UG = underground

TABLE 1.13
Reserves in Representative Porphyry Copper Deposits in Europe

DEPOSIT	RESERVES	TONNAGE (s.t. × 10^6)	GRADE				CUT-OFF GRADE (% Cu)	RATIO W:O	SOURCES
			Cu %	Mo %	Au oz./s.t.	Ag oz./s.t.			
WALES, U.K.									
Coed-y-Brenin	Drill-indicated mineralization	—	0.2+	0.0030–0.0050	0.0029	—	—	—	Rice and Sharp, 1976, p. B10–11
YUGOSLAVIA									
Bor (Krivelj)	"Feasibility" reserves, 1972	422.0	0.428	0.2–0.015	0.0023	0.012–0.29	0.27	1.5:1–4.15:1	Internat. Geol. Rev., v. 12, 1970, p. 370 & 374; Min. Mag., May 1973, p. 342–355
Majdanpek	Interim res., 1957	145.0	0.7	0.006	—	0.029	0.3	1.1:1	E&MJ, Sept. 1962, p. 77–80
	Reserves, 1961–1962	330.0	0.69 (rec)	Yes	—	—	—	—	Internat. Geol. Rev., v. 12, 1970, p. 376; Min. Mag., Sept. 1973, p. 182–187

NOTE: Countries are given in all capitals; names of the principal deposits are shown in boldface; and alternative names are in parentheses.

KEY: rec = recovered, as distinct from indicated or estimated, grade geography. The amount of capital required to equip a mine, mill, smelter, and so on, in a remote location is so large that the additional sums required to supply infrastructure, if it is lacking, are relatively unimportant. This fact helps to explain why it is feasible to exploit porphyry copper deposits from the mountains of South America to the tropical islands of the southwest Pacific and from British Columbia to the arid lands of Asia Minor. Some very informative figures on operating, capital, and financing costs have been provided by Winters (1978).

Needless to say, the capital cost of a plant depends on, among other things, size. Since it is common to express the size of a mine in terms of its daily ore-handling capacity, engineers are wont to employ as a rough measure of capital cost the cost of 1 ton of daily mine/mill capacity. During the years with relatively low inflation in the 1960s and early 1970s this figure was around $2,000; thus a mine and mill with a capacity of 20,000 t.p.d. would have cost (very roughly) 20,000 x $2,000—for a total of $40 million. In the late 1970s the unit cost was more like $5,000 or $6,000 per ton of daily capacity (and it was still rising very rapidly), so the same 20,000 t.p.d. mine and mill plant would have cost (again, very roughly) between $100 and $120 million. This is a very crude yardstick, however, which fails both to accommodate the critical factor of grade and to relate the capital outlay to the cost of producing a unit of metal.

Another simple yardstick of the capacity of a mine/mill/smelter complex is the number of tons of copper metal it produces each year. An economic factor which is derived from this property, the cost of 1 ton p.a. of installed copper capacity, does have the desirable ability of reflecting the grade of a deposit. In early 1979 this figure was around $6,000 to $7,000 in the United States. Thus, if the example cited above recovered 10 pounds of copper per ton for 300 working days, it would produce 30,000 tons of metal per annum (neglecting smelter losses, etc.) and the capital cost would be 30,000 x $6,000 or $7,000: between $180 and $210 million. The principal difference between these figures and the previous $100 to $120 million is the added cost of the smelter, refinery, etc., which is necessarily included in the "per unit of refined copper capacity" figures. This difference shows why the "installed refined copper" yardstick is useful in relation to projects where an integrated mine/mill/smelter operation must be built in order to ensure that the chief product, which must be shipped great distances, is 99.9 percent copper and not 30 to 35 percent copper, with the balance iron, sulphur, moisture, etc. In areas where fully integrated units are not normally built (e.g., the southwestern United States and British Columbia), a different measure of unit cost is indicated.

A third, fairly simple, cost index may be used. If the capital cost (estimated or actual) of a given development is divided by the number of pounds of copper in the estimated reserves, the capital cost per pound of metal (or metal equivalent) may be derived. This measure has the advantage of relating the capital costs to the amount of copper in deposits, although it says nothing about the distribution of copper or the relationship between grade and tonnage. This index can refer to a unit consisting only of mine and mill or to a fully integrated mine, mill, smelter, and refinery. If costs are being figured for a mine and mill plant, the addition of operating, general, administrative, and financing costs plus local taxes gives the cost of producing copper in concentrate. Further addition of the costs of freight (of concentrate from mine to smelter), smelting, refining, marketing, and additional taxes gives the total cost of producing the metallic copper.

Table 1.14 shows a few representative examples of total capital costs in Arizona. These costs are also expressed in terms of dollars per ton of daily mine/mill capacity and of cents per pound of contained copper. Both estimated and actual cost figures were used, as available. To be strictly comparable, the costs should be brought to a uniform time base. Even the "raw" figures, however, reveal significant relationships between costs, capacity, grade, and size: for example, even though the estimated cost of a ton of capacity at Miami East is high, the cost per pound is moderate, because of the relatively high grade. The figures for Lakeshore show a high cost per ton, but a below-average cost per pound, owing principally to the very large tonnage in the reserves.

As before, some representative figures for undertakings elsewhere (during approximately the same time period) are shown for purposes of comparison (see Tables 1.15 [British Columbia] and 1.16 [Central and South America]). Among these are examples of mine/mill units—producing only concentrates—and fully integrated (mine/concentrator/smelter, etc.) complexes—producing refined copper.

THE FUTURE OF MINABLE GRADES

Apart from relatively short-term fluctuations with a "wave length" of some five or six years, it seems reasonable to believe that economically minable grades will generally continue to fall. Lowell (1970) and Prokop (1975) have both suggested that by the end of this century the average copper equivalent grade (copper, plus recoverable minor metals) will have declined to approximately 0.2 to 0.25 percent. Page and Creasey (1975), on the other hand, have argued that the diminution in grade observed in the past cannot go on much longer because the rising cost of energy per unit of metal produced will place a floor under grade reduction. They predict that deposits with grades below 0.2 to 0.25 percent will not be mined for common use in the foreseeable future. While not apparently in conflict, the first prediction is positive, or permissive, while the second is restrictive. Both assertions rest on the assumption that conditions will remain constant. There are three areas, however, in which changes have the potential to affect such projections: (a) metal prices, (b) the fraction of production costs reflecting the price of energy, and (c) other production costs.

Many authors have emphasized that, compared to the costs of other goods and services, most metal prices have declined in the last few decades; and the mid- to late-1970s recession exacerbated rather than alleviated that situation. In 1978 copper was selling for 71 to 72¢ per pound in the U.S. and 54 to 66¢ in Western Europe. In December of that year, George Munro, Chairman of the Phelps Dodge Corporation, noted that considering the effects of inflation, cost of production, etc., the price in the early 1970s should have been 90¢ to $1.00 and that by the late 1970s it should have risen to $1.20. In short, there was room for the price of copper to

TABLE 1.14
Representative Capital Costs of Porphyry Copper Mines and Plants in Arizona

PORPHYRY COPPER MINE/PLANT	RESERVES		TOTAL Cu CONTENT (s.t. × 10^6)	TYPE MINE & PLANT	RATED CAPACITY (s.t.p.d. ore)	CAPITAL COST (U.S. $ × 10^6)	CONDITIONS (Year)	COSTS		SOURCES
	s.t. × 10^6	% Cu						U.S. $/s.t.p.d. capacity	U.S. ¢/lb Cu in reserves	
Bagdad-Cyprus	±300	±0.50	1.5	OP M & M	40,000	$ 200	Estimate (1973–75)	$ 5,000	6.67¢	E&MJ, Jun. 1974, p. 205; E&MJ, Mar. 1975, p. 252
	±300	±0.50	1.5	OP M & M	40,000	240	Actual (1978)	6,000	8.00	E&MJ, Apr. 1978, p. 45; Min. Eng., Apr. 1978, p. 351 & 352
Kalamazoo	440	0.67	2.98	UG M	63,000	150	Estimate (1968)	2,381	2.5	Author's estimate
Lakeshore	500 25	0.70 1.70	3.93	UG M & M & RLE	17,400	±200	Actual (1978)	11,490	2.5	Min. Mag., May 1975, p. 335; Min. Mag., May 1976, p. 355–361; Min. Mag., Jun. 1977, p. 431
Metcalf (King Peak)[a]	400	0.75	3.00	OP M(?)	20,000	±100	Estimate (1972)	5,000	±1.7	Author's estimate
Miami East	50	1.95	0.97	UG M & M	5,000	100	Estimate (1975)	20,000	5.1	Min. Eng., May 1975, p. 8; Min. Mag., Sept. 1975, p. 157
Pinto Valley	350	0.44	1.54	OP M & M	40,000	±100	Actual (1975)	2,500	3.2	Min. Eng., Jun. 1975, p. 25–33; Min. Mag., Nov. 1975, p. 344–359
Sacaton West	34	0.76	0.26	OP M & M	9,000	±40	Actual (1974)	4,444	7.8	Min. Mag., Feb. 1975, p. 90–97
Sierrita	414	0.35	1.45	OP M & M	72,000	±190	Actual (1970)	2,639	6.5	Min. Mag., Mar. 1971, p. 192–199
Average Open Pit								$ 4,042	3.8¢	
Average Under-ground								$11,290	3.4¢	

[a]alternative name

KEY: M = mine (alone)
M & M = mine and mill
OP = open pit
RLE = roast-leach electrowin
UG = underground

TABLE 1.15
Representative Capital Costs of Porphyry Copper Mines and Plants in British Columbia

PORPHYRY COPPER MINE/PLANT	RESERVES		TOTAL Cu CONTENT (s.t. × 10^6)	TYPE MINE & PLANT	RATED CAPACITY (s.t.p.d. ore)	CAPITAL COST (U.S. \$ × 10^6)	CONDITIONS (Year)	COSTS		SOURCES
	s.t. × 10^6	% Cu						U.S. \$/s.t.p.d. capacity	U.S. ¢/lb Cu in reserves	
Afton	34	1.00	0.34	OP MM & S	7,000	\$±90	Estimate (1975)	\$12,857	13.2¢	Min. Mag., Dec. 1975, p. 419 & 421
Brenda	193	0.48 (eCu)	0.93	OP M & M	24,000	62.3	Actual (1971)	2,596	3.3 (eCu)	Min. Mag., Apr. 1971, p. 269; Min. Mag., Jun. 1972, p. 416–423
Gibraltar	358	0.37	1.33	OP M & M	36,000	±74	Estimate (1974)	2,055	2.8	Min. Mag., Feb. 1972, p. 81 & 83; Min. Mag., Jul. 1972, p. 37–41; Min. Eng., Jul. 1972, p. 84–90
Highmont	147	0.28	0.42	OP M & M	25,000	±70	Estimate (±1973)	2,800	8.4	E&MJ, Aug. 1973, p. 140
Island Copper	283	0.52	1.47	OP M & M	33,000	70+	Estimate (1970)	±2,275	2.5	Min. Mag., May 1970, p. 339; Min. Mag., Oct. 1972, p. 334–349; E&MJ, Jul. 1972, p. 8
Lornex	500	0.41	2.05	OP M & M	38,000	143 (Can. \$)	Actual (1973)	3,763	3.5	Min. Mag., Mar. 1973, p. 154–163
Copper Mountain-Ingerbelle (Similkameen)[a]	84	0.53	0.45	OP M & M	15,000	±76 (Can. \$)	Estimate (1972)	5,067	8.3	Author's estimate
Valley Copper	940	0.48	4.51	OP M & M	75,000	300	Estimate (1971)	4,000	3.3	Min. Mag., Aug. 1971, p. 150
					40,000	180	Estimate (1971)	4,500	2.1	Min. Mag., Aug. 1971, p. 143
					50,000	250	Estimate (1976)	5,000	2.8	Min. Jour., Jun. 4, 1976, p. 457

[a] alternative name

KEY: eCu = copper equivalent
M = mine (alone)
M & M = mine and mill
MM & S = mine, mill, and smelter
OP = open pit

TABLE 1.16
Representative Capital Costs of Porphyry Copper Mines and Plants in Central and South America

PORPHYRY COPPER MINE/PLANT	RESERVES		TOTAL Cu CONTENT (s.t. × 10^6)	TYPE MINE & PLANT	RATED CAPACITY (s.t.p.d. ore)	CAPITAL COST (U.S.$ × 10^6)	CONDITIONS (Year)	COSTS		SOURCES
	s.t. × 10^6	% Cu						U.S. $/s.t.p.d. capacity	U.S. ¢/lb Cu in reserves	
CHILE										
Andacollo	350	0.69	2.41	OP MM&S	35,000(?)	$ 350	Estimate (1970)	$10,000	7.3¢	Min. Jour., Jun. 22, 1977; E&MJ, Sept. 1977
Andina (Rio Blanco)	320	1.17	3.74	UG M & M	11,000	157	Estimate (1970)	14,272	2.1	Min. Eng., Nov. 1969, p. 59–90; Min. Mag., May 1972, p. 333; Min. Mag., Oct. 1974, p. 259
MEXICO										
La Caridad	700	0.70	4.90	OP MM&S	40,000	600	Actual (1979)	8,571	6.1	E&MJ, Jan. 1979, p. 41; E&MJ, Oct. 1979, p. 72–88
La Verde	81	0.70	0.56	OP M & M	15,000	121	Actual (1976)	8,066	10.7	Min. Jour., May 7, 1976, p. 373
Nacozari	130	0.83	1.08	OP M & M	15,000	128	Estimate (1974)	8,533	5.9	Min. Mag., Dec. 1974, p. 431
PANAMA										
Cerro Colorado	2,000	0.6	12.00	OP MM&S	80,000(?)	±800	Estimate (1975)	10,000	3.5	Min. Jour., Oct. 10, 1975, p. 281
	2,046	0.67	13.71	OP MM&S	100,000	±1,600	Estimate (1979)	16,000	5.9	E&MJ, May 1979, p. 202; Min. Mag., May 1979, p. 395[a]
PERU										
Cuajone	492	1.00	4.92	OP MM&S	30,000	280	Estimate (1960)	—	—	E&MJ, July 1968, p. 11
					45,000	730	Actual (1977)	16,222	7.4	Min. Mag., Aug. 1976, p. 110–115; E&MJ, Jan. 1977, p. 23
Michiquillay	±630	0.72	±4.54	OP M & M	48,400	570	Estimate (1976)	11,777	6.3	Min. Jour., June 18, 1976; E&MJ, Oct. 1976, p. 141
Toquepala	470	1.00	4.7	OP MM&S	42,000	240	Actual (1960)	5,714	2.5	E&MJ, Apr. 1960, p. 81–116; Min. Eng., Nov. 1969, p. 79–83

NOTE: Countries are given in all capitals; names of principal deposits are shown in boldface; and alternative names are in parentheses.

[a]Comparison of these two references indicates the uncertainty of estimates based on published data.

KEY: M = mine (only)
M & M = mine and mill
MM&S = mine, mill, and smelter
OP = open pit
UG = underground

have moved upward without exceeding a fair price relative to the costs of other goods and services. However, due to an oversupply relative to demand, the price of copper remained in the 70¢ range. If the price had moved up, some—perhaps most—of the producers who were still staying alive at 71 to 72¢ per pound could have reduced their cut-off and mill-head grades and the trend toward lower copper grades would have continued.

The chief limitations on the supply—and therefore on prices—of established sources of energy (coal, oil, gas, nuclear and hydroelectric power) are man-made (political, social, legal), while the chief obstacles to the adoption of potential alternative sources (solar, fusion, etc.) are scientific, technological and economic. In theory, at least, it should be possible to resolve or alleviate the former before the latter; in practice the reverse may be true. Energy prices will almost certainly not come down, even relative to the cost of other items, but they need not (they *may,* but they *need* not) rise as rapidly in the early 1980s as they have in the late 1970s. If they do not, then the cost of the other components of prices charged for goods and services, including metals, should be able to catch up and restore the fraction attributable to energy to a more nearly typical (in historical terms) proportion of the total.

Whether or not energy costs continue to climb disproportionately in relation to other costs, technical advances can be expected to reduce mining costs either in constant terms or relative to other prices. Even the reference to high energy costs suggests ways in which this might come about. One of the largest contributions to the high energy costs of which Page and Creasey (1975) have written is made by comminution—crushing and grinding. The compressive strength of rocks is generally much higher than the tensile strength, yet conventional crushing and grinding techniques attack the former; they represent the mechanical equivalent of crushing rock with a hammer. Research into ways of breaking rocks by applying tensile stress has the potential for considerable savings. Examples of other advances which will work toward a reduction in costs include new explosives and blast-hole patterns, impact rock-breaking, hydraulic drilling equipment, drilled mine openings, and electrical energy to break rocks (elecro-fracturing). Metal processing (smelting and refining) is liable to move to areas where cheap energy, e.g., hydroelectric power, is to be found, and this move will reduce the proportion attributable to energy in the total cost of production. Thus, both adaptations of established mining methods (e.g., *in situ* leaching of copper mineralization) and completely new approaches can be expected to contribute to an absolute or relative reduction or production costs. Therefore, it is to be expected that the trend toward lower acceptable grades will continue into the foreseeable future.

ACKNOWLEDGMENTS

I would like to acknowledge the help of J. M. Newell and C. H. Laughton who supplied me with references on occurrences in, respectively, British Columbia (Alaska and Yukon), and southeast Asia and the southwest Pacific. I am also indebted to S. R. Titley for his help and encouragement at various stages in the preparation of the foregoing. Last, but not least, I would like to thank my wife for typing more drafts than either of us cares to remember.

REFERENCES CITED

Aiken, D. M., and West, R. J., 1978, Some geologic aspects of the Sierrita-Esperanza copper-molybdenum deposit, Pima County, Arizona: Ariz. Geol. Soc. Digest, v. 11, p. 117–128.

Allen, D. G.; Panteleyev, Andrejs; and Armstrong, A. T., 1976, Galore Creek, *in* Sutherland Brown, A., ed., Porphyry Copper Deposits of the Canadian Cordillera: CIM, Spec. Vol. 15, p. 402–414.

Bauer, H. L.; Cooper, J. J.; and Breitrick, R. A., 1960, Porphyry copper deposits in the Robinson mining district, White Pine County, Nevada: Intermontane Assoc. Petroleum Geologists, Guidebook Eleventh Annual Field Conference, p. 220–229.

Blecha, Matthew, 1974, Batchawana area—a possible Precambrian porphyry copper district: Can. Inst. Min. Bull., v. 67, n. 748 (Aug.), p. 71–76.

Briskey, J. A., and Bellamy, J. R., 1976, Bethlehem Copper's Jersey, East Jersey, Heustis and Iona deposits, *in* Sutherland Brown, A., ed., Porphyry Copper Deposits of the Canadian Cordillera: CIM, Spec. Vol. 15, p. 105–119.

Bryner, Leonid, 1969, Ore deposits of the Philippines—an introduction to their geology: Econ. Geol., v. 64, n. 6, p. 644–666.

Canadian Mines Handbook 1978–1979: Northern Miner Press Limited, Toronto, 404 p.

Cargill, D. G.; Lamb, John; Young, M. J.; and Rugg, E. S., 1976, Island Copper; *in* Sutherland Brown, A., ed., Porphyry Copper Deposits of the Canadian Cordillera: CIM, Spec. Vol. 15, p. 206–218.

Carr, J. M., 1966, Geology of the Bethlehem and Craigmont copper deposits, *in* Tectonic History and Mineral Deposits of the Western Cordillera: CIM, Spec. Vol. No. 8, p. 321–328.

Carr, J. M., and Reed, A. J., 1976, Afton, *in* Sutherland Brown, A., ed., Porphyry Copper Deposits of the Canadian Cordillera: CIM, Spec. Vol. 15, p. 376–387.

Carson, D. J. T., and Jambor, J. L., 1976, Morrison: geology and evolution of a bisected annular porphyry copper deposit, *in* Sutherland Brown, A., ed., Porphyry Copper Deposits of the Canadian Cordillera: CIM, Spec. Vol. 15, p. 264–273.

Carson, D. J. T.; Jambor, J. L.; Ogryzlo, P. L.; and Richards, T. A., 1976, Bell copper: geology, geochemistry and genesis of a supergene-enriched, biotized porphyry copper deposit with a superimposed phyllic zone, *in* Sutherland Brown, A., ed., Porphyry Copper Deposits of the Canadian Cordillera: CIM, Spec. Vol. 15, p. 245–263.

Christie, J. S., 1976, Krain, *in* Sutherland Brown, A., ed., Porphyry Copper Deposits of the Canadian Cordillera: CIM Spec. Vol. 15, p. 182–185.

Dixon, D. W., 1966, Geology of the New Cornelia mine, Ajo, Arizona, *in* Titley, S. R., and Hicks, C. L., eds., Geology of the Porphyry Copper Deposits, Southwestern North America: Tucson, Univ. Ariz. Press, p. 123–142.

Ellis, R. A., 1977, Disseminated copper in a Caledonian calc-alkaline intrusion, Argyllshire, Scotland: Trans. Instn. Min. Metall., v. 86, p. B52–54.

Evans, A. M., 1977, Copper-molybdenum mineralization in the Ballachulish Granite, Argyllshire, Scotland: Trans. Instn. Min. Metall., v. 86, p. B152–153.

Fahrni, K. C., Kim, Hun; Klein, G. A.; and Carter, N. C., 1976*a*, Granisle, *in* Sutherland Brown, A., ed., Porphyry Copper Deposits of the Canadian Cordillera: CIM, Spec. Vol. 15, p. 239–244.

Fahrni, K. C.; Macauley, T. N.; and Preto, V. A., 1976*b*, Copper Mountain and Ingerbelle, *in* Sutherland Brown, A., ed., Prophyry Copper Deposits of the Canadian Cordillera: CIM, Spec. Vol. 15, p. 368–375.

Ford, R. E., 1959, Geology of the Gaspé Copper mine: Can. Inst. Min. Metall. Bull., v. 52, n. 567, p. 425–429.

Fountain, R. J., 1972, Geological relationships in the Panguna porphyry copper deposit, Bougainville Island, New Guinea: Econ. Geol., v. 67, n. 8, p. 1049–1064.

Fox, P. E.; Grove, E. W.; Seraphim, R. H.; and Sutherland Brown, A., 1976, Schaft Creek, *in* Sutherland Brown, A., ed., Porphyry Copper Deposits of the Canadian Cordillera: CIM, Spec. Vol. 15, p. 219–226.

Gallagher, M. J.; Michie, U. McL.; Smith, R. T.; and Haynes, L., 1971, New evidence of uranium mineralization in Scotland: Trans. Instn. Min. Metall., v. 80, p. B150–B173.

Gambell, N. A., 1978, Geology and mineralization of the Ray silicate orebody, Pinal County, Arizona: Ariz. Geol. Soc. Digest 11, p. 35.

Gilluly, James, 1946, The Ajo mining district, Arizona: U.S. Geol. Surv. Prof. Paper 219, 112 p.

Gilmour, Paul, 1962, Notes on a non-genetic classification of copper deposits: Econ. Geol., v. 57, n. 3, p. 450–455.

Godwin, C. I., 1976, Casino, *in* Sutherland Brown, A., ed., Porphyry Copper Deposits of the Canadian Cordillera: CIM, Spec. Vol. 15, p. 344–354.

Greeley, M. N., 1978, The primary copper industry of Arizona in 1975 and 1976: Ariz. Dep. Mineral. Res., Spec. Rept. No. 2, 87 p.

Hammond, E. D., 1961, History of mining in the Bingham district, *in* Cook, D. R., ed., Geology of the Bingham mining district and northern Oquirrh Mountains: Utah Geol. Soc., Guidebook to the Geol. of Utah, No. 16, p. 120–129.

Himes, M. D., 1972. Mineralization and alteration at the Pima mine—a complex porphyry copper deposit, Arizona: Soc. of Mining Engineers of AIME, Preprint No. 72-I-57, 47 p.

Hodgson, C. J.; Bailes, R. J.; and Verzosa, R. S., 1976, Cariboo-Bell, *in* Sutherland Brown, A., ed., Porphyry Copper Deposits of the Canadian Cordillera: CIM, Spec. Vol. 15, p. 388–396.

Hollister, V. F., 1973, Regional characteristics of porphyry copper deposits of South America: Min. Eng., v. 25, n. 8 (Aug.) p. 51–56.

———, 1979, Porphyry copper-type deposits of the Cascade volcanic arc, Washington: Minerals Sci. Engng, v. 11, n. 1 (January), p. 22–35.

Hollister, V. F.; Potter, R. R.; and Barker, R. L., 1974, Porphyry-type deposits of the Appalachian orogen: Econ. Geol., v. 69, n. 5, p. 618–630.

James, D. H., 1976, Huckleberry, *in* Sutherland Brown, A., ed., Porphyry Copper Deposits of the Canadian Cordillera: CIM, Spec. Vol. 15, p. 284–287.

James, L. P., 1978, The Bingham copper deposits, Utah, as an exploration target: history and pre-excavation geology: Econ. Geol. v. 73, p. 1218–1227.

Kirkham, R. V., and Soregaroli, A. E., 1975, Preliminary assessment of porphyry deposits in the Canadian Appalachians: Geol. Surv. Can., Paper 75-1, pt. A, p. 249–252.

Langton, J. M., 1972. Ore genesis in the Morenci-Metcalf district: AIME Annual Meeting, San Francisco, Feb. 20–24, Preprint 72-I-47, 38 p.

Laznicka, Peter, 1976, Porphyry copper and molybdenum deposits of the U.S.S.R. and their plate tectonic settings: Trans. Instn. Min. Metall. (London), v. 85, p. B14–32.

Lindgren, Waldenar, 1905, The copper deposits of the Clifton-Morenci district, Arizona: U.S. Geol. Surv. Prof. Paper, 43, 375 p.

Lowell, J. D., 1970, Copper resources in 1970 (1970 Jackling Lecture): Min. Eng., v. 22, n. 4 (Apr.), p. 67–73.

———, 1975, Geology and economics of South American prophyry Cu deposits: World Mining, v. 37, n. 7 (June.), p. 32–37.

———, 1978, Thirty-year evolution of porphyry copper exploration in southwest U.S.A.; Pt. 2, Case histories of discoveries: Ariz. Geol. Soc. Digest, v. 11, p. 175–178.

Lowell, J. D., and Guilbert, J. M., 1970, Lateral and vertical alteration-mineralization zoning in porphyry ore deposits: Econ. Geol., v. 65, n. 4, p. 373–408.

Lynch, D. W., 1966, The economic geology of the Esperanza mine and vicinity *in* Titley, S. R., and Hicks, C. L., eds., Geology of the Porphyry Copper Deposits, Southwestern North America: Tucson, Univ. Ariz. Press, p. 267–279.

McMillan, W. J., 1976, J. A., *in* Sutherland Brown, A., ed., Porphyry Copper Deposits of the Canadian Cordillera: CIM, Spec. Vol. 15, p. 144–162.

Meyer, William; Gale, R. E.; and Randall, A. W., 1976, O.K., *in* Sutherland Brown, A., ed., Porphyry Copper Deposits of the Canadian Cordillera: CIM, Spec. Vol. 15, p. 311–316.

Millar, D. C., 1976, Maggie, *in* Sutherland Brown, A., ed., Porphyry Copper Deposits of the Canadian Cordillera: CIM, Spec. Vol. 15, p. 329–335.

Mining Magazine (Anon.), 1971, Duval Sierrita: v. 124, n. 3 (Mar.), p. 192–199.

———, 1978, Saindak porphyry copper—Pakistan's integrated mineral project: Nov., p. 484–493.

National Academy of Science, 1975, Mineral resources and the environment: Rept. prepared by Comm. Mineral Resources and Environment, Natl. Research Council, 345 pp.

Olmstead, H. W., and Johnson, D. W., 1966, Inspiration geology, *in* Titley, S. R., and Hicks, C. L., eds., Geology of the Porphyry Copper Deposits, Southwestern North America: Tucson, Univ. Ariz. Press, p. 143–156.

Osatenko, M. J., and Jones, M. B., 1976, Valley Copper, *in* Sutherland Brown, A., ed., Porphyry Copper Deposits of the Canadian Cordillera: CIM, Spec. Vol. 15, p. 130–143.

Page, N. J., and Creasey, S. C., 1975, Ore grade, metal production and energy: Journ. Research U.S. Geol. Surv., v. 3. n. 1 (Jan–Feb.), p. 9–13.

Panteleyev, Andrejs; Drummond, A. D.; and Beaudoin, P. G., 1976, Berg, *in* Sutherland Brown, A., Ed., Porphyry Copper Deposits of the Canadian Cordillera: CIM, Spec. Vol. 15, p. 275–283.

Parsons, A. B., 1933, The Porphyry Coppers: New York, Amer. Inst. Min. Metall. and Petroleum Engineers, Rocky Mountain Fund Ser., 581 p.

———, 1957, The Porphyry Coppers in 1956: New York, Amer. Inst. Min. Metall. and Petroleum Engineers, Rocky Mountain Fund Ser., 270 p.

Perret, F. A., 1937, The eruption of Mt. Pelee 1929–32: Carnegie Institution of Washington, Pub. no. 458, 126 p.

Peterson, N. P., 1962, Geology and ore deposits of the Globe-Miami district, Arizona: U.S. Geol. Surv. Prof. Paper, 342, 151 p.

Prigogine, Alexandre, 1975, Mamut mine and mill—newest southeast Asian porphyry development: World Mining, v. 37, n. 10 (Oct.), p. 42–48.

Prokop, F. W., 1975, The future economic significance of large lowgrade copper and nickel deposits: Monograph Series on Mineral Deposits (H. Borchert, Chief Editor), No. 13, Gebrüder Borntraeger, Berlin, 67 p.

Ransome, F. L., 1919, The copper deposits of Ray and Miami, Arizona: U.S. Geol. Surv. Prof. Paper, 115, 192 p.

Reed, A. J., and Jambor, J. L., 1976, Highmont: linearly zoned copper-molybdenum porphyry deposits and their significance in the genesis of the Highland Valley ores, *in* Sutherland Brown, A., ed., Porphyry Copper Deposits of the Canadian Cordillera: CIM, Spec. Vol. 15, p. 163–181.

Rennie, C. C.; Pentland, W. S.; and Sheng, C. C., 1961, Geology of the Craigmont mine: Trans. Can. Inst. Min. Metall., v. 64, p. 199–203.

Rice, C. M., and Davies, B., 1979, Copper mineralization associated with an appinite pipe in Argyll, Scotland: Trans. Instn. Min. Metall., v. 88, p. B154–160.

Rice, Robert, and Sharp, C. J., 1976, Copper mineralization in the forest of Coed-y-Brenin, North Wales: Trans. Instn. Min. Metall. v. 85, p. B1–B13.

Richards, Gordon, 1976, Ox Lake, *in* Sutherland Brown, A., ed., Porphyry Copper Deposits of the Canadian Cordillera: CIM, Spec. Vol. 15, p. 289–298.

Saegart, W. E.; Sell, J. D.; and Kilpatrick, B. E., 1974, Geology and mineralization of La Caridad porphyry copper deposit, Sonora, Mexico: Econ. Geol., v. 69, p. 1060–1077.

Sawyer, J. B. P., and Dickinson, R. A., 1976, Mount Nansen, *in* Sutherland Brown, A., ed., Porphyry Copper Deposits in the Canadian Cordillera: CIM, Spec. Vol. 15, p. 336–343.

Sayers, R. W.; Tippett, M. C.; and Fields, E. D., 1968, Duval's new copper mines show complex geologic history: Min. Engr., v. 20, n. 3 (Mar.), p. 55–62.

Schwartz, G. M., 1953, Geology of the San Manuel copper deposit, Arizona: U.S. Geol. Surv. Prof. Paper 256, 65 p.

Seraphim, R. H., and Rainboth, W., 1976, Poison Mountain, *in* Sutherland Brown, A., ed., Porphyry Copper Deposits in the Canadian Cordillera: CIM, Spec. Vol. 15, p. 323–328.

Sillitoe, R. H., 1976, A reconnaissance of the Mexican porphyry copper belt: Trans. Instn. Min. Metall., v. 85, p. B170–189.

Soregaroli, A. E., and Whitford, D. F., 1976, Brenda, *in* Sutherland Brown, A., ed., Porphyry Copper Deposits in the Canadian Cordillera: CIM, Spec. Vol. 15, p. 186–194.

Sutulov, Alexander, 1973, Mineral Resources and the Economy of the U.S.S.R.: New York, McGraw Hill, 192 p.

Thurmond, R. E.; Olk, J. F.; Komadina, G. A.; Journeay, J. A.; Spaulding, E. D.; and Hernlund, R. W., 1958, Pima: a three-part story: Min. Engr., v. 10, n. 4 (April), p. 453–462.

Titley, S. R., 1972, Intrusion, and wall rock, porphyry copper deposits: Econ. Geol., v. 67, n. 1, p. 122–123.

———, 1978, Copper, molybdenum and gold content of some porphyry copper systems of the southwestern and western Pacific: Econ. Geol., v. 73, n. 5, p. 977–981.

Titley, S. R., and Hicks, C. L., eds., 1966, Geology of the Porphyry Copper Deposits, Southwestern North America: Tucson, Univ. Ariz. Press., 287 p.

Waterman, G. C., and Hamilton, R. L., 1975, The Sar Cheshmeh porphyry copper deposit: Econ. Geol., v. 70, p. 568–576.

Wilkinson, W. J.; Stevenson, R. W.; and Garnett, J. A., 1976, Lorraine, *in* Sutherland Brown, A., ed., Porphyry Copper Deposits in the Canadian Cordillera: CIM, Spec. Vol. 15, p. 397–401.

Winters, H. J., 1978, Production costs, porphyry copper mines, Western United States, *in* Proceedings of the Porphyry Copper Symposium (Tucson March 18–20, 1976): Ariz. Geol. Soc. Digest, v. 11, p. 139–142.

Wolfhard, M. R., 1976, Fish Lake, *in* Sutherland Brown, A., ed., Porphyry Copper Deposits in the Canadian Cordillera: CIM, Spec. Vol. 15, p. 317–322.

World Mining (Anon.), 1963, Palabora—why it's the most exciting new copper mine in the 1960's: (Sept.), p. 30–36, 92.

2

Geologic Setting of Porphyry Copper Deposits

SOUTHEASTERN ARIZONA

Spencer R. Titley

The porphyry copper deposits of southeastern Arizona and contiguous regions compose one of the richest copper metallogenic provinces on earth and perhaps the richest of some seven separate porphyry copper provinces which surround the Pacific Basin. At least thirty-five separately named significant occurrences of porphyry-intrusion-related concentrations of copper occur here (Fig. 2.1), and the record of discovery suggests that more will be found.

With the exception of only a few deposits of pre-Laramide age, the deposits were formed during an interval (ca. 75–55 m.y. ago) within Laramide time (Table 2.1). Why they occur here in such numbers and in such a restricted region and why they evolved in such a short period of geologic time are not clear. It is also not clear what features of the crust or mantle may have controlled their specific positions. Although there have been well-considered hypotheses advanced on many of these matters, the evidence remains obscure or equivocal.

The deposits occur in a part of North America in which many episodes of intrusive and extrusive igneous activity and mountain building took place. These events span the time from the oldest recorded rocks in the region, volcanic units some 1,800 m.y. old, to Late Tertiary volcanism, with major episodes of igneous activity during the Precambrian, the Mesozoic, and the mid-Tertiary. Each igneous-orogenic episode has acted to obliterate some evidence of prior episodes. The late Tertiary Basin and Range episode resulted in widescale destruction and scattering of pieces of the puzzle. The copper deposits, which represent the products of a remarkably widespread but remarkably temporally restricted igneous event of Laramide age, are themselves centers of local destruction of the record. They have obliterated the original character of wall rocks of intrusions and have imposed the effects of stress on these walls to an extent which makes determination of local stratigraphic and structural settings difficult in many instances. These effects of intense hydrothermal activity, which attended deposition of the metals, have modified not only the walls, but the intrusions as well, to a degree that makes assessment of primary petrology extremely difficult. It is thus necessary to view the deposits in a broader, more regionally oriented context in order to search for any order or control which may have been important in the epicrustal environment. This chapter outlines the differing styles of geologic evolution which affected the American Southwest, particularly southeastern Arizona and adjoining regions, during the Precambrian, the Paleozoic, and Mesozoic eras, and during Laramide time. Its purpose is to attempt to show geologic data, largely in the form of outcrop maps, on which the locations of the porphyry systems are also shown and from which many potentially important associations can be further interpreted.

The synthesis of geological characteristics of this region is based on the integration of stratigraphy, radiometric ages, structural geology, and outcrop distribution and draws heavily upon the work of many geologists. Butler (1933) showed broad relationships of ore deposits to regional geology in the western United States, and Schmitt (1933) examined the relationship of deposits (which included the porphyry systems of the Southwest) in the context of their geologic setting. Anderson (1966, 1968*a*) summarized the areal geology of the region and the relationship of the copper deposits to that setting, and Schmitt (1966) reviewed their association with continental scale tectonics. Billingsley and Locke (1941) and Mayo (1958) examined western ore districts and their place in the tectonic evolution of the region, and Jerome and Cook (1967) reviewed regional tectonic environments as related to

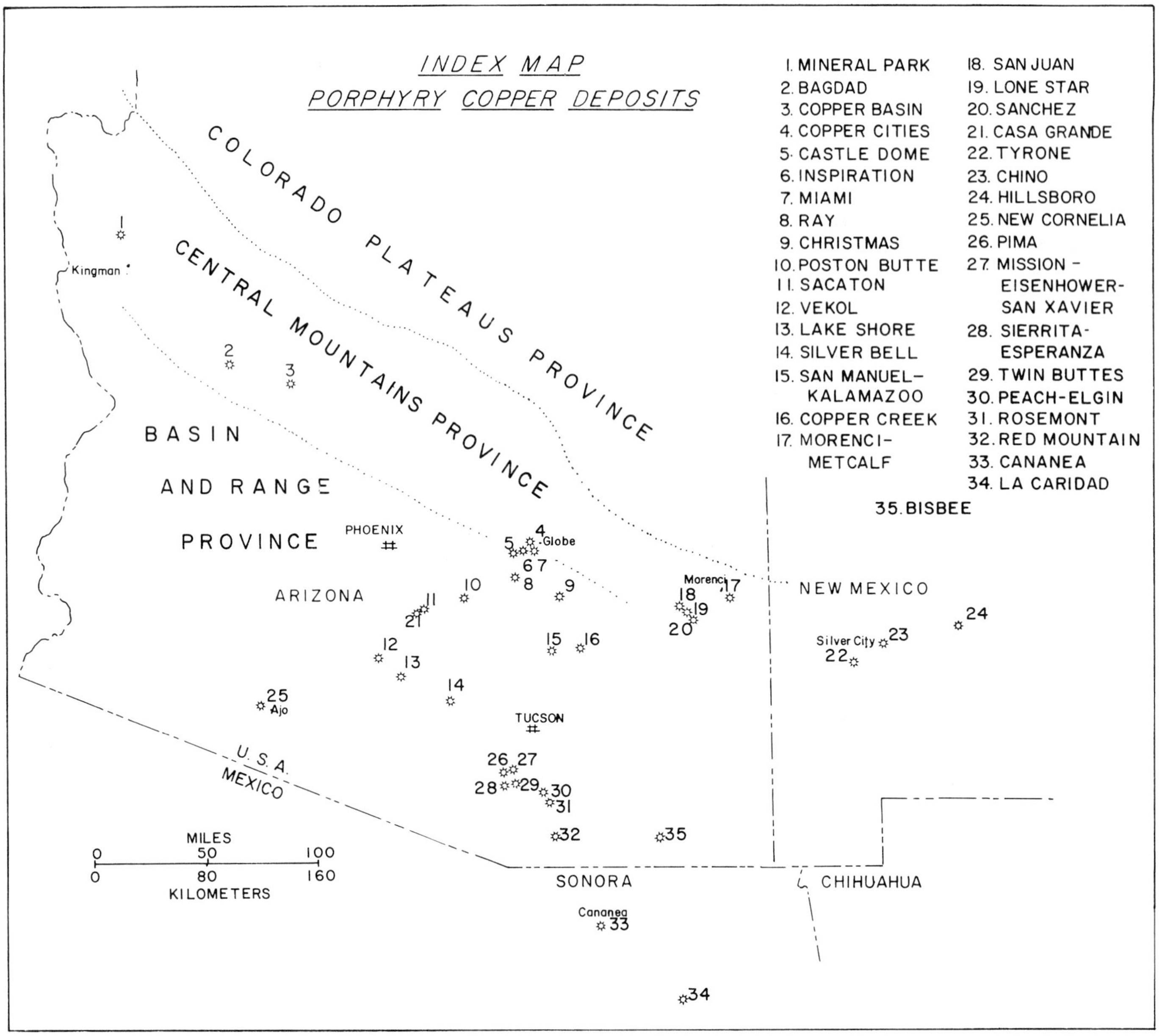

Figure 2.1. Index map to principal named porphyry copper deposits in Arizona, New Mexico, and Sonora, Mexico

ore districts. Lowell (1974) reported studies of the deposits as they related to regional stratigraphy and structure. The study of this problem—the relationship of porphyry copper deposits to regional geology and geologic history—is complex and continues. The results of each study provide new data and interpretations, and each successive study builds upon what has been discovered before. These prior summaries, therefore, remain of major importance and, together with newer information, constitute the basis upon which the work of this chapter is presented and interpreted.

THE NATURE AND HABITS OF PORPHYRY COPPER DEPOSITS

Laramide tectonic events and the Late-Tertiary episode of mountain building have segmented much of the geologic record of the Southwest. It is nonetheless possible, in some places, to reconstruct some Laramide geology and to deduce something of the nature of evolution of these systems. There appear to be important features and characteristics common to the porphyry systems, and there also appear to be habits of occurrence and geologic association which may be related to their origin. Most porphyry systems of the Southwest are still recognizable as intrusion-related mineralized systems of large size (generally greater than 1.5 km in diameter). The rare exceptions to this generalization are some large copper systems in skarn, such as Mission-Pima, but even in this complex, events of Laramide age or of mid- or Late-Tertiary age may have displaced large volumes of rock from their intrusion centers. Porphyries compose the hearts of systems and commonly the porphyritic rocks comprise many textural and compositional variations as part of intrusive complexes. Mineralization of the porphyry copper deposit is localized in fractures and veins which transect the igneous rocks and their wall rock hosts. The effects of hydrothermal processes

TABLE 2.1
Radiometric Age Dates of Some Porphyry Copper Systems of the North American Southwest

Porphyry Copper System	Age (in m.y.)
Arizona	
1. Mineral Park	71.5
2. Bagdad	70.9
3. Copper Basin	64
4. Copper Cities	63.0
5. Castle Dome	57.8
6. Inspiration	57.8
7. Miami	—
8. Ray	65.4
9. Christmas	62.0
10. Poston Butte	62.0
11. Sacaton	64.5
12. Vekol	—
13. Lake Shore	64.1
14. Silver Bell	67.1
15. San Manuel-Kalamazoo	67
16. Copper Creek	67.5
17. Morenci-Metcalf	55.2
18. San Juan	—
19. Lone Star (Safford)	62.4
20. Sanchez	—
21. Casa Grande	—
25. New Cornelia	63.0
26. Pima	56.7
27. Mission, et al.	56.7
28. Sierrita-Esperanza	61.6
29. Twin Buttes	58.6
30. Peach-Elgin	—
31. Rosemont	—
32. Red Mountain	—
35. Bisbee	163–178
New Mexico	
22. Tyrone	56.2
23. Chino	59.0
24. Hillsboro	73.4
Sonora, Mexico	
33. Cananea	58.5
34. La Caridad	53.0

Sources: Creasey and Kistler (1962), #35; Damon and Mauger (1966), #33; Hedlund (1974), #24; Kelley (1977), #29; Langlois (1978), #26; Livingston (1973), #1–6, 8–11. 13–17, 19, 22, 25, 28, 34.

NOTE: Numbers of systems are keyed to the location map in Figure 2.1.

have been to produce zoned mineralization and alteration, although in many deposits such zoning is extremely complex.

Porphyry copper deposits tend to occur in clusters. As can be observed from the distribution shown in Figure 2.1, clusters occur in the Globe-Miami area or, depending on scale, the Globe-Miami-Ray-Christmas area. Clustering is present at Safford, perhaps at Copper Creek, and in the Pima district, south of Tucson. Not all of the clustering of deposits, however, can be considered as primary in origin; rather, some is the result of post-ore fragmentation by faulting. Together with the Pima-Mission-San Xavier orebodies—believed to be displaced parts of the Twin Buttes system (Cooper, 1960; Jansen, 1978)—there is also the well-described fault-offset of the San Manuel orebody, Kalamazoo (Lowell, 1968). Future work in many districts may well result in discoveries based on structural studies and further documentation of post-ore separation of porphyry systems.

There appears to be a close correspondence on a regional scale between the copper deposits and dated or inferred Laramide volcanic rocks and associated clastic units. Although these rocks have been scattered or eroded since the Laramide, there still remain many exposures of them in some districts and in and near some deposits. This association in time and space leads to fundamental inquiries about volcanogenic processes and their relationship to porphyry copper systems.

Most of the deposits of the region occur in areas where the pre-ore, Phanerozoic column was comparatively thin. The major component of thick Phanerozoic columns in southeastern Arizona is a section of Lower Cretaceous sedimentary rocks which was possibly as thick as 5,000 m. These strata were either eroded prior to Laramide time or not deposited in the environment of occurrence of most porphyry systems here. Geologic reconstructions lead to the interpretation that, if undisturbed, the section which the intrusions crossed above the basement could have consisted of Paleozoic strata, possibly a thin (1,200 m) Mesozoic column, and a column of Laramide volcanic rocks of unknown thickness. Not all deposits occur in contact with Paleozoic or younger rocks, but where the evidence remains, it suggests that the stocks crossed most of the pre-ore Phanerozoic column. It can be concluded from this association that the level of emplacement of many deposits was to shallow crustal levels, as the reconstructions suggest only a few kilometers or less of cover must have existed above the stocks.

PRECAMBRIAN

Rocks of Proterozoic age compose the basement of Phanerozoic rocks of Arizona and contiguous regions. In many Laramide-aged copper deposits of this region (Bagdad, Globe-Miami, Ray, Ithaca Peak, and others) present levels of erosion reveal that these rocks have been important hosts to hypogene ores. They have been closely involved with, and have possibly influenced, some aspects of evolution of the hydrothermal systems. In some localities of the region copper-related stocks of Laramide and Jurassic age have been localized along contacts between Precambrian rocks of sharply contrasting lithologies, and their shapes and internal structures appear to be grossly concordant with recognizable Precambrian structural elements. Precambrian rocks in contact with copper-related stocks, at the levels observed, are also strikingly similar in mineralogical-chemical composition to widespread, late alteration mineral assemblages present within the systems. Thus, although no porphyry copper occurrence of Precambrian age has yet been recognized in the region, consideration of Precambrian geology, particularly its structure and lithology, is relevant to further discussion of the regional geologic environment. The discussion of Precambrian geology in this chapter follows the convention—suggested by Butler and Wilson (1938)—of separate recognition of "Older Precambrian" and "Younger Precambrian" time rock groups. The dichotomy used is based upon the recognition of two distinctive rock successions with contrasting lithologies, ages, and structural histories which are separated by a profound unconformity.

Older Precambrian Rocks

Intrusive, volcanic, and sedimentary rocks—and their probable metamorphic equivalents—assigned to the Older

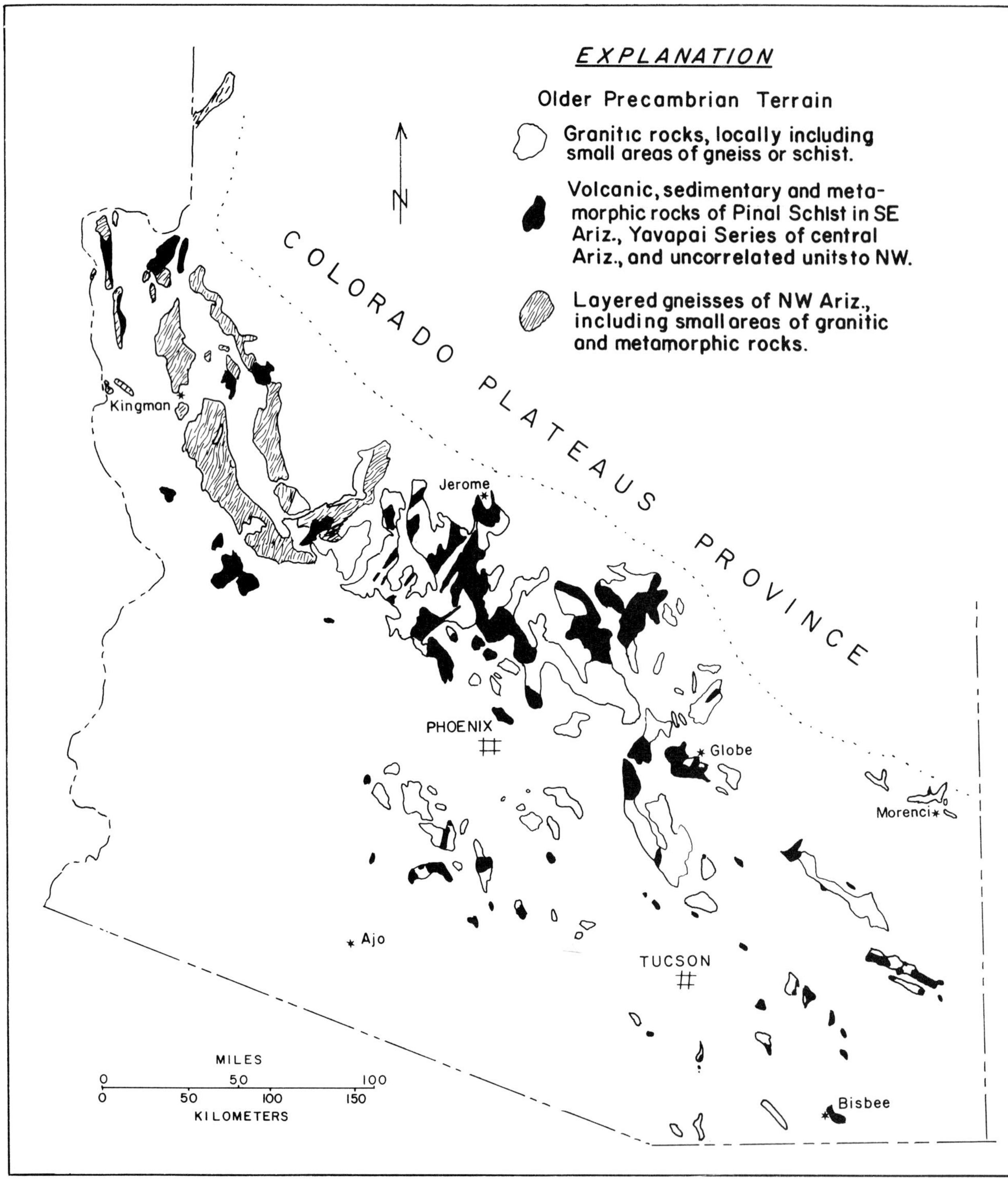

Figure 2.2. Outcrop map of principal Older Precambrian exposures in the Central Mountains and the Basin and Range provinces of Arizona. Major exposures occupy a northwest-trending belt across the state. South of the belt isolated exposures are the result of Basin and Range mountain building.

Precambrian are widely and extensively exposed in a northwest-trending belt across central Arizona (Fig. 2.2). It is within this terrain that the most thorough studies of Precambrian rocks have been carried out. Particularly noteworthy among such reports are those on Bagdad (Anderson et al., 1955), the Jerome-Prescott area (Anderson, 1951, 1968*b*, 1972; Anderson and Creasey, 1958; Anderson and Blacet, 1972), the Mazatzal Mountains (Wilson, 1939), the Johnny Lyon Hills (Cooper and Silver, 1964), and the Dos Cabezas Mountains (Erickson, 1968). Regional syntheses concerned with Precambrian rocks have been reported by Anderson (1966), Anderson and Silver (1976), and Silver (1978).

In the Basin and Range province, the environment of the preponderance of the known porphyry copper deposits, Precambrian rocks are present in abundance but in widely scattered and restricted outcrops. With the exceptions of only the Johnny Lyon Hills and Dos Cabezas Mountains, the stratigraphic sequences, structural features, and intrusive histories

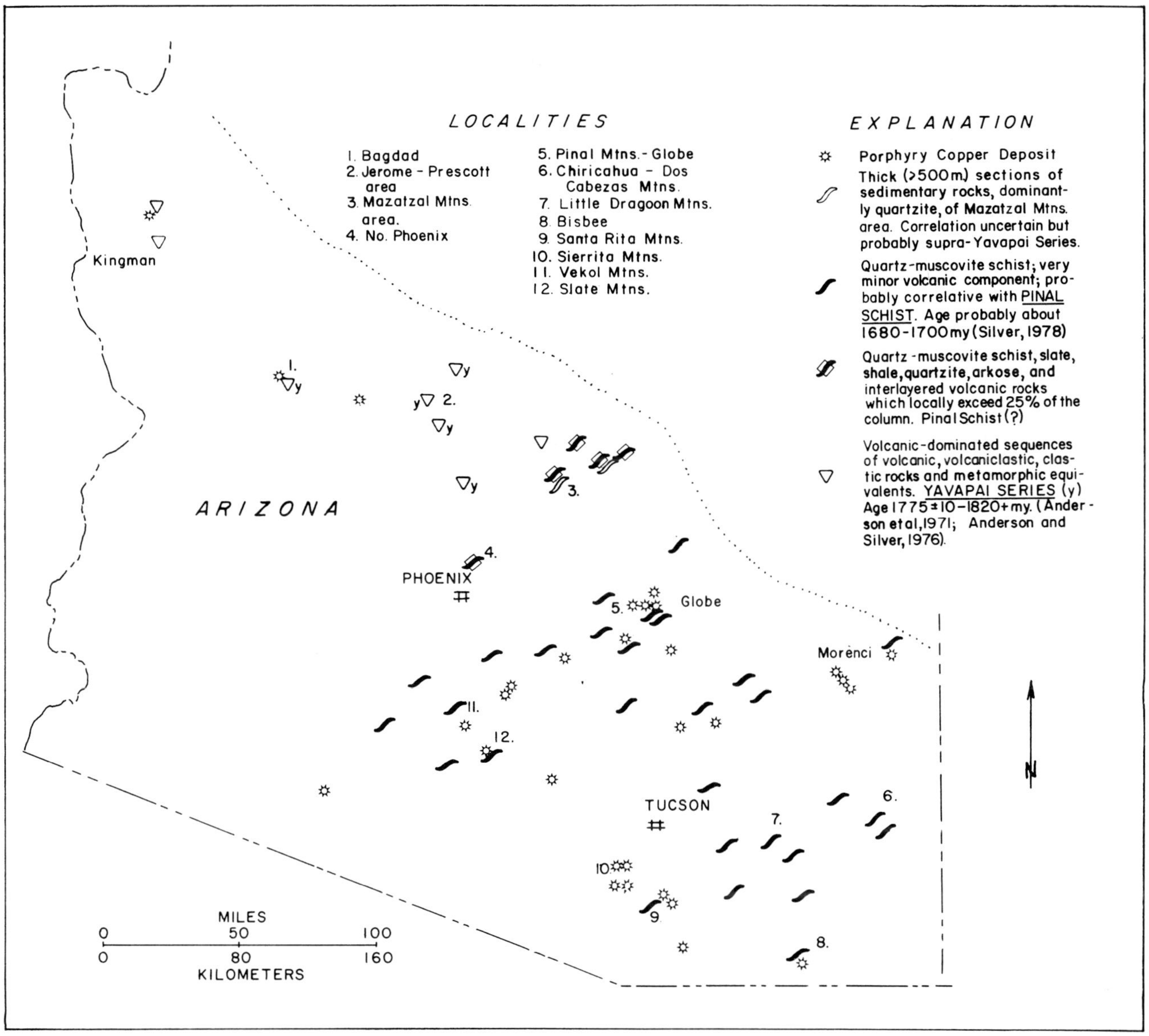

Figure 2.3. Map of central and southern Arizona showing distribution of principal volcanic and sedimentary rock types, or their metamorphic equivalents, of Older Precambrian age. Pinal Schist is the dominant non-granitic lithology in southeastern Arizona. These rocks, together with an increased volcanic component, lie in contact with thick sections of Precambrian sedimentary rocks and greenstones of central Arizona.

of the Older Precambrian in this region have not been well studied.

General Characteristics, Age, and Correlations. In a very general way, the Older Precambrian of Arizona can be grouped into two categories of rocks in most regions of occurrence. The older of the two groups comprises volcanic, volcaniclastic, or clastic rocks, or their metamorphic equivalents, in various proportions. This group is usually associated with slightly younger crystalline rocks which range from granitoid intrusions through layered gneisses. Throughout Arizona and in large parts of the western United States, this older basement was invaded by a somewhat younger group of granites during a short interval at about 1,420–1,450 m.y. ago (Silver et al., 1977). Metamorphic and intrusive events predate the evolution of a major unconformity during the Proterozoic at about 1,100 m.y. ago. Distribution of lithologies is shown on Figure 2.3.

In Arizona, the lithologic groups of different known ages can be separated into at least three distinctive associations, which occur in specific parts of the central belt across the state. The three regions considered can be defined as (1) extending northwestward from about the location of Bagdad, (2) the interval from Bagdad to about the Mazatzal Mountains, and (3) an interval extending from the Mazatzal Mountains an unknown distance southeastward into New Mexico and Mexico.

In the northwest interval, lithologies are characterized by a dominance of layered gneisses and metamorphic rocks interpretable as metavolcanics. In the Cerbat Mountains the lithologies consist of hornblende–diopside schist, amphibolite, biotite schist, and quartzite (Thomas, 1949). The dominant lithology is *lit-par-lit* gneiss that makes up the mass of the Cerbat, Hualapai, and other lesser ranges of northwestern Arizona. The age of these rocks is imperfectly known, but in the northern Hualapai Mountains Rb/Sr ages of about 1,800 m.y. for gneiss have been reported (Kessler, 1976).

The interval from Bagdad to the Mazatzal Mountains includes the Jerome–Prescott area, where the Precambrian has been studied extensively. In this interval there occur thick sections of recognizable Older Precambrian rocks which are volcanic dominated. Probably in excess of 6,700m of strata, composed of interlayered dacite to rhyolite flows and pyroclastic rocks and clastic sedimentary rocks, have been mapped. These strata, which were invaded by Older Precambrian intrusions, have been assigned to the Yavapai Series, representing the interval 1,775 ± 10 m.y. to > 1,820 m.y. ago (Anderson et al., 1971). The younger age was assigned from the age of a cross-cutting intrusion. Rocks of the Yavapai Series have been compared to and correlated with the lithologies of greenstone belts (Lausen, 1930; Anderson and Silver, 1976), and Anderson and Silver have suggested that the sequence of Yavapai rocks at Jerome correlates with lithologically similar and stratigraphically equivalent units at Bagdad.

From the Mazatzal Mountains southeastward (see Fig. 2.3) lithologies contrast sharply with those to the northwest, and the area in which Precambrian strata are exposed is considerably widened. The layered rocks—the Pinal Schist—are dominated by quartz-muscovite schists, fine-grained arkoses, and quartzites, with only rare and thin interlayered volcanic units. Sections specifically correlated with the Pinal Schist of central Arizona (Ransome, 1903) include the sections at Bisbee (Ransome, 1904), Morenci (Lindgren, 1905), the Dos Cabezas Mountains (Erikson, 1968), the Chiricahua Mountains (Sabins, 1957), the Little Dragoon Mountains, and the Johnny Lyon Hills (Cooper and Silver, 1964). The lithology, however, is widespread in many other ranges of southeastern and southern Arizona, and outcrops of probable Pinal Schist are present as far west as the Vekol Mountains and the Javelina Mountains near Black Gap. The correlations are less certain in the Mazatzal Mountains—where lithologies are less volcanic-dominated than in the Yavapai Series and consist of great thicknesses of slate, quartzite, and greenstone—and in the Diamond Butte Quadrangle—where similar lithologies exist (Gastil, 1958). Anderson and Silver (1976) have suggested that these metasedimentary sections, which overlie a volcanic succession of possible Yavapai Series equivalence, may be correlative with the Pinal Schist further to the southeast. The section located at Squaw Peak (Thorpe and Burt, 1978) is quite probably correlative.

Reliable radiometric ages documenting the history of the Pinal Schist are reported from only one locality. In the Johnny Lyon Hills and the nearby Little Dragoon Mountains (see Fig. 2.3), Silver (1978) and Silver and Deutsch (1963) report ages of accumulation for rocks of the Pinal at between 1,680 and 1,700 m.y. ago. Metamorphism of the strata took place in the interval 1,625–1,680 m.y. ago (Silver, 1978). The next major event to be recorded was emplacement of granite at 1,420 m.y. ago, reported by Silver (1978) in the Johnny Lyon Hills and by Livingston and Damon (1968) in the Winkelman area. Data reported by Livingston and Damon (1968) permit an interpretation of a similar history of accumulation of Pinal Schist and younger intrusion in the Pinal Mountains, Ray, and the Mammoth area.

There is, thus, at least a threefold separation of lithologies and ages of Older Precambrian terrain in Arizona. Although the dating is imprecise, probably the oldest of the three terrain units occurs in northwesternmost Arizona as layered gneisses and metavolcanic terrain. Younger belts or terrain units occur southeastward and consist successively of the volcanic and metavolcanic rocks of the Yavapai Series in central Arizona and the sedimentary and metasedimentary rocks of the Pinal Schist in the southeastern third of the state. Possible overlap of Pinal Schist equivalents on older volcanic and metavolcanic units is present in the Mazatzal Mountains and nearby ranges. Chronostratigraphic Precambrian rocks have been described for the southwestern and far western United States (Silver et al., 1977). The Precambrian rocks described for Arizona have been included in their discussion in a general way and the belts have been suggested to have a northeast strike with progressive younging in the southeast.

Aeromagnetic Expression. The northeast trend of Precambrian belts described by Silver and others (1977) can be interpreted for the Precambrian of Arizona on the basis of aeromagnetic data. The residual aeromagnetic map of Arizona (Sauck and Sumner, 1970) is shown in Figure 2.4. Precambrian rocks of the southwestern half of Arizona disappear to the north below the younger cover of the Colorado Plateaus. However, beneath that screen of younger rocks, two pronounced magnetic lineaments are present which appear to separate the three terrain types exposed in the central mountains. It is noteworthy that a group of lithologies similar to the Precambrian of the Yavapai Series and the sections of the Mazatzal Mountains reappears from beneath the cover of the Plateaus in the Needle Mountains of Colorado. These rocks may be correlative with those of the central belt of Yavapai Series rocks shown in central Arizona. The Precambrian of the San Juans is alluded to as 1.8-b.y.-old rocks (Lipman et al, 1978), and ages and interpretations suggested by Barker (1969) and Bickford and others (1969) lend credence to the belt-like distributions of certain Precambrian terrains. It seems additionally noteworthy that the two magnetic lineaments would, if extended, border the Colorado Mineral Belt on the northwest and southeast.

The northernmost of the two lineaments has been discussed by Shoemaker and others (1974, 1978) in the context of the Mesa Butte fault system of northern Arizona and has been described by those authors as turning easterly and lying within the San Juan Mountains. The total intensity map for Colorado (Zeitz and Kirby, 1972) does not lend itself to easy interpretation, but it is suggested here that the northwestern lineament may continue on the trend seen in Arizona. The southeastern line corresponds roughly to the Holbrook Granitic Ridge, a basement feature of northeast trend (Huddle and Dobrovolny, 1952), and to the edge of the Defiance Positive area.

The reason for the magnetic expression shown by these two lineaments is not certain. Shoemaker and others (1978) have suggested that movement along the northwestern line juxtaposed amphibolites against rocks of different magnetic susceptibility. A similar suggestion might be advanced for the southeastern line, but this line may also simply express a contrast in susceptibility of adjacent rock types along the

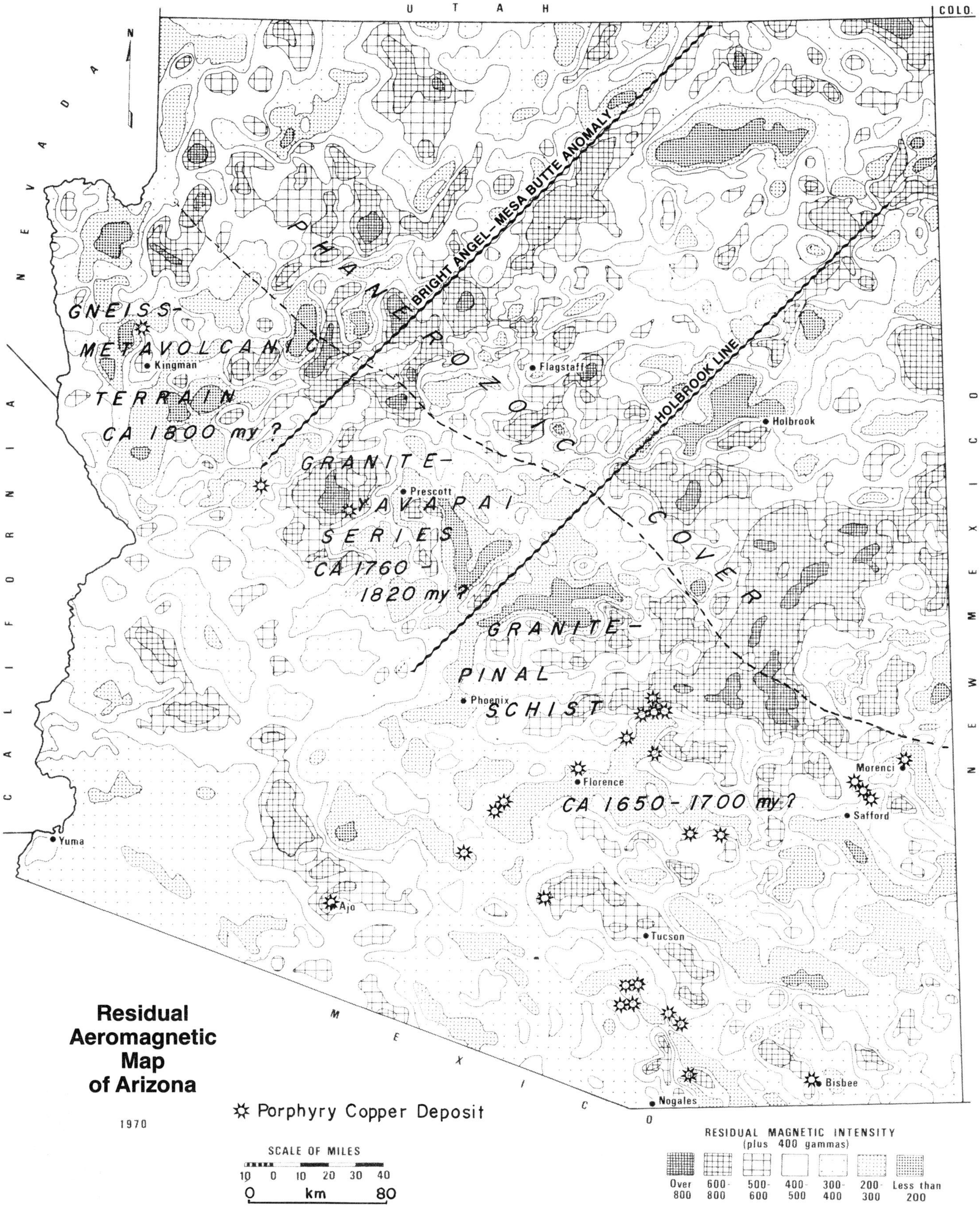

Figure 2.4. Residual aeromagnetic map of Arizona from Sauck and Sumner (1970). Northeast-trending lines show approximate trend of aeromagnetic basement anomalies, which are broader than the lines imply. Lines separate distinctive types of Precambrian terrain in central Arizona. Porphyry copper deposits—except for Ithaca Peak, Copper Basin, and Bagdad—are seen as floored by a basement of Pinal Schist or, in the case of Ajo, by gneiss, in southern Arizona. Lines enclosing the Yavapai Series metavolcanics also project to enclose the Colorado Mineral Belt to the northeast.

anomaly. Notwithstanding such uncertainties, the lines appear to be the expression of basement phenomena and there is cause to suggest that they separate Precambrian terrains of different lithologies and age. The southwestern (Holbrook) line appears particularly important in its relationship to the porphyry copper deposits of southeastern Arizona.

The southwestern projection of the Holbrook line marks the western and northwestern limit of known porphyry copper deposits of southeastern Arizona; the line also marks the northwestern boundary of recognized Pinal Schist lithologies. Except for Ajo, the deposit at Kingman, and the deposits at Bagdad and Copper Basin, all of the known deposits of the southeastern province are sited in the region characterized by Precambrian terrain composed of Pinal Schist and younger granite intrusions and lie southeast of the projected extension of the Holbrook line (see Fig. 2.4).

Nature of the Association. Many geologists have noted the predominant northeast to east-northeast structural grain of the Pinal Schist and younger granites of southeastern Arizona. In the Globe-Miami district Peterson (1962) has commented upon a control exerted by this grain over both the direction of elongation of intrusions and their location along northeast-trending contacts between granite and schist. This association is strikingly shown in Figure 2.5. In the Casa Grande area of Arizona Balla (1972) has suggested a similar relationship for intrusions of Laramide age which appear to be localized along Precambrian rock contacts of northeast trend. This characteristic cannot be documented everywhere, and it is clearly not the case at Ajo, for example, where the orientation of the intrusion is indistinct and where gneiss of Precambrian age (Gilluly, 1946) composes the basement. It is, nonetheless, important to emphasize that such an association between copper-related intrusions and contacts of Precambrian rocks exists and to suggest that the northeast-trending structural anisotropy of the basement may in some way exert important control over emplacement.

A second important association is common. Many copper deposits of the region reveal a major late stage of hydrothermal activity, characterized by late fractures which guided an intense stage of quartz-sericite alteration. In view of the fact that in many deposits where Pinal Schist wall rocks to intrusions are known or can be inferred, there is unequivocal evidence of fluid interaction with the Schist wall rocks. For example, Ray, the deposits of Globe-Miami, and Bisbee all reveal this late stage of alteration, and all are closely associated with the Pinal Schist host rocks. It seems very reasonable to suggest that there may be a genetic association between the alteration and the quartz-muscovite mineralogy of the walls.

Younger Precambrian Rocks

Following the metamorphism and folding of the old basement, a succession of marine and continentally derived sediments was deposited. This column, probably not more than about 850 m thick, consists of two separately recognized stratigraphic types. At the base rocks of the Apache Group (consisting of conglomerate, shales, interbedded basalt, limestone, and quartzite) up to about 500 m thick are exposed south of the Colorado Plateaus in a narrow belt in central

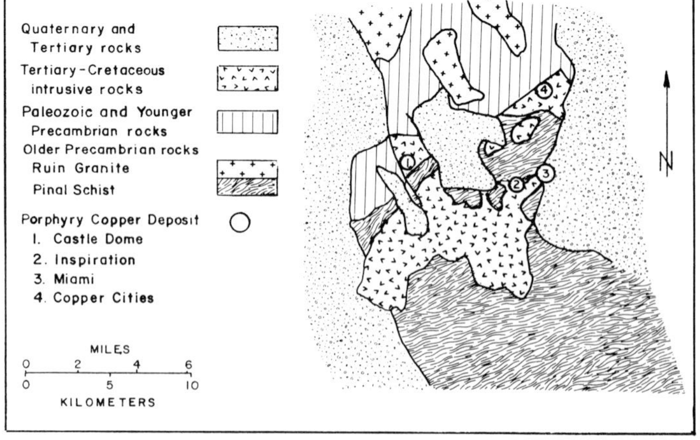

Figure 2.5. Geologic map of the Globe-Miami area, showing relationships of Laramide intrusions and Older Precambrian rocks. Porphyry copper deposits are localized along or near northeast-trending contacts. Modified from Peterson (1962, Figure 14).

Arizona. These strata, exposed about as far south as the Johnny Lyon Hills (Shride, 1967) and as far southwest as the Vekol Mountains (Carpenter, 1947), are interpreted to have been deposited at some time during the interval 1,100–1,420 m.y. ago (Silver, 1978). The Troy Quartzite of Younger Precambrian age overlies the Apache Group on a surface which represents a slight regional unconformity (Shride, 1967). Strata of the Apache Group were gently warped and eroded during the pre-Troy interval. The Troy Quartzite, which consists of arkose, sandstone, and quartzite, attains a maximum reported thickness of about 400 m and is restricted to the region of southern Arizona where the Apache Group is present. Following deposition of the Troy Quartzite, the Younger Precambrian strata were folded on a local scale; Shride (1967) has noted that this folding occupied widely separated belts of north and northwest trend. After folding, the Younger Precambrian strata were intruded on a remarkably wide scale by diabase, which formed extensive sills. An age of 1,100 ± 15 m.y. or earlier has been reported by Silver (1978) for the diabase of southeastern and central Arizona. Figure 2.6 shows the distribution of Younger Precambrian strata in relationship to the Holbrook magnetic lineament. It is noteworthy that the strata of Younger Precambrian age lie to the southeast of that feature. Although diabase is present further west at Bagdad, it is not clear that the rock there is of the same age and affinity as the diabase of the Younger Precambrian terrain considered here.

Younger Precambrian rocks, including the diabase, are present in and near the porphyry systems of the Globe-Miami, Ray, and Christmas regions, where they locally lie in contact with the younger intrusions. Because the evidence for interaction between the hydrothermal processes and these wall rocks is clear and unequivocal, further comment on their properties is warranted. Certain of the units within the Apache Group have unusual and potentially important compositions. The section comprises limestone, dolomite, shale, arkose, sandstone, conglomerate, and basalt, as well as the diabase. Within this highly varied lithology, there are units, such as the Mescal Limestone, in which salt casts occur. The presence of salt casts and the dolomitic composition indicate

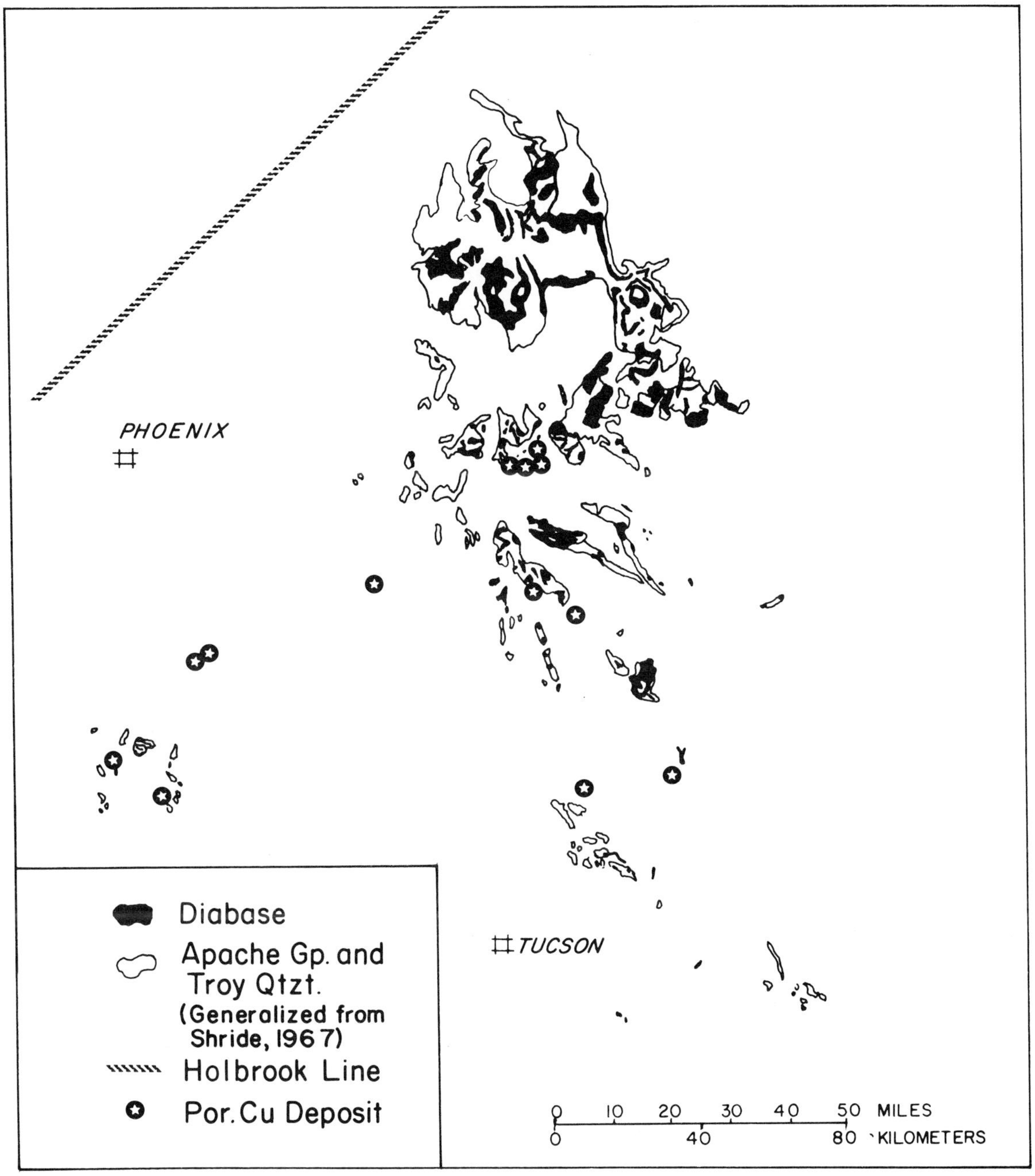

Figure 2.6. Map of Younger Precambrian outcrops in central Arizona. Part of the southeastern aeromagnetic lineament is shown to the northwest of Phoenix. Modified from Shride (1967).

evaporite environments of deposition. There occur as well algal reefs and, in the Dripping Spring Quartzite, locally abundant pyrite or hematite. Metz and others (1968) suggest that diabase has been an important host to ore at Ray because the rock has been both chemically reactive and strongly fractured. In the deposits of Globe-Miami (see Fig. 2.5) Apache Group strata and diabase are exposed near the deposits, so interaction at higher, now eroded, levels in the system can only be inferred.

Following deposition of the Troy Quartzite and emplacement of the diabase, a long interval of erosion ensued, during which the surface was reduced to a nearly featureless landscape. Notable exceptions to this existed, however: a northwest-trending granitic ridge remained a positive feature until the Mississippian (the Holbrook Granitic Ridge), and an additional landmass extending southwestward along that line was not covered until the Devonian. In northeasternmost Arizona, the Defiance Positive area also stood above Paleozoic seas until the Pennsylvanian. The record in southwestern Arizona is obscure.

PALEOZOIC

The Paleozoic section, dominated by carbonate rocks, is an important host to copper ores in many of the southeastern Arizona and southwestern New Mexico deposits. At Silver Bell, Vekol, Lake Shore, Christmas, and the Twin Buttes, Mission, and Pima deposits of the Pima district calc-silicate

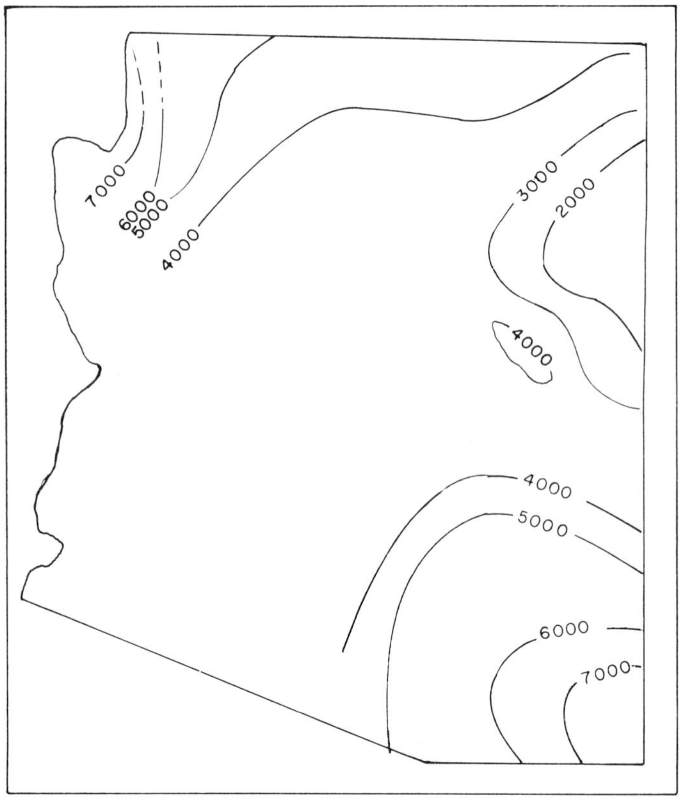

Figure 2.7. Paleozoic isopachs of Arizona. Contour interval shown is 1,000 ft. (305 m). Adapted from Peirce and Wilt (1970).

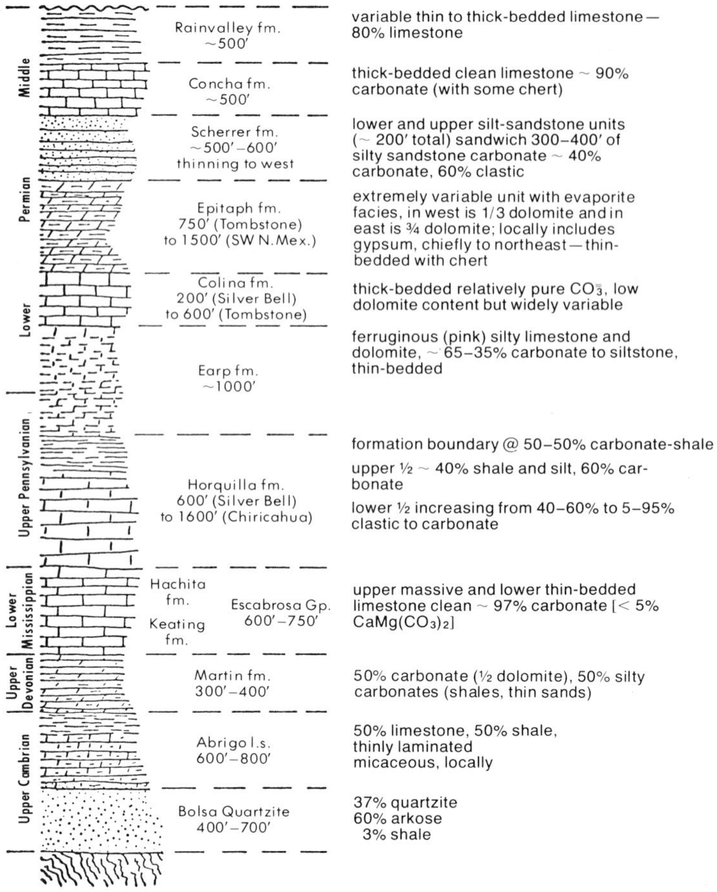

Figure 2.8. Stratigraphic column of principal Paleozoic formations of southeastern Arizona. Not included are Ordovician, Silurian, and upper Mississippian formations from the southeasternmost corner of the state. Lithologies shown are approximate averages of units in southeastern Arizona and vary from place to place in this region.

altered carbonates of the Paleozoic may exceed 50 percent of the total mineralized rock volume. For this reason and because the depositional patterns of some Paleozoic Systems appear to mirror the deeper and more fundamental structure of the region, some aspects of Paleozoic history in Arizona are considered here.

There is no record of igneous activity during this time; the section is entirely sedimentary rocks. The record of Paleozoic sedimentation in southwestern Arizona is largely incomplete; thus, its nature and distribution in this part of the region remains a matter of speculation. In central, northern, and southeastern Arizona, however, the pattern of isopachs (Fig. 2.7) reveals cratonic conditions of sedimentation which existed between the Cordilleran Geosyncline to the northwest and the Pedregosa Basin and its antecedents to the southeast. Sedimentation probably occurred across the area of missing isopachs. Sufficient scattered outcrops occur across the central part of Arizona to indicate that, at least at some times and places, seaways were continuous between these two basins. Notwithstanding this cratonic environment and the relative thinness of the section (1,700 m) compared to the sections outside of Arizona to the northwest and southeast, the depositional conditions were complex at times, and the lithologies are diverse.

General Stratigraphy

Much detailed study of the Paleozoic in southeastern Arizona and adjoining New Mexico has been reported since the column was first described in a general way by Ransome (1904) from studies at Bisbee. Results of continuing studies of the column and its geologic history have been reported successively by Darton (1925), Stoyanow (1936), and Gilluly (1956). Paleogeography has been outlined by McKee (1951), Peirce and Wilt (1970), and, for part of the region, by Kottlowski (1963). Works describing the Lower Paleozoic include Hayes (1975), Huddle and Dobrovolny (1952), and Schumacher (1978). Studies of the Upper Paleozoic have been reported by Gilluly, and others (1954), Bryant and McClymonds (1961), Armstrong (1962), and Ross (1973). The names, thicknesses, and general lithologies of principal Paleozoic formations of southeastern Arizona are shown in Figure 2.8.

Middle Cambrian sandstones and arkoses form the base of the section and may have been derived from erosion of a generally north- to northwest-trending shore line which moved eastward through much of the Cambrian (Lochman-Balk, 1972). Upper Cambrian strata in southeastern Arizona reflect marine conditions in the deposition of carbonate-rich shales and sandstones with fetid, thinly laminated limestones. The influence of land masses on Cambrian sedimentation is also expressed in Ordovican strata and in the Martin Formation of Upper Devonian age. Although much of southeastern Arizona appears to have been covered by Lower Paleozoic strata, parts of central Arizona remained emergent until the Upper Devonian. The apparent wedging out of successively

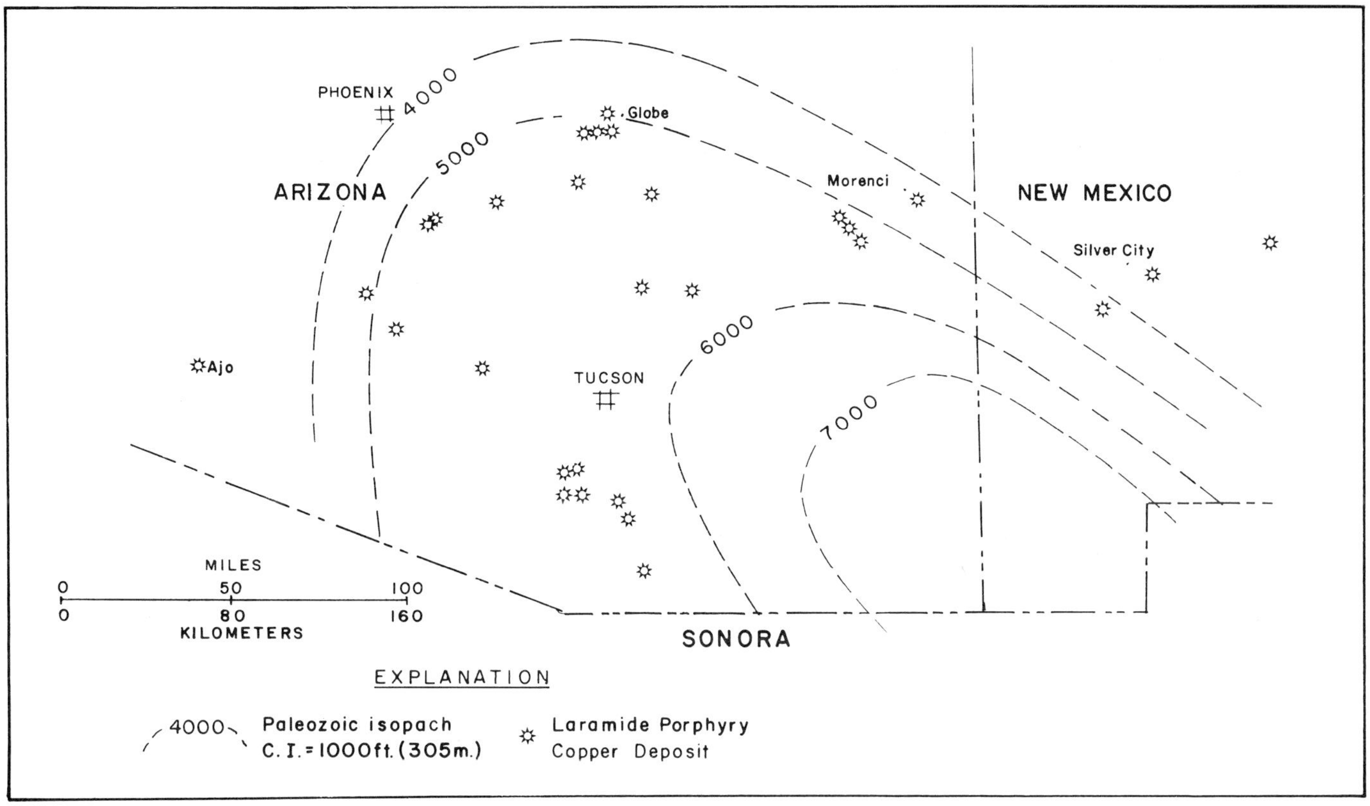

Figure 2.9. Paleozoic isopachs of southeastern Arizona, with principal porphyry copper deposits superimposed. Adapted from Peirce and Wilt (1970).

younger rock systems to the southeast and northwest in central Arizona during the Lower Paleozoic has led Peirce (1976) to suggest that deposition was controlled—at least in part—by the Transcontinental Arch, whose northeast axis and nose trend through central Arizona.

The sandstones, thin carbonates, and shaly limestones of the Lower Paleozoic give way at the base of Mississippian rocks to increasingly limestone-dominated sections of the Upper Paleozoic. Not only is there a change in conditions of deposition, but there appears to have emerged during the Devonian the first outlines of a structurally controlled basin in southeastern Arizona whose influence seems to have endured, at least intermittently, through the Mesozoic (Peirce, 1976). Isopach patterns change from the forms interpreted for the Lower Paleozoic to patterns which reflect the influence of a narrow (200 km), northwest-trending basin, which deepens over short distances to the southeast out of Arizona and New Mexico (Armstrong and Mamet, 1978). This basin is interpreted to lie south of the Deming Axis described by Turner (1962) and to have influenced the nature of sedimentation during the Mississippian, Pennsylvanian, and Permian periods.

The relatively thick sequences of upper Paleozoic strata (up to 2,200 m in southeasternmost Arizona) reflect deposition under marine environments during the Mississippian, but with more complex conditions prevailing during the Pennsylvanian and Permian periods. During these latter two periods, the influence of structurally controlled basins became more pronounced (Ross, 1973, 1978), and lithologies characteristic of environments ranging from basins, through shelves, lagoons, tidal flats, and river bars are present in southeastern Arizona. In southeastern Arizona the section is dominantly carbonate, but within some units, such as the Earp Formation, silts and mudstones become dominant and within others, such as the Epitaph Dolomite, gypsiferous and dolomitic units prodominate over limestone. Within this upper part of the Paleozoic some disconformities exist, and there is evidence of epeirogenic unrest, with alternate emergence and submergence. There are also indications that the positions of positive areas were controlled by northwest- to north-northwest–trending structures.

Paleozoic Characteristics and Porphyry Copper Deposits

Paleozoic isopachs are shown in their relationships to the distribution of porphyry copper systems in Figure 2.9. There seems to be a clear association between the deposits and the location of thinner parts of the section, but cause and effect, if such exists, cannot be demonstrated with any confidence. Although poorly defined on the basis of early Paleozoic sedimentational patterns, the structural framework which is revealed during the upper Paleozoic appears not only to have exerted control on thicknesses and lithologies but also to have been rejuvenated in later geologic periods, perhaps acting in some way as a structural control during the time of copper porphyry emplacement.

The nature of such control is shown on Figure 2.10. Butler (1971) demonstrated a profound northwest orientation of the distribution of the evaporite facies (dolomite and gypsum) of the Epitaph and Colina formations in southeast-

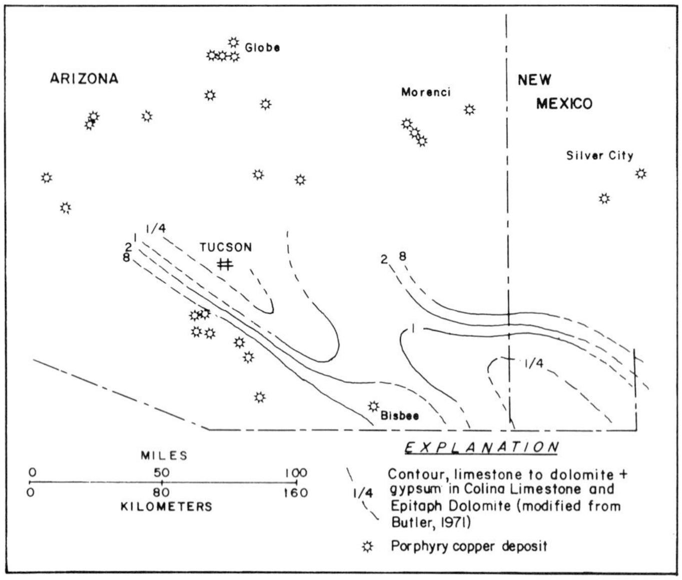

Figure 2.10. Porphyry copper deposits in relation to distribution of Permian evaporite facies in southeastern Arizona and adjoining New Mexico. Contours show approximate position and trend of the more extensive Pedregosa Basin of Upper Paleozoic age. Data from Butler (1971).

ern Arizona. This northwest trend and the southwestern boundary of the evaporites, as defined, parallel other major northwest-trending structures in southern Arizona. Further, many deposits not only are aligned along that structural direction, but also appear to lie on the flanks of the late Paleozoic basin. Lithologies have influenced, to varying degrees, the expression of porphyry copper alteration and mineralization. The presence of the carbonate-rich section in much of southeastern Arizona has resulted in many porphyry systems in which calc-silicate alteration around intrusions is the dominant type.

MESOZOIC

The Mesozoic Era in southeastern Arizona represents a pronounced change in the style of geologic evolution. At the end of the Paleozoic the comparatively uniform evolution of rocks over the region and the geology of northern and southern Arizona evolved in different ways. In southern Arizona the quiet and stable conditions of sedimentation on a craton during the Paleozoic, which gave rise to the thin column of basin and shelf marine sedimentary rocks, came to an end. The evidence suggests that much of the southern part of the region was differentially uplifted and began to contribute debris to the Colorado Plateaus region.

During the early Mesozoic, volcanism replaced marine sedimentation as the dominant rock-forming process. As a further contrast with the Paleozoic, the Mesozoic was marked by heightened structural disruption—characterized by block faulting—and the greater variety of geologic processes resulted in a much more complex geologic record. Volcanic activity was widespread and recurrent during the early and late Mesozoic, and the region was also subjected to further effects of erosion and deposition of sediment in structurally controlled basins. In southeastern Arizona well over twice the thickness of sedimentary rocks was formed than is

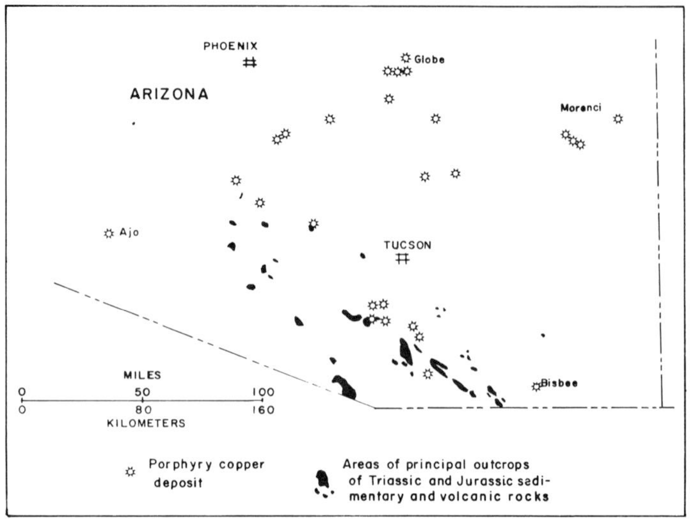

Figure 2.11. Porphyry copper deposits of southeastern Arizona shown in relationship to principal outcrops of Triassic and Jurassic strata. Data to the southeast in Mesozoic rocks from Hayes and Drewes (1978); to the northwest and west of Tucson, from Titley (1976).

recorded for the Paleozoic. The Mesozoic Era culminated in the Laramide Revolution, during which most porphyry copper deposits of the region were formed.

Studies of the Mesozoic and its definition in southern Arizona stem largely from the results of field investigations and of radiometric age dating. A summary of this work particularly applicable to the Triassic and Jurassic has been reported by Hayes and Drewes (1978). The great thickness of Lower Cretaceous sedimentary rocks in southeastern Arizona has been the object of much study since the rocks were first defined by Ransome (1904) at Bisbee. The Cretaceous System in the region has been further described and interpreted by Hayes (1970*b*). The Mesozoic has been described in the Sierrita Mountains by Cooper (1971), in the Santa Rita Mountains by Drewes (1971), in the Mule and Huachuca Mountains by Hayes (1970*a*), and in the Patagonia Mountains by Simons (1972).

Triassic and Jurassic Characteristics, Distribution, and Depositional Framework

On the Colorado Plateaus, rocks of the Triassic and Jurassic thicken northward from an east-trending zero isopach across the middle of Arizona (McKee, 1951). In southern Arizona this part of the column is characterized by widely scattered outcrops of various rock types. The column is best known and studied in southeastern Arizona, but it is likely that the Lower Mesozoic is present (although unrecognized) in many ranges of southwestern Arizona. The distribution of outcrops of Triassic-Jurassic rocks and their relationship to porphyry copper deposits in southeastern Arizona are shown in Figure 2.11.

Hayes and Drewes (1978) recognized a threefold separation of rock types in this part of the section. A lower unit of up to 3,000 m of volcanic rocks is successively overlain by redbeds and other clastic rocks about 600 m thick and by an upper group of volcanics 2,000 m thick. The lower unit comprises andesite and rhyodacite flows and pyroclastic units and has been dated in the Santa Rita Mountains at about 220

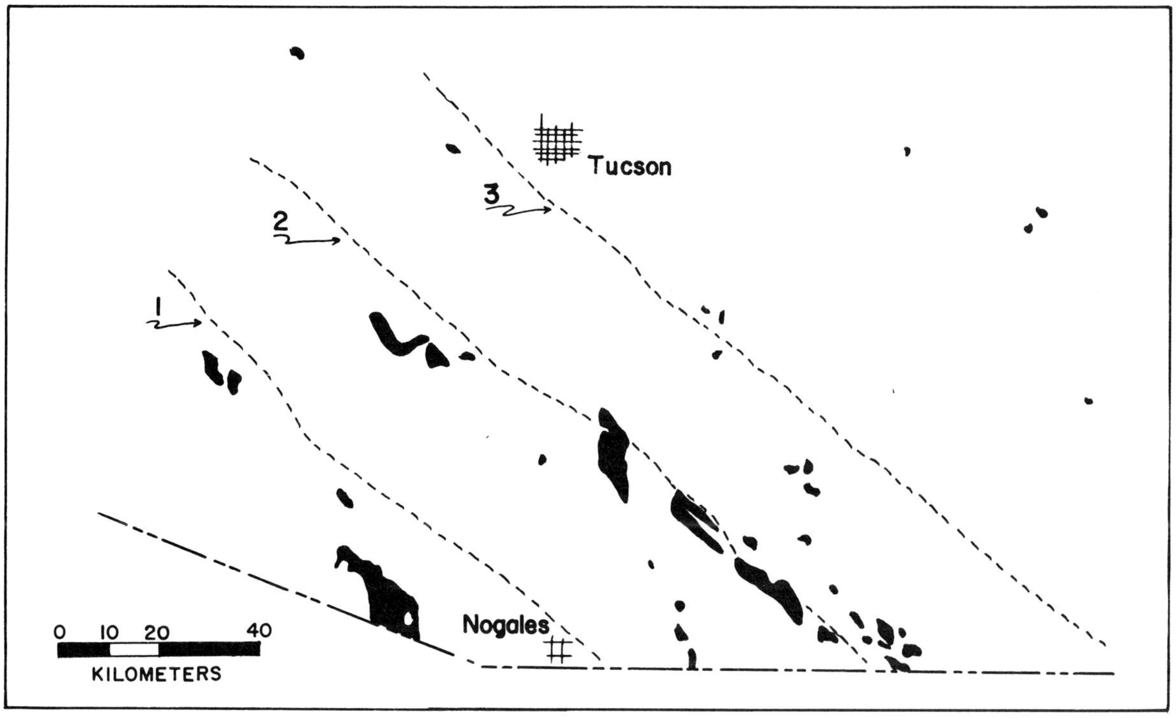

Figure 2.12. Interpreted trace of major structural discontinuities in southern Arizona: (1) the Comobabi-Nogales discontinuity, (2) the Sawmill Canyon fault, (3) the Silver Bell-Bisbee discontinuity. The discontinuities separate distinctive Paleozoic and Mesozoic rock associations. Outcrops of Triassic-Jurassic rocks of Figure 2.11 lie immediately south of the Sawmill Canyon fault. From Titley (1976).

m.y. old. Various lithologies and combinations of them make up the medial sedimentary rock unit. Rocks of this group appear more widely distributed than the lower volcanic unit and are present in the Tucson mountains, the Canelo Hills, Vekol Mountains, possibly in the Silver Bell Mountains, and in scattered exposures in southeasternmost Arizona. The lithologies consist of quartz cobble or chert pebble conglomerates, massive and thick-bedded mudstones, red shales, sandstones, and local interbeds of volcanic rocks. Age is inferred in many places by lithologic correlation and stratigraphic position below known Lower Cretaceous strata. In the Tucson Mountains the redbed unit is cut by a 150 million-year-old dike (Damon et al., 1967). The upper volcanic unit is composed chiefly of siliceous volcanic rocks, which, so far as known, are restricted to a small area in the Canelo Hills and Huachuca Mountains.

The most extensive exposures of these rocks and the greatest reported thicknesses are found southwest of the Sawmill Canyon Fault. This fault is one of three northwest-trending, regional breaks that appear to have influenced distribution of rocks during the late Paleozoic and Mesozoic (Fig. 2.12). North of the Fault the lower volcanic unit is not present and the medial sedimentary unit is deposited on Paleozoic rocks. Although the fault is not obviously a control of volcanic centers, the distribution of Paleozoic rocks and Triassic and Jurassic strata are influenced by it (Titley, 1976) and thus the fault must have been intermittently active during the early Mesozoic (Drewes, 1972).

Triassic-Jurassic Intrusions

Pre-Cretaceous intrusions have been recognized and mapped in several ranges of southeastern Arizona. These areas include the Dragoon Mountains (Gilluly, 1956), the Patagonia Mountains (Simons, 1972), the Santa Rita Mountains (Drewes, 1971), the Sierrita Mountains (Cooper, 1971), and Bisbee (Ransome, 1904). The range of radiometric ages for the bodies extends from about 190 m.y. ago to about 140 m.y. ago, and indicates widespread and intermittent but continuous intrusive activity in the region during the Jurassic. Many of the intrusions, which range from monzonite to granite compositions, occur in ranges and are near or in contact with lower Mesozoic strata; exceptions are Bisbee and the Dragoon Mountains, where the older rocks are not known.

At the level viewed only a few of the intrusions are clearly related to copper mineralization of Jurassic age. The most important of these is the Juniper Flat Granite at Bisbee, which is ca. 180 m.y. old (Marvin et al., 1973). The mineralization there has been assigned by many students since Ransome to a pre-Cretaceous age, based on the fact that various ore-bearing rocks and capping fragments are present in the conglomerates at the base of the Lower Cretaceous section. Jurassic intrusions of the Dragoon Mountains are associated with some weak copper and pyritic mineralization, but since a suite of Laramide rocks occurs in close association, it has not yet been possible to discover whether the mineralization is indigenous to the Jurassic rocks or represents a younger overprint. Such overprinting is present in the Sierrita Mountains, where a Jurassic intrusion is a host rock to Laramide-aged porphyry copper mineralization in the Esperanza-Sierrita complex (West and Aiken, 1982). Notwithstanding such uncertainties, the evidence from Bisbee clearly reveals that the Jurassic represents a metallogenic epoch in the Southwest, and the search for lower Mesozoic mineralization remains an important exploration activity.

Cretaceous

At some time or times during the Triassic and Jurassic, structural relief—possibly as great as several thousand meters—developed, and Lower Cretaceous volcanic and sedimentary rocks were deposited across a land surface of highly varied age and lithology. Relief on this surface at the time the oldest of the Cretaceous rocks were laid down has been suggested to be as great as 300 meters (Hayes and Drewes, 1978). Several hundreds of meters of relief were present at Bisbee on a surface which exposed juxtaposed rocks revealing at least 2,000 meters of structural separation. Just as there is evidence for development of some structural relief during the Triassic and Jurassic (Titley, 1976), there is also evidence from sedimentary rock types that some structural and topographic relief evolved during Lower Cretaceous time. This topography appears to have been reduced during the Lower Cretaceous, and southeastern Arizona was once again the site of evolution of a northwest-trending basin—the Sonoran Embayment—which received at least 4,000 m of sediment in some places. This trough, which extended southeastward into Mexico, had its terminus in southeastern Arizona. Although other possible Lower Cretaceous rocks may occur to the west across southern Arizona, there is no evidence at this time to associate them with the strata of the Sonoran trough to the southeast.

The Lower Cretaceous reflects a profound shift from the volcanic-dominated processes and strata of the earlier part of the Mesozoic, to processes characterized by shallow marine and deltaic sedimentation. Except in the Santa Rita Mountains, where minor volcanic components are present in some Lower Cretaceous units (Drewes, 1971), the Lower Cretaceous succession consists of sedimentary rocks. These rocks —the Bisbee Group or its correlatives—were first described at Bisbee and in the Mule Mountains (Ransome, 1904). They are chiefly clastic rocks, although in the southernmost part of the region they include one persistent and thick marine limestone unit. The base of the Bisbee Group consists of a fanglomerate which is only locally present and which is interpreted as derived from block-fault mountains (Titley, 1976; Bilodeau, 1978). Above this basal conglomerate a thick column of conglomerate, sandstone, arkose, and shale is present. Deposition locally persisted into earliest Upper Cretaceous (Schafroth, 1968).

The distribution of Lower Cretaceous rocks is on Figure 2.13. The pattern of outcrops reflects the position of the basin terminus, and it is noteworthy that, if Lower Cretaceous strata of Bisbee Formation affinity were at one time more widespread than shown, they were removed prior to deposition of rocks of Upper Cretaceous age, which are scattered but widely present outside of the region of outcrop shown. A second noteworthy association is shown in Figure 2.13. Porphyry copper deposits of Laramide age occur around the basin edge, but only rarely within it. This observation was made by Anderson (1966) and was based on the distribution of nine deposits. The addition of about twenty-five deposits to Anderson's list has not substantially changed the general validity of the observation, although the Rosemont-Helvetia complex and copper mineralization at Johnson Camp both occur within the interpreted basin boundary. In this southeastern part of Arizona some Laramide intrusions (e.g. in the Empire, Whetstone Mountains, Tombstone Hills) occur within the suggested basin boundary, but seldom are they more than weakly, if at all, mineralized or altered at the level viewed. Reasons for the great number of deposits on the basin edge remain obscure, but the observation has been detailed further (Titley, 1972*a*).

LATE CRETACEOUS—EARLY TERTIARY (LARAMIDE)

A hiatus of 25 to 30 million years exists between deposition of the youngest Bisbee Group rocks and formation of the youngest Cretaceous rocks. These strata reveal that once again a pronounced shift in style of geological evolution took place and that volcanic activity again became dominant. It was during a period of time between about 80 m.y. ago and 50 m.y. ago (a time that spans the last of the Mesozoic and earliest Cenozoic) that the great numbers of porphyry copper systems in this part of North America came into being. Although knowledge of the geology of previous eras is considerable, little is known of the geomorphology, the structural geology, and the rock distribution patterns of Laramide time. While the association of certain geologic structures with rocks can be shown for earlier periods, and interpretations can be drawn for those associations, considerable uncertainty attends interpretations of Laramide history on the same bases. Extensive volcanic activity, with mostly subaerial deposition of rocks, morphologically unstable volcanic superstructures, and widescale disruption and destruction of the rock column by early Tertiary erosion and Late-Tertiary mountain building have all served to obliterate much of the record. There remain the porphyry copper plutons and, in some locations, associated volcanic and volcaniclastic rocks.

Rocks of Laramide Age

In southwestern New Mexico and southeastern Arizona rocks of the Laramide include the porphyry copper stocks, many small stocks and other intrusive igneous bodies which are not mineralized, and remnants of probably large and extensive blankets of volcanic and volcaniclastic rocks. Because of close spatial relationships between some stocks and volcanic units, and because of closely similar ages of intrusions and volcanic rocks where they have been measured and compared, a genetic relationship is inferred. In areas where the two types of rock occur together the volcanic units can be shown to be older than the stocks, from either radiometric age dates or from cross-cutting relationships. There exist as well volcanic units in many of these regions which are clearly post-mineral in age and are of known or inferred mid-Tertiary age. Where the Laramide volcanic units have been radiometrically dated, the ages extend from about 72 m.y. old, as in the Santa Rita Mountains, Tombstone Hills, Mustang Mountains, and the Tucson Mountains (Hayes and Drewes, 1978) to about 80 m.y. old in the Williamson Canyon Formation at Christmas (Koski and Cook, 1982).

The distribution of Laramide volcanic rock units and their spatial relation to the porphyry copper systems is shown

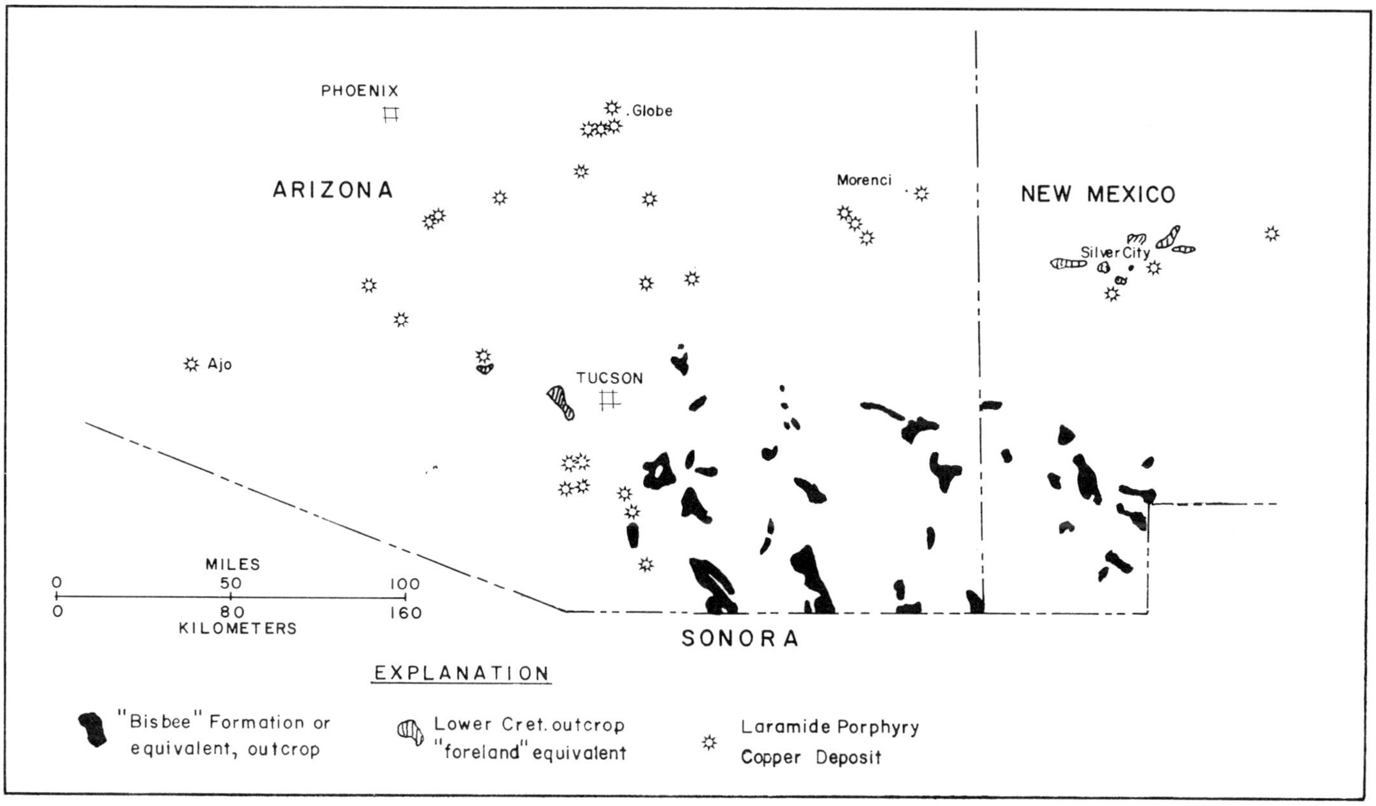

Figure 2.13. Porphyry copper deposits of southeastern Arizona and contiguous New Mexico shown in relationship to exposures of Lower Cretaceous strata. Foreland equivalents include possible and probable uppermost Lower Cretaceous strata of the Silver City area, and the Tucson, Silver Bell, and Sierrita Mountains. Data from Titley (1972*a*, 1976).

on the outcrop map in Figure 2.14. Some exposures shown as Laramide have been identified on the basis of distinctive lithologic types and stratigraphic position rather than by radiometric age dates. Important localities where intrusions of porphyry, associated ore deposits, and the volcanic units are all present include Safford (Robinson and Cook, 1966), Silver Bell (Richard and Courtright, 1966), the Sierrita Mountains (Cooper, 1971), Hillsboro (Dunn, 1982), and Lakeshore. Less certainty attends the assignment of pre-ore volcanics to the Laramide in the deposits of Sonora, Mexico, but rocks closely similar to those in the United States and in similar stratigraphic positions occur at Cananea (Velasco, 1966) and in the Nacozari district (Wade and Wandke, 1920; Saegart et al., 1974).

Considerable variation in lithology is present on a regional scale and within individual sequences. At Silver Bell, where Courtright (1958) first recognized the nature and importance of these units, the lithology is dominated by andesite, andesitic breccias and mud flows (lahars). Much greater diversity has been reported for the Laramide units in the Santa Rita Mountains, where Drewes (1971) has described a 1,200-m sequence of dacitic to andesitic flows and tuff breccia, dacite breccias, welded tuffs, arkose, and mixed volcanic-sedimentary and agglomerate units. A common feature of most sequences is the presence of volcanic breccias, which in some localities contain fragments many meters in size—described in the Tucson Mountains as "Chaos" (Kinnison, 1959) and in the Santa Rita Mountains as "Exotic Block Member" (Drewes, 1971). Although several interpretations of the origin of these units have been proposed, their inclusion within volcanic sequences and their nature suggests explosive volcanism.

Following the deposition of the volcanic units, and in a span of time ranging from about 72 m.y. ago to about 53 m.y. ago, many stocks were emplaced and cooled in this region. As at Hillsboro and Safford, at least some succeeded in penetrating the volcanic pile above them, and Laramide volcanic rocks are hosts to mineralization in some systems. A great variety of rocks is present in this group of intrusions, and a common hallmark of a porphyry copper system is an intrusive porphyry complex which reveals many textural and sometimes compositional characteristics. The area of exposure of the common Laramide pluton is small (cf. Norton, 1982), seldom over 3 km wide at the level exposed, and usually about 1.5 km. The shape of the complex is sometimes circular, but many show northwest or northeast elongation. Many stocks are crosscut by still younger dikes or irregular intrusions, but, where the radiometric data are available, the younger bodies are still of Laramide age and many are mineralized. An important feature of the region is that not all Laramide intrusions present are known to be progenitors of porphyry copper systems at the level observed.

The modal composition of stocks includes many variants between granodiorite and quartz monzonite—terms and descriptions of rocks which have been long used in this region. Many equigranular, Laramide intrusions are present and are, in some instances, hosts to copper ores in the porphyry systems. It is important to emphasize, however, that without

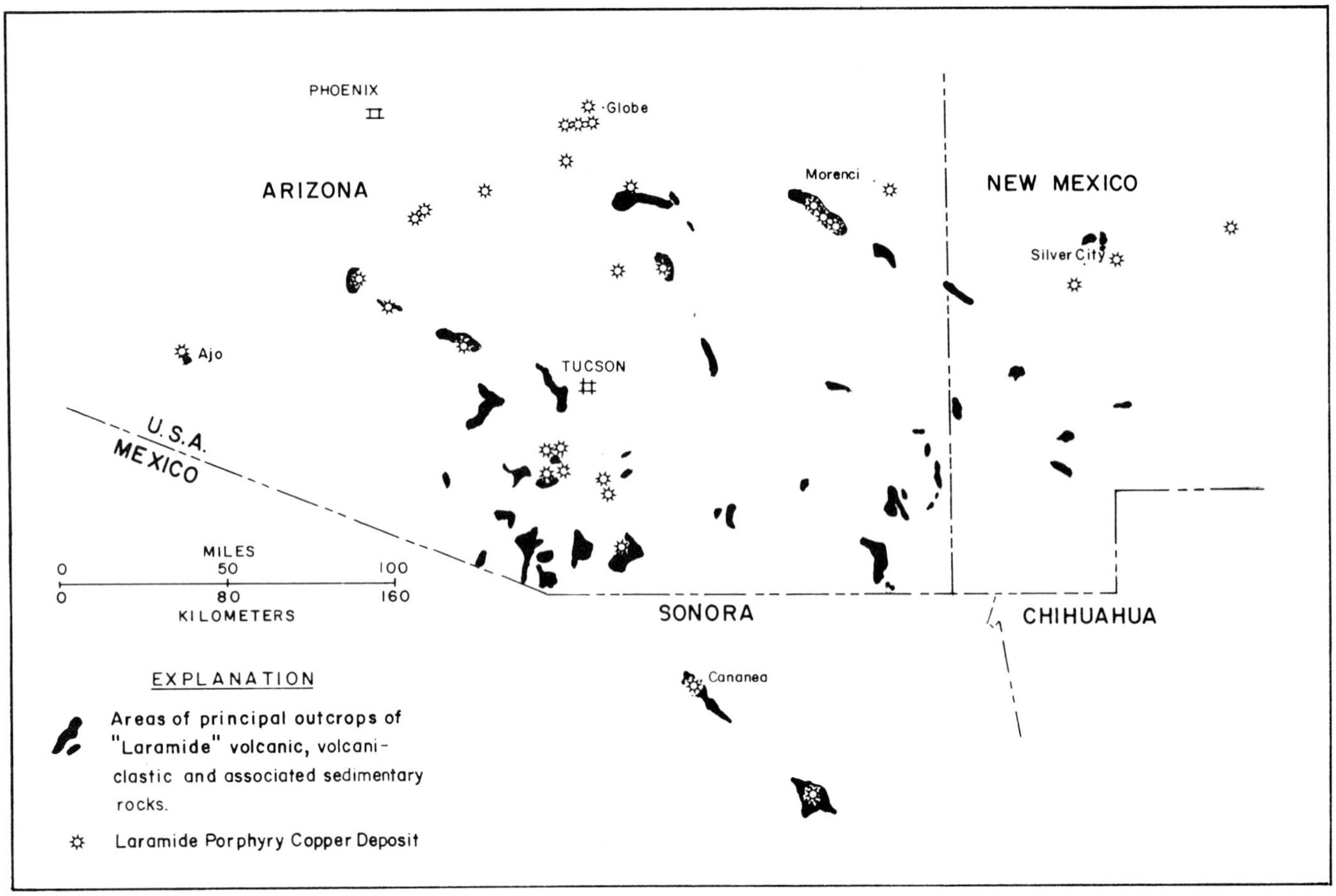

Figure 2.14. Porphyry copper deposits of southeastern Arizona and contiguous regions shown in relationship to exposures of Laramide-aged volcanic and volcaniclastic rocks

known exception the hydrothermal systems are centered on porphyry plutons.

Compared with other porphyry copper deposit provinces, such as the southwestern Pacific (Gustafson and Titley, 1978) or many deposits of the Canadian Cordillera (Sutherland Brown, 1976), there are only sparse chemical data on rocks from deposits of the American Southwest upon which petrogenetic interpretations can be based. Several factors contribute to this situation. The deposits are old (ca. 60 m.y.) and have undergone a protracted and complex history of modification during the Tertiary. There is evidence that some, if not most, were intermittently oxidized, covered, uncovered, re-oxidized, and covered again. Erosion has not been sufficient to remove the oxidized caps (nor, fortunately, the secondary sulfide-enriched blankets upon which the economic viability of so many has depended), and rocks showing the effects of supergene activity are widely present in many orebodies. Supergene effects have plunged deeply into some orebodies: after some 70 years of operation, secondarily enriched ores are still being mined in some systems. In many porphyry copper systems the supergene effects are imposed upon host rocks and porphyry which have been extensively altered by quartz-sericite-pyrite in densely fractured rocks. For these reasons, rocks suitable for analysis are difficult, if not impossible, to find in the porphyry centers of many deposits. As mining progresses into hypogene-altered parts of systems, and as the nature of that alteration becomes better understood in particular deposits, a clearer idea of rock chemistry may evolve than that now recognized.

Interpretations of chemical data for parts of some porphyry systems of this region have been published. Creasey (1966) reported compositions of some unaltered igneous rocks from several deposits of the Southwest on Q-P1-Kspar diagrams which revealed the granodiorite-quartz monzonite range of composition. He also compared rock compositions of porphyry systems from various provinces around the Pacific Basin (Creasey, 1977). Moore (1973) presented data for some unaltered rocks on the fringe of mineralization at Bingham. In the present volume data for rocks from around the Ray deposit are presented (Cornwall, Chapter 11) and are compared with rocks from other deposits; Koski and Cook (Chapter 17) report chemical data for Christmas; and West and Aiken (Chapter 21) report the results of various analyses of rocks from Sierrita. In their interpretations of rock compositions Cornwall and Koski and Cook note the essential calc-alkaline nature of the differentiation series. The "alkaline suite" noted for the western Canadian Province (Barr et al., 1976) is not widely present in the Southwest, although small volumes of undersaturated volcanics and plugs are present in a few districts, such as Santa Rita and Sierrita.

In summary, habits of occurrence of the Laramide rocks are those of isolated exposures of sequences of volcanic and volcaniclastic rocks and of plutons or pluton complexes. One particularly noteworthy habit is the clustering of plutons in small areas, such as the Globe-Miami area, the Sierrita Mountains, and Copper Creek. Distribution of some, such as the deposits at Safford, those in the interval from Red

Mountain to Lake Shore, and those in the interval from Vekol to Globe-Miami, occur as groups of aligned deposits, suggesting fundamental structural controls.

Laramide Structure

Profound overprinting of earlier structures in this region by those of Late-Tertiary mountain building in the Basin and Range Province results in complex geology that is difficult to interpret. The structural geology of this region has been the subject of much study, and many papers have been devoted to results of that work. Most of the Laramide districts of the American Southwest occur within the "Texas Zone" (Schmitt, 1966), a west-northwest-trending belt of major structural deformation. The nature of this belt and the habit of ore deposits within it have been described by Mayo (1958), who suggests control of intrusion centers within the belt by fault intersections, and on a broader scale by Schmitt (1966), who interprets the location of groups of districts to be related to the intersection of the Texas Zone and the Wasatch Orogen. While it remains clear that there is coincidence of porphyry copper deposits and the "Texas Zone," no clear picture of the cause and effect relationships has been developed. The uniquely Laramide age of structural activity within the belt remains an elusive fact to document, and there is no clear concurrence on the style of Laramide structural deformation which took place within it. Long studied, the nature of Laramide deformation remains an important object of scientific inquiry.

Davis (1979) has succinctly reviewed various models of Laramide deformation, such as: differential vertical uplift (Jones, 1966); compression-induced regional overthrusting (Ransome, 1904; Cooper and Silver, 1964; Drewes, 1978); crustal extension (Lowell, 1974); and gravity gliding (Jones, 1963). Davis (1979) has based his research on extensive field investigations of rock distribution and the character of folds. Using determinations of transport direction interpreted on the basis of structural geometry, he has shown that northwest-aligned fold axes and southeastward transport are widely present in southeastern Arizona. These Laramide features are best explained by a "basement-cored uplift" model in which Laramide compressional stresses were directed northeast-southwest. The result of these stresses was initiation of "major reverse-slip and thrust-slip faulting along zones of weakness in the region" (Davis, 1979, p. 563). One of the lines of weakness described by Davis is the Sawmill Canyon fault zone (see Fig. 2.12).

Although the style of tectonics described by Davis (1979) was worked out in southeasternmost Arizona, the lines bordering these blocks extend northwestward into the region of porphyry copper deposits. In that region, however, Rehrig and Heidrich (1976) proposed a mechanism of uplift along northwest-trending axes to explain the consistent and region-wide fracture patterns and styles in Laramide intrusions. There is, thus, the indication that Laramide structural evolution in the region to the porphyries was that of basement-cored uplift, but clear evidence for its existence during the Laramide, and outside of the area of Davis's study has not been developed. It is clear, however, that the deposits at Twin Buttes, Sierrita, Silver Bell, Lake Shore, and Vekol border the projection of the basement uplift shown by Davis (1979).

Various estimates of the levels to which the porphyry plutons were emplaced have been made, most of which are based upon stratigraphic reconstructions. While a fair estimate of anywhere from 1,300 m to 3,300 m of pre-Laramide rocks can be made for some locations in the region, the great unknown is the thickness of pre-ore, Laramide-aged volcanic and sedimentary strata which may have existed. About 1,000 m of such rocks (locally, greater) have been measured in some sections; notwithstanding such thicknesses, there is evidence (e.g., deposits at Safford, Hillsboro, Christmas, and perhaps Silver Bell) that intrusions may have made their way, at least in some instances, several hundreds of meters into the volcanic piles. From such stratigraphic evidence depths of burial as little as 500 m have been proposed (Titley, 1972*a*), and ranges of depths from 1.5 to 3 km to the original tops of intrusions have been suggested by Sillitoe (1973). Cornwall (1982) suggests a range of from 1.5 to a maximum of 5 km for depths of burial of plutons at Ray. A different line of evidence for depths of burial has been developed from fluid inclusion studies at Red Mountain (Bodnar and Beane, 1977). There an intrusion, still buried, is interpreted from evidence of boiling and salinities to have been emplaced at least 4 km beneath the surface. The evidence ranges from permissive to at least strongly suggestive for emplacement to shallow depths in the crust of many porphyry plutons of this region, and while their total vertical extent is largely unknown, their tops may have ranged from less than 1 to about 4 km beneath the surface.

The porphyritic texture of the stocks (suggestive of rapid cooling), their suspected emplacement to very shallow levels, and the absence of xenoliths point to an environment of intrusion in which forces impeding a rapid rise to shallow levels were minimized. It would follow that some unique structural preparation existed or developed throughout this restricted region. Likely structural controls would include fault intersections (Mayo, 1958), which have been interpreted to have controlled the localization of the stock at Bagdad (Anderson et al., 1955), and strike deviations in regional wrench fault systems, which have been suggested for deposits in some southwestern Pacific environments (Titley and Heidrick, 1978). Although such regional breaks probably were present in the southwestern North American environment, their effects on controlling emplacement have not yet been documented.

Many individual porphyry plutons or groups of plutons are elongated. The direction of elongation in the American Southwest is either northeast or northwest. Groups of northeast-elongated plutons occur as a well-defined, northeast-trending belt of bodies at Bagdad (Anderson et al., 1955), and separate northeast-aligned bodies occur at Globe-Miami (Peterson, 1962). A northwest-trending belt of northwesterly-aligned plutons occurs in the Sierrita Mine area. East-northeast-trending plutons occur at Safford (Dunn, 1978), but they are aligned *en echelon* to the northwest. There is, thus, clear evidence for profound structural anisotropy during the Laramide and for well-established directions of regional stress (Heidrick and Titley, 1982).

Further evidence for preferred directions of stress orientations has been established by Rehrig and Heidrick (1972, 1976) and Heidrick and Titley (1981). Measurements of directions of Laramide dikes, faults, fault veins, and veins from many intrusion centers reveal a pronounced east-northeast (±20°) orientation of these features. Such directions were revealed in the work at Bagdad by Anderson and others (1955), and these directions have been shown to occur in almost every porphyry copper system studied (Heidrick and Titley, 1981). The direction and the stresses necessary to produce it have been interpreted as southwest- to west-southwest–directed compression during the Laramide, an orientation consistent with that interpreted by Davis (1979) as necessary to explain evolution of the larger scale structural features.

Laramide-Age and Tertiary Plate Tectonics

Many features of the porphyry copper deposits and of regional geology have been interpreted in the context of plate tectonic history. Coney (1976, 1978*a*, 1978*b*) has outlined the path of plate history as it has affected the American Southwest, particularly southeastern Arizona. A change in direction of motion of the North American plate about 80 m.y. ago (Coney, 1972) resulted in near-normal convergence with the Farallon plate at high convergence rates. Results of this convergence have been interpreted as a strong northeastward-directed compression, uplift, intrusion, and volcanism. These effects swept northeastward across Arizona and into Colorado and are interpreted to have been the result of flattening of the Benioff Zone (Lipman et al., 1972; Heidrick and Titley, 1976; Coney and Reynolds, 1977). During this time of high convergence rates porphyry copper plutons were emplaced. It has been suggested that the effects of high rates of normal convergence resulted in structural preparation by producing epicrustal extension, which may have aided emplacement of plutons at high crustal levels (Heidrick and Titley, 1976).

The possible slowing of convergence rates brought about by a change in the type of plate interaction (Coney, 1976) corresponds in a general way to the time of cessation of Laramide activity. There is clearly a change in the nature of mid-Tertiary plutons, which only rarely are related to porphyry copper deposition. Rehrig and Heidrick (1976) have documented a region-wide, north-trending orientation of dikes, faults, and veins in some mid-Tertiary plutons which contrasts sharply with the pronounced east-northeast trends determined for the Laramide (Fig. 2.15). It is possible to interpret, therefore, some cause and effect relationships between the styles of deformation and intrusion of the Laramide and mid-Tertiary and the interpreted nature of plate interactions in the American Southwest.

POST-MINERALIZATION HISTORY

In southeastern Arizona and the adjoining regions, there is little evidence to interpret the nature of Eocene (Lower Tertiary) history. The history of the Cenozoic, however, has been discussed by Scarborough and Peirce (1978). Presumably much erosion took place, and there is evidence that at least some oxidation and enrichment of the Laramide por-

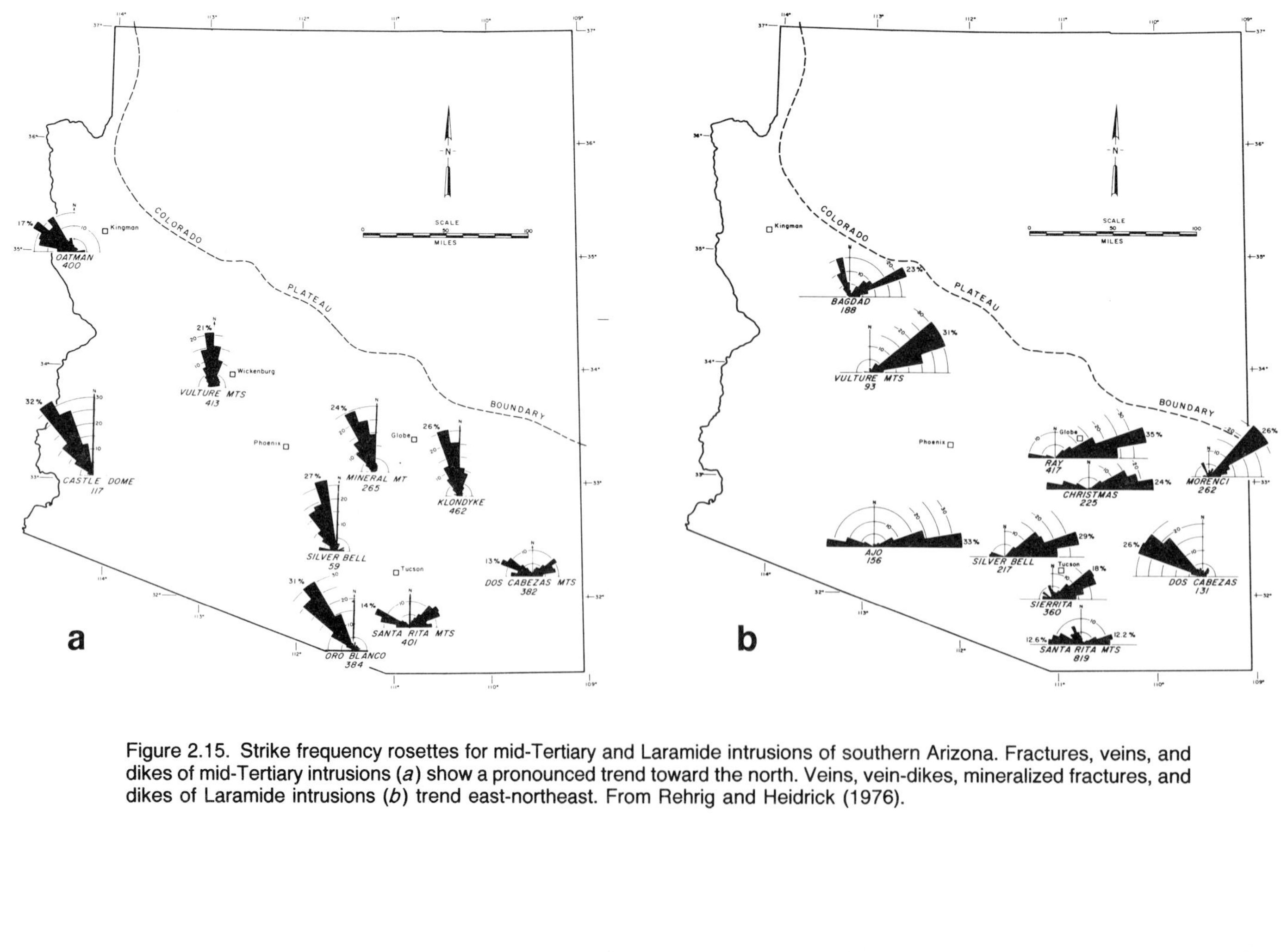

Figure 2.15. Strike frequency rosettes for mid-Tertiary and Laramide intrusions of southern Arizona. Fractures, veins, and dikes of mid-Tertiary intrusions (*a*) show a pronounced trend toward the north. Veins, vein-dikes, mineralized fractures, and dikes of Laramide intrusions (*b*) trend east-northeast. From Rehrig and Heidrick (1976).

phyry copper systems also took place. Much of this early, post-primary-mineralization history has been discussed by Livingston and others (1968). In at least one deposit of the region there is evidence of early Tertiary oxidation and leaching. At Silver Bell, Richard and Courtright (1966) report the presence of oxidized fragments of ore in the basal conglomerate of a unit beneath dated volcanic rocks about 30 m.y. in age. Elsewhere, at Morenci (Moolick and Durek, 1966) and at Safford (Robinson and Cook, 1966) mid-Tertiary volcanic rocks overlie oxidized Laramide ores. Livingston and others (1968) have shown this phenomenon to be of widespread occurrence in the southeastern Arizona Province. It should be noted further, however, that evidence from Silver Bell (Graybeal, 1982) and from Twin Buttes (Barter and Kelly, 1982) indicates that there is at least locally post-mid-Tertiary oxidation with some enrichment in those systems.

By mid-Tertiary times (33 m.y. ago at Safford and Clifton) volcanic rocks covered the deposits and either slowed or stopped the oxidation and enrichment process. With the development of the Basin and Range landforms in the Late Tertiary, deposits were fragmented with some, or parts of some, uplifted and others depressed. These various and complex events of the Tertiary are of major importance, and understanding them is critical to exploration. Without a period of tectonic quiescence the deposits would probably not have been as deeply enriched as they were. Were it not for a protective volcanic cap put upon them, they could have been eroded away, and they may have been further protected by being locally down-dropped during the time of Late-Tertiary mountain building. Only localized volcanic activity has taken place since about 20 m.y. ago, and the deposits have been undergoing a regime characterized by their weathering and destruction. For some which may still be buried, oxidation and enrichment may still be proceeding.

SUMMARY

Many associations of bedrock geology, geologic events, and aspects of geologic history with the Laramide porphyry copper deposits of the Southwest have been observed and have been discussed here. As noted at the outset, establishment of geologic cause and effect is commonly difficult. Nonetheless, some of these associations merit a final summary and analysis and are set forth as follows:

1. There is a clear association of some deposits with a basement characterized by Pinal Schist and granites (ca. 1, 400 m.y. old) which intrude it. There is documentation of control exerted by an east-northeast-trending grain within the Precambrian upon the position of emplacement of plutons. Many intrusion sites of plutons are along old Schist-granite contacts. It is at least a curious coincidence that this old east-northeast grain is the same as the pronounced Laramide east-northeast grain which can be interpreted in the context of south-southwest-directed compression during the Laramide. It seems reasonable to suggest that this coincidence between the old basement anisotropy and younger stresses which were sympathetic with and superimposed upon it was in some way responsible for the widespread structural preparation believed to be necessary for intrusions of porphyry copper systems (Heidrick and Titley, 1976).

2. There is also a pronounced northwest structural grain characterized by faults, possibly as old as the Precambrian, but certainly active during the upper Paleozoic and through the Mesozoic. Consideration of the existence of these regional breaks and the block fault mountains believed to have evolved during the middle and upper Mesozoic, together with the basement anisotropy, leads to a suggestion that the basement of the southeastern Arizona Province was in a very weakened state, so that magmas which developed beneath it found a very permeable crust through which to move.

3. Most porphyry copper systems evolved in an environment of thin (4–5 km), pre-Laramide Phanerozoic cover. Where that thickness is doubled in southeastern Arizona, Laramide plutons are not recognized to be copper-related. Cause and effect, if any, are not by any means clear, but the association is real with few exceptions.

4. There is no clear association with Triassic-Jurassic volcanism, although that period of time represents a metallogenic epoch in its own right. In the Sierrita Mountains, the Patagonia Mountains, the Dragoon Mountains, and at Bisbee, both Jurassic and Jurassic(?), and Laramide or Tertiary intrusions and volcanic rocks are present. Repetitious igneous activity in these particular regions suggests the possibility of reactivation of controls on magma emplacement by Jurassic or older structures. Further analysis and study of pre-Laramide structural evolution of the region is certainly warranted.

5. The distribution of porphyry copper systems in southeastern Arizona and the adjoining regions around the distal end of the Sonoran trough (Lower Cretaceous) remains an unexplained phenomenon. If thinned, post-Precambrian rock columns and structural control are prerequisites to emplacement and generation of a porphyry copper system, the basin edge is certainly ideally suited.

6. In many places it is clear that Laramide volcanic activity preceded or accompanied emplacement of the porphyry copper plutons, although it can only be inferred that the plutons represent the immediate subvolcanic intrusions. The volcanic and volcaniclastic columns present are remnants of once larger, locally derived, volcanic piles. Rocks which remain suggest that volcanic piles which may have existed above the systems were not more than a few kilometers thick, but the depths of cover beneath which presently exposed levels of porphyry copper deposits evolved remain speculative. They may have been as great as 4–5 km or as little as 1–2 km.

ACKNOWLEDGMENTS

Many people have had a part, directly or indirectly, in developing the approach to regional geology which is presented here. An early appreciation of the geology of the Southwest and the nature of many problems was inspired by the late Eldred D. Wilson, and by John F. Lance and Evans B. Mayo. I am indebted to John S. Sumner for providing both the geophysical base map used here and for discussions concerning the interpretation presented. Discussions over a period of many years on various aspects of the geology in this region and the relationship of ore deposits to that geologic framework with Tom L. Heidrick, Donald L. Bryant, Joseph

F. Schreiber, Frederick T. Graybeal, and Denis L. Norton, are gratefully acknowledged. S. J. Reynolds supplied some data for western Arizona. Early versions of the manuscript benefitted from critical reviews by and discussions with Peter J. Coney, George H. Davis, and H. Wesley Peirce. I thank them for their interest in this subject and for their efforts. The manuscript was prepared with help from J. A. Woodward and J. Lekawa.

REFERENCES CITED

Anderson, C. A., 1951, Older Precambrian structure in Arizona: Geol. Soc. America Bull., v. 62, p. 1331–1346.

———, 1966, Areal geology of the Southwest, *in* Titley, S. R., and Hicks, C. L., eds., Geology of the Porphyry Copper Deposits, Southwestern North America: Tucson, Univ. Ariz. Press, p. 3–16.

———, 1968*a*, Arizona and adjacent New Mexico, *in* Ridge, J. D., ed., Ore Deposits of the United States, 1933–1967: New York, AIME, p. 1163–1190.

———, 1968*b*, Metamorphosed Precambrian silicic volcanic rocks in central Arizona, *in* Coats, R. R.; Hay, R. L.; and Anderson, C. A., eds., Studies in Volcanology: Geol. Soc. America, Mem. 116, p. 9–44.

———, 1972, Precambrian rocks in the Cordes area, Yavapai County, Arizona: U.S. Geol. Survey Bull. 1345, 36 p.

Anderson, C. A.; Scholz, E. A.; and Strobell, J. D., Jr., 1955, Geology and ore deposits of the Bagdad area, Yavapai County, Arizona: U.S. Geol. Survey Prof. Paper 278, 103 p.

Anderson, C. A., and Creasey, S. C., 1958, Geology and ore deposits of the Jerome area, Yavapai County, Arizona: U.S. Geol. Survey Prof. Paper 308, 185 p.

Anderson, C. A.; Blacet, P. M.; Silver, L. T.; and Stern, T. W., 1971, Revision of Precambrian stratigraphy in the Prescott-Jerome area, Yavapai County, Arizona: U.S. Geol. Survey Bull. 1324-C, 15 p.

Anderson, C. A., and Blacet, P. M., 1972, Precambrian geology of the Northern Bradshaw Mountains, Yavapai County, Arizona: U.S. Geol. Survey Bull. 1336, 82 p.

Anderson, C. A., and Silver, L. T., 1976, Yavapai Series—A greenstone belt: Ariz. Geol. Soc. Digest X, p. 13–26.

Armstrong, A. K., 1962, Stratigraphy and paleontology of the Mississippian System in southwestern New Mexico and adjacent southeastern Arizona: New Mexico Bur. Mines and Min. Resources Mem. 8, 95 p.

Armstrong, A. K., and Mamet, B. L., 1978, The Mississippian System of southwestern New Mexico and southeastern Arizona: New Mexico Geol. Soc., Ariz. Geol. Soc., 29th Field Conf. Guidebook, p. 183–192.

Balla, J. C., 1972, The relationship of Laramide stocks to regional structure in central Arizona: Unpub. Ph.D. Diss., Univ. of Ariz., 132 p.

Barker, F., 1969, Precambrian geology of the Needle Mountains, southwestern Colorado: U.S. Geol. Survey Prof. Paper 644A, 35 p.

Barr, D. A.; Fox, P. E.; Northcote, K. E.; and Preto, V. A., 1976, The alkaline suite porphyry deposits: A summary, *in* Sutherland Brown, A., ed., Porphyry Deposits of the Canadian Cordillera: CIM Spec. Vol. 15, p. 359–367.

Barter, C. G., and Kelly, J. L., 1982, Geology of the Twin Buttes mineral deposit, Pima mining district, Pima County, Arizona, *in* Titley, S. R., ed., Advances in Geology of the Porphyry Copper Deposits, Southwestern North America: Tucson, Univ. Ariz. Press, Chap. 20.

Bickford, M. E.; Wetherill, G. W.; Barker, F.; and Lee-Hu, C. N., 1969, Precambrian Rb-Sr chronology in the Needle Mountains, southwestern Colorado: Jour. Geophys. Research, v. 74, p. 1660–1676.

Billingsley, P., and Locke, A., 1941, Structure of ore districts in the continental framework: AIME Trans., v. 144, p. 9–64.

Bilodeau, W. L., 1978, The Glance Conglomerate, a Lower Cretaceous syntectonic deposit in southeastern Arizona, *in* Land of Cochise, Southeastern Arizona: New Mex. Geol. Soc., Ariz. Geol. Soc. Guidebook, 29th Field Conf., p. 209–214.

Bodnar, R. J., and Beane, R. E., 1977, Temperature variations in pre-intrusive cover over a buried pluton (abs.): Geol. Soc. America, Ann. Mtg., Abs. with Prog., p. 903–904.

Bryant, D. L., and McClymonds, N. E., 1961, Permian Concha Limestone and Rainvalley Formation, southeastern Arizona: Amer. Assoc. Petroleum Geologists Bull., v. 45, p. 1324–1333.

Butler, B. S., 1933, Ore deposits as related to stratigraphic, structural and igneous geology in the western United States: Part I, Summary, *in* Ore Deposits of the Western States: New York, AIME, p. 198–240.

Butler, B. S., and Wilson, E. D., 1938, General features of some Arizona ore deposits: Ariz. Bur. Mines Bull. 145, p. 9–25.

Butler, W. C., 1971, Permian sedimentary environments in southwestern Arizona: Ariz. Geol. Soc. Digest IX, p. 71–93.

Carpenter, R. H., 1947, The geology and ore deposits of the Vekol Mountains, Pinal County, Arizona: Unpub. Ph.D. Diss., Stanford Univ., 110 p.

Coney, P. J. 1972, Cordilleran tectonics and North America Plate motion: Am. Jour. Science, v. 272, p. 603–628.

———, 1976, Plate tectonics and the Laramide orogeny: New Mex. Geol. Soc. Pub. 6, p. 5–10.

———, 1978*a*, Mesozoic cordilleran plate tectonics: Geol. Soc. America Mem. 152, p. 33–50.

———, 1978*b*, The plate tectonic setting of southeastern Arizona: New Mex. Geol. Soc., Ariz. Geol. Soc. Guidebook, 29th Field Conf., p. 285–290.

Coney, P. J., and Reynolds, S. J., 1977, Cordilleran Benioff Zones: Nature, v. 270, p. 403–406.

Cooper, J. R., 1960, Some geologic features of the Pima mining district, Pima County, Arizona: U.S. Geol. Survey Bull. 1112-C, 103 p.

———, 1971, Mesozoic stratigraphy of the Sierrita Mountains, Pima County, Arizona: U.S. Geol. Survey Prof. Paper 658-D, 42 p.

Cooper, J. R., and Silver, L. T., 1964, Geology and ore deposits of the Dragoon Quadrangle, Cochise County, Arizona: U.S. Geol. Survey Prof. Paper 416, 196 p.

Cornwall, H. R., 1982, Petrology and chemistry of igneous rocks, Ray porphyry copper district, Pinal County, Arizona, *in* Titley, S. R., ed., Advances in Geology of the Porphyry Copper Deposits, Southwestern North America: Tucson, Univ. Ariz. Press, Chap. 11.

Courtright, J. H., 1958, Progress report on investigation of some Cretaceous-Tertiary formations in southeastern Arizona: Ariz. Geol. Soc. Digest I, Tucson, p. 7–9.

Creasey, S. C., 1966, Hydrothermal alteration, *in* Titley, S. R., and Hicks, C. L., eds., Geology of the Porphyry Copper Deposits, Southwestern North America: Tucson, Univ. Ariz. Press, p. 51–74.

———, 1977, Intrusives associated with porphyry copper deposits: Geol. Soc. Malaysia Bull. 9, p. 51–66.

Creasey, S. C., and Kistler, R. W., 1962, Age of some copper-bearing porphyries and other igneous rocks in southeastern Arizona: U.S. Geol. Survey Prof. Paper 450D, Art. 120, p. 1–5.

Damon, P. E., and Mauger, R. L., 1966, Epeirogeny-orogeny viewed from the Basin and Range province: AIME Trans., v. 235, p. 99–112.

Damon, P. E., and others, 1967, Correlation and chronology of ore deposits and volcanic rocks, Ann. Prog. Rept. No. C00-689-76 to Research Div., U.S. Atomic Energy Comm.: Unpub. Rept. by Geochemical Section, Geochron. Labs., Tucson, Univ. of Ariz., 82 p.

Darton, N. H., 1925, A resume of Arizona Geology: Ariz. Bur. Mines Bull. 119, Ser. No. 3, 298 p.

Davis, G. H., 1977, Characteristics of metamorphic core complexes, southern Arizona (abs.): Geol. Soc. America Ann. Mtg., Abs. with Program, p. 944.

———, 1979, Laramide folding and faulting in southeastern Arizona: Am. Jour. Sci., v. 273, p. 543–569.

Drewes, H. L., 1971, Mesozoic stratigraphy of the Santa Rita Mountains, southeast of Tucson, Arizona: U.S. Geol. Survey Prof. Paper 658-C, 81 p.

———, 1972, Structural geology of the Santa Rita Mountains, southeast of Tucson, Arizona: U.S. Geol. Survey Prof. Paper 748, 35 p.

———, 1978, The Cordilleran orogenic belt between Nevada and Chihuahua: Geol. Soc. America Bull., v. 89, p. 641–657.

Dunn, P. G., 1978, Regional structure of the Safford district, Arizona: Ariz. Geol. Soc. Digest XI, p. 9–15.

———, 1982, Geology of the Copper Flat Porphyry Copper Deposit, Hillsboro, Sierra County, New Mexico, *in* Titley, S. R., ed., Advances in Geology of the Porphyry Copper Deposits, Southwestern North America: Tucson, Univ. Ariz. Press, Chap. 14.

Erickson, R. C., 1968, Geology and geochronology of the Dos Cabezas Mountains, Cochise County, Arizona, *in* Southern Arizona Guidebook III: Tucson, Ariz. Geol. Soc., p. 192–198.

Gastil, G., 1958, Older Precambrian rocks of the Diamond Butte Quadrangle, Gila County, Arizona: Geol. Soc. America Bull., v. 69, p. 1495–1514.

Gilluly, J., 1946, The Ajo mining district, Arizona: U.S. Geol. Survey Prof. Paper 209, 112 p.

———, 1956, General geology of central Cochise County, Arizona: U.S. Geol. Survey Prof. Paper 281, 169 p.

Gilluly, J.; Cooper, J. R.; and Williams, J. S., 1954, Late Paleozoic stratigraphy of central Cochise County, Arizona: U.S. Geol. Survey Prof. Paper 266, 49 p.

Graybeal, F. T., 1982, Geology of the El Tiro area, Silver Bell mining district, Pima County, Arizona, *in* Titley, S. R., ed., Advances in Geology of the Porphyry Copper Deposits, Southwestern North America: Tucson, Univ. Ariz. Press, Chap. 24.

Gustafson, L. B., and Titley, S. R., 1978, Porphyry copper deposits of the southwestern Pacific islands and Australia, Preface: Econ. Geol., v. 73, p. 597–599.

Hayes, P. T., 1970*a*, Mesozoic stratigraphy of the Mule and Huachuca Mountains, Arizona: U.S. Geol. Survey Prof. Paper 658-A, 28 p.

———, 1970*b*, Cretaceous paleogeography of southeastern Arizona and adjacent areas: U.S. Geol. Survey Prof. Paper 658-B, 42 p.

———, 1975, Cambrian and Ordovician rocks of southern Arizona and New Mexico and westernmost Texas: U.S. Geol. Survey Prof. Paper 873, 98 p.

Hayes, P. T., and Drewes, H., 1978, Mesozoic depositional history of southeastern Arizona, *in* Land of Cochise, Southeastern Arizona: New Mex. Geol. Soc., Ariz. Geol. Soc. Guidebook, 29th Field Conf., p. 201–207.

Hedlund, D. C., 1974, Age and structural setting of base-metal mineralization in the Hillsboro-San Lorenzo area, southwestern New Mexico (abs.), *in* Ghost Ranch: New Mexico Geol. Soc. Guidebook 25, p. 378–379.

Heidrick, T. L., and Titley, S. R., 1976, Structural evolution of southwestern North American Laramide porphyry copper deposits and its relationship to the history of plate interactions (abs.): Int. Geol. Congr., 25th, Sydney, Abstracts Vol. 3, p. 740.

———, 1982, Fracture and dike patterns in Laramide plutons and their structural and tectonic implications, American Southwest *in* Titley, S. R., ed., Advances in Geology of the Porphyry Copper Deposits, Southwestern North America: Tucson, Univ. Ariz. Press, Chap. 4.

Huddle, J. W., and Dobrovolny, E., 1952, Devonian and Mississippian rocks of central Arizona: U.S. Geol. Survey Prof. Paper 233-D, 112 p.

Jansen, L. J., 1978, The San Xavier fault, Pima mining district, Arizona: Ariz. Geol. Soc. Digest XI, p. 99–100.

Jerome, S. E., and Cook, D. R., 1967, Relation of some metal mining districts in the western United States to regional tectonic environments and igneous activity: Nevada Bur. Mines Bull. 69, 35 p.

Jones, R. W., 1963, Structural evolution of part of southeastern Arizona: Am. Assoc. Petroleum Geologists Mem., No. 2, p. 140–151.

———, 1966, Differential vertical uplift—a major factor in the structural evolution of southeastern Arizona: Ariz. Geol. Soc. Digest VIII, p. 97–124.

Kelly, J. L., 1977, Geology of the Twin Buttes copper deposit, Pima County, Arizona; AIME Trans., v. 262, p. 110–116.

Kessler, E. J., 1976, Rubidium-Strontium geochronology and trace element geochemistry of Precambrian rocks in the northern Hualapai Mountains, Mohave County, Arizona: Unpub. M.S. Thesis, Univ. Ariz., 73 p.

Kinnison, J. E., 1959, Chaotic breccias in the Tucson Mountains, Arizona, *in* Southern Arizona Guidebook II: Ariz. Geol. Soc., p. 49–57.

Koski, R. A., and Cook, D. S., 1982, Geology of the Christmas porphyry copper deposit, Gila County, Arizona, *in* Titley, S. R., ed., Advances in Geology of the Porphyry Copper Deposits, Southwestern North America: Tucson, Univ. Ariz. Press, Chap. 17.

Kottlowski, F. E., 1963, Paleozoic and Mesozoic strata of southwestern and south-central New Mexico: New Mexico Bur. Mines and Min. Res. Bull. 79, 100 p.

Langlois, J. D., 1978, Geology of the Cyprus Pima mine, Pima County, Arizona: Ariz. Geol. Soc. Digest XI, p. 103–113.

Lausen, C., 1930, The Pre-Cambrian greenstone complex of the Jerome Quadrangle: Jour. Geol. v. 38, p. 174–183.

Lindgren, W., 1905, The copper deposits of the Clifton-Morenci district, Arizona: U.S. Geol. Survey Prof. Paper 43, 375 p.

Lipman, P. W.; Prostka, H. J.; and Christiansen, R. L., 1972, Cenozoic volcanism and plate-tectonic evolution of the Western United States, I. Early and Middle Cenozoic: Phil. Trans. Roy. Soc. Lond., v. A271, p. 217–248.

Lipman, P. W., Doe, B.; Hedge, C. E.; and Steven, T. A., 1978, Petrologic evolution of the San Juan volcanic field, southwestern Colorado—Pb and Sr isotope evidence: Geol. Soc. America Bull., v. 89, p. 59–82.

Livingston, D. E., 1973, A plate tectonic hypothesis for the genesis of porphyry copper deposits of the southern Basin and Range province: Earth Planet. Sci. Letters, v. 20, p. 171–179.

Livingston, D. E., and Damon, P. E., 1968, The ages of stratified Precambrian rock sequences in central Arizona and northern Sonora: Can. Jour. Earth Sci., v. 5, p. 763–772.

Livingston, D. E.; Mauger, R. L.; and Damon, P. E., 1968, Geochronology of the emplacement, enrichment, and preservation of Arizona porphyry copper deposits: Econ. Geol., v. 63, p. 30–36.

Lochman-Balk, Christina, 1972, Cambrian System, *in* Geologic Atlas of the Rocky Mountain Region: Denver, Colo., Rocky Mtn. Assoc. of Geol., p. 60–75.

Lowell, J. D., 1968, Geology of the Kalamazoo orebody, San Manuel district, Arizona: Econ. Geol., v. 63, p. 645–654.

———, 1974, Regional characteristics of porphyry copper deposits of the southwest: Econ. Geol., v. 69, p. 601–617.

Marvin, R. F.; Stern, T. W.; Creasey, S. C.; and Mehnert, H. H., 1973, Radiometric ages of igneous rocks from Pima, Santa Cruz, and Cochise Counties, southeastern Arizona: U.S. Geol. Survey Bull. 1379, 27 p.

Mayo, E. B., 1958, Lineament tectonics and some ore districts of the southwest: Min. Eng., Nov., p. 1169–1175.

McKee, E. D., 1951, Sedimentary basins of Arizona and adjoining areas: Geol. Soc. America Bull., v. 62, p. 481–506.

Metz, R. A.; Phillips, C. H.; and Caviness, C. R., 1968, Recent developments in the geology of the Ray area, *in* Southern Arizona Guidebook III: Ariz. Geol. Soc., p. 137–146.

Moolick, R. T., and Durek, J. J., 1966, The Morenci district, *in* Titley, S. R., and Hicks, C. L., eds., Geology of the Prophyry Copper Deposits, Southwestern North America: Tucson, Univ. Ariz. Press, p. 221–231.

Moore, W. J., 1973, Igneous rocks in the Bingham mining district, Utah: U.S. Geol. Survey Prof. Paper 629B, 42 p.

Norton, D., 1982, Fluid and heat transport phenomena typical of copper-bearing pluton environments, southeastern Arizona, *in* Titley, S. R., ed., Advances in Geology of the Porphyry Copper Deposits, Southwestern North America: Tucson, Univ. Ariz. Press, Chap. 3.

Paige, Sidney. 1916, Silver City folio: U.S. Geol. Survey, Geol. Atlas (no. 199).

Peirce, H. W., 1976, Elements of Paleozoic tectonics in Arizona: Ariz. Geol. Soc. Digest X, p. 37–58.

Peirce, H. W., and Wilt, J. C., 1970, Oil, natural gas, and helium, *in* Peirce, H. W., Keith, S. B., and Wilt, J. C., eds., Coal, oil, natural gas, helium, and uranium in Arizona: Ariz. Bur. Mines Bull. 182, p. 43–101.

Peterson, N. P., 1962, Geology and ore deposits of the Globe-Miami district, Arizona: U.S. Geol. Survey Prof. Paper 342, 151 p.

Ransome, F. L., 1903, Geology of the Globe copper district, Arizona: U.S. Geol. Survey Prof. Paper 12, 168 p.

———, 1904, The geology and ore deposits of the Bisbee quadrangle, Arizona: U.S. Geol. Survey Paper 21, 168 p.

Rehrig, W. A., and Heidrick, T. L., 1972, Regional fracturing in Laramide stocks of Arizona and its relationship to porphyry copper mineralization: Econ. Geol., v. 67, p. 198–213.

———, 1976, Regional stress during the Laramide and Late Tertiary intrusive periods, Basin and Range Province, Arizona: Ariz. Geol. Soc. Digest X, p. 205–228.

Richard, K., and Courtright, J. H., 1966, Structure and mineralization at Silver Bell, Arizona, *in* Titley, S. R., and Hicks, C. L., eds., Geology of the Porphyry Copper Deposits, Southwestern North America: Tucson, Univ. Ariz. Press, p. 157–163.

Robinson, R. F., and Cook, A., 1966, The Safford copper deposit, Lone Star mining district, Graham County, Arizona, *in* Titley, S. R., and Hicks, C. L., eds., Geology of the Porphyry Copper Deposits, Southwestern North America: Tucson, Univ. Ariz. Press, p. 251–266.

Ross, C. A., 1973, Pennsylvanian and Early Permian depositional history, southeastern Arizona: Am. Assoc. Petroleum Geologists Bull., v. 57, p. 887–912.

———, 1978, Pennsylvanian and Early Permian depositional framework, southeastern Arizona, *in* Land of Cochise, Southeastern Arizona: New Mex. Geol. Soc., Ariz. Geol. Soc. Guidebook, 29th Field Conf., p. 193–200.

Sabins, F. F., Jr., 1957, Geology of the Cochise Head and western part of the Vanar quadrangles, Arizona: Geol. Soc. America Bull., v. 68, p. 1315–1342.

Saegart, W. E.; Sell, J. D.; and Kilpatrick, B. E., 1974, Geology and mineralization of La Caridad porphyry copper deposit, Sonora, Mexico: Econ. Geol., v. 69, p. 1060–1077.

Sauck, W. A., and Sumner, J. S., 1970, Residual aeromagnetic map of Arizona: Univ. Ariz., Dept. of Geosciences, 1:1,000,000.

Scarborough, R. B., and Peirce, H. W., 1978, Late Cenozoic basins of Arizona, *in* Land of Cochise, Southeastern Arizona, New Mex. Geol. Soc., Ariz. Geol. Soc. Guidebook, 29th Field Conf., p. 209–214.

Schafroth, D. W., 1968, Stratigraphy of some Cretaceous formations of southeastern Arizona, *in* Southern Arizona Guidebook III: Ariz. Geol. Soc., p. 59–67.

Schmitt, H. A., 1933, Summary of the geological and metallogenic history of Arizona and New Mexico, *in* Ore Deposits of the Western States: New York, AIME p. 316–326.

———, 1966, The porphyry copper deposits in their regional setting, *in* Titley, S. R., and Hicks, C. L., eds., Geology of the Porphyry Copper Deposits, southwestern North America: Tucson, Univ. Ariz. Press, p. 17–33.

Schumacher, D., 1978, Devonian stratigraphy and correlations in southeastern Arizona, *in* Land of Cochise, Southeastern Arizona: New Mex. Geol. Soc., Ariz. Geol. Soc. Guidebook, 29th Field Conf., p. 175–181.

Shoemaker, E. M.; Squires, R. L.; and Abrams, M. J., 1974, The Bright Angel and Mesa Butte fault systems of northern Arizona, *in* Geology of Northern Arizona, Part I—Regional Studies: Geol. Soc. Am. Rky. Mtn. Sect. Mtg., Flagstaff, p. 355–391

———, 1978, Bright Angel and Mesa Butte fault systems of northern Arizona: Geol. Soc. America Mem. 152, p. 341–368.

Shride, A. F., 1967, Younger Precambrian geology in southern Arizona: U.S. Geol. Survey Prof. Paper 566, 89 p.

Sillitoe, R. H., 1973, The tops and bottoms of porphyry copper deposits: Econ. Geol., v. 68, p. 799–815.

Silver, L. T., 1964, Mazatzal orogeny and tectonic episodicity (abs.): Geol. Soc. Am. Ann. Mtg., Abs. With Programs, p. 185.

———, 1978, Precambrian formations and Precambrian history in Cochise County, southeastern Arizona, *in* Land of Cochise, Southeastern Arizona: New Mex. Geol. Soc., Ariz. Geol. Soc. Guidebook, 29th Field Conf., p. 157–163.

Silver, L. T., and Deutsch, S., 1963, Uranium-lead isotopic variations in zircons, a case study: Jour. Geol., v. 71, p. 721–758.

Silver, L. T.; Anderson, C. A.; Crittenden, M.; and Robertson, J. M., 1977, Chronostratigraphic elements of the Precambrian rocks of the southwestern and far western United States (abs.): Geol. Soc. Am. Ann. Mtg., Seattle, 1977, Abs. With Program, p. 1176.

Simons, F. S., 1972, Mesozoic stratigraphy of the Patagonia Mountains and adjoining areas, Santa Cruz County, Arizona: U.S. Geol. Survey Prof. Paper 658-E, 23 p.

Stoyanow, A. A., 1936, Correlation of Arizona Paleozoic formations: Geol. Soc. America Bull., v. 47, p. 459–540.

Sutherland Brown, A., 1976, ed., Porphyry deposits of the Canadian Cordillera: CIM Spec. Vol. 15, 510 p.

Thomas, B. E., 1949, Ore deposits of the Wallapai district, Arizona: Econ. Geol., v. 44, p. 663–705.

Thorpe, D. G., and Burt, D. M., 1978, Precambrian metavolcanic rocks of the Squaw Peak Area, Maricopa County, Arizona: Tucson, State of Ariz. Bur. Geol. Mineral Tech., Guidebook to the geology of central Arizona, Special Paper No. 2, p. 101–104.

Titley, S. R., 1972*a*, Pre-ore environment of southwestern North American porphyry copper deposits: Int. Geol. Cong. 24th, Montreal, Proc. Sect. 4, p. 252–260.

———, 1972*b*, Some geological criteria applicable to the search for southwestern North American porphyry copper deposits: MMIJ-AIME Joint Mtg., Tokyo, May 24–27, Preprint G I 2.

———, 1976, Evidence for a Mesozoic linear tectonic pattern in southeastern Arizona: Ariz. Geol. Soc. Digest X, p. 71–101.

Titley, S. R., and Heidrick, T. L., 1978, Intrusion and fracture styles of some mineralized porphyry systems of the southwestern Pacific and their relationship to plate interactions: Econ. Geol., v. 73, p. 891–903.

Turner, G. L., 1962, The Deming Axis, southeastern Arizona, New Mexico and Trans-Pecos, Texas, *in* New Mex. Geol. Soc. Guidebook, 13th Field Conf., p. 59–71.

Velasco, J. R., 1966, Geology of the Cananea district, *in* Titley, S. R., and Hicks, C. L., eds., Geology of the Porphyry Copper Deposits, Southwestern North American: Tucson, Univ. Ariz. Press, p. 245–249.

Wade, W. R., and Wandke, A., 1920, Geology and mining methods at Pilares mine: AIME Trans., v. 63, p. 382–407.

West, R. J., and Aiken, D. M., 1982, Geology of the Sierrita-Esperanza deposit, Pima mining district, Pima County, Arizona, *in* Titley, S. R., ed., Advances in Geology of the Porphyry Copper Deposits, Southwestern North America: Tucson, Univ. Ariz. Press, Chap. 21.

Wilson, E. D., 1939, Pre-Cambrian Mazatzal revolution in central Arizona: Geol. Soc. America Bull., v. 50, p. 1113–1164.

Zeitz, I., and Kirby, J. R., Jr., 1972, Aeromagnetic map of Colorado: U.S. Geol. Survey Map GP-836, 1:500,000.

3

Fluid and Heat Transport Phenomena Typical of Copper-Bearing Pluton Environments

SOUTHEASTERN ARIZONA

Denis L. Norton

In southeastern Arizona, copper deposits which are closely associated with fractured porphyritic plutons occur within large, sulfide-bearing systems. Anomalous concentrations of sulfide minerals occur throughout tens of cubic kilometers of rock, but they are genetically related to relatively small porphyritic intrusions, generally two kilometers or less in diameter. These deposits appear to have been formed by extensive circulation of fluids which redistributed components, reacted with rocks along their flow paths, and produced alteration mineral assemblages. The time duration and nature of this ore-forming process depends on the cooling history of the intrusives, which lasts for a few hundred thousand years. Although the complete igneous history of these environments usually includes repeated intrusion of magmas whose cooling times are on the order of several hundred thousand years, mineral alteration and concentration of ore appear to be more closely associated with smaller intrusives.

The nature of hydrothermal processes has been deduced from modern analogs of systems found in regions of active volcanism (Naboko, 1964); from very young deposits in regions of rapid erosion (Sillitoe, 1973); from restorations of complexly faulted deposits (Lowell, 1968); and from deep drill-hole information, which has provided system characteristics at depth. Modern and fossil hydrothermal systems contain the products of processes integrated over thousands of years; however, quantitative aspects of the hydrothermal processes are not well documented because of the complexities of interpreting such data.

The purpose of this chapter is to summarize the nature of the hydrothermal fluid circulation which is believed to have occurred during formation of large sulfide systems in the southeastern Arizona copper porphyry province. Numerical simulation of the transport of thermal energy and mass in these environments has been used, together with field and laboratory data, to define quantitatively the temporal and spatial variation of temperature, pressure, and fluid flux, as well as the pathlines and sourcelines of fluids in these systems.

GEOLOGIC ENVIRONMENT

In porphyry copper systems rocks containing anomalous quantities of sulfur, predominantly as pyrite, occur in regions intruded by dikes, sills, and stocks. However, sulfides are usually spatially distributed with respect to one particular pluton—or portion of a pluton—and occur in granite, schist, clastic and carbonate sedimentary, and volcanic host rocks.

An extensive geologic data base is a necessary prerequisite for analyzing the nature of hydrothermal systems. In particular, size and shape of the pluton, permeability of the pluton and host rocks, and thickness of host rocks over the pluton must be known. Since permeability of host rocks often relates closely to rock type, the distribution of various lithologic units is necessary information. Accordingly, such data have been compiled for ~ 15 sulfide systems in Arizona and New Mexico. Extensive data reported in the literature attests to the insight of field geologists and to the quality of field and laboratory studies they have conducted on hydrothermal deposits. Several of the features relevant to this study are summarized by the sections in Figure 3.1.

Plutons

Plutons most closely related to ore include closely spaced dikes near the pre-intrusive surface, as is evident at Safford (Robinson and Cook, 1966) and Red Mountain (Corn, 1975). Relatively small diameter (≤ 1 km) stocks are typical of Ray (Banks et al., 1972; Metz and Rose, 1966), Christmas (Eastlick, 1968), Helvetia (Drewes, 1971*a,* 1971*b*), Silverbell

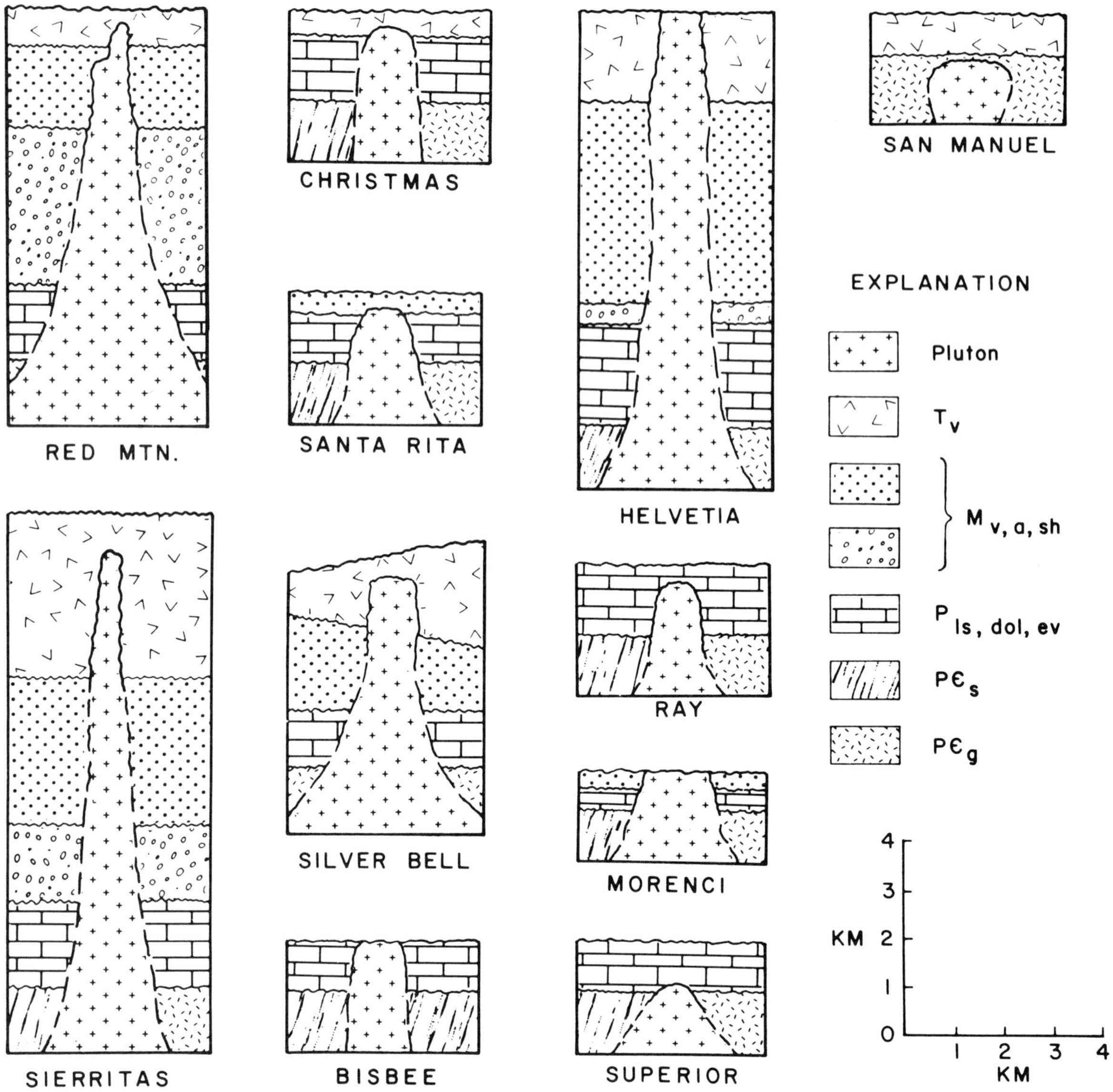

Figure 3.1. Schematic geological cross sections for several representative areas showing the geometry of plutons and their contact relationships with host rocks, as inferred from the literature and structural-mechanical considerations. Pluton compositions range from granodiorite to quartz monzonite, and host rock compositions include felsic volcanics, arkose, shale, limestone, dolomite, evaporites, schist, and granite. Key: T = Tertiary, M = Mesozoic, P = Paleozoic, v = volcanics, a = arkose, sh = shale, ls = limestone, dol = dolomite, ev = evaporite, s = schist, g = granite.

(Richard and Courtright, 1966; Clarke, 1965), and Bisbee (Bryant and Metz, 1966; Ransome, 1904*a,* 1904*b*). These stocks are interpreted to represent the intermediate depths of the systems. Larger diameter ($1 \geq 2$ km) stocks can be seen at Morenci (Moolick and Durek, 1966), San Manuel (Creasey, 1965, 1967), Santa Rita (Jones et al., 1967), and Superior (Peterson, 1969). These stocks suggest that deeper portions of the intrusive mass are exposed. The total depth extent of plutons can be inferred from the geology of host rocks, continuous vertical exposures of systems (Sillitoe, 1973; Naboko, 1964; Etminan, 1977; Förster et al., 1972), mechanical theory of magma emplacement (Weertman, 1971*a*, 1971*b*), and mining depths. Virtually all the stocks are systematically fractured (Rehrig and Heidrick, 1972; Heidrick and Titley, 1982), but the abundance of continuous fractures varies between deposits. The total mass and type of alteration and mineralization are functions of fracture abundance and continuity (Villas and Norton, 1977) and of fracture age (Titley et al., 1978; Haynes and Titley, 1980).

Portions of the sulfide systems anomalous in copper have vertical extents on the order of 3 to 5 km (Sillitoe, 1973), and, although sulfides were probably deposited near the original surface, the plutons apparently intruded at depths as shallow as 1 to 3 km. Although the distribution of igneous rocks at depths below the economically viable portion of the sulfide system is poorly documented, a total depth extent of 10 km appears to be consistent with the field data available. The depth extent of both the copper resource portion of the system and continuous fractures, spaced less than a meter or two apart, would be included in this interval.

Data relating to pluton geometry, reported in the literature, form the basis for construction of a two-dimensional cross-section of a "typical" pluton (Fig. 3.2), in which the pluton was constricted at depth to be consistent with shapes of viscous materials penetrating into elastic plates (Weertman, 1971*b*). Aeromagnetic and geologic data indicate that batholithic igneous masses occur beneath many shallow porphyritic plutons, but textural evidence is lacking which would suggest continued magma circulation between the shallow porphyritic plutons and the deeper batholithic size masses. Because the transition from stocks to batholiths, at ~ 10 km, also coincides with a transition from relatively large permeabilities to permeabilities $< 10^{-14}$ cm^2, this region is a convenient lower physical boundary for the system. Also, thermal energy derived from the batholith portion of the igneous system can be represented by appropriate heat fluxes along this boundary. At intermediate depths (6 to 9 km) the pluton has a bulbous shape, but at shallow depths (3 to 5 km) it is a relatively narrow (0.5 km wide) apophysis. Numerous dikes and sills are generally present but usually have relatively small widths and thicknesses, and at the map scale used in Figure 3.2 they do not appear.

Host Rocks

Host rocks into which the plutons intruded are similar over most of the region, as can be seen in figure 3.1. Metamorphic, igneous, and volcanic rocks, and both clastic and carbonate sedimentary rocks that range in age from Precambrian through Mesozoic occur in contact with plutons or in close proximity to them. The principal difference between types of host rocks is that portions of the sedimentary sections are not present over the entire region (Titley, 1972). Typically, the intrusives occur along or adjacent to the contact between metamorphic and granitic rocks of Precambrian age. These old granitic masses generally contain continuous fractures spaced several to tens of meters apart and, therefore, were apparently relatively impervious to hydrothermal fluids (Norton and Knapp, 1977).

Either Paleozoic or Mesozoic sedimentary rocks are present, except at San Manuel, and they vary in thickness over the Cretaceous foreland and the Paleozoic basin margin (Titley, 1972). A few examples of systems occurring in volcanic host rocks are present, e.g., Christmas, Safford, Red Mountain, Silverbell, and the Sierrita Mountains. However, where the shallow portions of porphyry intrusive systems are exposed, several kilometers of volcanic rocks which formed during the intrusion of stocks analogous to the ones considered herein are present (Förster et al., 1972; Lipman and Steven, 1970; Bazin and Hübner, 1969; Crittenden et al., 1973).

The two-dimensional cross-section that summarizes many of the relevant features of these systems (see Fig. 3.2) was constructed on the basis of the above data. These geologic conditions, together with fluid properties, initial temperatures, permeabilities, and volumetric heat sources, form the basis for simulating the nature of hydrothermal systems in these environments. This summary does not necessarily represent all features or the correct, detailed features of any one particular system, but it is sufficient for a first order approximation.

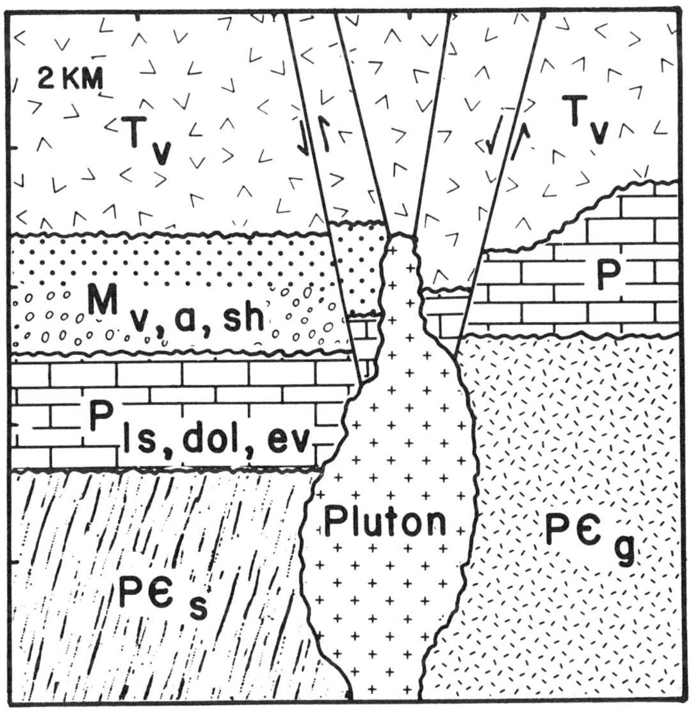

Figure 3.2. This generalized geological cross section 10 km by 10 km of a porphyry copper pluton and host rocks represents a first approximation to the characteristics of porphyry copper systems. Distribution of rock types and structure are based on those in Figure 3.1; key also as shown in Figure 3.1.

TRANSPORT PROPERTIES

Properties of rocks and fluids in active hydrothermal systems affect the style of energy and mass transport. These properties are generally well known and are represented by equations of state. However, properties such as permeability must be estimated.

Fluids

Fluids in this environment include groundwaters that were present in the host rocks prior to intrusion and fluids which have exsolved from crystallizing magma. Those which occur in the flow porosity of the rocks amount to a small fraction of the total fluid in the pluton and in the host rocks (Norton and Knapp, 1977). Although fluids from both these environments are often saline and have ionic strengths which range up to 4 molal (Beane, 1982), the system considered here will use the transport properties for phases in the H_2O-system (Helgeson and Kirkham, 1974).

Temperatures

Temperatures of host rocks are slightly higher than normal, probably as a result of earlier igneous intrusives, which are evident in most sulfide systems, or because the host rocks themselves are volcanic rocks that formed contemporaneously with the intrusives and have not cooled to ambient conditions. In either situation a 50 percent perturbation in the local geothermal gradient is likely; therefore, a 30°C km^{-1}

gradient seems reasonable (Bodnar and Beane, 1977). Initial temperatures of 800°C in the intrusive body are consistent with a quartz monzonite magma containing 4 weight percent H_2O at 1 kb pressure; heat generated by the crystallization of this body would be ~ 10 cal/gr (Burnham and Davis, 1971, 1974; Kesler and Heath, 1968). The completely liquid magma is presumed to have been emplaced rapidly with respect to its cooling time. Properties of magmas which form the parent stocks of sulfide systems are clearly more complex than is inferred by these simple parameters; these properties are, however, reasonable averages.

Permeabilities

Permeabilities of igneous rocks and their surroundings are known only to within orders of magnitude of their true values, but relative values have been estimated to perhaps an order of magnitude (Villas and Norton, 1977; Norton and Knapp, 1977; Norton and Knight, 1977; Norton and Taylor, 1979; Brace, 1977; and Brace et al., 1968). Circulation of large quantities of fluid through hydrothermal ore deposits is evident from the extensive exchange of stable light isotopes between meteoric waters and rocks (Taylor, 1974) and from gains and losses of ore-forming components caused by irreversible mass transfer between aqueous fluids and rocks (Helgeson, 1970). These data indicate that relatively large, $> 10^{-14}$ cm^2, permeabilities existed during the alteration process (Norton, 1978) and suggest that the distribution of permeabilities depicted in Figure 3.3 is reasonable. Boundary conditions are set on the basis of geological data which suggest that the sides and top of the system are open to fluid flow, but at 10 km depth permeabilities become very small, and fluid fluxes are insignificant. Thermal energy is conducted across all boundaries. An anomalous heat flux is provided for through the pluton's base in order to simulate contribution of heat from sub-system sources. Discretization interval is ~ 0.5 km, and domain includes 400 discrete points.

Principal flow channels are considered to be the continuous fractures which are ubiquitous in plutons (Fig. 3.4). The significance of fractures can also be seen in the distribution of alteration and sulfide minerals along veins. Fractures, joints, and bedding planes in the host rocks, augmented by fractures produced during emplacement of the magma and subsequent heating of pore fluids in host rocks, provide flow channels for transport of thermal energy away from the cooling magma body. Solidification of the magma and thermal contraction of igneous rocks, as well as increase in pore fluid pressure within the melt + crystals + fluid portion, can contribute to the formation of systematic fracture sets (Burnham and Davis, 1971; Villas and Norton, 1977; Knapp and Norton, 1981). Values of fracture permeability for large volumes of host rocks can be estimated on the basis of values measured on analogous rock types (Norton and Knapp, 1977; Brace, 1977) or can be estimated from fracture frequency, aperture data, and the distribution of fractures with respect to contacts between plutons and host rocks (Villas and Norton, 1977; Snow, 1965, 1970; Bianchi and Snow, 1969).

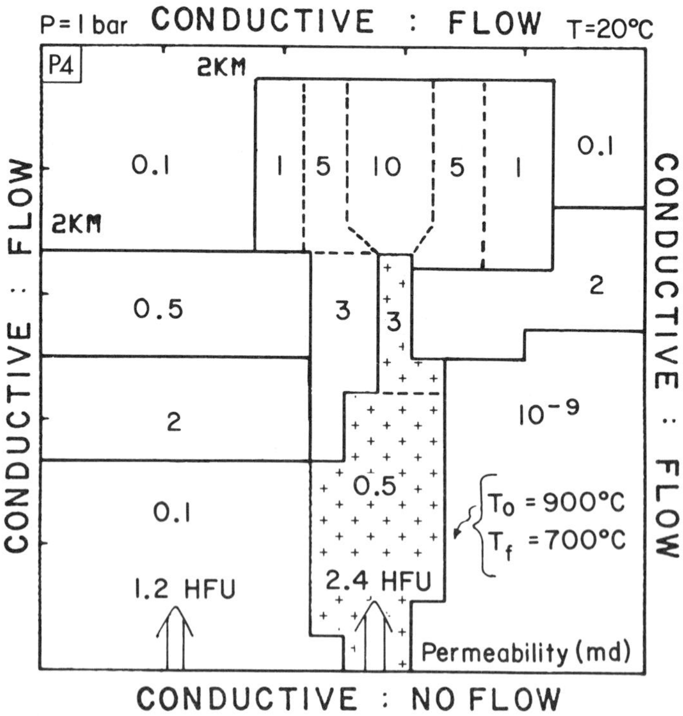

Figure 3.3. Numerical approximation of geological conditions in Figure 3.2 for magma at $T_{initial}$ = 900°C instantaneously emplaced into host rocks. The numbers represent permeabilities in millidarcys (md) for the rock units and fracture zones depicted in figure 3.2. Key: T_o = initial temperature, T_f = final temperature, *HFU* = heat flow units.

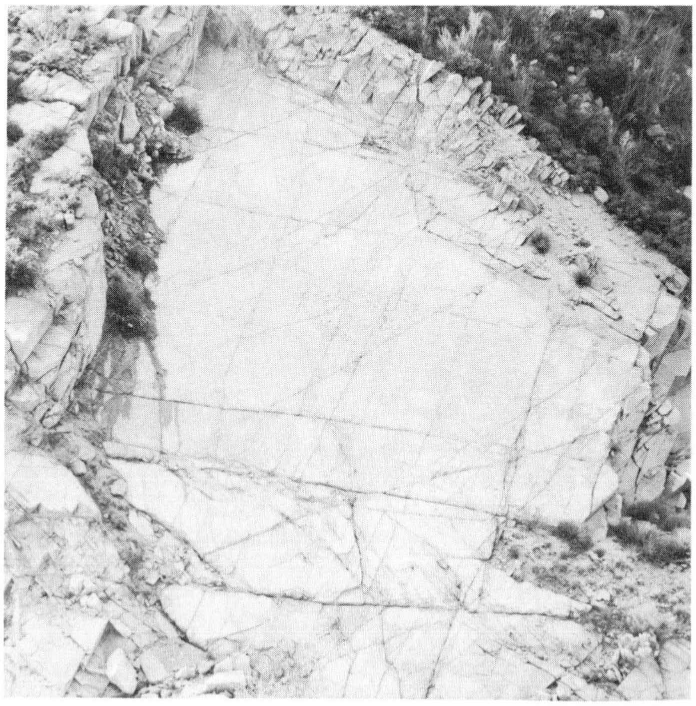

Figure 3.4. Continuous fractures in the Schultze granodiorite spaced about 2 m apart. This type of fracture constitutes the main flow channels for hydrothermal fluid circulation. In ore deposits the spacing of these fractures is usually less, e.g., ≤ 1 cm at Bingham. Discontinuous fractures interconnect the flow channels with interior regions of the matrix blocks, thereby facilitating the development of alteration and sulfide phases by diffusional transport of components away from flow channels (Norton and Knapp, 1977).

Fracture formation in plutons is hypothesized to occur in portions of the magma where temperature decreases to ~ 700°C, or about 100°C below the solidus, 800°C for the magma. Fracturing of rocks in response to the differential changes in pore fluid pressure is the primary cause of rock failure in the host rocks when temperature increases. Differential increases in fluid volume, rock, and magma are the primary causes of rock failure in the pluton when volume and fluid mass increase. At the "fracture" temperature, the region around the discrete point, where $T \leq 700$°C, assumes the original permeability value.

Because permeability is the most significant but poorest-known parameter, several hydrothermal systems differing only in permeability distributions have been studied in order to examine the effect of this property on the systems. The common occurrence of high-angle normal faults in rocks overlying plutons is caused by a distribution of permeabilities across a zone where values decrease from 10 md (millidarcies) directly above the pluton to 0.1 md at background values. Permeability of the rock unit analogous to schist (see Figs. 3.1 and 3.2) was set at 0.1 md (see Fig. 3.3).

HYDROTHERMAL PROCESSES

Magmas intruded into permeable, water-bearing rocks inevitably cause large quantities of groundwater to circulate if the intrinsic host rock permeability is greater than about 10^{-14} cm^2 (10^{-3} md). Fluid circulation results from conductive thermal energy transfer from the magma to the adjacent host rocks; fluids in the rocks become heated, their density decreases relative to those laterally away from the contact, and, as a result, the low-density fluids flow upward along the contact. Extensive fluid circulation occurs only in the host rocks until the magma has cooled and solidified; then fluids circulate into the pluton until it has cooled further to ambient conditions. Igneous rocks appear to fracture close to their respective solidus temperatures; consequently, fluids may circulate through crystalline igneous rocks at high temperatures (Norton and Knight, 1977). However, the differing extents of fracture formation noted in plutons suggest a wide range of *in-situ* permeabilities.

Fluids produced during the crystallization of the melt contribute to large pore-fluid pressures within the unfractured portion of the pluton (Burnham and Davis, 1971). These pore-fluid pressures ultimately cause fracture failure of the solidified pluton, and the abnormal pressures diffuse away from the point of fracture. Pore fluids released from the magma in this manner begin to circulate in accord with their density relative to that of fluids in the adjacent rocks. The crystallization process produces relatively small amounts of fluid, and, although the fluid flux from these regions may initially be very large, it decreases rapidly with time and distance from the source.

Convective and conductive heat transfer processes are closely linked because the driving force for fluid flow is caused by perturbations in fluid density, and the transport of thermal energy away from the anomaly decreases the magnitude of this perturbation. Temperature and pressure variations through the system affect, in turn, fluid viscosity, density, and heat content, and changes in these transport parameters cause fluid flux and conductive heat flux to change. Values of transport properties in the supercritical region of the water system change considerably with small fluctuations in temperature, particularly in the temperature interval 250–450°C (Norton and Knight, 1977; and Norton, 1977).

Mass and energy transport, together with variation in transport properties of fluids and rocks, is conveniently summarized by partial differential equations, which form statements on the conservation of energy, mass, and momentum for the system. The conservation of thermal energy equation, written in terms of temperature, T, and fluid heat content, H,

$$\rho_m c_m \frac{\partial T}{\partial t} + \overline{\nabla} \cdot K_m \overline{\nabla T} + \bar{u} \cdot \overline{\nabla H} + A = 0 \qquad (1)$$

(change) + (conductive) + (convective) + (source) = 0,

states that the conductive, convective, and source, A, rates are equal to the overall rate of change in energy in the system. The conductance rate is derived from the heat transfer flux, caused by thermal gradients, $\overline{\nabla T}$, in a medium with thermal conductivity, K_m. These thermal energy fluxes are, in turn, converted to volumetric rates by the divergence operator, $\overline{\nabla}\cdot$. Convective rate is derived from the vector product of the fluid mass flux, $\bar{u}$, and the gradient, ∇, in enthalpy, H, of the fluid. These terms, plus the volumetric source of energy—e.g., endothermic or exothermic heats of reaction—equal the overall rate of change in energy, $\rho_m c_m T$, of the system, where ρ_m and c_m are the volume averaged density and heat capacity, respectively, of the rock-fluid system.

Conservation of momentum and mass are derived from Darcy's Law for fluid flux:

$$\bar{u} = -\frac{k}{\nu} (\overline{\nabla P} - \rho g), \qquad (2)$$

where the permeability, k, and fluid viscosity, ν, are intrinsic properties of the rock and fluid, respectively. $\overline{\nabla P}$ is pressure gradient, ρ is fluid density, and $\bar{g}$ is gravitational acceleration. For convenience, the streamfunction, Ψ, is introduced to represent the circulation tendency of fluid:

$$u_x = \frac{\partial \Psi}{\partial y}\,;\; u_y = -\frac{\partial \Psi}{\partial x}\,, \qquad (3)$$

where the fluid fluxes, u_x and u_y, are defined by the respective gradients in the streamfunction normal to the flow direction. A steady state equation in terms of the streamfunction can then be derived:

$$\nabla \frac{\nu}{k} \overline{\nabla \Psi} = R_a \nabla_x \rho\,, \qquad (4)$$

where the magnitude and variation in fluid properties, viscosity, ν, and density, ρ, and rock permeability, k, together with the Rayleigh number, R_a, represent the circulation tendency of the fluid as caused by the fluid density perturbations in the horizontal plane, $\nabla_x \rho$.

Numerical approximation of equations 1–4 permits computations of the variation of temperature, T, streamfunction, Ψ, and—through equations 2 and 3—the mass flux, u, of fluid as a function of space and time for systems in which permeability, thermal conductivity, fluid density, viscosity, heat content, and geometry of the thermal source also vary in space and time. Calculations are made at discrete points throughout the system of interest so that the results represent averages of a finite region around each point, i.e., discrete points represent 0.5 by 0.5 km regions in the systems reported here. The numerical approximations represent the partial differential equations within < 10 percent and represent their natural analogs to within the reliability of the geological observations used to define the initial conditions.

COOLING HISTORY OF PLUTONS

The style of fluid circulation and temperature variations expected in natural systems is demonstrated by numerical simulation of the cooling history of the system, summarized in Figure 3.3 and henceforth referred to as P4. The coupling between fluid flow and temperature variations suggested by the transport equations can be seen in Figure 3.5, which illustrates a time sequence of calculations showing temperature and streamfunction values. Fluid fluxes are proportional to the gradient in the streamfunction, as defined by equation 3; therefore, fluid flux is greater where streamlines are more closely spaced. Dimensionless streamfunction, Ψ, used to depict the fluid circulation, may be converted to dimensioned values, $\hat{\Psi}$, by $\hat{\Psi} = 8.6 \times 10^{-6}\ \Psi$.

Plutons Related to Porphyry Copper Deposits

Apophyses and margins of plutons related to porphyry coppers are expected to cool to subsolidus temperatures, < 800 °C, during the initial 10^4 years, while host rock temperatures increase to $\geq$ 200 °C at distances of 0.5 to 1 km from the pluton's sides and 2 km above the pluton's top (Fig. 3.5*a*). During the initial cooling period 70 percent of the magma

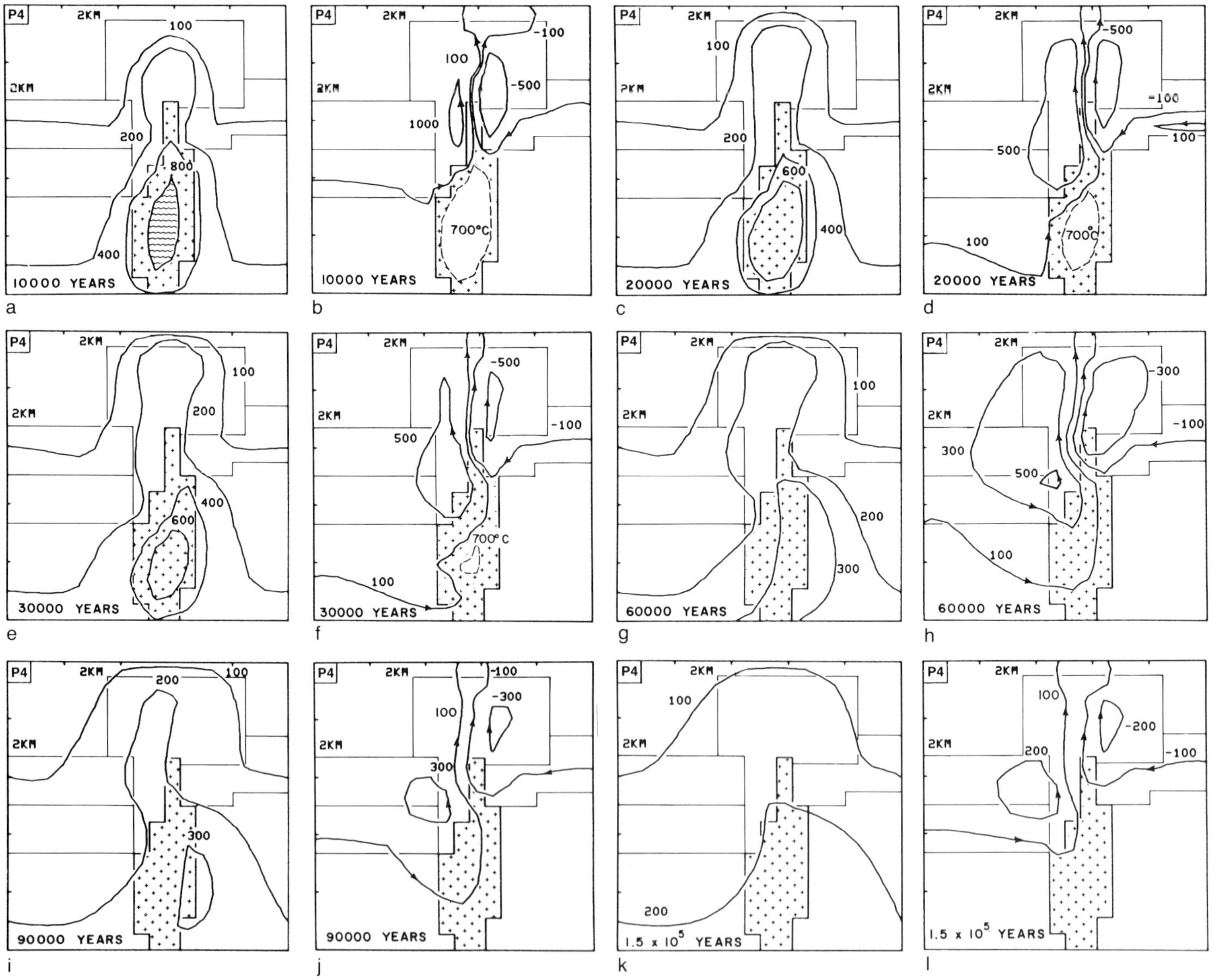

Figure 3.5. Two-dimensional numerical cross sections of porphyry copper system P4, depicting temperature in °C on the left (*a, c, e, g, i, k*) and steady state dimensionless streamfunction on the right, (*b, d, f, h, j, l*) at 10^4, 2×10^4, 3×10^4, 6×10^4, 9×10^4, and 1.5×10^5 years. Unfractured portion of pluton is shown by 700°C isotherm (*dashed line*). The region between 700°C and 800°C isotherm is analogous to crystalline but unfractured igneous rock in natural systems. Fluid formed by crystallization process is released at surface of 700°C isotherm.

has crystallized, at an average rate of 0.06 gr/sec. Presuming that the initial magma contained .04 wt percent volatile fluids and that they would all be released through the solidified-fractured zone around the magma, the average flux normal to this interface would be 1×10^{-8} gr cm^{-2} sec^{-1}, about 10 percent of the groundwater flux at the corresponding location. Fluids in the host rocks adjoining the pluton flow inward toward it. The largest fluid fluxes ($u_y = 10^{-6}$ gr cm^{-2} sec^{-1}) occur within relatively permeable Paleozoic rocks, where cool groundwaters flow toward the pluton from the host rocks. These groundwaters keep the 200 °C isotherm closer to the pluton-host rock contact near the apophyses base than at other contacts; those in the fractured margins of the pluton, $T \leq 700$ °C, flow upward toward the overlying fractured volcanics, where fluids either flow toward the surface or tend to recirculate (Fig. 3.5*b*). Overall fluid circulation is centered around the pluton's apophyses, and, as indicated by the large horizontal gradients in the streamfunction, the largest fluid fluxes in the entire system, 2×10^{-6} gr cm^{-2} sec^{-1}, occur near the top of the pluton in the host rocks.

The magma is completely crystallized after 2×10^4 years, but since the temperature of 2.5 km^3 of the intrusive is still greater than the fracture temperature, inflowing fluids are diverted around the impermeable zone (Fig. 3.5*c,d*). Temperatures in the fracture zone near the surface are > 200 °C, even within the fluid inflow zone on the left of the pluton. However, flow inward from the Paleozoic rocks on the right side of the pluton keeps the 200 °C isotherm against the pluton. Fluid circulation remains centered in the same position as at 10^4 years, but fluids within the schist are now flowing toward the pluton, as indicated by the downward shift of the $\Psi = 100$ streamline into the schist. Fluid fluxes have decreased to a maximum of 1.5×10^{-6} gr cm^{-2} sec^{-1}, as is evident from the decrease in magnitude and gradient of the streamfunction.

Temperatures within the upper portions of the pluton have decreased to ~ 300 °C after 3×10^4 years, but 0.75 km^3 of the pluton remains unfractured (Fig. 3.5*e, f*). Host rocks have now been heated to ≥ 200 °C over most of the zone where the permeability is ≥ 3 md, except for the inflow region coincident with the Paleozoic rocks on the right side. Fluid circulation in the fractured host rocks on the left side of the pluton has shifted downward, whereas circulation on the pluton's right side remains about in the same position, largely because of the low permeability of the granite, but it decreases in magnitude. Diversion of fluids around the last remaining portion of unfractured pluton can be seen in the $\Psi = 100$ streamline. Maximum fluid flux is at the same position as at previous times but has decreased to 1.1×10^{-6} gr cm^{-2} sec^{-1}.

During the next 3×10^4 years of cooling, isotherms within the host rocks do not shift appreciably, except that temperature increases in portions of the Mesozoic and Paleozoic sections on the left side of the pluton result in an asymmetric isotherm pattern (Fig. 3.5*g*). This asymmetry is further accentuated by temperatures in deeper portions of the pluton, where inflow of groundwaters from the schist has cooled its left side considerably faster than conductive heat transfer has cooled its right side. A substantial decrease in fluid circulation can be seen at 6×10^4 years (Fig. 3.5*h*), and within the pluton the circulation has shifted toward the granite contact where $u_x = 5 \times 10^{-7}$ gr cm^{-2} sec^{-1}. Within the host rocks on the left side of the pluton apophyses, fluid flux has decreased, $u_x = 8 \times 10^{-7}$ gr cm^{-2} sec^{-1}. The circulation center has shifted toward the Mesozoic-Paleozoic contact on the left side of the pluton, but it remains virtually in the same position on the right side. Circulation of fluids in the schist decreases, as indicated by the $\Psi = 100$ streamline which has shifted upward.

During the next 3×10^4 years temperatures decrease to less than 300 °C throughout the system; the 200 °C isotherm starts to move downward away from the surface and becomes displaced from the right to left side of the stock (Fig. 3.5*i*). Contributions of thermal energy from sources below the system have been decreased to regional values, 1.2 HFU (heat flow unit). Fluid circulation remains centered at the same locations as at 6×10^4 years, but the $\Psi = 100$ streamline continues to shift upward and out of the pluton (Fig. 3.5*j*). Again, the magnitude of circulation decreases markedly throughout the domain, and maximum fluid flux is 5×10^{-7} gr cm^{-2} sec^{-1} near the very top of the system.

The thermal anomaly is effectively dispersed by 1.5×10^5 years; temperatures have decreased to < 200 °C in the upper 5 km of the system, and the highest temperature, 260 °C, now occurs at the pluton-granite contact, ~ 8 km deep in the system (Fig. 3.5*k*). Fluid circulation has decreased appreciably in the lower portion of the pluton, as can be seen by the shift of the $\Psi = 100$ contour almost completely out of the pluton (Fig. 3.5*l*). Maximum fluid flux again occurs near the pluton's top but has decreased to 3×10^{-7} gr cm^{-2} sec^{-1}.

By 2×10^5 years elapsed time the thermal anomaly consists only of a slight (3 km) upward perturbation in the 200 °C isotherm, which is centered on the pluton-granite contact, and a broad (3 km) upward perturbation in the 100 °C isotherm. Fluid flux has decreased to a maximum of 1×10^{-7} gr cm^{-2} sec^{-1} but is generally $< 5 \times 10^{-8}$ gr cm^{-2} sec^{-1} everywhere in the system.

Relatively Impermeable Plutons

Relatively impermeable plutons, similar in size to the pluton discussed above, also occur in the Arizona province. Although these plutons are typically unmineralized and contain few continuous fractures and only minor alteration effects, the surrounding host rocks are both altered and mineralized. Host rocks in contact with both permeable and impermeable plutons are similar in composition and permeability; this similarity implies that fluids have circulated through the host rocks adjacent to the pluton contact, but not in appreciable quantities through the pluton.

In order to compare the style of fluid circulation one would expect to find around plutons of relatively low permeability, a system similar to the one previously discussed is simulated in Figure 3.6. This system is referred to as P2 in the following discussion and is similar to the one shown in Figure 3.3 (P4), except for an impermeable pluton of 10^{-6} md, lower permeability values of 0.01 md in the schist, and reversed permeabilities in the Mesozoic and Paleozoic rocks.

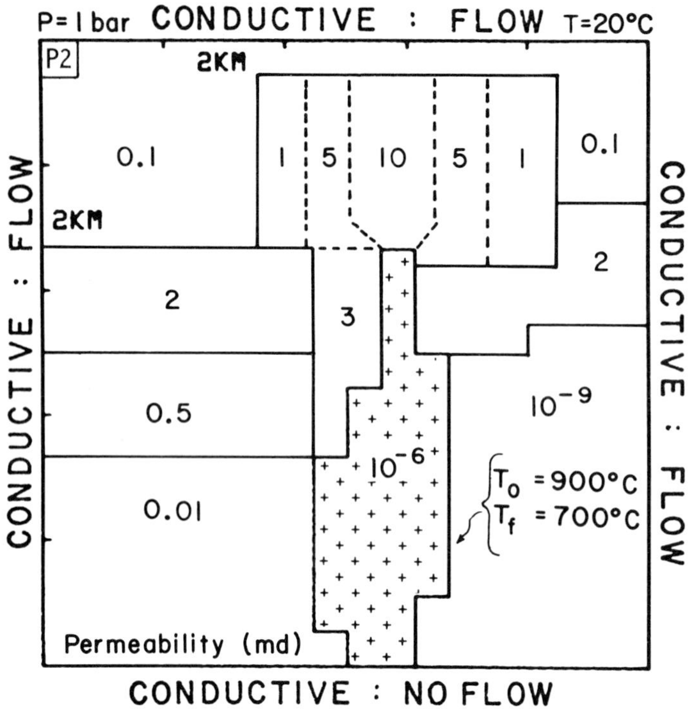

Figure 3.6. Numerical approximation of geological conditions for impermeable pluton (P2) at 10^{-6} md. Compare with system P4 (see Fig. 3.3), which is similar, except for a permeable pluton and different permeabilities in the Mesozoic and Paleozoic rocks. Key: T_o = initial temperature, T_f = fracture temperature.

Temperature decreases more slowly within the impermeable pluton than in the permeable pluton. Figure 3.7*a* shows that, after cooling for 2 X 10^4 years, approximately 1 km^3 of the pluton is still at temperatures greater than the solidus value. Host rock temperatures have increased to > 200 °C over a relatively small region, which extends into the permeable Mesozoic rocks (cf. Figs. 3.5*c* and 3.7*a*). Fluid circulation is centered in rocks along the intrusion and is comparable in style to the circulation pattern realized at 10^4 years in P4 (see Fig. 3.5*b*), although the fluid fluxes are slightly less. However, circulation does not extend significantly into the lower permeability schist, as indicated by the $\Psi = 100$ streamline (Fig. 3.7*b*).

An additional 7 X 10^5 years of cooling results in somewhat more symmetrically distributed temperature values in the pluton (Fig. 3.7*c*); these values are also greater by ~ 100 °C than those in P4 at 9 X 10^5 years (see Fig. 3.5*i*). Host rock temperatures > 200 °C extend 2 to 3 km outward from the pluton in the Mesozoic and Tertiary volcanic rocks. Fluid circulation remains centered at the same position at which it was during earlier times; also, some recirculation in the Mesozoic rocks has developed (Fig. 3.7*d*). Fluid fluxes have decreased to a maximum of 5 X 10^{-7} gr cm^{-2} sec^{-1}. This system requires 2 X 10^5 years to cool to temperature values similar to those in P4 at 1.5 X 10^5 years (see Fig. 3.5*k*).

These two systems depict some of the more significant characteristics of differences in pluton cooling styles and history. Temperature decreases as a function of time within the P2 pluton are typical conductive cooling curves (Fig. 3.8*a*, location points 2 and 3), as are the local temperature changes within the apophyses (location point 1). The latter temperature variation, though, is slightly more concave upward than typically observed in conductive processes, as a result of the large convective cooling rate at the host-pluton contact. The cooling style of analogous locations in the P4 pluton can be seen in Figure 3.8*b*. Whereas the temperature changes at times before 4 X 10^4 years for location 3 are identical to those for the same location in P2, at times after 4 X 10^4 years, all locations in P4 have temperature changes characteristic of a progressively fracturing pluton. The permeability at these locations is suddenly increased to values shown in Figure 3.3 as they cool below 700 °C; the temperature then decreases rapidly to the 300 to 400 °C range, but decreases more slowly for the remaining time. The sequence of fracturing is first at location 1, then at 2, and then at 3, as can be seen by the sudden decrease in temperatures at these points. Fluctuations in temperature at location 1 are caused by changes in convective flux associated with progressive fracture development with depth in the pluton. Temperature changes at 1 km over the pluton's top are similar for both systems, except that temperature increases more rapidly and attains a larger value above the P4 pluton (cf. Fig. 3.8*a* and *b*, curve 4).

Fluid flow rates in the P2 pluton are very small (Fig. 3.8 *c*); flow rates in the P4 system increase rapidly to a maximum, fluctuate in response to fracturing of locations within the pluton, and then decrease gradually (Fig. 3.8*d*). In both P2 and P4 systems flow rates at the host rock location initially increase, decrease, increase slightly, and then decay gradually.

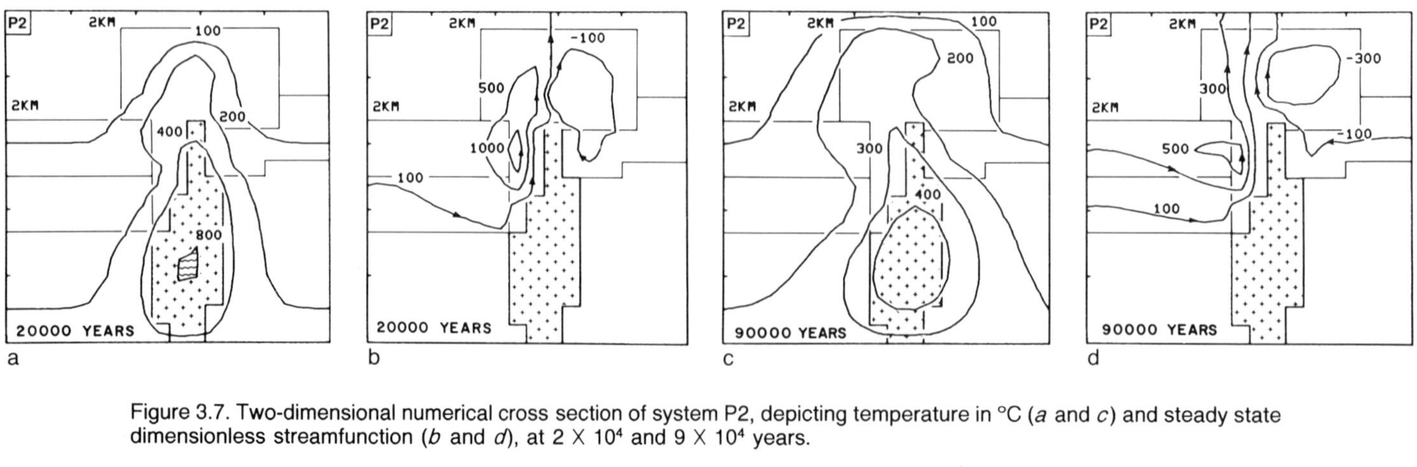

Figure 3.7. Two-dimensional numerical cross section of system P2, depicting temperature in °C (*a* and *c*) and steady state dimensionless streamfunction (*b* and *d*), at 2 X 10^4 and 9 X 10^4 years.

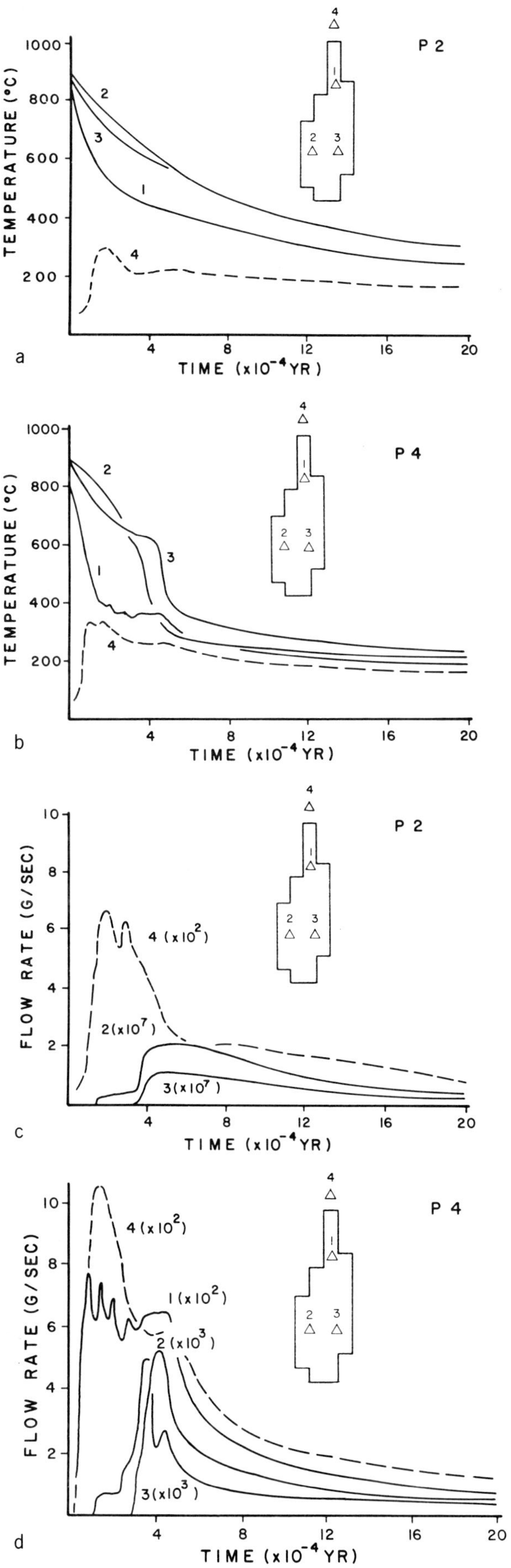

Figure 3.8. Temperature in °C, and fluid flow rate, gr sec^{-1}, as functions of time for P2 and P4 systems, at the locations shown by small triangles in pluton outline: *a,* temperatures for system P2; *b,* temperatures for system P4; *c,* flow rates for system P2; *d,* flow rates for system P4.

REDISTRIBUTION OF FLUIDS

Fluid pathlines describe the actual path followed by a fluid packet during the duration of the hydrothermal system (Norton, 1978). Transfer of chemical components between the fluid and rocks along the flow path determine the fluid's composition; therefore, definition of pathlines for each of these components in a system is essential if one wishes to study the effect of reactions between fluids and the pluton (Parmentier, 1980; Norton, 1980). However, only the case for a fluid moving at the Darcy velocity will be discussed.

Fluids that were initially in the P4 pluton flow upward through the pluton in the initial 3×10^4 years (Fig. 3.9*a*, pathline 6), continue flowing upward through the near-surface fracture zone, and flow out the top surface at $\sim 5 \times 10^4$ years. Pathlines for fluids initially in the schist adjacent to the pluton (Fig. 3.9*a,* pathline 5) flow into the pluton and then follow a path similar to 6. Pathlines for fluids initially in the permeable fracture zone, 1, or sedimentary section, 2, cross through the pluton and ultimately flow out through the surface. However, pathlines for fluids that are initially $>$ 2 km away from the pluton (Fig. 3.9*a,* pathlines 3 and 4) circulate toward the pluton and then upward toward the surface but remain within the system boundaries for the entire cooling period.

Fluid redistribution in systems with impermeable plutons is similar to the permeable pluton case, except the pathlines do not enter the pluton, pore fluids initially in the pluton remain there, and reactions between fluids from the host rocks and the pluton are restricted to the contact region (Fig. 3.9*b*).

Sources of Fluids and Components

Circulation of large masses of fluids from sources throughout the host rocks and pluton indicates the complexity of the question regarding ultimate sources for ore-forming components. However, the concept of fluid sourcelines permits the sourceregions of components to be quantitatively defined for the numerical systems. A fluid sourceline is the locus of points connecting the initial positions of fluids which circulate along pathlines and pass through a position of interest in the system. A sourceline can be defined for each location of interest in the system; for locations encompassing relatively large regions a family of sourcelines is obtained which, in turn, defines a sourceregion (Norton, 1978).

Fluid packets in the system flow the full length of a pathline; however, concentrations of aqueous components change significantly as a function of distance along a pathline as a consequence of non-equilibrium and equilibrium mass transfer between the fluids and rocks (Helgeson, 1970; Norton and Taylor, 1978). Therefore, sourcelines defined for the bulk fluid probably represent the maximum distance away from a location from which components could have been derived.

Sourcelines calculated for locations in the plutons considered in this study indicate that fluids were derived from at least 4 km laterally away from the pluton and 4 km vertically above the pluton (Fig. 3.10). The fluids derived from the sources farthest away flow through the rocks with largest

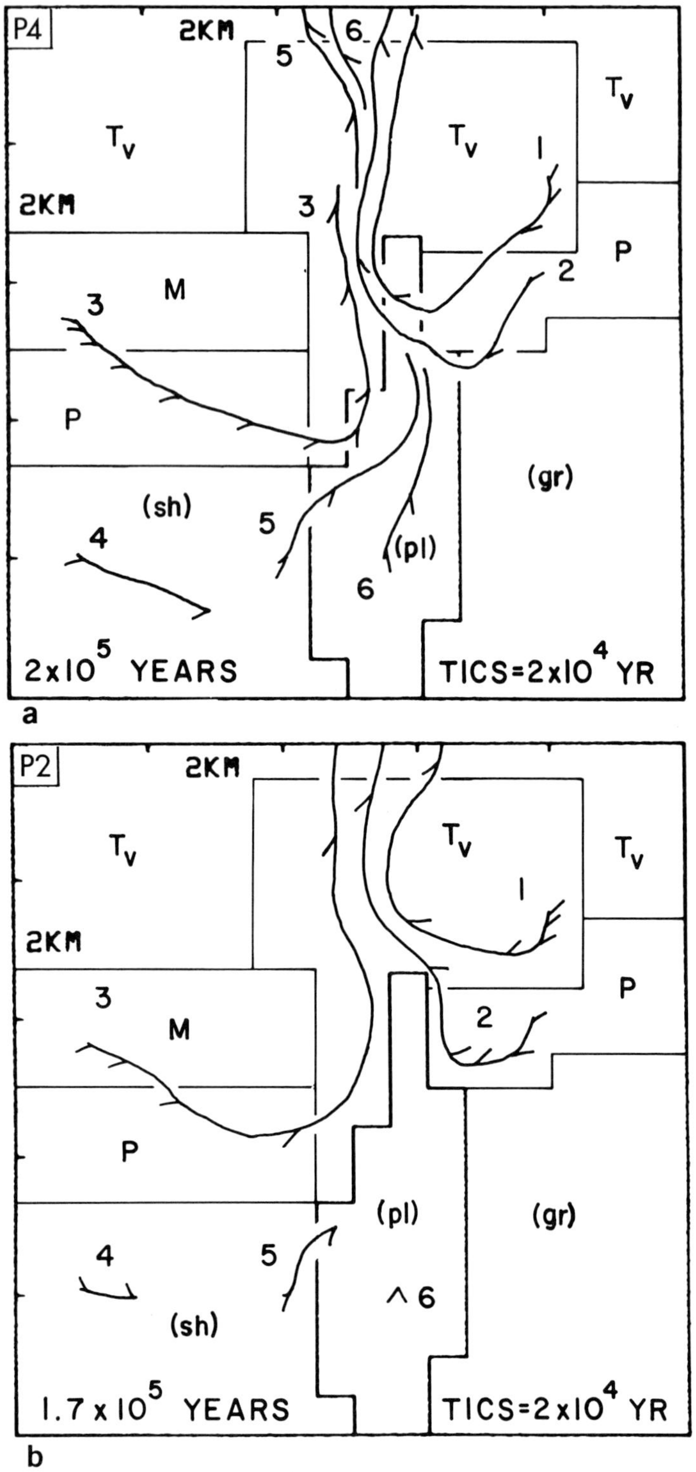

Figure 3.9. Two-dimensional numerical cross sections of pluton systems showing pathlines for 6 fluid packets: *a,* pluton system P4; *b,* pluton system P2. Tics on lines show direction of flow and occur every 2 X 10^4 years, except on short pathlines, where only initial and final tics are shown.

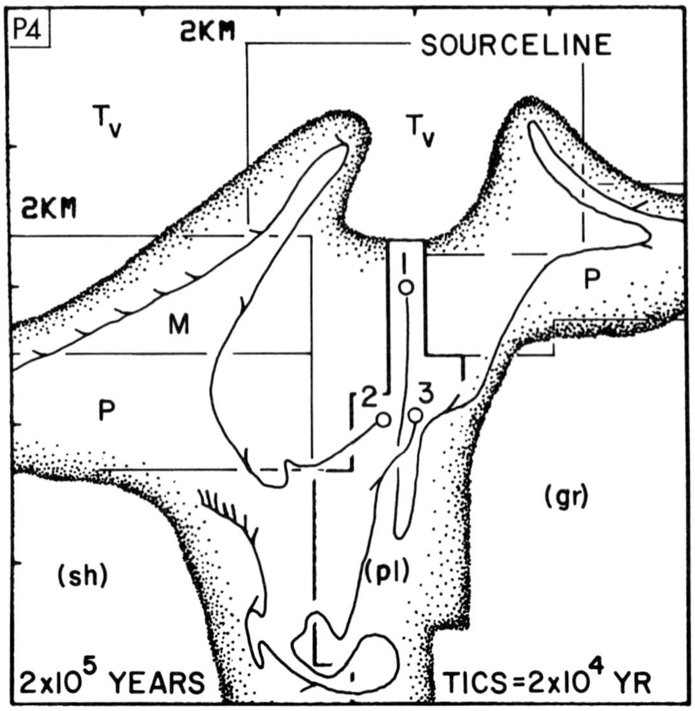

Figure 3.10. Two-dimensional numerical cross section of pluton system P4, showing sourcelines of fluid for 3 locations. Sourcelines have tics every 2 X 10^4 years which represent the transit time for fluid originally at the respective position on the sourceline to reach the location of interest. Shaded line represents outer boundary of sourceregion of fluids for pluton. Key: T_v = Tertiary volcanics, M = Mesozoic rocks, P = Paleozoic rocks, sh = schist, gr = granite, pl = pluton.

permeabilities for a major portion of their path, and, hence, sourceregions are dominated by these same rock units. At each location in the P4 pluton sources of the fluids are predominantly in the adjacent and overlying host rocks. Such domination occurs because only during the first few thousand years after the pluton cools below its solidus, fractures, and is capable of transmitting fluids are the fluids derived from sources within the pluton. If all the fluid exsolved from plutons composed of quartz monzonite magma, initially at 1 kb and 900°C and containing 4 weight percent at these conditions (Whitney, 1975*a*; Burnham and Davis, 1971, 1974), were to flow through the pluton apophysis, it would compose only 4 weight percent of the total fluid which would ultimately flow through this region during the thermal history of the system. The sources of fluids for positions 1 and 2 in Figure 3.10 are in host rocks above these positions. The source lines corresponding to positions lower in the pluton, or more toward the granite contact—e.g., position 3—indicate that fluid sources are predominantly from the schist, with minor contributions from the pluton.

Likely sources for components which have been concentrated in sulfide systems include both pluton and surrounding host-rock environments. Many components appear to be leached, transported, and redeposited within the limits of anomalous sulfide occurrences, e.g., iron in skarn magnetite zones can be accounted for by iron leached from adjacent host rocks. However, sources of sulfur, potassium, sodium, copper, lead, zinc, molybdenum, rhenium, and other transition elements have not been well established. Many components, particularly sulfur, might be derived from the Mesozoic or Paleozoic evaporites or saline pore fluids in the marine carbonate and clastic rocks, or from sulfide minerals in the Precambrian Pinal Schist.

Derivation of at least some components from host-rock sources is further supported by consideration of the masses of components available in the sourceregions. Consider the pluton to be cylindrical; if the radius is 1 km, then the sourceregion radius, as indicated by the P4 system, is ~ 4 km, and its height is ~ 5 km. The ore zone tonnages in porphyry deposits are on the order of 10^{12} kg, ~ 1 km^3 in volume, which is approximately equivalent in size to the apophyses on the pluton. The concentration factor, volume of sourceregion: volume of ore deposit, for any component leached from the sourceregion and deposited in the ore zone is 300:1. An 0.8 percent Cu deposit would require leaching 25 ppm from the surroundings and redepositing this amount in the ore zone. Anomalous sulfur-bearing rocks extend beyond the ore zone and include a volume ~ 5 times larger; sulfur has a concentration factor of ~ 50:1. Deposition of 2 weight percent pyrite throughout the larger volume of rock requires leaching 0.04 weight percent sulfur from the sourceregions and depositing it as pyrite.

Sourceregions for the valuable metals in these deposits are traditionally considered to be the pluton and/or its parent magma. Mass balance considerations, which require initial concentrations of 400 ppm through the pluton and thorough leaching of all this metal, indicate that the concentration factor for deriving copper only from the pluton is ~ 18:1. Alternatively, sources within igneous bodies below the pluton considered here require 100 km^3 of rock with 50 ppm copper content *and* permeable channels along which the leached copper can be transported into the shallow pluton. The latter condition contravenes the geologic observations that fracture abundances decrease substantially with depth. The feasibility of transfering components to near-surface environments by magmatic processes, such as magma circulation or anomalous fluid phase contents of the magma, is not known. More precise determination of the relative contributions of components from hydrothermal and magmatic sourceregions in these systems requires quantitative field and laboratory data on the distribution of components and fractures in sourceregion rocks, as well as within the sulfide systems, and quantitative simulation of magmatic processes believed to be active in these systems.

GEOLOGIC REALITY

The degree to which numerical systems approximate their natural analogs depends mostly on the degree to which the initial and boundary conditions and the values of transport parameters represent the natural system; the quality of the simulated systems depends directly on geological and geochemical data.

Transport properties of H_2O are known to better than 1 percent of their actual value; however, no natural systems contain a pure H_2O fluid. In particular, variations in dissolved components can produce fluid density gradients which may increase or decrease thermally induced buoyancy effects. Although salinity effects appear to be relatively insignificant for NaCl-H_2O fluids up to 2 m NaCl, the stratigraphic section into which the Arizona plutons were emplaced contains Permian evaporites (in the Epitaph Dolomite) and carbonate rocks which contained formation waters (seawater). Concentrated fluids are evident from fluid inclusions in the fossil system, which often contain $>$ 3 m NaCl equivalent fluids (Bodnar and Beane, 1977). The details of the effect of such fluids on the simulated systems are not known, but on the basis of preliminary calculations it is apparent that the style of fluid circulation is more sensitive to an order of magnitude change in permeability than to plausible variations in salinity. Also, the amount of fluid circulated will probably be within a few percent of that predicted for the system using properties of the phases in the H_2O system. Increasing salt content causes the critical end-point on the system to shift to higher pressures and temperatures, and anomalous variations in supercritical fluid properties (density, heat content, and viscosity) become shifted in a similar manner (Norton and Knight, 1977).

Values of rock parameters used in numerical simulation —in particular, permeability—are the source of the greatest potential differences between the numerical system and reality, as can be seen in the system discussed above. One challenge of field mapping is to develop methods useful in measuring permeabilities of rocks in hydrothermal systems, since this parameter is significant to the ore-forming process. There appears to be a fundamental difference between natural systems which contain ore and those that do not; this is particularly evident in comparisons of Laramide and mid-Tertiary age plutons, i.e., P4 vs. P2. Each of the different-age plutons is systematically fractured (Heidrick and Titley, 1982); however, the barren plutons of both ages appear to have far fewer continuous fractures and, therefore, lower permeabilities than ore-bearing plutons of these ages.

These numerical systems summarize our general understanding of the variations in temperature, pressure, and fluid circulation in hydrothermal systems and present a mapping challenge to the ore-deposit geologist. The fluids which compose hydrothermal systems are predominantly from host-rock environments; they flow along fractures, concentrate components from sourceregions into ore deposits, and produce various zones of alteration assemblages. Sourcelines regarding ore-forming components require an analogous study of reactive fluid circulation through reactive rocks (Norton, 1979).

ACKNOWLEDGMENTS

Professor S. R. Titley has contributed many hours of discussion and references that have greatly helped in defining the geologic environment of porphyry systems. Professors H. P. Taylor, R. E. Beane, H. C. Helgeson, and Dr. D. K. Bird have provided valuable criticism of the studies and manuscript. Janis Blainer compiled and helped interpret the almost endless geologic data on these systems, and Lynn McLean edited and typed the manuscript. I wish to thank each of them for their time and thoughts.

This chapter was derived from studies funded by NSF GA41136 and EAR74-03515-AO1 to the author.

REFERENCES CITED AND BIBLIOGRAPHY

Banks, N. G., 1976, Reconnaissance geologic map of the Mount Lemmon quadrangle, Arizona: U.S. Geol. Survey Map MF-747, 1:64500.

Banks, N. G.; Cornwall, H. R.; Silberman, M. L.; Creasey, S. C.; and Marvin, R. F., 1972, Chronology of intrusion and ore deposition at Ray, Arizona: Econ. Geol., v. 67, p. 864–878.

Bazin, Dominique, and Hübner, Helmuth, 1969, La région cuprifère à gisements porphyriques de Kerman (Iran): Mineral. Deposita, v. 4, p. 200–212.

Beane, R. E., 1982, Hydrothermal alteration in silicate rocks, southwestern North America *in* Titley, S. R., ed., Advances in Geology of the Porphyry Copper Deposits, Southwestern North America: Tucson, Univ. Arizona Press, Chapter 6.

Bianchi, L., and Snow, D. T., 1969, Permeability of crystalline rocks interpreted from measured orientations and apertures of fractures: Jodphur, Rajasthan, Arid Zone Research Assoc. of India, Annals of Arid Zone, v. 8, p. 231–245.

Bodnar, R. J., and Beane, R. E., 1977, Temperature variations in pre-intrusive cover over a buried pluton (abs.): Geol. Soc. America., Abs. with Program, v. 9, no. 7, p. 903.

Brace, W. F., 1977, Permeability from resistivity and pore shape: Jour. Geophys. Res., v. 82, p. 3343–3347.

Brace, W. F.; Walsh, J. B.; and Frangoes, W. F., 1968, Permeability of granite under high pressure: Jour. Geophys. Res., v. 73, no. 6, p. 2225–2236.

Braun, E. R., 1969, Geology and ore deposits of the Marble Peak area, Santa Catalina Mountains, Pima County, Arizona: Unpub. M.S. Thesis, Univ. Arizona, 75 p.

Bryant, D. G., and Metz, H. E., 1966, Geology and ore deposits of the Warren Mining District, *in* Titley, S. R., and Hicks, C. L., eds., Geology of the Prophyry Copper Deposits, Southwestern North America: Tucson, Univ. Arizona Press, p. 189–203.

Bryant, D. L., 1968, Diagnostic characteristics of the Paleozoic formations of southeastern Arizona, *in* Titley, S. R., ed., Southern Arizona Guidebook III: Ariz. Geol. Soc. p. 33–47.

Burnham, C. W., and Davis, N. F., 1971, The role of H_2O in silicate melts: I. P-V-T relations in the system $NaAlSi_3O_8$-H_2O to 10 kilobars and 1000°C: Am. Jour. Sci., v. 270, p. 54–79.

———, 1974, The role of H_2O in silicate melts: II. Thermodynamic and phase relations in the system $NaAlSi_3O_8$-H_2O to 10 kilobars, 700° to 1100°C: Am. Jour. Sci., v. 274, p. 902–940.

Chakarun, J. D., 1973, Mineralization and alteration of the Jhus Canyon area, Cochise County, Arizona: Unpub. M.S. Thesis, Univ. Arizona, 60 p.

Clarke, C. W., 1965, The geology of the El Tiro Hills, west Silver Bell Mountains, Pima County, Arizona: Unpub. M.S. Thesis, Univ. Arizona.

Cooper, J. R., 1960, Some geologic features of the Pima mining district, Pima County, Arizona: U.S. Geol. Survey Bull. 1112-C, p. 63–103.

———, 1971, Mesozoic stratigraphy of the Sierrita Mountains, Pima County, Arizona: U.S. Geol. Survey Prof. Paper 658-D, 42 p.

———, 1973, Geologic map of the Twin Buttes quadrangle, southwest of Tucson, Pima County, Arizona: U.S. Geol. Survey Map I-745, 1:48000.

Corn, R. M., 1975, Alteration-mineralization zoning, Red Mountain, Arizona: Econ. Geol., v. 70, p. 1437–1447.

Creasey, S. C., 1965, Geology of the San Manuel Area, Pinal County, Arizona: U.S. Geol. Survey Prof. Paper 471, 64 p.

———, 1967, General geology of the Mammoth quadrangle, Pinal County, Arizona: U.S. Geol. Survey Bull. 1218, 94 p.

———, 1975, Preliminary geologic map of Teapot Mountain quadrangle: U.S. Geol. Survey, Open File Rept. 75-314.

Crittenden, M. D., Jr.; Stackless, J. S.; Kistler, R. W.; and Stern, T. W., 1973, Radiometric dating of intrusive rocks in the Cottonwood area, Utah: U.S. Geol. Survey Jour. Res., v. 1, p. 173–178.

Drewes, Harald, 1971*a,* Geologic map of the Sahuarita quadrangle, southeast of Tucson, Pima County, Arizona: U.S. Geol. Survey Map I-613, 1:48000.

———, 1971*b,* Mesozoic stratigraphy of the Santa Rita Mountains, southeast of Tucson, Arizona: U.S. Geol. Survey Prof. Paper 658-C, 78 p.

Drewes, Harald, and Finnell, T. L., 1968, Mesozoic stratigraphy and Laramide tectonics of part of the Santa Rita and Empire mountains, southeast of Tucson, Arizona, Field Trip II, *in* Titley, S. R., ed., Southern Arizona Guidebook III: Ariz. Geol. Soc., p. 315–324.

Drewes, Harald, and Cooper, J. R., 1973, Reconnaissance geologic map of the west side of the Sierrita Mountains, Palo Alto Ranch quadrangle, Pima County, Arizona: U.S. Geol. Survey Map MF-538, 1:24000.

Eastlick, J. E., 1968, Geology of the Christmas mine and vicinity, Banner Mining District, Arizona, *in* Ridge, J. D., ed., Ore Deposits of the United States, 1933–1967: AIME, New York, p. 1191–1210.

Etminan, Hachem, 1977, Le porphyre cuprifère de Sar Cheshmeh (Iran). Rôle des phases fluides dans les mécanismes d'altération et de minéralisation: Unpub. Ph.D. Diss., L'Institut National Polytechnique de Lorraine, 249 p.

Finnell, T. L., 1970, Formations of the Bisbee Group, Empire Mountains quadrangle, Pima County, Arizona, *in* Changes in Stratigraphic Nomenclature by the U.S. Geol. Survey: U.S. Geol. Survey Bull. 1294-1, p. 28–35.

———, 1971, Preliminary geologic map of the Empire Mountain quadrangle, Pima County, Arizona: U.S. Geol. Survey, Open File Rept.

Förster, H.; Fesefeldt, K.; and Kursten, M., 1972, Magmatic and orogenic evolution of the Central Iranian Volcanic Belt: Internat. Geol. Conf., 24th, Section 2, p. 198–210.

Hayes, P. T., 1970*a,* Mesozoic stratigraphy of the Mule and Huachuca mountains, Arizona: U.S. Geol. Survey Prof. Paper 658-A, 28 p.

———, 1970*b,* Cretaceous paleogeography of southeastern Arizona and adjacent areas: U.S. Geol. Survey Prof. Paper 658-B, 42 p.

Hayes, P. T., and Landis, E. R., 1964, Geologic map of the southern part of the Mule Mountains, Cochise County, Arizona: U.S. Geol. Survey Map I-418, 1:48000.

Hayes, P. T., and Drewes, Harald, 1968, Mesozoic sedimentary and volcanic rocks of southeastern Arizona, *in* Titley, S. R., ed., Southern Arizona Guidebook III: Arizona Geol. Soc., p. 49–58.

Haynes, F. M., and Titley, S. R., 1980, The evolution of fracture-related permeability within the Ruby Star Granodiorite, Sierrita porphyry copper deposit, Pima County, Arizona: Econ. Geol., v. 75, p. 673–683.

Heidrick, T. L., and Titley, S. R., 1982, Fracture and dike patterns in Laramide plutons and their structural and tectonic implications, American Southwest, *in* Titley, S. R., ed., Advances in Geology of the Porphyry Copper Deposits, Southwestern North America: Tucson, Univ. Arizona Press, Chapter 4.

Helgeson, H. C., 1970, A chemical and thermodynamic model of ore deposition in hydrothermal systems: Mineral. Soc. America Spec. Paper 3, p. 155–186.

Helgeson, H. C., and Kirkham, D. H., 1974, Theoretical predictions of the thermodynamic behavior of aqueous electrolytes at high pressures and temperatures: I. Summary of the thermodynamic/electrostatic properties of the solvent: Am. Jour. Sci., v. 274, p. 1098–1198.

Jinks, J. E., 1961, The Margaret Wash section of the Mogul Fault, Pinal County, Arizona: Unpub. M.S. Thesis, Univ. Arizona, 19 p.

Jones, W. R.; Hernon, R. M.; and Moore, S. L., 1967, General geology of Santa Rita Quadrangle, Grant County, New Mexico: U.S. Geol. Survey Prof. Paper 555, 144 p.

Keith, S. B., and Barrett, L. F., 1976, Tectonics of the central Dragoon Mountains: A new look: Ariz. Geol. Soc. Digest, X, p. 169–204.

Kesler, S. E., and Heath, S. A., 1968, The effect of dissolved volatiles on magmatic heat sources at intrusive contacts: Am. Jour. Sci., v. 266, p. 824–839.

Knapp, R. B., 1978, Thermal-mechanical aspects of cooling pluton environments: Unpub. Ph.D. Diss., Univ. Arizona, 117 p.

Knapp, R. B., and Knight, J. E., 1977, Differential thermal expansion of pore fluids: Fracture propagation and microearthquake production in hot pluton environments: Jour. Geophys. Res., v. 82, p. 2515–2522.

Knapp, R. B., and Norton, D. L., 1981, Preliminary numerical analysis of processes related to magma crystallization and stress evolution in cooling pluton environments: Amer. Jour. Sci., v. 281, p. 35–68.

Krieger, M. H., 1974, Generalized geology and structure of the Winkleman 15' quadrangle and vicinity, Arizona: U.S. Geol. Survey, Jour. of Res., v. 2, p. 311–321.

Lacy, W. C., 1959, Structure and ore deposits of the east Sierrita area, *in* Heindl, L. A., ed., Southern Arizona. Guidebook II: Ariz. Geol. Soc., p. 184–192.

Lacy, W. C., and Titley, S. R., 1962, Geological development in the Twin Buttes District: Min. Cong. Jour., v. 48, p. 62–65.

Lipman, P. W., and Steven, T. A., 1970, Reconnaissance geology and economic significance of the Platoro Caldera, Southeastern San Juan Mountains, Colorado: U.S. Geol. Survey Prof. Paper 700-C, p. C19–C29.

Lootens, O. J., 1965, Geology and structural environment of the Sierrita Mountains, Pima County, Arizona: Arizona Geol. Soc. Digest, VIII, p. 33–56.

Lowell, J. D., 1968, Geology of the Kalamazoo Ore Body, San Manuel District, Arizona: Econ. Geol., v. 63, p. 645–654.

McClymonds, N. E., 1957, Stratigraphy and structure of the southern portion of the Waterman Mountains, Pima County, Arizona: Unpub. M.S. Thesis, Univ. Arizona, 98 p.

———, 1959, Paleozoic stratigraphy of the Waterman Mountains, Pima County, Arizona, *in* Heindl, L. A., ed., Southern Arizona Guidebook II: Ariz. Geol. Soc., p. 67–76.

Metz, R. A., and Rose, A. W., 1966, Geology of the Ray Copper Deposit, Ray, Arizona, *in* Titley, S. R., and Hicks, C. L., eds., Geology of the Porphyry Copper Deposits, Southwestern North America: Tucson, Univ. Arizona Press, p. 177–188.

Moolick, R. T., and Durek, J. J., 1966, The Morenci District, *in* Titley, S. R., and Hicks, C. L., eds., Geology of the Porphyry Copper Deposits, Southwestern North America: Tucson, Univ. Arizona Press, p. 221–231.

Naboko, S. I., 1959, Volcanic exhalations and products of their reactions as exemplified by Kamchatka-Kuriles volcanoes: Bulletin Volcanologique, Serie II, Tome XX, p. 121–136.

———, 1964, Modern volcanoes and fumarolic-hydrothermal activity [on Kamchatka] in Geologiya SSSR, Tom 31: Kamchatka, Kurilśkie j Komandorskie Ostrova, Chast 1., p. 303–371.

Neilsen, R. L., 1968, Hypogene texture and mineral zoning in a copper-bearing granodiorite porphyry stock, Santa Rita, New Mexico: Econ. Geol., v. 62, p. 37–50.

Norton, D. L., 1977, Fluid circulation in the earth's crust, *in* Heacock, John, ed., The Earth's Crust: Washington, D.C., Am. Geophys. Union Mono. 20, p. 693–704.

———, 1978, Sourcelines, sourceregions, and pathlines for fluids in hydrothermal systems related to cooling plutons: Econ. Geol., v. 73, p. 21–28.

———, 1979, Transport phenomena in hydrothermal systems: The redistribution of chemical components around cooling magmas: Bull. Mineral. v. 102, p. 471–486.

———, 1980, Transport phenomena in hydrothermal systems: Cooling plutons—the pathline concept in application to the study of transport processes in hydrothermal systems: Reply: Amer. Jour. Sci., v. 280, no. 8, p. 829–830.

Norton, D. L., and Knapp, R. B., 1977, Transport phenomena in hydrothermal systems: nature of porosity: Am. Jour. Sci., v. 277, p. 913–936.

Norton, D. L., and Knight, J. E., 1977, Transport phenomena in hydrothermal systems: Cooling plutons: Am. Jour. Sci., v. 277, p. 937–981.

Norton, D. L., and Taylor, H. P., Jr., 1979, Quantitative-simulation of the thermal history of igneous intrusives on the basis of oxygen isotope data and transport theory: An analysis of the hydrothermal system associated with the skaergaard intrusion: Jour. Petrology, v. 20, no. 3, p. 421–486.

Parmentier, E. M., 1980, Transport phenomena in hydrothermal systems: Cooling plutons—the pathline concept in application to the study of transport processes in hydrothermal systems: Discussion: Amer. Jour. Sci., v. 280, no. 8, p. 826–829.

Peterson, D. W., 1969, Geologic map of the Superior quadrangle, Pinal County, Arizona: U.S. Geol. Survey Map GQ-818, 1:24,-000.

Peterson, N. P., 1954, Geologic map of the Globe quadrangle, Arizona: U.S. Geol. Survey Map GQ-41, 1:24000.

———, 1962, Geology and ore deposits of the Globe-Miami district, Arizona: U.S. Geol. Survey Prof. Paper 342, 151 p.

Ransome, F. L., 1904*a,* Geology and ore deposits of the Bisbee quadrangle, Arizona: U.S. Geol. Survey Prof. Paper 21, 168 p.

———, 1904*b,* Description of the Globe quadrangle, Arizona: U.S. Geol. Survey Folio III, 17 p.

Rehrig, W. A., and Heidrick, T. L., 1972, Regional fracturing in Laramide stocks of Arizona and its relationship to porphyry copper mineralization: Econ. Geol., v. 67, p. 198–213.

Richard, K. E., and Courtright, J. H., 1966, Structure and mineralization at Silver Bell, Arizona, *in* Titley, S. R., and Hicks, C. L., eds., Geology of the Porphyry Copper Deposits, Southwestern North America: Tucson, Univ. Arizona Press, p. 157–162.

Richardson, C. B., 1976, Cross sections of southern Arizona and adjacent parts of California and New Mexico: Ariz. Geol. Soc. Digest, X, p. 1–6.

Robinson, R. F., and Cook, Annan, 1966, The Safford Copper Deposit, Lone Star Mining District, Graham County, Arizona, *in* Titley, S. R., and Hicks, C. L., eds., Geology of the Porphyry Copper Deposits, Southwestern North America: Tucson, Univ. Arizona Press, p. 251–266.

Schafroth, D. W., 1965, Structure and stratigraphy of the Cretaceous rocks south of the Empire Mountains, Pima and Santa Cruz counties, Arizona: Unpub. Ph.D. Dissertation, Univ. Arizona, 150 p.

———, 1968, Stratigraphy of some Cretaceous formations of southeastern Arizona, *in* Titley, S. R., ed., Southern Arizona Guidebook III: Ariz. Geol. Soc., p. 59–67.

Shafiqullah, M.; Langlois, J. D.; and Damon, P. E., 1976, Chronology of tectonic events in the Pima mining district, southern Arizona (abs.): Geol. Soc. America, Program with Abs., v. 8, no. 6, p. 1100.

Sillitoe, R. H., 1973, The tops and bottoms of porphyry copper deposits: Econ. Geol., v. 68, p. 799–815.

Simons, F. S., 1964, Geology of the Klondyke quadrangle, Graham and Pinal counties, Arizona: U.S. Geol. Survey Prof. Paper 461, 173 p.

———, 1972, Mesozoic stratigraphy of the Patagonia Mountains and adjoining areas, Santa Cruz County, Arizona: U.S. Geol. Survey Prof. Paper 658-E, 23 p.

———, 1974, Geologic map and sections of the Nogales and Lochiel quadrangles, Santa Cruz County, Arizona: U.S. Geol. Survey Map I-762.

Snow, D. T., 1965, A parallel plate model of fractured permeable media: Unpub. Ph.D. Dissertation, Univ. California, Berkeley, 331 p.

———, 1970, The frequency and aperture of fractures in rocks: Jour. Rock Mech., v. 7, p. 23–40.

Taylor, H. P., Jr., 1974, The application of oxygen and hydrogen isotope studies to problems of hydrothermal alteration and ore deposition: Econ. Geol., v. 69, p. 843–883.

Thoms, J. A., 1966, The geology and ore deposits of the Tascuela area, Sierrita Mountains, Pima County, Arizona: Unpub. Ph.D. Diss., Univ. Michigan, 87 p.

Titley, S. R., 1972, Pre-ore environment of southwestern North American porphyry copper deposits: Internat. Geol. Conf. 24th, Section 4, p. 252–260.

———, 1973, Pre-ore tectonic framework of southeastern Arizona porphyry coppers: Colorado Mining Assoc. Yearbook, p. 79–80.

Titley, S. R., and Hicks, C. L., eds., 1966, Geology of the Porphyry Copper Deposits, Southwestern North America: Tucson, Univ. Arizona Press, 287 p.

Titley, S. R.; Fleming, A. W.; and Neale, T. I., 1978, Tectonic evolution of the porphyry copper system at Yandera, Papua New Guinea: Econ. Geol., v. 73, p. 768–784.

Villas, R. N., and Norton, D. L., 1977, Irreversible mass transfer between circulating hydrothermal fluids and the Mayflower Stock: Econ. Geol., v. 72, p. 1471–1504.

Watson, B. N., 1964, Structure and petrology of the eastern portion of the Silver Bell Mountains, Pima County, Arizona: Unpub. Ph.D. Diss. Univ. Arizona, 101 p.

Weertman, J., 1971*a*, Theory of water-filled crevasses in glaciers applied to vertical magma transport beneath oceanic ridges: Jour. Geophys. Res., v. 76, p. 1171–1183.

———, 1971*b*, Velocity at which liquid-filled cracks move in the earth's crust or in glaciers: Jour. Geophys. Res., v. 76, p. 8544–8553.

Whitney, J. A., 1975*a*, The effects of pressure, temperature, and X_{H_2O} on phase assemblage in four synthetic rock compositions: Jour. Geol., v. 83, p. 1–31.

———, 1975*b*, Vapor generation in a quartz monzonite magma: a synthetic model with application to porphyry copper deposits: Econ. Geol., v. 70, p. 346–358.

———, 1977, A synthetic model for vapor generation in tonalite magmas and its economic ramifications: Econ. Geol., v. 72, p. 686–690.

Wilson, E. D.; Moore, R. T.; and Cooper, J. R., 1969, Geologic map of Arizona: Ariz. Bur. Mines and U.S. Geol. Survey Map, 1:1,000,000.

4

Fracture and Dike Patterns in Laramide Plutons and Their Structural and Tectonic Implications

AMERICAN SOUTHWEST

Tom L. Heidrick and Spencer R. Titley

Abundant fractures with varying physical, temporal, alteration, and mineralization characteristics are a prominent and ubiquitous phenomenon in porphyry copper plutons of the southwestern United States. The fractures typically carry the preponderance of economic mineralization and occur at scales ranging from megascopic, through-going, dike-filled joints and fault-veins down to microfractures that pervade the central portion of the deposits. The presence and importance of these fractures in porphyry copper systems has long been known (Lindgren, 1905; Ransome, 1919), but few attempts at documenting their systematics were reported in the literature prior to the early 1940s, when Pennebaker (1942) wrote that no dominant trend of fractures was recognizable at Ely. Gilluly (1946) reported that attempts to resolve fracture systematics at Ajo had been "fruitless." However, in a remarkable prediction, Butler and Wilson (1938, p. 74) noted that fractures in the porphyry at Morenci "would doubtless fall into definite systems if mapped in detail." In his studies at Bagdad, Anderson (1948) discovered that the minor mineralized fractures were not random but showed three preferred orientations. Such was the general scope of knowledge when McKinstry (1955) summarized the problem in a review that considered both the nature and cause of fracturing in porphyry plutons of the Southwest. At that time the nature and systematics of fractures in rocks from these systems were poorly known, and the mechanisms that produced the fractures were almost solely in the realm of educated speculation. McKinstry, however, observed that the fractured rocks of the deposits were not rotated (transported); he thus recognized and reported an important genetic constraint that obviated explosive (per se) processes.

By the late 1970s some advances had been made in attempts to further understand the geometric and dynamic nature of fractures in porphyry systems. The great number of porphyry copper deposits discovered, developed, and studied in the decades following McKinstry's review provided numerous field laboratories where many studies concerned with the orientation of fractures were carried out, not only in the American Southwest but in other porphyry copper clusters of the Pacific Basin margin. By the early 1980s the systematic nature of fractures in many porphyry copper systems in the southwestern United States, as well as in other regions, was a widely documented fact; advances had also been made in geology, petrology, and geophysics, which provided a much more rigorous foundation upon which dynamic aspects of the fracturing mechanism could be based. The synoptic fabric data presented and discussed in this chapter place many geometrical constraints on the nature and origin of stresses controlling the orientation and distribution of fractures and dikes observed in southwestern porphyry copper systems. Moreover, reasonable extrapolations of field-based data have allowed tentative definitions of likely sources of ambient stress at both the local pluton (emplacement-cooling energetics) and geotectonic scales of observations.

This chapter presents the results of field studies in the American Southwest in which the nature of fractures in porphyry copper systems was analyzed. Studies in 20 pluton environments and 24 mining districts included: (1) productive porphyry copper centers (pits), (2) non-productive portions of intrusive centers spatially and temporally related to porphyry copper deposits, and (3) non-productive (barren) plutons. The results indicate that there are systematic (preferentially oriented) fracture systems which pervade all plutons and their wall rocks. Further, the preferred orientations are virtually the same for all sites studied. Areas of more abundant and less systematic fracturing are closely centered on altered and mineralized portions of porphyry systems. Fractures extend well away from these productive centers and decrease in abundance and randomness outward into superjacent volcanic, plutonic, metamorphic, and sedimentary wall rocks where they eventually become regional-tectonic in nature or completely disappear. For these reasons, we view the porphyry centers as local energy *loci* capable of producing large volumes of fractured rocks; the orientations of the more areally widespread fractures are believed to be related to regional Laramide stress fields.

DEFINITIONS AND CLASSIFICATIONS

Structural elements present in porphyry copper systems include mineralized and unmineralized joint sets, veins, faults, fault-veins, dikes, and fault-dikes. Figure 4.1 presents in synoptic form the basic characteristics of these different features. Joint and joint set terminology in this chapter follows the classifications proposed by Heidrick and Rehrig (1972). Each respective joint type (J_1, J_2, and J_3) is present at most locations analyzed and varies only in relative abundance in different portions of the pluton–wall rock environment in which it occurs. Figure 4.2 schematically summarizes combinations of different common mesoscopic structural elements present in typical pluton environments. All elements are readily recognized in outcrop or working face without the aid of a microscope or hand lens and are large enough that direct observation can accurately establish their overall structural geometry.

J_1 Joints and Joint Sets

J_1 joint sets consist of smooth-surfaced, continuous planar, and through-going mesoscopic structures. They have had a pronounced effect on controlling and localizing both alteration and mineralization in all barren, ore-related, and productive Laramide porphyry systems examined. They range from structures with narrow (ca. 1 mm) to, more commonly, thicker (ca. 1 cm) alteration selvages and are the most

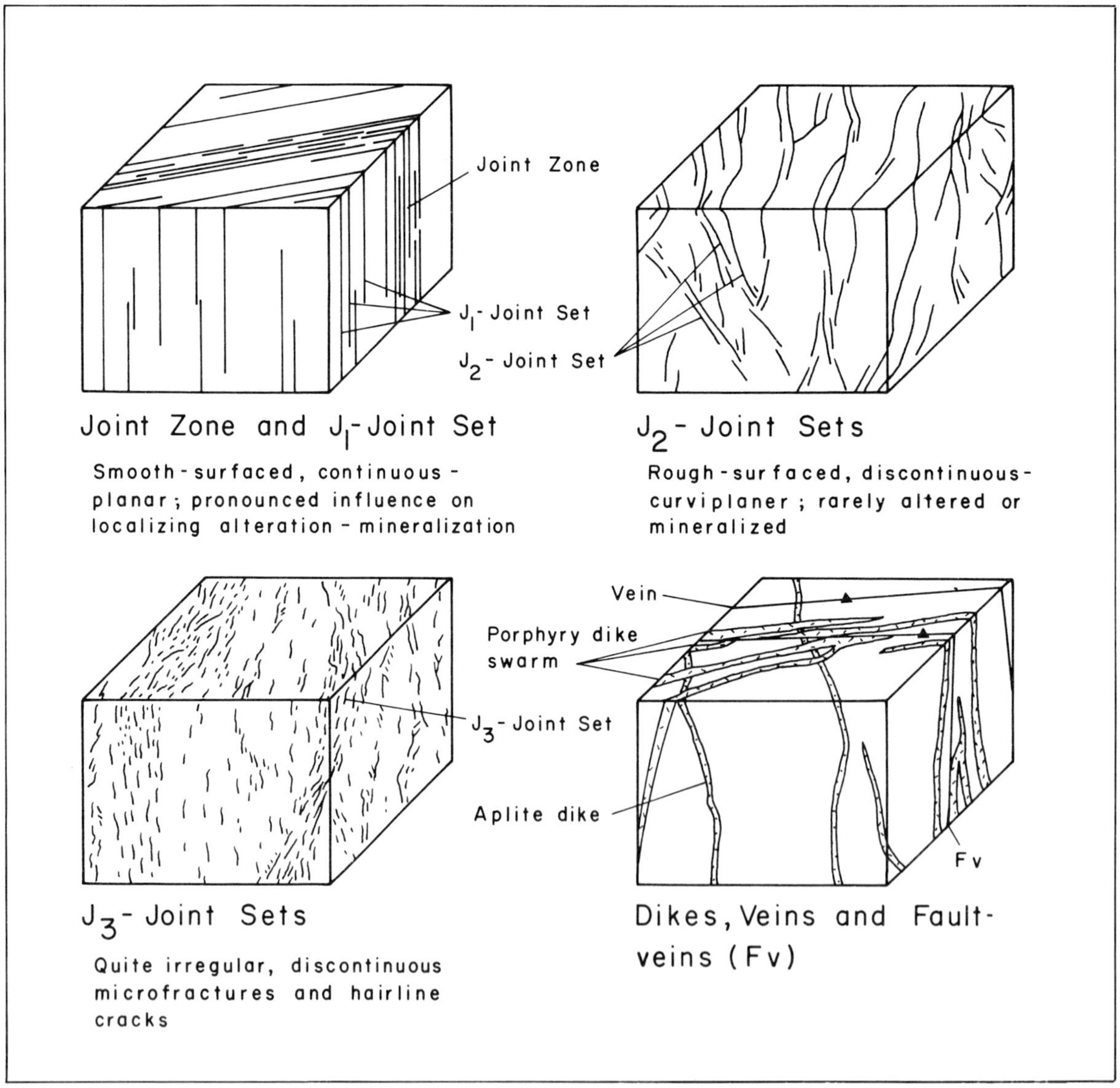

Figure 4.1. Schematic block diagrams characterize the three fundamental types of mesoscopic joint sets (J_1, J_2, and J_3), dikes, veins, and fault-veins repeatedly encountered cutting Laramide plutons of the American Southwest.

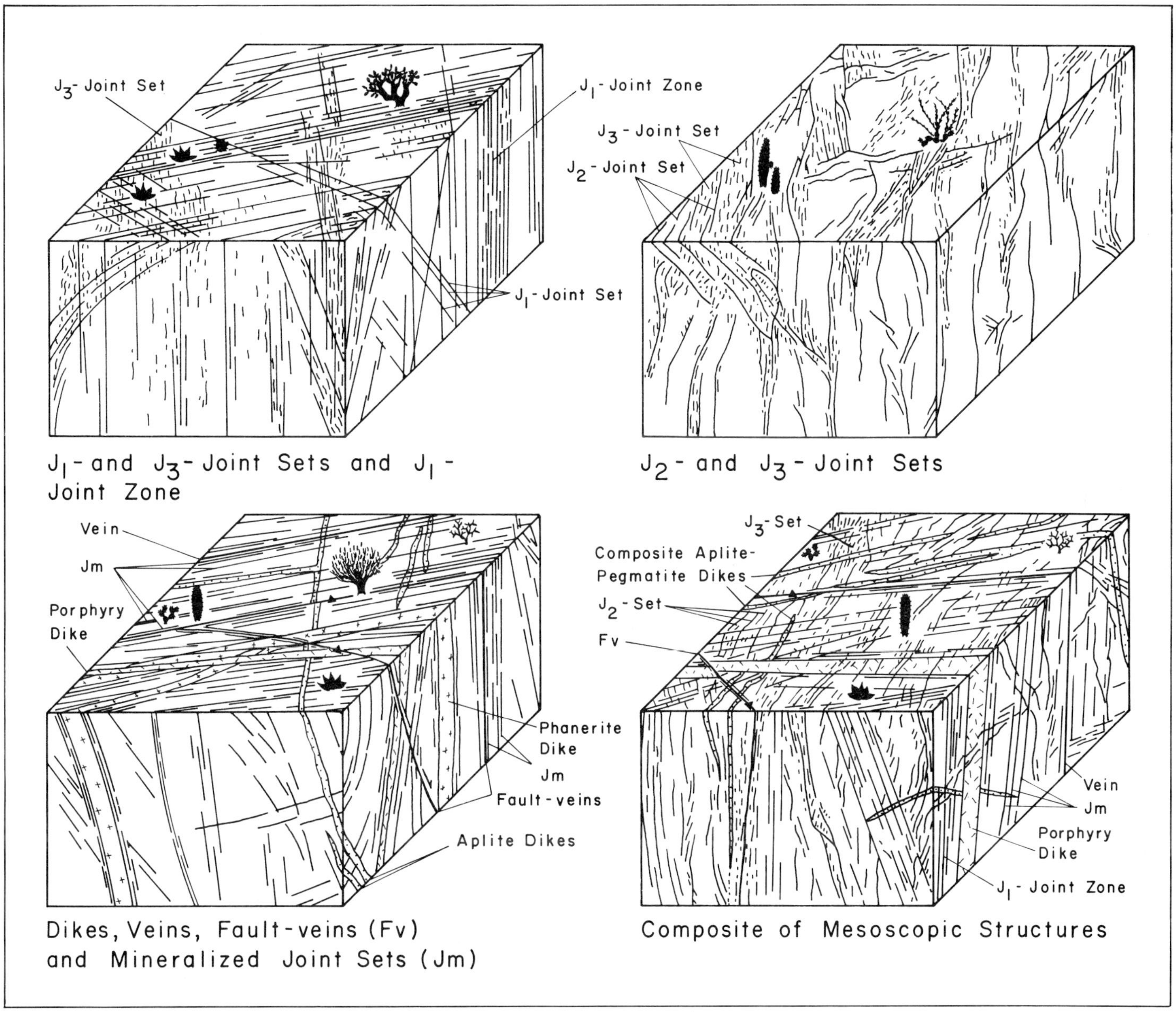

Figure 4.2. Schematic block diagrams characterize the physical, spatial, and temporal relationships between mesoscopic structures commonly observed cutting Laramide plutonic rocks of the American Southwest.

prominent structural elements in productive systems. J_1 joints in conjunction with co-planar veins may occur singly, with normal wall-to-wall spacings of up to several meters in width, or in sets having separations of 10 cm or less. Their abundance is correspondingly quite variable, but where ore grade mineralization is attained, fracture densities are often on the order of 0.2 to 0.4 cm^{-1} (Haynes and Titley, 1980). Their nature is indicated schematically on Figure 4.1.

J_2 Joints and Joint Sets

Rarer than the J_1 class, the J_2 joints are rough-surfaced, discontinuous, and curviplanar (see Fig. 4.1). They may be mineralized and altered, but only rarely. They occur paragenetically within the sequence of altered and mineralized veins and are, therefore, considered phenomena of intermineral fracturing of the pluton intrusion systems. Although present at the centers of porphyry copper mineralization, they are also present and are locally more abundant in areas of unmineralized, less structurally isotropic, non-intrusive wall rocks.

J_3 Joints and Joint Sets

J_3 joints and joint sets (see Fig. 4.1) are invariably the most abundant fracture type observed in Laramide porphyry systems and constitute all irregular, discontinuous microfractures, fracture cleavages, and hairline cracks. Individual J_3 joints have not been measured, and little detail has been reported concerning their nature. They are clearly related in time to J_1, and possibly to some J_2, fractures, since their alteration-mineralization products occur as specific and distinct paragenetic hierarchies; because of this relationship, they are considered to be lower-ordered elements of the more through-going structural features. Within porphyry copper deposits, they commonly carry sulfide minerals and reveal very thin (ca. 0.1 mm) alteration selvages. They persist away from centers of porphyry mineralization to the limits of fracturing several kilometers away, where they may be *loci* of alteration without accompanying sulfide minerals (Haynes and Titley, 1980). Their habit is typically discontinuous and sometimes irregularly sinuous; upon close inspection, however, they usually form sets of intersecting, hairline microveinlets possessing different alteration products within the same small volume of rock. Limited statistical fabric studies of J_3 elements reported here reveal systematic fracture distributions over relatively small volumes of host rocks. Viewed from the standpoint of fluid flow, and contrasted with major channels of fluid flow (J_1 elements), J_3 sets appear to have been channels that controlled much of the diffusion porosity for hydrothermal fluids.

Dikes and Veins

Dikes, fault-dikes, veins, fault-veins, and vein-dikes constitute some of the most persistent, through-going structural elements found in porphyry copper systems. In the American Southwest, where intermediate calc-alkaline compositions are prevalent, consanguineous dikes typically reveal rhyodacite-rhyolite and granitic aplite compositions. Their habit is characterized as that of continuous-planar to local curviplanar elements, with lateral extents measured in hundreds of meters (see Figs. 4.1 and 4.2). The dikes present in the deposits of the Southwest are of intermediate composition and have normal wall-to-wall widths of 2 to 15 m; they often occur as ill-defined *en echelon* sets and swarms. Aplite, composite aplite-pegmatite, and aplite porphyry dikes are prevalent in most plutons but are uncommon in adjacent wall rocks. Within the porphyry copper deposits, it is uncertain whether all aplite dikes and dikelets are intrusive in the strict sense. A metasomatic origin seems likely in some instances in which the "dikes" formed in response to brittle fracturing and concomitant channeling of metasomatizing fluids along early-formed continuous breaks within the host intrusion.

Lateral offset along mesoscopic structural elements that cut Laramide plutons is uncommon. However, statistical analyses of striae from crushed, brecciated, and sheared faults, fault-veins, fault-dikes and from along J_1 sets show that, when present, separations are predominantly the product of strike-slip and, less commonly, dip-slip or oblique-slip movements. Strike separations are commonly measured in centimeters, occasionally in meters, and rarely in tens of meters. Several of the common modes of lateral separations are shown schematically in Figure 4.2.

Other comparable, but less common, structural elements of the Laramide porphyry copper deposits include pre- or inter-mineral calc-alkaline porphyry dikes and, more rarely, concordant planar veins within porphyry dikes. Some dikes, particularly the rhyodacite-rhyolite porphyries, are crossed by J_1 and related J_3 sets, both of which carry sulfide mineralization. Such dikes are clearly pre-fracture and pre-mineralization in age, spatially restricted to specific intrusive centers, and systematically oriented.

Summary

The composite of Laramide fractures, dikes, marked variance in fracture characteristics, and frequencies are portrayed schematically on the diagrams in Figure 4.2. Large volumes of rock within, and peripheral to, centers of porphyry copper mineralization mirror the compound effects of repeated overprinting, as shown in this figure; the composite diagram of all fractures conveys the impression of stockworks so commonly ascribed to this deposit type. Notwithstanding such an abundance of fractures, the studies and observations reported here have revealed, unequivocally, that physical, temporal, and geometrical order pervades the systems analyzed. The results of these studies are based primarily upon the geometries of mineralized and unmineralized J_1 sets and of pre- and inter-mineral porphyry dikes, veins, and fault-veins. The overall scarcity of J_2 sets and our interpretation of microfractures (J_3) as representing lower orders of J_1 sets (as suggested both geometrically and paragenetically) preclude their statistical consideration in any major way in this analysis.

MESOSCOPIC FABRIC DATA

Mesoscopic fabric data—including unmineralized and mineralized joint sets, veins, fault-veins, dikes, and dike-veins—have been examined for numerous Laramide plutons scattered throughout the Basin and Range province of Arizona and New Mexico. Results of an initial structural analysis of mesoscopic structures from 8 non-productive and ore-related plutons and 3 porphyry copper deposits in Arizona were reported by Rehrig and Heidrick (1972). This preliminary analysis entailed the statistical treatment of about 15,000 high-angle, mesoscopic structures and employed conventional Schmidt equal-area projections and corresponding strike histograms. That data base is expanded here to include 7 additional, widely separated, non-productive and ore-related systems in Arizona and New Mexico; the new data bring the total number of mesoscopic elements measured to over 50,000 in 18 pluton-related systems, as reported in this chapter. The geographic distribution of the 20 intrusive complexes examined and discussed is illustrated on Figure 4.3, and their classification is indicated on Table 4.1, which shows 3 productive porphyry copper systems, 10 ore-related intrusions, and 7 non-productive plutons. As listed on Table 4.1, all pluton systems analyzed have Laramide (75–50 m.y.) radiometric ages *(sensu stricto)* or ages unequivocally interpreted from geologic relationships as Laramide.

Fabric data reported in this chapter were collected by employing criteria and techniques described by Rehrig and Heidrick (1972). Fracture and dike type, orientation, frequency, and dominant alteration-mineralization were recorded directly on mark-sense data cards, which were subsequently computer processed. Data for joints include those for sets in which three or more parallel to sub-parallel fracture surfaces occur. Single averages for joints and sets are based upon 5 or more measurements. Sub-parallel sets, veins, faults, or dikes with strike differentials in excess of $\pm 5°$ are included as individual measurements. Mesoscopic dikes,

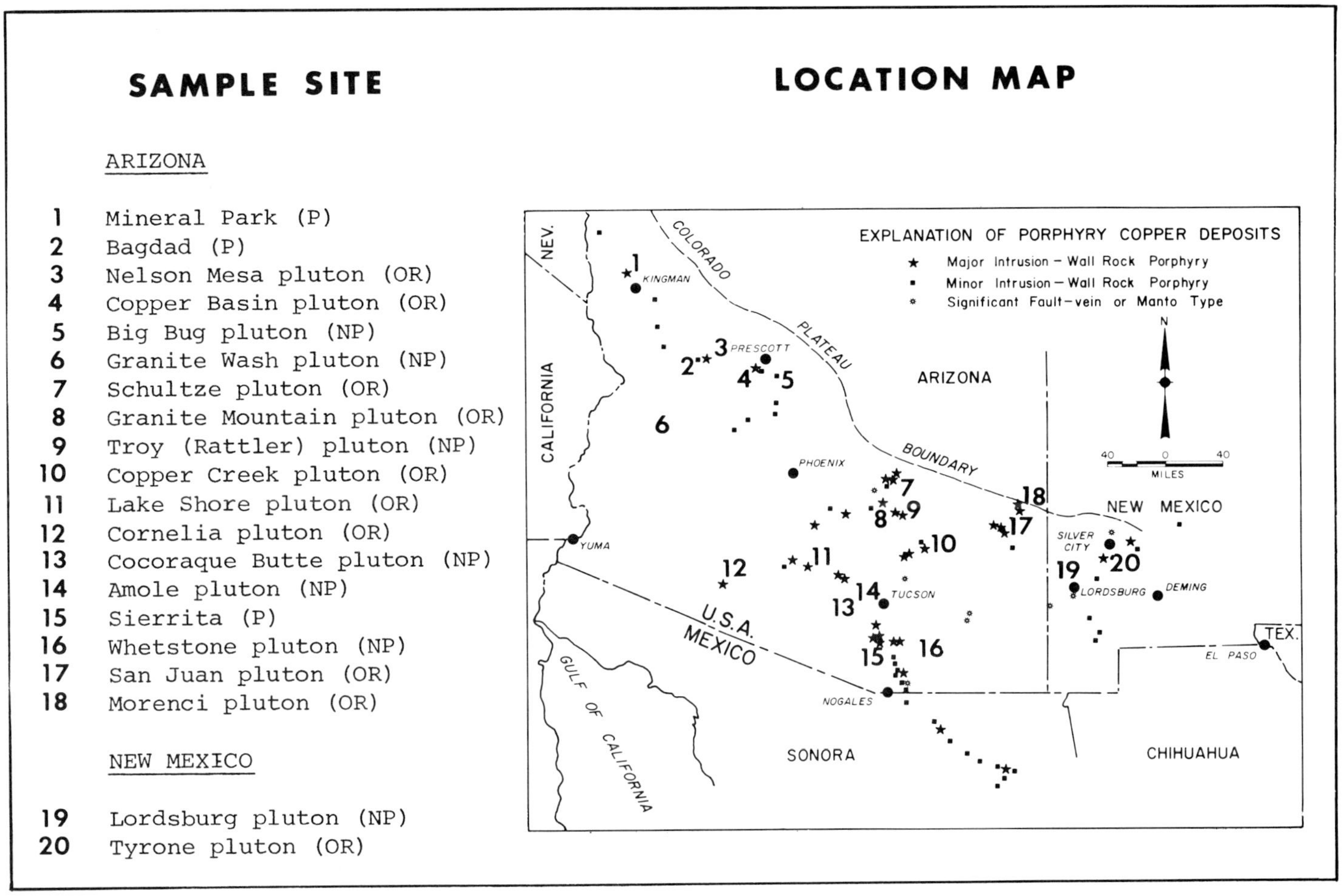

Figure 4.3. Index map shows the location of 20 Laramide plutons where detailed mesoscopic fabric studies were conducted. Each respective location is classified as follows: *NP* = non-productive pluton; *OR* = non–ore-grade intrusion that is spatially and temporally related to a known porphyry copper system; *P* = producing porphyry copper system.

veins, faults, or fault-veins are shown as separate measurements if they occur as single features. At sites studied, exposures in arroyos, creeks, road cuts, and benches reveal that only a small porportion (<15%) of the total fractures dip less than 45°. The results summarized here are, therefore, of high-angle fractures and dikes.

The fabric data shown are the result of computer processing to a final form as lower hemisphere Schmidt equal-area nets; they are contoured in the probability of being randomly distributed, utilizing a 1 percent counting circle. As only high-angle (>45° dip) fractures and dikes have been measured, the open central portion of each respective net is void of contoured data and is utilized here to portray the corresponding strike frequency rosette of plotted data employing 10° arc class intervals.

Figure 4.4 synthesizes and combines total poles (N) to fractures and includes unmineralized J_1, J_2, and J_3 sets *(A–C)*, mineralized J_1, J_2, and J_3 sets *(D–F)*, and veins, fault-veins, and faults *(G–I)* in categories for non-productive, ore-related, and productive plutonic settings. In a similar fashion, Figure 4.5 provides nets and rosettes for high-angle, mesoscopic dikes, including aplites, pegmatites, and composite aplite-pegmatites *(A–C)*; calc-alkaline porphyries *(D–F)*; and their summation *(G–I)* for the same non-productive and ore-related plutons. The grand total of all mesoscopic structures recorded for each respective geologic-mineralogic setting is given on Figure 4.6. These fabric data lead to several important conclusions concerning the nature and origin of Laramide stress in relation to pluton environments in the American Southwest; among these conclusions are the following:

1. Unmineralized joint sets and total dikes from non-productive and ore-related plutons are systematically oriented in a relatively simple motif. This motif is dominated by a sub-vertical system of orthogonal fractures and dikes striking ENE±15° and NNW±15° (see Figs. 4.4*A–C* and 4.5*A, D, G*).
2. Mineralized joint sets within both non-productive and ore-related plutons are systematically oriented in a statistically monotonous pattern dominated by sub-vertical double maxima striking N60°E±5° and N80°E±5°. These double maxima are particularly apparent on the synoptic strike frequency rosettes shown on Figure 4.4*D, E.*
3. In marked contrast to the above, the analysis of fabric in 3 productive porphyry copper deposits (Sierrita, Bagdad, and Mineral Park) defines a somewhat diffuse, NNW±15° maximum for unmineralized joint sets (see Fig.

TABLE 4.1
Radiometric K-Ar Age Dates for Plutons Studied in Arizona and New Mexico

Number Code[a]	Name of Pluton	K-Ar Date (m.y.)	Sources
1	Mineral Park, Ithaca Peak Pit (P)[b]	72	Anderson, 1968
2	Bagdad Pit (P)	71	Damon and Mauger, 1966
3	Nelson Mesa pluton (Bagdad) (OR)[c]	71	Damon and Mauger, 1966
4	Copper Basin pluton (OR)	64	Anderson, 1968
5	Big Bug pluton (NP)[d]	70	Anderson, 1968
6	Granite Wash pluton (NP)	65	Damon, 1969
7	Schultze Granite (OR)	58–66	Damon and Mauger, 1966; Livingston et al., 1968
8	Granite Mountain pluton, Ray (OR)	61	Banks and Stuckless, 1973
9	Troy (Rattler) pluton (NP)	70	Banks et al., 1972
10	Copper Creek pluton (OR)	66	Creasey, 1967
11	Lake Shore pluton (OR)	67	Johnston, 1972
12	Cornelia pluton, Ajo (OR)	63	McDowell, 1971
13	Cocoraque Butte pluton (NP)	68	Bikerman, 1967
14	Amole pluton (NP)	75	Bikerman and Damon, 1966
15	Sierrita pit (P)	58	Creasey and Kistler, 1962
16	Whetstone Mts. pluton (NP)	74	Marvin et al., 1973
17	San Juan pluton (OR)	58	Rose and Cook, 1965
18	Morenci pluton (OR)	62	McDowell, 1971
19	Lordsburg pluton (NP)	58	Marvin et al., 1978
20	Tyrone pluton (OR)	56	McDowell, 1971

[a] Numbers are coded to locations shown in Figure 4.3.
[b] *P* = productive pluton; studies were carried out in porphyry copper orebody.
[c] *OR* = ore-related intrusion; studies were conducted in sub-ore—grade portion of intrusive complex.
[d] *NP* = nonproductive pluton; studies were conducted on a weakly altered and mineralized pluton not known to be productive at the level viewed.

4.4*C*), while mineralized joint sets are dominated by a sub-vertical, orthogonal system striking ENE±10° and NNW±10° (see Fig. 4.4*F*).

4. Synoptic plots for veins, multiple veins, fault-veins, and faults show maxima of N70°E±10° (dominant) and N75°W±10° (moderate) in non-productive plutons (see Fig. 4.4*G*). In contrast, ore-related plutons show the monotonous, repetitive, east-northeast–striking double maxima (see Fig. 4.4*H*), while the productive porphyry copper deposits are pervaded by fault and vein patterns striking ENE±10°, with subordinate maxima of N70°W ±5° and N10°W±10° (see Fig. 4.4*I*).
5. Dikes made up 12 percent of all mesoscopic elements recorded during this study, and of this total over 70% were aplites and pegmatites having widths of 15 cm or less. As evidenced by the synoptic nets and rosettes on Figure 4.5, dikes cutting non-productive and ore-related plutons are not set at random. Non-productive plutons are pervaded by a near-perfect orthogonal system of aplite-pegmatite dikes striking N10°W±10° (dominant) and N80°E±10° (moderate) (see Fig. 4.5*A*), whereas the ore-related plutons reveal a perfect N75°E±15° unidirectional strike for both aplite-pegmatite and porphyry dikes (see Fig. 4.5*B, E, H*). Porphyry dikes in nonproductive plutons, however, are slightly off the above-mentioned direction and strike N30°W±5° (see Fig. 4.5*D*).
6. As has been frequently emphasized in the literature, rocks of porphyry copper deposits are typically broken on a very fine scale. The Schmidt plots and strike histograms show that mineralized fractures within the 3 productive plutons (see Fig. 4.4*F, I*) reveal a less pronounced systematic orientation than those present in barren and ore-related plutons (see Fig. 4.4*D, G,* and *E, H*). This characteristic suggests to us that fractures of local derivation do exist as systematic radial and concentric patterns or as non-systematic random patterns that have been overprinted by the regional unidirectional swarms and bidirectional systems.

The repetitious, orthogonal east-northeast and west-northwest fracture and dike system is clearly regional in extent and not restricted temporally or spatially to specific plutons or local domains within the southwestern province. In most instances, the ENE±20° set has exerted by far the dominant influence over ore localization at mesoscopic levels of observation. This remarkable structural persistence over such a broad geographic area and in plutons spanning nearly 20 m.y. has been the subject of previous study (e.g., Rehrig and Heidrick, 1972, 1976; Heidrick and Titley, 1976), and a review of published accounts by other authors provides supporting evidence for similar systematically oriented structures in many other southwestern porphyry copper deposits.

From the mesoscopic data assembled, it is clear that a long-lived, fixed-stress field directly or indirectly controlled the orientation of fractures and dikes that evolved during the emplacement, crystallization, and cooling cycle of the plutons studied. Furthermore, it is apparent that a consideration of these geometrical data, brittle-fracture criteria, and experimental-theoretical rock mechanics would seriously limit the number of possible unambiguous definitions of Late Cretaceous-early Tertiary principal stress directions. The following observations, extrapolations, and deductions, which draw upon studies by Heidrick (1974) and Heidrick and Titley (1976), help to outline the logic followed in arriving at a unique definition of the stress field under which the Laramide porphyry copper deposits were localized:

1. Wholesale NNW to SSE±20° extension was present across the porphyry copper province during the crystallization-mineralization of each respective pluton examined. The qualitative significance of this direction of extension is particularly apparent in the synoptic rosettes and nets for all dilatant structural elements, including mineralized joint sets, veins, multiple veins, dike swarms, and fault-veins. The pronounced preference of these sub-vertical elements to trend ENE±20° is ubiquitous to all environments analyzed (see Fig. 4.6). This plane of maxi-

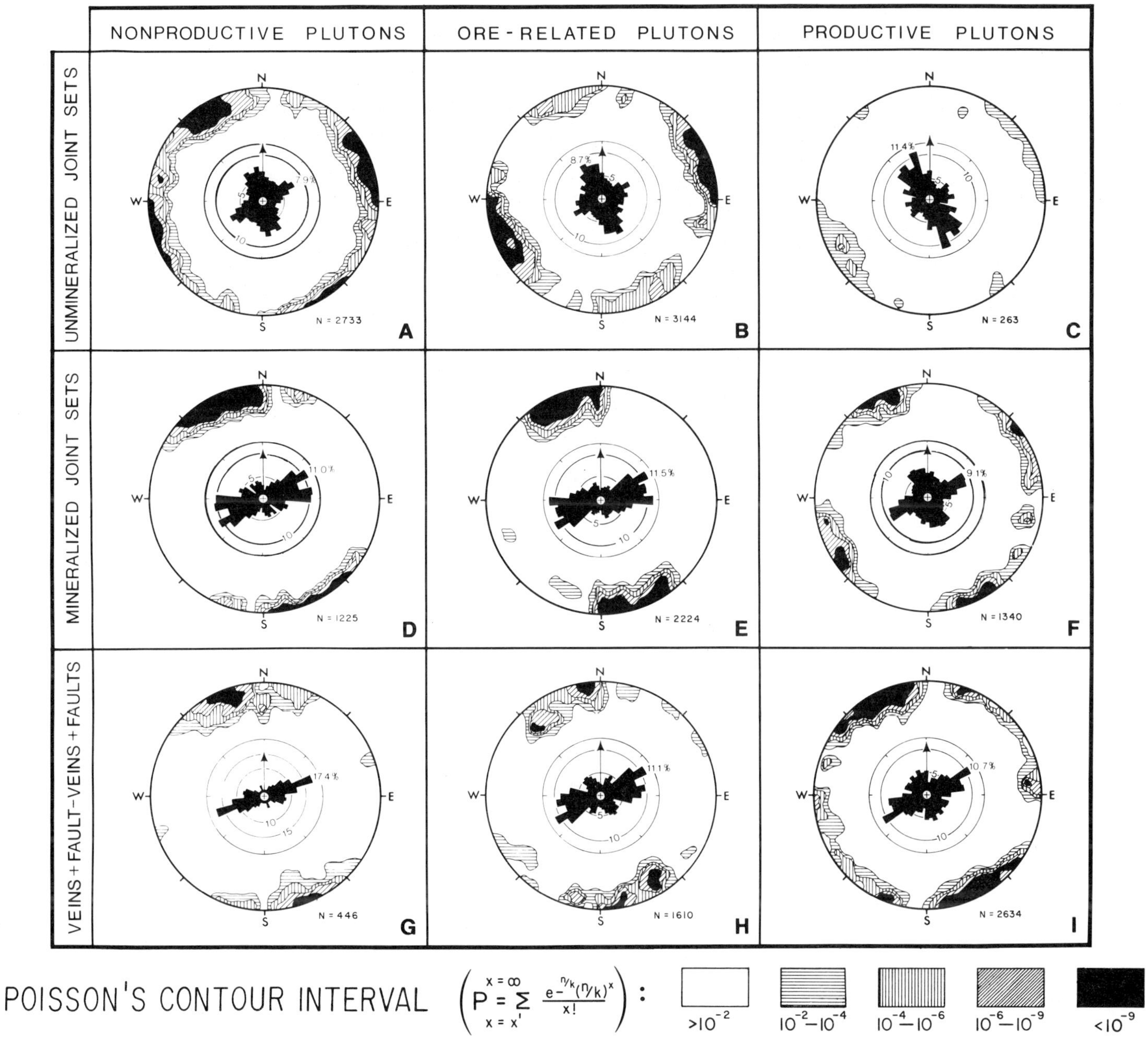

$$P = \sum_{x = x'}^{x = \infty} \frac{e^{-n/k}(n/k)^x}{x!}$$

Figure 4.4. Synoptic, lower hemisphere Schmidt equal-area nets, and strike histograms of N poles to joint sets (unmineralized, *A–C*; mineralized, *D–F*) and veins, fault-veins, and faults (*G–I*) were measured in 6 non-productive, 9 ore-related, and 3 productive Laramide plutons in the American Southwest.

mum extension fixes the minimum principal stress (σ_3) as horizontal or sub-horizontal and oriented NNW-SSE ±20° throughout main-stage porphyry copper metalization (75–50 m.y.). This orientation of σ_3, in turn, fixes the maximum (σ_1) and intermediate (σ_2) principal stresses in a vertical plane striking ENE±20° during Laramide time.

2. The recurrence of nearly perfect distributions of mutually perpendicular, dilatant mineralized joint (Fig. 4.4*A, B, F*) and dike (Fig. 4.5*A, C, G, I*) systems prohibits a conjugate shear origin for these brittle (extensional) fracture and dike systems.

3. In conjunction with mutually perpendicular, dilatant mineralized joint and dike systems, field relationships within phaneritic host rocks typically preclude the quantitative definition of strike-, dip-, or oblique-slip components along measured mineralized and unmineralized elements. However, Rehrig and Heidrick (1972) have noted that the repeated presence of horizontal to sub-horizontal slickensides along elements trending east-northeast was evident in every pluton studied. In this context, the persistent double maxima of N80°E±5°- and N60° E±5°-striking fractures with sub-horizontal slickensides, are almost certainly a direct product of conjugate shearing under conditions conducive to the development of small (10–25°), dihedral shear angles (see Fig. 4.4*D, E, H*). The weighted average of the acute bisectrix of the statistically defined east-northeast–striking double maxima uniquely defines the mean orientation of σ_1. The calculated trend for the acute bisectrix (σ_1) is N72°E-S72°W.

4. Provided that the mesoscopic, intra-plutonic structures mirror larger-scale elements of the Laramide framework and that established dynamics of faulting hold, wrench tectonics should pervade the porphyry province when σ_2 is vertical. However, during those periods when σ_1 is vertical, differential vertical uplift and normal fault tectonics should dominate. Low-angle, compressional thrust faulting is not expected under the proposed Laramide stress field, unless driven laterally as a

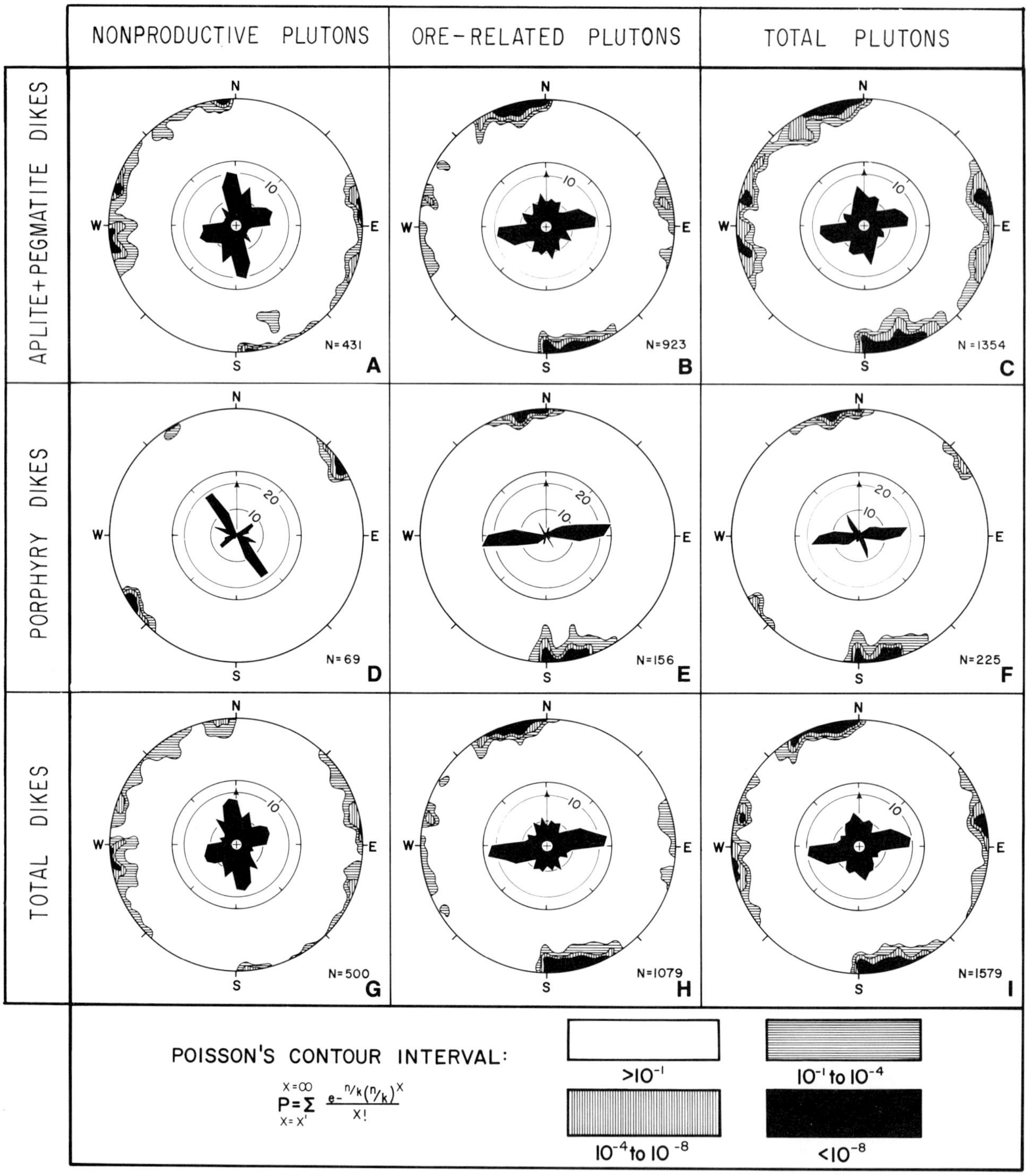

Figure 4.5. Synoptic, lower hemisphere Schmidt equal-area nets, and strike histograms of N poles to aplite and pegmatite dikes (*A–C*), calc-aklaline porphyry dikes (*D–F*), and their summation (*G–I*) were measured in non-productive and ore-related Laramide plutons in the American Southwest.

secondary consequence of convergent wrenching, differential vertical uplifting (upthrusting), or propelling off of prominent uplifts under the influence of gravity.

RESULTS OF STUDIES IN PLUTON-CENTERED DISTRICTS

Studies documenting pluton-centered, radial and concentric fracture patterns in the Southwest are few, although many workers have suspected the existence of such patterns. Initial fabric studies in three productive plutons have demonstrated that fractures at Ithaca Peak (Mineral Park) are generally more complex than those found at Sierrita or Bagdad. The diffuse, ill-defined, and relatively haphazard fracture distribution at Ithaca Peak has been "tentatively interpreted as an expression of radial and possibly concentric fractures . . ." (Rehrig and Heidrick, 1972, p. 208). A subsequent study on fractures by Wilkinson and others (1982) has likewise failed to reveal dominant systematic orientations at Mineral Park; these workers explain the apparent randomness of the fractures as the result of various controls acting at different times.

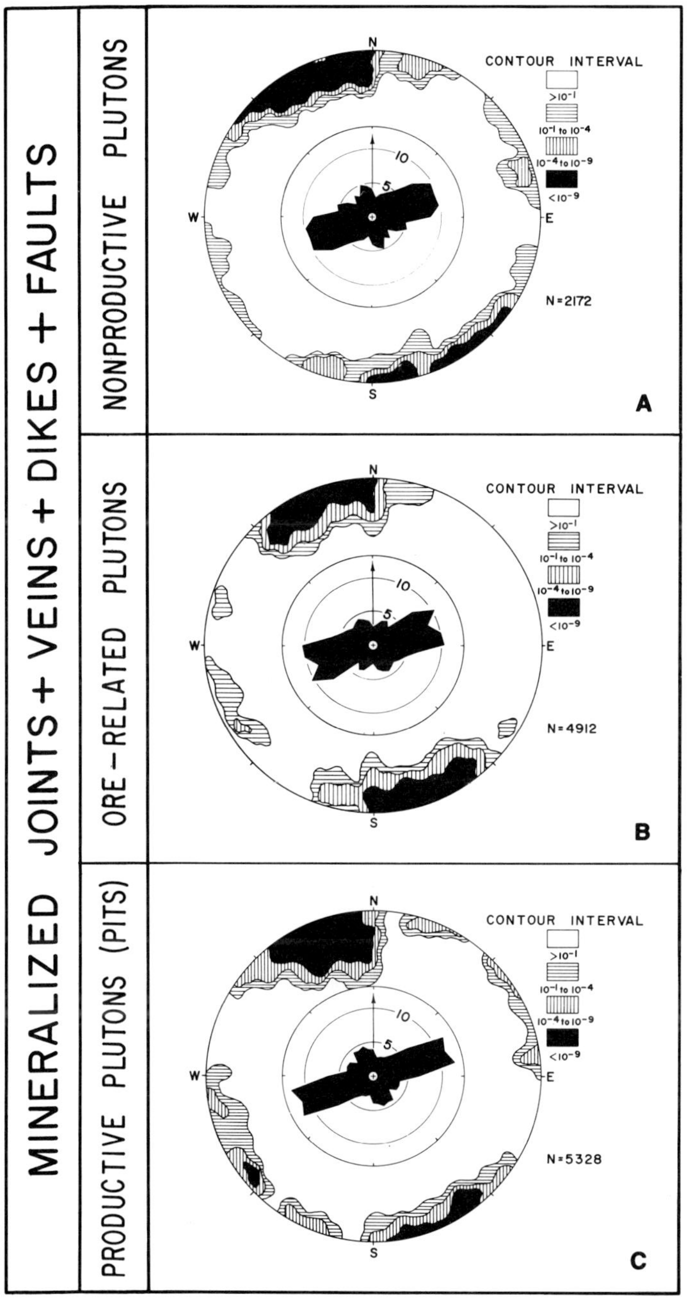

Figure 4.6. Synoptic, lower hemisphere Schmidt equal-area nets, and strike histograms of N poles to all mineralized joint sets, veins, dikes, and faults were measured in non-productive, ore-related, and productive Laramide plutons in the American Southwest.

Detailed mapping in the Safford (San Juan mine area) and Troy districts in Arizona and in the Hillsboro district in New Mexico (Dunn, 1982) demonstrates in a most convincing manner that pluton-centered radial and concentric fracture patterns are present in the Southwest. The location of the Troy district is shown in Figure 4.3, while those of the Lone Star (San Juan) and Hillsboro districts are given in Figure 4.7, along with 22 other districts, mountain ranges, and regions considered in our analysis of Laramide megascopic structures. As indicated in Table 4.2, each megascopic sample location shown in Figure 4.7 is spatially associated in some way with Laramide-aged plutons or pluton complexes.

Known porphyry copper deposits of the Safford district (see Fig. 4.7*Q*) include Dos Pobres, San Juan, Lone Star, and Sanchez. These deposits are aligned along a 24-km-long, northwest-trending belt of exhumed pre-mineral bedrock exposed along the upthrown side of the Butte fault, a regional discontinuity bordering the northeast edge of Safford Valley (Dunn, 1978). The general setting and nature of these 4 deposits are quite similar. All are directly related to a comagmatic suite of granodiorite and quartz monzonite porphyry plutons, latite to quartz latite dike swarms, and breccia pipes. All are localized within major transverse fracture zones which trend northeast to east-northeast and which repeatedly influenced the localization of copper mineralization at each respective deposit.

Our geologic sketch map of the San Juan mine area is included here as an example of a Laramide, porphyry-centered, fracture-dike system (Fig. 4.8). It shows in a generalized fashion the distribution of Laramide breccia pipes, porphyry dikes, and the San Juan quartz monzonite porphyry plug, along with major faults, fault-veins, and mineralized J_1 sets. Two superimposed fracture-dike patterns are apparent. The more obvious is an intrusion-centered pattern distributed centro-symmetrically to the main mass of the San Juan plug and coeval breccia pipes. It consists of both radial and concentric fault-veins, mineralized J_1 sets, and some porphyry dikes (Blake, 1971). The intrusion-centered pattern extends as a structural aureole outward from the center for a distance of 1.5 km. The second pattern is recognized as a 0.5-km-wide zone pervaded by numerous sub-vertical fault-veins and mineralized J_1 sets which trend northeast to east-northeast. The east-northeast–striking zone is obvious, as is the perturbing effect of that orientation upon the earlier intrusive-centered structures.

Extensive drilling at the San Juan mine and the deeper tests at Dos Pobres and Lone Star show porphyry copper mineralization localized, in large part, within layered volcanic wall rocks that are spatially and, by inference, genetically centered on relatively narrow, near-vertical systems of granodiorite–quartz monzonite porphyry apophyses, breccia pipes, and/or east–northeast–striking dike swarms. These observations, coupled with detailed, district-wide, stratigraphic reconstructions, suggest that each occurrence was epizonal in character and was localized, under near-surface conditions, directly above upward-extending hypabyssal cupolas and volcanic plugs. Viewed in the context of such conditions, the near-perfect, centrosymmetric, fracture-dike pattern developed about the San Juan intrusions reflects the apical portion of a sub-volcanic pluton system. Near-vertical plug and pipe emplacement and coaxially distributed copper-molybdenum metallization occurred very high in the overlying volcanic carapace, where ambient Laramide differential stresses at near-surface conditions were quite small (relaxed) and, at times, hydrostatic (Heidrick, 1974). Resultant radial and concentric patterns may, therefore, be interpreted either as the dynamic consequence of hydraulic fracturing induced by cooling of residual calc-alkaline magmas, intrusive

ARIZONA

- **A** Cerbat Mts. (P)
- **B** Bagdad district (P)
- **C** Big Bug district (NP)
- **D** Vulture Mts. (NP)
- **E** Superior-Globe-Miami (P)
- **F** Ray district (P)
- **G** Christmas district (P)
- **H** Copper Creek-Christmas (P)
- **I** Tortilla Mts. (NP)
- **J** Silver Bell Mts. (P)
- **K** Little Ajo Mts. (P)
- **L** Tucson Mts. (NP)
- **M** Sierrita Mts. (P)
- **N** Santa Rita Mts. (P)
- **O** Little Dragoon Mts. (P)
- **P** Dos Cabezas Mts. (NP)
- **Q** Lone Star (Safford) district (P)
- **R** Morenci district (P)

NEW MEXICO

- **S** Little Hatchet Mts. (NP)
- **T** Victorio Mts. (NP)
- **U** Lordsburg-Leitendorf (NP)
- **V** White Signal-Tyrone (P)
- **W** Santa Rita district (P)
- **X** Hillsboro district (P)

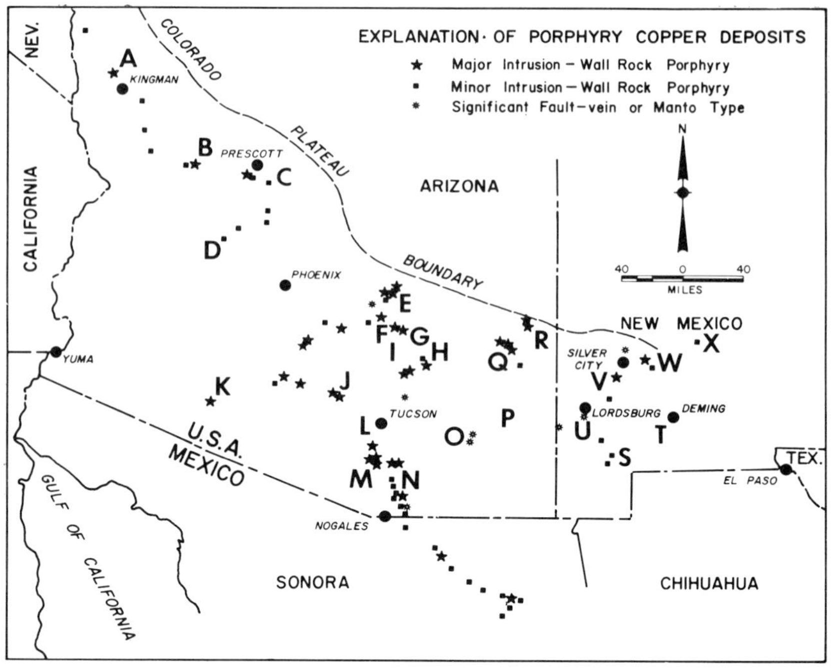

Figure 4.7. Index map shows the location of 24 districts, mountain ranges, or regions used in compiling Laramide megascopic fabric data. *P* = locality containing producing or established porphyry copper-molybdenum deposits; *NP* = nonproductive locality.

breccias, and ebullient excess volatiles, or as related to the dynamics of pluton emplacement and cooling. This structural style has counterparts in other areas of the Southwest, including Hillsboro (Dunn, 1982), Troy, and probably Red Mountain (Corn, 1975); it is also evident at Bougainville, Papua New Guinea (Baumer and Fraser, 1975), where subvolcanic plutons are characterized by both concentric and radial fracture patterns.

MEGASCOPIC FABRIC DATA

In an attempt to better characterize the distribution of large scale (megascopic) elements in the Laramide framework, strike frequency diagrams (rosettes) of mapped veins, fault-veins, dikes, and elongate intrusions were prepared from the results of systematic field analyses in 24 locations scattered throughout the Southwest (see Fig. 4.7 for geographic distribution). A Laramide age was documented at each sample location, either directly by radiometric methods or indirectly through stratigraphic superposition and crosscutting field relationships. Megascopic structural elements of questionable vintage were not incorporated in the synoptic rosettes. Table 4.2 shows the radiometric age, average age of several plutons or pluton complexes, or range of ages for each of the locations considered.

For the purpose of constructing individual rose diagrams, all available maps were normalized to an average scale, and each dike, vein, fault-vein, or elongate pluton of discernable Laramide age was divided into 1,000-ft. strike segments. The bearing of each segment was then measured, grouped into its respective 10° class interval, and plotted on percentage strike frequency diagrams. The number appearing beneath each respective rose shown on Figure 4.9 represents the total number of 1,000-ft. strike segments used in constructing each frequency diagram. To date, over 1,250 miles of Laramide strike segments in Arizona (Fig. 4.9, *A–R*) and 725 miles in New Mexico (Fig. 4.9, *S–X*) have been normalized, analyzed, and compiled. Details concerning data sources, structures incorporated, age relationships, etc., for 10 Arizona localities have been reported, along with some preliminary findings, by Rehrig and Heidrick (1976).

A comparison of mesoscopic structures (see Figs. 4.4–4.6) with those evident on the synoptic strike frequency rosettes for high-angle megascopic elements of Arizona and southwestern New Mexico (see Fig. 4.9) shows that both sets of data quantitatively share the same maxima in great detail. In particular, megascopic strike maxima show a

TABLE 4.2
Radiometric K-Ar Ages of Intrusions in Mountain Ranges, Mining Districts, and Other Regions Studied in Arizona and Southwestern New Mexico

Letter Code[a]	Location	K-Ar Age[d] (m.y.)	References
A	Cerbat Mts. (Chloride, Min. Park) (P)[b]	72	Anderson, 1968
B	Bagdad District (P)	71	Damon and Mauger, 1966
C	Big Bug District (NP)[c]	70	Anderson, 1968
D	Vulture Mts. (NP)	67	Rehrig et al., 1980
E	Superior-Globe Miami (P)	66–58	Damon and Mauger, 1966; Livingston et al., 1968
F	Ray District (P)	61	Banks and Stuckless, 1973
G	Christmas District (P)	62	Creasey and Kistler, 1962
H	Copper Creek, Christmas-Saddle Mtn. (P)	69–53	Guthrie and Moore, 1978
I	Tortilla Mts. (NP)	71–66	Damon, et al., 1964; Schmidt 1970; Krieger, 1974*a*, 1974*b*; Cornwall and Krieger, 1974
J	Silver Bell (P)	65	Mauger et al., 1965
K	Little Ajo Mts. (P)	63	Damon and Mauger, 1966
L	Tucson Mts. (NP)	75	Bikerman and Damon, 1966
M	Sierrita Mts. (P)	68–50	Creasey and Kistler, 1962; Shafiqullah and Langlois, 1978
N	Santa Rita Mts. (P)	74–56	Marvin et al., 1973
O	Little Dragoon Mts. (P)	50	Livingston et al., 1968
P	Dos Cabezas Mts. (NP)	62	Erickson, 1968
Q	Lone Star-Safford District (P)	70–48	Rose and Cook, 1965; Langton and Williams, 1982
R	Morenci District	62	McDowell, 1971
S	Little Hatchet Mts. (NP)	58	Loring and Loring, 1980
T	Victorio Mts. (NP)	—	No data
U	Lordsburg-Leitendorf District (NP)	58	Marvin et al., 1978
V	White Signal-Tyrone District (P)	56	McDowell, 1971
W	Santa Rita District (P)	59	Livingston, 1973
X	Hillsboro District (P)	74	Hedlund, 1974

[a] Letters are coded to locations shown on Figure 4.7.

[b] *P* = district or locality with producing or established porphyry copper-molybdenum deposits.

[c] *NP* = district or locality with no known producing or established porphyry copper-molybdenum deposits.

[d] Radiometric ages or interval indicated are selected from many dates reported for plutons and plutonic complexes throughout the region analyzed. Ages are averages for groups of dates or represent specific porphyry intrusions within the region or district examined.

marked statistical preference for northeast to east strikes over an area measuring tens of thousands of square miles. Regional stress that controlled the orientation of emplacement of plutons and dikes, as well as the orientation of mineralized structures, appears to have affected the entire southwestern porphyry province. Local perturbations and complexities exist; nevertheless, the Arizona and New Mexico synoptic rosettes portray an overriding predominance and consistency of N60 to 85°E(ENE) extensional phenomena not attained on a regional scale by other trends. This repetitious penetrative pattern is clearly shared by both mesoscopic and megascopic elements in the Laramide framework; the combination of those elements suggests an external regional tectonic control that uniformly affected the Arizona and New Mexico crust continuously from 75 to 50 m.y. ago. An unambiguous definition of this regional tectonic stress field is revealed from this analysis, which fixes the maximum Laramide principal stress axis (σ_1) as lying within the ENE to WSW±15° plane of maximum mesoscopic and megascopic extension-dilation. A horizontal orientation for σ_1 is indicated by the combined recurrence of sub-horizontal slickensides on the conjugate N60°E±5° and N80°E±5° double maxima for mineralized joints, veins, and fault-veins. At the shallow levels of emplacement considered here, however, lateral compression was not consistently profound, as shown by subordinate but statistically significant quantities of N10 to 30°W swarms of mesoscopic and megascopic dikes, as well as mineralized and unmineralized joint sets. Indeed, the data compiled suggest that Laramide porphyry copper localization favored structural sites dominated by tectonic relaxation, bidirectional extension, and strike-slip faulting.

INTERPRETATIONS AND IMPLICATIONS

Fabric data from Laramide plutons of this region and from all of the districts studied in which Laramide intrusions are present, clearly help establish regional tectonic stress directions which had a profound effect on delimited fracture and dike patterns. The close correspondence in habit and orientation of mesoscopic elements measured in both plutons and superjacent wall rocks point to a common origin. The tectogenetic development of fractures in the vicinity of plutons has been largely a matter of unrecorded observations; however, densities and orientation of fractures in the wall rocks at Sierrita (Haynes and Titley, 1980) and Silver Bell (Kanbergs, 1980) have been established. In these porphyry copper deposits the preponderance of mesoscopic elements measured near the centers of porphyry intrusions do not extend outward beyond distances of a few kilometers. This point is emphasized for a fundamental reason. Although observed J_1, J_2, and J_3 distributions and resulting composite fracture patterns reveal themselves on an areal or district-wide scale, regional tectonic stress is not believed directly responsible for the observed fractures. Those rock volumes with high densities of structural elements of the sort considered here are intrusion-centered, and the conclusion is forced that the energy responsible for their development is directly related to pluton tectonics and the cooling history of porphyry magmas. Sources of energy must, therefore, be sought

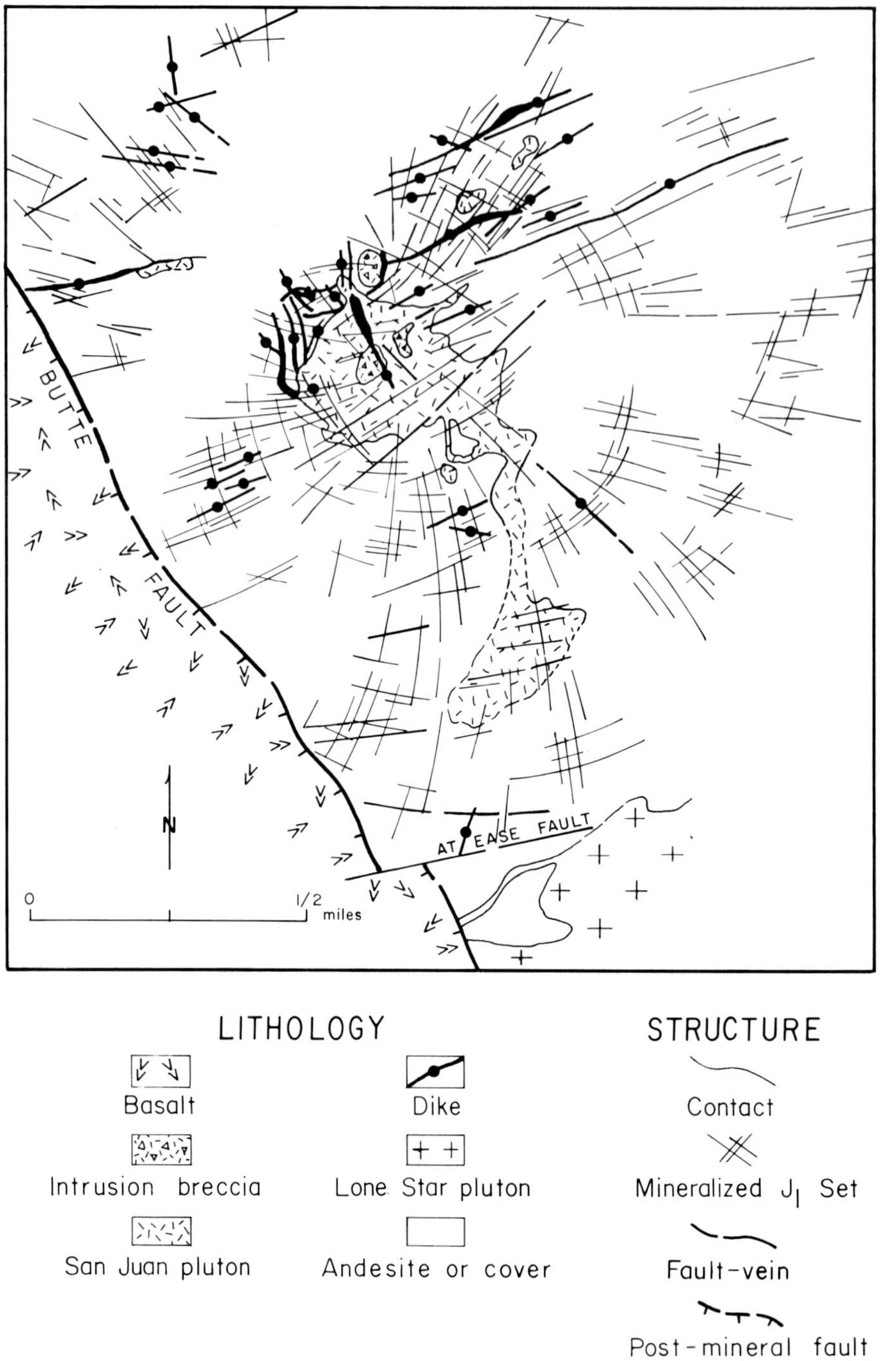

Figure 4.8. Geologic sketch map of the San Juan mine area, Safford district, Arizona

in processes of pluton emplacement and cooling, while resultant stress distributions about these centers are the composite effect of both regional-tectonic and local mechanical rock responses.

Plutons as Energy Sources

Pluton emplacement is an energetic process, and the cooling of magmas results in the transfer of great amounts of thermal energy. The effects of pluton cooling and energy transfer have been studied and are briefly reviewed here as they relate to the generation of fractures. Knapp and Norton (1981) have reported the results of a finite element analysis depicting the thermal history of a cooling tonalite magma in the shallow crust. Associated with the rapid development of a solid hood and general inward and downward crystallization of rest magma, heat is transferred from the hot pluton to the relatively cooler wall rocks. A "push-pull" phenomenon is interpreted as resulting from thermal contraction of the intrusion due to cooling with synchronous expansion of wall rocks due to heating. Magma pressure is interpreted to produce tension fractures within and near the pluton's top. Following crystallization, continued pressures from deeper magmas and from thermal processes acting on the wall rocks are believed to produce stresses that result in both radial and

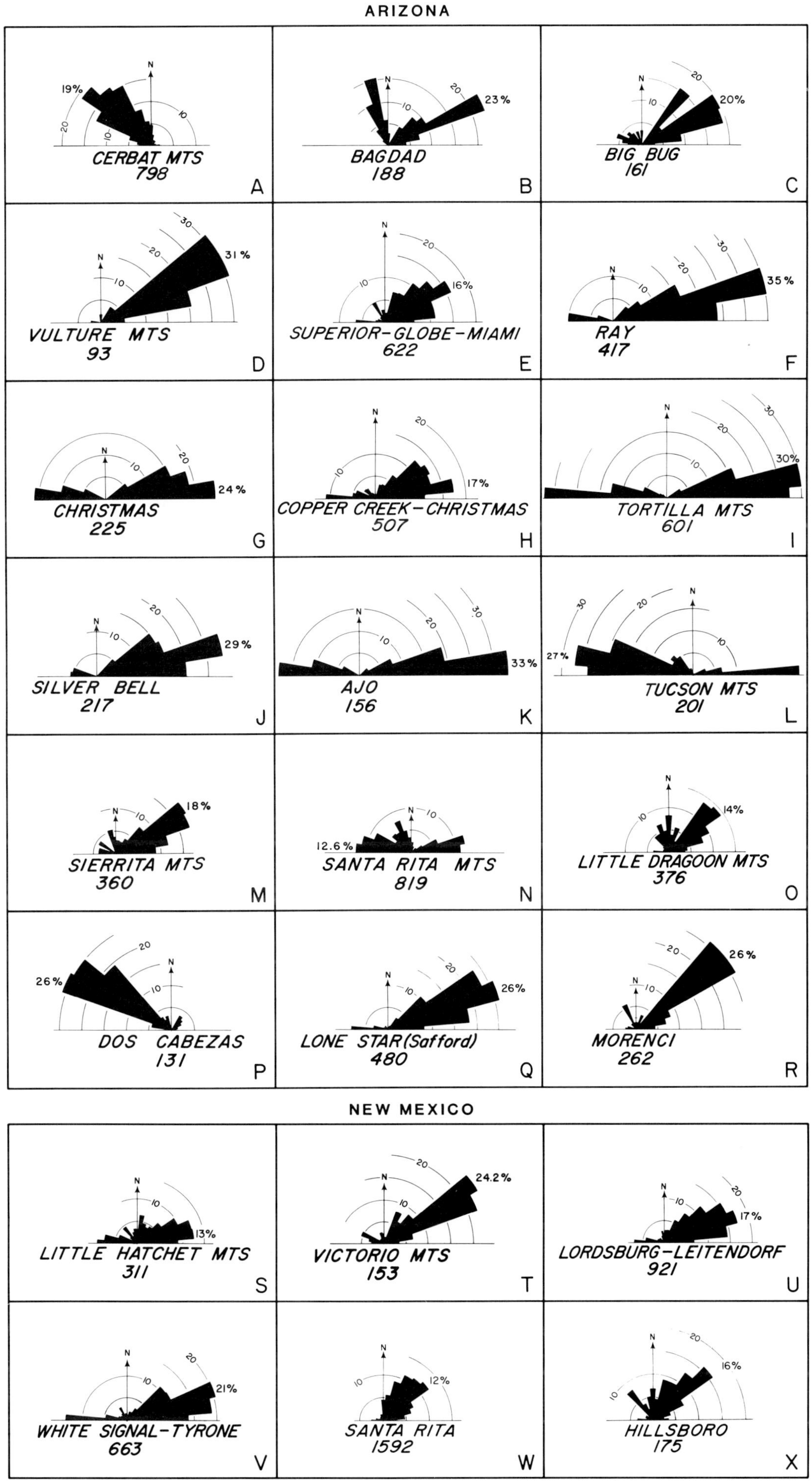

Figure 4.9. Strike rosettes for Laramide dikes, elongate plutons, veins, and fault-veins in Arizona and New Mexico. Rosette bars are constructed for 10° class intervals. Length of strike bars is proportional to percentage of total elements measured. The number of 1,000-ft.-long strike segments used to construct each frequency diagram is indicated beneath each respective plot.

concentric fracture patterns centered over those rock domains which experienced the greatest temperature differentials. Initial cooling of the pluton by conduction is subsequently enhanced by convection through the thermally expanded and fractured adjoining wall rocks.

From a study of stresses associated with emplacement and cooling of a pluton, Koide and Bhattacharji (1975) have also suggested an energy source related to magma emplacement that results in development of fractures with predictable geometry. With reference to high magma and hydrothermal fluid pressures, these workers have showed that concentric and radial fracture patterns develop when lithostatic pressures are exceeded. During the time of pluton emplacement, radial fracture patterns are interpreted to form above a pluton as a result of relatively low magma and hydrothermal fluid pressures. As these pressures increase during magma cooling, concentric and radial fractures are suggested to develop along with concentric tension fractures and normal faults. The resulting structural style is similar to that proposed by Knapp and Norton (1981), although the sequence of fracturing and the fracture types differ.

Burnham (1967, 1979) has analyzed the volatile history of a cooling pluton and has proposed an origin of fractures related to processes and consequences of the cooling of a hydrous magma. The mechanical energy which brings about fracturing of the hood of a pluton is suggested to result from a second boiling of water. Under certain conditions pressures in excess of lithostatic load develop, and the rigid tops of plutons fail by fracturing. This model of breaking by hydraulic fracturing is based on energies and water intrinsic to the pluton. Fracturing of wall rocks adjacent to plutons is, however, widespread, and it is not known whether the energy of waters intrinsic to the pluton is solely responsible for the ubiquitous fracturing of the large volumes of rocks in a porphyry copper system that extend well beyond the porphyry contacts.

Other fracturing mechanisms exist, including the heating of pore water in wall rocks. Knapp and Knight (1977) have considered the thermal history of pore waters in a hot pluton environment. A pluton cools by either convection or conduction of heat into cooler wall rocks. As the temperature of the wall rock increases from this transfer of heat, pore fluids in wall rocks are heated; with sufficient temperature increase, the effective pressure of these fluids becomes equal to the tensile strength of the rocks and results in fracture (Knapp and Knight, 1977). This process results in a front of fracturing corresponding to a thermal front that migrates away from the pluton. In view of the presence of multiple intrusions in many centers of porphyry copper mineralization, protracted times of cooling (resulting in widening aureoles of progressively higher rock temperatures [Norton and Knight, 1977]) may well be sufficient to develop the extensive fracturing present in so many systems.

It is probable that all three mechanisms—thermal effects, resurgent boiling of porphyry magmas, and heating of pore fluids in wall rocks—operate to induce fracturing of porphyry copper systems at different times and in different ways. A possible sequence of cause and effect is that of early but continuous rock failure from thermal effects followed by hydraulic fracturing in response to increased fluid pressures through crystallization. This mechanism may act intermittently, as successively lower levels of cooling magmas produce concentrations of volatiles, and it may, in turn, overlap with effects of the heating of pore fluids. Because a given volume of wall rock near a pluton undergoes heating and then cooling, multiple causes are reasonably sought. Multiple fracturing events are present in many porphyry copper systems. At Sierrita (Preece and Beane, in press; Haynes and Titley, 1980) and Silver Bell (Kanbergs, 1980) successive fracturing events became restricted in space to rock volumes progressively closer to parent plutons. Furthermore, the data from fluid inclusions studies in those two systems have revealed that the fluids which deposited minerals in each of the younger fracture sets became progressively cooler. Thus, a fundamental energy source in plutons appears to exist and to act intermittently as cooling proceeds.

Sources of Stress

Two fundamental styles of fracture orientation occur in porphyry copper deposits of the American Southwest. One, which appears to occur early in the intrusion history and particularly at high levels, is intrusion-centered and consists of concentric and radial fractures. This fracture style has also been recognized in some high-level intrusions of the southwestern Pacific (Titley and Heidrick, 1978). The other style is characterized by nearly monotonous strike directions and is revealed in much of the data from plutons in the American Southwest. The existing fracture geometries require contrasting stress distributions and, thus, differing sources of stress are sought.

Stresses related solely to thermal effects and energetics of pluton emplacement are dominated near pluton tops by vertical principal stress (σ_1). Intermediate and least principal stresses (σ_2 and σ_3) are horizontal and, under conditions which produce radial and concentric fractures, equal. This distribution of principal stresses is most likely at high levels in an intrusion system (for example, within a volcanic pile) or, as Knapp and Norton (1981) have suggested, at high levels around a pluton (when thermal effects from the initial results of pluton emplacement are pronounced).

The origin of the stresses which controlled the pronounced east-northeast direction of fracturing of Laramide porphyry plutons in the American Southwest is properly sought in geotectonic phenomena. The results of studies in many plutons in Arizona and New Mexico, which have been outlined earlier in this chapter, reveal unequivocally that the preferred orientation is region-wide. The direction is also temporally restricted, as shown in the results of studies of the same phenomena in post-Laramide intrusions of this same region (Rehrig and Heidrick, 1976). The east-northeast strike of fractures, veins, and dikes, so prominent during the Laramide, is absent in mid-Tertiary and younger (<30 m.y. old) districts and is replaced by a similarly profound north–north-northwest direction.

The nature of Laramide (e.g., 80–40 m.y. *sensu latus*) tectonics has been an object of many studies since the turn of the century. Many different interpretations of style and, consequently, of origin have been proposed. Structure-tectonic interpretations in many parts of southern Arizona have led workers to proposals of regional overthrusting, driven by regional compression (Ransome, 1904; Gilluly, 1956; Cooper and Silver, 1964; and Drewes, 1978). The sources of stress that produced the overthrusting have been interpreted in different ways. The low-angle "thrust" faults present in southern Arizona have been suggested to be low-angle normal faults or gravity glide faults localized along the flanks of uplifts (Jones, 1963, 1966). Vertical tectonics suggested by Jones have also been considered by Mayo (1966) and Mayo and Davis (1976) to be responsible for developing low-angle glide-faults and folds. Davis (1979) has proposed that basement-cored uplift, produced by regional compression, resulted in a tectonic style characterized by northwest-trending belts of deformation. The belts reveal uplift and folding of Paleozoic strata with northeast- and southwest-directed transport. Results of earlier studies of fractured plutons, in which the dominant east-northeast strike of structural elements was recognized, led Rehrig and Heidrick (1976) to the suggestion of east-northeast–directed compression that resulted in development of north-northwest–trending arches across Arizona. The delineated fracture and dike patterns were attributed to differential vertical uplift and concomitant extension in the shallow crust.

A synthesis of these many ideas into one regionally applicable model for Laramide tectonism awaits the results of much additional work. The region has been the site of many prior episodes of igneous and tectonic activity, each with its particular effect and signature. There is growing acceptance, however, of the existence of a Laramide compressive stress, directed west-southwest to east-northeast, that affected the tectonism of the southwestern Cordillera. Additional evidence for compressive stress of this orientation comes from consideration of plate tectonic phenomena.

The porphyry copper deposits of the Southwest developed over a remarkably narrow span of geologic time (see Tables 4.1 and 4.2.). Essentially all major productive districts were localized during Late Cretaceous-early Tertiary time. The oldest productive system (c. 75 m.y. old) signals the culmination of tectonism, magmatism, and metamorphism associated with the Franciscan, Sierra Nevada, and Sevier terrains to the west. Moreover, the older productive systems (70 to 75 m.y. old) are essentially synchronous with suggested major reorganizations in plate motions of the ocean basins surrounding North America (Coney, 1971, 1972, and 1973). Unfortunately, the quantification of the direction and rate of relative motions between North America and various Pacific Ocean plates during copper metallization is difficult to establish and requires the construction of either (a) relative motion vector circuits across seven different plate boundaries (Atwater and Molnar, 1973) or (b) "absolute motion" vectors using the Hawaii and Tristan de Cunha "hot spot" frame of reference (Morgan, 1972).

As demonstrated by Coney (1976), either construction shows southwestern North America interacting with the Farallon plate during the Laramide orogeny. Furthermore, both methods suggest very high rates of Farallon–North America convergent motion. The gross interaction of north-northeast to east-northeast underthrusting of the Farallon plate with the west to west-southwest movement of the North American plate away from Europe and spreading centers in the North Atlantic produced the profound east-northeast to west-southwest compression that characterizes the Laramide orogeny of the southwestern Cordillera. In addition to producing regional lateral compression, the resultant high convergence rates (12–20 cm/yr.), in concert with North American plate impingement on the youthful, warm, hydrated east flank of the Farallon-Pacific rise, produced the shallow, east-dipping Laramide Benioff zone (Lipman et al., 1972; Coney and Reynolds, 1977). This shallow, and at times probably sub-horizontal, attitude promoted an unusually wide belt of interspersed centers of intra-arc volcanic and plutonic activity, north to northwest–striking elongate basement-cored uplifts, flanking intermontane basins, and marginal upthrusts along ranges. These features are believed to have characterized the Laramide style of mountain building in this region. Several of the more significant elements of the Laramide tectonic framework, inferred relative motion vectors of the Farallon and North American plates, and suggested geometry of subduction at the peak of porphyry copper pluton emplacement are shown schematically in a paleotectonic reconstruction in Figure 4.10.

As has been shown and discussed here, the geometrical consequence of the proposed plate tectonic model is statistically evident in the fracture and dike patterns at many scales of observation—outcrop (bench face), mine, and district. Although ambiguous in some respects, the influence of the style of plate interactions is apparently provincial, in that most known porphyry copper systems of the Southwest appear to be systematically distributed, either along the axis of a north-northwest–trending arc orogen, or along sympathetic transverse belts of northeast strike. This interpretation is shown, together with the strain ellipsoid suggested from our synthesis for the Laramide, in Figure 4.11. As shown on this figure, the sum of fracture and dike orientations fixes the direction of maximum principal stress *(B–B')* and the major arc orogen is seen to lie within a belt corresponding to the orientation of the axis of greatest strain *(A–A')*. The subordinate northeast-trending belts of deposits correspond to transverse direction parallel to maximum crustal extension.

One effect of Laramide stress as we view it here was to produce a northwest-striking left-lateral couple. Such a stress and the evolution of northwest-striking, left-lateral faults is consistent with many interpretations, commencing with those of Schmitt (1966), of this style of Laramide faulting in the Southwest. The orientation of this shear couple of N50°W (see Fig. 4.11, *X–X'*) is, coincidently, parallel to the orientation of a group of older structural features believed to have influenced patterns of sedimentation during the late Paleozoic and Mesozoic in southeastern Arizona (Titley, 1976). These structures, or discontinuities, are shown by numbered lines in Figure 4.11, and one of them, the Sawmill Canyon Fault (2), has been interpreted to have undergone left lateral movement during the Laramide (Drewes, 1972).

Thus, in our view a pattern has emerged involving Laramide structural elements of diverse nature and histories that is at least partially consistent with more broadly interpreted geotectonic phenomena. The driving force that produced the

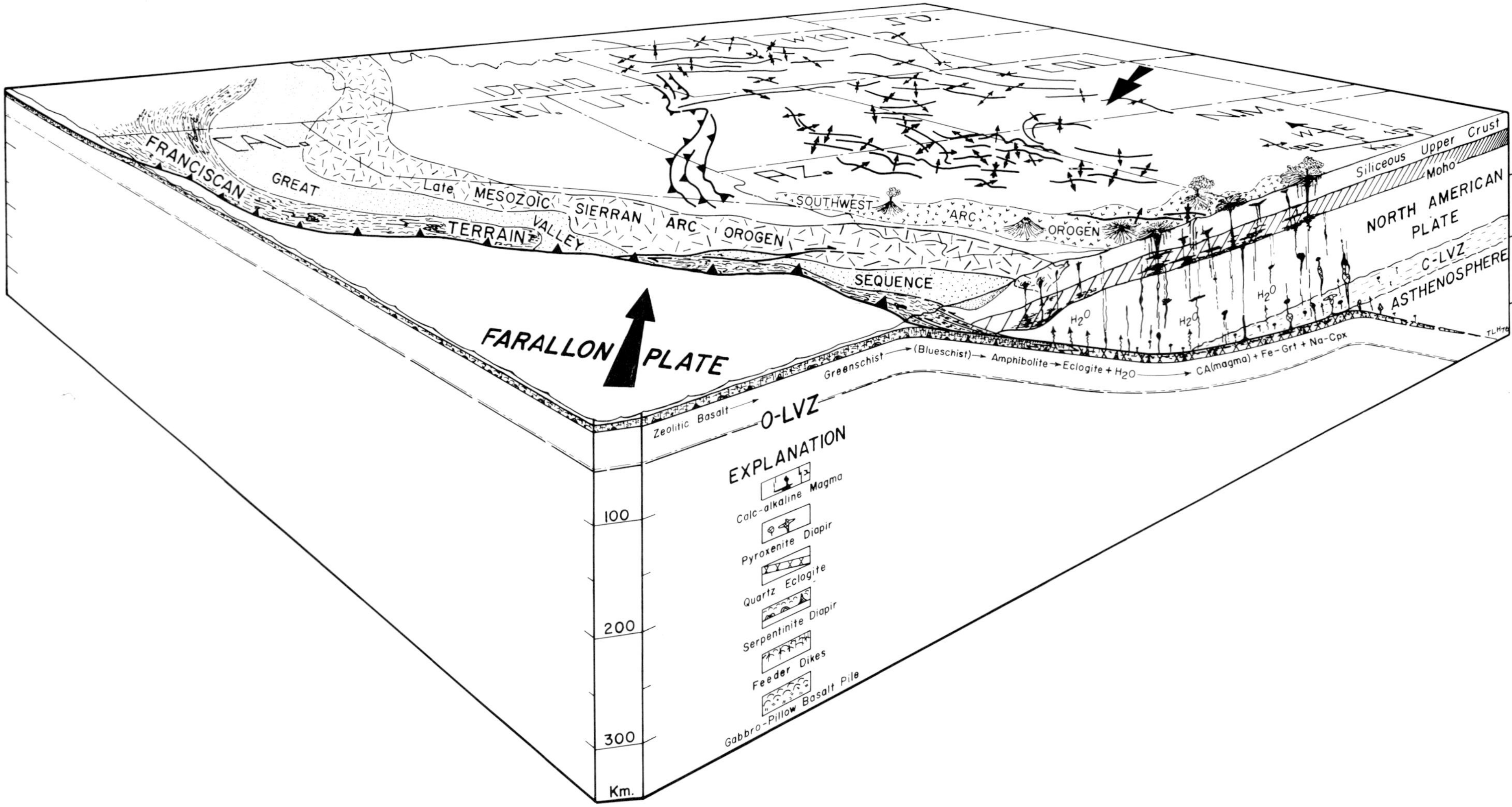

Figure 4.10. Partial paleotectonic model of the southwestern United States during Laramide time. Middle and late Tertiary distortions resulting from wrench faulting along the San Andreas system and Basin and Range rifting are not removed. Heavy black arrows show accepted "absolute motion" vectors for the North American and Farallon plates during early Laramide porphyry copper metallization.

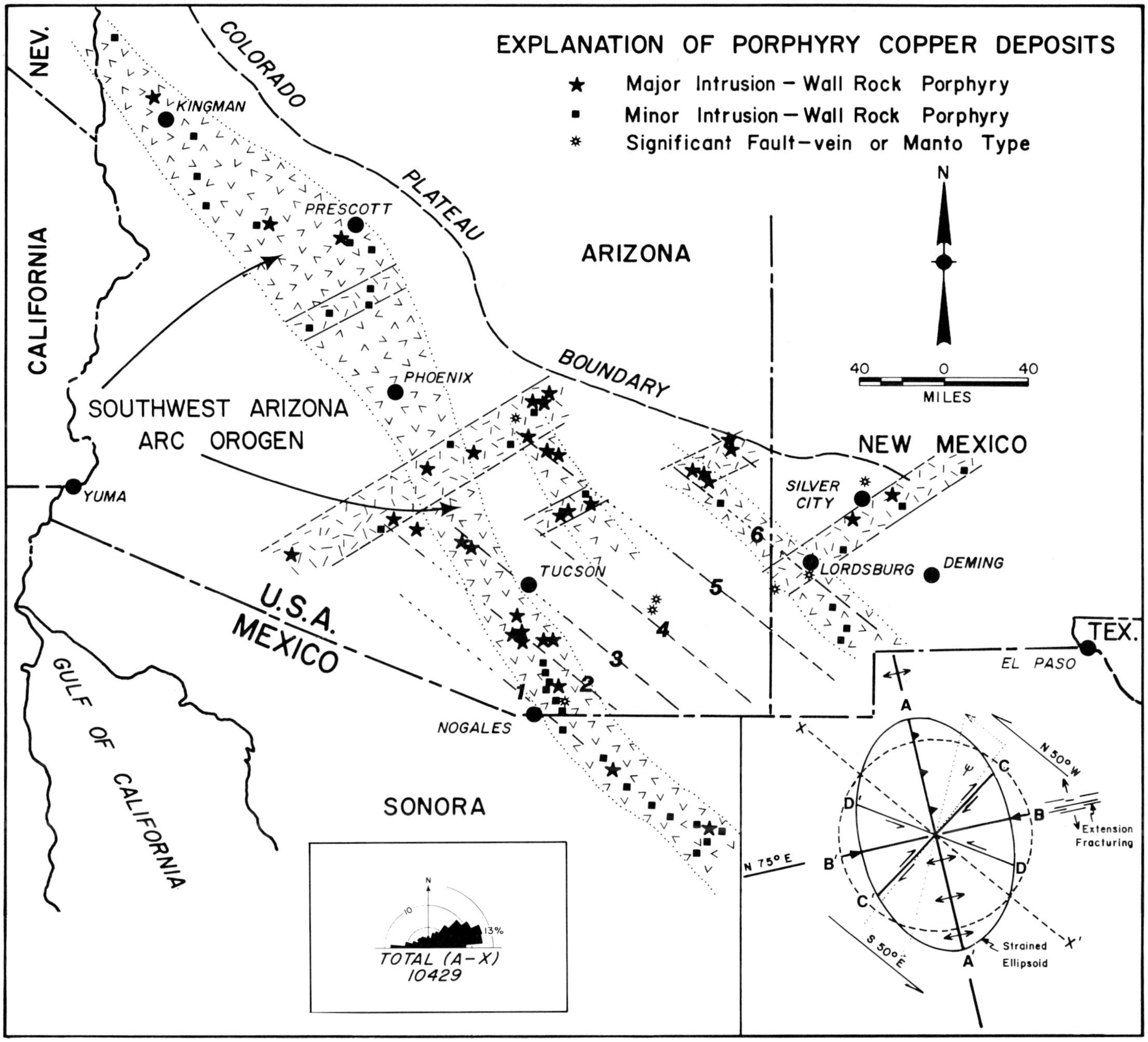

Figure 4.11. Laramide volcano-tectonic framework of southwestern New Mexico and southern Arizona shows the distribution of major and minor porphyry deposits, summation of megascopic strike rosettes (see Fig. 4.9), derived inter-mineral paleostrain field, position of inferred composite Andean arc orogen, and several transverse east-northeast–trending porphyry breaks. The northwest-trending linear discontinuities (1–6) are adapted from Titley (1976). The discontinuities have influenced Permian and Cretaceous depositional patterns and include, from south to north, (1) the Comobabi-Nogales discontinuity, (2) the Sawmill Canyon fault zone, (3) the Bisbee discontinuity, (4) the Dragoon discontinuity, (5) the Dos Cabezas discontinuity, and (6) the Gila discontinuity.

features present may be considered in great part related to plate interactions and may reflect long-lived and profound regional compressive stresses oriented east-northeast to west-southwest. Such stresses, active during the entire Laramide orogeny, are reflected in the close similarity of dike and fracture patterns among many deposits of the region, whose ages span a time of nearly 20 m.y. We should further emphasize the fact that interpretations of geotectonic phenomena on the scale considered here appear to be reflected in the responses of rocks observed on the largest scale of mapping and interpretation. Consequently, other regions may be considered potentially responsive to similar investigations and may yield similarly useful data amenable to regional tectonic synthesis.

ACKNOWLEDGMENTS

The interpretations of field data presented here have benefitted from discussions with many colleagues in industry, academia, and the U.S. Geological Survey. Professor Evans

B. Mayo was a source of many ideas from which the study of fractures evolved and his continued interest in this work is gratefully acknowledged. W. H. Rehrig was involved in the early stages of some of the work and his continued interest is appreciated. D. L. Norton has been a constructive critic of many of our ideas concerning the origin of fractures. Access to and study of many of the districts and deposits of this region were aided by many mining companies and geologists; without this freedom of access, the study would not have been possible.

Funds made available by the Department of Geosciences of the University of Arizona were used to support both field work and some computer analysis. Computer facilities used were those at the University of Arizona. Additional funding for some of the work was made available through AMAX, Inc., and ASARCO, Inc. Mrs. Georgia Recchio typed the manuscript. We acknowledge with thanks reviews of the chapter by Joe Wilkins and Professor G. H. Davis. Permission to publish results of this study was given by Gulf Mineral Resources Co.

REFERENCES CITED

Anderson, C. A., 1948, Structural control of copper mineralization, Bagdad, Arizona: AIME Trans., v. 178, p. 170–180.

———, 1968, Arizona and adjacent New Mexico, *in* Ore deposits of the United States, 1933–1967, v. 2: New York, Am. Inst. Mining, Metall. and Petrol. Eng., p. 1163–1190.

Atwater, T., and Molnar, P., 1973, Relative motion of the Pacific and North American plates deduced from sea-floor spreading in the Atlantic, Indian, and South Pacific Oceans: Stanford Univ. Publ. in Geol. Sci., v. 13, p. 136–148.

Banks, N. G.; Cornwall, H. R.; Silberman, M. L.; Creasey, S. C.; and Marvin, R. F., 1972, Chronology of intrusion and ore deposition at Ray, Arizona: Part I, K-Ar ages: Econ. Geol. v. 67, p. 864–878.

Banks, N. G. and Stuckless, J. S., 1973, Chronology of intrusion and ore deposition at Ray, Arizona: Part II, Fission-track ages: Econ. Geol. v. 68, p. 657–664.

Baumer, A., and Fraser, R. B., 1975, Paguna porphyry copper deposit, Bougainville, *in* Knight, C. L., ed., Economic geology of Australia and Papua New Guinea, 1: Metals: Australasian Inst. Mining Metallurgy Mon. 5, p. 855–866.

Bikerman, M., 1967, Isotopic studies in the Roskruge Mountains, Pima County, Arizona: Geol. Soc. America Bull., v. 78, p. 1029–1036.

Bikerman, M. and Damon, P. E., 1966, K-Ar chronology of the Tucson Mountains, Pima County, Arizona: Geol. Soc. America Bull., v. 77, p. 1225–1234.

Blake, S. W., 1971, Geology, alteration, and mineralization of the San Juan mine area, Graham County, Arizona: Unpub. M.S. Thesis, Univ. Ariz., 85 p.

Burnham, C. W., 1967, Hydrothermal fluids at the magmatic stage, *in* Barnes, H. L., ed., Geochemistry of Hydrothermal Ore Deposits: New York, Holt, Rinehart and Winston, Inc., p. 34–76.

———, 1979, Magmas and hydrothermal fluids, *in* Barnes, H. L., ed., Geochemistry of Hydrothermal Ore Deposits, 2nd Ed.: New York, J. Wiley & Sons, p. 71–136.

Butler, B. S., and Wilson, E. D., 1938, Clifton Morenci district: Ariz. Bur. Mines, Geol. Ser. no. 12, Bull. 145, p. 72–80.

Coney, P. J., 1971, Cordilleran tectonic transitions and motion of the North American plate: Nature, v. 233, p. 462–465.

———, 1972, Cordilleran tectonics and North American plate motion: Am. Jour. Sci., v. 292, p. 603–628.

———, 1973, Mesozoic-Cenozoic Cordilleran plate tectonics: Geol. Soc. America, Mem. 152.

———, 1976, Plate tectonics and Laramide orogeny: New Mexico Geol. Soc. Spec. Pub. 6, p. 5–10.

Coney, P. J., and Reynolds, S. J., 1977, Cordilleran Benioff zones: Nature, v. 270, p. 403–406.

Cooper, J. R., and Silver, L. T., 1964, Geology and ore deposits of the Dragoon quadrangle, Cochise County, Arizona: U.S. Geol. Survey Prof. Paper 416, 196 p.

Corn, R. M., 1975, Alteration-mineralization zoning, Red Mountain, Arizona: Econ. Geol. v. 70, p. 1437–1447.

Cornwall, H. R., and Krieger, M. H., 1974, Geologic map of the Kearny quadrangle, Pinal County, Arizona: U.S. Geol. Survey Map GQ-1188, scale 1:24,000.

Creasey, S. C., 1967, General geology of the Mammoth quadrangle, Pinal County, Arizona: U.S. Geol. Survey Bull. 1218, 95 p.

Creasey, S. C., and Kistler, R. W., 1962, Age of some copper-bearing porphyries and other igneous rocks in southeastern Arizona, *in* Geological Survey Research 1962, U.S. Geol. Survey Prof. Paper 450-D, p. D1–D5.

Damon, P. E., (compiler), 1969, Correlation and chronology of ore deposits and volcanic rocks—U.S. Atomic Energy Comm. Contract AT(11–1)-689, Ann. Prog. Rept. C00–689–120: Tucson, Univ. Ariz. Geochronology Laboratory.

Damon, P. E.; Mauger, R. L.; and Bikerman, M., 1964, K-Ar dating of Laramide plutonic and volcanic rocks within the Basin and Range province of Arizona and Sonora: Internat. Geol. Cong. 22d, India, Part 3, Proc. Sec. 3, p. 45–55.

Damon, P. E., and Mauger, R. L., 1966, Epeirogeny-orogeny viewed from the Basin and Range Province: AIME Trans., v. 235, no. 1, p. 99–112.

Davis, G. H., 1979, Laramide folding and faulting in southeastern Arizona: Am. Jour. Sci., v. 279, p. 543–569.

Drewes, Harald, 1972, Structural geology of the Santa Rita Mountains, southeast of Tucson, Arizona: U.S. Geol. Survey Prof. Paper 748, 35 p.

———, 1978, The Cordilleran orogenic belt between Nevada and Chihuahua: Geol. Soc. America Bull., v. 89, p. 641–657.

Dunn, P. G., 1978, Regional structure of the Safford district, Arizona: Ariz. Geol. Soc. Digest XI, p. 9–15.

———, 1982, Geology of the Copper Flat Porphyry Copper Deposit, Hillsboro, Sierra County, New Mexico: *in* Titley, S. R., ed., Advances in Geology of the Porphyry Copper Deposits, Southwestern North America: Tucson, Univ. Ariz. Press, Chapter 14.

Erickson, R. C., 1968, Geology and geochronology of the Dos Cabezas Mountains, Cochise County, Arizona, *in* Southern Arizona Guidebook III: Ariz. Geol. Soc. Tucson, p. 192–198.

Gilluly, James, 1956, The Ajo mining district, Arizona: U.S. Geol. Survey Prof. Paper 209, 112 p.

Guthrie, J. O., and Moore, D. G., 1978, The geology of the Copper Creek area, Bunker Hill mining district, Galliuro Mountains, Arizona: Ariz. Geol. Soc. Digest XI, p. 25–31.

Haynes, F. M., and Titley, S. R., 1980, The evolution of fracture-related permeability within the Ruby Star Granodiorite, Sierrita porphyry copper deposit, Pima County, Arizona: Econ. Geol., v. 75, p. 673–683.

Hedlund, D. C., 1974, Age and structural setting of base-metal mineralization in the Hillsboro-San Lorenzo area, southwestern New Mexico (abs.), *in* Ghost Ranch: New Mexico Geol. Soc. Guidebook 25, p. 378–379.

Heidrick, T. L., 1974, A dynamic model for fracturing and diking in Laramide plutons of Arizona (abs.): Geol. Soc. Am., Rocky Mtn. Sect. Mtg., Program with Abstracts, p. 445–446.

Heidrick, T. L., and W. A. Rehrig, 1972, Mesoscopic fracturing in nonproductive Laramide stocks and porphyry copper deposits of Arizona (abs.): Geol. Soc. Am., Program with Abstracts, v. 3, no. 6, p. 387.

Heidrick, T. L., and Titley, S. R., 1976, Structural evolution of southwestern North American Laramide porphyry copper deposits and its relationship to the history of plate interactions: Int. Geol. Congr., 25th, Sydney, Abstracts, v. 3, p. 740.

Johnston, W. P., 1972, K-Ar dates on intrusive rocks and alteration associated with the Lakeshore porphyry copper deposit, Pinal County, Arizona: Isochron/West, no. 4, p. 29–30.

Jones, R. W., 1963, Structural evolution of part of southeastern Arizona: Am. Assoc. Petrol. Geol., Mem. 2, p. 140–151.

———, 1966, Differential vertical uplift—a major factor in the structural evolution of southeastern Arizona: Ariz. Geol. Soc. Digest VIII, p. 97–124.

Kanbergs, Karlis, 1980, Fracturing along the margins of a porphyry copper system, Silver Bell District, Pima County, Arizona: Unpub. M.S. Thesis, Univ. Ariz., 90 p.

Knapp, R. B., and Knight, J. E., 1977, Differential thermal expansion of pore fluids: Fracture propagation and microearthquake production in hot pluton environments: Jour. Geophys. Res., v. 82, p. 2515–2522.

Knapp, R. B., and Norton, D. L., 1981, Preliminary numerical analysis of processes related to magma crystallization and stress evaluation in cooling pluton environments: Am. Jour. Sci., v. 281, p. 35–68.

Koide, H., and Bhattacharji, S., 1975, Formation of fractures around magmatic intrusions and their role in ore localization: Econ. Geology, v. 70, p. 781–799.

Krieger, M. H., 1974*a,* Geologic map of the Winkelman quadrangle, Pinal and Gila Counties, Arizona: U.S. Geol. Survey, Geol. Map GQ-1106, scale 1:24,000.

———, 1974*b,* Geologic map of the Crozier Peak quadrangle, Pinal County, Arizona: U.S. Geol. Survey, Map GQ-1107, scale 1:24,000.

Langton, J. M., and Williams, S. A., 1982, Structural, petrological, and mineralogical controls for the Dos Pobres orebody, Lone Star mining district, Graham County, Arizona: *in* Titley, S. R., ed., Advances in Geology of the Porphyry Copper Deposits, Southwestern North America: Tucson, Univ. Ariz. Press., Chapter 16.

Lindgren, W., 1905, The copper deposits of the Clifton, Morenci district, Arizona: U.S. Geol. Survey Prof. Paper 43, 412 p.

Lipman, P. W.; Prostka, H. J.; and Christiansen, R. L., 1972, Cenozoic volcanism and plate-tectonic evolution of the western United States, I: Early and middle Cenozoic: Royal Soc. London Phil. Trans., v. 271, p. 217–248.

Livingston, D. E., 1973, A plate tectonic hypothesis for the genesis of porphyry copper deposits of the southern Basin and Range province: Earth and Planet. Ltrs., v. 20, p. 171–179.

Livingston, D. E.; Mauger, R. L.; and Damon, P. E., 1968, Geochronology of the emplacement, enrichment, and preservation of Arizona porphyry copper deposits: Econ. Geol., v. 63, p. 30–36.

Loring, A., and Loring, R., 1980, Age of thrust faulting—Little Hatchet Mountains, southwestern New Mexico: Isochron/West, no. 27, p. 29–30.

Marvin, R. F.; Stern, T. W.; Creasey, S. C.; and Mehnert, H. H., 1973, Radiometric ages of igneous rocks, Pima, Santa Cruz, and Cochise counties, southeast Arizona: U.S. Geol. Survey Bull. 1379, 27 p.

Marvin, R. F.; Naeser, C. W.; and Mehnert, H. H., 1978, Tabulation of radiometric ages—including unpublished K-Ar and fission-track ages for rocks in southeastern Arizona and southwestern New Mexico: New Mexico Geol. Soc. Guidebook 29, p. 243–252.

Mauger, R. L.; Damon, P. E.; and Giletti, B. J., 1965, Isotopic dating of Arizona ore deposits: AIME Trans. v. 232, p. 81–87.

Mayo, E. B., 1966, Preliminary report on a structural study in the Museum Embayment, Tucson Mountains, Arizona: Ariz. Geol. Soc. Digest VIII, p. 1–32.

Mayo, E. B., and Davis, G. H., 1976, Origin of the Red Hills—Piedmontite Hills uplift: Ariz. Geol. Soc. Digest X, p. 103–131.

McDowell, F. W., 1971, K-Ar ages of igneous rocks from the western United States: Isochron/West, no. 2, p. 1–17.

McKinstry, H. E., 1955, Structure of hydrothermal ore deposits: Econ. Geol., 50th Anniv. Vol., p. 170–225.

Morgan, W. J., 1972, Plate motions and deep mantle convection, *in* Shagam, R., and others, eds., Studies in Earth and Space Sciences (Hess Volume): Geol. Soc. America Mem. 132, p. 7–22.

Norton, D. L., and Knight, J. E., 1977, Transport phenomena in hydrothermal systems: Cooling plutons: Amer. Jour. Sci., v. 277, p. 937–981.

Pennebaker, E. N., 1942, Robinson mining district, Nevada, *in* Newhouse, W. H., ed., Ore Deposits as Related to Structural Features: Princeton, Princeton Univ. Press, p. 128–131.

Preece, R. K. III, and Beane, R. E., in press, Contrasting evolutions of hydrothermal alteration in quartz monzonite and quartz diorite at the Sierrita porphyry copper deposit, Arizona: Econ. Geol. v. 76.

Ransome, F. L., 1904, The geology and ore deposits of the Bisbee quadrangle, Arizona: U.S. Geol. Survey Prof. Paper 12, 168 p.

———, 1919, Copper deposits of Ray and Miami, Arizona: U.S. Geol. Survey Prof. Paper 115, 192 p.

Rehrig, W. A., and Heidrick, T. L., 1972, Regional fracturing in Laramide stocks of Arizona and its relationship to porphyry copper mineralization: Econ. Geol., v. 67, p. 198–213.

———, 1976, Regional tectonic stress during the Laramide and late Tertiary intrusive periods, Basin and Range province, Arizona: Ariz. Geol. Soc. Digest X, p. 205–228.

Rehrig, W. A.; Shafiqullah, M.; and Damon, P. E., 1980, Geochronology, geology, and listric normal faulting of the Vulture Mountains, Maricopa County, Arizona: Ariz. Geol. Soc. Digest XII, p. 89–110.

Rose, A. W., and Cook, D. R., 1965, Radioactive age dates of porphyry copper deposits in western United States (abs.): Geol. Soc. Amer. Ann. Mtg. Kansas City, Mo., Program with Abstracts, p. 141–142.

Schmidt, E. A., 1970, A belt of Laramide intrusive rocks in southeast Arizona, *in* Correlation and Chronology of Ore Deposits and Volcanic Rocks, U.S. Atomic Energy Comm., Ann. Prog. Report C00–689–1301, p. 29–32.

Schmitt, H. A., 1966, The porphyry copper deposits in their regional setting, *in* Titley, S. R., and Hicks, C. L., eds., Geology of the Porphyry Copper Deposits, Southwestern North America: Tucson, Univ. Ariz. Press, p. 17–33.

Shafiqullah, M., and Langlois, J. D., 1978, The Pima mining district, Arizona—a geochronologic update: New Mexico Geol. Soc. Guidebook, 29th Field Conf., p. 321–327.

Titley, S. R., 1976, Evidence for a Mesozoic linear tectonic pattern in southeastern Arizona: Ariz. Geol. Soc. Digest X, p. 71–101.

Titley, S. R., and Heidrick, T. L., 1978, Intrusion and fracture styles of some mineralized porphyry systems of the southwestern Pacific and their relationship to plate interactions: Econ. Geol., v. 73, p. 891–903.

Wilkinson, W. H., Jr.; Vega, L. A.; and Titley, S. R., 1982, The geology and ore deposits at Mineral Park, Mohave County, Arizona, *in* Titley, S. R., ed., Advances in Geology of the Porphyry Copper Deposits, Southwestern North America: Tucson, Univ. Ariz. Press, Chapter 26.

5

The Style and Progress of Mineralization and Alteration in Porphyry Copper Systems

AMERICAN SOUTHWEST

Spencer R. Titley

The manifestations of alteration and mineralization in many porphyry copper systems result from complex mechanical and hydrothermal processes and the ensuing effects of weathering. The rocks of these deposits reveal that they have been repeatedly fractured and altered and that the physical and chemical conditions of ore and alteration mineral deposition have changed through the geologic history of the system. It is the purpose of this chapter to describe the nature of manifestations of different kinds of alteration of porphyry copper systems and to review the interpretations of alteration types in the context of the way in which the alteration and mineralization evolve.

Results of many studies of porphyry copper systems, commencing with those of Peterson and others at Castle Dome in 1949, have shown that alteration of porphyry copper deposits is a complex phenomenon; it involves not only changes of alteration types in space but also changes of composition of alteration products in time. The process results in rock volumes within porphyry copper deposits in which many alteration types may be present and separable on the basis of crosscutting veinlet relationships and on the assessment of the stability of mineral assemblages with respect to one another. Alteration paragenesis as deduced from studies of altered rocks and vein alteration assemblages indicates that, in the range of compositions of igneous rocks common to many porphyry deposits of the southwestern North American province, a persistent sequence of alteration types and styles is commonly present. Felsic igneous host rocks from within the mineralized parts of deposits usually record an early potassic alteration characterized first by precipitation of biotite, then by precipitation of orthoclase. These alteration mineral types may be synchronous with development of minerals of the propylitic assemblage (epidote, chlorite, calcite) at the fringe of the system. Propylitic alteration may proceed inward with time but appears to pre-date evolution of clay mineral assemblages and development of the phyllic assemblage (quartz, sericite, and pyrite). Variations in this sequence or in the stable assemblages may be present in different deposits, in different parts of the same deposit, or in rocks with differing compositions in the same deposit. As a result, the definition of discrete zones of alteration in porphyry copper systems, characterized by single specific alteration assemblages, is not ordinarily possible unless paragenesis is also considered. The type of veinlet alteration cannot ordinarily be used as a criterion for identification of the alteration type affecting the rock as a whole because of superposition of alteration types.

The chemical and mineralogical composition of host rocks exerts a profound control on the alteration minerals produced under changing thermochemical conditions. Similarly, mechanical properties of rocks, together with compositional characteristics, influence the evolutionary style of alteration and mineralization. When the rocks are ultimately exposed to the effects of weathering, the style of alteration and mineralization further influences the nature and expression of the weathered zone which results. Because of the many permutations of primary and secondary alteration features which evolve, an awareness of such variation is important to the proper understanding and assessment of the evolution of a particular system and of outcrop studies.

GENERAL CHARACTERISTICS AND ENVIRONMENTS OF ALTERATION AND METALLIZATION

The hydrothermal processes which produce the large metallized and altered copper systems include the effects of mechanical and thermal energy changes, changes in chemical energy, and the effects of changing patterns of fluid transport and flow. The process results in three generally distinguishable manifestations of alteration: selectively pervasive alteration, pervasive alteration, and the alteration along veins and veinlets. A common result of selectively pervasive alteration, which affects specific minerals of rocks, is enhancement of rock texture. This alteration is commonly the most widely distributed type present in these systems. Pervasive alteration, as used here, is that which results in destruction of original rock textures because of its apparent non-selective nature. Such alteration is most commonly present within or near the mineralized centers. Vein-veinlet alteration attends deposition of most of the volume of ore minerals. The alteration type progresses from fractures into the walls of veins, and, although some sulfide mineralization extends into veinlet walls, such mineralization is most commonly and most abundantly localized along vein-veinlet centers. Vein-veinlet alteration develops in fractures, which may occur in all rocks of a system.

Porphyry copper deposits are commonly described as disseminated, in allusion to the nature of distribution of ore minerals. Such a description and its implications, however, are correct only at scales which consider the deposits in their entirety. At the scale of mining, mineralization is accurately referred to as disseminated because large volumes of rock contain relatively uniformly distributed values of metal. In actual fact, the disseminated mineralization is the product of alteration along vein walls, with concurrent deposition of sulfide minerals in the vein or within the vein alteration selvage. These characteristics of mineralization were recognized at Globe-Miami in the zone of supergene enrichment by Ransome (1919) and have been succinctly summarized by Parsons (1957). This aspect of porphyry copper metallization has long been known, but the characteristic requires re-emphasis in the context of the increased understanding of the metallizing process. Minor amounts of disseminated mineralization occur in most deposits and are characterized most commonly by grains of sulfide localized chiefly in the sites of mafic minerals. Close study of the habit of occurrence of sulfides in many deposits nonetheless reveals that, even where apparently disseminated, sulfide grains can be seen to occur in linear or sinuous microfractures of host rocks. An excellent description of this habit has been presented by Anderson and others (1955) from their study at Bagdad, where it was noted that isolated euhedral crystals of sulfides occur in chain-like distribution in host rocks. This distribution suggests that mineralization was fracture guided but that associated quartz and orthoclase alteration healed the controlling fracture. An example of mineralization controlled by veins, microveinlets and mafic sites is shown on Figure 5.1.

Porphyry copper deposits are mineralized systems related to plutons and, consequently, are the result of the emplacement and cooling history of magmas. In most instances the intrusive rocks are porphyries emplaced at relatively shallow crustal levels. Exceptions to this generalization may be some deposits of the Canadian Cordillera, where a porphyry association is less certain and the deposits are interpreted as genetically related to equigranular intrusions—the "plutonic porphyry deposits" of Sutherland Brown (1976).

A general concept, by no means documented for all porphyry copper systems, holds that the deposits are parts of sub-volcanic plutons. Such a genesis has been inferred or suggested for the Pacific Basin Rim—particularly South America (Sillitoe, 1973), for island arcs in general (Mitchell and Bell, 1973), for the southwestern Pacific islands (Branch, 1976; Mason and McDonald, 1978), for the Philippines (Wolfe, 1973), and for the Caribbean islands and Central America (Kesler et al., 1977). In the American Southwest, pre-ore Laramide volcanic rocks are hosts to some intrusions which are centers to copper mineralization. The volcanogenic association of some porphyry copper deposits of the Canadian Cordillera is less certain, except that Lower Mesozoic volcanic rocks are hosts to much younger plutons. Where a volcanogenic association can be shown for a porphyry copper deposit, however, there is seldom adequate radiometric age data to establish a common genesis of volcanic rocks, plutons, and metals. Notwithstanding many uncertainties concerning the sub-volcanic nature of porphyry copper plutons, the evidence from rock textures and from interpretations based upon restoration of pre-ore geologic cover in the southwestern United States (Titley, 1972*a*, 1982; Heidrick and Titley, 1982) suggests emplacement of the porphyry plutons to relatively shallow crustal levels (tops at 1–5 km depth).

Porphyry copper systems encompass far greater volumes of rock than solely that of the pluton or the porphyry intrusion complexes. In some instances it is clear from the geologic evidence in the American Southwest that pre-mineral cover above the intrusions was an important host for primary copper mineralization. Within intrusions and intrusive complexes, mineralization and alteration may occur across several kilometers of height. Although known initially only from the results of drill hole data, and although the geometry of the porphyry progenitor has not been reported, mineralization of the Kalamazoo orebody (Lowell, 1968) occurs over an original vertical interval of more than 3 km. Norton (1982) has shown generalized geological cross sections of several important porphyry systems of this region in which the environments of alteration within the plutons and their hosts can be interpreted as extending over many vertical kilometers. Geological relationships reported from three major porphyry copper systems of this region further indicate that the tops of some intrusions have not been penetrated or may lie at depths beyond the limit of exploration. These include the San Juan orebody at Safford (Robinson and Cook, 1966) and the Dos Pobres orebody, also at Safford, where Langton and Williams (1982) have suggested that deep drilling may have just penetrated a pluton 1 km below the surface. At Red Mountain (Corn, 1975), exploration to depths of 2 km has not revealed a pluton, notwithstanding the presence of porphyry copper type mineralization across that interval. In these three systems copper mineralization occurs in pre-ore volcanic rocks, in close association with dike and sill swarms, presumably above a parent pluton. Generalized geological relationships, assuming a sub-volcanic emplacement of porphyry copper plutons, are shown for the geologic setting of some porphyry copper deposits in southeastern Arizona in Figure 5.2. This figure is composited

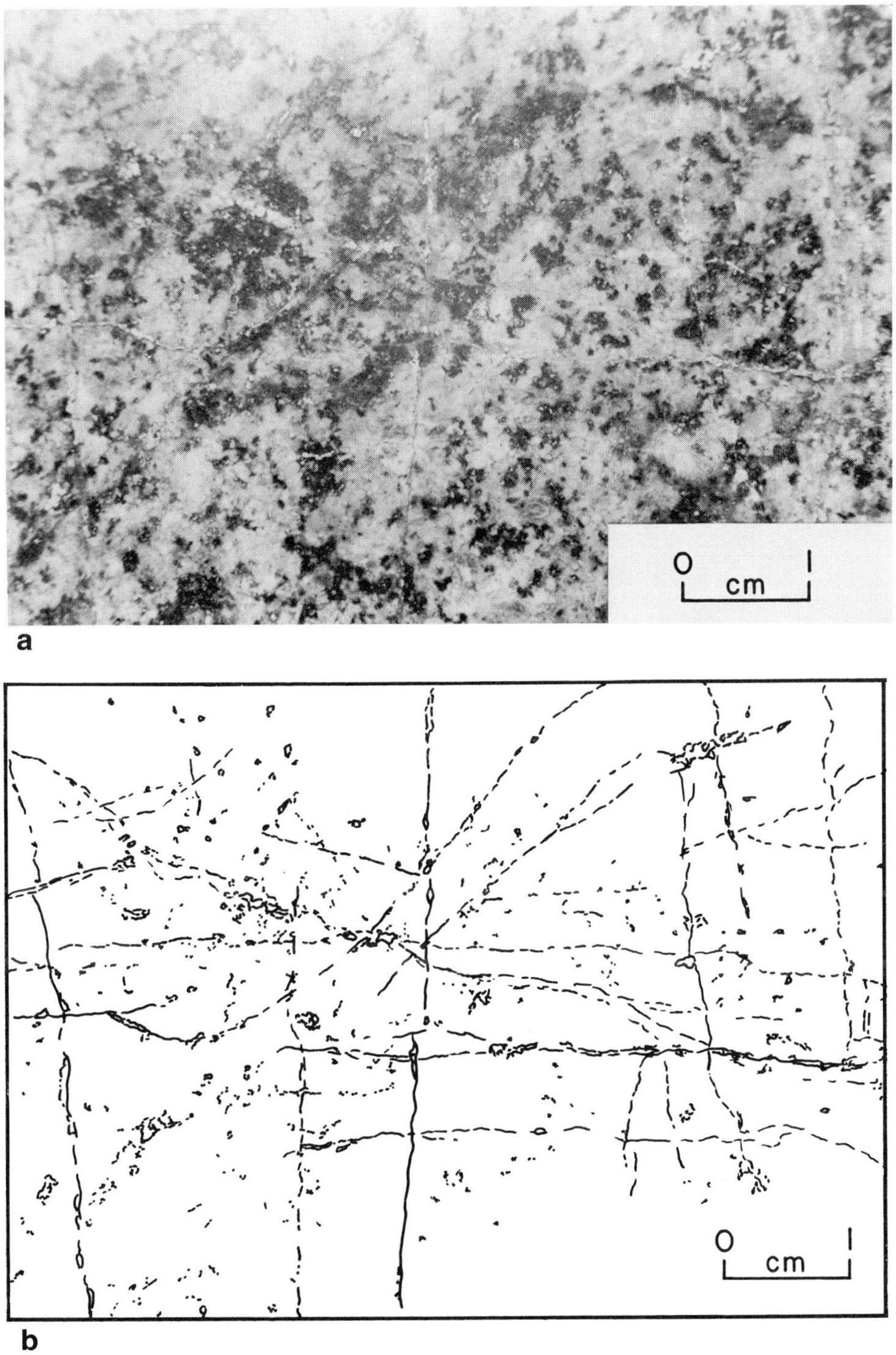

Figure 5.1. Fracture and veinlet-microveinlet control of mineralization in Harris Ranch Quartz Monzonite, an igneous host rock at Sierrita: *a*, photograph of the surface showing the commonplace nature of fracture and veinlet-microveinlet control of sulfide mineralization; *b*, an artist's emphasis of the distribution of sulfide minerals showing the typical chains of isolated sulfide grains evolved along micro-fractures and further controlled by positions of interstitial biotite in the host rock.

from many systems and shows the range of hydrothermal effects at deep and shallow levels as they have been interpreted from Silver Bell, Sierrita, Red Mountain, and Twin Buttes.

Viewed in the context of a volcanic system many kilometers in height, extending from parts of a sub-aerial volcanic pile to the plutonic environment at many kilometers of depth, and based upon geologic evidence that the hydrothermal systems were active over much of that area, it can be inferred that many different chemical and mechanical environments influenced the evolutionary style of porphyry copper systems at different times. At the time of porphyry emplacement, lithostatic loads across the system may have ranged from 0.5 to 3 or 4 kb. Host rocks to the plutons heated and then cooled during the dying stages of pluton cooling. Fracturing of the pluton and its hosts lowered pressures on the hydrothermal system and, with the passing of time, oxidizing conditions appear in some instances to have penetrated into the deeper

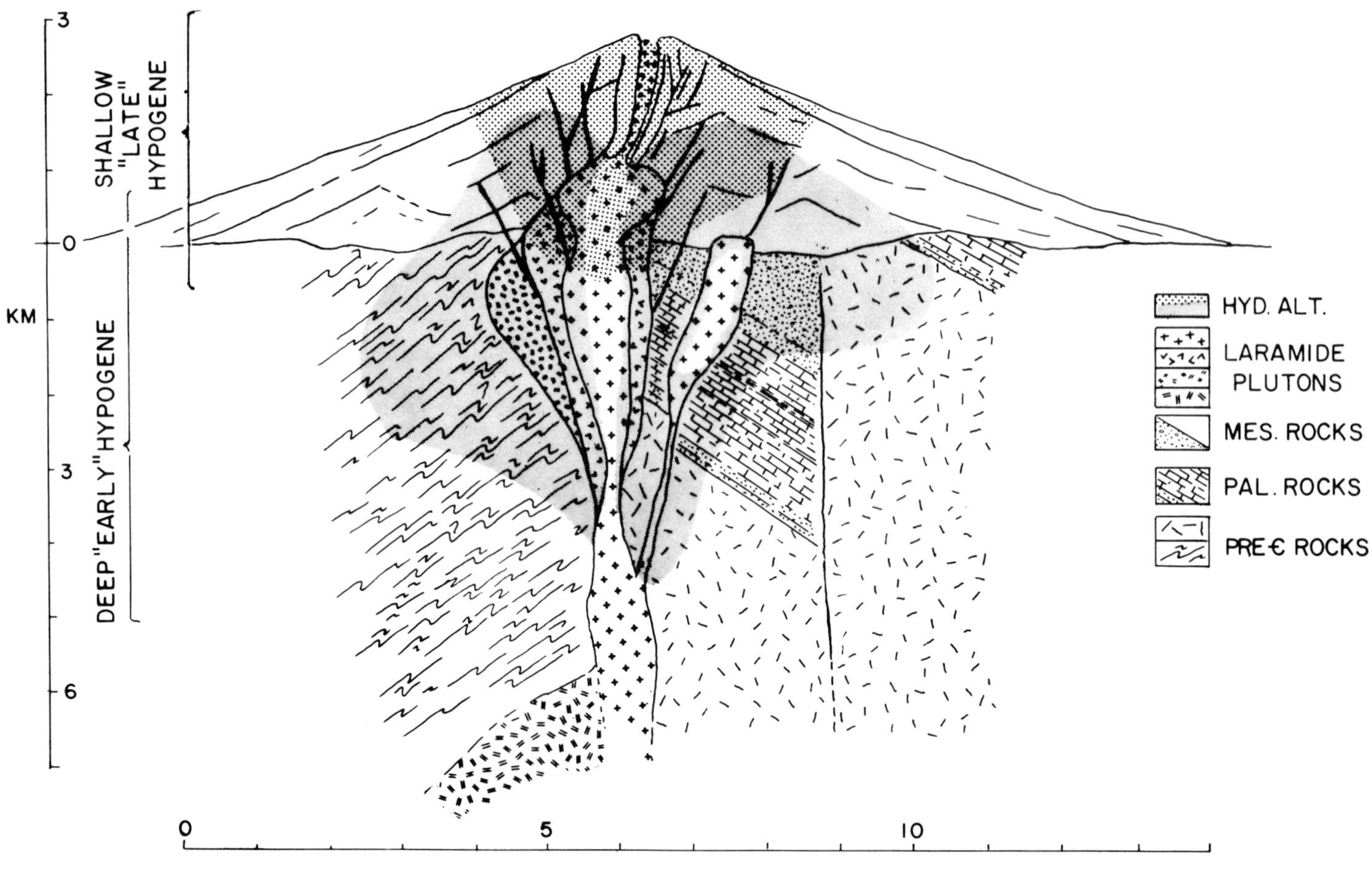

Figure 5.2. Generalized geological cross section of a composited porphyry copper system in southeastern Arizona. The cross section assumes a sub-volcanic origin of plutons, emplaced within a stratovolcanic system. Features at the top of the pluton are interpreted from data from Red Mountain and the Safford deposits. At depth, geological features are composited from Silver Bell and from basement relationships in the Globe-Miami district. Deep hypogene alteration is scaled from effects at Sierrita, and shallow hypogene relationships are suggested from features at Red Mountain.

hypogene reducing environments. The variation in lithostatic load, as a function of depth, together with changed stress orientations and magnitudes, resulted in different fracture-vein orientations and styles.

The view across porphyry systems is probably only a fraction of that of the total height of the original system, for there are few data at this time for most deposits which allow accurate or, in some cases, even approximate placing of the level at its original position within the deposit. Consequently no values can be assigned to terms such as deep, intermediate, or shallow when applied to relative depths. In some instances fracture patterns and the nature of alteration assemblages allow a subjective approximation of the environment studied to relatively deep or relatively shallow; changes from reducing to oxidizing enviroments with time can also sometimes be assessed.

HYPOGENE ENVIRONMENT

With few exceptions, the exposures of porphyry copper deposits are at levels within the deeper hypogene environment. At these levels the style and sequence of alteration types are broadly similar within those deposits for which detailed studies have been reported. These similarities include both an early widespread selectively pervasive alteration and a late, more restricted pervasive alteration; the two types of alteration are separated by episodes of fracturing and evolution of numerous types of vein alteration assemblages, usually in a consistent sequence. During the time of hydrothermal activity the compositions and textures of rocks within a system may be completely changed by pervasive alteration. These alteration styles can be recognized in rocks of contrasting compositions (for example, granitic host rocks and carbonate host rocks).

Selectively Pervasive Alteration

Selectively pervasive alteration is that in which only specific minerals of host rocks and porphyry have been altered in great volumes of rock. Consideration of this kind of alteration stems from the fact that, since large volumes of rock are involved (well beyond mineralized parts of deposits), its occurrence is one criterion by which proximity to a mineralized system may be recognized. The result of such alteration may be only subtle changes in, or enhancement of, rock texture. This alteration type commonly occurs closely peripheral to centers of systems, although it is likely that its effects, some of which are paragenetically early, are widespread. The most common manifestation is the selective conversion of igneous hornblende or igneous book biotite to secondary, recrystallized biotite. Other manifestations include selective alteration of feldspar phenocrysts to different minerals such as clay (kaolinite) chlorite, or epidote and, in progressively later hydrothermal stages, selective conversion of biotite or hornblende to chlorite. For most kinds of selectively pervasive alteration, it appears that minerals of the host rock, rather than composition of solutions, controlled the alteration.

Biotite Alteration. Many porphyry systems which evolved within igneous host rocks or within rocks of igneous lithologies (e.g., arkose) appear to occur within a broad aureole characterized by the presence of secondary biotite. The mineral develops as a replacement of pre-existing mafic minerals, usually hornblende. The alteration transects rock types and may involve a wide variety of volcanic and granitoid hosts, as well as some sedimentary clastic rocks. The occurrence of the alteration beyond mineralized centers has been described at some deposits, but, owing to lack of outcrop, to post-ore cover, or simply to lack of knowledge of district-wide alteration phenomena, the extent of that occurrence is generally poorly known. The most thoroughly described examples are those of the Babine Lake region of British Columbia, where Carson and Jambor (1974) have noted the character and distribution of selective biotite alteration with respect to copper deposits centered on biotite feldspar porphyries. In the United States, this alteration type is reported at Bingham (Peters et al., 1966; Moore, 1978), at Christmas (Eastlick, 1968; Koski and Cook, 1982), at the Safford district (Robinson and Cook, 1966; Langton and Williams, 1982), at Silver Bell (Graybeal, 1982), and at Butte (Roberts, 1973). Selective alteration of hornblende or recrystallization of biotite is present within a large area of outcrop which extends more than 3 km north of the Sierrita orebody, although a complete picture of the distribution of such alteration has not yet been developed. Many of the irregularly shaped patches of biotite shown in Figure 5.1 consist of very finely granular biotite which is recrystallized from "shreds" of original interstitial rock biotite. This rock, from the Sierrita deposit, is typical in its expression of selective biotite alteration. The alteration type is also present at Ray (Phillips et al., 1974), although its distribution is imperfectly known. In other parts of the world it is reported from El Salvador, Chile (Gustafson and Hunt, 1975); Yandera, Papua New Guinea (Watmuff, 1978); Panguna, Papua New Guinea (Ford, 1978); and Plesyumi, Papua New Guinea (Titley, 1978).

Igneous host rocks are volumetrically the most important host for occurrences described above but the presence of biotite as an alteration fringe is reported for some systems in which sedimentary rocks make up the hosts. In sedimentary rocks secondary biotite occurs as an outer fringe to skarn alteration at Copper Canyon (Theodore et al., 1982). The mineral is also present in the skarns at Christmas (Perry, 1968; Koski and Cook, 1982), and it is reported to occur in sedimentary rocks at Bingham-Carr Fork by Atkinson and Einaudi (1978). Clastic sedimentary rocks of the porphyry copper deposit at Mamut, Malaysia (Kosaka and Wakita, 1978) contain secondary biotite, and the alteration extends into rocks beyond the limits of ore. It is reported as an alteration of arenaceous rocks at Copper Canyon (Theodore et al., 1982) and as an interstitial mineral in quartzites at Carr Fork (Atkinson and Einaudi, 1978).

In igneous host rocks, biotite alteration may be subtle and recognizable only after careful study and comparison based upon knowledge of district-wide alteration mineral habits. Both hornblende and biotite are affected, and, for most occurrences reported, hornblende is apparently most susceptible. Very fine grained biotite is often observed pseudomorphing hornblende. Original book biotite is susceptible, but less so, and often reveals only recrystallization of edges of books to shreds of biotite. The subtle nature of occurrence of the alteration type has been described by Anderson and others (1955) at Bagdad. They note (p. 52) that there, "Much of the quartz monzonite . . . appears unaltered. However, . . . the biotite is leafy and pale. In the unaltered quartz monzonite, biotite occurs in book-habit." Similar textural changes have been reported and described at Bingham by Lanier and others (1978), and Carson and Jambor (1974) describe a wide variety of textural, mineralogical, and chemical characteristics for some Canadian occurrences. The widespread distribution of secondary biotite in some well-documented deposits (and its probable similar occurrence in many less well studied ones) reveals the large size of the hydrothermal systems in which porphyry copper deposits occur—commonly many kilometers in diameter. It is important to underscore again the habits of occurrence of biotite alteration upon which this interpretation is based: that of transecting contacts of many different kinds of rocks and that of being centered on porphyry copper mineralization.

There seems no clear consensus concerning the time or conditions under which biotite alteration took place. Many workers report an early time of formation. In view of the general instability of biotite with respect to younger (and cooler) alteration phases, it appears that biotite may be a product of alteration processes at relatively higher temperatures, although there is little direct data to assess such temperatures. Beane (1974), who has determined biotite temperatures on the basis of chemical compositions, suggests temperatures ranging between 350°C and 550°C for the examples which he illustrates. Roberts (1973) has suggested a temperature range of between 550°C and 700°C for the early pervasive biotite at Butte on the basis of the melting curve of quartz monzonite and the Fe-Ti compositions of biotite. Brimhall (1977) has suggested temperatures of 650 ±100°C for development of pre-Main Stage mineralization at Butte, an event which he has suggested correlates with development of Roberts' pervasive biotite. Jacobs and Parry (1979) have recognized early hydrothermal biotite at Santa Rita and, reasoning from an assumption of continuity between igneous and hydrothermal processes, they have proposed that compositions of secondary biotites there indicate a temperature of formation between 650°C and 580°C.

Although some workers have suggested deuteric conditions as causative factors for biotite formation, the meaning and implications of this term are seldom clear. Early secondary biotite (recrystallization) is obviously in part related to the presence of microfractures, and even younger biotite in microveinlets is obviously fracture related. Where the alteration is pervasive, it is reported in many cases to occur in extensively fractured rock and is obviously related to hydrothermal processes.

Major relevant points which may be drawn from the results of reported studies are:

1. Development of selectively pervasive biotite alteration is of pre-ore age and is one of the earliest (if not the earliest) recognized alteration events in a large number of porphyry copper systems.
2. The effects of the alteration type are seen in large volumes of rock which are centered on porphyry plutons and on a much more restricted metallized center. Porphyry copper deposits very commonly occur within a large biotite alteration aureole.
3. The alteration appears to progress away from micro-fractures and veinlets into the rock and appears to take place at relatively high (>500°C) temperatures. The development of the controlling fractures took place throughout very large volumes of rock and may represent the first stages of a long and continuous process of rock fracturing in these deposits.

Chlorite Alteration. In contrast with the interpreted early alteration characterized by the development of biotite, the development of selectively pervasive chlorite is late in the history of the hydrothermal process and appears somewhat less selective than early biotite. The igneous mafic minerals are always affected, but, to a lesser degree, so is feldspar. In further contrast with the monomineralic nature of biotite alteration, chlorite alteration may sometimes be accompanied by the development of additional obvious phases, which include epidote minerals, clays, carbonates, zeolites, and—in some rock types—orthoclase feldspar. Variations in solution chemistry and rock compositions which control composition of alteration assemblages associated with chlorite are discussed in some detail by Beane (1982).

The rocks in which selective chlorite alteration is important extend from within the area of sulfide mineralization to the farthest extent of the hydrothermal system, as defined by altered veins and veinlets. In some systems the alteration may even extend beyond the limits of fracturing; in such cases it may be interpreted to correspond to greenschist facies metamorphism.

The time of formation of chlorite is not unequivocally clear. It is a widely observed and recorded fact that much chlorite selectively replaces the earlier secondary biotite; consequently, at least some is younger than the biotite and coextensive with it in part of the large volume of rocks in which the biotite was developed. Chloritization may actually be the result of a cooling process involving changes in solution chemistry, with the alteration moving inward as conditions in the hydrothermal system change. The selective nature of chlorite alteration produces rocks in which original textures may be only slightly modified. The most common habit is that of replacement of hornblende or biotites of various origins, and the alteration progresses from weak replacement of edges of crystals to complete replacement of original minerals. It appears to be controlled by the same types of features which controlled selective biotite alteration: microfractures and grain boundary openings that extend from larger fractures in the rock.

Selective Alteration of Feldspar. Within the more centrally restricted parts of some porphyry copper deposits, particularly in porphyritic rocks, pervasive selective alteration of feldspars has occurred. Rocks that appear particularly susceptible have fine-grained goundmasses, but reasons for this association are not obvious. Large volumes of porphyry may reveal the alteration style by the pronounced textural enhancement of phenocrysts. Such enhancement results from conversion of phenocrysts to mixtures of clays, sericite, and —in some instances—carbonate minerals and epidote. The alteration type develops at a time during the hydrothermal process when temperatures are considerably lower than those which attend early selective biotite alteration, although no measurements or interpretations for temperatures of formation have been reported. It appears to develop in rocks more densely fractured than those found at the periphery of porphyry copper systems.

The conversion of phenocrysts of some porphyries to mixtures of epidote and clay is evident in parts of some deposits, but it is uncommon. This alteration also develops in porphyritic rocks with extremely fine grained groundmasses, but—unlike the clay alteration of feldspars described above—it tends to occur in rocks at the periphery of deposits and is seldom correlated with mineralization. The rocks which have been altered are commonly fractured, but not densely so, and it appears that the alteration progresses from microfractures across or around mineral grains and through the rock groundmass in a fashion similar to that which guides clay and chlorite alteration.

Summary. Selectively pervasive alteration is restricted to specific minerals and results either in recrystallization of these minerals or in their conversion to new ones. The development of secondary biotite, the chloritic alteration of biotite, and the modification of phenocrysts point to alteration processes more strongly controlled by minerals of the host rock than by variations in fluid composition. Where developed, rock minerals other than biotite or feldspars appear unaffected by solutions which produced the alteration. Temperatures assigned to selectively pervasive alteration appear to range from the very high ones assigned to some biotite formation to the probable lower temperatures of the selective conversion of biotite and hornblende to chlorite. There is some evidence to suggest that selectively pervasive biotite and some chlorite alteration may be synchronous in the early history of the hydrothermal system and that they may represent early thermal zoning. Biotite may evolve relatively close to the thermal center of a system and chlorite alteration of primary biotite may proceed at a greater distance. However, it also seems clear that with gradual cooling of the system or with a lowering aK^+/aH^+ in the solutions (Beane, 1982), together with increases in fracture permeability, conditions of chlorite stability move toward the centers of systems. Such movement produces the superposition of chlorite alteration on secondary biotite that is commonly reported. The early potassic aureole, represented by biotite, may be accompanied by development of a still broader aureole of propylitic alteration (characterized by chlorite) which formed under different conditions of temperature and solution composition; as the system cools, the front of the zone of propylitic alteration retreats toward the center of the system. No evidence has been reported to suggest that the inward encroachment took place during the heating of the system. However, the history of the development of alteration patterns during the initial heating and outward movement of the isotherms is not known.

An important aspect of the selective style of alteration of porphyry copper deposits is that some major changes in chemical composition may take place in the conversion of hornblende to biotite and of biotite to chlorite. This aspect is often overlooked because it does not result in obvious textural change. Especially noteworthy are the changes in silica and potash content in the hornblende-to-biotite conversion and, for some compositions, changes in lime. Also significant are the possible large changes in iron and magnesium content. No chemical gain or loss evaluations have been reported to assess the importance of such changes, but the fact that solutions gain access to rocks through fractures and change the composition of these rocks should constrain interpretations based upon whole rock chemistry. Further, the large area beyond the porphyry copper deposits in which selectively pervasive alteration is now increasingly recognized and the very subtle nature of the textural changes which take place establish a point of caution in the collection, analysis, and interpretation of data from fresh-appearing igneous rocks from these large hydrothermal systems.

Pervasive Alteration

As used in the context of this discussion, pervasive alteration is an extensive type of alteration which has resulted in the complete change of rock compositions and textures. This use differs from that of some authors (Brimhall, 1977; Roberts, 1973), who use the term to describe some of the selectively pervasive phenomena outlined above. The process that produces this alteration has often been alluded to as flooding (an informal term, sometimes also used to describe the resulting texture), and it results in conversion of all minerals in a host rock to a new, usually monomineralic, assemblage. Examples include conversion of rock masses to orthoclase, to quartz and sericite, to biotite, to tourmaline and, in carbonate rocks, to calc-silicate minerals. Pervasive alteration is pre-ore or inter-ore in age and results in rocks which may be hosts to ore minerals. The alteration type may present major problems in lithologic interpretations; Spatz (1979) and Clark (1979) have discussed such problems in relation to the Cerro Colorado deposit in Panama.

Unlike selective alteration, in which host rock mineralogy appears to exert a strong control on the effects of altering solutions, pervasive alteration takes place under conditions in which rocks have become overwhelmed by the effects of large shifts in the chemical composition of fluids. In many occurrences it appears to be localized in volumes of rock where fractures were abundant; the resulting overlap of minerals of vein alteration selvages produced homogenization of alteration products. The alteration is non-selective and may transgress rock contacts. In the case of biotite or orthoclase flooding, which usually occurs near the mineralized centers of systems, rock volumes affected may be on the order of hundreds of cubic meters, more commonly less; contacts may be knife sharp or, more commonly, diffuse across tens of centimeters of rock. Rock masses produced are usually irregular in form; an exception is massive replacement of parts of breccia columns by quartz, tourmaline, or biotite, which results in columnar bodies of metasomatic rock. A further exception is quartz-sericite alteration, which may be imposed on large rock volumes and over considerable depth, and which produces geometrically regular zones of alteration.

Biotite Alteration. The habit of pervasive biotite alteration ranges from complete alteration of rock volumes to extensive replacement of the groundmass mineral assemblage in porphyries. Although widespread, the habit has not been widely reported. At Ray, however, Phillips and others (1974, p. 1246) have reported that diabase is "totally altered for tens of feet" where closely spaced fractures are present. At Bingham (Johns, 1978, p. 1255), "hydrothermal biotite is pervasive in the highly fractured center of the deposit and becomes restricted to envelopes along sulfide-bearing veinlets outward and downward." At Sierrita there occur small (cubic meter) masses of an originally biotite-rich igneous rock altered nearly completely to secondary biotite, and at Twin Buttes, masses of arkose have been pervasively altered to biotite. In the occurrences at Ray and Sierrita the alteration has acted on a rock originally high in ferromagnesian mineral content, while at Twin Buttes it has affected a sedimentary section with a possibly high original content of red beds.

Another style of the alteration appears to affect porphyry groundmasses; although pervasive in the sense considered here, this type does not destructively alter rock textures. At Bingham (Peters et al., 1966) hydrothermal biotite exceeds 35 percent (volume) of igneous rocks exclusive of the original biotite, and at Kalamazoo, (Lowell and Guilbert, 1970) pervasive biotite locally replaces groundmass feldspar of Type A porphyries.

Orthoclase Alteration. Potash metasomatism within porphyry systems sometimes results in the formation of orthoclase or orthoclase-quartz rocks. The aplitic texture which sometimes results may be misleading and the alteration interpreted as an intrusion, rather than rock of metasomatic origin. While it is not always possible to prove that such is the case, there are some well-studied instances which indicate the metasomatic nature of these rocks. In one such study, Gilluly (1946, p. 92) has described the nature of orthoclase at Ajo, noting in some instances there was "clear microscopic evidence of . . . replacement of the groundmass [of the monzonite] by orthoclase." At Santa Rita, Rose and Baltosser (1966) have noted evidence in the South Pit for a time of widespread stability of orthoclase as an alteration product; small masses of finely granular orthoclase rock are present there in which relict textures strongly suggest its derivation from the granodiorite porphyry (Fig. 5.3). At Yandera, Grant and Nielsen (1975) have recorded the presence of pink aplitic quartz monzonite within the ore zone; this rock has been subsequently interpreted as an alteration product (Titley et al., 1978). A large mass of orthoclase rock, contained within porphyry and a pre-ore intrusion, was mined out at Sierrita (Daniel Aiken, 1978, personal communication) and was probably of replacement origin; it occured in the Harris Ranch Quartz Monzonite, a rock particularly susceptible to orthoclase flooding in this deposit. As with pervasive biotite

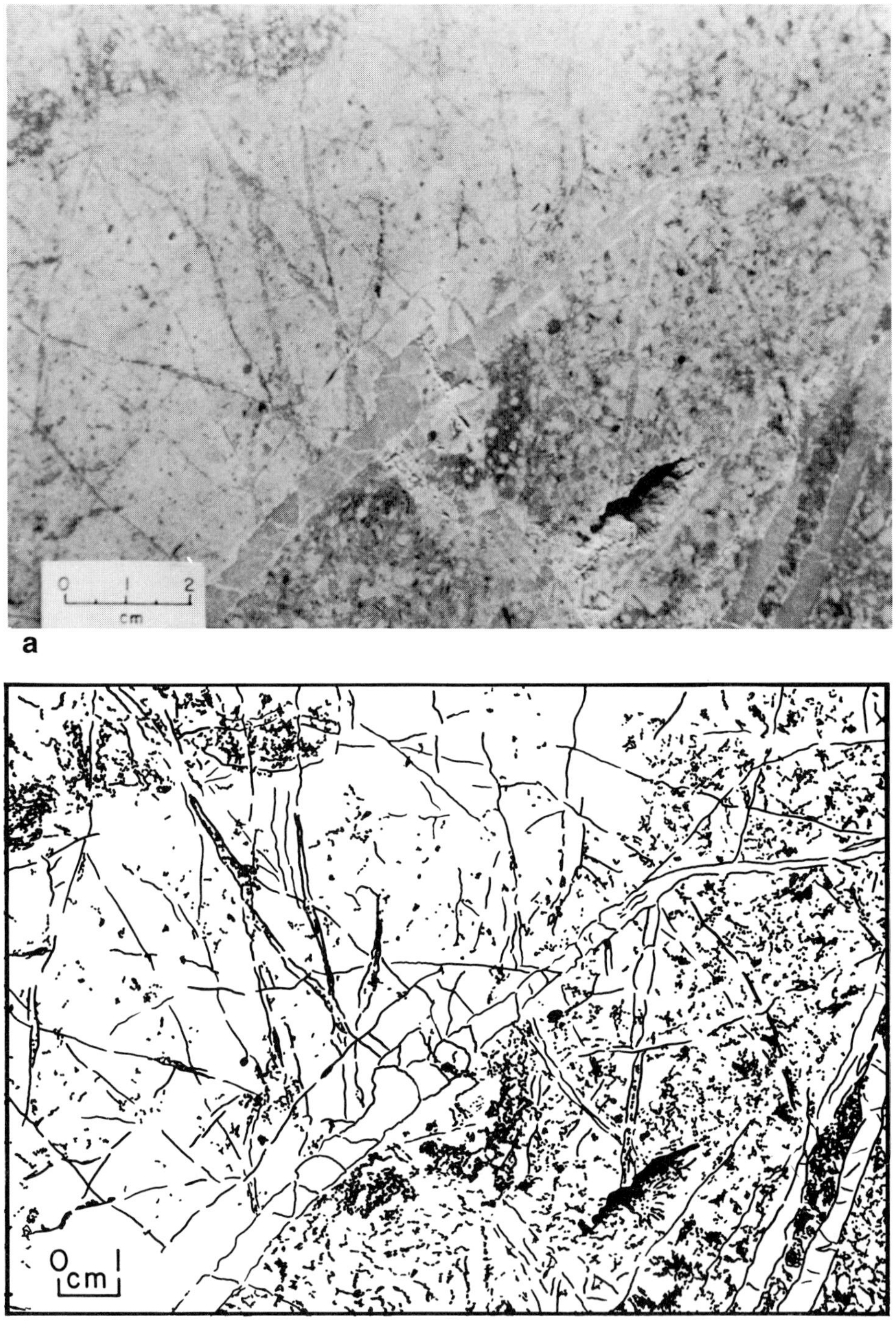

Figure 5.3. Pervasive orthoclase alteration in granodiorite porphyry from Santa Rita. Photograph of the surface (*a*), shows the nature of pervasive development of orthoclase as an alteration product, progressing from the diagonal quartz vein in the center of the photograph. Within the orthoclase mass, quartz phenocrysts of the same size and distribution as those in the unaltered granodiorite establish a firm basis for interpreting the metasomatic nature of the rock. Numerous small quartz veinlets extending into the orthoclase mass suggest the orientation of the original lines of permeability, which were responsible for solution flow through the original rock. In the lower right corner is a vitreous grey quartz vein which Neilsen (1968) has interpreted as very early and of high-temperature formation. Artist's sketch (*b*) emphasizes veins and alteration.

alteration, there have likely been many unreported occurrences of small volumes (tens of cubic meters) of metasomatic orthoclase rock in other porphyry systems.

Quartz-Sericite-(Pyrite) Alteration. Second only to the effects of supergene activity, alteration of igneous rocks to quartz-sericite, usually accompanied by pyrite, is the most widespread, most volumetrically important, and most texturally destructive type of alteration. Very commonly this alteration, one of the last recorded hypogene alteration phenomena, has so obliterated earlier alteration effects that the early alteration history of rocks involved can be interpreted only with difficulty. The alteration usually progresses from closely spaced fractures which develop in the late history of cooling of the porphyry system.

Viewed on a broader geographic scale than the American Southwest, where it is abundant, the distribution of quartz-sericite alteration ranges from virtually absent (e.g., Brenda, Morrison, and deposits in skarn—although in such deposits it may have a chemical-temporal counterpart) to well-developed, but discretely positioned, as in some of the Babine Lake deposits, Kalamazoo, Silver Bell, and other deposits where pyritic aureoles have been described. The alteration also is reported as an overprint of earlier alteration types at El Salvador (Gustafson and Hunt, 1975). Deep oxidation and leaching of sulfide-bearing rocks in porphyry copper deposits of the Southwest have usually taken place within the volumes of rock originally altered to quartz and sericite.

As with pervasive alteration of other kinds described here, quartz-sericite alteration results from profound shifts in the chemical contrasts between rocks and solutions, enhanced by the development of abundant fractures and resulting high flow porosity. The alteration is the result of strong acid attack, with fixing of alumina and potash, and the leaching of other components. When exposed to supergene solutions, the mineral assemblage undergoes further destruction, largely as a consequence of the evolution of acid by oxidation of pyrite, and the assemblage which results is rich in quartz, clay, and hydromica. It is thus difficult in many deposits to assess accurately the nature and extent of hypogene alteration types present. Early studies of alteration in porphyry systems (e.g., Kerr, 1951, at Silver Bell) interpreted supergene effects superimposed upon quartz-sericite alteration as hypogene argillic alteration. Deeper development by mining and a broader understanding of the effects of different kinds of alteration have combined to interpret more accurately supergene effects on this alteration type (Anderson, 1982).

A widely held interpretation, based upon suggested models of alteration zoning (for example that of Lowell and Guilbert, 1970), is that quartz-sericite alteration occurs between, and is synchronous with, an inner potassic and an outer propylitic alteration aureole. The intermediate zonal position of quartz-sericite is present in many deposits; however, as revealed in the examples discussed above, this position is not consistent. The alteration type is correlative with a late time of development, when great numbers of new fractures form near the thermal center of a porphyry copper system. By virtue of this relatively late time of evolution, it overprints earlier alteration types. Quartz-sericite alteration augments the sulfide content of the earlier stages of alteration of porphyry copper deposits, although the copper concentration which it appears to bring about is considerably less than that of the earlier potassic alteration.

Calc-Silicate Alteration. Carbonate-bearing sedimentary rocks in contact with intrusive porphyries undergo pervasive alteration to calcium-magnesium-silicate mineral assemblages. Einaudi (1982*a*, 1982*b*) has discussed the nature and details of mineralogy and the occurrence of such rocks (see Chapters 7 and 8). In the context of considerations of alteration styles, however, calc-silicate alteration is viewed as the pervasive, texturally destructive alteration of certain types of reactive sedimentary rocks. Although solution-dominated in great part, calc-silicate alteration results in a much greater diversity of mineral assemblages and rock textures than do the other alteration types heretofore considered. The alteration results from processes which range from solely thermal ones to those in which extensive metasomatism takes place. It is because of this latter manifestation that formation of calc-silicates is considered a type of alteration of porphyry copper deposits involving different wall rocks to intrusions (Titley, 1973).

Large volumes of rock adjacent to intrusions or to major structures are commonly replaced by calc-silicate minerals; this process involves loss of CO_2. Although solutions dominate the process, original carbonate rock compositions (which reflect variations in CaO, MgO, Al_2O_3, SiO_2, and sometimes iron) exert subtle influences on calc-silicate compositions. Unlike the alteration of K-silicate rocks, which results in aureoles of alteration many kilometers wide, the alteration of carbonate rocks is restricted to rock volumes immediately adjacent to porphyry centers and produces aureoles usually only hundreds of meters wide.

Summary. Contrasted with the wide aureoles of selectively pervasive potassic alteration (orthoclase and biotite), the pervasive alteration of rocks to orthoclase or to biotite in porphyry copper systems is much more restricted and involves only minor rock volumes. The alteration is non-selective and, in some reported instances, progresses from volumes of rock where fractures are closely spaced. Rock types involved are generally those with igneous rock mineralogies; some kinds of clastic sedimentary rocks may also be affected, but only in restricted volumes.

As the potassic types are closely related to volumes of fractured rock, so too is the pervasive alteration of rocks to masses of quartz, sericite, and pyrite. However, the rock volumes affected by pervasive quartz-sericite alteration are large and are commonly quite varied in composition. Pervasive quartz-sericite alteration appears to post-date pervasive potassic alteration and accompanies or shortly follows a time during which large volumes of rock, usually close to a porphyry center, are intensely fractured. Development of calc-silicate alteration in carbonate host rocks involves both contact effects and—presumably later—metasomatic effects. Although large bodies of altered rocks may be produced, the effects of calc-silicate alteration are restricted to much smaller rock volumes than those of early selective alteration by biotite and chlorite.

Vein-Veinlet Alteration

The pervasive alteration types described above progress from closely spaced fractures in many reported instances. Thus, the breaking of porphyry and host rocks has locally influenced alteration patterns; because of changing conditions of solution chemistry and episodic fracturing, it has also influenced alteration mineral assemblages. Of comparable importance is the fact that it is fracture-guided mineralization that has resulted in the concentrations of copper and other metals which are present in the porphyry copper system. The deposit type is almost invariably characterized by an abundance of fractures, which range from wide (tens of centimeters), through-going veins to mesoscopic and microscopic veins and veinlets (Heidrick and Titley, 1982). The evolution of fractures appears to proceed from the earliest times at which the porphyries and host rocks are sufficiently competent to undergo brittle failure to the latest stages of cooling.

The Nature and Distribution of Fractures. Detailed studies of the nature, abundance, and distribution of fractures in porphyry copper deposits have been few and reports of such studies are scant. Fractures have long been recognized as a dominating control of mineralization and alteration in these systems (McKinstry, 1955), but the destructive effects of both hypogene quartz-sericite alteration and supergene processes have obliterated much of the mineralogical information necessary for a proper interpretation of the history of their evolution. The literature contains abundant reports on fracture orientation studies which have been directed almost solely toward interpretation of structural history; the extensive data collected in Arizona and New Mexico (Rehrig and Heidrick, 1972, 1976) have been important in this respect. A major result of such work has been the recognition that, in the region considered, fracture orientations are not random but generally systematic (Heidrick and Titley, 1982).

Careful studies at a number of deposits have shown many stages of fracturing, each recognizable because of consistent sequences of vein alteration assemblages developed along distinct fracture sets. The habit is observable in oxidized outcrops (Fig. 5.4) as well as in unoxidized rocks from within orebodies. Separation of different alteration types and an interpretation of the changes in orientation of stress as determined in the context of paragenetic time were outlined on the basis of such outcrops by Titley and others (1978) and Titley and Heidrick (1978). In a parallel study fracture abundances were correlated with different vein alteration types at prospects in New Britain, Papua New Guinea (Titley, 1978). Integration of measurements of fracture density, fracture (alteration) sequence, fracture location, and vein-filling temperatures has been reported for a part of the Sierrita, porphyry copper deposit (Haynes and Titley, 1980).

Results of the studies at Sierrita reveal that, in general, fracturing of porphyry and host rocks is episodic. This interpretation stems from the fact that a persistent sequence of different vein-alteration types occurs in this large hydrothermal system. The fracturing progressed from an early event which extended over a large area and produced fractures up to 4 km from the porphyry center; it became more centrally restricted with each subsequent stage of fracture evolution. Solutions which deposited quartz in each episode were progressively cooler for each episode. These data are shown in Figure 5.5 for a portion of the pre-porphyry Laramide granodiorite host rock north of the porphyry center.

From the field and laboratory data obtained on the Sierrita deposit, as well as from the studies in the southwestern Pacific regions, it is apparent that there is a close similarity in the way in which porphyry copper hydrothermal systems evolve. Further, studies of the Canadian deposits (Carson and Jambor, 1974), together with the observations in the American Southwest, suggest that zones of permeability for ore fluids become progressively more restricted laterally with time; however, for some alteration types—particularly the evolution of late quartz and sericite—the permeability of more centrally (laterally) located rocks increases appreciably. Little can be stated with certainty concerning the evolution of fractures in pre-ore rocks above a pluton, but the evidence from Safford (Robinson and Cook, 1966) indicates extensive fracturing of pre-ore andesite host rocks in a large rock volume characterized by numerous dikes; the parent pluton is presumably still undiscovered at depth.

The Nature of Fracture-Localized Alteration. Alteration and metal zoning in many porphyry copper deposits is now recognized to be composed of many different alteration types which developed in veins that formed continuously in porphyry and host rock. It is noteworthy that this characteristic was reported long ago in some deposits. Recognized vein paragenesis of alteration mineral assemblages within deposits and stated or implied superposition of the alteration types have been reported from Ajo (Gilluly, 1946), Castle Dome (Peterson et al., 1951), and Bagdad (Anderson et al., 1955). Other studies in the Southwest have detailed the paragenesis of alteration at Santa Rita (Nielsen, 1968) and Ray (Phillips et al., 1974). Published maps of deposits depicting superposition of different alteration mineral assemblages include those from Bingham (Peters et al., 1966; Lanier et al., 1978; Moore, 1978); Safford (Robinson and Cook, 1966); Sierrita (West and Aiken, 1982); Silver Bell (Graybeal, 1982); and Christmas (Koski and Cook, 1982). Additional descriptions of superposed alteration types have been provided for many deposits of the Canadian Cordillera (Sutherland Brown, 1976) and for some deposits of the southwestern Pacific and Australia (Gustafson and Titley 1978). The progress of superposition has been especially well-documented and described at El Salvador by Gustafson and Hunt (1975).

In many descriptions of alteration zoning, the basis for designation of zone composition is not always specified. As it is becoming increasingly recognized that alteration mineral assemblages in the rocks of these deposits reflect changes in the course of chemical and mechanical events, reporting of such criteria becomes an increasingly important aspect of study. The most casual observation of rocks within porphyry copper deposits or of drill core from them is sufficient to reveal the fact that veinlet alteration is abundant, highly varied, and commonly manifests a consistent and generally predictable sequence of formation. With the exception of alteration types which are pervasive and texturally destructive, most rocks within deposits reveal a sequence of overprinted vein-alteration types and, thus, the basis for designation of alteration zones is sometimes uncertain.

The descriptions of different types of vein alteration mineralogies and their habits have been outlined and discussed by Meyer and Hemley (1967). The paragenetic relations and alteration sequences from a number of porphyry systems have been summarized by Beane (1982). Most paragenetic data are reported from studies within strongly altered and mineralized systems. There are few reported studies of alteration at distal parts of porphyry copper systems; however, where reported, some characteristic veinlet alteration assemblages appear to persist from their occurrence in orebodies to the limits of fracture-localized alteration. In central ore-related parts of intrusions and wall rocks and in

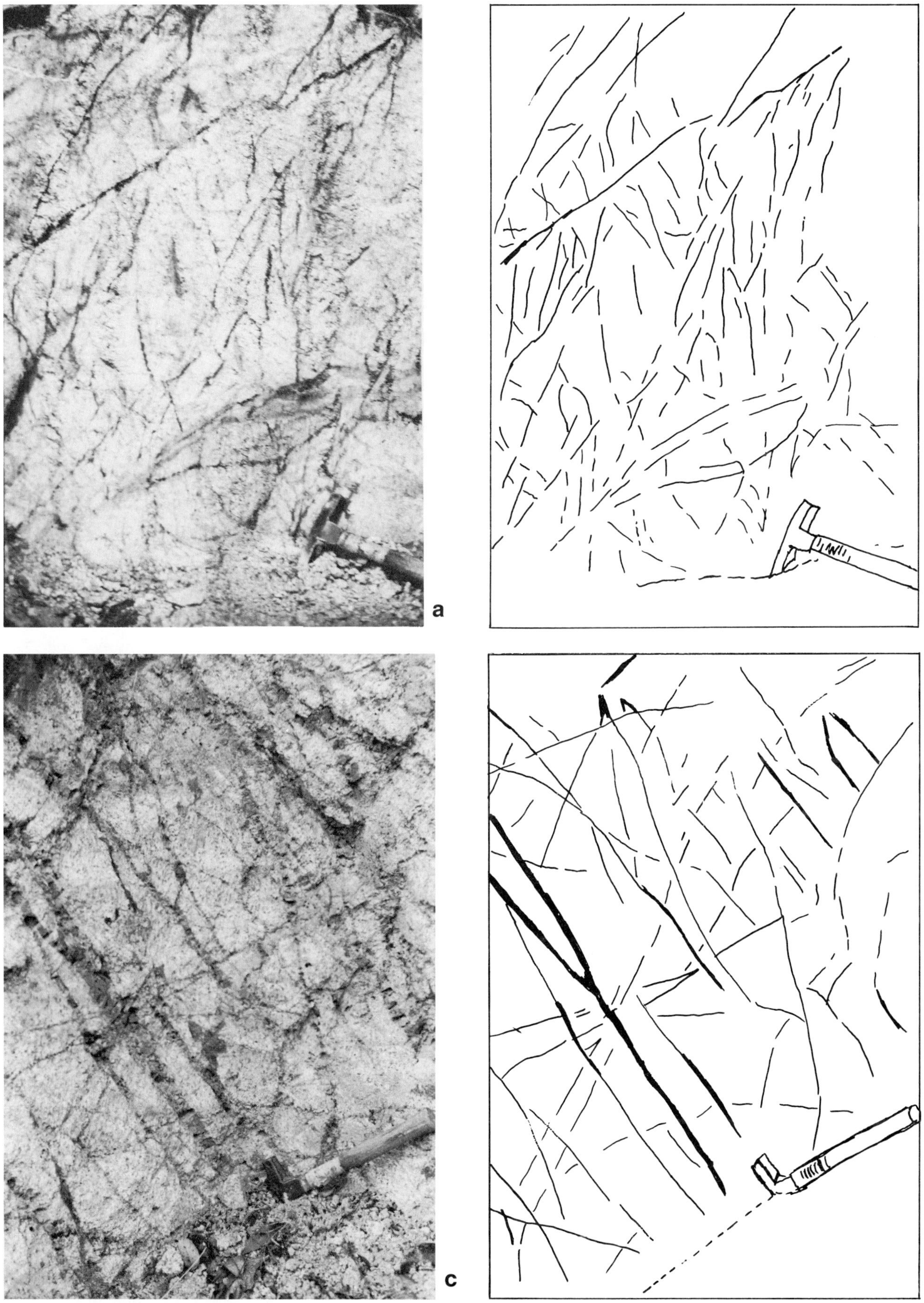

Figure 5.4. Outcrop exposures of granodiorite and porphyry at Yandera, Papua New Guinea, showing typical densities of fractures within the central parts of many porphyry copper systems. Photograph of sample (*a*) shows fractures enhanced by traces of oxidized products in saprolite. Two different vein types, quartz-sericite-chlorite-pyrite and quartz-orthoclase-chalcopyrite, are exposed in crosscutting relationships. The fracture density (n = measured fracture length ÷ area of measurement) is about 0.6^{-1} for each alteration type and 1.2 cm^{-1} for all fractures. Artist's sketch (*b*) of sample in *a* shows fractures on overlay. Photograph (*c*) shows quartz-pyrite veins cutting younger quartz-orthoclase-chalcopyrite veins, each with a fracture density of about 0.5 cm^{-1}. Artist's sketch (*d*) of sample in *c* shows fractures on overlay.

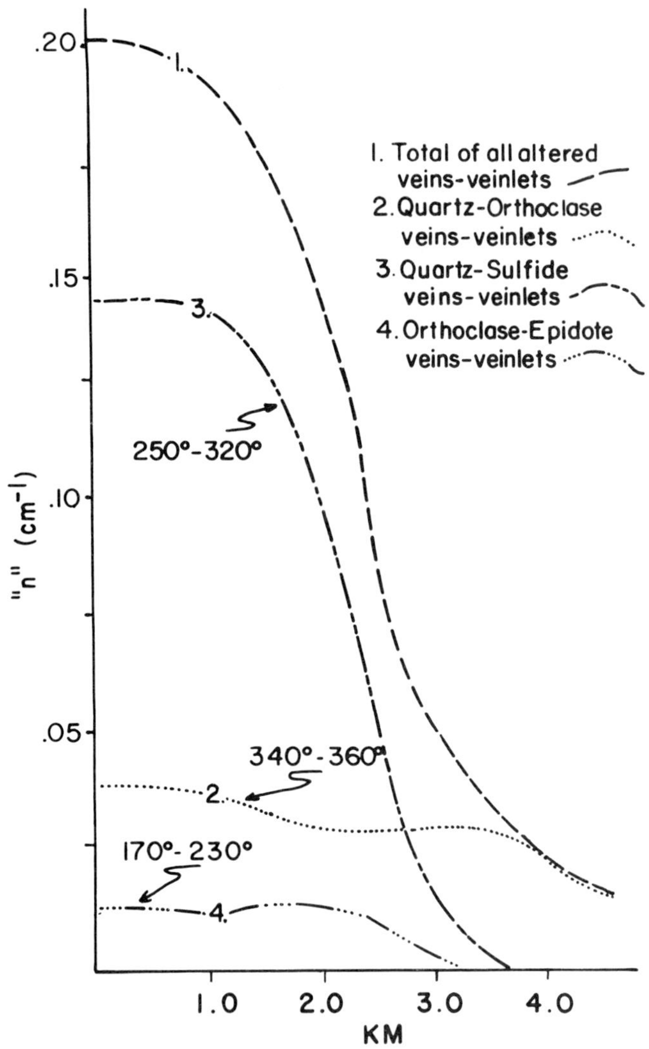

Figure 5.5. Separate and integrated fracture densities for three types of altered veins in the Ruby Star Granodiorite near the Sierrita orebody. Temperatures shown for the different vein types are from fluid inclusions collected at sample sites 1.9 and 2.8 km from the quartz monzonite porphyry center of the orebody (0 km on the horizontal axis). Fracture density (*n*) determined from total length of fractures in a sample area, divided by that area. Data modified from Haynes and Titley (1980).

concentrator intrusions and closely adjacent wall rocks with igneous mineralogies a generalized veinlet alteration sequence is commonly as follows:

1. Early barren quartz veins, sometimes ptygmatic
2. Biotite precipitation/recrystallization in veins and vein walls (biotite-quartz-magnetite sulfide veins)
3. Orthoclase precipitation in veins and vein walls (orthoclase-quartz ±sericite ±sulfide veins)
4. Quartz-sulfide precipitation in and along veins
5. Quartz-sericite-pyrite (texturally destructive) alteration of vein selvages
6. Quartz-pyrite-alunite-pyrophylite veins, possibly synchronous at high levels with no. 5 above
7. Clay-sericite-carbonate-sulfate-zeolite alteration of vein walls or precipitation in open spaces
8. Chlorite-epidote-montmorillonite-carbonate veins

These simplified assemblages and the sequence are characteristic of those found in felsic igneous host rocks and porphyries or in sedimentary host rocks, such as arkose. Variations in compositions appear to be controlled in great part by host rock compositions. Thus, plagioclase-bearing rocks (diorites, quartz diorites) tend to be altered to assemblages relatively richer in soda than in potash.

Early Quartz Veins. The oldest veins recognized (found in a few deposits and possibly more widespread than has been reported) are a generation of distinctive quartz veins. They are the "vitreous grey quartz veins" of Santa Rita (Neilsen, 1968) and the "*A*-veins" of El Salvador (Gustafson and Hunt, 1975). They may also be represented in some of the early "Pre–Main Stage" veins of Butte (Brimhall, 1977). High temperatures of formation of the veins have been interpreted from compositional data at Butte (Brimhall, 1977), from isotope geothermometry (Sheppard et al., 1971), from fluid inclusion studies at Santa Rita (Reynolds and Beane, 1979), and from interpretations of minimum filling temperatures of fluid inclusions at El Salvador (Gustafson and Hunt, 1975).

Characteristically, the veins are sinuous, with irregular curving walls which give rise to traces that pinch and swell. In marked contrast to later generations of quartz veins, which express sharp planar walls and sometimes reaction selvages in these same deposits, the early veins are crackled, folded, and discontinuous, with local anastomosing and branching parts. Quartz is the dominant mineral but sulfides, biotite, and orthoclase may be present locally; anhydrite is reported to occur with the early veins at El Salvador and Santa Rita. One such vein from Santa Rita is shown in Figure 5.3; filling temperatures of inclusions from this particular vein are in excess of 800°C (Reynolds and Beane, 1979)

There is little certainty concerning the origin of this early vein type, but some speculations have been advanced. Its confinement to intrusive porphyries rather than to wall rocks suggests that its origin may be linked with events related to emplacement and to early cooling of intrusive rock hosts. Gustafson and Hunt (1975) have suggested that the vein type represents non-brittle fracturing. Neilsen (1968) has suggested that the veins at Santa Rita formed following an early stage of crystallization of the porphyry when failure took place. The porphyry was subsequently remobilized and intruded into a still earlier stage of consolidated stock. Results of a numerical analysis of the cooling history of plutons and the concomitant history of stress (Knapp and Norton, 1980) suggest a means of formation not too dissimilar from that proposed by Neilsen (1968). Post-emplacement cooling of plutons is determined to be a complex process involving domains of rock which crystallize and remelt, and then recrystallize at still later times. It is thus tempting to suggest that these early, high temperature veins, with inclusion-filling temperatures near the solidus, represent the effects of early crystallization; brittle failure; vein-filling; sufficient re-heating to lower viscosity or to partially melt and move a domain of porphyry; recrystallization; and entrapment of the contorted veins.

Potassium Silicate Alteration. Potassium silicate veins, which include within them specific stages of copper

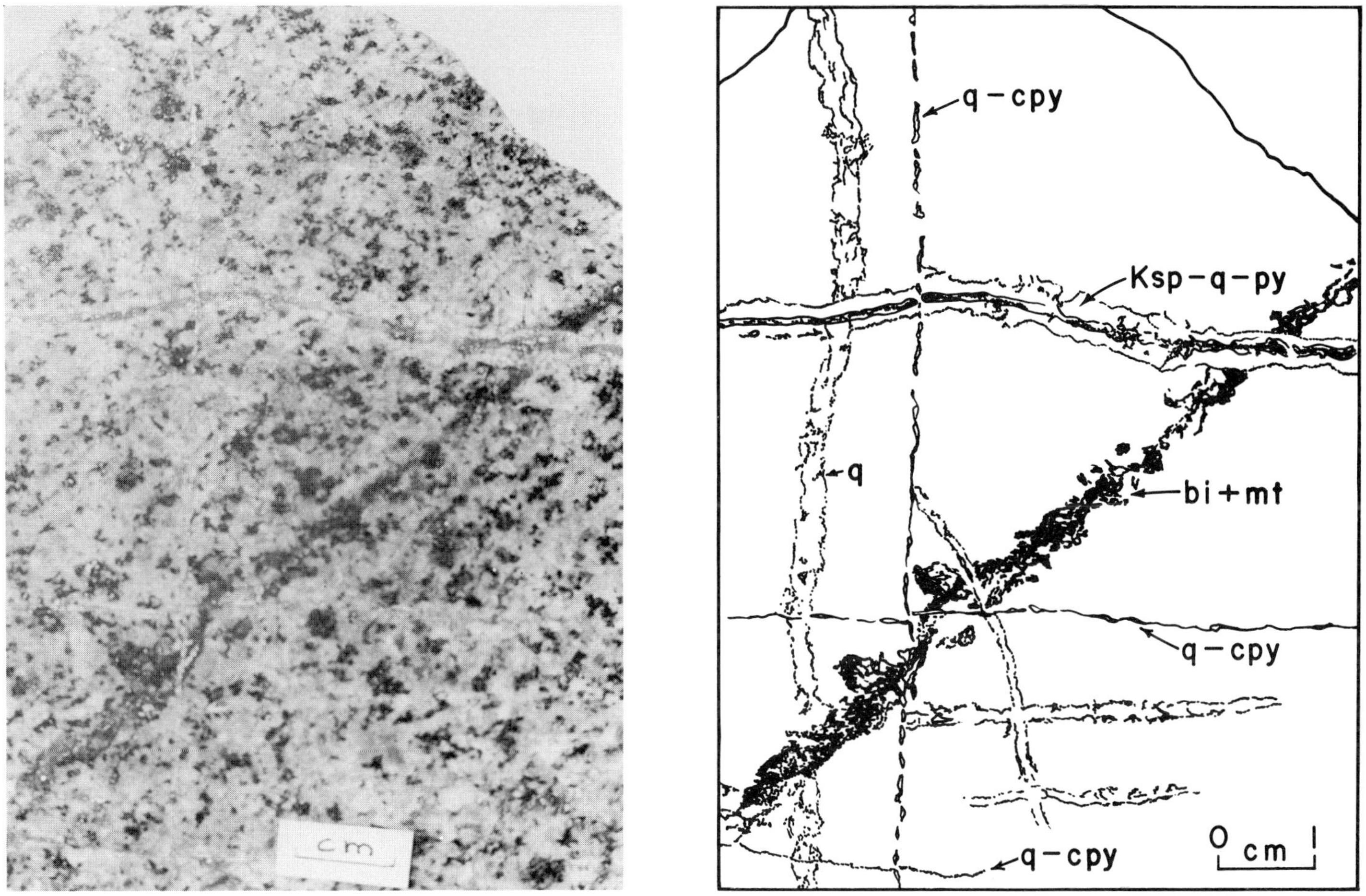

a b

Figure 5.6. Typical sequence of potassium silicate veins in Harris Ranch Quartz Monzonite at Sierrita. Presence of biotite and orthoclase veins, together with stability of interstitial rock biotite, shown in photograph of surface (*a*) indicates stability of potassium silicate alteration phases. Artist's sketch (*b*) shows nature of principal vein types and sequence of biotite veins, quartz veins, orthoclase-quartz veins, and latest quartz-chalcopyrite veins, the principal stage of copper mineralization. Key: *bi* = biotite, *cpy* = chalcopyrite, *Ksp* = Kspar, *mt* = magnetite, *py* = pyrite, *q* = quartz.

and molybdenum deposition, consist generally of biotite-stable, orthoclase-stable, and quartz-sericite alteration assemblages. A typical sequence of veins from a granitic host rock at Sierrita is shown on Figure 5.6. Because of the presence of biotite in some veins and of orthoclase selvages in others and because of the stability of interstitial biotite in the rock, a designation of potassic alteration is applied to this alteration type. The sample shows the typical complexity of veining which occurs and illustrates the temporal discreteness of sulfide deposition—pyrite and chalcopyrite occur within their own specific alteration types.

In the zone of potassic-altered veins, host rock compositions commonly exert a strong control on resulting alteration assemblages. Although the effects are commonly more subtle, a striking example of such control is shown in Figure 5.7, also from the Sierrita Mine. An early, biotite-cemented breccia vein is shown crosscut by a younger vein and its associated alteration products. Where solutions moving through the younger vein interacted with biotite, the vein alteration products produced reflect the original abundance of potash and iron in the vein wall; these products consist of orthoclase, quartz, and pyrite and grade through coarse muscovite to a selvage of sericite and chlorite. Orthoclase is sparse or absent in the vein wall at the edges of the photograph, and alteration minerals are dominated by sericite, quartz, and pyrite.

Characteristics of host rock mineral control of alteration are common in the early biotite and orthoclase vein assemblages, but they contrast with those of younger kinds of potassic alteration, chiefly in the development of widespread quartz, sericite and pyrite. Yet, even in this younger alteration assemblage there may be local wall rock control of mineral assemblages. For the most part, the phyllic assemblage is strongly corrosive, commonly extends from closely spaced veins, and results in wholesale transfer of chemical components. An example is shown in Figure 5.8, a metamorphic wall rock to mineralization at Ithaca Peak, Arizona. Quartz-sericite veins have wide selvages of sericite but unaltered domains exist between veins. Wall rock control is shown along the vein extending from the upper left corner diagonally across the sample. In the schist wall rock, chalcopyrite and pyrite are the principal vein sulfides. Where the fracture crosses the feldspar-aplite part of the host rock, the metallic assemblage is molybdenite and sparse pyrite.

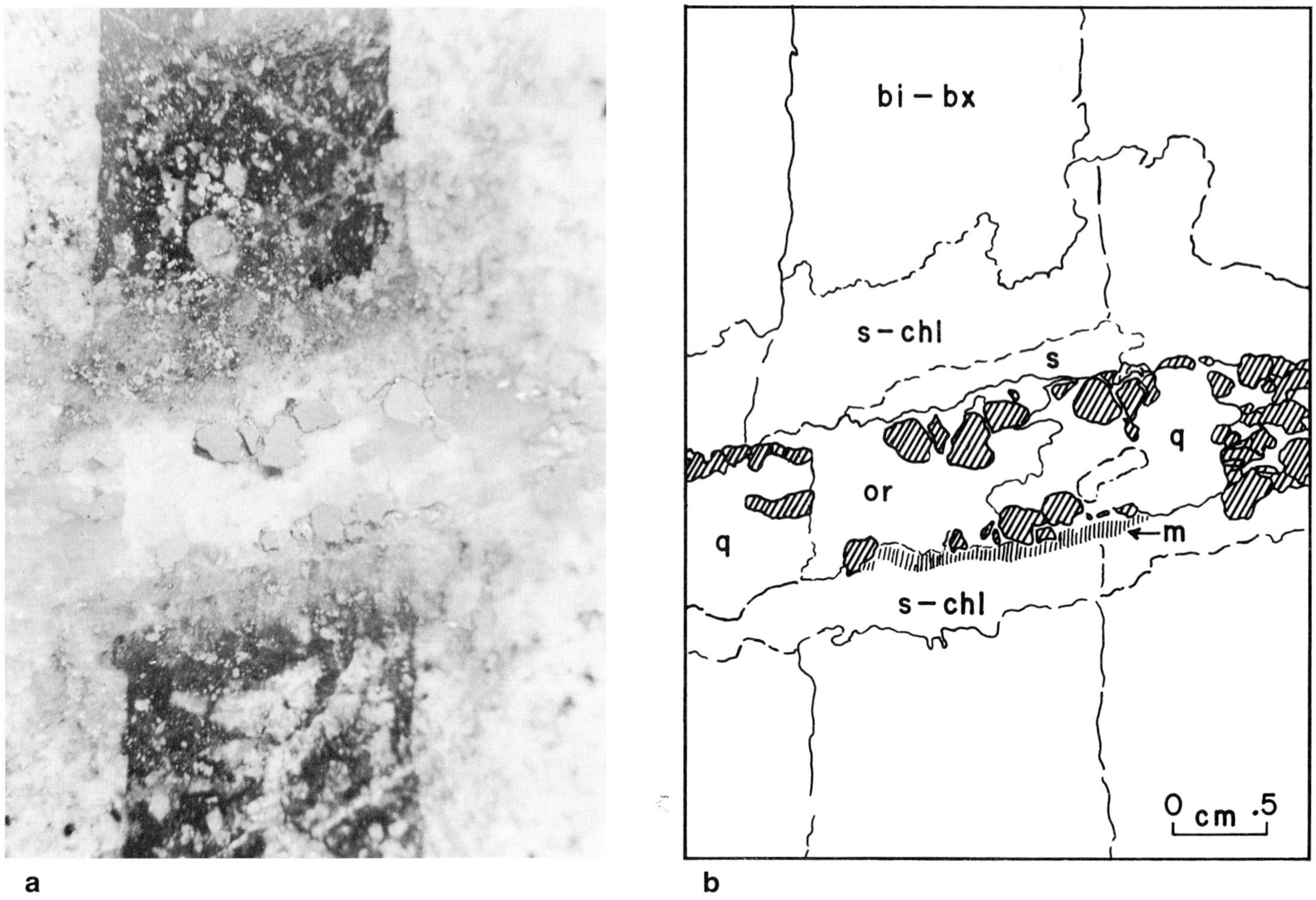

Figure 5.7. Wall rock control of alteration mineralogy in Harris Ranch Quartz Monzonite host rock at Sierrita: *a,* photograph of surface of sample; *b,* artist's sketch emphasizing the mineralization. A biotite cemented breccia (*bi-bx*) is crossed by a younger vein. Where the biotite breccia is a wall to the vein, orthoclase (*or*), together with coarse muscovite (*m*), sericite-chlorite (*s-chl*), and pyrite (*hatched*) form a zoned vein-wall selvage. Beyond limits of the breccia, alteration products are quartz (*q*), sericite-chlorite, and pyrite.

A composite of the potassic alteration types considered here is shown in another example from Sierrita, Figure 5.9. The original rock textures characterized by interstitial biotite gradually disappear under the influence of conversion of the rock to orthoclase. Younger orthoclase-sulfide veins are imposed upon the orthoclase rock, and still younger quartz-sericite-pyrite vein alteration is imposed on the less-altered part of the sample. The figure illustrates the relationships and effects of several different vein types and, even more importantly, serves to show common features of the evolutionary style of porphyry copper deposit alteration and the difficulties in assessing the spatial distribution of alteration types solely from the characteristics of veinlet alteration assemblages.

Argillic Alteration. Much argillic alteration in porphyry copper systems is either late, supergene, and pervasive in nature or is hypogene and the result of a selective attack on feldspars and sericite. In a few instances it is restricted to veinlets, where it appears to be a result of continued alteration of vein walls following development of sericite-like minerals. Production of a variety of clay types and associated quartz may progress from earlier alteration of feldspars. The distinction between argillic alteration and some manifestations of quartz-sericite alteration is not clear, and the problem has not been closely studied in porphyry deposits of the Southwest. In the deep hypogene zone considered here, evolution of significant amounts of clays—of a kind and on a scale which clearly establish zones or times of argillic alteration—suggests conditions which may be correlative with evolution of the advanced argillic alteration at high levels of the hypogene environment (cf. Beane, 1982).

Quartz-Clay-Pyrophyllite-Alunite-Pyrite Alteration. In the shallow hypogene environment (Fig. 5.2) of some porphyry copper systems—such as Red Mountain (Corn, 1975), El Salvador, Chile (Gustafson and Hunt, 1975), and some deposits of the Celebes, Indonesia (Lowder and Dow, 1978)—hypogene alteration assemblages dominated by quartz and alunite are reported to occur with copper mineralization. This assemblage, or important elements of it, is a veinward alteration type at Butte (Meyer et al., 1968), where it occurs in a central portion of the system but below a level of sericite alteration.

In porphyry copper deposits, the assemblage may occur along veins or veinlets which, if closely spaced, effect wholesale replacement of the host rock in the same fashion as

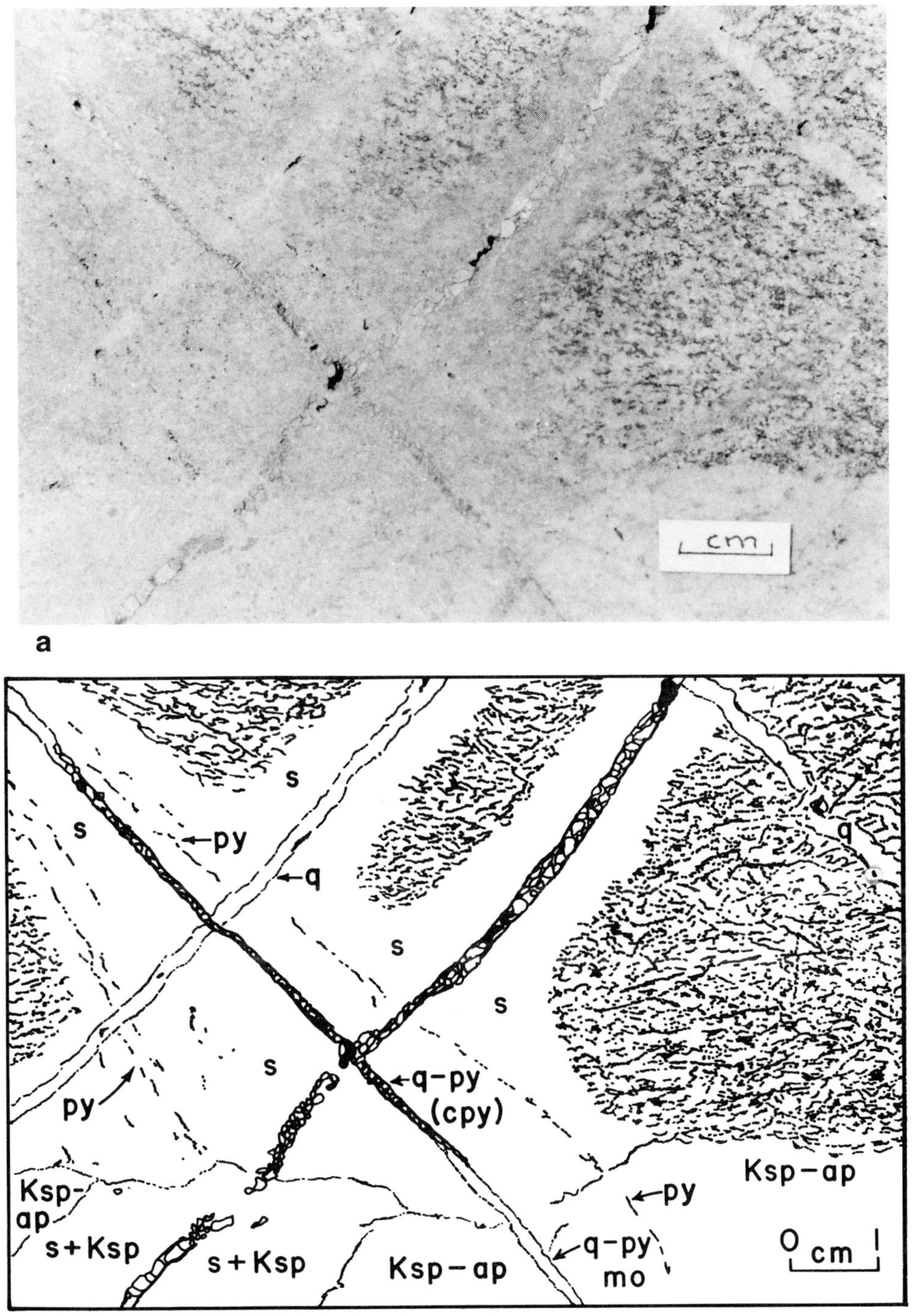

Figure 5.8. Quartz-sericite alteration of schist at Ithaca Peak: *a,* photograph of surface of sample; *b,* artist's sketch of sample showing quartz-sericite (*q, s*) veins with wide alteration selvages. Sulfide veins (*q-py-cpy*) change composition crossing from schist to aplite (*Ksp-ap*) to quartz-pyrite-molybdenite (northwest to southeast) and from quartz-pyrite to pyrite (northeast to southwest).

quartz sericite. Thus, quartz-alunite-pyrophyllite flooding may result. This interpretation is given to the Red Mountain occurrence, where narrow (1 mm), closely spaced (2 cm) quartz veinlets in some volumes of wall rock appear to have resulted in nearly complete silicification and alunitization. There remains doubt in some instances about the timing of the alteration type and what, if any, earlier alteration types may have been present at the high levels at which it is sometimes seen. Gustafson and Hunt (1975) report that the alteration assemblage appears to encroach downward and that it overprints earlier quartz-sericite–altered rocks at El Salvador. In that location, the alteration type is reported not to be an apparent direct alteration of either potassium silicate rocks or biotite-orthoclase types of hypogene alteration. Rather the alteration type mineral assemblage, which may include diaspore and andalusite as well, has been identified as advanced argillic (Meyer and Hemley, 1967; Gustafson and Hunt, 1975). The temperatures at which it formed may

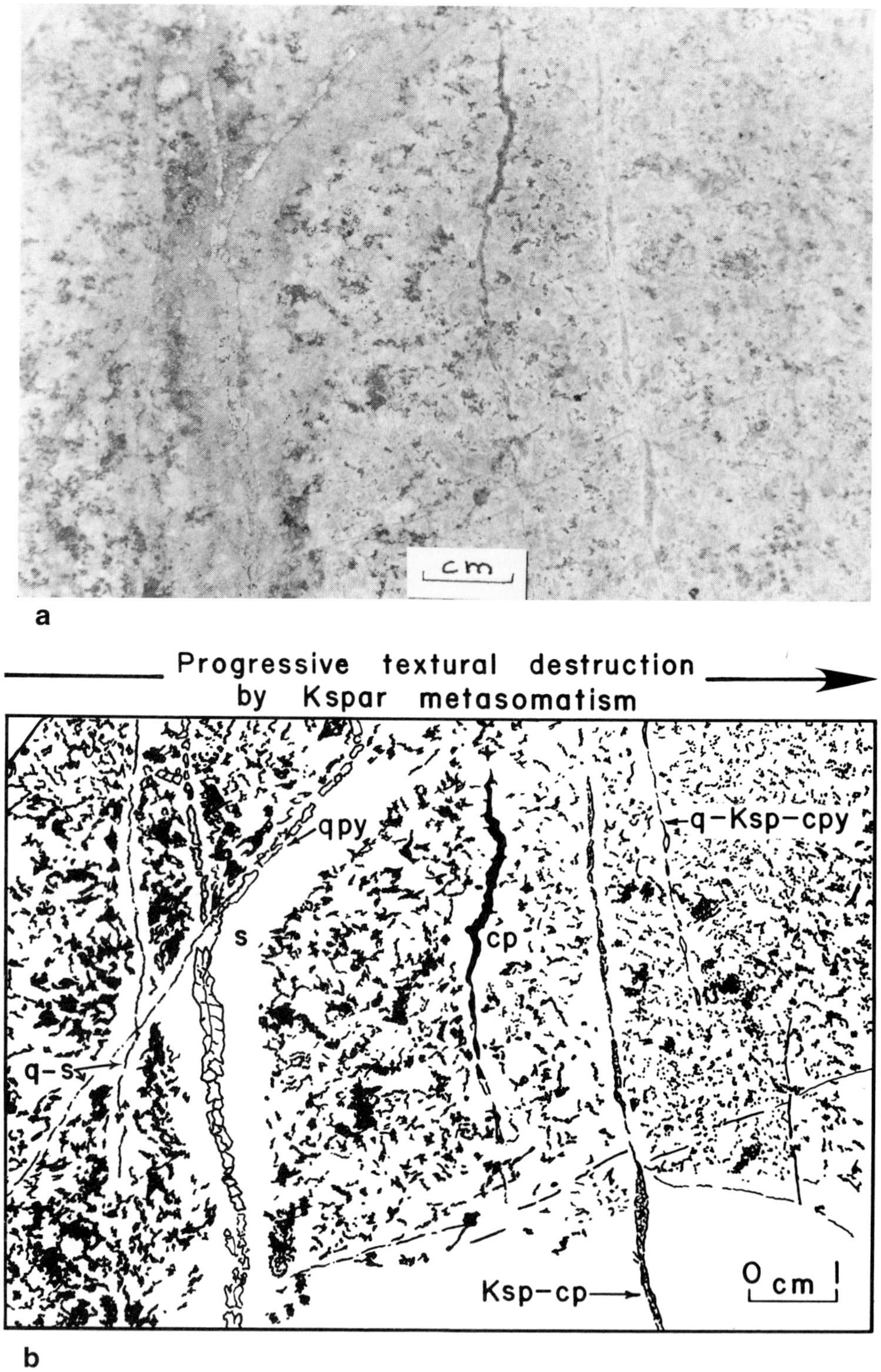

Figure 5.9. Complex of vein alteration types and the results of progressive orthoclase alteration in Harris Ranch Quartz Monzonite host rock at Sierrita: *a,* photograph of sample; *b,* artist's sketch showing how interstitial biotite of relatively fresh rock (left part of sample) is gradually destroyed under effects of orthoclase alteration. Late quartz-sericite-pyrite (*q, s, py*) alteration destroys the original texture along the vein selvage. Quartz-K-feldspar-chalcopyrite (*q, Ksp, cpy*) veins cross early orthoclase alteration.

have been high, and at kilometers of inferred height above intrusions, where fluid inclusion thermometry indicates temperatures above 300°C at Red Mountain. (Bodnar and Beane, 1977). Somewhat lower temperatures, on the order of 200°C, are inferred for the alteration at El Salvador (Gustafson and Hunt, 1975).

Chlorite-Epidote-Montmorillonite Alteration. In the fringe areas of many systems, an alteration assemblage of chlorite-epidote-montmorillonite-carbonate-(albite) is present and is representative of the propylitic assemblage. Although some parts of deposits contain rock volumes where it is pervasive, it is nonetheless closely vein-related. For some of the members of the assemblage, the alteration is selective; an example is the chloritization of biotite. A separate episode of fracturing of rocks, a phenomenon which appears to attend development of earlier vein alteration assemblages, is not obvious for this alteration, and much of it appears to be parasitic, following earlier fractures and altering earlier alteration minerals.

The timing of the alteration type is less certain than for other vein alteration types. In the context of zoning it has been shown by most workers to lie at the outermost edge of hydrothermal systems and to occupy its own distinct and unique volume of space. It appears, thus, to be synchronous with some argillic alteration types, but it may commence at an early time in the cooling history of a pluton. The assemblage is characteristic of greenschist metamorphism, and at deposit fringes it may represent closed-system metamorphism. However, the minerals are in some instances clearly alteration products of earlier alteration minerals, and they are consequently interpreted to represent an alteration type which encroaches upon the centers of systems as wall rocks to plutons cool.

Alteration Paragenesis and Zoning

Recognition of the fact that diagnostic alteration minerals in porphyry copper systems are systematically arranged in space stems from observations at least as early as those of Peterson (1948) and Peterson and others (1951) at Castle Dome. Additional information gathered during the next 20 years led to elaborate descriptions of lateral and vertical zoning by Lowell and Guilbert (1970), Rose (1970), and James (1971). Modifications of these views of zoning, based upon the recognition of the influence of different kinds of host rocks and plutons, were later presented by Guilbert and Lowell (1974) and Hollister (1975). The essentially static nature of these alteration zones has been the subject of comment by Gustafson (1978). Vein sequences within many porphyry copper systems have been described for many deposits, beginning at least as early as the descriptions at Bagdad by Anderson and others (1955), and such studies have led to more detailed investigation of the phenomenon by many workers since that time. An increased awareness of the importance of both alteration paragenesis, and of the distribution in space of the alteration types has begun to broaden the understanding of the nature of evolution of these large systems. Our understanding is far from perfect, but some aspects of the nature of alteration as developed in the preceding sections of this chapter may be worked into an understanding of the way in which alteration zones evolve.

Two important aspects of the evolution of hypogene alteration in porphyry copper deposits, as revealed by field data, form the basis of the interpretations presented here. First, episodic fracturing of host rocks and porphyry appears to take place in most systems studied and reported. The basis for this interpretation is that different alteration mineral assemblages are consistently developed, in generally consistent sequences, in their own sets of cross-cutting veins or veinlets. Second, by virtue of the fact that different alteration mineral assemblages develop sequentially, consideration of changes in either the composition of solutions or the physical conditions of mineral stabilities—or both—is virtually forced. That physical conditions have changed is revealed from an overwhelming mass of evidence from studies of fluid inclusion thermometry. The trend toward cooling temperatures is generally consistent with the observed sequence of progressively younger vein alteration assemblages superimposed on older types. Therefore, fracturing events take place during the cooling history of plutons and stable alteration assemblages change during that same cooling history. These observations and interpretations form the basis for the interpretation of alteration progress diagrammed in Figure 5.10. The figure separates each alteration event in the hypogene zone and shows the course and extent of each fracturing event. It also illustrates the progress from high to low temperatures, although minor reversals of the trend may be present within some of the alteration types in some deposits. From bottom to top it traces the place of evolution of fractures and concommitant alteration. The progress of hypogene alteration (with references to Fig. 5.10) is summarized as follows:

1. Sinuous quartz veins evolve in the early history of cooling of the pluton and are commonly restricted to the intrusion.
2. Widespread secondary biotite develops at greatly lowered temperatures or through a temperature decline from about 800°C to about 550°C in most deposits. Simultaneously, propylitic alteration—interpreted here as metamorphism—moves away with outward movement of heat.
3. Following the development of selective biotite alteration, an early fracturing event takes place and biotite is precipitated in microfractures and veinlets. The selective biotite alteration and veinlet biotite compose the biotite aureole within which many deposits lie. As temperatures in the wall rock fall, propylitic alteration, manifested prominently by chloritization of secondary biotite, encroaches across earlier alteration types.
4. Subsequent fracturing events, at apparently successively lower wall rock temperatures, retreat toward the pluton. Each event is followed by development of discrete stable alteration assemblages. During this time specific stages of alteration are interpreted as responsible for precipitation of metal sulfides. Propylitic alteration is interpreted as continuing to progress toward the pluton.
5. The last major fracturing event results, in almost every instance reported, in fracture abundances many times greater than any previous episode; phyllic alteration attends this event, and its destructive effects result in the obliteration of most earlier types which evolved (cf. Drummond and Godwin, 1976).

SUPERGENE ENVIRONMENT

Supergene alteration has been profoundly important in the evolution of economic porphyry copper deposits. This alteration has resulted in the development of secondarily enriched copper mineralization at shallow and mineable depths—mineralization which has provided the necessary grade and tonnage of accessible copper ore in the early stages of mining. Although in the late 1970s some porphyry copper deposits were being mined for hypogene ores, other deposits with decades of production—notably Ray, Morenci, and Santa Rita—were still being mined for significant tonnages of

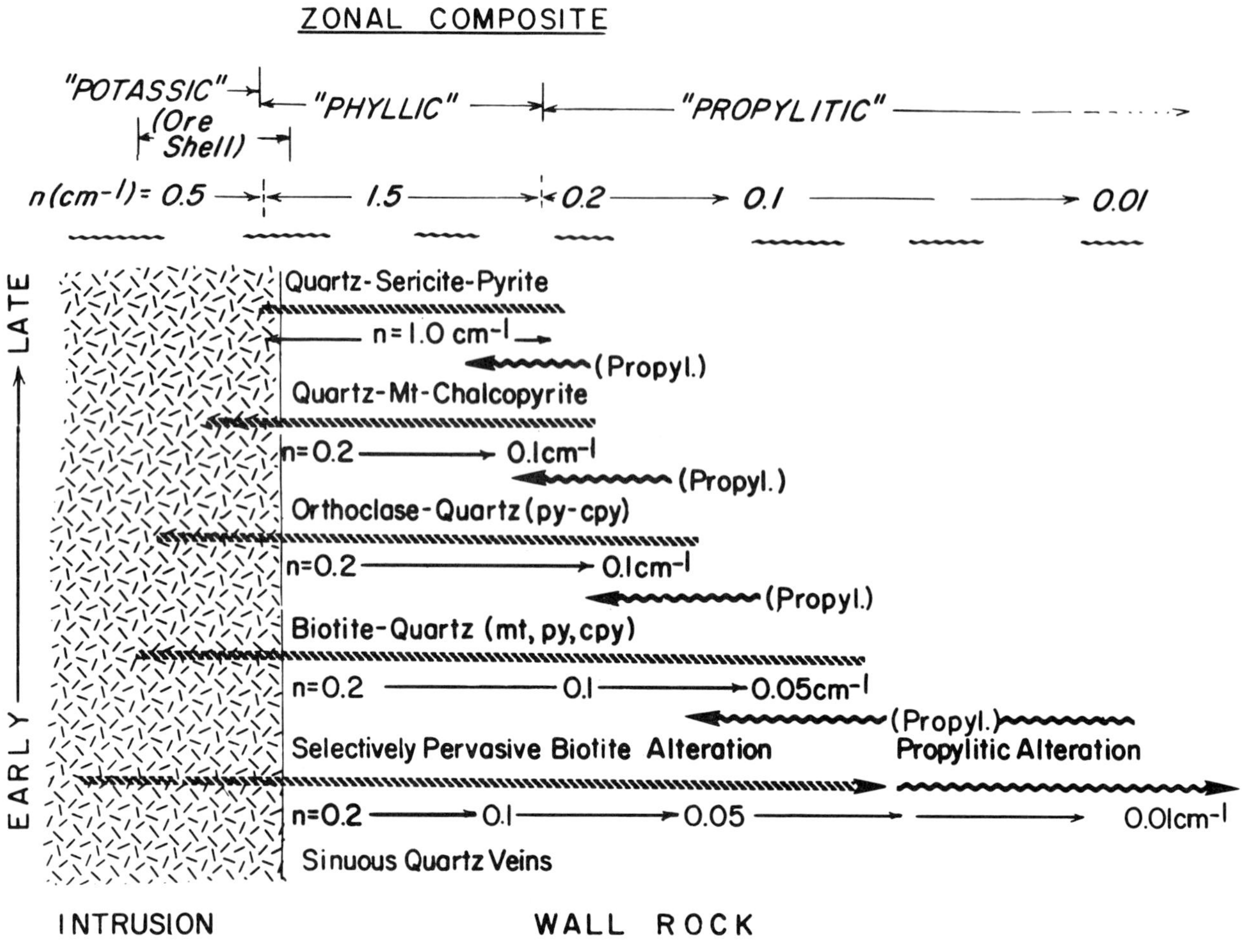

Figure 5.10. Alteration progress diagram of the hypogene environment showing the relative positions and times of formation of some principal types of vein alteration in a porphyry copper deposit formed in plutons and wall rocks of potassium silicate mineralogy. Temperature ranges shown are only approximate and are intended to indicate general cooling. Propylitic alteration is interpreted as a cooling and retrograde phenomenon that encroaches on the system. Fracture densities are shown as $n = \text{cm}^{-1}$. Compositing of alteration types results in quartz-sericite alteration superimposed on most earlier types and flanked by potassic alteration in the intrusion and by potassic and then propylitic alteration away from it.

secondarily enriched copper. Other deposits with less lengthy records of production were also being mined for secondary ores. The nature of supergene processes and their effects are, thus, of major importance in the scope of studies of porphyry copper genesis. Much literature of the period 1900 through 1955 was given over to study of supergene alteration, largely in the context of the chemistry of oxidation of sulfide minerals. Much of this literature was reviewed by Anderson (1955). Since that time the subject has received only scattered study, as judged by the infrequency of published reports; however, the nature and problems of supergene alteration remain extremely important.

The results of hypogene processes influence supergene alteration in many ways. Hypogene alteration mineralogy, host rock compositions, fracture abundance, and original primary pyrite content combine in many ways to influence the effects and manifestation of weathering. Thus, interpretation of leached outcrops involves a knowledge or presumption of some aspects of these primary parameters (Anderson, 1982). Climatic factors, pyrite content, fracture permeability, original copper content, and host rock mineralogy combine to influence the path and nature of secondary enrichment. Further, post-mineralization geologic events—such as geomorphic changes, faulting and volcanic activity—also combine with climate to act as controls or modifiers of the weathering and enrichment processes (Livingston et al., 1968). The effects of weather are thus complex and controlled by a variety of factors; many permutations of the factors listed acted to control and modify supergene alteration of deposits in the American Southwest.

Supergene Alteration in Potassium Silicate Rocks

Weathering of porphyry copper deposits is enhanced by the presence of permeability (fractures) and by a high pyrite content. In rocks containing potassium silicate alteration minerals the effects of oxidation bring about the development of supergene copper sulfide enrichment under proper conditions of climate and physiography. The chemistry of sulfide dissolution and precipitation of copper sulfides has been outlined by Emmons (1913), Locke (1926) and Blanchard (1968). These workers have stressed the requirement for large volumes of pyrite to promote the process of sulfide enrichment. As is shown on Figure 5.10, large pyrite volumes and large fracture densities are characteristic of the zone of phyllic alteration. The zone is particularly susceptible to weathering, and it is in this zone where deep oxidation produces the blankets of secondarily enriched copper sulfide ores. In those instances where detailed descriptions of secondary sulfide enrichment have been outlined, the characteristics of pyrite content and fracturing are those of the phyllic zone. There are few reports of secondary sulfide enrichment of consequence above the zone of potassic alteration and high hypogene grades or above hypogene propylitic altered rocks.

Early descriptions of the ores of Ray and Miami, Arizona (Ransome, 1919), have reported the presence of kaolin minerals and sericite with enriched sulfides in rocks strongly fractured and containing high sulfide contents. Peterson (1948) has described mineralized rocks at Castle Dome, Arizona, that contain abundant, closely spaced fractures and an abundance of sericite and clay. The enrichment blanket there was developed above a zone of hypogene mineralization that carried moderate pyrite and 0.1 to 0.3 percent copper. Higher primary grades beneath secondary enrichment are reported for Bagdad (Anderson et al., 1955), but insufficient data have been reported to assess the distribution of alteration types or the sulfide content of rocks at Bagdad; however, pyrite-bearing quartz-sericite-orthoclase veins are present (Anderson et al., 1955). At Mineral Park, Arizona, nearly pervasive quartz-sericite alteration occurs with secondarily enriched copper above primary hypogene grades of 0.1 to 0.15 percent copper (Eidel et al., 1968; Wilkinson et al., 1982). Saegart and others (1974) have reported phyllic alteration within and beneath the zone of oxidation and enrichment at La Caridad, Mexico, and have noted that, although rocks within the supergene zone appear megascopically more strongly altered than those beneath, there is no diminishment of phyllic alteration beneath the blanket when the rocks are observed microscopically. Their description of hypogene mineralization corresponds with general characteristics of phyllic zone alteration; 3 to 4 percent total sulfides, pyrite:chalcopyrite ratios on the order of 10:1, and low (ca. 0.2–0.25%) primary copper grades.

The presence of large volumes of supergene altered rocks superimposed upon the volume of hypogene quartz-sericite-altered rocks poses major problems in study and interpretation. Beane (1982) has noted that the products of acid weathering of potassium silicate rocks are similar in many respects to those same products produced by the relatively strong acid effects that produce quartz-sericite alteration (Figs. 5.11 and 5.12). The effects of the oxidizing process on altered potassium silicate rocks are poorly known; however, there exist some kinds of data that allow an attempt to generalize the results of leaching and enrichment.

Figure 5.13 shows a composited cross section through the primary alteration zone of a porphyry copper deposit in potassium silicate rocks, suggested by the data from Kalamazoo (Lowell, 1968). Sulfide content and compositions of the particular zones are shown, as is the integrated fracture density (suggested from many observations; see Fig. 5.10). The position of an enriched blanket which would form is shown above the zone of phyllic alteration. Included on the section is a sequence of vertical zones developed within the range of supergene activity. From bottom to top, they consist of chlorite; a mixture of sericite and other clays, chiefly kaolinite; and within and above the blanket, a zone dominated by kaolinite. The zones represent the effects of the downward

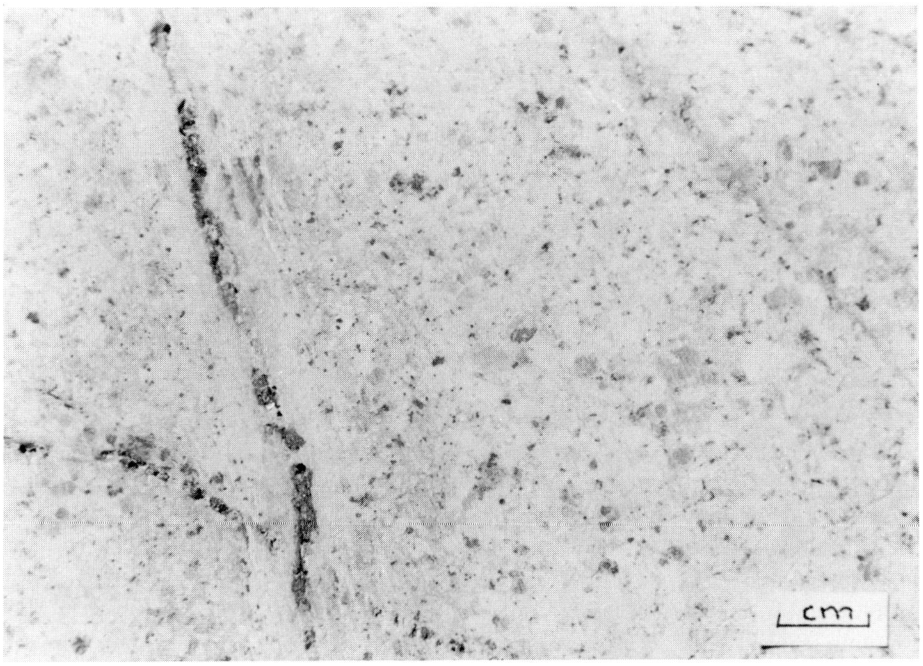

Figure 5.11. Supergene alteration in porphyry from Morenci. Diagonal vein at upper-right of sample is an orthoclase-quartz-sulfide vein. Thicker veins at left are original pyrite veins with destructive quartz-sericite selvages. Dark patches are chalcocite replacement of pyrite. The rock is strongly overprinted by supergene alteration effects that have nearly destroyed the original rock texture by converting it to fine-grained clay-mica mixtures.

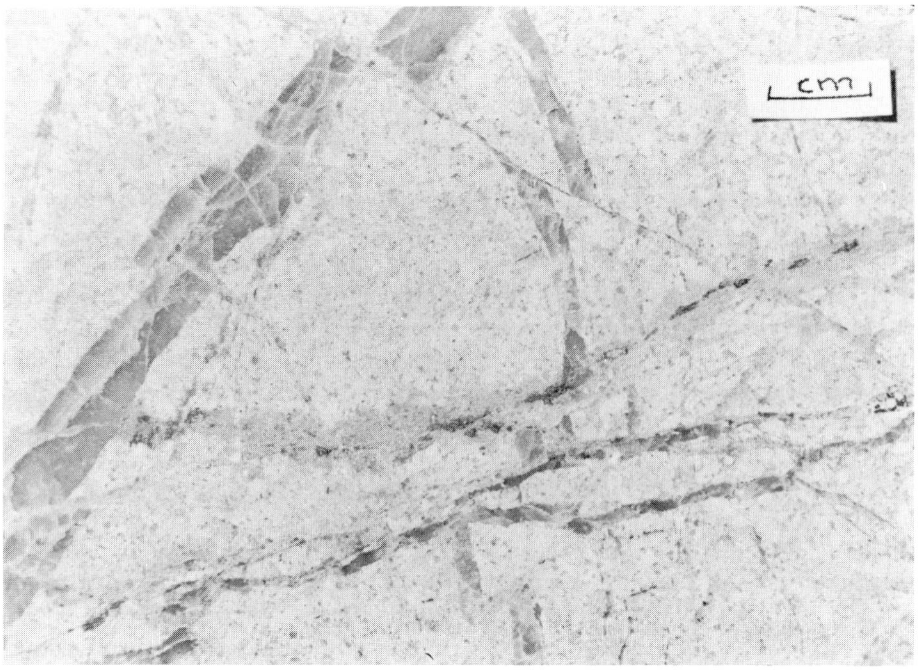

Figure 5.12. Supergene altered host rock from the zone of secondary sulfide enrichment, Santa Rita. The original rock was probably the granodiorite porphyry, as evidenced by the existence of original(?) quartz phenocrysts and similar styles of quartz veining (cf., Fig. 5.3). Quartz veins (dark) and alunite veins (light) cross the specimen; alunite veins with dark centers (chalcocite) are at center-right in the photograph and may represent original quartz-pyrite veins.

movement of acid-sulfate solutions through potassium silicate altered rocks; such effects are eventually neutralized beneath the blanket. The evidence is based on scattered observations by the author and some reports that have been cited above. Chorite as a product of supergene alteration has been suggested at Santa Rita by Rose and Baltosser (1966). Smectites with exchangeable iron have been reported beneath sulfide enrichment at Morenci (Moolick and Durek, 1966), and montmorillonite has been reported to occur in abundance only beneath the enrichment blanket at North San Xavier (Koenig, 1978). Both sericite and clay minerals have been reported to occur within enrichment blankets and kaolinite has been widely reported to occur within higher parts of enriched zones and in rocks above them. It is important to emphasize the point that supergene effects produce vertically zoned mineral assemblages which are superimposed upon laterally distributed zones of primary alteration products in many porphyry copper deposits.

Development of the enriched blanket shown in Figure 5.12 progresses in stages. Ransome (1919) has suggested that the process may have gone through stages in which enrichment blankets were created and then destroyed. The presence of limonites after chalcocite (Anderson, 1982) at the present surface in many porphyry copper deposits reveals the former presence of chalcocite at these and formerly higher levels. In some deposits (Red Mountain, Silver Bell) the presence of limonites after chalcocite at widely separated levels in host rocks indicates that multi-cycle enrichment has taken place. In regions such as the Basin and Range province, complex post-ore tectonic histories indicate periods of uplift and subsidence, together with intermittent covering of land surfaces by volcanic and sedimentary strata since the Laramide; it is, thus, not surprising that several, if not many, separate stages of oxidation and enrichment may have taken place.

Lowering of zones of enrichment appears to progress in a series of steps represented by abrupt and significant changes in elevation or in some base level, rather than by gradual lowering of such base level controls. Evidence for this stems from the wide separation of capping after sulfides, and the present levels of enriched sulfides. Maturity of enrichment can qualitatively be assessed from the extent of replacement of chalcopyrite and pyrite by chalcocite. In first or early stages this is seldom complete because of the relatively high pyrite:chalcopyrite ratios, which reflect low primary copper values. As the process continues, with successive lowering of the base level control, the concentration of copper in each successive blanket is probably increased because of the greater amount of copper available from superjacent blankets. Continued downward concentration of copper in successive enrichment cycles appears to result in increasing maturity (more complete replacement of primary sulfides) of enriched blankets. Such mature blankets are represented by those formerly present at Gobe-Miami, Ray, Morenci, and La Caridad, Mexico. The evolution of enrichment has been described for deposits in New Britain, Papua New Guinea (Titley, 1978), where multi-cycle but still immature enrichment has been recognized and separate pyrite grains have been replaced only to about 10 percent of their original volume by chalcocite.

Supergene Alteration in Calc-Silicate Rocks

Few studies report the nature of weathering of the calc-silicate alteration assemblage. The habit of primary alteration and mineralization is that of pervasive calc-silicate

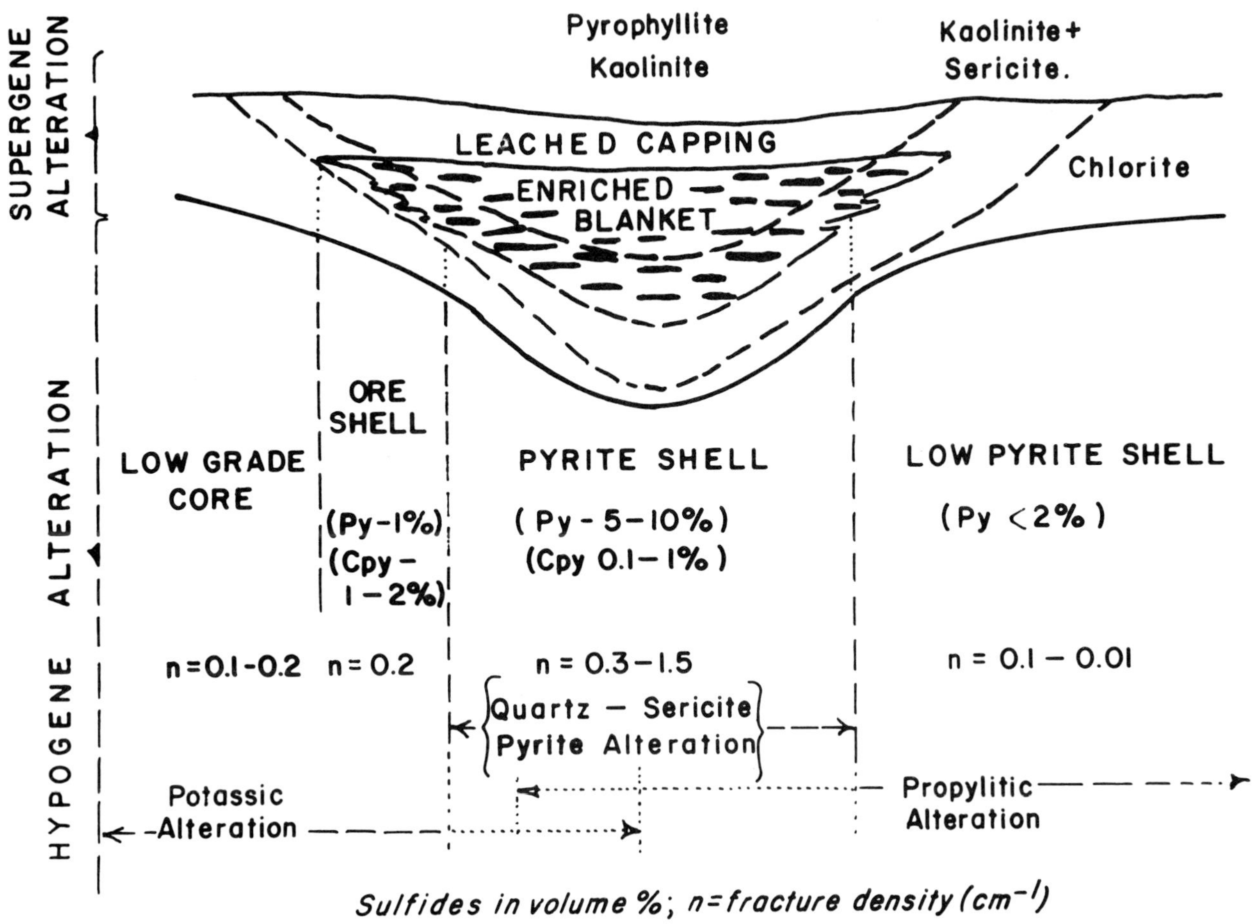

Figure 5.13. Composited cross section diagram of primary alteration zones in a porphyry copper deposit in potassium silicate host rocks and porphyry. Potassic alteration and propylitic alteration are shown as partially co-extensive and overprinted by quartz-sericite alteration of the pyrite shell. Primary alteration zones are shown from the porphyry center (*left*) to limits of mineralization in wall rocks (*right*). Sulfide mineral values shown are in volume percent. Section suggested from Lowell (1968). Supergene alteration and the enriched blanket are shown superimposed mostly on volume of high pyrite, densely fractured rocks. Fracture densities suggested from studies of Sierrita and Silver Bell. Diagram based on Titley (1972*a*).

alteration, together with younger vein and veinlet control of hydrous calc-magnesium silicates and sulfide minerals. Yet there are few reported instances of development of any significant grade or tonnage of secondary sulfides within such orebodies. Copper enriches, nonetheless, but most commonly as a mixture of various manganese, iron, and copper oxides, as well as chrysocolla and melaconite.

Silver Bell provides an important case in point. Much of the ore mined there before and during the 1970s was secondarily enriched sulfide ore from alaskite and quartz monzonite. Within the mass of igneous rocks, however, significant tonnages of copper ore occur in skarns. These ores, which occur at about the same topographic level as the enriched ores in igneous rocks, consist of primary, rather than secondary, sulfides. Graybeal (1982) has observed that the skarns at the contact of the Imperial stock were not significantly enriched by chalcocite but that copper liberated by oxidation was fixed as malachite. He has attributed this phenomenon to the neutralizing effects of calcite in the skarns on acid solutions formed by oxidation. He has also noted that the enrichment present within the skarns is dominated by chrysocolla.

At Twin Buttes, some enrichment occurs in skarns, and Barter and Kelly (1982) have described three recognizable levels within the supergene zone. The deepest is one in which anhydrite has been removed but in which sulfides are unaffected; in the intermediate zone formation of alteration clays after some calc-silicates, with minor immature enrichment by chalcocite near its top, took place; the upper zone of oxidation and leaching is also a zone of precipitation of considerable quantities of secondary copper oxides and chrysocolla. In the Mission orebody only insignificant amounts of chalcocite were produced from weathering; these are confined to the highest topographic levels in the skarn and are overlain at the paleosurface by copper oxides and silicates (Louis Jansen, 1978, personal communication).

From examples studied and cited in the American Southwest, it is, thus, apparent that there exists an environment within skarn-altered rocks which is not favorable to the development of the same extensive and rich secondary sulfide blankets that occur in potassium silicate rocks. The process has been poorly studied, however, and reasons for such differences are not clearly described or understood.

SUMMARY

The summary presented below includes salient points concerning different kinds of alteration and the way in which they are interpreted to have evolved. It is restricted to examples of alteration cited in this chapter and is dominated by observations from the American Southwest.

1. Porphyry copper deposits are large hydrothermal systems that involve both porphyry plutons and great volumes of wall rock. The hydrothermal systems, as defined by the presence of intrusion-related fracturing and alteration minerals, commonly extend a kilometer or more from porphyry contacts.
2. Copper mineralization is, in great part, fracture- or veinlet-localized and is apparently synchronous with the development of some kinds of non-sulfide alteration products.
3. Hydrothermal alteration is a complex process that evolves with time in large volumes of rock. Both pluton and wall rocks are extensively involved in the process, and many kinds of alteration transgress lithologic contacts. The evolution of alteration results in the superposition of many different kinds of alteration products, at different times, on rock volumes within the system.
4. In great part the alteration of porphyry copper deposits appears to progress along with, and may possibly be contingent upon, the continuous evolution of fracture permeability in host rocks and porphyry plutons.
5. The mineralogical compositions of host rocks and plutons exert a pronounced control on the composition of alteration minerals during times of early hydrothermal activity. During later times, when aided by extensive fracturing of rocks, solution compositions appear to control compositions of alteration assemblages.

It is obvious that alteration is a complex subject and that continuing detailed observations will greatly augment the somewhat generalized interpretations of alteration progress and types presented here for porphyry copper deposits in the Southwest. Such detailed studies will help to solve the broader problems of the nature of ore solutions, the changes which they undergo with time, and the provenance of copper, associated metals, and sulfur in these deposits.

ACKNOWLEDGMENTS

A synthesis of data such as presented in this chapter reflects the accumulation of many ideas and the observations of many years. It is difficult to acknowledge adequately the discussions with many geologists with whom I have worked in many deposits around the Pacific Basin Rim, and to acknowledge adequately the continuing stimulus of many present and former students and colleagues, many of whom have helped crystallize some of the ideas presented here. T. L. Heidrick, N. E. Lehman, and F. M. Haynes have provided many hours of critical discussions. Colleagues R. E. Beane, D. L. Norton, and J. M. Guilbert have helped sort out many of the complex problems which were initially recognized in this work. I am grateful to all for their continuous interest and constructive as well as destructive criticisms during the evolution of some concepts suggested here. However, the interpretations suggested in this work are my own responsibility; my colleagues and associates are not responsible for errors or controversial interpretations of data. A part of this work was carried out under NSF Grant EAR 78-22897.

REFERENCES CITED

Anderson, C. A., 1955, Oxidation of copper sulfides and secondary sulfide enrichment: Econ. Geol., 50th Anniv. Vol., pt. 1, p. 324–340.

Anderson, C. A.; Scholz, E. A.; and Strobell, J. J., Jr., 1955, Geology and ore deposits of the Bagdad area, Yavapai County, Arizona: U.S. Geol. Survey Prof. Paper 278, 103 p.

Anderson, J. A., 1982, Characteristics of leached capping and techniques of appraisal: *in* Titley, S. R., ed., Advances in Geology of the Porphyry Copper Deposits, Southwestern North America: Tucson, Univ. Ariz. Press, Chapter 12.

Atkinson, W. W., Jr., and Einaudi, M. T., 1978, Skarn formation and mineralization in the contact aureole at Carr Fork, Bingham, Utah: Econ. Geol., v. 73, p. 1326–1365.

Barter, C. F., and Kelly, J. L., 1982, Geology of the Twin Buttes mineral deposit, Pima mining district, Pima County, Arizona: *in* Titley, S. R., ed., Advances in Geology of the Porphyry Copper Deposits, Southwestern North America: Tucson, Univ. Ariz. Press, Chapter 20.

Beane, R. E., 1974, Biotite stability in the porphyry copper environment: Econ. Geol., v. 69, p. 241–256.

———, 1982, Hydrothermal alteration in silicate rocks, southwestern North America *in* Titley, S. R., ed., Advances in Geology of the Porphyry Copper Deposits, Southwestern North America: Tucson, Univ. Ariz. Press, Chapter 6.

Blanchard, Roland, 1968, Interpretation of leached outcrops: Nev. Bur. Mines Bull. 66, 196 p.

Bodnar, R. J., and Beane, R. E., 1977, Temperature variations in pre-intrusive cover over a buried pluton: Geol. Soc. American Ann. Mtg., Prog. with Abs., p. 903–904 (abs.)

Branch, C. D., 1976, Development of porphyry copper and stratiform volcanogenic ore bodies during the life cycle of andesitic stratovolcanoes: *in* Johnson, R. W., ed., Volcanism in Australasia: New York, London, Amsterdam, p. 337–342.

Brimhall, G. H., Jr., 1977, Early fracture-controlled disseminated mineralization at Butte, Montana: Econ. Geol., v. 72, p. 37–59.

Carson, D. J. T., and Jambor, J. L., 1974, Mineralogy, zonal relationships and economic significance of hydrothermal alteration at porphyry copper deposits, Babine Lake area, British Columbia: CIM Bull., v. 67, no. 742, p. 1–24.

Clark, A. H., 1979, Potassium-argon age of the Cerro Colorado porphyry copper deposit, Panama—a reply: Econ. Geol., v. 74, p. 695.

Corn, R. M., 1975, Alteration-mineralization zoning, Red Mountain, Arizona: Econ. Geol., v. 70, p. 1437–1447.

Drummond, A. D., and Godwin, C. I., 1976, Hypogene mineralization: an empirical evaluation of alteration zoning: *in* Sutherland Brown, A., ed., Porphyry Deposits of the Canadian Cordillera: CIM Spec. Vol. 15, p. 52–63.

Eastlick, J. T., 1968, Geology of the Christmas mine and vicinity, Banner mining district, Arizona: *in* Ridge, J. D., ed., Ore Deposits of the United States, 1933–1967 (Graton-Sales Volume), New York, AIME, p. 1189–1210.

Eidel, J. J.; Frost, J. E.; and Clippinger, D. M., 1968, Copper-molybdenum mineralization at Mineral Park, Mohave County, Arizona: *in* Ridge, J. D., ed., Ore Deposits of the United States, 1933–1967 (Graton-Sales Volume): New York, AIME, p. 1258–1281.

Einaudi, M. T., 1982*a*, Description of skarns associated with porphyry copper plutons, southwestern North America: *in* Titley, S. R., ed., Advances in Geology of the Porphyry Copper Deposits, Southwestern North America: Tucson, Univ. Ariz. Press, Chapter 7.

———, 1982*b*, General features and origin of skarns associated with porphyry copper plutons, southwestern North America: *in* Titley, S. R., ed., Advances in Geology of the Porphyry Copper Deposits, Southwestern North America: Tucson, Univ. Ariz. Press, Chapter 8.

Emmons, W. H., 1913, The enrichment of sulphide ores: U.S. Geol. Survey Bull. 529, 260 p.

Ford, J. H., 1978, A chemical study of alteration at the Panguna porphyry copper deposit, Bougainville, Papua New Guinea: Econ. Geol., v. 73, p. 703–720.

Gilluly, James, 1946, The Ajo mining district, Arizona: U.S. Geol. Survey Prof. Paper 109, 112 p.

Grant, J. N., and Nielsen, R. L., 1975, Geology and geochronology of the Yandera porphyry copper deposit, Papua New Guinea: Econ. Geol., v. 70, p. 1157–1174.

Graybeal, F. T., 1982, Geology of the El Tiro area, Silver Bell mining district, Pima County, Arizona: *in* Titley, S. R., ed., Advances in Geology of the Porphyry Copper Deposits, Southwestern North America: Tucson, Univ. Ariz. Press, Chapter 24.

Guilbert, J. M., and Lowell, J. D., 1974, Variations in zoning patterns in porphyry ore deposits: CIM Bull., v. 67, p. 99–109.

Gustafson, L. B., 1978, Some major factors of porphyry copper genesis: Econ. Geol., v. 73, p. 600–607.

Gustafson, L. B., and Hunt, J. P., 1975, The porphyry copper deposit at El Salvador, Chile: Econ. Geol., v. 70, p. 857–912.

Gustafson, L. B., and Titley, S. R., eds., 1978, Porphyry copper deposits of the southwestern Pacific islands and Australia: Econ. Geol., Spec. Issue, v. 73, no. 5., p. 597–985.

Haynes, F. M., and Titley, S. R., 1980, The evolution of fracture-related permeability within the Ruby Star Granodiorite, Sierrita porphyry copper deposit, Pima County, Arizona: Econ. Geol., v. 75, no. 5, in press.

Heidrick, T. L., and Titley, S. R., 1982, Fracture and dike patterns in Laramide plutons and their structural and tectonic implications, American Southwest *in* Titley, S. R., ed., Advances in Geology of the Porphyry Copper Deposits of the American Southwest: Tucson, Univ. Ariz. Press. Chapter 4.

Hollister, V. F., 1975, An appraisal of the nature and source of porphyry copper deposits: Minerals Sci. Eng., v. 7, p. 225–233.

Jacobs, D. C., and Parry, W. T., 1979, Geochemistry of biotite in the Santa Rita porphyry copper deposit, New Mexico: Econ. Geol., v. 74, p. 860–887.

James, A. H., 1971, Hypothetical diagrams of several porphyry copper deposits: Econ. Geol., v. 66, p. 43–47.

Johns, E. C., 1978, Mineral zones in the Utah copper orebody: Econ. Geol., v. 73, p. 1250–1259.

Kerr, P. F., 1951, Alteration features at Silver Bell, Arizona: Bull. Geol. Soc. America, v. 62, p. 457–480.

Kesler, S. E.; Sutter, J. F.; Issigonis, M. J.; Jones, L. M.; and Walker, R. L., 1977, Evolution of porphyry copper mineralization in an oceanic island arc: Panama: Econ. Geol., v. 72, p. 1142–1153.

Knapp, Richard, and Norton, D. L., 1980, Preliminary numerical analysis of processes related to magma crystallization and stress evolution in cooling pluton environments: Am. Jour. Sci., in press.

Koenig, B. A., 1978, Oxidation-leaching and enrichment zones of a porphyry copper deposit—a mineralogic and quantitative chemical study: Univ. Ariz. Unpub. M.S. Thesis, 57 p.

Kosaka, H., and Wakita, Kenji, 1978, Some geologic features of the Mamut porphyry copper deposit, Sabah, Malaysia: Econ. Geol., v. 73, p. 618–627.

Koski, R. A., and Cook, D. S., 1982, Geology of the Christmas porphyry copper deposit, Gila County, Arizona: *in* Titley, S. R., ed., Advances in Geology of the Porphyry Copper Deposits, Southwestern North America: Tucson, Univ. Ariz. Press, Chapter 17.

Langton, J. M., and Williams, S. A., 1982, Structural, petrological and mineralogical controls for the Dos Pobres orebody, Lone Star mining district, Graham County, Arizona: *in* Titley, S. R., ed., Advances in Geology of the Porphyry Copper Deposits, Southwestern North America: Tucson, Univ. Ariz. Press, Chapter 16.

Lanier, George; Raab, W. J.; Folsom, R. B., and Cone, S., 1978, Alteration of equigranular monzonite, Bingham mining district, Utah: Econ. Geol., v. 73, p. 1270–1286.

Livingston, D. E.; Mauger, R. L.; and Damon, P. E., 1968, Geochronology of the emplacement, enrichment, and preservation of Arizona porphyry copper deposits: Econ. Geol., v. 63, p. 30–36.

Locke, Augustus, 1926, Leached Outcrops as Guides to Copper Ore: Baltimore, Williams and Wilkins, 175 p.

Lowder, G. G., and Dow, J. A. S., 1978, Geology and exploration of porphyry copper deposits in North Sulawesi, Indonesia: Econ. Geol., v. 73, p. 628–644.

Lowell, J. D., 1968, Geology of the Kalamazoo orebody, San Manuel district, Arizona: Econ. Geol., v. 63, p. 645–654.

Lowell, J. D., and Guilbert, J. M., 1970, Lateral and vertical alteration mineralization zoning in porphyry ore deposits: Econ. Geol., v. 65, p. 373–408.

Mason, D. R., and McDonald, J. A., 1978, Intrusive rocks and porphyry copper occurrences of the Papua New Guinea–Solomon Islands region: a reconnaissance study: Econ. Geol., v. 73, p. 857–877.

McKinstry, H. E., 1955, Structure of hydrothermal ore deposits: Econ Geol., 50th Anniv. Vol., p. 170–225.

Meyer, Charles, and Hemley, J. J., 1967, Wall rock alteration: *in* Barnes, H. L., ed., Geochemistry of Hydrothermal Ore Deposits: Holt, Rinehart and Winston, p. 166–235.

Meyer, Charles; Shea, E. P.; Goddard, C. C.; Jr.; Staff, 1968, Ore deposits at Butte, Montana: *in,* Ridge, J. D., ed., Ore Deposits of the United States, 1933–1967 (Graton-Sales Volume): New York, AIME, p. 1375–1416.

Mitchell, A. H., and Bell, J. D., 1973, Island-arc evolution and related mineral deposits: Jour. Geol., v. 81, p. 381–405.

Moolick, R. T., and Durek, J. J., 1966, The Morenci district: *in* Titley, S. R., and Hicks, C. L., eds., Geology of the Porphyry Copper Deposits, Southwestern North America: Tucson, Univ. Ariz. Press, p. 221–231.

Moore, W. J., 1978, Chemical characteristics of hydrothermal alteration at Bingham, Utah: Econ. Geol., v. 73, p. 1260–1269.

Nielsen, R. L., 1968, Hypogene texture and mineral zoning in a copper-bearing granodiorite porphyry stock, Santa Rita, New Mexico: Econ. Geol., v. 63, p. 37–50.

Norton, D. L., 1982, Fluid and heat transport phenomena typical of copper-bearing pluton environments, southeastern Arizona: *in* Titley, S. R., ed., Advances in Geology of the Porphyry Copper Deposits, Southwestern North America: Tucson, Univ. Ariz. Press, Chapter 3.

Parsons, A. B., 1957, The Porphyry Coppers in 1956: New York, AIME, 270 p.

Perry, D. V., 1968, Skarn genesis at the Christmas mine, Gila County, Arizona: Econ. Geol., v. 64, p. 255–270.

Peters, W. C.; James, A. H.; and Field, C. W., 1966, Geology of the Bingham Canyon porphyry copper deposit, Utah: *in* Titley, S. R., and Hicks, C. L., eds., Geology of the Porphyry Copper Deposits, Southwestern North America: Tucson, Univ. Ariz. Press, p. 165–175.

Peterson, N. P., 1948, Geology of the Castle Dome Copper deposit, Arizona: AIME, Min. Tech., v. 12, no. 2, TP2302, 11 p.

Peterson, N. P.; Gilbert, C. M.; and Quick, G. L., 1951, Geology and ore deposits of the Castle Dome area, Gila County, Arizona: U.S. Geol. Survey Bull. 971, 134 p.

Phillips, C. H.; Gambell, N. A.; and Fountain, D. S., 1974, Hydrothermal alteration, mineralization, and zoning in the Ray deposit: Econ. Geol., v. 69, p. 1237–1250.

Ransome, F. L., 1919, The copper deposits of Ray and Miami, Arizona: U.S. Geol. Survey Prof. Paper 115, 192 p.

Rehrig, W. A., and Heidrick, T. L., 1972, Regional fracturing in Laramide stocks of Arizona and its relationship to porphyry copper mineralization: Econ. Geo., v. 67, p. 198–213.

———, 1976, Regional stress during the Laramide and Late Tertiary intrusive periods, Basin and Range Province, Arizona: Ariz. Geol. Soc. Digest X, p. 205–228.

Reynolds, T. J., and Beane, R. E., 1979, The evolution of hydrothermal fluid characteristics through time at the Santa Rita, New

Mexico, porphyry copper deposit: Geol. Soc. America Ann. Mtg., Prog. with Abs., v. 11, no. 7, p. 502 (abs.).

Roberts, S. A., 1973, Pervasive early alteration in the Butte district, Montana: Soc. Econ. Geol. Guidebook, Butte Field Mtg., Butte, Montana, Anaconda Co., p. HH1–HH8.

Robinson, R. F., and Cook, Annan, 1966, The Safford copper deposit, Lone Star mining district, Graham County, Arizona: *in* Titley, S. R., and Hicks, C. L., eds., Geology of the Porphyry Copper Deposits, Southwestern North America: Tucson, Univ. Ariz. Press, p. 251–266.

Rose, A. W., 1970, Zonal relations of wallrock alteration and sulfide distribution at porphyry copper deposits: Econ. Geol., v. 63, p. 920–936.

Rose, A. W., and Baltosser, W. W., 1966, The porphyry copper deposit at Santa Rita, New Mexico: *in* Titley, S. R., and Hicks, C. L., eds., Geology of the Porphyry Copper Deposits, Southwestern North America: Tucson, Univ. Ariz. Press, p. 205–220.

Saegart, W. E.; Sell, J. D.; and Kilpatrick, B. E., 1974, Geology and mineralization of La Caridad porphyry copper deposit, Sonora, Mexico: Econ. Geol., v. 69, p. 1060–1077.

Sheppard, S. M. F.; Nielsen, R. L.; and Taylor, H. P., Jr., 1971, Hydrogen and oxygen isotope ratios in minerals from porphyry copper deposits: Econ. Geol., v. 66, p. 515–542.

Sillitoe, H., 1973, The tops and bottoms of porphyry copper deposits: Econ. Geol., v. 68, p. 799–815.

Spatz, D. M., 1979, Potassium-argon age of the Cerro Colorado porphyry copper deposit, Panama—a discussion: Econ. Geol., v. 74, p. 693–695.

Sutherland Brown, A., ed., 1976, Porphyry Copper Deposits of the Canadian Cordillera: CIM Spec. Vol. 15, 510 p.

Theodore, T. G.; Blake, D. W., and Kretschmer, E. L., 1982, Geology of the Copper Canyon porphyry copper deposits, Lander County, Nevada: *in* Titley, S. R., ed., Advances in Geology of the Porphyry Copper Deposits, Southwestern North America: Tucson, Univ. Ariz. Press, Chapter 27.

Titley, S. R., 1972*a,* Some geological criteria applicable to the search for southwestern North American porphyry copper deposits: AIME-MMIJ Joint Mtg., Tokyo, May, Preprint G I 2, 16 p.

———, 1972*b,* Intrusion and wall rock porphyry copper deposits: Econ. Geol., v. 67, p. 122–123.

———, 1973, "Pyrometasomatic"—an alteration type: Econ. Geol., v. 68, p. 1326–1329.

———, 1976, Characteristics of some telescoped alteration patterns in southwestern Pacific porphyry copper deposits: Econ. Geol., v. 71, p. 703 (abs.).

———, 1978, Geologic history, hypogene features, and processes of secondary sulfide enrichment at the Plesyumi copper prospect, New Britain, Papua New Guinea: Econ. Geol., v. 73, p. 768–784.

———, 1982, The geologic setting of porphyry copper deposits, southeastern Arizona: *in* Titley, S. R., ed., Advances in Geology of the Porphyry Copper Deposits, Southwestern North America: Tucson, Univ. Ariz. Press, Chapter 2.

Titley, S. R.; Fleming, A. W.; and Neale, T. I., 1978, Tectonic evolution of the porphyry copper system at Yandera, Papua New Guinea: Econ. Geol., v. 73, p. 810–828.

Titley, S. R., and Heidrick, T. L., 1978, Intrusion and fracture styles of some mineralized porphyry systems of the southwestern Pacific and their relationship to plate interactions: Econ. Geol., v. 73, p. 891–903.

Watmuff, I. G., 1978, Geology and alteration-mineralization zoning in the central portion of the Yandera porphyry copper prospect, Papua New Guinea: Econ. Geol., v. 73, p. 829–856.

West, R. J., and Aiken, D. M., Geology of the Sierrita-Esperanza Deposit, Pima County, Arizona: *in* Titley, S. R., ed., Advances in Geology of the Pophyry Copper Deposits, Southwestern North America: Tucson, Univ. Ariz. Press, Chapter 21.

Wilkinson, W. H., Jr.; Vega, Luis; and Titley, S. R., 1982, Geology and ore deposits at Mineral Park, Mohave County, Arizona: *in* Titley, S. R., ed., Advances in Geology of the Porphyry Copper Deposits, Southwestern North America: Tucson, Univ. Ariz. Press, Chapter 26.

Wolfe, J. A., 1973, Tectonic fingerprint in Philippine porphyry deposits: AIME, Preprint 73–5–37, 31 p.

6

Hydrothermal Alteration in Silicate Rocks

SOUTHWESTERN NORTH AMERICA

Richard E. Beane

Porphyry copper mineralization in southwestern North America occurs in close spatial and chronologic association with intrusive rocks ranging in composition from quartz diorite to quartz monzonite. Upon close examination it is seen that sulfide mineralization is, for the most part, demonstrably epigenetic in the sense that it occurs in close association with post-crystallization fractures in the associated igneous rock. In these mineralized systems, original rock-forming minerals contiguous to sulfide veinlets commonly undergo alteration, apparently in conjunction with the mineralization process, and the overall effects of hydrothermal mineralization and alteration are superimposed upon both the intrusive porphyry and the varied host rocks intruded.

Several lines of evidence point to the fact that mineralization and wall-rock alteration evolve in the presence of hot aqueous fluids which are responsible for the introduction and removal of chemical components from large rock volumes. This chapter is designed to examine the effects of interaction between hydrothermal fluids and silicate rocks in the porphyry copper environment. Analogous considerations regarding carbonate wall rocks are described by Einaudi in Chapter 8 of this volume. Much of the present review will build upon and extend the discussion of hydrothermal alteration by Creasey (1966), recognizing that at that time detailed geologic information on hypogene characteristics was available for only a few of the porphyry copper deposits in southwestern North America. Up to 1966 many of these deposits had been exploited largely for higher-grade, supergene ore (Gilmour, 1982). The processes attending supergene enrichment often obliterated original igneous and hypogene characteristics and made recognition and study of these features difficult, if not impossible. Subsequent mining and drilling below the level of pervasive supergene alteration in the last decade has enabled significant expansion of the bank of available field and laboratory data on various aspects of hypogene alteration in or pertaining to porphyry copper deposits.

The diagrams that accompany the text to illustrate mineral stability relations at elevated temperatures were calculated using thermodynamic data recently compiled for minerals (Helgeson et al., 1978), aqueous species (Helgeson and Kirkham, 1976), and H_2O (Helgeson and Kirkham, 1974). Such data were derived, for the most part, from results of laboratory studies (e.g., Montoya and Hemley, 1975) and hence the calculated stability diagrams can be considered to be compatible with experimental work. In recent years, numerous reports have revealed the results of detailed alteration studies of deposits in regions other than southwestern North America (e.g., Gustafson and Hunt, 1975; Carson and Jambor, 1974; Hollister, 1978; numerous articles in Gustafson and Titley, 1978). This chapter will center attention on studies pertaining to deposits located in the area upon which this volume is focused, and relevant information from other regions will be called upon only when necessary to clarify observations from southwestern North America.

ALTERATION MINERALS AND ASSEMBLAGES

Hydrothermal alteration reflects the response of preexisting, rock-forming minerals to thermal and/or chemical conditions different than those under which they originally formed. The level of alteration ranges from selected individual phases to that of the composite rock mineralogy, and extends from narrow selvages along vein walls through increasing halo widths, until the entire rock mass between pairs of adjacent veins is pervaded (Titley, 1982). In certain instances hydrothermal, vein-filling fluids were apparently at or near equilibrium with enclosing wall rocks, because no alteration is observed along vein margins. In such instances vein-filling minerals may be indistinguishable from those of the enclosing rock mass upon casual observation, and sulfides in such veins may appear to be disseminated in wall rocks. For the most part, however, porphyry copper deposits are characterized by widespread development of new silicate mineralogies which differ in aspect both within individual deposits—as a function of host-rock composition, space, and time—and between deposits which occur in similar rock types.

Types of Alteration Assemblages

Early detailed studies of hypogene alteration revealed that distinct, recognizably different mineral assemblages could be separated spatially and chronologically within single deposits (Schwartz, 1947; Stringham, 1953; Anderson, 1950). As such data began to accumulate, it was recognized that certain assemblages of minerals were recurrent across the porphyry copper deposits as a group (Creasey, 1959, 1966; Burnham, 1962). Table 6.1 shows comparative classifications of alteration mineral assemblages from porphyry copper deposits set forth by Creasey (1959), Lowell and Guilbert (1970), Rose (1970), and Meyer and Hemley (1967). Because the classification of alteration assemblages is based on observed minerals, the various schemes in Table 6.1 should, and do, closely resemble one another.

K-Silicate or Potassic Assemblage. K-silicate (Creasey, 1959; Meyer and Hemley, 1957), or potassic (Lowell and Guilbert, 1970), alteration is normally characterized by the presence of K-feldspar in the rock of interest and hence is equivalent to the orthoclase-bearing groups of Rose (1970). Persistence or formation of two of the three characteristic minerals—K-feldspar, biotite, and muscovite (or sericite)—might define this assemblage. K-feldspar and quartz are stable as original rock-forming minerals and as vein-filling constituents. K-feldspar also occurs as an alteration product after plagioclase in wall rocks. Original igneous biotite and K-feldspar are not stable in the strict sense of the word during potassic alteration, because these minerals undergo compositional readjustment. Hydrothermal K-feldspar contains less Na than the original igneous counterpart. Biotite shows increasing Mg:Fe (Beane, 1974; Jacobs and Parry, 1976; Moore and Czamanske, 1973) and loss of Ti, which appears as ilmenite or sphene; intergrown sulfides indicate sulfur fixation of the extracted iron. While the composition of igneous biotite is modified, other mafic silicates, chiefly amphibole and hornblende, are converted to alteration biotite by potassium addition. Also, magnesian biotite may be precipitated in veins or as a selvage along vein walls. It is not uncommon to find vein-related, hydrothermal biotite in varying degrees of alteration to chlorite with approximate Mg:Fe conservation, while K-feldspar remains apparently stable. Sericite or, less commonly, montmorillonite is seen as an alteration product in the sites of original rock-forming plagioclase, while K-feldspar is unaffected. This alteration may attack only the calcic plagioclase component

TABLE 6.1
Comparative Classifications of Porphyry Copper Assemblages

Creasey (1959, 1966)	Lowell and Guilbert (1970)	Rose (1970)	Meyer and Hemley (1967)
K-silicate K-feldspar biotite muscovite	*Potassic* K-feldspar biotite sericite chlorite quartz	*Orthoclase-Sericite-Quartz* *Orthoclase-Biotite-Quartz* *Orthoclase-Sericite-Biotite-Quartz*	*K-silicate* K-feldspar biotite muscovite anhydrite
(*Sericite-Quartz-Pyrite*)	*Phyllic* quartz sericite pyrite hydromica chlorite	*Sericite-Quartz*	*Sericitic* sericite quartz pyrite ± chlorite
Argillic kaolinite muscovite	*Argillic* kaolinite montmorillonite chlorite	*Sericite-Kaolinite-Quartz*	*Argillic* 1) Advanced kaolinite/dickite pyrophyllite 2) Intermediate kaolinite group montmorillonite ± chlorite
Propylitic muscovite (sericite) epidote chlorite carbonate	*Propylitic* chlorite epidote	*Propylitic* epidote albite calcite chlorite	*Propylitic* epidote albite chlorite septachlorite carbonate

and leave an apparently stable albitic residual product. Accessory minerals in the potassic assemblage include anhydrite, apatite, magnetite, siderite, pyrite, and chalcopyrite. In many of the porphyry copper deposits of southwestern North America, the occurrence of potassic phases in both veins and wall rocks is coincident in space with the hypogene, ore-forming minerals. Chalcopyrite and pyrite, in approximately equal, relatively low abundance ($\leq$ 1 volume % total sulfides), form in veins and in the sites of wall-rock mafic silicates accompanying their alteration to magnesian biotite.

Propylitic Assemblage. The propylitic mineral assemblage, in its most common mode of occurrence, is one characterized chiefly by development of new calcium and magnesium minerals by rearrangement of original rock-forming components. Here the anorthitic component of plagioclase is converted to epidote and calcite, while the albitic component is preserved. Original mafic minerals are most commonly altered to chlorite, although at Bingham (Bray, 1969) an intermediate step has been observed in which augite is altered to actinolite. Propylitic alteration, also referred to as saussuritization, can be characterized by the presence and stability of two of the following three mineral groups: (1) sodic plagioclase (albite-oligoclase), (2) 7- or 14-Å chlorite, (3) epidote-zoisite or calcite. Non-essential accessory minerals include sericite, montmorillonite, and hematite. Pyrite, with or without chalcopyrite, may also be present, but never in significant amounts. The essential minerals in this assemblage can be produced from original rock-forming minerals by addition of minor amounts of CO_2 and H_2O.

Phyllic Assemblage. The main difference between Creasey's classification and the others in Table 6.1 is that the former includes muscovite (sericite) as a member of both the K-silicate and argillic assemblages, rather than creating a separate subdivision characterized by this phase alone. However, "Quartz-sericite-pyrite without either a clay mineral or K-feldspar" has been noted by Creasey (1966, p. 62) to represent a potentially distinct alteration assemblage. Thus quartz-sericite-pyrite, or phyllic, alteration must be defined by intense development of these phases with accompanying destruction of minerals characteristic of other alteration assemblages (e.g., K-feldspar and biotite). With this assemblage, quartz and sericite occur in alteration envelopes adjacent to veins consisting almost entirely of quartz and pyrite, and they replace all original rock-forming silicates or their pre-existing alteration products. This group of minerals, unlike either the K-silicate or propylitic assemblages, is texturally destructive when introduced in igneous rocks. Local development of large volumes of pyrite with the quartz-sericite assemblage (up to 15–20 volume %) indicates addition of significant amounts of sulfur, plus iron in excess of that initially present in mafic minerals; minor amounts of chalcopyrite may also be present. As discussed by Meyer and Hemley (1967), the term "sericite" permits considerable latitude in chemical composition; it has been used largely for convenience in describing light-colored (but not necessarily white), fine-grained, mica-like minerals which may include sericite, illite, hydromica, hydromuscovite, phengite, paragonite, pyrophyllite, phlogopite, and a profusion of mixed layer phases, in addition to simple muscovite.

Argillic Assemblage. Kaolinite or related phases of like composition (halloysite, dickite), pyrophyllite, and montmorillonite characterize the argillic alteration assemblage and have been identified in abundance at a number of the porphyry copper deposits during early stages of development. But as mining and drilling extended below the zone of supergene enrichment, these phases were generally found to decrease significantly in abundance. Thus, in the porphyry copper environment, development of the clay minerals alone appears to be largely related to supergene processes. However, oxygen isotope data point to a hydrothermal origin for clays from several of these deposits (Taylor, 1974); these clays occur most commonly as high-level alterations in the evolving hypogene system and are accompanied by abundant pyrite and, less commonly, by hematite, chalcopyrite, and enargite. Such effects are observed at Butte, Montana (Brimhall, 1979) and Red Mountain, Arizona (Corn, 1975) and are associated with large veins having zoned alteration haloes (Meyer and Hemley, 1967). Clay minerals are sometimes seen to occur as alteration products in the sites of original plagioclase in the company of K-feldspar and biotite of the potassic assemblage (Bingham, Santa Rita, Ray, Ruth-Ely, Globe-Miami) or with sericite (Bingham, San Manuel, Bisbee, Silver Bell, Morenci).

Chemical Changes Attending Alteration

Hydrothermal minerals in porphyry copper deposits occur both within veins and in the rocks crosscut by these structures. Minerals within veins often contain chemical components not found within pre-existing rocks, and, thus, it may be concluded that fluids moving through fractures served as transport media for endogenous materials. The most obvious of the introduced elements are copper and sulfur, but mineral alterations and chemical gains and losses in wall rocks bordering veins show that other major rock-forming components were also transported by migrating hydrothermal fluids.

Hydrothermal alteration is interpreted petrologically in terms of addition and subtraction of chemical components from a rock mass having a certain initial composition and mineralogy. The compositions of essential silicate minerals of igneous and hydrothermal origin in porphyry copper deposits are defined by the following chemical components: K_2O, Na_2O, CaO, MgO, FeO, Fe_2O_3, Al_2O_3, SiO_2, and H_2O. Combinations of these may be used as endmembers on modified *AKF* and *ACF* diagrams (Fig. 6.1) upon which compositions of silicate minerals are plotted. The *AKF* diagram contains the following as chemical components: $A = Al_2O_3 + Fe_2O_3$, $K = K_2O + Na_2O$, and $F = MgO + FeO$, with SiO_2 and H_2O in excess. The complementary *ACF* diagram introduces another component, C=CaO, which combines with CO_2 or SO_3 as calcite or anhydrite, respectively, at the appropriate apex. Several of the phases displayed on these diagrams exhibit compositional ranges concomitant with coupled solid solution among components or with mixed layering of phyllosilicates. Compositions of original igneous rocks lie along the alkali feldspar-biotite join on the *AKF*

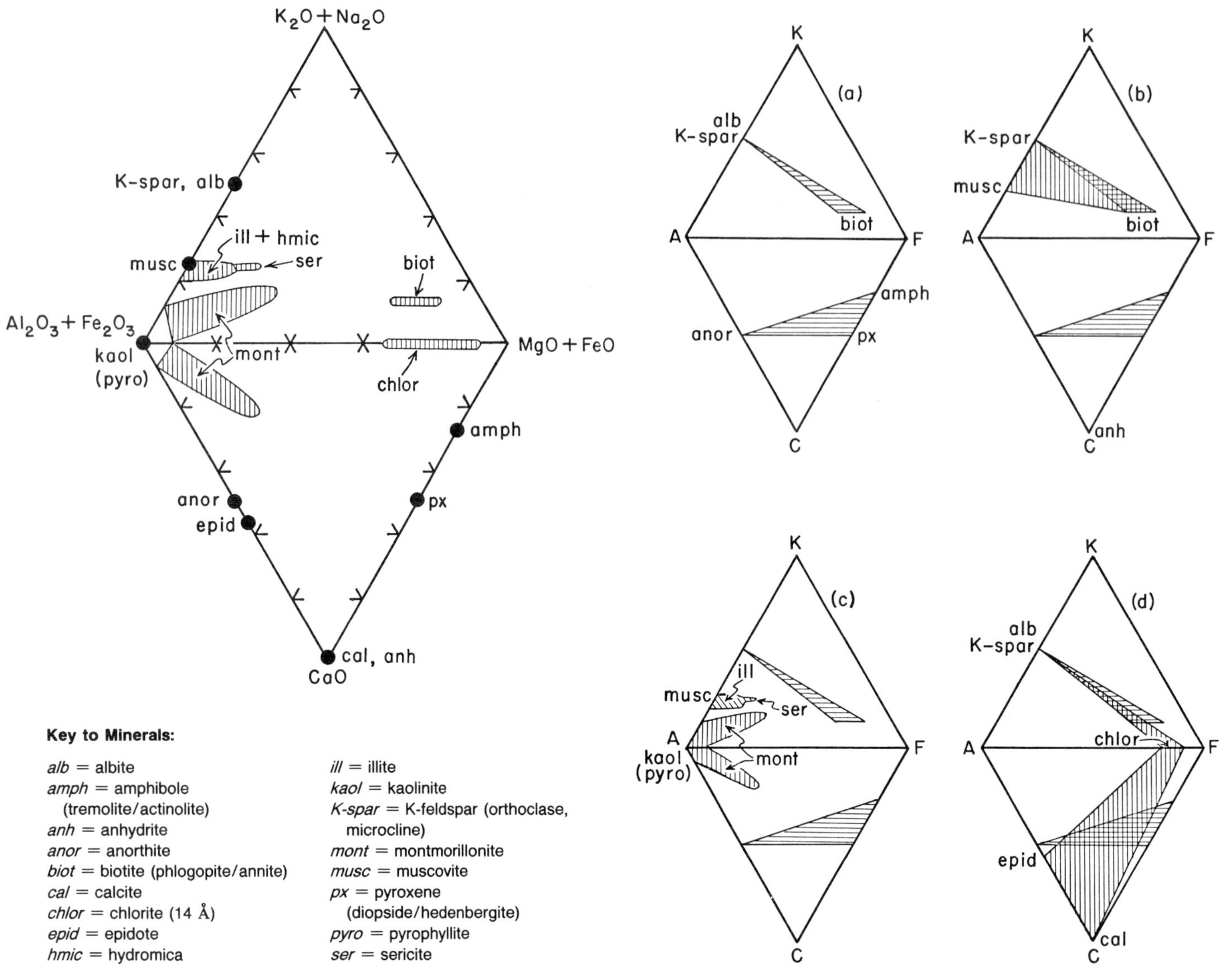

Figure 6.1. *AKF* and *ACF* composition diagrams, showing mineral compositions (*left*) and alteration assemblages (*right*) commonly found in the porphyry copper deposits of southwestern North America: *a,* minerals originally present in igneous rocks of quartz dioritic to granitic composition (horizontal hatching); *b,* original igneous minerals (horizontal hatching) and potassic alteration assemblage (vertical hatching); *c,* original igneous minerals (horizontal hatching) and phyllic (diagonal hatching) and argillic (vertical hatching) alteration assemblages; *d,* original igneous minerals (horizontal hatching) and propylitic alteration assemblage (vertical hatching). Alteration assemblages from, and diagrams modified after, Meyer and Hemley (1967).

diagram and move from the feldspar endmember toward biotite as affinities change from granitic to dioritic. On the *ACF* diagram igneous rock-forming minerals include amphibole, pyroxene, and the anorthitic component of plagioclase, all of which occupy the central portion of the diagram. Potassically altered rocks lie on the *AKF* diagram in a region bounded by K-feldspar, biotite, and muscovite-sericite (using the criteria presented by Creasey [1966]). This alteration type reflects generally strong K-metasomatism and conversion of original igneous amphibole and plagioclase to biotite and K-feldspar, with or without muscovite. Potassic alteration can essentially be thought of as an ion exchange process of potassium for calcium and sodium. The phyllic assemblage generally lies in a restricted region close to the K_2O-Al_2O_3 edge of the *AKF* triangle. Development of this alteration type is characterized by the wholesale removal of sodium, calcium, and magnesium from rock volumes during intense hydrogen and weaker potassium metasomatism. Original iron is usually conserved in the rock mass as pyrite, and some new iron may be introduced as well, but it does not occur in silicate phases. Argillic alteration is represented by rock compositions lying at or near the Al_2O_3 apex of the diagram. Montmorillonites, when present as hypogene minerals, tend to be of the calcian or magnesian variety and, hence, lie on the *ACF* diagram. This alteration assemblage is generally characterized by strong leaching of alkalis, particularly sodium and potassium. As noted above, however, instances have been recorded in which the argillic minerals occur with the potassic phases K-feldspar or biotite. As a general rule, the argillic alteration assemblage lies only on the

ACF diagram. Propylitic alteration, characterized by calcite, epidote, and chlorite, forms a region which overlaps that of unaltered igneous rocks on the *ACF* diagram, reflecting the nearly isochemical rearrangement of original rock-forming components. On the *AKF* diagram, propylitic alteration would correspond to a tie-line between chlorite and K-feldspar when adularia is present, and by necessity this tie-line would shift toward the Al_2O_3 apex (away from the K_2O-MgO side) so as to avoid intersecting biotite. Thus, propylitic alteration may involve minor leaching of potassium and magnesium + iron from the rock mass.

Alteration Mineral Zoning and Paragenesis

Both Lowell and Guilbert (1970) and Rose (1970) have established a geometric relationship among the various alteration types in which potassic alteration is centrally located and the phyllic, argillic, and propylitic assemblages are circumferentially arranged at increasingly greater lateral distances from the potassic core. The model set forth by Lowell and Guilbert, which is based heavily on petrographic studies of alteration mineralogy of the Kalamazoo deposit, is shown in Figure 6.2. These authors feel that the spatial relationship among alteration types is sufficiently systematic and recurrent to warrant definition as "typical" alteration zoning for porphyry copper deposits. This spatial arrangement has been widely accepted for use in exploration since presentation of the model, but certain constraints must be recognized in its use. In the first place, the Kalamazoo deposit occurs in wall rocks and in an intrusive of similar, quartz monzonitic composition (Lowell, 1968). Variations in alteration mineralogy can be expected when different silicate rock types are acted upon by the alteration process (cf., Guilbert and Lowell, 1974; Meyer and Hemley, 1967; Hollister, 1978). Furthermore, while the model is based on observed or recorded characteristics from 27 porphyry copper deposits, few of these adhere to the "average" in every respect. Detailed examination of alteration data reveals numerous exceptions to the suggested rule in terms of absence, rearrangement, and mixing of specific alteration types. The latter feature is, in part, responsible for Creasey's (1966) hesitation to define a distinct muscovite + quartz alteration assemblage.

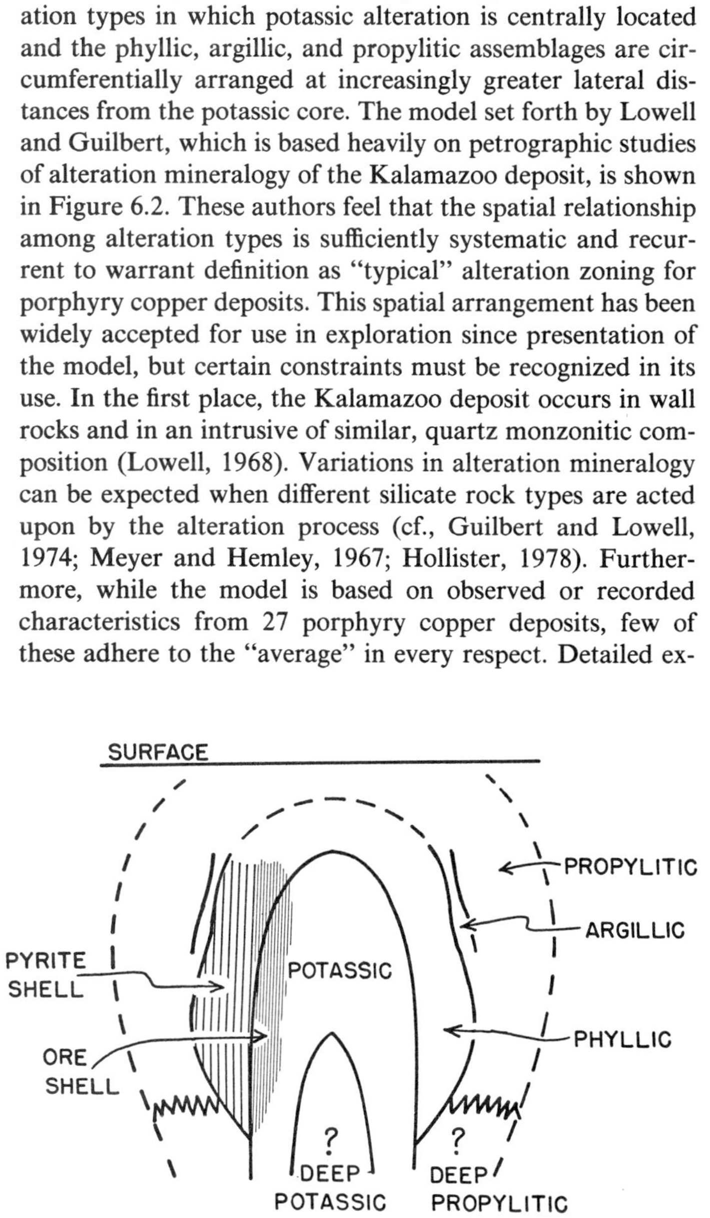

Figure 6.2. Vertical cross section of a "typical" porphyry copper deposit, showing zonal relationships among hydrothermal mineral assemblages: *left,* the ore shell (with low total sulfides, chalcopyrite ≥ pyrite) and the pyrite shell (with high total sulfides, low Cu, pyrite >> chalcopyrite); *right,* alteration assemblages. Modified from Lowell and Guilbert (1970), Figure 3.

The zonal alteration patterns described by Lowell and Guilbert (1970) and Rose (1970) have not made provision for chronologic relations among mineral assemblages, features which supply information concerning evolving environments of alteration and mineralization. Meyer and Hemley (1967) have discussed problems associated with definition of unequivocal age relationships among alteration types—particularly between the phyllic and argillic assemblages and between the argillic assemblage and supergene processes. However, some reasonably definitive relations may be derived from petrography, cross-cutting veins, and field relationships (Gustafson and Hunt, 1975). Available paragenetic data for alteration minerals from the porphyry copper deposits of southwestern North America are compiled in Table 6.2. These data indicate almost unanimously that quartz-sericite-pyrite (phyllic) alteration is a late stage or terminal event in the sulfide-generating hydrothermal process, although hypogene argillic and hypogene acid sulfate alteration, when they occur, may be even later. At Ajo and Sierrita, where mineralization is hosted by both quartz monzonite and quartz diorite rock types, phyllic alteration is more abundant in the former (West and Aiken, 1982; Gilluly, 1946; and personal observations). Also at Ray, Phillips and others (1974, p. 1249) have noted that ". . . biotized diabase is only inches away from sericitized schists or quartzite, strongly suggesting biotite must have formed in diabase from the same solutions that produced sericite in the silicic rocks." While the occurrence of phyllic alteration may, in part, reflect original wall-rock composition, I suggest that the degree of development of phyllic alteration relative to the potassic and propyllitic types may also indicate an "extent-of-evolution" of hydrothermal alteration in the porphyry copper deposits. Apparently, potassic (K-feldspar, biotite) and propylitic (albite, chlorite, epidote, calcite) assemblages mark the onset of hydrothermal alteration in these systems, but the relative age relationship between the two is variable. In some cases (Castle Dome, Tyrone, Bisbee), potassic alteration is not reported, but this may simply reflect depth or position of exposure relative to supergene enrichment as has been shown by reports of alteration at Morenci (compare Moolick and Durek, 1966, with Langton, 1973) and Pinto Valley adjacent to Castle Dome (Creasey, 1979, personal communication). The intermediate position of phyllic alteration relative to the potassic and propylitic zones results from the fact that the latter alteration types develop in intrusive rocks and wall rocks, respectively, while phyllic alteration is closely tied to a late stage of fracturing that is concentrated in the contact zone between these two rock types (Titley, 1982; Beane and Titley, in press).

MINERAL STABILITIES IN ALTERATION ENVIRONMENTS

Stabilities of minerals, defined in terms of the variables temperature, pressure, and chemical composition of a given

TABLE 6.2
Paragenetic Sequences of Alteration Assemblages in Silicate Rocks from Porphyry Copper Deposits in the Southwestern United States

Name of Deposit	Alteration Sequences				References
	Early Alteration			Late Alteration	
Ajo	K-feldspar biotite	K-feldspar chlorite	chlorite zoisite albite ankerite	epidote sericite calcite	Gilluly (1946)
Bagdad	K-feldspar biotite albite	K-feldspar sericite	—	—	Anderson (1950); Anderson et al. (1955)
Bingham	K-feldspar biotite	(?) chlorite calcite	sericite kaolinite montmorillonite	—	Stringham (1953); Bray (1969); Moore and Nash (1974); Moore (1975)
Bisbee	chlorite epidote calcite	sericite clay	—	—	Bryant and Metz (1966)
Castle Dome	chlorite epidote calcite	montmorillonite	sericite	—	Peterson et al. (1951)
Ely	K-feldspar biotite "carbonate"	K-feldspar biotite kaolinite montmorillonite	sericite	—	Bauer et al. (1966); Fournier (1967*a*, 1967*b*), James (1976)
Esperanza	biotite albite	K-feldspar chlorite epidote sericite	chlorite albite sericite	sericite	Smith (1975); Aiken and West (1978)
Globe-Miami	chlorite epidote sericite K-feldspar calcite	montmorillonite sericite K-feldspar biotite	sericite	—	Peterson (1962)
Mineral Park	K-feldspar biotite	K-feldspar	K-feldspar chlorite epidote	sericite chlorite	Wilkinson et al. (1982)
Ray	K-feldspar epidote calcite	K-feldspar biotite calcite	sericite	—	Phillips et al. (1974)
Safford	epidote chlorite	K-feldspar biotite albite	chlorite sericite calcite	sericite	Robinson and Cook (1966)
San Manuel	chlorite albite epidote calcite sericite	K-feldspar biotite albite sericite	sericite kaolinite	—	Schwartz (1953)
Santa Rita	K-feldspar biotite siderite	K-feldspar chlorite montmorillonite kaolinite	sericite	—	Nielsen (1968); Reynolds and Beane (1979)
Sierrita	K-feldspar biotite ± albite	chlorite epidote	sericite	—	West and Aiken (1982); Preece and Beane (in press)
Silver Bell	K-feldspar biotite	chlorite epidote calcite	sericite	—	Galey (1979); Graybeal (1982)

NOTE: Quartz is usually ubiquitous. The order in which minerals appear at a given stage in any deposit generally indicates their decreasing order of abundance.

rock volume, provide a framework within which to examine mineralization and alteration environments. A growing body of experimental data is available to define stability limits of minerals in terms of thermal decomposition at hydrostatic pressures. In addition, hydrothermal experiments coupled with thermodynamic data are being used increasingly to study mineral stability relations as a function of fluid composition at fixed temperature and pressures. Determination of conditions under which alteration minerals are stable serves the important purpose of defining the general environment of porphyry copper–type alteration and mineralization.

Decomposition of Silicate Minerals

The single most effective means of defining the temperature of formation of a given mineral is to establish the temperature-pressure boundary conditions outside of which that phase will decompose. In some cases in which a mineral is stable at relatively high temperatures, it may decompose by melting or partial melting. Such would be the case, for instance, for the alkali feldspars. Other minerals which contain component H_2O, such as kaolinite, muscovite, biotite, epidote, and chlorite, decompose by dehydration upon heating. Thermal stabilities of hydrous minerals may be further limited if other phases are present with which they may react. Quartz, which is commonly present with other hydrothermal minerals in porphyry copper alteration assemblages, serves as a potential reactant phase for dehydration reactions. The presence of reactive SiO_2 has a significant effect upon the thermal stabilities of kaolinite, muscovite, and zoisite that can lower their dehydration curves at hydrostatic pressure by as much as 50 to 100°C.

An important example of a limiting dehydration reaction involves co-existence and compatibility of muscovite, phlogopite, and quartz, as permitted by Creasey's (1959, 1966) definition of K-silicate alteration. A lower limit to the temperature of formation of this assemblage is defined because these three phases make up the reaction products for the dehydration of chlinochlore (Mg-chlorite) in the presence of K-feldspar:

$$3Mg_5Al_2Si_3O_{10}(OH)_8 + 8KAlSi_3O_8 = 5KMg_3AlSi_3O_{10}(OH)_2 + 3KAl_3Si_3O_{10}(OH)_2 + 9SiO_2 + 4H_2O \quad (1)$$

Unfortunately, the equilibrium curve for this reaction has not been defined experimentally, and the thermodynamic data for the two magnesian phases are not sufficiently accurate to warrant calculation of the reaction boundary. The position of this boundary in natural assemblages is also significantly affected by Fe-Mg solid solution in biotite and chlorite. Preliminary data by Hoschek (1973) indicate that at 4,000 bars pressure the reaction occurs at temperatures on the order of 475°C in the Mg system, while the same reaction occurs at 425°C in the Fe system. A reliable determination of the dehydration curve for this reaction would prove valuable in establishing an upper temperature limit for formation of the K-feldspar + chlorite assemblage, provided that solid solution effects in biotite and chlorite can be taken into account.

Most naturally occurring minerals are capable of, and frequently exhibit, some degree of compositional variation. The effect of diluting a phase through formation of a solid solution generally has the effect of stabilizing that compound. Certain silicate minerals observed in porphyry copper deposits exhibit limited solid solution restricted by miscibility gaps. Minerals displaying this type of solid solution include alkali feldspar and muscovite-paragonite, compositions of which Brimhall (1977) has used for geothermometry at Butte. Other common phases, including biotite, chlorite, epidote, sericite, and montmorillonite, show extensive compositional variation (cf., Moore and Czmanske, 1973; Beane, 1974; Fellows, 1976). This variability allows such phases, when they become unstable under certain conditions of temperature and pressure, to re-establish stability by appropriate compositional readjustment in the solid solution, providing suitable components are available.

Plagioclase and biotite, both of which are common minerals in original igneous rocks, provide excellent examples of such compositional readjustment under hydrothermal conditions. Primary plagioclase in rocks of quartz monzonite to granodiorite composition is normally andesine, whereas the alteration or vein-filling counterpart is commonly oligoclase or albite. Calcium liberated by compositional adjustment during propylitic alteration may remain in close proximity in the form of epidote or calcite. The compositional change exhibited by igneous biotite when exposed to hydrothermal solutions appears to play an important role in deposition of sulfides. Alteration and hydrothermal biotite are commonly highly magnesian, in contrast to the igneous progenitor which typically contains on the order of 40 mole percent Fe in octahedral coordination (Beane, 1974). The decomposition of the igneous biotite often appears to be a result of sulfurization of the iron component; this process produces pyrite, which remains intimately intergrown with the magnesium-enriched alteration biotite:

$$K(Mg_{0.6}Fe^{2+}_{0.4})_3AlSi_3O_{10}(OH)_2 + 1.2S_2 = 0.6KMg_3AlSi_3O_{10}(OH)_2 + 1.2FeS_2 + 0.4KAlSi_3O_8 + 0.4H_2O + 0.6O_2 \quad (2)$$

The K-feldspar produced from this reaction supplements that formed by potassic alteration of plagioclase.

Decomposition of Non-Silicate Minerals

Pressure in porphyry copper environments is exerted predominantly by H_2O, but other gases—such as O_2, S_2, CO_2, and SO_3—are present in minor amounts, as indicated, for example, by Reaction (2) above. Interpretation of the activities (~ partial pressures) of these minor gas components can supply important information concerning environmental favorability for formation of copper-bearing sulfide minerals and of oxide, sulfide, sulfate, and carbonate gangue minerals. Simple relationships among oxide and sulfide minerals are commonly used as geochemical indicators of activities of gas species (Barton and Skinner, 1967; Holland, 1959, 1965). Examples of such relationships are:

$$6Fe_2O_3 = 4Fe_3O_4 + O_2 \quad (3)$$

$$Cu_5FeS_4 + 4FeS_2 = 5CuFeS_2 + S_2 \quad (4)$$

$$2FeS_2 = 2FeS + S_2 \quad (5)$$

Both hematite and magnetite occur in the potassic alteration zone, and although they are rarely found together, the occurrence of one or the other suggests that oxygen fugacity in the porphyry copper deposits is probably close to values defined by Reaction (3). Sulfur fugacities must lie between the equilibrium values for Reactions (4) and (5) if chalcopyrite and pyrite are to co-exist (Fig. 6.3). Between ~ 350 and 625°C, a lower limit to sulfur activity is further provided by formation of an intermediate solid solution from chalcopyrite, with or without pyrite (Barton, 1973). The presence of calcite in the propylitic assemblage and the occurrence of anhydrite in the potassic zone serve to establish lower limits to the fugacities of CO_2 and SO_3 gases based on the respective stabilities of these phases relative to wollastonite in the presence of quartz (see Fig. 6.3).

MINERAL STABILITIES IN HYDROTHERMAL SYSTEMS

The preceding reactions defining mineral stabilities as a function of temperature and activity, or pressure, of a volatile component were all written to reflect conservation of rock-forming cation oxide components among solid phases. Viewed in this context alone, variations in alteration mineralogy would result only from rearrangement of cation oxides within a fixed rock volume. Considerable data exist, however, to show clearly that significant gains and losses of material accompany the processes of alteration and mineralization in the porphyry copper environment. Such additions and subtractions of oxide components were clearly evident when the compositions of various alteration assemblages were plotted on *AKF* and *ACF* diagrams (see Fig. 6.1). During hydrothermal alteration, cation oxide components are mobilized as aqueous species, with the hydrothermal fluid acting as the transfer medium. Changes in mineral stability relations attending gains or losses of a specific cation oxide relative to a given rock volume are conveniently linked to the co-existing aqueous phase using the ratio $a_{z^+}/a^{z}_{H^+}$ where € is the cation of interest having charge *z*, and *a* denotes the thermodynamic activity of the subscripted aqueous species.

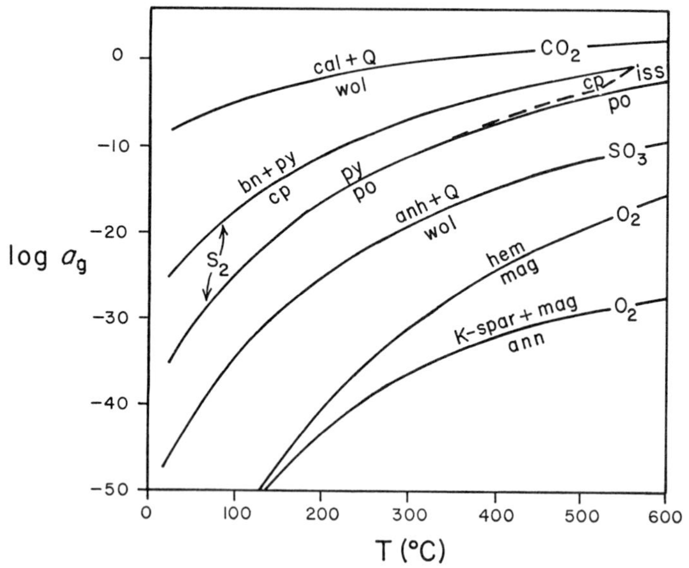

Key to Minerals:

anh = anydrite
ann = annite (Fe^{2+}-biotite)
bn = bornite
cal = calcite
cp = chalcopyrite
hem = hematite
K-spar = K-feldspar (orthoclase/microcline)
mag = magnetite
po = pyrrhotite
py = pyrite
Q = quartz
wol = wollastonite

Figure 6.3. Gas activity–temperature curves for reactions limiting stability of minerals characteristic of porphyry copper deposits. Dashed line shows transition of chalcopyrite to intermediate solid solution (iss) with or without pyrite (Barton, 1973).

Solution-Mineral Equilibria

In order for a mineral to be stable within an alteration environment, it must not only satisfy requirements regarding thermal decomposition, but must also be compatible with the composition of the co-existing hydrothermal fluid. Although hydrothermal mineral assemblages commonly contain several potential compositional variables of the form given above (i.e., one for every cation oxide component present), certain simplifications can be incorporated for the porphyry copper environment which are justified by geologic observations and practical considerations. In the first place, alteration at a given level in the earth's crust may be considered to proceed at essentially constant pressure. Also, the presence of free SiO_2, in the form of quartz, and a high density aqueous phase indicate that the components SiO_2 and H_2O are present in excess and, hence, cannot be considered to be compositional variables. Finally, owing to the relatively insoluble nature of aluminum in moderately acid solutions, component Al_2O_3 is conventionally considered to be conserved among solid phases during alteration (Hemley et al., 1980).

Thus the stability relations of minerals in the system $K_2O + Al_2O_3 + SiO_2 + H_2O$ can be examined in terms of the variables: temperature and a_{K^+}/a_{H^+} of the aqueous phase. Equilibrium relations among minerals in this system and a hydrothermal fluid are well understood from an experimental standpoint (Hemley and Jones, 1964; Montoya and Hemley, 1975; Shade, 1974). The diagram which graphically illustrates the results of these experimental studies (Fig. 6.4*a*) is generally familiar to geologists working with porphyry copper alteration, because three of the included minerals (K-feldspar, muscovite, and kaolinite) are characteristic of the potassic, phyllic, and argillic assemblages, respectively. At low temperatures, the ion activity ratio used on this diagram is very nearly equal to the total chemical concentration ratio between potassium and hydrogen, but at elevated temperatures, these two parameters diverge in value as a consequence of ion association effects which will be discussed below. The dashed lines on the figure illustrate a modification which may be introduced by limiting the concentration of dissolved silica by amorphous silica saturation, rather than by quartz saturation. This alternate assumption has been discussed by Fournier (1967*b*) in the context of alteration at Ely, and is based upon the facts that quartz nucleates slowly and that the

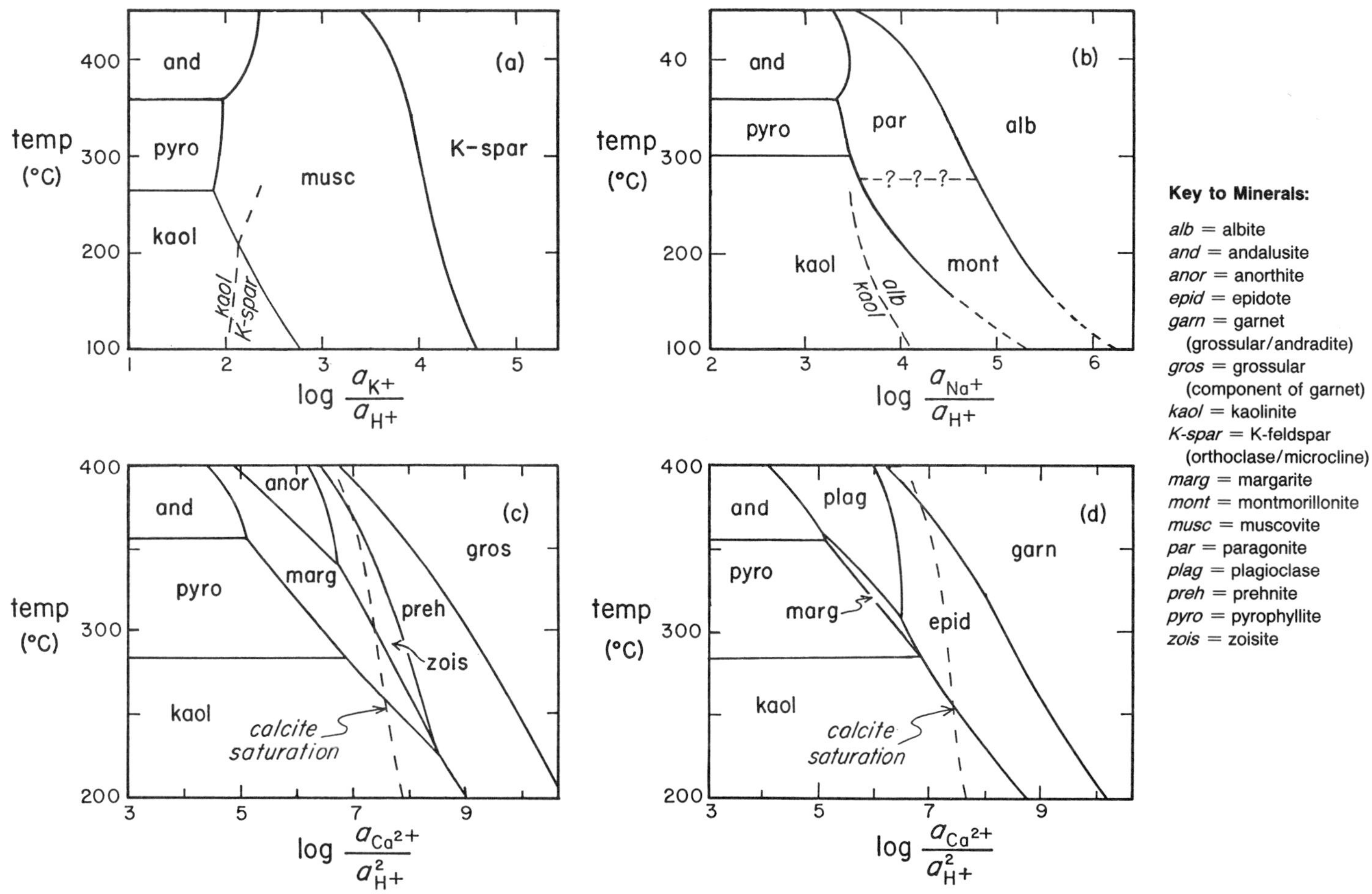

Figure 6.4. Calculated stability relations among minerals as a function of temperature and cation activity ratios in a co-existing aqueous phase at 500 bars. All systems conserve Al_2O_3 among solids and contain excess SiO_2 and H_2O. In diagrams of potassium-bearing phases (*a*) and sodium-bearing phases (*b*) solid lines denote quartz saturation, while dashed lines show the effects of limiting dissolved silica by amorphous silica saturation. The calcium-bearing phases (*c*) show stoichiometric compositions at quartz saturation. In calcium-bearing phases with provision for solid solution (*d*), compositions of phases are representative of porphyry copper occurrences. Activity-concentration relations from Saxena (1973) for plagioclase, from Bird and Helgeson (1980) for epidote and garnet. Calcite saturation curve is for $a_{CO_2} = 40$.

aqueous phase may be supersaturated relative to this mineral during vigorous hydrothermal alteration of plagioclase. A comparable diagram (Fig. 6.4*b*) showing stability relations in the system $Na_2O + Al_2O_3 + SiO_2 + H_2O$ is geometrically similar to Figure 6.4*a* because paragonite and albite are sodium analogues to muscovite and K-feldspar. The only difference between these diagrams, other than the compositional variable, is that at temperatures below about 300°C, sodium montmorillonite replaces paragonite in the Na_2O system (Hemley et al., 1971).

The $CaO + Al_2O_3 + SiO_2 + H_2O$ system (Fig. 6.4*c*) differs significantly from the K_2O and Na_2O counterparts. With increasing values of $a_{Ca^{2+}}/a^2_{H^+}$, the aluminosilicates (kaolinite, pyrophyllite) give way to interrelated stability fields of margarite (an endmember for Ca-montmorillonite), clinozoisite (an endmember for epidote), prehnite, and anorthite (an endmember for plagioclase). Finally, under extremes of $a_{Ca^{2+}}/a^2_{H^+}$ and temperature, the garnet endmember (grossular) is stable. When compared to the K_2O and Na_2O diagrams, the phases margarite, clinozoisite, prehnite, and anorthite, occurring at intermediate values of $a_{Ca^{2+}}/a^2_{H^+}$, are seen to occupy a position analogous to the dioctahedral micas and to Na montmorillonite, while the grossular stability field is comparable to that of the alkali feldspars. With the exception of prehnite, all of the calcium aluminosilicates appearing as stable phases on Figure 6.4*c* show significant compositional variation in natural occurrences. Analyses of epidotes from several porphyry copper deposits indicate approximately 0.3 mole fraction Fe typically substituting for Al (Fellows, 1976). The extent of Fe substitution for Al in garnet equilibrated with such epidote is determined to be approximately $Al_{0.3}$-$Fe_{0.7}$ using partition coefficients given by Bird and Helgeson (1980). Also hydrothermal and alteration plagioclases are highly sodic and are commonly of oligoclase ($Na_{0.8}$) or albite composition. The enhanced stability of minerals resulting from solid solution is exhibited by expansion of the size of the stability fields of the phases exhibiting non-stoichiometric behavior on mineral stability diagrams. When these compositional variations are added, the stability relations shown by Figure 6.4*c* are modified appreciably to those shown in Figure 6.4*d*. Expansion of the stability fields of clinozoisite and grossular deletes that of prehnite, which does not undergo extensive compositional variation, and the combined effects of plagioclase and epidote solid solution serve to collapse the area occupied by margarite to a small region adjacent to that of pyrophyllite in Figure 6.4*d.* While margarite itself does not appear in porphyry copper alteration, this phase can be considered a component of Ca-montmorillonite (Helgeson and Aagaard, in press). As such, margarite in solid solution occupies a larger stability field on the diagram than that which is shown for the pure phase. Owing to solid solution in plagioclase and epidote, these phases may co-exist at temperatures in the approximate range 300 to 425°C. By assigning a more sodic composition to plagioclase, the stability field of this phase may be further expanded to even lower temperatures.

Unlike K^+ and Na^+, which are very soluble in silicate systems lacking aluminum, Ca^{2+} solubility is commonly limited by saturation of the aqueous phase with respect to wollastonite, calcite, or anhydrite. Thus the reaction

$$CaCO_3 + 2H^+ = Ca^{2+} + CO_2 + H_2O \qquad (6)$$

provides an upper limit to the compositional variable $a_{Ca^{2+}}/a^2_{H^+}$ at a given temperature and activity of CO_2. The usual absence of grossular in porphyry copper alteration assemblages in igneous rocks suggests that calcite or anhydrite limits values of $a_{Ca^{2+}}/a^2_{H^+}$ to less than are necessary for the formation of garnet. Bird and Helgeson (1981) have discussed additional constraints and detailed compositional interrelationships for the calcium aluminosilicates.

The important role played by variation in aqueous solution composition within each of the simple chemical systems described above may be expanded graphically to include interrelationships between various pairs of the alkali and alkali-earth cations, but, in order to do this, temperature must be specified. For example, combination of the sodium and potassium systems at 350°C, with the previous assumptions regarding pressure, conservation of aluminum, and excess SiO_2 and H_2O (see Figs. 6.4*a,b*), provides the stability diagram shown in Figure 6.5*a*. On this diagram, slight curvature of the paragonite stability field near the paragonite + muscovite stability boundary is a result of limited solid solution between potassium and sodium in the micas. Stability relations in the potassium and calcium systems are similarly combined in Figure 6.5*b,* with provisions for solid solution discussed earlier taken into account. Combination of the potassium and magnesium systems provides an additional

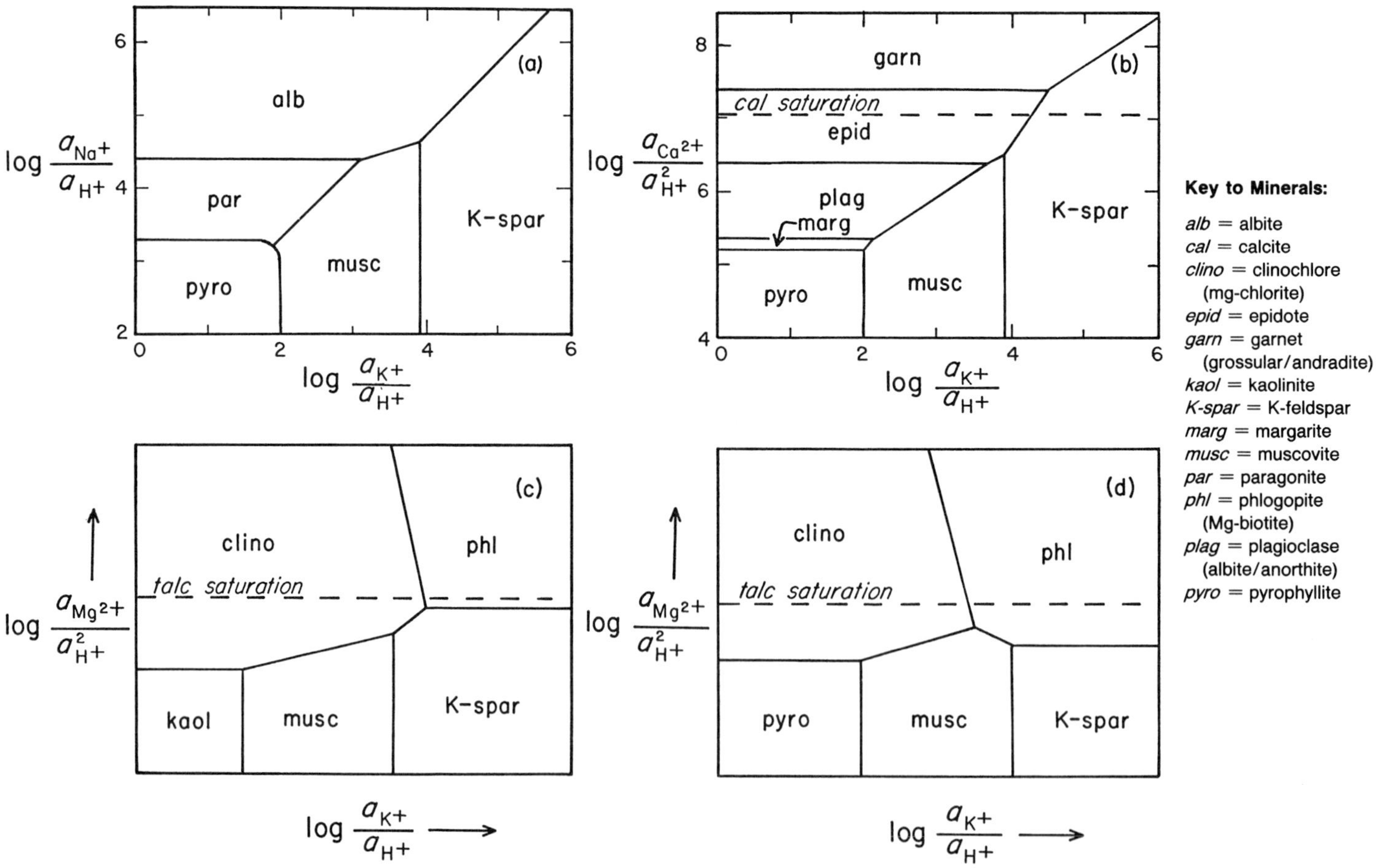

Figure 6.5. Stability relations among minerals as a function of various pairs of cation activity ratios in a co-existing aqueous phase at 500 bars. All diagrams conserve Al_2O_3 among solids and contain excess SiO_2 and H_2O. Quartz saturation is defined in all cases. In diagram (*a*), mixed potassium and sodium systems at 350°C, the curved portion of the pyrophyllite stability field schematically illustrates limited solid solution in the micas. Diagram (*b*) shows mixed potassium and calcium systems at 350°C and $a_{CO_2} = 20$. In diagram (*c*), mixed potassium and magnesium systems, the stability field of biotite takes account of solid solution to permit stability with K-feldspar at a temperature near 300°C; the chlorite stability field is schematically drawn to depict compatibility with K-feldspar, as suggested for pure phases at 300°C. Diagram (*d*) is a schematic representation of mixed potassium and magnesium systems at a temperature above the equilibrium value for muscovite biotite compatibility at a given pressure.

feature, namely, formation of a mixed-cation silicate, phlogopite. Two variations of this diagram are shown (Fig. 6.5*c,d*) in order to illustrate schematic phase relations above and below the equilibrium temperature for Reaction 1. In natural systems, the K-feldspar and chlorite fields can be joined at temperatures higher than those of Figure 6.5*d*, if provision is made for Fe-Mg substitution in chlorite, because solid solution can be shown to have a strong stabilizing effect on this mineral. Like Ca^{2+}, solubility of Mg^{2+} is restricted in the absence of aluminum. In this case, an upper limit to $a_{Mg^{2+}}/a^2_{H^+}$ in the presence of quartz is provided by talc saturation, and the appropriate boundary is drawn on Figure 6.5*c,d.* At 350°C, talc saturation limits $a_{Mg^{2+}}/a^2_{H^+}$ to a value less than is necessary for equilibrium between phlogopite and K-feldspar. However, by allowing for Fe-Mg substitution in the mica, the stability field of phlogopite can be expanded sufficiently to permit K-feldspar and biotite as a stable assemblage at this temperature.

Applications to Porphyry Copper Alteration

Several observations can be made concerning development of different alteration minerals and assemblages in the porphyry copper environment in light of the stability relations shown in Figures 6.4 and 6.5. Decreases in both temperature and the ratio $a_{Є^{z+}}/a^z_{H^+}$ of the aqueous phase lead to stability of minerals with progressively lower Є : Al ratios in all systems (see Fig. 6.4). With decreasing temperature in the $K_2O + Al_2O_3 + SiO_2 + H_2O$ system, the progression of stable phases (K-feldspar→muscovite→kaolinite) corresponds to the zonal arrangement of critical minerals for the potassic, phyllic, and argillic alteration assemblages (see Fig. 6.2) as they are indicated to occur by Lowell and Guilbert (1970) and Rose (1970). At quartz saturation, K-feldspar and kaolinite are not compatible because of the intervening muscovite stability field (see Fig. 6.4*a*). However, if dissolved silica exceeds quartz saturation, these two phases may coexist in equilibrium (e.g., Ely, Santa Rita) up to a temperature of about 200°C, depending upon the degree to which the solution is supersaturated with respect to quartz. The presence of kaolinite in an alteration assemblage indicates a maximum temperature of formation of about 265°C, if equilibrium quartz is present, or lower, if the aqueous phase is supersaturated with respect to quartz (Hemley et al., 1980). The apparent absence of paragonite in porphyry copper alteration assemblages suggests (1) preclusion of this phase, due to a_{Na^+}/a_{K^+} ratios insufficient for its stabilization; (2) dissolved silica significantly in excess of quartz saturation (leading to kaolinite-albite stability); or (3) alteration below 300°C, at which temperature Na-montmorillonite becomes stable instead of the Na-mica (Montoya and Hemley, 1975).

Oligoclase and epidote in the propylitic assemblage may co-exist compatibly down to temperatures of approximately 250 to 300°C (see Fig. 6.4*d*). The presence of calcite with high-Fe epidote in altered silicate rocks lacking garnet indicates temperatures below about 350°C with CO_2 pressure (P_{CO_2}) as follows: $P_{CO_2} \approx 10$ bars ($a_{CO_2} = 10$). This temperature is lowered with decreased CO_2 pressure reaching about 260°C at $a_{CO_2} = 1$ ($P_{CO_2} \approx 1$ bar). In order to stabilize plagioclase and hydrothermal epidote at this lower temperature, the feldspar must have a Na content in excess of approximately Ab_{92}. At 300°C, albite is seen to be compatible with both muscovite and K-feldspar (see Fig. 6.5*a*). With increasing temperature, stability of the sodic phase is promoted so that increasingly higher ratios of a_{K^+}/a_{Na^+} in the aqueous phase are necessary in order to stabilize K-feldspar relative to albite. The stability field of Ab_{80} plagioclase is restricted sufficiently by those of muscovite and epidote solid solution at 300°C to exclude K-feldspar from this assemblage (see Fig. 5*b*). However, Na- and K-feldspar may co-exist if the plagioclase composition is changed to about Ab_{87} at this temperature. Phase relations in the mixed potassium + magnesium system shown schematically in Figure 6.5*c,d,* coupled with the rarity of the biotite + muscovite assemblage in porphyry copper deposits, suggest relatively low temperatures of formation for the Ajo pegmatites, the cementing stage in Whim Hill breccia pipe at Santa Rita, and other examples of the K-feldspar + chlorite assemblage.

Mineral stability relations in mixed cation systems (see Fig. 6.5) permit important interpretations of alteration phenomona in rock types of contrasting composition. Potassic alteration, characterized chiefly by K-feldspar addition, is essentially the result of potassium exchange for the sodium and calcium that were originally present in igneous plagioclase. Such alteration is produced by introducing a solution having a relatively high value of a_{K^+}/a_{H^+} into a given rock mass. However, in high-magnesium environments, corresponding to high values of $a_{Mg^{2+}}/a^2_{H^+}$ in Figure 6.5*c,* potassium addition results in biotization, so that on the scale of mineral grains within a given rock volume, biotite replaces amphibole, while K-feldspar replaces plagioclase during potassium metasomatism. At slightly lower values of a_{K^+}/a_{H^+} an aqueous solution may produce K-feldspar + muscovite, but only at high temperatures can the high magnesium analogue, biotite + muscovite, form (as discussed earlier in the context of Reaction 1); at lower temperatures these two phases react to form K-feldspar + chlorite. Chloritization of early alteration biotite in the presence of stable alteration K-feldspar is commonly observed in porphyry copper deposits (e.g., in the pegmatitic bodies at Ajo), and such a mineral paragenesis can be interpreted to represent waning potassium metasomatism reflected in decreased a_{K^+}/a_{H^+} of the hydrothermal fluid. Continued decrease in this parameter of fluids interacting with rocks of granitic and quartz monzonitic composition can lead to development of muscovite in place of K-feldspar. In rocks with relatively high calcium and magnesium contents, however, decreased a_{K^+}/a_{H^+} below K-feldspar stability can be expected to produce chlorite and epidote instead of muscovite, as is seen, for example, in dioritic rocks at Sierrita (Preece and Beane, in press; West and Aiken, 1982). Chlorite and epidote serve to define propylitic alteration, and this assemblage in dioritic rocks can be thought of as an analogue to phyllic alteration in rocks of more quartz monzonitic affinity. Strong phyllic alteration, therefore, might be expected in these latter rock types only when magnesium is relatively low and when calcium and sodium have been effectively replaced by development of early K-feldspar. In a diorite, early potassium addition can be absorbed by large percentages of original magnesium-bearing minerals, so that it does not displace other cations so effectively. These cations, in turn, inhibit development of later phyllic alteration as solutions decrease in a_{K^+}/a_{H^+}.

An important conclusion which must be drawn from this brief consideration of hydrothermal stabilities of silicate minerals is that over reasonably wide temperature ranges and aqueous solution compositions, virtually any combination of the phases observed in association with porphyry copper alteration can co-exist in equilibrium. This co-existence is made possible chiefly by the fact that many of the phases observed or originally present in silicate rock masses can have extensive compositional variations. The fact that certain phases persist in composition, association, and paragenesis across the porphyry copper deposits as a group suggests that some combination of environmental conditions is common to the deposits and is optimal for development of economic sulfide mineralization. But because mineral compatibilities can change with relatively minor variations in compositional parameters, it is important to keep in mind that the absence of alteration assemblages defined as "typical" does not necessarily preclude the presence of copper mineralization. The critical problem is to define and understand those parameters which are diagnostic of hydrothermal conditions necessary for development of economic grades of metalization.

THE HYDROTHERMAL FLUID

Although hydrothermal minerals are still present in porphyry copper deposits, the aqueous fluids responsible for their formation have long since been dissipated. Nevertheless, several techniques are available which can be used to broadly define the physicochemical characteristics of the hydrothermal fluid responsible for alteration and mineralization in these now extinct geothermal systems.

Geothermometry

Using a variety of techniques (all of which give similar results), researchers have identified the temperatures attending mineralization and alteration. Fluid inclusion homogenization studies provide the most widely applicable means for determining temperatures of hydrothermal activity. Temperatures determined by fluid inclusion homogenization may require an upward pressure correction, but this is generally small (<100°C) for the epizonal deposits of southwestern North America, as concluded from evidence of boiling or from reconstruction of geologic overburden (Norton, 1982; Nash, 1976). Drawing upon a review of fluid inclusion data from numerous sources, Nash (p. D5) concludes: ". . . in most porphyry copper deposits temperatures were typically about 400° ± 100°C. Higher temperature pulses, when present, probably were of brief duration. . . ." Temperatures in excess of 500°C are reported from Bingham (Roedder, 1971; Moore and Nash, 1974), San Manuel-Kalamazoo (Davis, 1974), Santa Rita (Reynolds and Beane, 1979), and Copper Creek (Walker, 1979), but only at Bingham, where homogenization temperatures as high as 725°C were measured by Roedder (1971), is mineralization associated with such fluids. A number of different geothermometric techniques have been applied to the porphyry copper deposit at Santa Rita. Early veins of potassic-assemblage minerals contain hypersaline fluid inclusions for which uncorrected homogenization temperatures in excess of 800°C have been determined (Reynolds and Beane, 1979). Minor amounts of chalcopyrite present in these veins occur in later, crosscutting microveinlets having moderately saline fluid inclusions that homogenize at significantly lower temperatures (~300–350°C). Such dilute fluids are seen in association with later K-feldspar–chlorite–chalcopyrite–pyrite and quartz-sericite-pyrite vein types. An intermediate generation of hypersaline fluids associated with potassic minerals has also been defined as having homogenization temperatures on the order of 300 to 500°C, but like their high-temperature counterparts, such fluids apparently did not deposit sulfide minerals. Oxygen isotope ratios of co-existing minerals indicate temperature ranges of 390 to 580°C and 285 to 390°C for potassic and phyllic assemblages, respectively (Sheppard et al., 1971); alteration kaolinite appearing paragenetically between these two alteration types (Nielsen, 1968) has an upper stability limit of slightly less than 265°C at quartz saturation (Hemley et al., 1980). Compositional variation in biotite also furnishes a means of geothermometry using either the F:OH ratio (Jacobs and Parry, 1976, 1979), or the Fe-Mg content of the mica if magnetite and K-feldspar are present (Beane, 1974). The first of these compositional geothermometers yields formation temperatures in the range of 580 to 670°C for potassic vein alteration. The latter technique renders a lower temperature range of 350 to 425°C for the potassic phases in association with sulfide mineralization. (Additional compositional data for biotite from Jacobs and Parry [1979] provide a temperature of about 530°C using the Fe-Mg geothermometer).

Fluid Composition

The character of the mineralizing fluids which attended formation of the porphyry copper deposits of southwestern North America may be determined in part from microscopic samples which were trapped within structural defects or growth defects of minerals originally in contact with hydrothermal solutions. Visual and thermal analysis of these fluid inclusions provide either direct or circumstantial evidence that hydrothermal solutions consisted chiefly of NaCl + KCl brines having NaCl-equivalent salinities ranging from moderate (~1 molal) to very concentrated (10 to > 30 molal), and contained sporadically significant concentrations of calcium, copper, iron, sulfur, and carbonate.

Roedder (1971) and Moore and Nash (1974) have made use of the halite and sylvite daughter products in fluid inclusions to establish an atomic ratio of K:Na in the range 0.26 to 0.59 for highly saline fluids at Bingham. Reynolds (1980) has determined similar ratios for hypersaline fluid inclusions in veins and higher values (up to 1.12) for the Whim Hill breccia pipe at Santa Rita. A slightly lower value for this ratio (~0.1) was determined for moderately saline solutions at Sierrita using crushing and leaching techniques (Denis, 1974), halite-sylvite dissolution (Preece, 1979), and stability relations between alkali feldspars (Beane, unpublished data). Higher ratios (0.52–1.76) were determined at Red Mountain,

Arizona, by Bodnar and Beane (1980). Scanning electron microscopy, electron microprobe analysis, and optical microscopy have suggested or established the presence of a variety of other daughter products in fluid inclusions from southwestern North American porphyry copper deposits (Nash, 1976; Metzger et al., 1977; E. Anthony, 1980, personal communication). Among these phases are most of those observed in vein and altered rocks, including alkali feldspars, muscovite, chalcopyrite, pyrite, magnetite, hematite, anhydrite, and calcite, although others not occurring as rock forming minerals are also observed (e.g., dawsonite). In spite of the occurrence of carbonate minerals in some inclusions, cooling and crushing tests indicate that CO_2 generally makes up less than 3 mole percent of fluids, although larger amounts have been detected at Battle Mountain, Bagdad, and Yerrington (Nash, 1976; Ypma, 1968).

From the results of geothermometric studies of mineral assemblages, equilibrium constants may be calculated for reactions describing stability relations among minerals observed in altered rocks. From these equilibrium constants, compositional characteristics of aqueous solutions responsible for alteration and mineralization may be calculated. Activities of individual dissolved species determined in this manner are obtained only for electrically neutral species, however. When the species of interest is electrically charged, the characterizing reaction must contain some other ion or ions for charge compensation. Some examples are:

$$NaAlSi_3O_8 + K^+ = KAlSi_3O_8 + Na^+ \quad (7)$$

$$3KAlSi_3O_8 + 2H^+ = KAlSi_3O_{10}(OH)_2 + 2K^+ + 6SiO_2 \quad (8)$$

$$KFe_3AlSi_3O_{10}(OH)_2 + 6H^+ = KAlSi_3O_8 + 3Fe^{2+} + 4H_2O \quad (9)$$

As shown in reactions (8) and (9), the ion commonly present for charge compensation in solution-silicate equilibrium reactions is H^+. When this ion is present, the equilibrium constant is numerically equal to an expression of the form $a_{C^{z+}}/a^z_{H^+}$ used earlier (see Figs. 6.4 and 6.5). Thus, in order to employ solution-mineral equilibrium relations to uniquely define activities of dissolved species, it is usually necesssary to know the value of solution pH. Based on available fluid inclusion data (homogenization temperatures, salinities, K : Na ratios) and solution mineral equilibrium considerations, it can be concluded that at temperatures in the range 300 to 350°C, K-feldspar and muscovite co-exist at pH values of approximately 4 to 5 in porphyry copper alteration environments. Also, because hypogene advanced argillic phases (kaolinite, pyrophyllite) are generally not found without accompanying sericite, it is likely that solution pH values below about 3 are uncommon. When a value of solution pH and a temperature for a given alteration environment are known, silicate mineral stability relations, such as those shown diagrammatically in Figures 6.4 and 6.5, can be used to define, or delimit, activities of individual cations and anion in the altering hydrothermal fluid.

Conversion of thermodynamic activities to total chemical concentration of species of interest is reasonably straightforward to approximately 300 to 350°C in solutions having NaCl concentrations of 3 molal, based on calculations described by Helgeson (1969) and Helgeson and Kirkham (1974, 1976). At higher temperatures and in more concentrated solutions, however, conversion of activities to concentrations is subject to significant uncertainty. The discrepancy between total concentration of dissolved species and the corresponding thermodynamic activity of individual ions is largely a consequence of the phenomenon of ion association, an aspect which plays an important role in material transport and deposition in porphyry copper systems. At standard conditions (25°C, 1 atm), aqueous solutions of strong electrolytes, such as NaCl, consist almost entirely of free ions. But with rising temperature, chloride and sulfate solutions of the alkali metals and hydrogen undergo ion pairing to form aqueous species, such as KCl, NaCl, and HSO_4^-, which are held together chiefly by electrostatic forces (Helgeson, 1964). As temperature exceeds 300°C, free ions constitute an increasingly smaller portion of total dissolved material in aqueous electrolyte solutions. Dissolved metals in these solutions, such as copper and zinc, also associate with the chloride iron to form complex species which differ from ion pairs in that the chemical character of the bond is largely covalent. Experimental studies (e.g., Crerar and Barnes, 1976) and theoretical considerations (Helgeson, 1964) show that this phenomenon contributes significantly to the solubilities of base metal sulfides in hydrothermal systems. Weakly acid solutions having oxygen fugacities compatible with mineral phases observed in porphyry copper deposits (see Fig. 6.3) carry dissolved copper and iron predominantly in the reduced states of Cu^+ and Fe^{2+} respectively. These base-metal ions each complex with chloride, although iron does so to a considerably lesser extent than does copper at temperatures on the order of 350°C (Crerar and Barnes, 1976). Various complexes of copper with HS^- and H_2S and of iron with HS^-, H_2S, and OH^- have been studied experimentally at elevated temperatures (see summary by Crerar and Barnes, 1976), but these species appear, for the most part, to be present in insignificant amounts compared to the chloride complexes in weakly acid NaCl + KCl brines correlated with porphyry copper formation.

Sulfur dissolved in hydrothermal solutions occurs in two oxidation states as both sulfide and sulfate. Under standard conditions the strong acid H_2SO_4 is largely dissociated into the free ions, except at low pH values (<2) where HSO_4^- predominates over SO_4^{2-}. Like the chloride ion, SO_4^{2-} becomes increasingly associated with H^+, Na^+, and K^+ at elevated temperatures. In concentrated brines of Na^+ and K^+, the sulfate ion may exhibit significant ion pairing, even at low temperatures. In contrast, the sulfide ion is strongly associated with H^+ as HS^- and H_2S under mildly acid conditions at 25°C, but undergoes minimal interaction with Na^+ and K^+ (Herr and Helz, 1978). With increasing temperature, the intermediate HS^- species becomes associated with H^+, Na^+, and presumably K^+. Further, the S^{2-} species contributes minimally to the concentration of total dissolved sulfide in moderately acid solutions. In mildly acid brine solutions having temperatures in excess of 300°C, the predominant dissolved sulfur species appear to be HSO_4^-, H_2S, and possibly $NaSO_4^-$.

Boundaries for dissolved sulfur concentrations compatible with pyrite, chalcopyrite, K-feldspar, and anhydrite at 300°C and pH = 5, as well as a similar set of relations involving muscovite instead of K-feldspar at pH = 3, are shown in Figure 6.6. Also depicted on these diagrams are the oxygen fugacities defining magnetite + hematite equilibrium (Reaction 3) and the sulfide vs. sulfate dominant regions at the two different pH values. An examination of Figure 6.6 shows that a considerable range in concentrations of dissolved sulfur is permitted in the presence of pyrite + chalcopyrite + K-feldspar, but when oxygen fugacity is fixed, the tolerance in sulfur concentrations afforded by this mineral assemblage is rather small. If biotite is present as an additional phase, the range of sulfur concentrations and oxygen fugacities are restricted to the segment of the line forming the lower boundary of the shaded area in the H_2S-predominant region. Within the potassic alteration zone, the phases K-feldspar, biotite, quartz, pyrite, and chalcopyrite are commonly accompanied by minor amounts of magnetite. Occasionally, hematite may either be present instead of, or be replaced by, magnetite. At an oxygen fugacity generally compatible with this group of phases at 300°C and pH = 5, dissolved sulfur concentrations would be in the range of about 0.001 to 0.02 molal. With rising temperature, increasingly larger and more restricted concentrations of dissolved sulfur are necessary to stabilize the mineral assemblage under consideration, which is commonly observed in the ore zone of porphyry copper deposits.

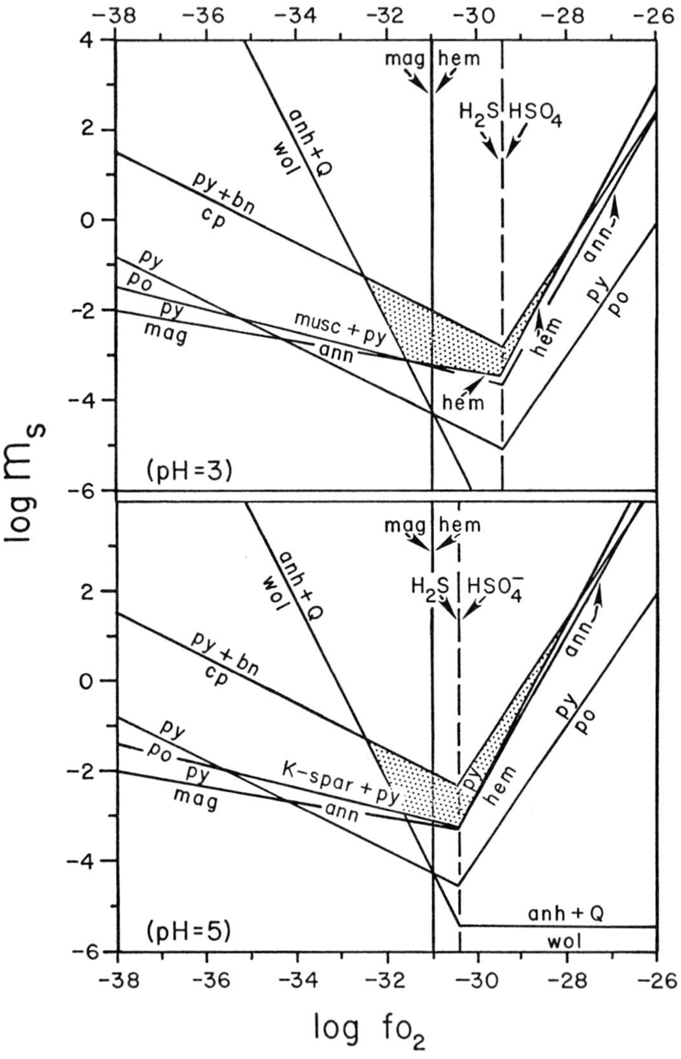

Key to Minerals:

anh = anhydrite
ann = annite (Fe^{2+}-biotite)
bn = bornite
cp = chalcopyrite
hem = hematite
K-spar = K-feldspar (orthoclase/microcline)
mag = magnetite
musc = muscovite
po = pyrrhotite
py = pyrite
Q = quartz
wol = wollastonite

Figure 6.6. Equilibrium boundaries for reactions at 300°C, defining stability relations of minerals commonly observed in porphyry copper deposits of southwestern North America as a function of oxygen fugacity and total dissolved sulfur (sulfide + sulfate) at pH values of 3 (*upper*) and 5 (*lower*). The stippled portion of each diagram indicates environments compatible with the assemblages quartz + anhydrite + chalcopyrite + pyrite + muscovite (pH = 3) or quartz + anhydrite + chalcopyrite + K-feldspar (pH = 5) in solutions having $a_{K^+} = 0.3$.

Like sulfur, total concentrations of copper and iron in the ore-forming solution are reasonably approximated from solution-mineral equilibrium considerations. Crerar and Barnes (1976) experimentally studied the solubility of coexisting chalcopyrite + bornite + pyrite to temperatures of 350°C and found that, in excess of 1,000 ppm, Cu and Fe could be dissolved in mildly acid NaCl solutions containing 0.1 molal H_2S. This study did not, however, account for silicate control of iron solubility (e.g., Reaction 9), which provides an upper limit to the ratio $a_{Fe^{2+}}/a^2_{H^+}$ in solution because of annite saturation. If annite co-exists with K-feldspar, the maximum activity of Fe^{2+} occurs at the lowest pH at which this phase is stable, as defined by temperature and the activity of K^+ in solution. At 300°C and pH = 3.0, dissolved iron as Fe^{2+} may reach, but not exceed, a concentration of about 150 ppm (~0.003 molal), as long as muscovite is present. If the $FeCl^+$ complex is included in this calculation (Crerar and Barnes, 1976), the solubility of iron is increased by about 70 ppm. When pH increases to 5.0 and K-feldspar stability is substituted for that of muscovite, the activity of Fe^{2+} decreases and hydroxide complexes of both Fe^{2+} and Fe^{3+} become predominant over the free ions (Sweeton and Baes, 1970). Although these hydroxide complexes partially offset the effects of rising pH, iron solubility is nevertheless depressed to slightly more than about 0.1 ppm. If the effects of solid solution on biotite are taken into account, the annite stability field expands and iron solubility is further suppressed to a level which is approximately 25 percent of that in equilibrium with pure annite.

The preceding calculations suggest that at temperatures on the order of 300°C, iron is essentially an immobile component in the potassic alteration zone, but it is soluble to a limited extent under the more acid conditions associated with argillic and phyllic alteration. With rising temperature, limiting values of $a_{Fe^{2+}}/a^2_{H^+}$ in the presence of muscovite and K-feldspar become progressively smaller, but total iron solubility increases due to the expanding stability of chloride and hydroxide complexes (Sweeton and Baes, 1970; Crerar et al., 1978; Whitney et al., 1979). Such effects may permit dissolved iron to reach levels of 4,000 to 12,000 ppm (0.07–0.2 molal), which have been calculated to be present in fluid inclusions from potassically altered rocks from Bingham, where temperatures were well in excess of 300°C (Roedder, 1971). Nevertheless, low calculated iron solubilities in the presence of minerals common to porphyry copper alteration at temperatures less than about 400°C indicate the importance of original iron-bearing minerals in the host rock as a center for deposition of sulfides from hydrothermal fluids at such temperatures. This solution behavior is compatible with numerous observations of only minor changes in total iron in hydrothermally altered and mineralized rocks as compared to unaltered rock values (McKinstry, 1957; Robinson and Cook, 1966; Galey, 1979).

Copper concentrations in the fluids responsible for mineralization in the porphyry copper deposits are generally expected to be significant, simply from consideration of the volumes of fluids required to produce the substantial tonnages of economic mineralization present. By analogy with sphalerite solubilities in solutions equilibrated with quartz + muscovite + K-feldspar at 300 to 500°C, Rose (1970) has suggested copper concentrations of 2,000 ppm (~0.03 molal) in mineralizing solutions. Crerar and Barnes (1976) have also suggested copper contents in the range 10 to 1,000 ppm, based on various lines of evidence, including solubility studies. Beane (1974) has used mineral equilibrium considerations to calculate hydrothermal fluid characteristics directly as a function of solution pH. This technique indicates about 800 ppm dissolved copper in a 3 molal chloride solution having pH = 4.0 and equilibrated with K-feldspar + biotite + magnetite + pyrite + chalcopyrite at 300°C. Parallel calculations using data extrapolated to 350°C indicate copper contents of several thousand ppm in the aqueous phase. Measurement of dimensions of chalcopyrite daughter minerals in fluid inclusions from Santa Rita reveal concentrations of Cu on the order of 7,000 ppm in saline fluids having temperatures in excess of 400°C (Reynolds and Beane, 1979); similar contents of Fe and S are also required of the fluids. Calculations point out that a major obstacle facing the theory of high-temperature mineralization is the large concentrations of copper required in concentrated chloride solutions to overcome the stability of chloride complexes before deposition of sulfide minerals is possible. The basic difference between the conclusions derived by Crerar and Barnes (1976) from experimental studies, and those obtained through calculations by Beane (1974) is that the former do not take into account the role of silicate phases in lowering iron solubility in the hydrothermal fluid. If iron concentrations are effectively suppressed by biotite or chlorite formation, then the aqueous phase can dissolve and transport correspondingly larger copper concentrations.

PROCESSES RESPONSIBLE FOR ALTERATION AND MINERALIZATION

Two fundamentally different mechanisms, decrease in temperature and evolving chemical reaction, are called upon to explain the variations with both time and space in alteration mineralogy of porphyry copper deposits. Although the rocks and hydrothermal fluids which formed these mineral deposits involve a considerable number of chemical components contributing to their overall compositions, mineral stability relations in the simple system $K_2O + Al_2O_3 + SiO_2 + H_2O$ may be used to illustrate the basic concepts of the two hypotheses of formation. The discussion will refer to Figure 6.7, a modification of Figure 6.4*a* that incorporates the general effects of ion association with increasing temperature. On this modified diagram, total molalities of dissolved KCl and HCl are employed in the composition ratio, rather than individual ion activities of K^+ and H^+ (Montoya and Hemley, 1975). The two geologic criteria which must be satisfied by any model for alteration in porphyry copper deposits are: (1) the zoning of potassic, phyllic, and (occasionally) argillic alteration at increasingly greater distances from the intrusive center (see Fig. 6.2), and (2) the paragenetic sequence of early K-feldspar–stable and subsequent muscovite-stable alteration observed at fixed points in these geothermal systems (see Table 6.2).

Temperature-Defined Alteration Assemblages

In the case of temperature-defined alteration assemblages, a high-temperature fluid derived from presumed magmatic processes (e.g., degassing) originates in the central portions of a partially solidified quartz monzonitic magma and moves upward and outward into cooler fractured igneous rock (Meyer and Hemley, 1967; Rose, 1970; Burnham, 1979). The fluid is generated by magmatic processes, so it has a composition in equilibrium with igneous minerals (in this case, K-feldspar). If the fluid has an initial temperature and KCl : HCl concentration ratio corresponding to point *A* in Figure 6.7, then, upon cooling along line *A-B,* the solution composition moves progressively through the stability fields of K-feldspar, muscovite, and kaolinite. When the fluid moves through a rock mass containing K-feldspar at continually decreasing temperature, it remains in equilibrium with this mineral until it cools to temperature T_1. With further

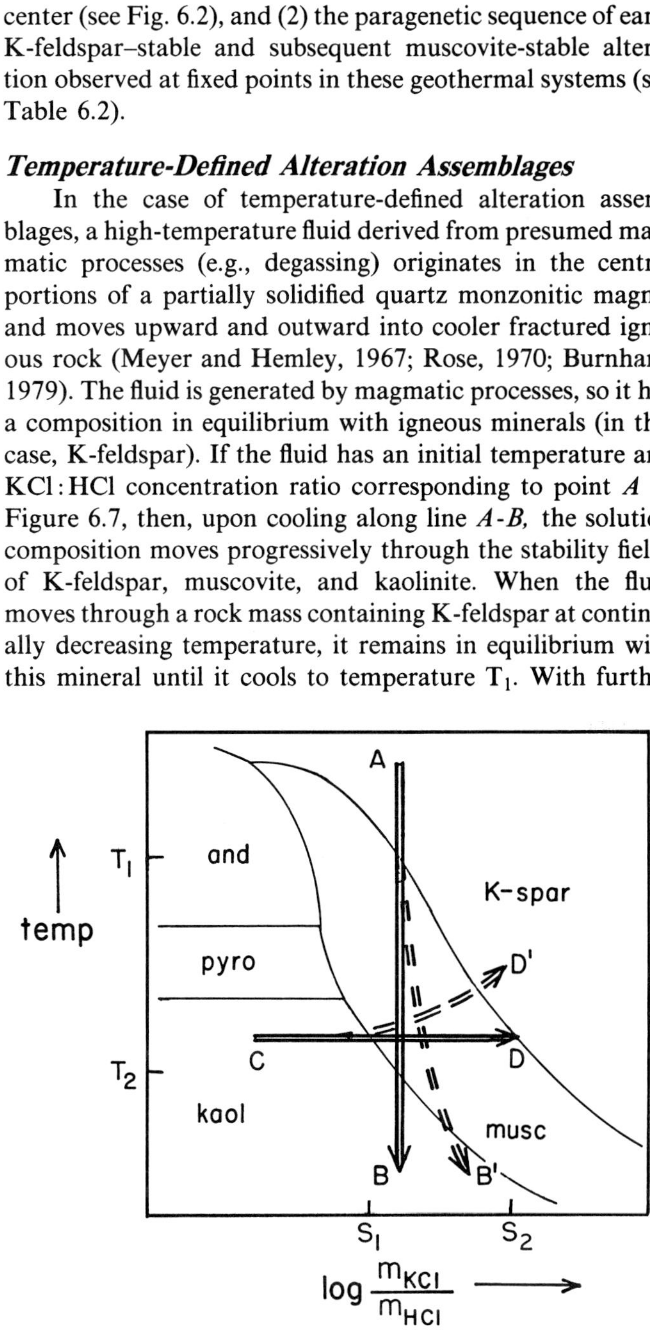

Key to Minerals:

and = andalusite *K-spar*= K-feldspar *musc* = muscovite
kaol = kaolinite (orthoclase/microcline) *pyro* = pyrophyllite

Figure 6.7. Schematic modification of Figure 6.4*a* to account for ion association at elevated temperatures (see Montoya and Hemley, 1975). The cation ratio on the horizontal axis correponds to total concentrations (*m*) of dissolved KCl and HCl. Reaction paths are shown by arrows.

temperature decrease, rock-forming feldspar will alter to muscovite from T_1 to T_2:

$$3KAlSi_3O_8 + 2H^+ \rightarrow KAl_3Si_3O_{10}(OH)_2 + 6SiO_2 + 2K^+ \quad (10)$$

It will alter to kaolinite below T_2:

$$2KAlSi_3O_8 + 2H^+ + H_2O \rightarrow Al_2Si_2O_5(OH)_4 + 4SiO_2 + 2K^+ \quad (11)$$

Each of these reactions consumes H^+ from the aqueous phase and contributes K^+ to it; thus, the concentration ratio KCl: HCl increases above the initial value point (*A*). The actual amount by which this parameter increases during the cooling and alteration process depends upon the initial solution composition, and upon the relative rates at which temperature decreases and reactions proceed. In addition, the solution composition is also changed by the deposition of silicates which results from cooling. The modified reaction path *A*–*B'* takes qualitative account of the effects of alteration reactions on solution composition. The general result of these reactions is to lengthen the temperature interval over which the solution composition corresponds to muscovite stability before it moves into the kaolinite stability field.

According to the temperature-controlled alteration model, paragenetic sequences result from retreat of the thermal source as deeper portions of the magma crystallize. Thus, at a given point in the rock mass, temperature decreases with time, and paragenetic sequences show early high-temperature phases (K-feldspar) which then progress to lower temperature minerals (muscovite). Mineralization, according to this model, is largely attributed to decreased chalcopyrite solubility and Cu-Cl complexing with decreasing temperature and, thus, can occur with any of the alteration assemblages.

Reaction-Defined Alteration Assemblages

In the case of reaction-defined alteration assemblages, a fluid having a relatively low pH, and, therefore, a low KCl: HCl concentration ratio, reacts with K-feldspar in fractured intrusive rock (Helgeson, 1970). Point *C* on Figure 6.7, for example, might represent the composition of an original fluid that is in equilibrium with kaolinite. Because the rock-forming feldspar is out of equilibrium with respect to the hydrothermal solution, it is converted to a clay mineral compatible with the solution composition, according to Reaction 11. The resulting consumption of H^+ and release of K^+ shift the solution composition along the line emanating from point *C*. When the muscovite-kaolinite boundary is reached at S_1, argillization of feldspar ceases, because the fluid is now in equilibrium with muscovite instead of kaolinite. Sericitization now proceeds (Reaction 10) and solution composition continues to evolve in the direction of the arrow until the KCl: HCl ratio has increased to a value corresponding to equilibrium between muscovite and K-feldspar at S_2. At this stage in the simple system, interaction between water and rock ceases because the fluid composition is compatible with rock-forming K-feldspar.

If the fluid moves while it is interacting with the rock-forming feldspar, then the relative locations of the kaolinite, muscovite, and K-feldspar stability regions correspond to early, intermediate, and late positions of the reacting fluid, respectively. The spatial relations of the alteration assemblages shown in Figure 6.2 require solution movement and concomitant interaction between water and rock from the periphery inward toward the center of the fractured intrusive. According to this model, therefore, the source of the fluid is the wall rocks to the altered intrusive, and the water is of meteoric origin.

Initial equilibrium of the hydrothermal fluid with respect to kaolinite (see Fig. 6.7, point *C*) would require either interaction between meteoric waters and argillaceous wall rocks or the operation of an acid-generating process due to the increase in temperatures of meteoric waters as the central intrusive is approached (Fig. 6.7, line *C*-*D'*). Later solutions following the same flow path and having the same initial composition as the preceding fluids would not begin reacting with the igneous rock until they passed through the zone containing kaolinite produced by earlier fluids, because they are in equilibrium with the mineral. Hence, a given position in the rock mass is exposed to progressively more acid solutions as a result of delayed reaction, and later minerals (e.g., muscovite) have a more acid-stable character than earlier phases (e.g., K-feldspar). Dissolution of iron-bearing silicates causes a reduction of dissolved sulfur and a progressive consumption of acid, which are responsible for deposition of sulfide minerals in the water/rock interaction model (Helgeson, 1970).

Theories of Alteration and Mineralization

Several lines of evidence may be examined to evaluate applicability of the two hypotheses discussed above to alteration and accompanying mineralization of the porphyry copper deposits in southwestern North America. Based on oxygen and hydrogen isotope analyses of hydrothermal minerals at Santa Rita and other deposits, Sheppard and others (1969, 1971) have proposed that waters of magmatic and meteoric origin might each be involved, at different times, in alteration within porphyry copper systems. These workers have suggested that the former are responsible for high temperature potassic phases, and that the latter produced phyllic and argillic assemblages at lower temperatures. Unfortunately, isotopic studies do not provide conclusive answers regarding sources of altering fluids for porphyry copper deposits of southwestern North America because the assumed D:H ratio of meteoric waters during the Laramide in that region is identical to that adopted for waters of magmatic origin (Taylor, 1974).

Rose (1970, p. 929) has adopted the premise that "... ore transport is outward from a magmatic source ...," and has concluded that the extent of cooling of magmatic fluids necessary to produce alteration and ore deposition requires at least one of the following three processes: (1) mixing with cool waters, (2) throttling due to pressure release, (3) "extremely slow" flow rates. Rose reached these conclusions after demonstrating that simple conductive cooling of initially high-temperature fluids (600°C) results in a sharp thermal front that migrates outward from the origin into relatively cold wall rocks and produces alteration phenomona not compatible with observations.

Numerical simulation of fluid flow in porphyry copper environments has led Norton (1982) to conclude that, while magmatic fluids may be present at an early stage of evolution, wall rocks adjacent to the intrusive are the source of the vast majority of fluids circulating through a fractured hypabyssal pluton during its cooling history. Thermal interaction between the hot, fractured pluton and convecting meteoric waters results in relatively rapid cooling of the intrusive and general smoothing of isotherms over much of the composite hydrothermal system. Fluid inclusion studies, accompanied by detailed paragenetic analyses, offer a reasonably reliable means of establishing thermal and chemical characteristics of fluids associated with development of specific alteration types in porphyry copper deposits. These techniques can often be used also to establish chronologic relations among fluids having different properties, although the task is not a simple one. Fluid inclusions homogenizing at or near magmatic temperatures ($>600°C$) and having high salinities have been observed in association with early generations of potassic alteration at Bingham (Roedder, 1971; Moore and Nash, 1974) and Santa Rita (Reynolds and Beane, 1979) and in the breccia pipes at Copper Creek (Walker, 1979). These high-temperature, high-salinity fluids are, according to the isotopic definition, magmatic (i.e., fluids which interact with magmas or igneous rocks at magmatic temperatures). All porphyry copper deposits studied in southwestern North America show evidence that fluids of intermediate temperature ($\sim$300–500°C), with both high and low salinity, were present at one time or another during their protracted evolutionary histories (Nash, 1976). The origins of these lower-temperature fluids of variable salinity are uncertain. In the late 1970s there evolved a tendency to label late, intermediate-temperature, low-salinity fluids as meteoric, but little firm evidence exists for such a designation or for implying that the more saline fluids of similar temperature are of magmatic origin. It is generally agreed that both endogenous and exogenous fluids were involved, at different times, in the alteration of plutons exhibiting porphyry copper characteristics, and that alteration may have been produced by both cooling and fluid reaction within these systems. However, the question still remains as to the source of introduced copper and sulfur, and the origin of the fluids responsible for their transport.

Field (1966) and Ohmoto and Rye (1979) concluded from sulfur isotope ratios in sulfide and sulfate minerals that this component in porphyry copper deposits could have been derived from an igneous and/or mantle source. Partitioning systematics have shown that several hydrothermal parameters must be evaluated before deposited minerals can be used to establish either the isotopic characteristics of sulfur transported by hydrothermal fluid or the source from which the sulfur was derived (Ohmoto, 1972; Rye and Ohmoto, 1974). Such data has not been integrated with sulfur isotope data for porphyry copper deposits of southwestern North America. No techniques are available to evaluate the source of copper found in large porphyry systems, but some evidence is available from fluid inclusion studies. Numerous reports based on microscopically observable properties have indicated that chalcopyrite is present as a daughter mineral in fluid inclusions. Scanning electron microscopy and semi-quantitative emission analysis have confirmed that chalcopyrite is present as one of the daughter products in fluid inclusions from Santa Rita which homogenized at magmatic temperatures (Reynolds and Beane, 1979). Microscopic estimates of the size of this daughter product in inclusions from Bingham (Roedder, 1971) and Santa Rita (Reynolds and Beane, 1979) indicate that concentrated fluids of complex chemistry apparently transported copper at levels on the order of several thousand parts per million at magmatic and sub-magmatic temperatures. The studies at Bingham indicate deposition of chalcopyrite from such fluids, but careful paragenetic analysis has shown this not to be the case at Santa Rita. Similar chalcopyrite daughter minerals and dissolved copper concentrations have been established for dilute fluid inclusions from Red Mountain, Arizona, although such fluids did not deposit chalcopyrite in enclosing rocks (Bodnar and Beane, 1980). Several workers have found that mineralization can be correlated with both high- and low-salinity fluids of intermediate temperature at different porphyry copper deposits in southwestern North America (e.g., Nash and Cunningham, 1974; Logsdon, 1969; Preece and Beane, in press; Bodnar and Beane, 1980). Definitive evidence for the origin of the two fluid types is lacking, however.

Correlation of Mineralization With Alteration

Deposition of chalcopyrite (and bornite) in the porphyry copper environment occurs both by open space (or vein) filling and by replacement (or alteration) of pre-existing minerals, and it may proceed according to the various mechanisms outlined in Table 6.3. Alteration selvages adjacent to veins containing mineralization indicate active chemical interaction between wall rocks and hydrothermal solutions. In only a few instances do wall rocks peripheral to mineralized veins show no evidence of alteration; such lack of alteration is indicative of sulfide deposition as a result of cooling of hydrothermal solutions that were apparently in chemical equilibrium with host rocks. Replacement chalcopyrite generally appears in close proximity to fluid channelways, which range from centimeters in width down to microscopic scale. Here, diffusion of copper and sulfur from fluid channelways into wall rocks produces disseminated mineralization, usually in the sites of pre-existing, iron-bearing minerals such as biotite and magnetite. The comprehensive analyses of porphyry copper deposits by Lowell and Guilbert (1970) and Rose (1970) place the "ore zone" in the outer portion of the potassic alteration zone; the ore zone extends to the potassic-phyllic interface, beyond which occurs the region of intense pyritization (see Fig. 6.2). The so-called "barren core" (interior to the ore zone) commonly contains relatively high, but still sub-ore–grade copper contents associated with potassic alteration minerals. Therefore, it might be concluded that the processes responsible for potassic alteration are the same as those responsible for copper mineralization. Detailed studies of mineral relationships at individual deposits, however, indicate that the extension of the spatial correlation to paragenetic equivalence does not necessarily follow.

TABLE 6.3
Mechanisms for Deposition of Chalcopyrite from Hydrothermal Solutions in Porphyry Copper Environments

Open-Space Filling in Veins, Veinlets, etc.

$(Cu^+ + Fe^{2+} + 2H_2S + \frac{1}{4}O_2 = CuFeS_2 + 3H^+ + \frac{1}{2}H_2O)$

Cooling of hydrothermal solutions
- Decreased solubility of sulfides
- Decreased stability of Cu-Cl complexes

Diffusion of Fe from wall rocks
- Combination with Cu and S in vein solutions

Dilution of concentrated solutions
- Dissociation of Cu-Cl complexes

Mixing of fluids transporting individual components

Neutralization of acid solutions
- Dissociation of H-S complexes

Replacement or Alteration of Pre-Existing Ferromagnesian Minerals

Fe-biotite → Fe-chlorite

$$2KFe_3AlSi_3O_{10}(OH)_2 + Cu^+ + 2H_2S + O_2 + H^+ = Fe_5Al_2Si_3O_{10}(OH)_8 + CuFeS_2 + 2K^+ + 6SiO_2 + \frac{1}{2}H_2O$$

Fe-biotite → K-feldspar

$$KFe_3AlSi_3O_{10}(OH)_2 + 3Cu^+ + 6H_2S + \frac{3}{4}O_2 = KAlSi_3O_8 + 3CuFeS_2 + 3H^+ + 1\frac{1}{2}H_2O$$

Magnetite

$$Fe_3O_4 + 3Cu^+ + 6H_2S + \frac{1}{4}O_2 = 3CuFeS_2 + 3H^+ + \frac{9}{2}H_2O$$

Pyrite

$$FeS_2 + Cu^+ + \frac{1}{2}H_2O = CuFeS_2 + H^+ + \frac{1}{4}O_2$$

Reduction of sulfate species in vein solutions

$$Cu^+ + Fe^{2+} + 2HSO_4^- = CuFeS_2 + H^+ + \frac{7}{2}O_2 + \frac{1}{2}H_2O$$

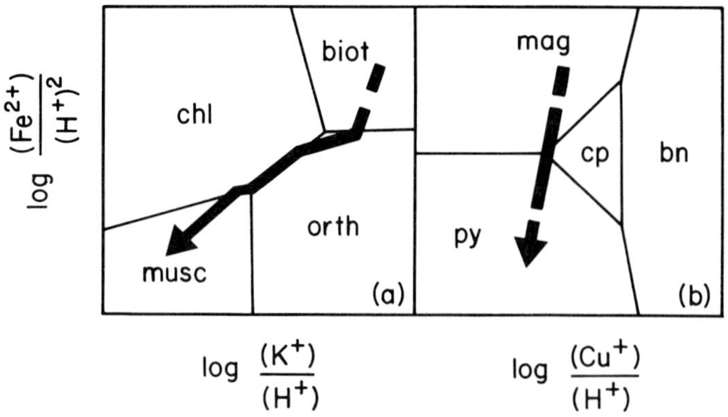

Key to Minerals:

biot = biotite	*cp* = chalcopyrite	*orth* = orthoclase
bn = bornite	*mag* = magnetite	*py* = pyrite
chl = chlorite (14Å)	*musc* = muscovite	

Figure 6.8. Schematic stability relations among (*a*) silicate minerals and (*b*) sulfides and oxides of Cu and Fe at unspecified temperature and activities of O_2 and H_2S in the presence of an aqueous solution. Chlorite and biotite represent the Fe component of solid solutions. Relative positions of the two diagrams in terms of the Fe^{2+} compositional variable are based on common mineral assemblages in porphyry copper deposits in the southwestern United States. Arrows indicate changing assemblages from early to late. From Beane and Titley (in press).

Figure 6.8*a* shows schematic stability relations among silicate minerals similar to those shown in Figure 6.5*c*, but with Fe^{2+} substituted for Mg^{2+} as a compositional variable to represent the Fe component in biotite and chlorite. Figure 6.8*b* is a complementary diagram which schematically shows hydrothermal stability relations among sulfide and oxide minerals of Cu and Fe. The arrows on these diagrams show the general paragenetic sequences of appropriate silicate and sulfide minerals seen in the porphyry copper deposits of southwestern North America (see also Table 6.2). While the transition from potassic to phyllic alteration might be attributed to decreasing temperature of the causative hydrothermal fluid, such a mechanism does not readily provide the observed sequence of magnetite → chalcopyrite → pyrite seen at most deposits (Helgeson et al., 1969). Fluid inclusion data from several locations further indicate that the observed mineral parageneses do not reflect a decrease in temperature, but rather can be reasonably explained from the standpoint of chemical reactions and their influence on hydrothermal fluid composition, as shown in Figure 6.8.

Close examination of the timing between mineralization and alteration reveals that, for the most part, chalcopyrite deposition occurs late in the evolution of potassic alteration or during a transitional stage between potassic and phyllic alteration when early hydrothermal biotite is altered to chlorite, while K-feldspar remains stable. This association provides the link in terms of $a_{Fe^{2+}}/a^2_{H^+}$ between silicate minerals (see Fig. 6.8*a*) and sulfide/oxide minerals (see Fig. 6.8*b*) in the porphyry copper deposits. The composite mineral assemblages in paragenetic sequence (as shown by the arrows on Fig. 6.8) are: K-feldspar + biotite + magnetite, K-feldspar + chlorite + chalcopyrite, and muscovite (sericite) + pyrite; quartz is ubiquitous. The stage at which biotite is altered to chlorite appears to represent an important transition in which evolving alteration mineralogy begins to be controlled by the hydrothermal fluid, rather than by the host rock (cf., Fig. 6.1). Helgeson (1970) has pointed out the important role played by ferromagnesian silicates and magnetite as sources of Fe for deposition of chalcopyrite and as potential reducing agents for dissolved sulfate. Paragenetic studies of hydrothermal minerals generally indicate that if mineralization has not developed prior to the point at which the ferromagnesian silicates begin to undergo quartz-sericite-pyrite alteration, it is not likely to develop with further evolution of the hydrothermal system.

Examination of hydrothermal alteration and mineralization at the abundant examples of economic, sub-economic, and barren porphyry copper-type systems of southwestern North America reveals numerous variations on the general patterns outlined here, but most show the same general styles of development. Different wall rock types, fluid characteristics, and crystallization histories of epizonal intrusions clearly have led to certain modes of mineralization and alteration and have precluded others; in the extremes such differences produced both economic and barren hydrothermal systems. A clear understanding, both of environments in which different hydrothermal mineral assemblages form and of paragenetic relations among silicate and sulfide minerals in the field, is critical to effective exploration for the large geothermal systems whose evolution has led to development of porphyry copper mineralization.

ACKNOWLEDGMENTS

I would like to extend my thanks to Drs. D. L. Norton, S. C. Creasey, J. J. Hemley, D. K. Bird, and particularly S. R. Titley for their many helpful comments and suggestions during the course of development of this chapter. Certain points in the final product are not universally agreed upon by these individuals, and the author accepts full responsibility for the content. Many of the concepts and details included have evolved from studies carried out by graduate students working with the author at the University of Arizona. I would particularly like to acknowledge contributions by T. J. Reynolds, R. K. Preece, III, R. J. Bodnar, W. W. Wilkinson, V. A. Walker, and F. M. Haynes. I am also grateful to Barb Beane, Jean Matthews, Debbie Church, and Dan Valenzuela for preparation of the manuscript and illustrations. This work was supported, in large part, by funds from National Science Foundation Grant EAR77-13642, with additional aid from the State of Arizona.

REFERENCES CITED

Aiken, D. M., and West, R. J., 1978, Some geologic aspects of the Sierrita-Esperanza copper-molybdenite deposit, Pima County, Arizona: Ariz. Geol. Soc. Digest, v. XI, p. 117–128.

Anderson, C. A., 1950, Alteration and metallization in the Bagdad porphyry copper deposit, Arizona: Econ. Geol., v. 45, p. 609–628.

Anderson, C. A.; Scholz, E. A.; and Strobell, J. D., 1955, Geology and ore deposits of the Bagdad area, Yavapai County, Arizona: U.S. Geol. Surv. Prof. Paper 278, 103 p.

Barton, P. B., Jr., 1973, Solid solutions in the system Cu-Fe-S, Part I: The Cu-S and CuFe-S joins: Econ. Geol., v. 68, p. 455–465.

Barton, P. B., and Skinner, B. J., 1967, Sulfide mineral stabilities: *in* Barnes, H. L., ed., Geochemistry of Hydrothermal Ore Deposits: New York, Holt, Rinehart, and Winston, p. 236–333.

Bauer, H. L., Jr.; Breitrick, R. A.; Cooper, J. J.; and Anderson, J. A., 1966, Porphyry copper deposits in the Robinson mining district, Nevada: *in* Titley, S. R., and Hicks, C. L., Geology of the Porphyry Copper Deposits: Tucson, Univ. of Ariz. Press, p. 232–244.

Beane, R. E., 1974, Biotite stability in the porphyry copper environment: Econ. Geol., v. 69, p. 241–256.

Beane, R. E., and Titley, S. R., in press, Geologic characteristics, environments, and genesis of porphyry copper deposits, Part II: Hydrothermal alteration and mineralization: Econ. Geol., 75th Anniv. Vol.

Bird, D. K., and Helgeson, H. C., 1980, Chemical interactions of aqueous solutions with epidote-feldspar mineral assemblages in geologic systems, 1: Thermodynamic analysis of phase relations in the system CaO-FeO-Fe_2O_3-Al_2O_3-SiO_2-H_2O-CO_2: Amer. Jour. Sci., v. 280, p. 907–941.

———, 1981, Chemical interaction of aqueous solutions with epidote-feldspar mineral assemblages in geologic systems, 2. Equilibrium constraints in metamorphic/geothermal processes: Amer. Jour. Sci., v. 281, p. 576–614.

Bodnar, R. J., and Beane, R. E., 1980, Temporal and spatial variations in hydrothermal fluid characteristics during vein filling in pre-ore cover overlying deeply buried porphyry copper mineralization at Red Mountain, Arizona: Econ. Geol., v. 75, p. 876–893.

Bray, R. E., 1969, Igneous rocks and hydrothermal alteration at Bingham, Utah: Econ. Geol., v. 64, p. 34–49.

Brimhall, G. H., Jr., 1977, Early fracture-controlled mineralization at Butte, Montana: Econ. Geol., v. 72, p. 37–59.

———, 1979, Lithologic determinations of mass transfer mechanisms of multiple-stage porphyry copper mineralization at Butte, Montana: Vein formation by hypogene leaching and enrichment of potassium-silicate protore: Econ. Geol., v. 74, p. 556–589.

Bryant, D. G., and Metz, H. E., 1966, Geology and ore deposits of the Warren mining district, *in* Titley, S. R., and Hicks, C. L., eds., Geology of the Porphyry Copper Deposits: Tucson, Univ. of Ariz. Press, p. 189–203.

Burnham, C. W., 1962, Facies and types of hydrothermal alteration: Econ. Geol., v. 57, p. 768–784.

———, 1979, Magmas and hydrothermal fluids: *in* Barnes, H. L., ed., Geochemistry of Hydrothermal Ore Deposits, 2nd ed.: New York, Wiley-Interscience, p. 71–136.

Carson, D. J. T., and Jambor, J. L., 1974, Mineralogy, zonal relationships and economic significance of hydrothermal alteration at porphyry copper deposits, Babine Lake area, British Columbia: CIM, v. 67, p. 1–24.

Corn, R. M., 1975, Alteration-mineralization zoning, Red Mountain, Arizona: Econ. Geol., v. 70, p. 1437–1447.

Creasey, S. C., 1959, Some phase relations in hydrothermally altered rocks of porphyry copper deposits: Econ. Geol., v. 54, pp. 353–373.

———, 1966, Hydrothermal alteration, *in* Titley, S. R., and Hicks, C. L., eds., Geology of the Porphyry Copper Deposits: Tucson, Univ. Ariz. Press, p. 51–75.

Crerar, D. A., and Barnes, H. L., 1976, Ore solution chemistry, V: Solubilities of chalcopyrite and chalcocite assemblages in hydrothermal solutions at 200°C–350°C: Econ. Geol., v. 71, p. 772–794.

Crerar, D. A.; Susak, N. J.; Borcsik, M.; and Schwartz, S., 1978, Solubility of the buffer assemblage pyrite + pyrrhotite + magnetite in NaCl solutions from 200°C–350°C: Geochim. Cosmochim. Acta, v. 42, p. 1427–1437.

Davis, J. D., 1974, Geothermometry, geochemistry, and alteration at the San Manuel porphyry copper ore body, San Manuel, Arizona: Unpub. Ph.D. Diss. Univ. Ariz., 250 p.

Denis, M., 1974, Altération et fluides associés dans le porphyre cuprifère de Sierrita: Unpub. Diss. University of Nancy I, France, 153 p.

Einaudi, M. T., 1982, General features and origin of skarns associated with porphyry copper plutons, southwestern North America, *in* Titley, S. R., ed., Advances in Geology of the Porphyry Copper Deposits, Southwestern North America: Tucson, Univ. Ariz. Press, Chapter 8.

Fellows, M. L., 1976, Composition of epidote from porphyry copper deposits: Unpub. M.S. Thesis, Univ. Ariz., 190 p.

Field, C. W., 1966, Sulfur isotope abundance data, Bingham District, Utah: Econ. Geol., v. 61, p. 850–871.

Fournier, R. O., 1967*a*, The porphyry copper deposit exposed in the Liberty pit mine near Ely, Nevada, I: Syngenetic formation: Econ. Geol., v. 62, p. 57–81.

———, 1967*b*, The porphyry copper deposit exposed in the Liberty pit mine near Ely, Nevada, II: The formation of hydrothermal alteration zones: Econ. Geol., v. 62, p. 207–227.

Galey, J. L., 1979, General geology and hydrothermal alteration of the Silver Bell porphyry copper deposit: Soc. Econ. Geol. Guidebook, 1979 Field Conf., 18 p.

Gilmour, Paul, 1982, Grades and tonnages of porphyry copper deposits, *in* Titley, S. R., ed., Advances in Geology of the Porphyry Copper Deposits: Tucson, Univ. Ariz. Press, Chapter 1.

Gilluly, J., 1946, The Ajo mining district, Arizona: U.S. Geol. Surv. Prof. Paper 209, 112 p.

Graybeal, F. T., 1982, Geology of the El Tiro area, Silver Bell mining district, Pima County, Arizona, *in* Titley, S. R., ed., Advances in Geology of the Porphyry Copper Deposits, Southwestern North America: Tucson, Univ. Ariz. Press, Chapter 24.

Guilbert, J. M., and Lowell, J. D., 1974, Variations in zoning patterns in porphyry ore deposits: Can. Min. and Pet. Bull., v. 67, p. 99–109.

Gustafson, L. B., and Hunt, J. P., 1975, The porphyry copper deposits at El Salvador, Chile: Econ. Geol., v. 70, p. 857–912.

Gustafson, L. B., and Titley, S. R., eds., 1978, Porphyry copper deposits of the southwestern Pacific islands and Australia: Econ. Geol., Spec. Issue v. 73, no. 5, p. 597–986.

Helgeson, H. C., 1964, Complexing and Hydrothermal Ore Deposition: New York, The Macmillan Co., 128 p.

———, 1969, Thermodynamics of hydrothermal systems at elevated temperatures and pressures: Amer. Jour. Sci., v. 267, p. 729–804.

———, 1970, A chemical and thermodynamic model of ore deposition in hydrothermal systems: Mineral. Soc. Amer. Spec. Paper 3, p. 155–186.

Helgeson, H. C.; Brown, T. H.; and Leeper, R. H., 1969, Handbook of Theoretical Activity Diagrams Depicting Chemical Equilibria in Geologic Systems Involving an Aqueous Phase at One Atm and 0° to 300°C: San Francisco, Freeman, Cooper and Co., 253 p.

Helgeson, H. C., and Kirkham, D. H., 1974, Theoretical predictions of the thermodynamic behavior of aqueous electrolytes at high pressures and temperatures, I: Summary of the thermodynamic/electrostatic properties of the solvent: Amer. Jour. Sci., v. 274, p. 1098–1198.

———, 1976, Theoretical predictions of the thermodynamic behavior of aqueous electrolytes at high pressures and temperatures, III: Equation of state for aqueous species at infinite dilution: Amer. Jour. Sci., v. 276, p. 96–240.

Helgeson, H. C.; Delaney, J. M.; Nesbitt, H. W.; and Bird, D. K., 1978, Summary and critique of the thermodynamic properties of rockforming minerals: Amer. Jour. Sci., v. 278-A, p. 1–229.

Helgeson, H. C., and Aagaard, P., in press, Activity/composition relations among silicates and aqueous solutions, 1: Thermodynamics of intercrystalline exchange reactions: Am. Jour. Sci., v. 281.

Hemley, J. J., and Jones, W. R., 1964, Chemical aspects of hydrothermal alteration with emphasis on hydrogen metasomatism: Econ. Geol., v. 59, p. 538–569.

Hemley, J. J.; Montoya, J. W.; Nigrini, A.; and Vincent, H. A., 1971, Some alteration reactions in the system CaO-Al_2O_3-SiO_2-H_2O: Joint Symp. Vol., IMA-IAGOD meetings, 1970, Tokyo, Soc. Min. Geol. of Japan, p. 58–63.

Hemley, J. J.; Montoya, J. W.; Marinenko, J. W.; and Luce, R. W., 1980, Mineral equilibria in the system Al_2O_3-SiO_2-H_2O and some implications of alteration/mineralization processes: Econ. Geol., v. 75, p. 210–228.

Herr, F. L., Jr., and Helz, G. R., 1978, On the possibility of bisulfide ion-pairs in natural brines and hydrothermal solutions: Econ. Geol., v. 73, p. 73–81.

Holland, H. D., 1959, Some applications of thermochemical data to problems of ore deposits, I: Stability relations among the oxides, sulfides, sulfates and carbonates of ore and gangue minerals: Econ. Geol., v. 54, p. 184–233.

———, 1965, Some applications of thermochemical data to problems of ore deposits, II: Mineral assemblages and the composition of ore-forming fluids: Econ. Geol., v. 60, p. 1101–1166.

Hollister, V. F., 1978, Geology of the Porphyry Copper Deposits of the Western Hemisphere: New York, AIME, SME, 219 p.

Hoschek, G., 1973, Zur stabilität metamorpher biotit-paragenesen: Tsch. Min. Petr. Mitt., v. 20, p. 48–58.

Jacobs, D. C., and Parry, W. T. 1976, A comparison of the geochemistry of biotite from some Basin and Range stocks: Econ. Geol., v. 71, p. 1029–1035.

———, 1979, Geochemistry of biotite in the Santa Rita porphyry copper deposit, New Mexico: Econ. Geol., v. 74, p. 860–887.

James, L. P., 1976, Zoned alteration in limestone at porphyry copper deposits, Ely, Nevada: Econ. Geol., v. 71, p. 488–512.

Langton, J. M., 1973, Ore genesis in the Morenci-Metcalf district: AIME Trans., v. 254, p. 247–257.

Logsdon, M. J., 1969, A fluid inclusion study of the porphyry copper deposits at Ray and San Manuel, Arizona (abs.): in Proc. of COFFI, Roedder, E., ed., v. 2, p. 20.

Lowell, J. D., 1968, Geology of the Kalamazoo orebody, San Manuel district, Arizona: Econ. Geol., v. 63, p. 645–654.

Lowell, J. D., and Guilbert, J. M., 1970, Lateral and vertical alteration-mineralization zoning in porphyry ore deposits: Econ. Geol., v. 65, p. 373–408.

McKinstry, H., 1957, Source of iron in pyritized wall rocks: Econ. Geol., v. 65, p. 373–408.

Metzger, F. W.; Kelly, W. C.; Nesbitt, B. E.; and Essene, E. J., 1977, Scanning electron microscopy of daughter minerals in fluid inclusions: Econ. Geol., v. 72, p. 141–152.

Meyer, C., and Hemley, J. J., 1967, Wall rock alteration, *in* Barnes, H. L. ed., Geochemistry of Hydrothermal Ore Deposits: New York, Holt, Rinehart and Winston, p. 166–235.

Montoya, J. W., and Hemley, J. J., 1975, Activity relations and stabilities in alkali feldspar and mica alteration reactions: Econ. Geol., v. 70, p. 577–582.

Moolick, R. T., and Durek, J. J., 1966, The Morenci district, *in* Titley, S. R., and Hicks, C. L., eds., Geology of the Porphyry Copper Deposits: Tucson, Univ. Ariz. Press, p. 221–231.

Moore, W. J., 1975, Chemical characteristics of hydrothermal alteration at Bingham, Utah (abs.): Abs. Ann. Mtg., Geol. Soc. America, v. 7, p. 1204–1205.

Moore, W. J., and Czamanske, G. K., 1973, Compositions of biotites from unaltered and altered monzonite rocks in the Bingham mining district: Econ. Geol., v. 68, p. 269–274.

Moore, W. J., and Nash, J. T., 1974, Alteration and fluid inclusion studies of the porphyry copper orebody at Bingham, Utah: Econ. Geol., v. 69, p. 31–45.

Nash, J. T., 1976, Fluid-inclusion petrology—Data from porphyry copper deposits and applications to exploration: U.S. Geol. Surv. Prof. Paper 907-D, 16 p.

Nash, J. T., and Cunningham, C. C., Jr., 1974, Fluid inclusion studies of the porphyry copper deposit at Bagdad, Arizona: U.S. Geol. Surv. Jour. Research, v. 2, p. 31–34.

Nielsen, R. L., 1968, Hypogene texture and mineral zoning in a copper-bearing granodiorite stock, Santa Rita, New Mexico: Econ. Geol., v. 63, p. 37–50.

Norton, D. L., 1982, Fluid and heat transport phenomena typical of copper-bearing pluton environments, southeastern Arizona, *in* Titley, S. R., ed., Advances in Geology of the Porphyry Copper Deposits, Southwestern North America: Tucson, Univ. Ariz. Press, Chapter 3.

Ohmoto, H., 1972, Systematics of sulfur and carbon isotopes in hydrothermal ore deposits: Econ. Geol. v. 67, p. 551–578.

Ohmoto, H., and Rye, R. O., 1979, Isotopes of sulfur and carbon, *in* Barnes, H. L., ed., Geochemistry of Hydrothermal Ore Deposits, 2nd ed.: New York, Wiley Interscience, p. 500–567.

Peterson, N. P., 1962, Geology and ore deposits, Globe-Miami district, Arizona. U.S. Geol. Survey Prof. Paper 342, 151 p.

Peterson, N. P.; Gilbert, C. M.; and Quick, G. L., 1951, Geology and ore deposits of the Castle Dome area, Gila County, Arizona: U.S. Geol. Survey Bull. 971, 134 p.

Phillips, C. H.; Gambell, N. A.; and Fountain, D. S., 1974, Hydrothermal alteration, mineralization, and zoning in the Ray deposit: Econ. Geol., v. 69, p. 1237–1250.

Preece, R. K. III, 1979, Paragenesis, geochemistry and temperatures of formation of alteration assemblages: Unpub. M. S. Thesis, Univ. Ariz., 106 p.

Preece, R. K. III, and Beane, R. E., in press, Contrasting evolutions of hydrothermal alteration in quartz monzonite and quartz diorite at the Sierrita porphyry copper deposit, Arizona: Econ. Geol., v. 76.

Reynolds, T. J., 1980, Variations in hydrothermal fluid characteristics through time at the Santa Rita porphyry copper deposit, New Mexico: Unpub. M.S. Thesis, Univ. Arizona.

Reynolds, T. J., and Beane, R. E., 1979, The evolution of hydrothermal fluid characteristics through time at the Santa Rita, New Mexico, porphyry copper deposit (abs.): Abs. Ann. Mtg. Geol. Soc. America, v. 11, p. 502.

Robinson, R. F., and Cook, A., 1966, The Safford Copper Deposit, Lone Star mining district, Graham County Arizona, *in* Titley, S. R., and Hicks, C. L., eds., Geology of the Porphyry Copper Deposits: Tucson, Univ. Ariz. Press, p. 251–266.

Roedder, E., 1971, Fluid inclusion studies on the porphyry-type ore deposits at Bingham, Utah: Butte, Montana; and Climax, Colorado: Econ. Geol., v. 66, p. 98–120.

Rose, A. W., 1970, Zonal relations of wallrock alteration and sulfide distribution at porphyry copper deposits: Econ. Geol., v. 65, p. 920–936.

Rye, R. O., and Ohmoto, H., 1974, Sulfur and carbon isotopes and ore genesis, A review: Econ. Geol., v. 69, p. 836–842.

Saxena, S. K., 1973, Thermodynamics of rock-forming crystalline solutions: New York, Springer-Verlag, 188 p.

Schwartz, G. M., 1947, Hydrothermal alteration in the "porphyry copper" deposits: Econ. Geol., v. 42, p. 319–352.

———, 1953, Geology of the San Manuel copper deposit, Arizona: U.S. Geol. Surv. Prof. Paper 256, 65 p.

Shade, J. W., 1974, Hydrolysis reactions in the SiO_2-excess portion of the system K_2O-Al_2O_3-SiO_2-H_2O in chloride fluids at magmatic conditions: Econ. Geol., v. 69, p. 218–229.

Sheppard, S. M. F.; Nielsen, R. L.; and Taylor, H. P., Jr., 1969, Oxygen and hydrogen isotope ratios of clay minerals from porphyry copper deposits: Econ. Geol. v. 64, p. 755–777.

———, 1971, Hydrogen and oxygen isotope ratios in minerals from porphyry copper deposits: Econ. Geol., v. 66, p. 515–542.

Smith, V. L., 1975, Hypogene alteration at the Esperanza mine, Pima County, Arizona: Unpub. M. S. Thesis, Univ. Ariz. 161 p.

Stringham, B., 1953, Granitization and hydrothermal alteration at Bingham, Utah: Geol. Soc. America Bull., v. 64, p. 945–991.

Sweeton, F. H., and Baes, C. F., Jr., 1970, The solubility of magnetite and hydrolysis of ferrous ion in aqueous solutions at elevated temperatures: J. Chem. Thermo., v. 2, p. 479–500.

Taylor, H. P., Jr., 1974, The application of oxygen and hydrogen isotope studies to problems of hydrothermal alteration and ore deposition: Econ. Geol., v. 69, p. 843–883.

Titley, S. R., 1982, The style and progress of mineralization and alteration in porphyry copper systems, American Southwest, *in* Titley, S. R., ed. Advances in Geology of the Porphyry Copper Deposits, Southwestern North America: Tucson, Univ. Ariz. Press, Chapter 5.

Walker, V. A., 1979, Relationship among several breccia pipes and a lead-silver vein in the Copper Creek mining district, Pinal County, Arizona: Unpub. M.S. Thesis, Univ. Ariz., 163 p.

West, R. J., and Aiken, D. M., 1982, Geology of the Sierrita-Esperanza deposit, Pima mining district, Pima County, Arizona, *in* Titley, S. R., ed., Advances in Geology of the Porphyry Copper Deposits, Southwestern North America: Tucson, Univ. Ariz. Press, Chapter 21.

Whitney, J. A.; Simon, F. O.; Hemley, J. J.; and Davis, N. F., 1979, Iron concentrations in chloride solutions equilibrated with synthetic quartz monzonite assemblages, Part I: Sulfur free systems (abs.): Abs. Ann. Mtg. Geol. Soc. America, v. 11, p. 540.

Wilkinson, W. W.; Vega, L. J.; and Titley, S. R., 1982, Geology and ore deposits at Mineral Park, Mohave County, Arizona, *in* Titley, S. R., ed., Advances in Geology of the Porphyry Copper Deposits, Southwestern North America: Tucson, Univ. Ariz. Press, Chapter 26.

Ypma, P. J. M., 1968, A fluid inclusion study of the role of volatiles in the formation of porphyry copper deposits, *in* Roedder, E., ed., Proceedings of COFFI, 1969, v. 2, p. 10.

7

Description of Skarns Associated With Porphyry Copper Plutons

SOUTHWESTERN NORTH AMERICA

Marco T. Einaudi

The invariable association of porphyry copper plutons emplaced in carbonate-rich sedimentary rocks with mineralized calc-silicate or siliceous replacement bodies is well known. Numerous examples of this association occur in southwestern North America; the importance of this type of deposit as an exploration target has increased over the years due to the fact that porphyry deposits with carbonate ores commonly display higher hypogene copper grades than those lacking carbonate wall rocks.

In spite of the economic importance and scientific interest of carbonate-hosted ores, knowledge of their critical field relations and petrology has lagged behind knowledge of these aspects in the porphyries themselves. Of the thirteen deposits summarized in this chapter, only three have had fairly extensive published coverage (Christmas, Bingham, and Ely) in which details of paragenesis, zoning, and approximate phase compositions have been laid out. This gap is only partially closed by the present volume; Twin Buttes is described for the first time by Barter and Kelly (see Chapter 20). One of the main aims of this chapter, then, is to summarize the better-known deposits and to describe the lesser-known occurrences. Unpublished data acquired by the author are presented for Yerington, Bingham, and Palo Verde; descriptions of Cananea, Silver Bell, Twin Buttes, Mission, Continental, and Ely are colored by knowledge gained during field visits and discussions with geologists who have extensive personal knowledge of these deposits; descriptions of Christmas, Santa Rita, Morenci, and Bisbee are based entirely on the published record. The general features and origin of ores in carbonate wall rocks of porphyry plutons are discussed in Chapter 8 of this book.

SKARN TERMINOLOGY

The terminology applied to altered and mineralized carbonate-bearing rocks often is misleading, and different terms have evolved to describe identical features. Descriptive and genetic terms must, therefore, be clearly differentiated. For a broader discussion, the reader is referred to Burt (1977).

Skarn refers to coarse-grained calc-silicates which replace carbonate-rich rocks during regional or contact metamorphism. Skarns tend to consist of a sequence of monomineralic or bimineralic layers which are zoned relative to sedimentary or igneous contacts and fissures or fractures. Two broad categories of skarn are recognized. Skarn formed over a few millimeters or meters along shale-limestone contacts during high-grade metamorphism, and whose bulk composition reflects that of the reacting rocks, is termed *reaction skarn.* Reaction skarns can be shown to be the result of bimetasomatic diffusion of locally derived components in a possibly stagnant, intergranular hydrothermal fluid. Of greater interest here are the larger *ore skarns,* which may contain significant quantities of ore minerals, and whose bulk composition bears no simple relation to the enclosing rocks. Ore skarns normally are thought to result from infiltration of an iron-rich hydrothermal fluid derived from dominantly magmatic processes. Clearly, gradations between reaction skarns and ore skarns are possible. However, a distinction often can be made within a given district on the basis of age relations (reaction skarn tends to be early) and composition of calc-silicates (reaction skarn tends to be more aluminous); this is an important point, and will be discussed in greater detail in later sections. In the present chapter, the term *skarn* is reserved for calc-silicate gangue which is spatially and temporally related to ore deposition. The term *tactite* would be roughly synonymous with this usage.

Metamorphism is commonly defined as recrystallization, often accompanied by mineralogical transformations, which involves no transfer of matter into or out of the system other than volatile components such as H_2O and CO_2. In contrast, *metasomatism* involves changes in the amounts of non-volatile components such as Fe, Mg, and Si. Whether a particular rock is considered to be of metamorphic or metasomatic origin may depend on how the system is defined; for example, reaction skarns may be considered metasomatic if only the carbonate bed is considered, or metamorphic if the system is defined as the total sequence of interbedded carbonate-shale. In terms of processes, however, reaction skarns display the hallmark of the metasomatic process: abrupt discontinuities in bulk composition across monomineralic or bimineralic zonal boundaries. Metamorphic rocks, on the other hand, show no such compositional discontinuities across mineral zoning boundaries; the boundaries simply reflect thermal or volatile fugacity gradients.

Skarns can be classified according to the type of rock replaced: *endoskarns* replace an intrusive or other aluminous rock; *exoskarns* replace carbonate rocks. Endoskarns generally are only weakly developed in porphyry-related deposits. In the present chapter the term "skarn" is synonymous with "exoskarn." Further classification of exoskarn can be based on the calc-silicate mineral association. *Calcic skarns,* which generally replace non-magnesian limestone, display relatively high Ca/Mg ratios and consist of garnet, clinopyroxene, and wollastonite; one or more iron-rich calc-silicates always are present. *Magnesian skarns,* which generally replace dolomitic rocks, display relatively low Ca/Mg ratios and consist of foresterite, talc, tremolite, and serpentine; iron-rich calc-silicates generally are absent and magnetite is abundant. Due to the paucity of dolomite in sedimentary strata associated with porphyry copper deposits in southwestern North America, magnesian skarns are less important than calcic skarns in the deposits considered here.

Hornfels is a term generally applied to massive, fine-grained rocks resulting from contact metamorphism. A qualifier may be used to denote the dominant mineralogy or composition: calc-silicate hornfels or biotite hornfels. Although the term "hornfels," as used in the literature, generally implies an origin through metamorphism, it is clear that some hornfelses in porphyry-copper districts are metasomatic rocks. In this chapter, the term "hornfels" is used in a descriptive sense only.

The distinction between metamorphism and metasomatism becomes increasingly difficult if a sequence of impure carbonate and shale beds is replaced on a large scale by garnet-rich assemblages. Such assemblages may consist of coalesced reaction skarns or bedded sequences of coarse reaction skarn and finger-grained garnet hornfels resulting from metamorphic recrystallization of calcareous shale or marl. The term *skarnoid* is used in the present chapter to denote such garnet-rich rocks of uncertain origin.

The carbonate-hosted ores considered here are associated with highly fractured, hypabyssal granodiorite to quartz monzonite porphyry stock complexes that exhibit varying degrees of potassium silicate and/or sericitic alteration associated with Cu-Fe sulfide mineralization. With regard to alteration types in the stocks, the terms "propylitic," "potassium-silicate," "intermediate argillic," "sericitic," and "advanced argillic" are used in the sense defined by Meyer and Hemley (1967, p. 171–178).

CHARACTERISTICS OF SEDIMENTARY ROCKS IN SOUTHWESTERN NORTH AMERICA

Sedimentary rocks of porphyry copper districts in southwestern North America range from the carbonate-dominated cratonic deposits of southeastern Arizona to the sandstone-dominated subsident basin deposits of western Utah and eastern Nevada, to the basinal marine volcanic-arc deposits of western Nevada. A brief summary of sedimentary environments and lithologies is given here to set the context for the section dealing with individual deposits.

Carbonate Rocks of Arizona, New Mexico, and Sonora

The Paleozoic strata of southern Arizona, western New Mexico, and northeastern Sonora consist of a thin (1–2 km) sequence of shallow marine cratonic shelf deposits in which carbonate typically constitutes 65 percent of the whole (Figs. 7.1 and 7.2). The section thickens abruptly in the northwestern corner of Arizona toward the Cordilleran miogeosyncline and more gradually to the southeast toward the Sonoran embayment. Minor warping, faulting and eustatic changes in sea level characterized the central Arizona shelf during much of Early and Middle Paleozoic time. Increasing tectonic activity during Late Paleozoic time is correlated by Ross (1978) with the final closure of the Marathon geosyncline during collision of Gondwana and Laurasia during Pennsylvanian and Early Permian time. Patterns of sedimentation were controlled in part by a positive region in central Arizona and by northwest-trending, fault-bounded basins in the south (Butler, 1971; Titley, 1976).

Pronounced facies changes compound the difficulties involved in determining the origin of skarn minerals. For example, the Colina Limestone and Epitaph Formation, of Permian age, consist of dark-colored limestone, dolomite, marl, and gypsum; considerable variation in the proportions of these lithologies reflects the abrupt changes from a shallow lagoonal-evaporating pan (dolomite and gypsum) to deeper water (limestone) environments in the Pedregosa basin (Butler, 1971). The Silver Bell-Mission-Twin Buttes-Bisbee trend lies parallel to the northwest-trending basin axis and near its southwestern shoreline (Fig. 7.1), where the limestone:dolomite + gypsum ratio defined by Butler (1971) varies from 1:1 to 8:1. In areas where fresh equivalents of altered strata are not exposed, the determination of the source of magnesium in skarn and of the sedimentary or metasomatic origin of anhydrite is difficult at best.

Broader facies variations in other formations yield more predictable variations in calc-silicate associations. Where the Martin Formation is dominantly sandy dolomite to dolom-

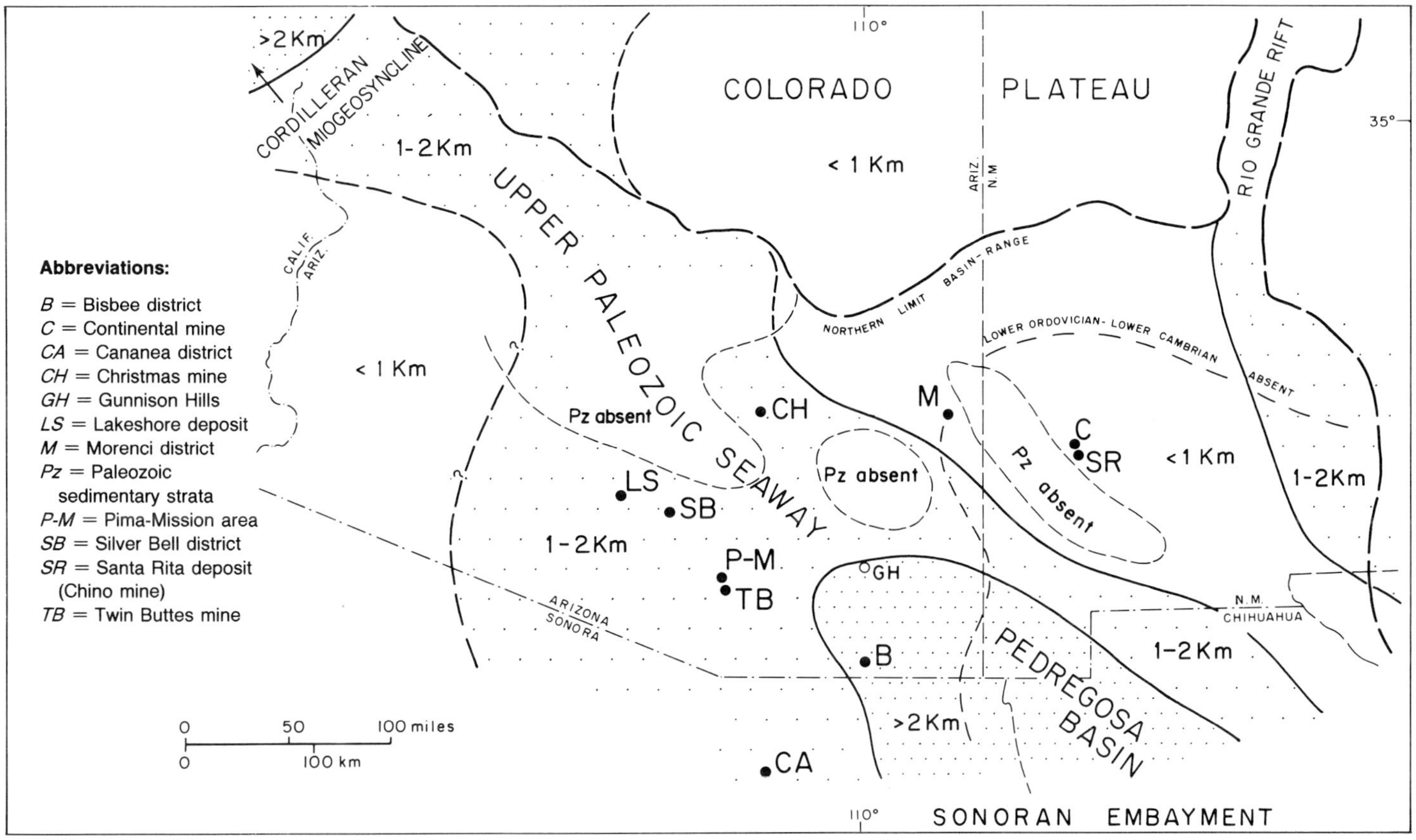

Figure 7.1. Paleothickness (in km) of Paleozoic sedimentary rocks in southeastern Arizona, southwestern New Mexico, and northernmost Sonora and Chihuahua. Porphyry-related skarn deposits are located mostly in areas of greatest thickness of carbonate-bearing strata that extend northwestward from the Pedregosa Basin. The absence of Paleozoic strata in some of the areas is due in part to non-deposition, in part to erosion. Information based on McKee (1951), Peirce (1976), and Greenwood and others (1977).

itic limestone, it yields magnetite-rich magnesian skarn at Christmas and Twin Buttes; to the southeast, toward the basin, the Martin consists of silty limestone and yields calcic skarn. The Abrigo and Earp formations consist of interstratified limestone, sandstone, siltstone, and shale; dolomitic members, which are characteristic of the Abrigo to the north and northeast are generally absent in southeastern Arizona (Hayes, 1978). During the early metamorphic stages of contact alteration, these formations typically yield layered hornfels-skarnoid-marble, which may be overprinted by calcic skarn; magnesian skarn generally is not developed. The Escabrosa, Horquilla, and Concha limestones consist of massive, thick-bedded cherty limestone, with shale and silty beds prominent only near the base of the Horquilla; during the metasomatic stages of alteration, these units typically yield massive calcic skarn.

Sandstone-Dominated Successions of Utah and Eastern Nevada

Farther north, in Utah and eastern Nevada, the Paleozoic section is more than an order of magnitude thicker than the shelf-margin of Arizona and includes thick sections of clastic rocks accumulated in subsident basins of Middle to Late Paleozoic age. Late Mississippian basins, forerunners of the Oquirrh basin, accumulated a thick section of black shales (Chainman Shale at Ely; Manning Canyon Formation near Bingham). In Pennsylvanian and Permian time extensive downwarping of the Cordilleran miogeosyncline occurred along the Cortez-Uinta trend from the Antler orogenic belt on the west to the Utah-Wyoming shelf margin (Roberts et al, 1965). The area of maximum sedimentation, near the Bingham district, received 8 km of predominantly sandy clastic deposits (Oquirrh Group). The middle portion of the Oquirrh Group constitutes the country rocks of the Bingham stock and locally is designated the Bingham Mine Formation (Fig. 7.3). The formation consists predominantly of quartz sandstone, with lesser amounts of clastic limestone and calcareous siltstone. Shaly interbeds constitute less than 1 percent of the whole and dolomite is virtually absent (Atkinson and Einaudi, 1978). The overall composition of the Pennsylvanian strata, thus, was not conducive to the generation of metamorphic calc-silicate hornfels with local skarnoid interbeds which, in contrast, characterize the Arizona-New Mexico-Sonora occurrences. Early metamorphic effects consist of recrystallization to orthoquartzite and local development of wollastonite-bearing marble.

To the southwest, the Oquirrh Group grades into a calcareous and silty facies, which in the Robinson district (Ely) is represented by the ore-bearing Ely Limestone. The thinner, ore-bearing limestone beds of the Bingham Mine Formation and the thicker Ely Limestone are very similar in overall composition: 25 to 30 percent SiO_2 (as chert and quartz silt),

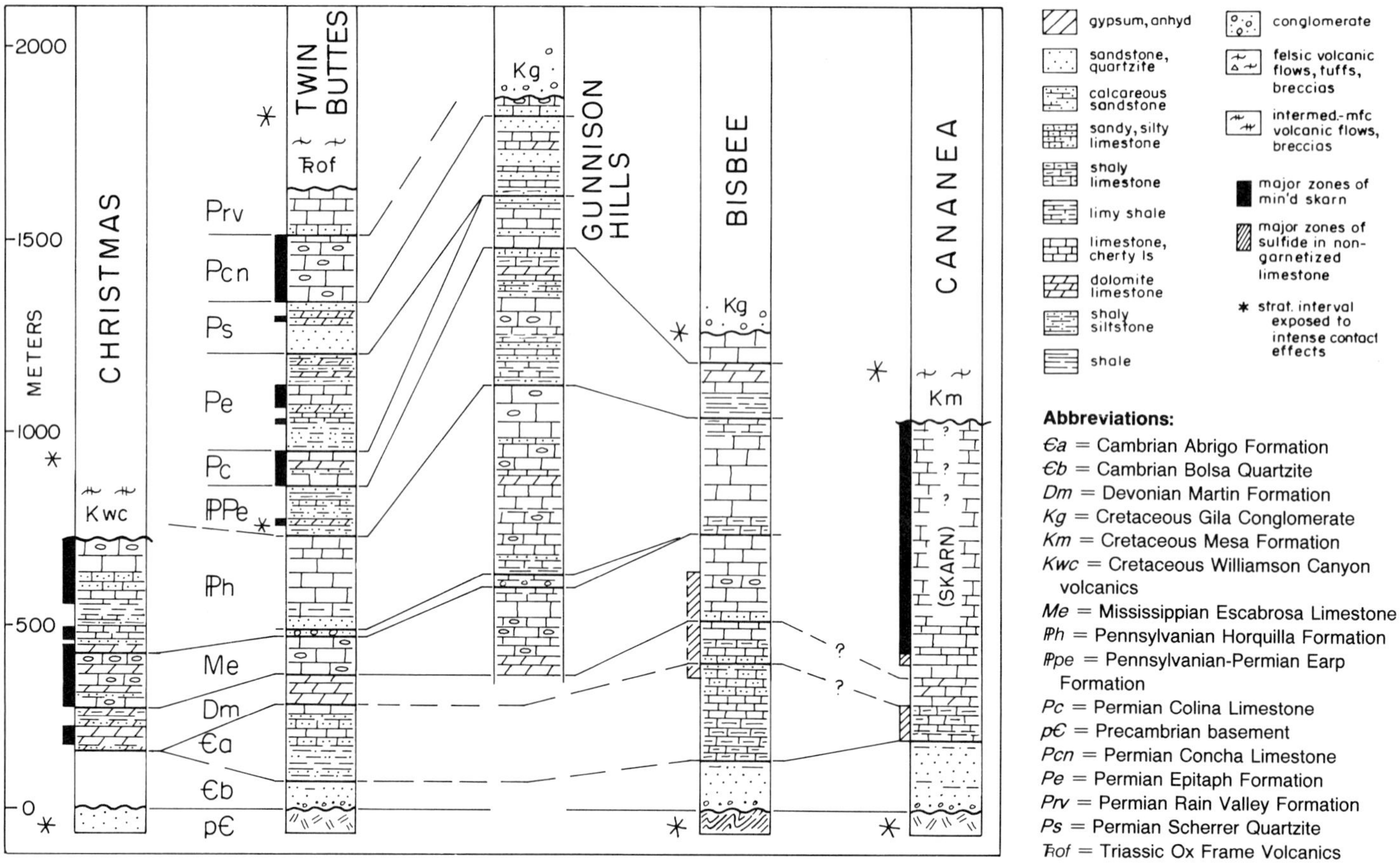

Figure 7.2. Paleozoic stratigraphic sections from southeastern Arizona and northernmost Sonora (localities shown in Fig. 7.1), illustrating lithologic variability within formations, dominance of carbonate lithology, and restriction of skarn (black bars) to purer carbonate beds. The stratigraphic interval occurring within the immediate contact aureole is indicated by stars for each locality. Source of data: Christmas (Perry, 1968); Twin Buttes (Barter and Kelly, 1982); Gunnison Hills (Gilluly et al., 1954); Bisbee (Bryant and Metz, 1966); Cananea (Mulchay and Velasco, 1954).

less than 1 percent MgO, and less than 1 percent Al_2O_3 (Reid, 1978; James, 1976).

Volcanic and Clastic Successions of Western Nevada

Further west, the strata of the western Great Basin consist of submarine volcanic arc deposits of Triassic age; lying west of the Paleozoic continental shelf, they are overlain by deposits which reflect the dominantly emergent continental margin terrain of Early to Middle Jurassic age (Speed, 1978). In the Yerington district, volcanic-sedimentary rocks consist of a Middle Triassic, andesite-rhyolite, volcanic-arc assemblage, which is overlain by Upper Triassic to Lower to Middle (?) Jurassic sedimentary rocks (Proffett, Livingstone, and Einaudi, in preparation). The sedimentary rocks consist of interstratified volcaniclastic rocks, black calcareous shale, argillite, and limestone of intermediate to shallow marine origin, overlain by evaporites and windblown (?) quartz sandstone (See Fig. 7.3). Middle Jurassic plutonism gave rise to dacite and quartz latite volcanic rocks, which unconformably overlie sandstone, and to porphyry copper and skarn deposits. The presence of intimately interbedded carbonate-argillaceous beds in the Triassic sedimentary section resulted in widespread development of calc-silicate hornfels and reaction skarns during the early metamorphic stages of Jurassic plutonism; metasomatic skarns were superimposed on this early metamorphic event and preferentially replaced pure limestone beds.

ALTERATION AND SKARN FORMATION

The correlation between potassium-silicate alteration in plutons and skarn formation, and between intense hydrolytic alteration in plutons and skarn destruction or silica-pyrite replacement of limestone has been documented at Santa Rita (Nielsen, 1970), Ely (James, 1976), and Bingham (Atkinson and Einaudi, 1978). In order to expand systematically on this theme, the twelve deposits considered in this chapter are discussed in a sequence which trends toward decreasing relative volumes of known potassium-silicate alteration and increasing relative volumes of known hydrolytic (sericitic and advanced argillic) alteration. Table 7.1 lays out this sequence for deposits where data are available; no implication as to relative depth of erosion is implied by the sequence. Two types of potassium-silicate alteration can be recognized in igneous rocks of most deposits. (1) Biotitization of hornblende and augite appears as a pervasive overprint on fresh rocks and is unrelated to distinct veinlets. Sulfide content is low (<1 wt. %) and grades of less than 0.2 percent Cu are typical. Where age/zonal relations are evident, this type predates and/or encompasses the second type. (2) Zones of sec-

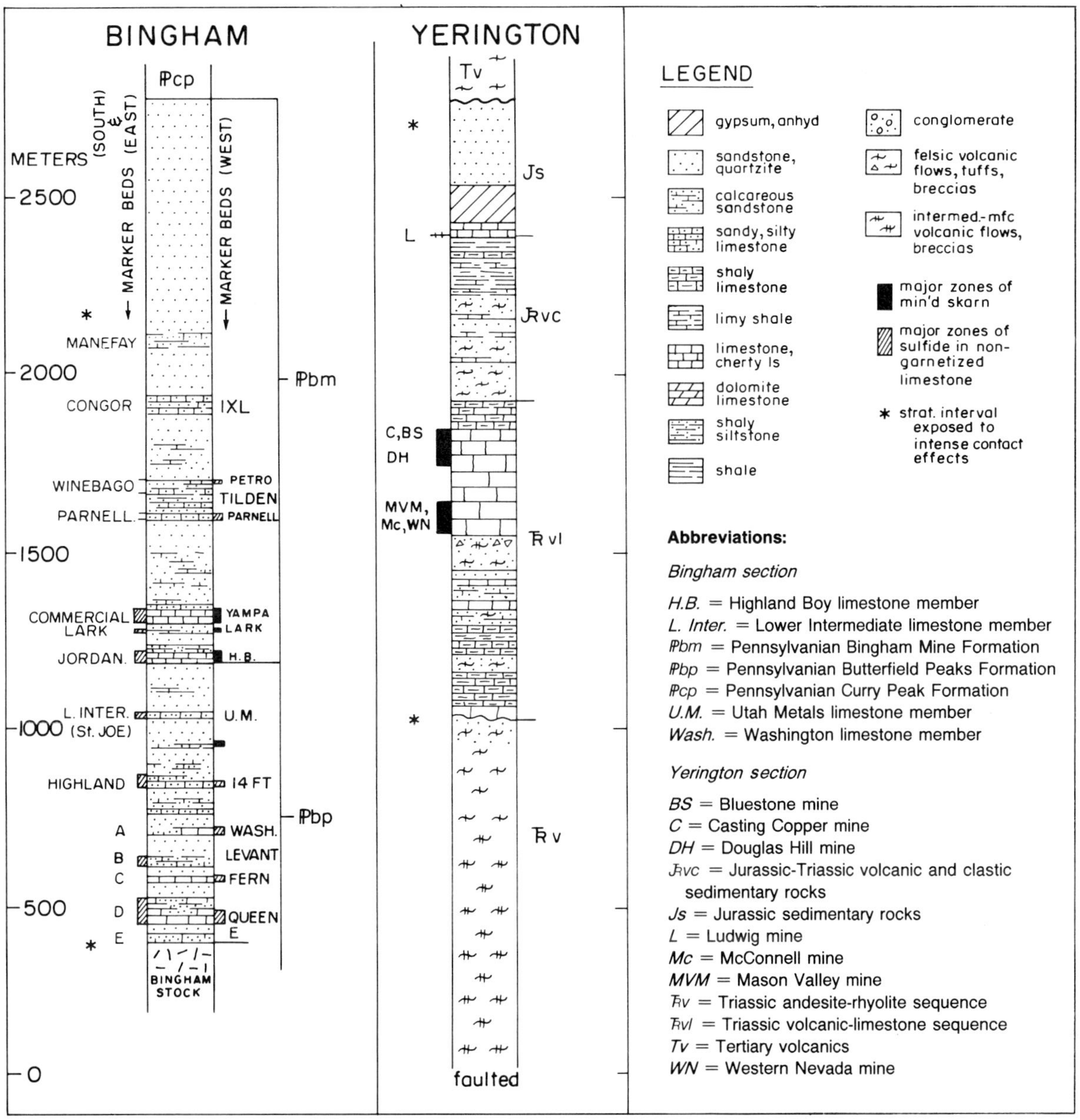

Figure 7.3. Stratigraphic sections at Bingham, Utah (based on Hansen, 1961; and Lanier, John, et al., 1978) and Yerington, Nevada (based on Proffett and Einaudi, unpublished). At Bingham, the skarn copper ores in the Carr Fork mine are localized in the Highland Boy and Yampa limestone members of the Bingham Mine Formation; these are the only major limestone beds in a sequence dominated by non-reactive quartzite. At Yerington, the skarn copper ores are localized at the lower and upper contacts of a thick-bedded limestone unit in a sequence of black shales, silicic tuffs, and siltstones.

ondary biotite and orthoclase are closely related to quartz-sulfide veinlets or microfractures and contain 1 to 4 weight percent sulfides displaying high Cu: Fe ratios and low sulfur (chalcopyrite + bornite, or pyrite:chalcopyrite <1). Grades range from 0.1 to 1.0 percent Cu. Magnesian and calcic skarn appear to be spatially and temporally related to both types of potassium-silicate alteration.

In Table 7.1, the column headed "sericitic" includes only quartz-sericite-pyrite alteration in which both orthoclase and plagioclase are replaced, and which in most cases forms as distinct envelopes on pyritic veins and veinlets. Where these envelopes coalesce, zones of pervasive sericite-quartz-pyrite develop, accompanied by 5 to 10 weight percent sulfides and very high pyrite:chalcopyrite ratios (10–40). This type of sericitic alteration is thought by many workers (e.g., Gustafson and Hunt, 1975) to represent the main influx of meteoric water into the cooling, sulfur-rich stock environment at hydrostatic pressures (<500 bars) and low temperatures ($<350°C$). Vein-related skarn destruction is the carbonate analogue of sericitic alteration superimposed on potassium silicate alteration. Silica-pyrite replacement of limestone is thought to be the carbonate analogue of pervasive sericite alteration superimposed on rocks not previously altered to potassium silicate assemblages. Minor lead-zinc-silver mineralization may accompany pyrite-quartz or occur as veins in peripheral limestone.

Not included in the sericite alteration type is the common, pervasive "wash" of sericitic-argillic alteration of

TABLE 7.1
Relative Volume of Alteration Types and Associated Mineralization in Ten Porphyry Copper Deposits

	Potassium Silicate Alteration					Sericitic (K-spar–destructive) Alteration				Advanced Argillic Alteration				Limestone	
Porphyry Copper Deposit	Pervasive Secondary Biotite	Biotite-Orthoclase Veinlets	Chalco-pyrite: Bornite	Pyrite: Chalco-pyrite	Weight % Total Sulfide	Vein-Related Quartz-Sericite-Pyrite	Pervasive Quartz-Sericite-Pyrite	Pyrite: Chalco-pyrite	Weight % Total Sulfide	Presence	Silicate Mineral Assemblage	Sulfide Mineral Assemblage (ratios)	Weight % Total Sulfide	Skarn	Silica-Pyrite
Christmas	XXX	X	>1	ND	<0.5	X	?	ND	ND	?				*XXX*	?
Twin Buttes	XX	X	rare bornite	<1	1–2	X	?	>1	1–3	?				*XXX*	?
Mission	XXX	X	rare bornite	ND	ND	XX	?	1.5–3	ND	?				*XXX*	?
Bingham	XXX	*XXX*	1 to >1	<<1	2.5	XX	?	2	3.5	?				*XXX*	?
Silver Bell	XXX	XXX	rare bornite	0.5–2	3–4	XX	X	4–15	5–9	?				*XXX*	X
Santa Rita	?	XXX	ND	3	1–5	XX	XX	40	4–8	?				*XXX*	?
Morenci	?	?	ND	ND	ND	XXX	XXX	7–25 (+sphalerite)	3.5–8	?				XX	?
Ely	XX	*XXX*	rare bornite	~1	1	XXX	XXX	4–10	5–10	X	kaolinite-gibbsite-zunyite	pyrite	ND	*XXX*	XXX
Cananea	present (?)	absent (?)	ND	>>1	<1	XX?	XXX	>>1	ND	XX	alunite-sericite-clay	pyrite-enargite	ND	??	*XXX*
Bisbee	present (?)	absent (?)	ND	ND	ND	X	XXX	>1 (+sphalerite)	ND	XXX	sericite-dickite-pyrophyllite-alunite	pyrite: chalcopyrite >20	15–18	absent (?)	*XXX*

Sources: Santa Rita (Nielson, 1970); Ely (James, 1976); Bingham (Atkinson and Einaudi, 1978).

KEY:
ND = no data
X = present in very minor (relative) volumes of rock
XX = present in moderate (relative) volumes of rock
XXX = constitutes a major portion of the total volume of altered and mineralized rocks
XXX = constitutes a major portion of the total volume and contains a significant tonnage of greater than 0.4 percent copper
? = not reported at present surface or in deeper exposures; no data on which presence or absence can be inferred for any level of the original pattern
absent (?) = some data available which imply absence of alteration type
present (?) = some data imply presence of the alteration type in deep exposures
?? = skarn in Capote Basin at Cananea may not be related to quartz porphyries

TABLE 7.2
Production and Mineralization in Porphyry, Skarn, and Breccia-Vein Deposits, Yerington District, Nevada

Deposit	Type	Years of Production	Production (In Thousands of Tons)	Percent Copper	Mineralization
Yerington	porphyry copper	1953–1978	162,400	0.55	oxide & sulfide; bornite-chalcopyrite-magnetite, chalcopyrite-pyrite
Ann Mason	porphyry copper	none	495,000 (resource)	0.40	sulfide: chalcopyrite, chalcopyrite-pyrite
Bear-Lagomarsino	porphyry copper	none	>500,000 (resource)	0.40	sulfide: chalcopyrite, chalcopyrite-pyrite
MacArthur	porphyry copper	none	13,000 (resource)	0.43	oxide: tenorite, chrysocolla
Bluestone	skarn-breccia pipe; garnet-epidote	1917–1930	~1,500	~1.5–3.5	sulfide: chalcopyrite >> pyrite
Douglas Hill	skarn; garnet	1911–1914?	~70	~5	oxide & sulfide: chalcopyrite >> pyrite
Mason Valley	skarn; garnet-pyroxene	1912–1930	~1,500	~1.5–3.5	sulfide: pyrite > chalcopyrite
McConnell	skarn; garnet-pyroxene	1912–1914, 1945	~20	~3	oxide & sulfide: pyrite > chalcopyrite
Casting Copper	skarn; garnet-pyroxene	1912– ?	~450	~3	oxide & sulfide: pyrite > chalcopyrite
Western Nevada	skarn; garnet-pyroxene	1944–1945	~4	~3	oxide & sulfide: pyrite > chalcopyrite (pyrrhotite)
Ludwig	replacement lode, breccia vein; quartz-pyrite	1906–1923	~200	~2–6	oxide: tenorite, malachite; sulfide: pyrite >> chalcopyrite

Source: Data from Knopf (1918); Stoddard and Carpenter (1950); Proxy Statement, The Anaconda Co. (1976); Einaudi, personal notes (1970–71).

plagioclase, sometimes accompanied by chloritization of biotite, in which orthoclase commonly is unaltered. This type of alteration generally is widespread in porphyry deposits and bears little obvious temporal or spatial relation to sulfides or other alteration types. This suggests that it is the result of many processes, including: (1) oxidation of H_2S by the dissociation of magmatic H_2O at the higher P-T conditions of potassium silicate alteration; (2) increase in K^+:H^+ ion activity ratio in fluids permeating the wall rocks beyond quartz-sericite-pyrite alteration envelopes developed during the main sericite stage; and (3) supergene processes.

Advanced argillic alteration as defined by Meyer and Hemley (1967) represents a greater degree of alkali-cation–leaching (thus, lower temperatures and/or lower K^+:H^+ activity ratios in the fluid) than sericitic alteration. The key mineralogical feature is the absence of feldspar, and the replacement of sericite by kaolinite, pyrophylite, or related aluminosilicates. Pyrite is ubiquitous and abundant, and if Cu-Fe sulfides are present, they represent sulfidation states higher than the chalcopyrite + S_2 = pyrite + bornite reaction; thus, pyrite-bornite, pyrite-digenite, or pyrite-covellite assemblages are characteristic, and enargite and low-Fe sphalerite are common associates. Relative to sericitic alteration, advanced argillic alteration is rare in porphyry copper deposits; this rarity may be due to the fact that advanced argillic alteration would be expected to occur at high structural levels which, in most cases, are removed by erosion. Alternatively, fluids in porphyry copper environments may only rarely evolve to the extremes of high sulfidation-oxidation states and low pH required. Of the deposits listed in Table 7.1, only Cananea and Bisbee contain important volumes of advanced argillic alteration. Both deposits contain the majority of ore in mineralized breccias associated with feldspar-destructive alteration. The carbonate analogue of advanced argillic alteration is massive sulfide ores associated with vein, manto, or pipe-like bodies of silica-pyrite breccias in limestone.

The relative volumes of alteration-mineralization types in known portions of individual deposits are relatively unambiguous in the deposits listed near the top of Table 7.1, but these volumes become difficult to evaluate as the degree of hydrolytic alteration increases. For example, the presence or absence of potassium silicate alteration in deeper portions of the Morenci, Cananea, and Bisbee deposits appears to be unknown, in spite of the fact that rocks with stable feldspar and biotite are known to occur at depth in underground mine workings or deep drill holes. Even if such rocks turn out not to show evidence of potassium-silicate alteration, the possibility must be considered that such alteration was present in upper levels, where hydrolytic alteration may have destroyed the evidence.

Yerington is not included in Table 7.1 because carbonate rocks—and hence skarn deposits—are located a considerable distance (3–4 km) from porphyry copper occurrences. The characteristics of Yerington skarns are similar to many "non-porphyry" skarns; thus, they serve to illustrate the link between such skarns and the larger, more complex skarns which are located at immediate contacts with mineralized porphyry copper stocks.

THE YERINGTON DISTRICT

The Yerington district, located in Lyon County, western Nevada, recently has been recognized as a major porphyry copper district with a future resource of greater than 1 billion tons of 0.4 percent Cu. Table 7.2 shows a breakdown of these figures by deposit. The Yerington mine, which closed in June 1978, produced about 162 million tons of 0.55 percent Cu. Skarn deposits represent a very minor portion of the district ore potential with recorded production of approximately 3.7 million tons of 1.5 to 6 percent Cu.

The geology of the Yerington district was first summarized in a comprehensive study by Knopf (1918). Since 1918, published accounts of district geology and mineral deposits have resulted from detailed studies by the geological staff of The Anaconda Company, including: Wilson (1963) on the Yerington porphyry copper deposit; Proffett and Proffett (1976) on the stratigraphy of the Tertiary ash-flow tuffs; Proffett (1977) on Basin and Range structure; and Einaudi (1977*a*) on skarn at the Mason Valley mine. The summary that follows is based on these and unpublished reports.

General Setting

The Yerington district is located 80 km east of the Sierra Nevada batholith in the western Great Basin province within a belt of Jurassic intrusives. One of these intrusives, the Yerington batholith, occupies much of the northern end of the Singatse Range. Strongly folded and faulted Lower Mesozoic volcanic and sedimentary rocks, with a total thickness of about 3,000 m, form an east-west–trending septum 8 km long and up to 3 km wide between the Yerington batholith and the batholith to the south (Fig. 7.4). The lower half of the volcanic-sedimentary section is composed of metamorphosed andesite and rhyolite flows, breccias, and sediments; the upper portion largely consists of massive limestone, thin-bedded black calcareous shale, and silicic volcaniclastic rocks (see Fig. 7.3). Limestone beds constitute the host rock for numerous, small, copper-bearing skarn deposits located on the outer fringe of a hornfels-skarnoid aureole extending 600 to 1,800 m from the Yerington batholith.

The Yerington batholith consists of granodiorite intruded by quartz monzonite and, later, by quartz monzonite porphyry dike swarms. Known porphyry copper mineralization is restricted to the core of the batholith and is associated with the porphyry dike swarms. Basin and Range normal faulting resulted in an average 70° westward tilt of all pre-Miocene rocks; the surface, therefore, approximates a series of fault-bounded cross sections, with their upper portions to the west.

Alteration of Sedimentary Rocks

The distribution of metasomatic and metamorphic rocks and the zoning of mineral assemblages indicate that the Yerington batholith, rather than the southern batholith, was responsible for the alteration. Alteration of sedimentary

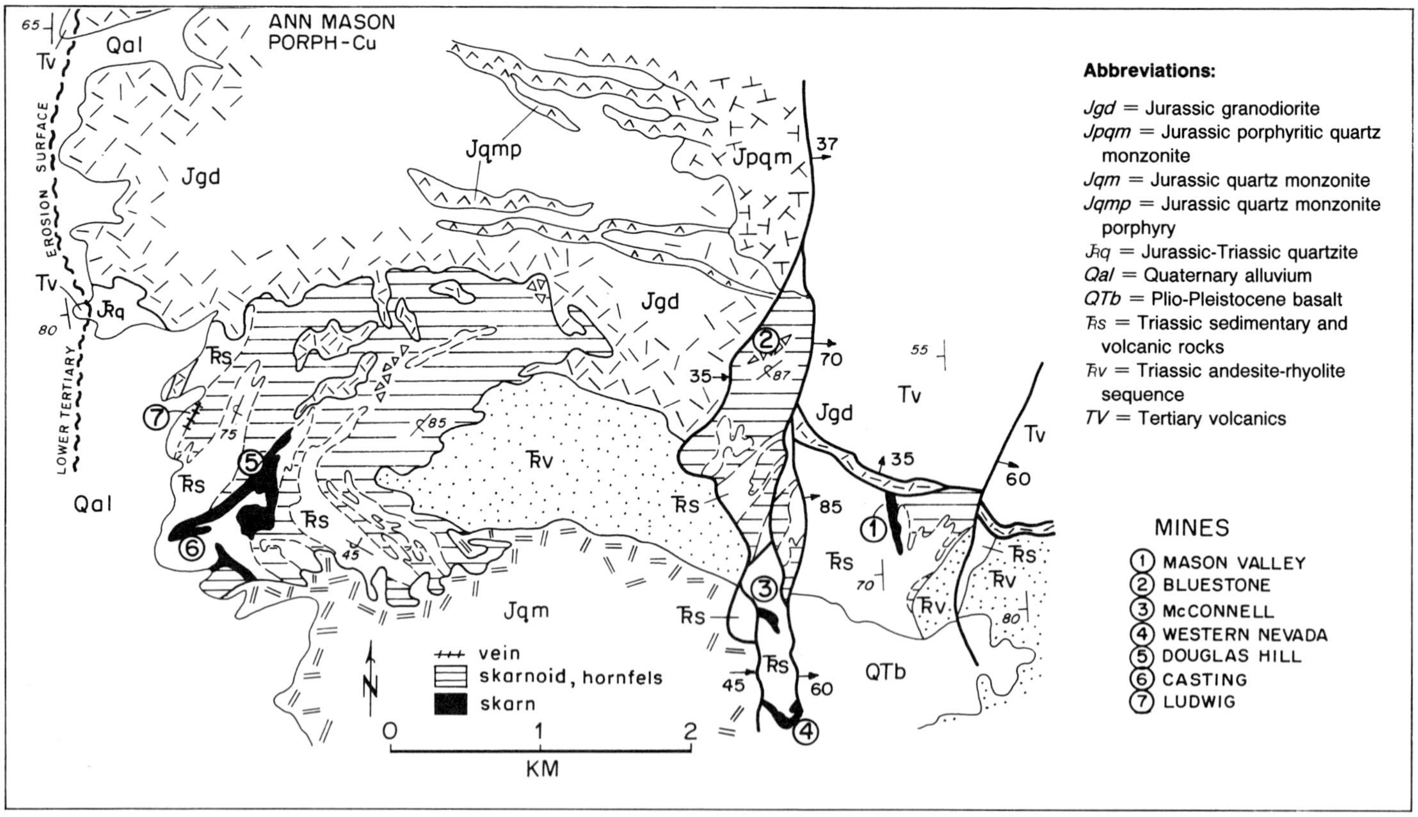

Figure 7.4. Geologic sketch map of the Yerington district, Nevada, showing septum of Triassic volcanic and Triassic-Jurassic volcaniclastic-sedimentary rocks between a southern quartz monzonite batholith and a northern granodiorite batholith. The Ann Mason and Yerington porphyry copper deposits are associated with quartz monzonite porphyry dikes and their porphyritic quartz monzonite roots within the granodiorite batholith. Yerington deposit is located 1 km northeast of the upper right corner of figure. Skarn copper deposits are located on the outer fringe of a skarnoid/garnet hornfels aureole. Based on mapping by J. M. Proffett and M. T. Einaudi.

rocks occurred in two episodes, as first documented by Knopf (1918).

Hornfels-Skarnoid. An early stage produced garnet (Ad_{25-70})*-pyroxene (Hd_{0-15}) hornfels and skarnoid near the batholith contact and recrystallization in hornblende hornfels facies rocks farther out. The district-wide formation of skarnoid probably represents a metamorphic event synchronous with the emplacement of the granodiorite batholith.

Skarn. Brecciation of early hornfels and skarnoid was followed by formation of chalcopyrite-pyrite–bearing skarns. Iron-rich garnets (Ad_{50-75}), locally accompanied by clinozoisite, formed near the batholith, and andradite (Ad_{80-100})-salite (Hd_{30-60}) skarns formed on the fringe of the skarnoid aureole in dolomitized marbles. Six skarn deposits are located in the Triassic septum west of Mason (see Fig. 7.4). Two of these, the Douglas Hill and Bluestone deposits, are located relatively close to the Yerington batholith, within the zone of early garnet-pyroxene skarnoid. Both are characterized by: (1) relatively low total sulfides, generally less than 5 volume percent; (2) relatively low pyrite:chalcopyrite ratios, generally less than 0.1; (3) absence of magnetite or hematite; (4) a gangue dominated by andradite, with minor epidote at the Bluestone mine; and (5) strong brecciation. A lack of zoning of calc-silicate and sulfide minerals is characteristic. Local limestone pods, which survived the earlier skarnoid stage, are replaced by massive andradite with disseminated chalcopyrite. In general, however, andradite was deposited as open-space fillings in veins or breccias, and it cemented skarnoid. The Bluestone mine shows evidence of several episodes of brecciation, with the final event forming a heterolithologic breccia composed of partially epidotized skarnoid, hornfels, and chalcopyrite fragments set in a matrix of finely comminuted garnet cemented by calcite and quartz. A quartz monozonite porphyry dike, intensely epidotized and broken into large blocks where it cuts the breccia zone, yields evidence that the porphyry cycle was broadly synchronous with breccia-skarn formation.

Four former producers (Mason Valley, Western Nevada, Casting Copper, and McConnell mines) are located in a fringe position relative to the andradite-chalcopyrite skarns. All four deposits formed in dolomitized marble in contact with skarnoid, 1 to 2 km from the Yerington batholith contact. These skarns are characterized by: (1) relatively high total sulfides, in the range 10 to 25 volume percent; (2) high pyrite:chalcopyrite ratios, generally greater than 1; (3) presence of trace quantities of magnetite, talc, and tremolite on the marble contact; (4) a gangue dominated by coarse, bladed salite and andradite, with salite near marble and andradite more centrally located; and (5) little or no evidence of large-scale brecciation. Zoning of calc-silicate and sulfide minerals is characteristic of these skarns; the general zonal sequence toward marble, as exemplified by the Mason Valley mine (Einaudi, 1977*a*) is: andradite, andradite-salite-chalcopyrite-pyrite, salite-actinolite-pyrite ± magnetite, chalcopyrite, tremolite-magnetite ± pyrite, talc-calcite ± magnetite, dolomite-calcite (Fig. 7.5). Cross-cutting vein and overgrowth

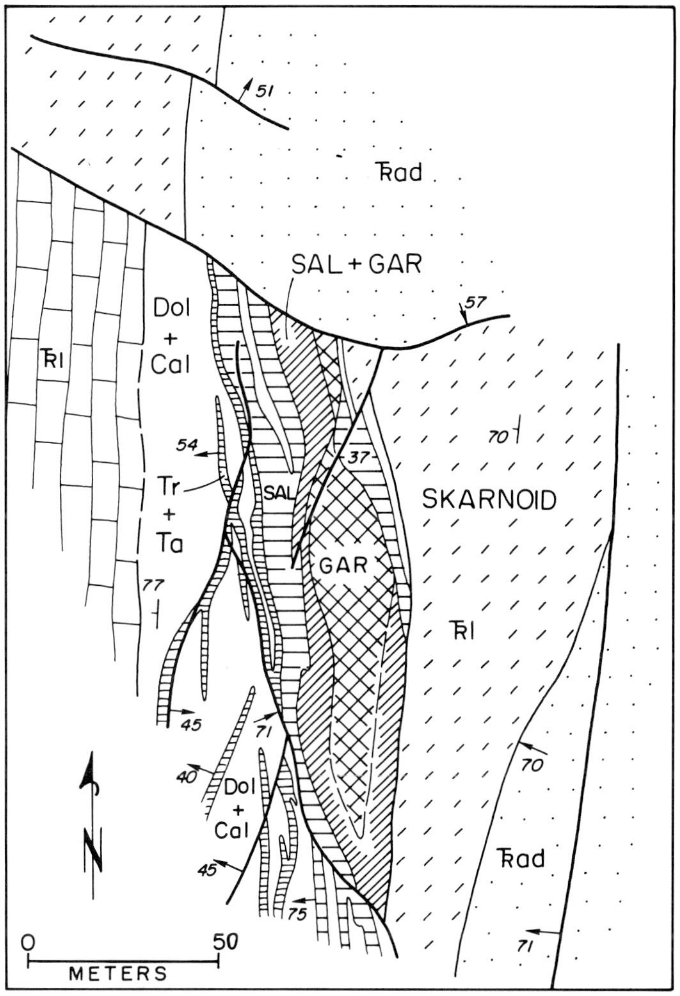

Abbreviations:

Cal = calcite	*Ta* = Talc
Dol = dolomite	*Tr* = tremolite
GAR = garnet	*R̄ad* = Triassic andesite-dacite tuff breccia
SAL = salitic pyroxene	*R̄l* = Triassic limestone

Figure 7.5. Plan map of 300-ft. level, Mason Valley mine, Yerington district, Nevada, illustrates zoning of skarn from garnet center to salite-garnet, salite, and tremolite-talc, toward dolomitic marble. Zones developed contemporaneously with garnet overgrowing salite, and salite overgrowing tremolite-talc. Skarnoid and dolomitization may represent an early event. Based on Einaudi (1977*a*).

relations indicate that inner zones encroached on outer zones during the process of skarn growth. However, in some localities, the process was not arrested at the end of pro-grade growth; at the Casting Copper mine, local brecciation of skarn was followed by the inward collapse of the above sequence. Actinolite-calcite-quartz ± magnetite, pyrite, chalcopyrite veins and breccia fillings cement rotated andradite blocks up to 1 m in diameter (Fig. 7.6); actinolite is separated from andradite by coarse-grained bladed salite, which grew outward from, and locally veined, the garnetite fragments.

Silica-Pyrite. In addition to skarn deposits, another type of ore occurrence in sedimentary rocks is illustrated by silica-pyrite rock at the Ludwig lode, located at a faulted contact between limestone and skarnoid north of the Casting Copper mine (see Fig. 7.4 for location). Intense supergene leaching resulted in a quartzose gossan at the surface and rich

*Mineral compositions are given as the mole percentage of iron endmembers.

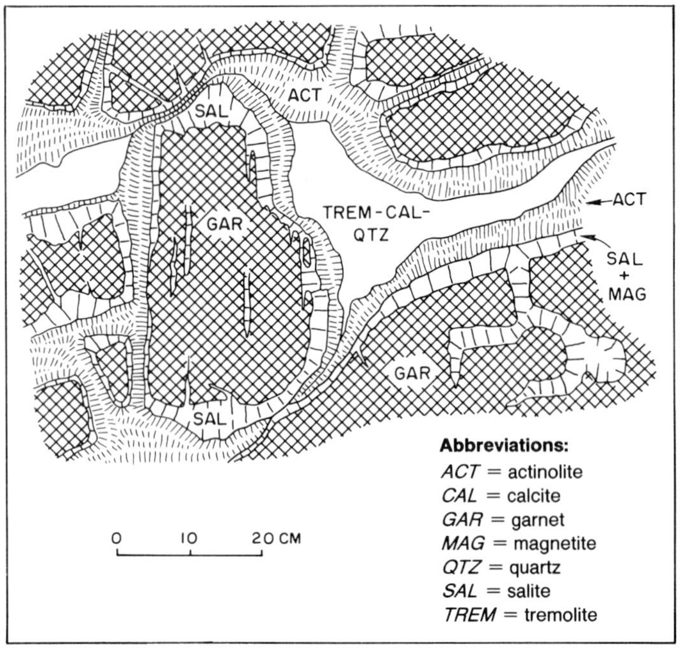

Figure 7.6. Sketch of skarn outcrop near Casting Copper mine, Yerington district, Nevada, illustrates reversal of mineral-age sequence following brecciation of garnet center.

tenorite ores up to 250 m thick below the surface. According to Knopf (1918), the protore at Ludwig below the 700-ft. level consists largely of pyrite and quartz which replaced a fault breccia consisting of marble and porphyry fragments cemented by carbonate. Large pyritic masses also occur in intensely silicified and quartz-veined porphyry dikes. The Ludwig deposit is the only known major sulfide accumulation in carbonate rocks of the Yerington district which is not directly associated with skarn minerals. The presence of brecciated, altered, and mineralized porphyry in the fissure zone, and of unaltered porphyry which cuts the fissure north of the mine area, indicates that the Ludwig mineralization was contemporaneous with the porphyry intrusive event.

Conclusions

An important aspect of the Yerington district, which contrasts with the southern Arizona-New Mexico-Sonora province, is the presence of a thick section of interbedded calcareous shale and felsic volcaniclastic rocks with relatively minor limestone. Intrusion of a batholith of granodiorite–quartz monzonite generated a metamorphic aureole which includes large volumes of garnet-rich skarnoid, a feature generally not present in other districts. Furthermore, the large mass of granodiorite effectively shielded the carbonate rocks from direct contact with the porphyry copper plutons; the ore-bearing skarns are located some 3 to 4 km distant from the outermost edge of significant porphyry copper alteration-mineralization in igneous rocks. The spatial separation of skarn and porphyry deposits resulted in a relatively mild retrograde event in the skarns, because these were not directly subjected to the long-lived hydrothermal activity and repeated fracturing which characterizes porphyry copper centers. Although there can be little doubt that the skarns and the porphyry copper deposits represent one metallogenic event, their extreme spatial separation introduces significant uncertainties in detailed correlation of alteration-mineralization events between igneous and sedimentary rocks.

THE CHRISTMAS MINE

The Christmas mine is located in the Banner mining district, southwestern Gila County, 43 km south of Globe, Arizona. It is a small porphyry-skarn copper deposit, which has produced 4.6 million tons of 2 percent Cu from underground ore in skarn from 1905 to 1966 and 15.8 million tons of open-pit ore averaging 0.6 percent Cu from 1965 to 1976. Ninety-five percent of the latter ore occurred in calc-silicate rocks. The ore zone presently being mined by open-pit methods contains an additional 80 million tons of ore reserves (Koski and Cook, 1982). The geological setting of the Christmas mine has been described by Ross (1925), Willden (1964), and Eastlick (1968); details of alteration-mineralization in igneous and sedimentary rocks have been provided by Koski (1978), Koski and Cook (1982), and D. V. Perry (1968, 1969).

General Setting

Ore-bearing skarns are associated with an elongate plug-dike complex of granodiorite and granodiorite porphyry, measuring 900 X 450 m in horizontal dimension. The stock, and an associated dike swarm of rhyodacite porphyry, intruded a 1,000-m-thick sequence of Precambrian, Paleozoic, and Cretaceous sedimentary and volcanic rocks (see Fig. 7.2) along an east-west–trending fault zone. The sedimentary rocks are broadly folded, forming a southeasterly-plunging anticline; in the ore zone west of the Christmas stock, the beds dip 15°S.

A major post-ore normal fault system (Christmas-Joker), striking north-northwest and dipping 75°E, bisects the stock (Fig. 7.7*A*); cumulative normal displacement is estimated to be approximately 1 km (Eastlick, 1968; Koski and Cook, 1982). As a result of this fault displacement, two different levels of exposure in the porphyry system are preserved: on the west, a relatively deep core environment with weakly altered and mineralized porphyry in contact with high-grade skarns in Paleozoic carbonate rocks; and, on the east, a relatively higher-level environment with potassium-silicate alteration and disseminated sulfides in porphyry and Cretaceous andesite (Fig. 7.7*B*).

Porphyry

Alteration-mineralization in the porphyry stock complex is described by Koski and Cook in Chapter 17 of this volume. Early potassium-silicate alteration, characterized by a stockwork of orthoclase-quartz-chalcopyrite-bornite veinlets, and partial to complete biotitization of hornblende, is best developed in the higher-level portion of the stock east of the Christmas-Joker fault. Quartz-sulfide veinlets and secondary biotite extend 100 to 200 m into the basaltic volcanic rocks; recent drilling indicates a large tonnage of 0.2 to 0.6 percent Cu mineralization. Fracture-controlled alteration of quartz-sericite and quartz-sericite-chlorite, accompanied by chalcopyrite and pyrite, is superimposed on the outer portion of the stockwork potassium-silicate zone.

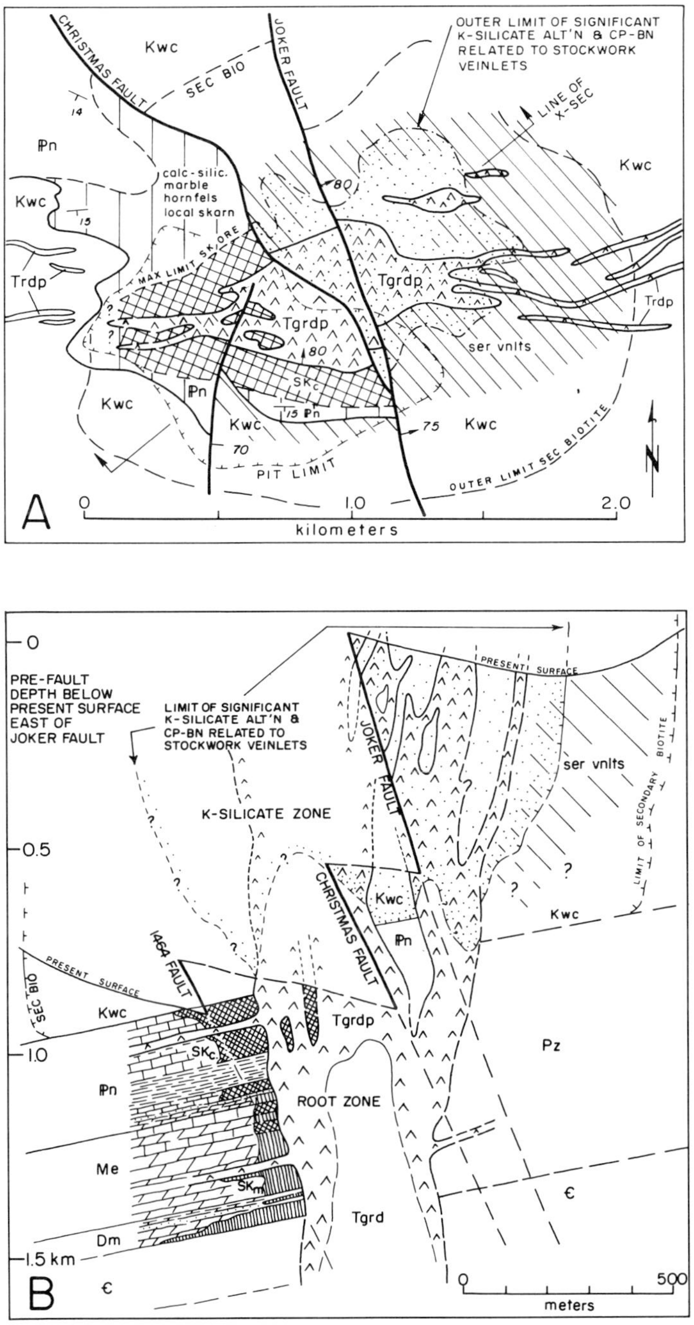

Abbreviations:

ALT'N = alteration
BN = bornite
Є = Cambrian Bolsa Quartzite
CP = chalcopyrite
calc. silic. = calc-silicate
Dm = Devonian Martin Formation
Kwc = Cretaceous Williamson Creek volcanics
Me = Mississippian Escabrosa Limestone
ℙn = Pennsylvanian Naco Group
Pz = Paleozoic sedimentary rocks
SEC BIO = secondary (hydrothermal) biotite
ser vnlts = sericite veinlets
SK_c = calcic skarn
SK_s = skarn, undifferentiated
SK_m = magnesian skarn
Tgrd = Tertiary granodiorite
Tgrdp = Tertiary granodiorite porphyry
Trdp = Tertiary rhyodacite porphyry

Figure 7.7. Christmas mine, Banner mining district, Arizona: *A*, surface geology and alteration; *B*, reconstructed cross section, looking northwest. The cross section illustrates location of mineralized skarn in contact with the deep root zone of the porphyry system and selective replacement of sedimentary strata. Based on Perry (1968), Eastlick (1968), Koski (1978), and Koski and Cook (1982).

According to Perry (1968, 1969) and Koski and Cook (1982), granodiorite porphyry west of the Joker fault also displays potassium-silicate alteration accompanied by sulfides, but the intensity of alteration-mineralization is lower than in the down-dropped block; copper grades range from 0.05 to 0.1 percent. Plagioclase is fresh and hornblende is only partially biotitized. The dominant opaque mineral assemblage is composed of less than 0.5 percent bornite and chalcopyrite, accompanied by 1 percent magnetite. Perry (1968) has described two types of sulfide-bearing veinlets: (1) thin, discontinuous, biotite veinlets that contain accessory quartz, K-feldspar and anhydrite; and (2) thicker, vuggy, quartz-lined veinlets that contain accessory K-feldspar, biotite, and rare molybdenite. Thus, the characteristics of alteration and mineralization in the westernmost fault block of the Christmas stock suggest a fairly deep exposure of a porphyry copper system.

Sedimentary Rocks

Copper-bearing skarn has been mined from the Martin Formation, Escabrosa Limestone, and Horquilla Formation in contact with porphyry west of the Joker fault. The following summary of contact metamorphism and metasomatism is based on descriptions by Perry (1968).

Contact Metamorphism. At distances greater than 1 km from the stock, hornfelses occur in shaly beds only at contacts with diorite-granodiorite sills. Within 750 m of the stock on the north, and 450 m on the west, shale, siltstone, and impure carbonate beds are converted to hornfels; cherty marble contains wollastonite with local garnet and diopside; sandy dolomitic marble is characterized by the assemblage tremolite-calcite; Martin dolomite locally contains brucite after periclase; and calcareous quartzite contains interstitial diopside-quartz with local wollastonite or phlogopite. Although Perry (1968, 1969) believes that these contact effects are largely metamorphic, he suggests that some local metasomatism must have occurred, particularly in the case of the monomineralic diopside hornfels beds which are characteristic of the Beckers Butte member of the lower Martin Formation.

Skarn. In general, skarn occurs in the purer carbonate units of the Paleozoic section (see Fig. 7.7) and extends farthest from the stock in carbonate beds which are interbedded with siltstone or shale. Thus, skarn in the thick-bedded, relatively pure Escabrosa Limestone extends only tens of meters from the stock, whereas skarn in the Martin and Horquilla Formations extends up to 120 to 200 m outward (see Fig. 7.7 *B*). Perry (1968) describes three dominant skarn types: (1) endoskarn in porphyry, (2) calcic skarn in limestone units of the Escabrosa and Horquilla Formations, and (3) magnesian skarn in dolomitic units of the Horquilla and Martin Formations. The major skarn orebodies occur in the upper Horquilla (calcic skarn) and lower Martin (magnesian skarn). The following summary is based on descriptions of these two ore zones; garnet compositions are based on cell-edge determinations. The zonal mineralogy of calcic skarn in the Horquilla Formation is summarized in Table 7.3.

Porphyry in contact with skarn is converted to endoskarn consisting of pale brown grossularitic garnet (Ad_{30-56})

TABLE 7.3
Zonal Mineralogy of Calcic Skarn and Endoskarn at Horquilla-Porphyry Contact, Christmas Mine

Rock Type	Distance From Igneous-Sedimentary Contact	Background Alteration	Veinlets, Veins	Late Alteration	Garnet Color	Volume Percent Magnetite	Volume Percent Sulfides	Major Sulfides	Minor Sulfides
limestone	>120 m	marble	garnet with local pyroxene envelopes	?	pale yellow-green	0	locally high	bornite, sphalerite	chalcopyrite, galena
exoskarn	variable (15–120 m)	garnet, calcite, minor pyroxene	calcite-sulfide	calcite	pale yellow-green	0	~3	bornite > chalcopyrite	sphalerite
exoskarn	erratic (near stock)	garnet	chalcopyrite-epidote-calcite-quartz	calcite	pale yellow-green	?	?	chalcopyrite, pyrite, magnetite	sphalerite
exoskarn	< 10 m	garnet, minor pyroxene & epidote	?	calcite	reddish brown	~3–8	5–10	pyrite > chalcopyrite	sphalerite
endoskarn	few cm to 1 m	local pyroxene in mafic sites; garnet (with minor pyroxene, idocrase, wollastonite) in plagioclase sites	calcite, zeolite	?	pale brown	0	"not common"	chalcopyrite > pyrite	?
endoskarn	few m	pyroxene, sphene (minor chlorite & epidote) in mafic sites; minor pyroxene, epidote in plagioclase sites	pyroxene	?	—	0	"not common"	?	?
granodiorite porphyry	>few m	minor biotite in hornblende	quartz-sulfide-biotite-anhydrite	?	—	1	<0.5	bornite-chalcopyrite, chalcopyrite-pyrite	molybdenite

Source: Data from Perry (1968).

and pale green clinopyroxene over widths of a few centimeters to several meters. Accessory minerals include wollastonite-idocrase or phlogopite-chlorite. Vugs and veinlets are filled with chalcopyrite, stilbite, and calcite; at greater depths, anhydrite-chalcopyrite veinlets with epidote alteration envelopes occur in endoskarn related to the Martin magnesian skarn.

Calcic exoskarn occurring as xenoliths in the stock, or within 10 m of the stock contact, consists of reddish-brown andradite (Ad_{92}) and minor diopside and epidote, with abundant magnetite and pyrite, lesser chalcopyrite, and magnetite pseudomorphous after specular hematite. Locally high chalcopyrite concentrations occur in irregular orbicular structures with calcite and garnet; these structures are cut by chalcopyrite-epidote-calcite-quartz veinlets and quartz-rich pods with disseminated sulfides. Copper grades are generally low in this zone and increase with distance from the stock (Petersen and Swanson, 1956; Eastlick, 1968). In the ore zones, granular, yellow-green garnetite (Ad_{72-91}), with local diopside, contains chert nodules; precursor wollastonite is suggested by local calcite-quartz textures. Bornite and lesser chalcopyrite occur interstitial to garnet, apparently as replacements of calcite, and in infrequent quartz veinlets. The outer skarn contact is marked by a zone of garnet veins (some with diopside-sulfide envelopes) cutting marble. Erratic concentrations of sphalerite-chalcopyrite, with traces of galena, are found along garnet-marble contacts and in veins.

Magnesian skarn is characterized by forsterite and abundant magnetite (5–25%) accompanied by brucite, anhydrite, and sulfides. Tremolite-talc masses and nodules of brown and green garnet (Ad_{85}, one sample)-diopside-anhydrite-sulfides occur locally. Perry (1968) describes orbicular growths and veinlet relations which indicate that forsterite, magnetite, anhydrite, and sulfides were broadly synchronous. Late serpentine replaces most of the forsterite.

Although the calc-silicates in magnesian skarn display no obvious zonal pattern, the sulfides are well zoned. The assemblage chalcopyrite-bornite (with local chalcocite) gives way laterally, toward the marble contact, to chalcopyrite-pyrite-pyrrhotite. Sphalerite abundance increases outward and toward the hanging wall and footwall of the skarn bed.

The hanging-wall contact of magnesian skarn with dolomitic marble reveals the fracture control of metasomatic fluid movement and of skarn growth; magnetite-calcite veinlets (with anhydrite, chalcopyrite, and sphalerite) are encased in zone envelopes consisting of (1) forsterite or forsterite-magnetite near the veinlet filling and (2) coarse calcite near the dolomitic marble wall.

Mineralization in Hornfels. Hornfelses locally are extensively veined and mineralized; they contain copper grades in the neighborhood of 1 percent, especially where they occur in contact with mineralized skarn. The Beckers Butte member of the Martin Formation, converted to light gray granular diopside hornfels in the early stages, is cut by veinlets of anhydrite-pyrite-chalcopyrite (± magnetite) that are 1 mm wide, with 0.5-mm-wide, dark green actinolite alteration envelopes. Other hornfelses higher in the Martin Formation contain similar veinlets, with epidote in addition to actinolite, or with biotite in inner zones near the sulfide veinlet-filling and with actinolite as an outer alteration product. Molybdenite, a rare mineral in skarn, occurs in quartz-rich hornfelses, containing interstitial actinolite and/or biotite.

Conclusions

The essentially synchronous development of skarn and magnetite-sulfide mineralization, in contrast with the multistage model of Eastlick (1968), is supported by observations reported by Perry (1968) and also by analogy with other porphyry skarn deposits. Some sulfide mineralization continued after main skarn formation, as evidenced by anhydrite-sulfide veinlets in calcic skarn, but Perry concludes that the quasi-pervasive serpentinization of magnesian skarn and the local replacement of calcic skarn minerals by calcite postdate most of the sulfide deposition.

The contemporaneity of the formation of both magnesian and calcic skarn with potassium-silicate alteration in the stock is suggested, but not proved, by the data. Sulfide-actinolite veining of hornfels is probably also synchronous with skarn formation and does not appear to represent a major retrograde event, such as might occur during hydrolytic alteration of the associated stock. This probability is supported not only by the fact that sericitic alteration is weak or absent at the relatively deep structural levels of the western fault block, but also by veinlet relations at contacts between hornfelses and biotite granodiorite porphyry dikes; here, veinlets with biotite alteration halos in porphyry cut into hornfels, where they display actinolite alteration halos (Einaudi, 1978, personal notes).

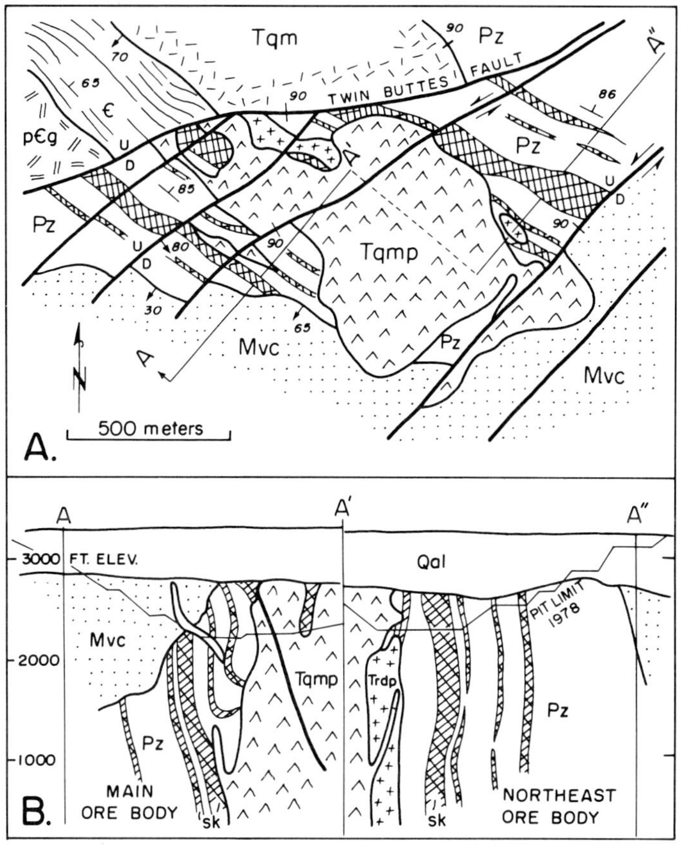

Є = Cambrian Abrigo Formation
Mvc = Mesozoic volcaniclastic rocks
pЄg = Precambrian granite
Pz = Paleozoic sedimentary rocks
Qal = Quaternary alluvium
sk = skarn
Trdp = Tertiary rhyodacite porphyry
Tqm = Tertiary quartz monzonite
Tqmp = Tertiary quartz monzonite porphyries

Figure 7.8. Twin Buttes mine, Pima mining district, Arizona: *A,* schematic geology at 2,100-ft. elevation; *B,* schematic cross section, looking northwest. Cross section illustrates steep bedding control of mineralized skarn. Based on Barter and Kelly (1982).

THE TWIN BUTTES MINE

The main and northeast ore zones at Twin Buttes are located in metasedimentary rocks of Permian age separated by a low-grade, northwest-trending quartz monzonite stock of Eocene age (Fig. 7.8). Ore reserves at the end of 1970 were approximately 475 million tons of 0.78 percent Cu; 20 percent of this reserve was oxide ore averaging 1.0 percent Cu and 80 percent was sulfide ore averaging 0.73 percent Cu and 0.03 percent Mo (Proxy Statement, The Anaconda Company, 1976). The following summary is based on Barter and Kelly (1982) and discussions with R. C. Baker and C. F. Barter, formerly of The Anaconda Company.

General Setting

The mineralized sedimentary rocks south of the Twin Buttes fault consist of a 400-m-thick section of Pennsylvanian and Permian strata correlated with the Earp, Colina, Epitaph, and Scherrer Formations; bedding is vertical and strikes N60°W. Arkosic siltstone, conglomerate, and interbedded rhyolitic flows and tuffs of Mesozoic age are exposed in the southern wall of the West Pit, where they unconformably overlie Paleozoic strata (see Fig. 7.8). A complex series of Eocene porphyries intrude the Paleozoic and Mesozoic strata. Mineralization and alteration of the sedimentary rocks is spatially related to these intrusions and to west-northwest–trending faults which also guided the emplacement of the intrusions.

Porphyry

Rhyodacite porphyry occurs as a dike-like body, 75 m wide, emplaced parallel to bedding. The rhyodacite porphyry is pervasively biotitized, displays pyrite:chalcopyrite ratios of less than 1, and contains 0.1 to 0.5 percent Cu; it is thought to represent the first of the Laramide porphyries and was emplaced either prior to, or during, the main period of mineralization.

A complex of quartz monzonite porphyries comprise the main mass of Laramide intrusive rocks; the porphyries form an irregular, steep-walled, northwest-trending stock up to 600 m wide, terminated at its southeast end by a steep northwest-striking fault zone. Potassium-silicate alteration of the porphyries locally is developed along quartz veinlets; sericitic alteration of feldspars and chloritic alteration of mafic minerals are also present. Pyrite, chalcopyrite, and molybdenite are the principal sulfides; pyrite:chalcopyrite ratios generally are greater than 1, and primary copper grades range from 0.01 to 0.25 percent.

Sedimentary Rocks

The bulk of the hypogene ore and zones of high sulfide content in the Twin Buttes pit occur in altered carbonate beds within the Colina Limestone and Epitaph Formation; lesser amounts of ore, generally of lower grade, occur in altered carbonate and siltstone beds of other Permian formations (see Fig. 7.2), in Mesozoic arkosic rocks, and in Eocene porphyries.

Hornfels. Hornfelses are present throughout the Permian section and are extremely variable in mineralogy. Some, representing original silty limestone or silty dolomitic limestone, consist of fine-grained, granular diopside-quartz hornfels with local patches of fine-grained garnet. In the higher sulfide zones near the center of the mine, diopside hornfelses contain 1.5 to 5 volume percent sulfides in abundant pyrite-chalcopyrite-quartz-epidote veinlets with dark green actinolite alteration envelopes. Flinty, aphanitic hornfelses containing recrystallized quartz, and variable amounts of diopside, tremolite, biotite, and feldspar are particularly common in the Earp and Abrigo Formations.

Quartzite and siltstone beds, with a variable but minor content of interstitial tremolite, biotite, sericite, and feldspar occur in the Earp, lowermost and uppermost Epitaph, and Scherrer formations. Sulfide-bearing fractures have sericitic envelopes in biotitic siltstones and biotite envelopes in tremolitic siltstones.

Calcic Skarn. Calcic skarn formed through metasomatic replacement of limestone beds in the lower Earp Formation, Colina Limestone, upper Epitaph Formation, and Concha Limestone. Near the stock and along contacts with interbedded siltstone, these limestone beds yielded granular to massive, dark reddish-brown garnet and clinopyroxene skarn with interstitial quartz, calcite, chalcopyrite, pyrite, and local magnetite. Dark brown garnet replaces both diopside and paler garnet, and forms overgrowths on pale garnet. Preliminary wet chemical analyses (Harold Vincent, 1973, personal communication) indicate that: (1) garnets are nearly pure endmember andradite, with 0.5 to 1.4 weight percent Al_2O_3, and (2) clinopyroxenes are nearly pure endmember diopside, with 1.9 to 2.1 weight percent total Fe as Fe_2O_3. The garnetite is cut by abundant quartz-sulfide and quartz-epidote-sulfide veinlets and patches, especially within 30 m of the stock. Sulfides in the quartz veins are pyrite, chalcopyrite, and molybdenite. The most persistent zones of +1.5 percent Cu occur in the Colina skarn; these contain 4 to 6 volume percent sulfides, with local zones containing up to 15 to 20 volume percent.

Garnetite pervasively replaces limestone beds in the center of the mine, but some limestone remnants are present farther from the stock. In these cases brown garnetite with chalcopyrite and pyrite replace limestone or an intervening wollastonite-bearing marble. In addition to wollastonite with local bornite-chalcocite, marble at the skarn contact contains: (1) pale brown and green garnet and idocrase in wollastonite with disseminated chalcopyrite, bornite, sphalerite, and local anhydrite; and (2) patches of massive sphalerite-chalcopyrite-pyrrhotite-magnetite in marble.

Magnesian Skarn. Magnesian skarn formed in dolomitic beds of the Colina Limestone, middle Epitaph Formation, and middle Scherrer Formation. It is characterized by the association of serpentine and tremolite, with high magnetite and high chalcopyrite contents. Forsterite, or serpentine after forsterite, are common in magnetite-rich zones, and coarse green mica is present in some areas. Farther from the central zone, unsilicated dolomitic beds contain magnetite-pyrite veinlets with serpentine envelopes.

Discussion

Barter and Kelly (1982) have implied that much of the anhydrous skarn and hornfels formation pre-dated the emplacement of the central porphyry complex. This early skarn-forming event may have been synchronous with the emplacement of the biotitized rhyodacite porphyry, and probably was accompanied by some copper mineralization. Local zoning in calcic skarn was developed primarily relative to sedimentary contacts or to northwest-striking bedding faults. Most of the molybdenite mineralization and, presumably, additional copper and pyritic hydrous alteration of skarn and hornfelses accompanied the later porphyries.

The overall zoning of sulfides in any given rock-alteration type appears to reflect distance from this late porphyry complex. Table 7.4, compiled on the basis of Figure 20.6 of Barter and Kelly (1982), presents the average copper and molybdenum grades, total sulfide content, and pyrite:chalcopyrite ratios of the four dominant rock-alteration types. Although calcic and magnesian skarn maintains a high level of total sulfides and copper grades irrespective of distance from the stock, a trend toward decreasing pyrite:chalcopyrite ratios with distance is clearly illustrated by all four rock types. Presumably, this reflects the late stage overprinting of pyrite near the stock.

THE MISSION AREA

It has been suggested that the Mission area represents a faulted upper portion of the Twin Buttes area, having moved relatively northward 10 km on a flat decollement structure—the San Xavier fault (Lacy, 1959; Cooper, 1960, 1971; Shafiqullah and Langlois, 1978). The stratigraphic section and the association of mineralized skarn, hornfelses, and arkoses with a relatively weakly mineralized quartz monzonite porphyry stock at Pima-Mission is virtually the same as just described for Twin Buttes.

General Setting

The structural setting at Pima-Mission is complex. As described by Gale (1965), the quartz monzonite was emplaced in the core of an east-plunging, asymmetrical, faulted antiform whose core consists of Paleozoic sedimentary rocks (Fig. 7.9). The flanks of the antiform consist of Mesozoic argillite and arkose resting unconformably or in fault contact with the underlying carbonate rocks. The fold is cut by steep, south-dipping faults which strike parallel to the fold axis and which pre-date mineralization. These structures are cut by

TABLE 7.4
Grade and Sulfide Content of Sedimentary Rocks at Twin Buttes
(In Weighted Means)

Alteration Type	Distance from Stock (m)	Length of Sample (m)	Weight % Cu	Weight % Mo	Cu:Mo	Volume % Chalcopyrite and Pyrite	Chalcopyrite: Pyrite
Magnesian Skarn[a]	< 200	41	1.55	0.050	31	5.5	0.6
	≥ 200	105	1.04	0.019	55	3.4	0.4
Weighted Average			1.18	0.028	42	4.0	0.5
Calcic Skarn[b]	< 200	212	1.30	0.053	25	6.8	1.1
	≥ 200	64	1.20	0.035	34	4.1	0.5
Weighted Average			1.28	0.049	27	6.2	1.0
Hornfels[c]	< 200	109	0.43	0.034	13	2.4	1.7
	≥ 200	47	0.70	0.023	30	2.4	0.8
Weighted Average			0.51	0.031	15	2.4	1.4
Quartzite[d]	< 200	299	0.17	0.032	5.3	1.0	2.1
	≥ 200	154	0.10	0.015	6.7	0.4	1.2
Weighted Average			0.15	0.026	5.8	0.8	1.8
Overall Average			0.65	0.033	18	2.9	1.3

Source: Data from Barter and Kelly (1982), Figure 20.6.

[a] Serpentine-tremolite-magnetite, minor diopside or forsterite.

[b] Garnet-diopside, minor quartz, actinolite, magnetite (wollastonite-bearing calcic skarn not included). Contains approximately 0.37 oz. Ag/ton.

[c] Diopside-quartz hornfels, with actinolite alteration, minor garnet; or, siliceous aphanitic hornfels.

[d] Siltstone and quartzite, with sericite-biotite or biotite-actinolite.

steeply dipping, north-northeast–striking faults which postdate the skarn-forming event (Fig. 7.10).

The stratigraphic identity of Paleozoic rocks at Mission is obscured by extensive faulting and alteration. Sedimentary rocks which underlie Mesozoic arkose consist of an upper section of quartzite, with interbedded diopside hornfels, and a lower section of skarn-bearing marble (see Fig. 7.10). Richard and Courtright (1959) and Gale (1965) have suggested a correlation of the quartzite with the Scherrer Formation and a tentative correlation of the marble with the Colina Limestone. However, further investigation has suggested that the section is overturned and that the skarn unit is developed in Concha Limestone (Einaudi, 1974; L. R. Jansen, 1976, quoted in Langlois, 1978). The limestone unit is separated from underlying volcaniclastic rocks and Precambrian granite by flat faults which belong to the San Xavier fault system (Richard and Courtright, 1959).

Large copper-bearing skarn bodies and disseminated lower-grade ore zones in hornfels, arkose, and porphyry are located within a 3-km-wide, northwest-trending zone of pyritic mineralization (see Fig. 7.9), which encompasses the porphyry stock, Pima and Mission pits, and Palo Verde Mine (Kinnison, 1966). At Mission mineralized skarn extends eastward 800 m from sill-like bodies of quartz monzonite porphyry largely emplaced along unconformable contacts between Paleozoic and Mesozoic rocks (Gale, 1965). North of the antiform axis the skarn beds dip 20 to 40° north under Mesozoic cover and are continuous with skarn exposed underground in the Palo Verde mine (MacKenzie, 1963; Einaudi, 1974). The Pima mine, which produced 146 million tons of copper ore between 1955 and 1978 (Langlois, 1978), is located in the southern limb of the fold. According to Journeay (1959) and Langlois (1978), southeast-dipping Mesozoic and Paleozoic rocks at Pima are in fault contact with underlying Tertiary granite. Ore-bearing skarn and hornfels in carbonate rocks, mineralized by fluids related to the emplacement of quartz monzonite porphyry (Himes, 1973; Langlois, 1978), extend over 500 m along strike, with an average thickness of 60 m. Although the average grade of skarn-hornfels is 0.81 percent Cu, 75 percent of the production in the late 1970s came from mineralized Mesozoic arkose which averaged 0.38 percent Cu (Langlois, 1978); the average grade of ore mined at Pima at that time was 0.47 percent Cu and 0.015 percent Mo (Parkinson, 1976).

Lesser ore occurrences located a few kilometers west and southwest of the Pima mine could be considered related to the same intrusion-mineralization episode. The Mineral Hill and Daisy Mines (see Fig. 7.9 for locations) described by MacKenzie (1959), occur along pre-ore, east-striking faults. These orebodies are small-scale duplications of the Pima-Mission-Palo Verde skarn ore zone: copper ore occurs dominantly in garnetite close to igneous contacts, molybdenite (and minor scheelite) is restricted to the porphyry or its immediate wall rocks, and sphalerite and galena occur at the marble contact. In contrast with the Pima-Mission orebodies, however, some ore at the Mineral Hill and Daisy mines occurs in manto replacement bodies. Although no details of the manto ores are published, massive replacement of limestone by sulfides, carbonates, and quartz can generally be taken to represent lower temperatures and/or higher sulfidation states (such as would dominate in areas peripheral to a major heat source).

A trend toward larger amounts of lead and zinc relative to copper is seen further south at the San Xavier mine (see Fig. 7.9 for location) which produced lead-zinc-silver ore with lesser amounts of copper (Irvin, 1959). Here,

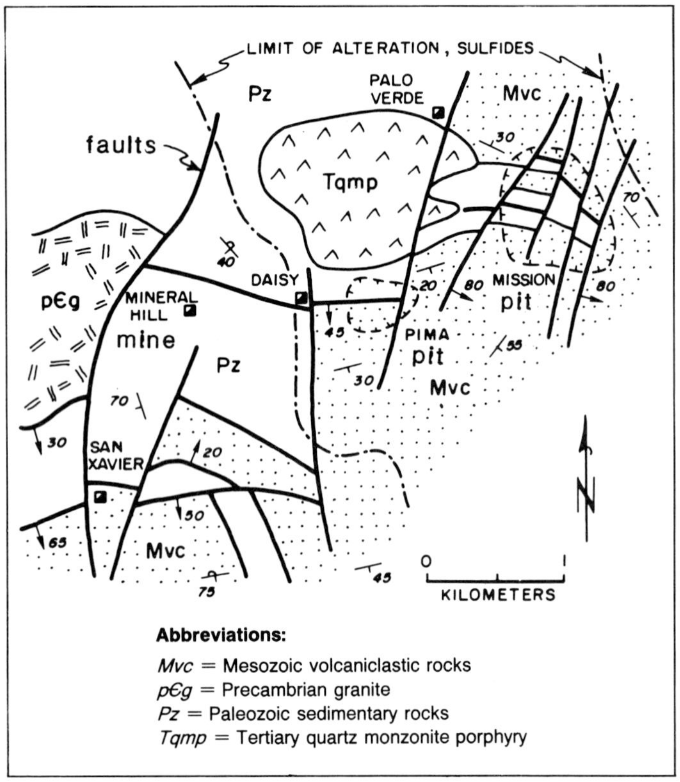

Figure 7.9. Location of Palo Verde shaft, Mission and Pima pits, and Daisy, Mineral Hill, and San Xavier mines relative to central porphyry complex of the Pima-Mission area, Pima mining district, Arizona. Generalized surface geology redrawn from Gale (1965). Limit of alteration and sulfides based on Kinnison (1966).

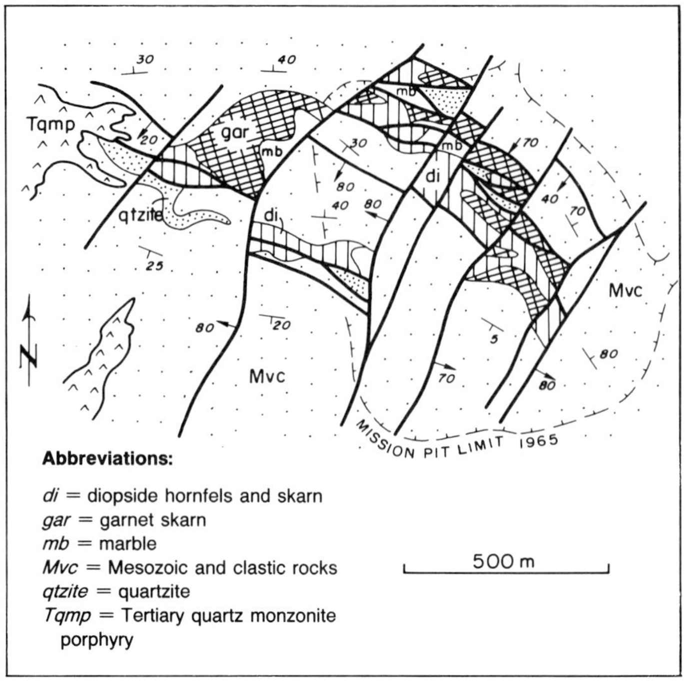

Figure 7.10. Distribution of garnet skarn, diopside hornfels, and marble in core of faulted antiform at Mission mine, Pima mining district, Arizona. Skarn extends down-dip under Mesozoic volcaniclastic rocks. Generalized surface geology redrawn from Gale (1965).

structurally controlled ore pipes and flat ore shoots consist of galena, sphalerite, and chalcopyrite with specularite, magnetite, pyrite, calcite and quartz. The ores are associated with some calc-silicate minerals, dominantly clinopyroxene.

Porphyry

The general setting of the Mission and related Palo Verde orebodies suggests that these are genetically related to the quartz monzonite porphyry stock exposed to the west. Detailed studies of calc-silicate and sulfide mineral zoning clearly support this contention (Gale, 1965; MacKenzie, 1963; Einaudi, 1974).

The quartz-monzonite at Mission is described by Gale (1965) as typical of porphyry copper plutons in general. Phenocrysts of 10 percent orthoclase, 30 percent plagioclase, and 5 percent biotite are set in a sub-graphic, fine-grained, K-feldspar-quartz groundmass. Potassium-silicate alteration generally is weakly developed, with ragged wisps of secondary biotite and replacement veinlets of quartz and K-feldspar. Gale (1965) has indicated that weak sericitic alteration is the most widespread alteration type: quartz-muscovite-pyrite-chalcopyrite veinlets locally are accompanied by pervasive replacement of plagioclase (but not of K-feldspar) by sericite; biotite remains fresh or is partly replaced by muscovite-chlorite-apatite-rutile and pyrite. Although primary copper grades and sulfide ratios have not been summarized by Gale, nor by Kinnison (1966), various lines of evidence indicate that overall the porphyry exposed at the Mission mine contains 0.15 to 0.3 percent Cu, rarely exceeds 0.4 percent Cu, and displays pyrite:chalcopyrite ratios of 3:2 to 3:1 (Gale, 1965, Table 12, p. 118; Kinnison, 1966, Figs. 5 and 6, p. 285). At Palo Verde (Einaudi, 1974) the copper grade in porphyry increases from 0.2 percent on the west to 0.4 percent on the east (Fig. 7.11). The average grade in porphyry at the Pima mine is 0.15 percent Cu (Langlois, 1978). Thus, rock type, alteration, copper grade, and sulfide ratios in the Pima-Mission area are strikingly similar to those exhibited by the porphyry stock complex at Twin Buttes.

Sedimentary Rocks at the Mission Pit

The major tonnage of ore-grade copper mineralization occurs in garnet and diopside skarn, with highest grades in skarn near marble contact and in west-northwest–striking fissures which contain massive sulfides. A lesser amount of open-pit ore occurs in Mesozoic argillite-arkose (Gale, 1965). Metal grades in three drill holes in the Mission pit are summarized in Table 7.5.

Alteration-mineralization in sedimentary rocks in the Mission pit has been studied by Gale (1965), who has suggested that early thermal metamorphism formed diopside in dolomitic siltstone and wollastonite in siliceous limestone. Later metasomatic alteration superimposed ore-bearing skarns. Gale has described three major types of skarn and their locations: (1) fine-grained, granular, diopside skarn (hornfels) largely occurs in a 10- to 30-m-thick bed within the Scherrer quartzite and in underlying carbonate beds at the contact with quartzite; (2) garnet (calcic) skarn, with variable garnet:pyroxene ratios and an outer wollastonite zone against marble, is zoned relative to quartzite-carbonate contacts or fissure zones; (3) epidote skarn (endoskarn), in Mesozoic argillite and arkose at contacts with calcic skarn, consists of epidote, K-feldspar, quartz, and tremolite, with lesser garnet and clinopyroxene.

According to Gale (1965) the major sulfide mineral associations and zonal distribution include: (1) pyrite-chalcopyrite-molybdenite in and near porphyry; (2) chalcopyrite-bornite dominant in skarn at the west end of the pit near porphyry; (3) chalcopyrite-pyrite as the dominant skarn sulfide assemblage, especially at the east end of the pit some distance from porphyry; (4) sphalerite most abundant at skarn-marble contacts; and (5) bornite-pyrite-sphalerite-galena-tetrahedrite in late quartz-calcite veins at the eastern periphery of the pit. On the basis of sulfide mineral zoning, Gale has concluded that there was a direct genetic link between the porphyries and mineralization.

Sedimentary Rocks at the Palo Verde Mine

The Palo Verde mine is a portion of the extensive Pima-Mission alteration zone, and, as in the Mission orebody, the majority of > 0.4 percent Cu mineralization is in Paleozoic and Mesozoic sedimentary rocks located east of and beneath a northwest-dipping, low-grade porphyry sill. High-grade zones are restricted to skarn in Paleozoic limestone on the contact with either Paleozoic quartzite or Mesozoic arkose. The skarn is separated from low-grade porphyry on the west by 30 to 60 m of quartzite and hornfels. The geology of the Palo Verde mine briefly has been described by MacKenzie (1963); the following is summarized from a more detailed study by Einaudi (1974). Rock type and alteration, copper grades, and sulfide assemblages are illustrated in Figure 7.11, an east-west cross section located north of the Mission pit, and summarized in Table 7.6.

Sedimentary rocks at Palo Verde are tentatively correlated with Scherrer Formation and Concha Limestone.

Quartzite-Hornfels. The bulk of the lower Scherrer Formation consists of glassy, white quartzite with very few impurities. The upper Scherrer Formation has a pale buff cast and contains 5 to 20 percent interstitial biotite, feldspar-mica, diopside-montmorillonite, or dolomite. Sulfide mineralization, with pyrite:chalcopyrite ratios ranging from 50:1 to 10:1, generally is fracture-controlled. Copper grades increase systematically from 0.1 percent on the west to 0.25 percent on the east.

The dominant rock type in the mid-Scherrer carbonate beds is diopside-quartz hornfels. Flinty to sandy, white to pinkish-white hornfels occurs at most contacts between quartzite and diopside hornfels. The white hornfelses consist largely of dolomite, with 5 to 20 percent recrystallized quartz; calcite is generally present in minor to trace amounts. Coarse green mica and white termolite may be present, especially near the contact with diopside hornfels. Very fine grained pyrite, chalcopyrite, and sphalerite are disseminated and in veinlets without visible alteration envelopes. Medium-grained, sugary-textured pale green diopside rock contains sparse, disseminated magnetite and pyrite. Chalcopyrite-pyrite (± quartz, magnetite) veinlets display dark green alteration envelopes which consist of actinolite-quartz with minor calcite. The intensity of veining is uniform from west to east and copper grades range from 0.4 to 0.6 percent.

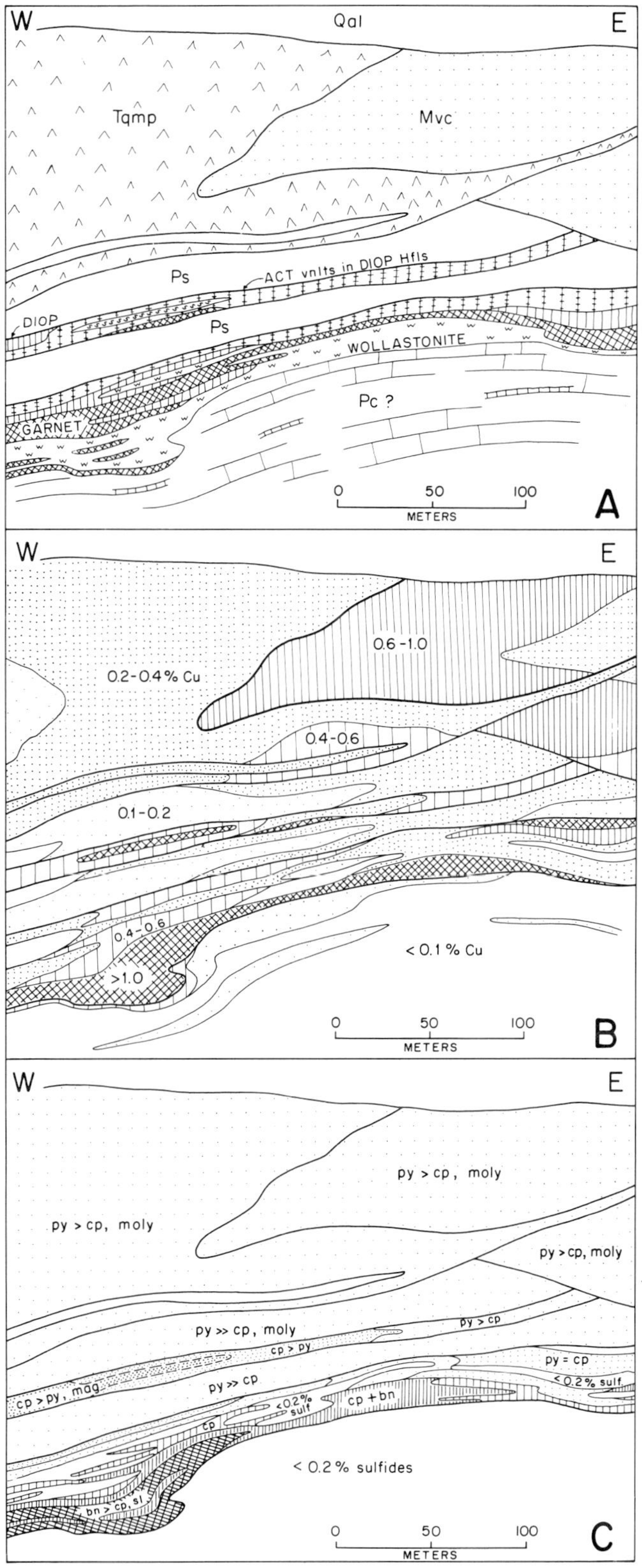

Abbreviations:

ACT vnlts = actinolite veinlets
bn = bornite
cp =chalcopyrite
DIOP Hfls = diopside hornfels
mag = magnetite
moly = molybdenite
Mvc = Mesozoic volcaniclastic rocks
Pc = Permian Concha Limestone
Ps = Permian Scherrer Formation
py = pyrite
Qal = Quaternary alluvium
sl = sphalerite
sulf = sulfides
Tqmp = Tertiary quartz monzonite porphyry

Figure 7.11. East-west cross section (looking north) of the Palo Verde mine in the Mission area of the Pima mining district, illustrating *A,* rock types and alteration; *B,* copper grades; and *C,* sulfide associations. Approximate pre-fault configuration is shown. Mid-Scherrer carbonate beds contain local serpentized magnesian skarn with magnetite. Concha Limestone contains calcic skarn. Based on diamond drill hole data (Einaudi, 1974).

TABLE 7.5
Grade of Skarn Ore in the Mission Pit

Drill Hole Number	Length of Sample (m)	Weight Percent			Oz./Ton	Cu:Mo	Cu:Pb
		Cu	Mo	Pb	Ag		
51	19	0.85	.013	.041	0.29	65	21
106	45	0.60	.008	.035	0.29	75	17
130	39	0.74	.009	.002	0.24	82	370

Source: Data from Gale (1965).

NOTE: Skarn type not specified.

Magnesian Skarn. The core of the mid-Scherrer diopside hornfels locally contains magnesian skarn characterized by patches and specks of brown serpentine rimmed with magnetite and set in a pale green, coarse tremolite-calcite matrix. Talc is a trace constituent in some areas. Chalcopyrite, with only minor pyrite, is disseminated throughout. No forsterite was noted in thin section, but the textures, and comparison with Twin Buttes samples, suggest that serpentine replaced original forsterite grains. Copper grades are generally greater than 1 percent.

Calcic Skarn. Immediately below the Scherrer quartzite in the western portion of Palo Verde, and below arkoses in the eastern portion, is a thick carbonate unit (Concha Limestone?) which consists largely of dark colored, locally cherty limestone. This unit is converted to garnet-diopside-wollastonite skarn along the contact with arkose and quartzite. The skarn zone varies in thickness from 20 to 45 m; post-skarn normal faulting has increased the thickness of skarn in some areas.

The metasomatic alteration of limestone may be described under three headings: (1) an inner zone, next to quartzite or arkose, consists dominantly of diopside hornfels; (2) an outer skarn zone consists of garnet-diopside-wollastonite; and (3) a marble zone consists largely of bleached and recrystallized limestone (see Fig. 7.11).

The inner skarn zone is similar in most respects to the mid-Scherrer carbonate unit, except that it lacks magnesian skarn; diopside constitutes over 80 percent of the rock. Disseminations and veinlets of chalcopyrite and pyrite are invariably rimmed with dark green actinolite halos. The contact of the inner skarn zone with the outer skarn zone is defined as the point at which actinolite halos disappear and garnet patches and veins appear in diopside. The contact generally is sharp; actinolite and garnet do not occur together, and no crosscutting relations between the two minerals were noted.

The outer skarn consists of garnet-diopside, garnet, and garnet-wollastonite, generally zoned toward marble in the order listed. Age relations between fine-grained diopside hornfels and garnet are generally lacking, but the presence of a number of garnet veins in diopside near the inner skarn zone suggests that garnet at any given point formed later than fine-grained diopside. In outer garnet-diopside zones, the two minerals show no discernable age relations. In wollastonite zones coarse, green diopside and garnet occur largely as patches, but veins of both diopside and garnet have been observed to cut wollastonite.

Garnet in the outer skarn zone varies from pale brown to green in color. There is a marked tendency for pale brown garnet to occur with diopside; locally this garnet is overgrown or veined by reddish brown garnet. Green garnet tends to occur on the marble side of the skarn zone and is associated with wollastonite.

An X-ray study of garnet compositions suggests a small, but systematic, increase in Al_2O_3 content with outward progression toward the marble contact. Eight garnet samples, selected from two drill holes, showed a change from 100 mole percent andradite to about 95 mole percent andradite in both sets of samples.

Sulfides consist of pyrite, chalcopyrite, bornite, and sphalerite; magnetite is absent. Fine hematite dusting in garnet is common, but probably is later than both andradite and sulfides. Pyrite and bornite do not occur in contact and generally do not occur in the same hand specimen. A general zoning is noted outward, from chalcopyrite-pyrite associated

TABLE 7.6
Grade and Sulfide Content in Sedimentary Rocks in the Palo Verde Mine, Pima-Mission Area
(Data in Weighted Means)

Drill Hole Sample Alteration Type	Length of Sample (m)	Weight % Copper	Volume % Sulfide (Chalcopyrite + Pyrite or Bornite)	Ore Assemblage
Quartzite[a]	—	0.15	1.5	pyrite : chalcopyrite = 5–10, molybdenite
Hornfels[b]	82	0.45	1.5	pyrite : chalcopyrite = 0.1–2, trace magnetite
Magnesian Skarn[c]	6	2.08	5.0	pyrite : chalcopyrite = 0.1, 5–10% magnetite
Calcic Skarn[d]	32	0.30	1.5	pyrite : chalcopyrite = 10
Calcic Skarn[d]	27	1.47	3.5	chalcopyrite, minor pyrrhotite
Calcic Skarn[d]	23	1.86	3.2	chalcopyrite, bornite; minor pyrrhotite
Calcic Skarn[e]	53	1.89	2.5	chalcopyrite, bornite, sphalerite; minor chalcocite, tennantite

Source: Data from Einaudi (1974).

[a] Scherrer quartzite.

[b] Diopside-quartz hornfels veined by sulfides-actinolite or sulfides-garnet, mid-Scherrer Formation.

[c] Serpentine-tremolite-calcite-magnetite skarn, mid-Scherrer Formation.

[d] Garnet-diopside skarn, Concha Limestone.

[e] Garnet-wollastonite skarn at marble contact, Concha Limestone.

with diopside and garnet-diopside to chalcopyrite-bornite (± sphalerite, pyrrhotite) associated with garnet-wollastonite. This relation is illustrated in Figures 7.11 and 7.12. Pyrite does not occur with wollastonite. Sulfides occur as streaks and disseminations in fresh garnet, diopside, and wollastonite. In massive garnet zones, sulfides—particularly chalcopyrite and bornite—preferentially replace calcite, which occurs as patches interstitial to garnet. Sphalerite and sphalerite-bornite (± chalcocite, tennanite) tend to occur with green garnet in wollastonite, whereas chalcopyrite-bornite tends to occur with brown garnet.

Within a few feet of the marble contact and within the marble itself, there is generally an increase in sulfide abundance. Chalcopyrite and chalcopyrite-sphalerite occur as

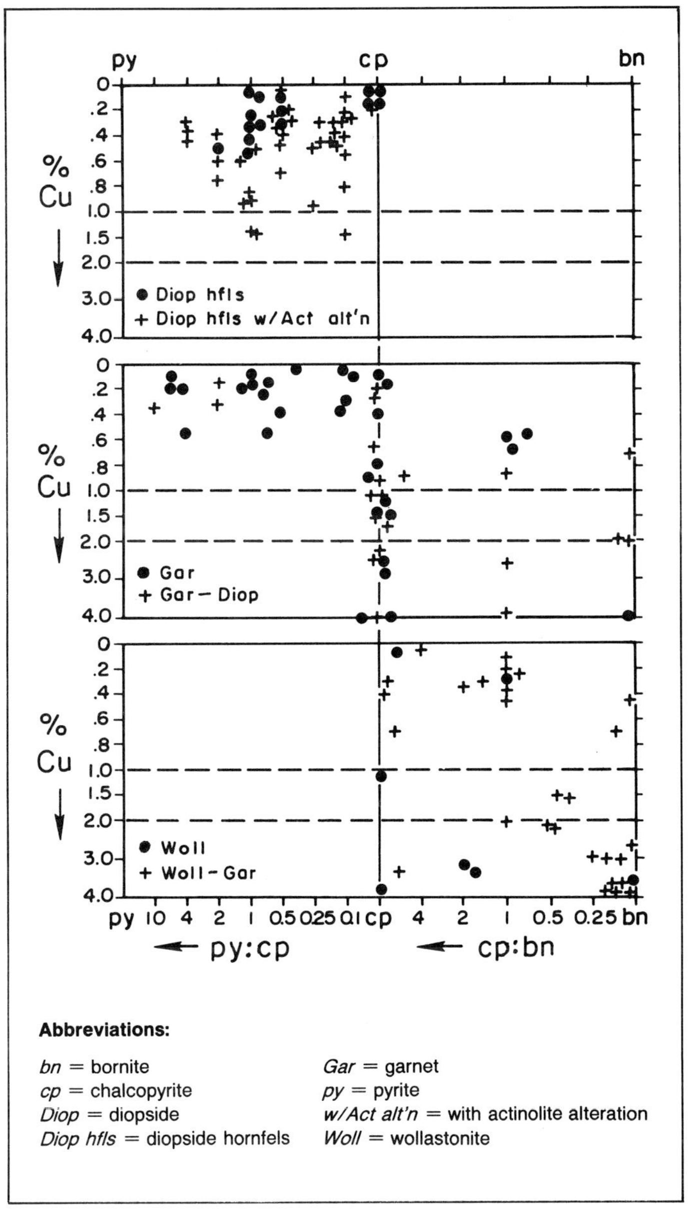

Figure 7.12. Plot of pyrite:chalcopyrite and chalcopyrite:bornite ratios, and copper grade as a function of calc-silicate assemblage at the Palo Verde mine, Pima mining district, Arizona. Each datum point represents visual estimate of sulfide ratio over core intervals of 1 to 2 m from cross section shown in Fig. 7.11. Plot shows decreasing Fe:Cu ratio in sulfides and increasing copper grades from diopside ± actinolite to garnet ± diopside and wollastonite ± garnet. Based on Einaudi (1974).

massive bedding streaks in white calcite marble, a few centimeters to 1 meter beyond wollastonite-garnet, or in dolomite-quartz envelopes in dolomitic marble beyond diopside-garnet.

Copper grades within the inner 7 to 15 m of the outer skarn zone average around 0.4 percent. In the outer 5 to 7 m, as the marble contact is approached, copper grades increase to 2.5 to 4.0 percent.

Marble Zone. The marble zone has a highly variable sulfide and silicate mineralogy, dependent to a large degree on original dolomite content. Wollastonite is not an abundant mineral; it characteristically occurs as rims on chert nodules; locally along fractures; and over short, apparently bedding-controlled intervals in calcite marbles. Idocrase is present in such intervals.

Two types of alteration envelope assemblages occur on sulfide veinlets in dolomite. Chalcopyrite-pyrite-magnetite veinlets have serpentine envelopes, and sphalerite-chalcopyrite (± pyrite) veinlets have white dolomite-quartz (± calcite) envelopes. The dolomite content in the envelopes is generally higher than in the enclosing marble. Similar veins with dolomite envelopes also occur in calcite marble.

The most abundant type of alteration in marbles consists of soft, pale buff to greenish, altered diopside hornfels, with minor garnet and idocrase. Talc-serpentine alteration of diopside is often pervasive and the enclosing rock may be partly replaced by talc-serpentine, which yields a pale yellowish marble. In thin section talc appears to replace both diopside and idocrase. Montmorillonite generally is less abundant than talc-serpentine, and tremolite is absent. Sulfides consist of pyrite-chalcopyrite and sphalerite-chalcopyrite; bornite is absent.

Late Alteration. Alteration of wollastonite and garnet to a variety of assemblages—including the minerals calcite, quartz, hematite, siderite, and chlorite—is widespread in the outer skarn zone. These late minerals occur in alteration envelopes on calcite-siderite veins and on post-skarn fault breccias cemented by calcite-hematite-siderite. Skarn fragments within fault breccias are pervasively altered to carbonate-hematite. Pervasive alteration extends up to 1 m beyond strong fault zones and into the skarn along fractures.

Wollastonite is the first mineral affected by late recarbonation; it is replaced by a pale gray mixture of calcite-quartz. Andradite is next affected; abundant thin fractures of calcite-hematite darken the color of garnet to a deep carmine red and any associated wollastonite is completely destroyed. Within and near breccia zones, andradite may be completely replaced by dark purple calcite-quartz-hematite, with local siderite and traces of chlorite. Skarn textures are preserved and the above assemblage pseudomorphously replaces andradite grains. Diopside associated with andradite appears to undergo the same alteration. Bornite does not survive this late alteration; it is converted to chalcopyrite.

THE LAKESHORE DEPOSIT

In May, 1968, El Paso Natural Gas Company announced the discovery of a major copper deposit on the Lakeshore property, located on the southwest flank of the

Slate Mountains in Pinal County, 28 miles south of Casa Grande, Arizona. The following summary of the geology is based on studies of the mine area by Harper and Reynolds (1969) and Barron (1969), as reported in Hallof and Winniski (1971), and by South (1972); discussions with J. J. Quinlan and Craig Hansen of Hecla Mining Company also were helpful.

General Setting

The southern end of the Slate Mountains consists largely of Precambrian Pinal Schist intruded by a large stock of equigranular quartz monzonite of Laramide age, known as the Lakeshore stock. This stock extends 4 km in a northwesterly direction and is bounded on the west by the Lakeshore fault, a major, west-dipping, range-front normal fault with a west-side-down normal displacement of several thousand meters.

West of the fault, in the block containing the Lakeshore deposit, are scattered pediment outcrops of younger Precambrian Apache Group rocks overlain disconformably, or in fault contact with, volcanic and sedimentary rocks of Cretaceous age. Irregular sills and stocks of quartz monzonite porphyry, presumably representing the preserved cupola portions of the Lakeshore stock, occur at depth. A plan view of the 400-ft. level and cross section at the Lakeshore mine are presented in Figure 7.13.

Primary copper mineralization is spatially associated with the upper portions of the porphyry bodies and includes: (1) lower grade (0.5–0.8% Cu), disseminated chalcopyrite in porphyry, Precambrian diabase, skarn, and Cretaceous volcanic sedimentary rocks; and (2) higher grade (~1.7% Cu) tabular bodies of chalcopyrite mineralization in skarn. The skarn ore occurs in a limestone unit which may be either Precambrian (Mescal Limestone?) or early Paleozoic in age.

Skarn

The skarn bed dips 20° west, has an average thickness of 20 m, and is terminated on the east and west by normal faults (see Fig. 7.13). Low-angle shears disrupt the bed on a local scale; many contacts between higher-grade and lower-grade mineralization and between differing calc-silicate assemblages are fault surfaces. The base of the skarn bed is also locally faulted.

In spite of the structural disruptions and local lithological controls of calc-silicate mineralogy within the limestone unit, the following dominant mineral associations are roughly arranged from northwest to southeast with increasing distance from the main porphyry mass: (1) garnet, with generally low sulfide content and high pyrite:chalcopyrite ratios; 2) diopside, with patches of garnet, relatively higher sulfide content and high pyrite:chalcopyrite ratios, containing abundant, sulfide-bearing fractures with dark green (actinolite?) alteration envelopes; and (3) talc-tremolite with relatively low pyrite:chalcopyrite ratios, and with magnetite ranging up to 25 percent. Zones dominated by garnet or tremolite-magnetite contain the highest copper grades; the most persistent zones of high-grade ore occur in the latter assemblage. Overall, the skarn contains 1 to 6 percent pyrite,

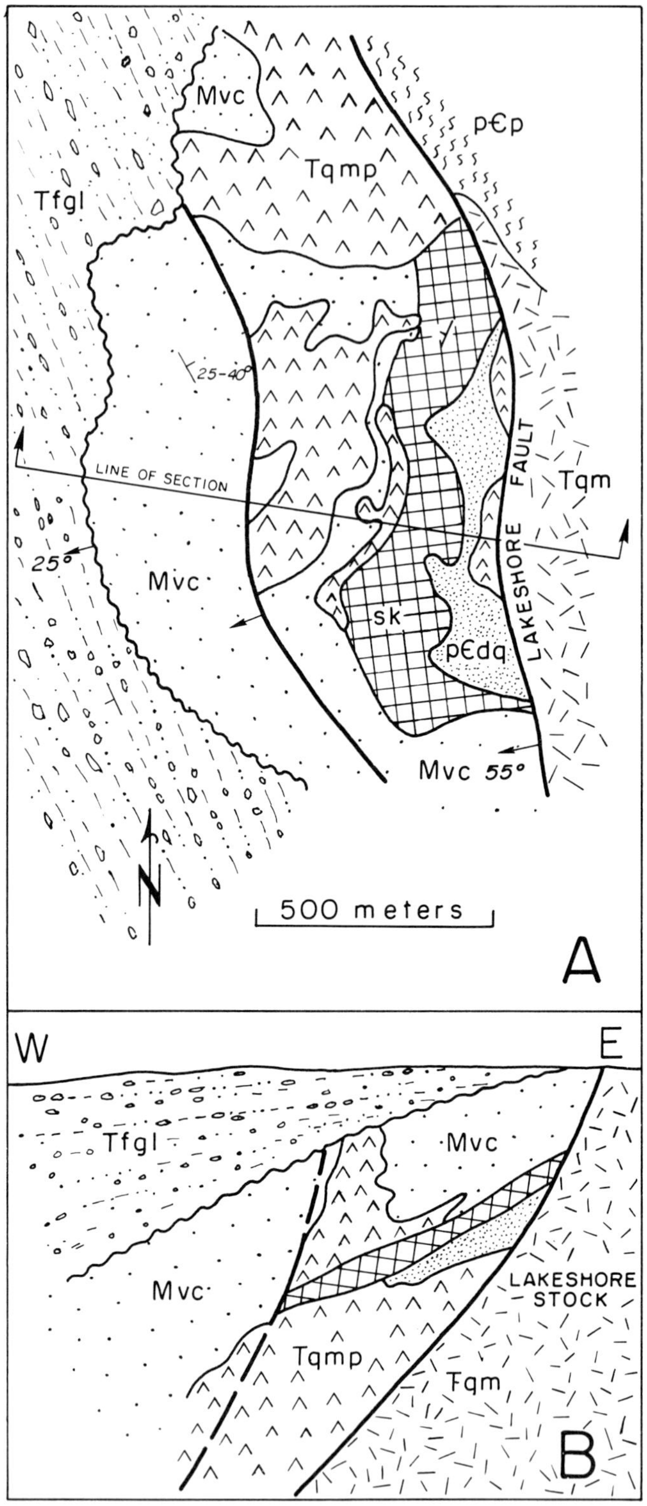

Abbreviations:

Mvc = Mesozoic volcaniclastic rocks
pЄdq = Precambrian diabase and quartzite
pЄp = Precambrian Pinal schist
sk = skarn
Tfgl = Tertiary fanglomerate
Tqm = Tertiary quartz monzonite
Tqmp = Tertiary quartz monzonite porphyry

Figure 7.13. Plan view of 400-ft. level (*A*) and cross section, looking north (*B*) at the Lakeshore mine, Slate Mountains, Arizona, illustrating the location of skarn and quartz monzonite porphyry stock in down-dropped block west of Lakeshore fault. Redrawn from South (1972).

1 to 4 percent chalcopyrite, and pyrite:chalcopyrite ratios range from 1:2 to 4:1.

THE BINGHAM MINING DISTRICT

The Bingham mining district has been the subject of intense geological study for many years; advances in geological knowledge are documented in *Economic Geology,* v. 73, no. 7 (1978). The Bingham district is unique; not only does it contain the largest known porphyry copper deposit in North America, with a production of 1.3 billion tons of 0.85 percent Cu ore from 1904 to 1976, but also it contains the world's largest known skarn Cu deposits and is the only porphyry copper system from which major lead-zinc-silver ore tonnages (47 million tons from 1870–1971) have been mined. With a high-grade skarn-ore preserve of greater than 60 million tons of approximately 2 percent Cu, a lower-grade skarn-ore resource of 150 million tons of 1.3 percent Cu (Proxy Statement, The Anaconda Co., 1976), and additional reserves for which tonnage and grade figures are unavailable, the district promises to maintain its premier position in metal production for many decades to come. In addition, 2 km of vertical exposure due to mining and deep drilling in an essentially continuous structural block is unparalleled in any other porphyry-skarn system. A unique opportunity exists, therefore, to document the changes in skarn mineralogy as a function of depth, from deep zones, spatially related to a low-grade root zone in igneous rocks, to relatively higher-level environments, spatially related to well-mineralized porphyry dominated by potassium silicate alteration (Table 7.7).

General Setting

Sedimentary rocks in the contact aureole are of Pennsylvanian age and consist of quartzite, with lesser amounts of calcareous siltstone and limestone (see Fig. 7.3). The relatively small volume of carbonate-rich rocks in the Pennsylvanian section at Bingham—in contrast with southern Arizona, New Mexico, and Sonora—is noteworthy and may be one of the key factors which led to the immense tonnage of highly mineralized skarn.

Compressive deformation from the southwest during Mesozoic time formed east-west–trending folds, bedding plane faults, and a set of northwest-striking, imbricated, thrust or right lateral, strike-slip faults. A system of northeast-striking faults, which were later to serve as major ore solution conduits (especially in the southwestern and southern portion of the district, Fig. 7.14*a*), originated largely as tension fissures parallel to the direction of maximum principal stress. Intrusion of quartz monzonite during mid-Tertiary time was controlled to a large degree by the zone of northeast faults and by steep bedding.

Porphyry

The Bingham stock—composed of a multiple intrusive sequence of early monzonite, followed by quartz monzonite porphyry and late quartz latite porphyry—contains a relatively high-grade primary ore assemblage ($\simeq$0.65% Cu) of chalcopyrite-bornite and chalcopyrite-pyrite associated with biotite-orthoclase alteration. Figure 7.14*b* shows that a late stage of quartz-sericite-montmorillonite alteration of plagioclase, with stable orthoclase and biotite, occurs along a structurally permeable zone along the northwestern contact of the stock (Moore and Nash 1974; Moore, 1978). The configuration of disseminated and stockwork copper mineralization has been described by James (1971) as an inverted, cup-shaped volume which is draped over a low-grade core zone. The alteration-mineralization pattern, clearly centered on the quartz monzonite porphyry phase, indicates that the hydrothermal activity responsible for this pattern was synchronous with the emplacement and cooling of the porphyry. This relation is particularly clear in the cross sections shown in Figure 7.15, which illustrate the assymetry of the pattern relative to the stock as a whole.

The contrast in alteration-mineralization in the stock near the surface and 1,000 m below the surface is largely one of intensity, rather than kind. At the surface (see Fig. 7.14) the copper ore zone is centered on the porphyry, and the outer limit of >0.35 percent Cu extends a few hundred meters eastward and westward beyond the monzonite stock contact into biotite and actinolite-bearing quartzite (John, 1978; Atkinson and Einaudi, 1978). Copper grade decreases southward in the monzonite stock as potassium-silicate alteration and stockwork veinlets decrease in intensity and grade out through secondary actinolite to unaltered augite-hornblende monzonite (Lanier, Raab, et al, 1978). At depths of 1,000 m below the surface (See Fig. 15), however, the porphyry contains less than 0.25 percent sulfides, although the intensity of potassium-silicate alteration remains high; at these depths the zone of >0.35 percent Cu is located 450 m from the porphyry contact on the south and east sides, where the wall rock is monzonite, containing only minor secondary biotite (John, 1978). On the west side of the porphyry, where the wall rock is quartzite, the better-grade zone appears as a mirror image of the eastern ore zone, although grades reach only 0.1 to 0.4 percent Cu (Atkinson and Einaudi, 1978).

Timing of Cu Versus Pb-Zn-Ag

The zonation of ores and alteration in the sedimentary wall rocks of the Bingham stock was first documented by R. N. Hunt (1924); Table 7.8 shows that copper ores are restricted to garnetized limestone beds near the intrusion, whereas lead-zinc-silver ores occur principally in limestone and monzonite outside the zone of skarn minerals (see also Fig. 7.14). Although there exists a clear zonal relation between the copper and lead-zinc-silver zones, the timing of these two zones relative to each other and relative to alteration-mineralization events in the stock is not so clear. Atkinson and Einaudi (1978) concluded that deposition of copper-iron sulfides was essentially synchronous with garnetization of limestone and with actinolite alteration of diopside in hornfels and quartzite; both were broadly synchronous with biotite-orthoclase alteration of igneous rocks. The contemporaneity of actinolite alteration of diopside and biotite-orthoclase alteration of igneous rocks is clearly documented by veinlet relations at igneous-sedimentary rock contacts.

TABLE 7.7
Changes in Alteration-Mineralization with Depth at Carr Fork, Bingham Mining District

	Alteration-Mineralization	Skarn		Quartzite		Porphyry	
		Surface	1 km Depth	Surface	1 km Depth	Surface	1 km Depth
<100 m from intrusive contact	% Copper	0.6–1.0	0.2–0.6	0.4	<0.1	0.65	<0.1 locally high molybdenum
	Volume % Sulfide	0.5–4	0.5–1	1–2	<0.25	1.5	0.5
	Sulfide Assemblage	chalcopyrite= pyrite	chalcopyrite > bornite	chalcopyrite > pyrite	molybdenite> chalcopyrite	chalcopyrite > bornite	molybdenite > chalcopyrite
	Volume % Iron Oxide	1–2	2–5	0	0	0	trace
	Iron Oxide Assemblage	magnetite, hematite	magnetite	—	—	—	magnetite
	Main Stage Alteration	garnet (clinopyroxene)	garnet (clinopyroxene)	interstitial actinolite; actinolite-biotite veinlets	interstitial biotite	(actinolite-epidote)[a] biotite-orthoclase	(actinolite-epidote?)[a] biotite-orthoclase
	Late Alteration	clay after clinopyroxene; opaline silica, pyrite	garnet (clinopyroxene) clay after clinopyroxene	chlorite, sericite, montmorillonite	local sericite	(chlorite) sericite, montmorillonite, pyrite	weak sericite, montmorillonite
100–400 m from intrusive contact	% Copper	1–4	1–4	0.2–0.4	0.1–0.4	↑	↑
	Volume % Sulfide	5–15	2–8	1	0.25–1		
	Sulfide Assemblage	pyrite > chalcopyrite	chalcopyrite >> bornite chalcopyrite= pyrite	chalcopyrite= pyrite	chalcopyrite > pyrite; chalcopyrite >> bornite		
	Volume % Iron Oxide	1–2	2–10	0	0	porphyry not found	prophyry not found
	Iron Oxide Assemblage	magnetite, hematite	magnetite	—	—		
	Main Stage Alteration	garnet-pyroxene	garnet-pyroxene	interstitial clinopyroxene, actinolite; actinolite-biotite veinlets	interstitial actinolite; actinolite-biotite veinlets		
	Late Alteration	clay after clinopyroxene; local opaline silica, pyrite	absent	chlorite; montmorillonite	absent	↓	↓
>400 m from intrusive contact	% Copper	<0.1	erratically very high	<0.1	<0.1	↑	↑
	Volume % Sulfide	trace–1	erratically very high	trace–1	trace–0.5		
	Sulfide Assemblage	bornite, chalcopyrite (sphalerite, galena)	pyrite > chalcopyrite	pyrite > chalcopyrite	pyrite= chalcopyrite		
	Volume % Iron Oxide	0	erratically very high	0	0	porphyry not found	porphyry not found
	Iron Oxide	—	magnetite	—	—		
	Main Stage Alteration	garnet replaces wollastonite	magnetite and sulfide replace marble	interstitial clinopyroxene; actinolite veinlets	interstitial clinopyroxene, actinolite; actinolite (biotite) veinlets		
	Late Alteration	clay, chalcedony replace limestone; pyrite-sphalerite-galena	?	only on north-east fissures	absent	↓	↓

[a] Endoskarn.

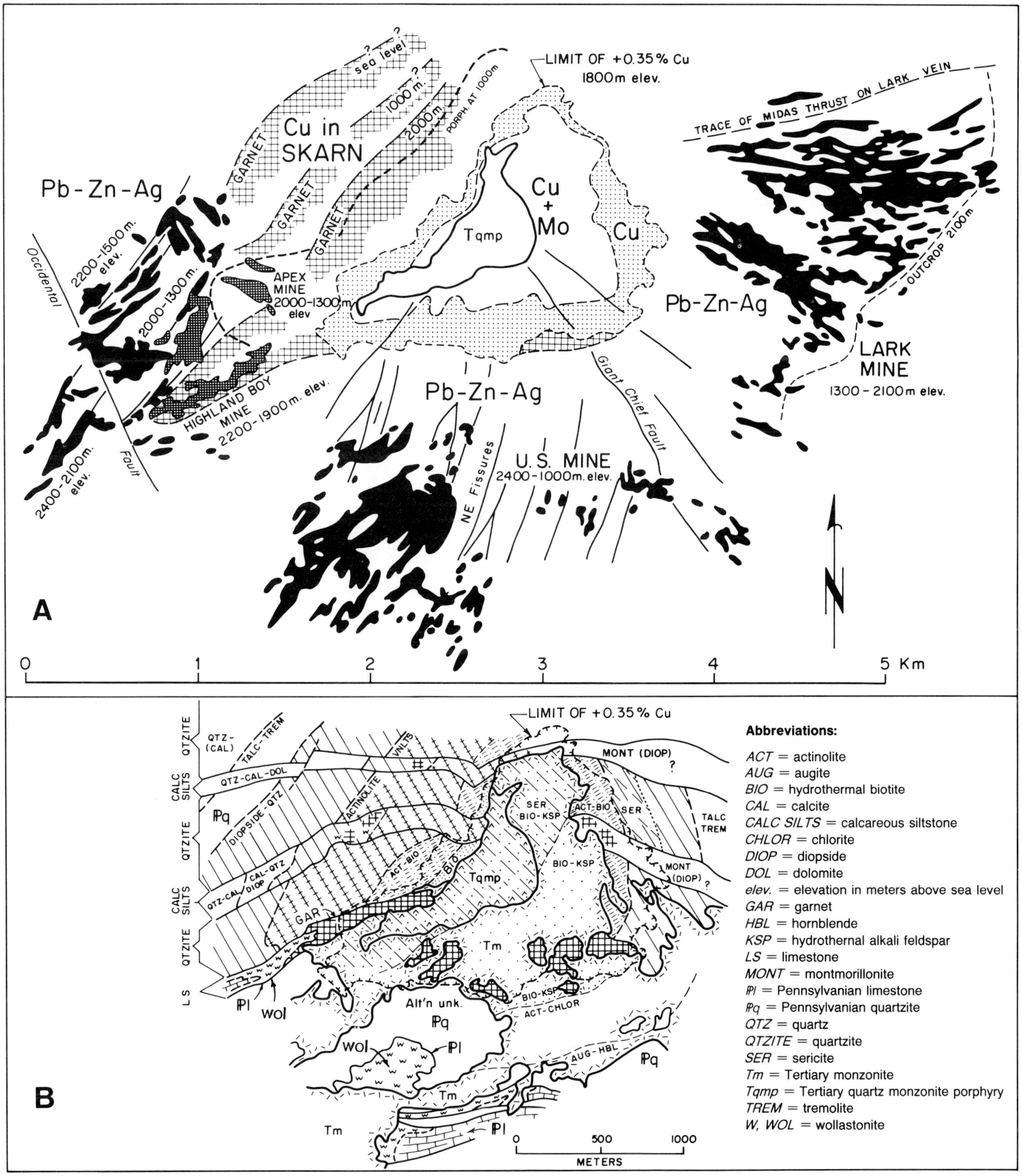

Figure 7.14. Mineral zoning and alteration in the Bingham mining district, Utah. *A,* metal zoning relative to central quartz monzonite porphyry projected to a horizontal plane: Cu + Mo and Cu disseminated in igneous rocks and peripheral sediments at 1,800-m elevation; Cu in skarn (garnet, cross-hatched) on west and northwest from 2,200- to 0-m elevation; Pb-Zn-Ag replacement and fissure ores (black) in limestone, quartzite, and monzonite from 2,400- to 1,000-m elevation. *B,* alteration in igneous and sedimentary rocks at the surface. Based on Lanier, John, and others (1978), John (1978), Moore (1978) Lanier, Raab, and others (1978), Atkinson and Einaudi (1978).

J. P. Hunt (1957) has concluded that much of the lead-zinc-silver mineralization was associated with a later hydrogen metasomatizing environment which produced sericite in igneous rocks, clays (not actinolite) in calc-silicate rocks, and carbonate-silica in limestone.

Sedimentary Rocks

The following summary of alteration-mineralization in sedimentary rocks is based on the study of the western contact aureole by Atkinson and Einaudi (1978). An early stage of magnesium-silica metasomatism produced diopside in quartzite and in silty limestone beds up to 1,500 m from the stock and wollastonite, with minor idocrase and garnet, in thick, cherty limestone up to 600 m from the porphyry (see Figs. 7.14 and 7.15). A trace amount of sulfides accompanied this early metasomatic-metamorphic event, which was synchronous with emplacement of monzonite and continued during the initial emplacement of quartz monzonite porphyry.

Actinolite-biotite alteration of diopside along sulfide-

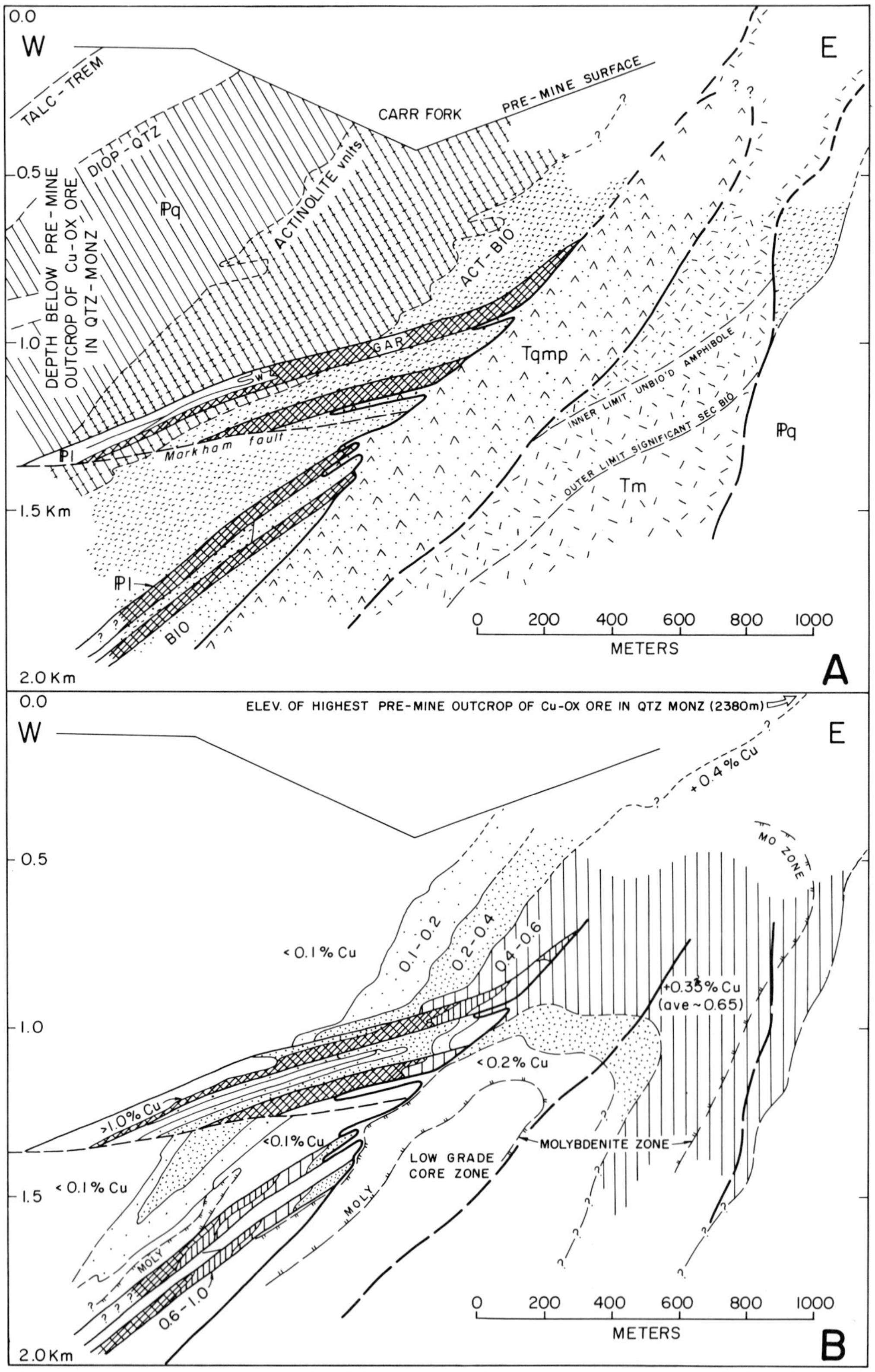

Figure 7.15. Cross section (looking north) of the Bingham mining district, Utah, illustrating alteration (*A*), copper grade (*B*), and sulfide ratios (*C*) in the western contact zone (Carr Fork area) of Bingham stock. Relations at depth east of the porphyry in monzonite and quartzite are semi-schematic and based on John (1978) and Lanier, John, and others (1978); relations at depth in porphyry and west of porphyry are based on Atkinson and Einaudi (1978) and Einaudi (unpublished data).

bearing fractures in quartzite, and garnetization of wollastonite-bearing marble, represent the beginning of main-stage mineralization and are synchronous with biotite-orthoclase alteration of igneous rocks. Pyrite:chalcopyrite ratios decrease toward the stock in the zone of actinolite envelopes. Crosscutting veinlet relations indicate that the biotite zone expanded from the stock onto the outer actinolite zone during a trend toward decreasing pyrite:chalcopyrite and Cu-Fe sulfide:molybdenite ratios. Late pyritic veinlets with actinolite envelopes represent the waning of main-stage mineralization in quartzite.

Two cherty limestone beds, 15 to 60 m thick and separated by 100 m of quartzite, contain the major copper-bearing skarns in the district. Zoning in these skarn beds is summarized in Table 7.9. Main-stage alteration consists of brown andradite (average Ad_{95} by chemical analysis), diopside, magnetite, and chalcopyrite superimposed on early-stage wollastonite up to 450 m from the porphyry. In the wollastonite zone, yellow-green garnet (average Ad_{72} by X-ray) is accompanied by chalcopyrite and bornite, with minor galena and sphalerite. Pyrite:chalcopyrite ratios decrease from the outer edge of the andradite-diopside zone toward the intrustive contact; they also decrease with depth. Massive magnetite locally replaces garnet at lower elevations; at higher elevations, the skarns have a lower iron-oxide content, hematite appears, and the hematite-magnetite ratio increases to unity near the surface.

The main stage of ore deposition in skarn culminated with alteration of andradite to variable mixtures of calcite, quartz, hematite, magnetite, siderite, and sulfides. In the more diopside-rich skarn of the outer zones, alteration assemblages accompanying some sulfide deposition include andradite-actinolite or actinolite in addition to the minerals listed above. These reactions may have been largely the result of declining temperatures; it is unclear whether any new copper, iron, or sulfur was introduced at this stage.

A late stage of alteration produced pyrite, chlorite, montmorillonite, sericite, talc, and opal from earlier calcsilicates and locally redistributed chalcopyrite. Lead-zinc and gold deposits, accompanied by arsenic-bearing minerals such as tennantite and arsenopyrite, also belong to this time frame. The late stage is believed to be contemporaneous with sericite-pyrite alteration of intrusive rocks, and largely is restricted to higher elevations.

THE SANTA RITA DEPOSIT

The Santa Rita deposit is located on the east side of the Central mining district, about 20 km east of Silver City, New Mexico. The general geology of the Santa Rita quadrangle has been described by Jones and others (1967). Copper-bearing skarns related to the Santa Rita stock, which have been described by Nielsen (1970), display the characteristic mineralogy of skarns related to porphyry copper intrusive systems: they are copper-dominant and contain an association of andraditic garnet and diopsidic clinopyroxene with zinc present in minor, uneconomic concentrations near the marble contact. These skarns are in marked contrast with the zinc-bearing skarns located north of Santa Rita (Fig. 7.16) on the southern fringe of the Hanover-Fierro stock at the Kearney, Oswaldo, Empire, and Pewabic mines (Schmitt, 1939; Hernon and Jones, 1978). The zinc-bearing skarns are characterized by the association of manganhedenbergite, bustamite, rhodonite, and local ilvaite located on the marble side of andraditic garnet zones. It is likely that this association, which has not been reported from porphyry-copper-related skarns, is unrelated to the emplacement of the Santa Rita stock and to the formation of its associated copper-bearing

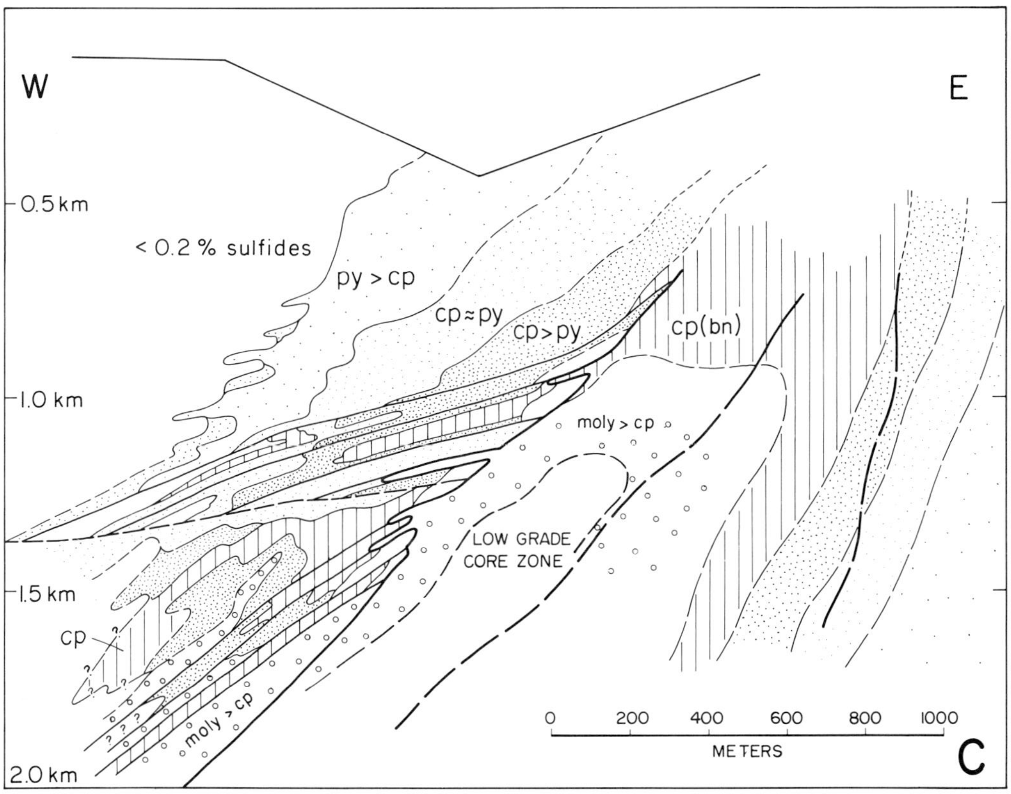

Abbreviations:

ACT = actinolite
BIO, SEC BIO = secondary (hydrothermal) biotite
bn = bornite
cp = chalcopyrite
DIOP = diopside
GAR = garnet
Mo = molybdenum
MOLY = molybdenite
IPl = Pennsylvanian limestone
IPq = Pennsylvanian quartzite
py = pyrite
QTZ = quartz
QTZ MONZ = quartz monzonite
Tm = Tertiary monzonite
Tqmp = Tertiary quartz monzonite porphyry
TREM = tremolite
UNBIO'D = unbiotized
vnlts = veinlets
w = wollastonite

TABLE 7.8
Metal Grades and Zones of Limestone Replacement-Fissure Ores and Skarn in the Bingham Mining District

Mineralization-Alteration Type	Location	Distance From Porphyry (m)	Elevation (m)	Weight % Cu	Weight % Mo	Weight % Pb	Weight % Zn	Oz./Ton Au	Oz./Ton Ag	Pb:Cu	Pb:Zn	Cu:Mo
Pb-Zn-Ag Fissure and Replacement	Carr Fork	2,300–500	2,190–1,860	1.0	ND	14.4	10.7	0.05	4.9	16.4	1.2	—
Pb-Zn-Ag Concordant and Replacement	Lark	2,700–900	2,120–1,300	0.7	ND	12.1	8.5	0.03	4.0	18.7	1.5	—
Pb-Cu Fissure Ore	Carr Fork	900–240	1,680–1,310	2.6	ND	3.9	(9.0)[a]	0.08	2.1	1.7	(1.0)[a]	—
Cu Ore, Garnet Skarn	Highland Boy Mine	670–0	2,200–1,910	2.2	ND	ND	ND	0.07	0.7	—	—	—
Wollastonite Skarn	Yampa Limestone outcrop, Carr Fork	750–300	2,240–2,075	0.017	0.0004	0.023	0.055	ND	0.04	1.4	.42	43
Open-Pit Cu Ore, Garnet Skarn	Yampa Limestone, Utah pit	300–0	2,000–1,820	0.65	0.009	0.002	0.02	ND	0.15	0.003	0.10	72
Cu Ore, Garnet Skarn	Carr Fork Mine[b]	450–120	1,760–970	1.9	0.008	ND	ND	0.02	0.4	—	—	238
Cu Ore, Garnet Skarn	Carr Fork Mine[b]	450–120	1,420–1,000	2.2	0.021	ND	ND	0.02	0.4	—	—	105
Cu Ore, Garnet Skarn	Carr Fork Mine[b]	600–270	1,240–300	2.4	0.057	ND	ND	0.02	0.4	—	—	42

Source: Data from The Anaconda Company; Atkinson and Einaudi (1978); Rubright and Hart (1967); Reid (1978).

NOTE: ND = no data; dash = no data on one of the elements in the ratio.

[a] Zn occurs sporadically; this value represents mean of Zn-rich ores.

[b] Grade of underground geological inventory.

TABLE 7.9
Main Stage Mineral Zoning in Deep Skarn at Carr Fork, Bingham, Utah

Distance From Bingham Stock (m)	Gangue	Garnet Color	Volume Fraction Garnet:Garnet + Diopside	Volume % Magnetite	Volume % Sulfides	Sulfide Associations	Volume Ratio Pyrite:Chalcopyrite
0–50	andradite-calcite-quartz-diopside	red-brown	0.7	1–2	1–2	chalcopyrite, minor chalcopyrite-bornite	0
50–100	andradite	red-brown	1.0	2–5	2–5	chalcopyrite-pyrite	0.2
100–300	andradite, diopside	red-brown, yellow in patches	0.9–0.8	5–10	15	chalcopyrite-pyrite	0.5–1.0
300–350	andradite, diopside	yellow, red in late veins	0.6	2	5	chalcopyrite-pyrite	5
350–400	wollastonite; veins, patches of garnet, diopside	yellow, yellow-green	highly variable	0	1	bornite-chalcopyrite-sphalerite, trace pyrite	0
400–600	wollastonite-diopside-quartz; wollastonite-calcite; marble	—	0	0	0.5	bornite, chalcopyrite, sphalerite, galena	0
>600	marble, limestone	—	—	0	trace	sphalerite, galena, pyrite	—

Source: Data from Atkinson and Einaudi (1978) and Einaudi (personal notes).

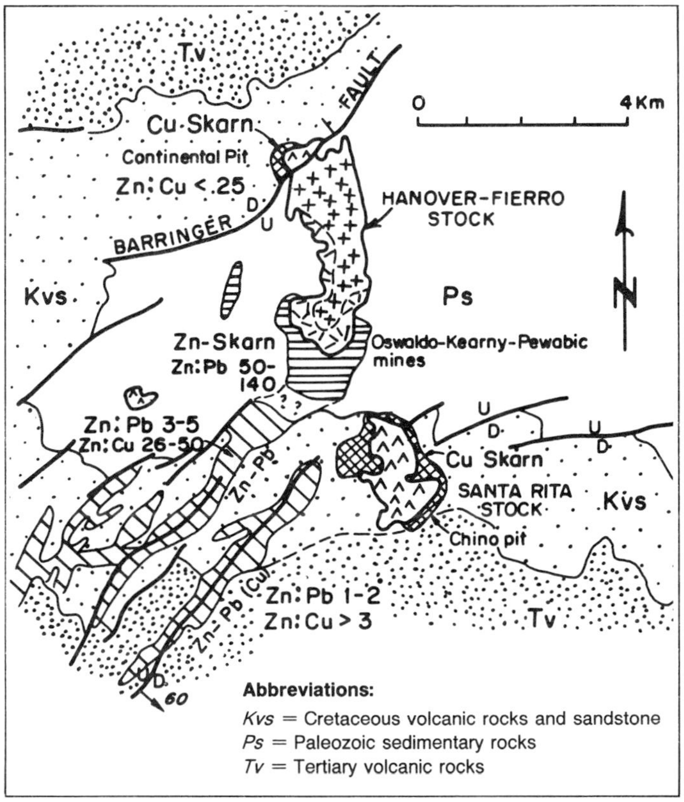

Figure 7.16. Generalized surface geology of the Central mining district, New Mexico, illustrating distribution of copper-bearing skarn (cross-hatched) in Paleozoic-carbonates at Chino pit (Santa Rita) and Continental pit, zinc-bearing skarn (horizontal ruling) near the southern lobe of Hanover-Fierro stock, and zinc-lead-(copper) veins (diagonal ruling) in a northeast-striking fault zone in the southwest portion of the district. Based on Jones and others (1967).

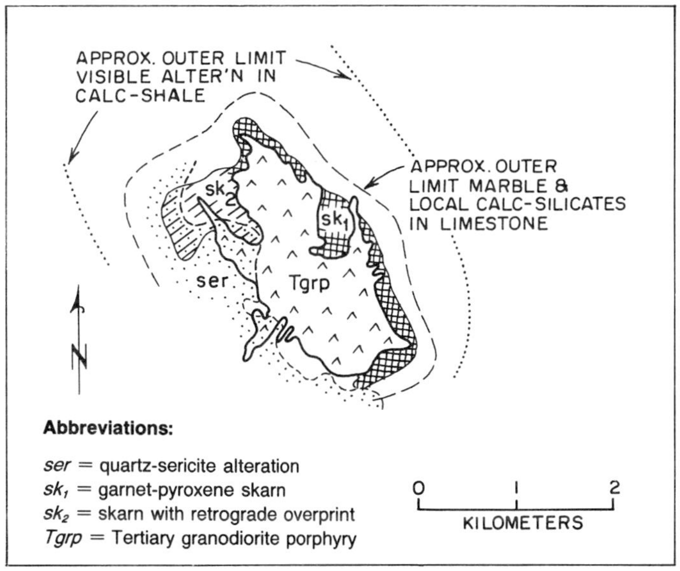

Figure 7.17. Sketch of the limits of alteration in limestone and calcareous shale and the distribution of the most intense sericitic alteration in igneous rocks at Santa Rita (Chino mine), Central mining district, New Mexico. The sketch illustrates the spatial relation between skarn and potassium-silicate alteration in stock on the east, and skarn destruction and sericitic alteration in stock on the west. Based on Nielsen (1970).

skarns. The relations between the contrasting environments of zinc- and copper-bearing skarn in the Central mining district remain an intriguing and unresolved question.

General Setting

The Oswaldo Formation of Pennsylvanian age, the principal host rock for Cu-bearing skarn in the district, consists of massive, non-dolomitic, cherty limestone, with thin shale partings and interbeds. The Syrena Formation, also Pennsylvanian in age, overlies the Oswaldo and consists of calcareous shale and interbedded impure limestone. The Santa Rita grandiorite and quartz monzonite porphyry stock and related dikes are elongated in a north-northwesterly direction parallel to the strike of bedding. Beds in the vicinity of the stock dip away from the stock at 20 to 40°.

Porphyry

Alteration-mineralization in the porphyry consists of an early potassium-silicate stage, which is best developed in the northern half of the stock, and a later stage of feldspar destructive alteration, which is, in part, superimposed on the potassium-silicate zone and appears to be structurally controlled by the western contact of the stock (Nielsen, 1968). The potassium-silicate stage is characterized by abundant quartz veining, secondary orthoclase and biotite, and a pyrite:chalcopyrite ratio of about 3. Total sulfides increase outwards from less than 1 weight percent in the core to 1 to 5 weight percent near the edge of the stock. The late stage consists of locally pervasive quartz-sericite alteration with 4 to 8 weight percent pyrite and a pyrite:chalcopyrite ratio of about 40. The hypogene grade is estimated to range from 0.1 to 0.3 percent Cu, with most of the potassium-silicate zone containing 0.1 percent Cu or less (Rose and Baltosser, 1966).

Sedimentary Rocks

The Oswaldo and Syrena Formations are intensely silicated or recrystallized within 60 to 900 m from the stock; hornfelses in calcareous shale extend outward an additional 600 m. Skarn considered to be ore grade (0.5–1% Cu?) occurs locally and erratically up to 600 m from the stock, although the most continuous areas of ore occur near the stock margins. The summary of zonal and paragenetic features that follows is based on Nielson (1970).

Hornfels. Recrystallization of calcareous shale is detected by X-ray analysis up to 2,400 m from the stock. Within 1,500 m, visible alteration consists of conversion to hornfelses containing quartz, calcite, actinolite, and plagioclase (Fig. 7.17). Fringing the ore zones closer to the stock, the hornfels takes on a mottled, greenish gray appearance and consists of epidote, quartz, actinolite, diopside, and albite, with minor garnet. Adjacent to potassium-silicate alteration in the stock, these hornfelses are cut by biotite-orthoclase veinlets; in the strong pyrite halo on the west margin of the stock, up to 10 percent pyrite occurs in veinlets with alteration envelopes containing variable mixtures of epidote, chlorite, montmorillonoids, calcite, siderite, and specular hematite.

Skarn. In the outmost zone of visible alteration, limestone beds contain thin reaction skarn at contacts with hornfelses (calcareous shales). Silication within relatively pure limestone beds is restricted to fractures of breccia zones; pale yellow-brown or green garnet veins with local sphalerite cut bleached marble. Closer to the stock massive, yellow-brown, garnet-diopside skarn, with interstitial magnetite and pyrite, replaces marble. Near the contact with porphyry, which contains potassium silicate alteration, magnetite (2–40%) and pyrite-chalcopyrite (4–18%) become more abundant as disseminations and cross-cutting veins in brown garnetite and in massive garnet-epidote-magnetite skarn. The pyrite:chalcopyrite ratio ranges from 1:1 to 10:1. Nielson (1970) concludes that this skarn assemblage (marked sk_1 on Figure 7.17) is synchronous with potassium-silicate alteration in the stock.

The early skarn assemblage is overprinted by hydrous silicates and carbonates near contacts with sericitized porphyry. Patches and veins of quartz-pyrite are bordered by a variety of late minerals, including actinolite, chlorite, montmorillonoids, epidote, siderite, pyrite and chalcopyrite. This type of alteration is associated with the highest grade of primary ore at Santa Rita and is particularly well developed at the northwest edge of the stock in the Lee Hill area (marked sk_2 on Figure 7.17). In this area, the skarn contains 20 to 75 percent magnetite and 10 to 25% total sulfides; the pyrite:chalcopyrite ratio is approximately 10:1 to 25:1.

THE CONTINENTAL MINE

A zone of secondary copper enrichment in Cretaceous sedimentary rocks was mined in the last century (1858 to 1861) at the Hanover Mountain mine, located on the north (down-thrown) side of the Barringer fault, near the northern lobe of the Hanover-Fierro stock (Spencer and Paige, 1935). From the turn of the century to approximately 1947, some 3 to 5 million tons of iron ore in skarn were mined from this same area at the Modoc, Republic, and Continental mines (Lindgren et al., 1910; Hernon, 1949). In 1947, interest shifted back to copper in the Continental mine area (see Fig. 7.16 for location), where significant mineralization in skarn had been discovered by surface diamond drilling (Forrester, 1972). Sporadic production ensued until 1962, when U.S. Smelting Refining and Mining Company substantiated a sufficient tonnage of copper ore to justify major development. The new Continental orebody, containing approximately 47 million tons of ore (W. T. Worthington, personal communication), was developed by open-pit and underground mining methods.

The following summary is based on discussions with W. T. Worthington, Chief Geologist at UV Industries' (formerly U. S. Smelting Refining and Mining Company) Continental mine, and on personal field notes.

Porphyry

The copper ore at the Continental mine occurs in skarn bordering the contact with the Hanover-Fierro stock. The igneous rock exposed in the east wall of the open pit consists largely of biotite quartz monzonite porphyry with a medium-grained aplitic groundmass. Chalcopyrite occurs almost exclusively in sparse pyritic quartz veins and veinlets which display sericitic alteration envelopes up to 0.3 m wide. Other quartz veinlets, generally lacking sulfides, but which are typical of potassium-silicate alteration, are encased in thin secondary biotite and magnetite alteration envelopes. Overall, the porphyry averages about 0.04 percent primary Cu, although some drill hole intercepts, up to 50 m in length, average as much as 0.1 percent Cu. Thus, the Hanover-Fierro porphyry exposed in the Continental pit has some characteristics of a weakly mineralized and altered porphyry copper pluton.

Sedimentary Rocks

Selective underground mining from the No. 3 Continental Shaft yields ore averaging approximately 2 percent Cu, 0.50 percent Zn, and 15 to 20% percent Fe as magnetite, largely from skarn in the Oswaldo formation. Open-pit copper ore in calcic skarn occurs dominantly in the Pennsylvanian Oswaldo Formation and the Mississippian Lake Valley Limestone. A minor portion of pit ore occurs in magnetite-rich magnesian skarn in the Montoya and El Paso dolomite of Ordovician age, which is separated from the upper Paleozoic strata by the Barringer fault. Open-pit ore averages approximately 0.85 percent Cu.

The Syrena formation overlying the Oswaldo skarn consists of flinty buff to green hornfels cut by a stockwork of thin pyrite veinlets with dark green alteration envelopes. Pale buff and red, massive garnet occurs as patches, veins, and veinlets. Magnetite is sparse to absent.

The Oswaldo skarn ore appears to be very similar to that exposed at the contact of the Santa Rita stock. On the outermost edge of silication, garnetite developed preferentially along the basal shale unit and overlying Syrena hornfels; locally garnetite at the marble contact is separated from marble by wollastonite and contains sphalerite, pyrite, and chalcopyrite. The main exposed ore-bearing skarn zone, some 200 m wide and extending along the stock contact approximately 1 km, consists of layers of dense, olive green, granular clinopyroxene (presumably salite) alternating with layers of red-brown garnet; the layering appears to be parallel to bedding, which dips 20 to 30° west. A lesser portion of the garnet occurs as irregular patches and crosscutting veins in the clinopyroxene. A large portion of the chalcopyrite, pyrite, magnetite, and hematite present in the skarn occur as disseminations in patches and veins of garnet, although garnet veins are cut by later quartz-chalcopyrite-pyrite veins. Within 30 m of the stock the grade drops to 0.15 percent Cu.

The skarn-marble contact in the Lake Valley Limestone is exposed in the south-central portion of the pit. A sketch of zoning and textures at the marble contact is presented in Figure 7.18. Beyond the skarn front, chert-nodules and lenses of white marble are rimmed with coarse wollastonite; the marble is cut by irregular, thick veins containing magnetite-pyrite or magnetite-sphalerite. Closer to the main skarn, wollastonite and most of the chert is replaced by pale green garnet and marble is replaced by massive magnetite with coarse patches of pyrite. Narrow pyrite-chalcopyrite veinlets with brown garnet envelopes cut green garnet and chert and appear to cut the massive magnetite. Veins and patches of brown garnet become more abundant toward the stock to the point where green garnet and chert become rare and the skarn consists of brown garnet, clinopyroxene, magnetite,

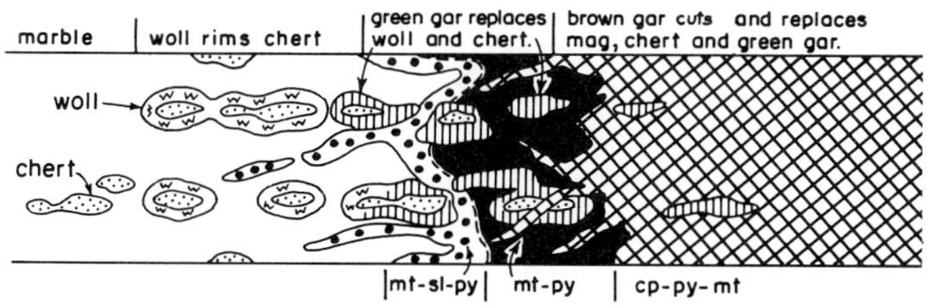

Abbreviations:

cp = chalcopyrite
gar = garnet
mt, mag = magnetite
py = pyrite
sl = sphalerite
w, woll = wollastonite

Figure 7.18. Sketch of zoning in calcic skarn of the Lake Valley Limestone at the Continental mine, Central mining district, New Mexico. Stock contact is toward the right. The scale is variable, on the order of tens of meters.

pyrite, and chalcopyrite in irregular, patchy, and complex vein textures.

The presence of green garnet in some magnetite-sphalerite veins suggests contemporaneity of these minerals. Also, in one magnetite-sphalerite vein that cut a wollastonite pod, the wollastonite was replaced by green garnet along the borders of the vein. These relations suggest that most of the sphalerite predated the formation of the main brown garnetite skarn and its associated chalcopyrite. However, the age relations between massive magnetite (lacking sphalerite) and brown garnet are ambiguous. Although brown garnet veins appear to cut massive magnetite, the magnetite may have preferentially replaced marble present between the brown garnet veins and green garnet pods.

THE SILVER BELL MINING DISTRICT

Mining activity in the Silver Bell mining district, located 56 km northwest of Tucson, was centered on local occurrences of copper-bearing skarn until 1930; after 1954, production largely came from supergene chalcocite ore in Laramide stocks, but during the 1970s hypogene copper ore in skarn was of increasing importance. The following summary is based on Stewart (1912), Richard and Courtright (1966), Graybeal (1982), and discussions with F. T. Graybeal and J. L. Galey of ASARCO Incorporated.

General Setting

According to Richard and Courtright (1966), a northwest-trending fault zone—which separates Paleozoic carbonate rocks on the northeast from Mesozoic arkosic sandstone on the southwest—served as the locus of magmatic activity in Laramide time. Emplacement of an elongate pluton of equigranular alaskite, (7 X 2 km in horizontal dimensions) and of later, sill-like bodies of dacite porphyry predated, by an unknown time interval, the intrusion of quartz monzonite porphyry stocks and the generation of the porphyry-skarn copper deposits. The porphyry stocks, which are irregular, steep-walled, and average 500 m in diameter, largely were emplaced along the northeast border of the alaskite batholith (Fig. 7.19). Graybeal (1982) has estimated that the Laramide surface was 1.8 km above the present surface.

Porphyry

The main zone of potassium-silicate alteration and mineralization is fairly symmetrical about a north-south line joining the El Tiro, Daisy, and North Silver Bell stocks (see Fig. 7.19). As described by Graybeal (1982), the highest grade of hypogene copper in igneous rocks (0.35% Cu) is associated with quartz-biotite-chalcopyrite ± pyrite veinlets in the central portion of the El Tiro stock. Copper grade decreases toward the outer portions of the stock and drops to less than 0.1 percent toward the east in the Imperial stock and surrounding dacite porphyry. Parallel changes in alteration-mineralization include the disappearance of veinlet biotite and an increase in the pyrite:chalcopyrite ratio from 1:2 to 4:1. Total sulfide content averages 2 volume percent. Bornite is rare and magnetite is absent. Beyond the outer edge of disseminated hydrothermal biotite, which defines the limit of potassium-silicate alteration (see Fig. 7.19), the pyrite:chalcopyrite ratio increases to 20:1 in the propylitic zone.

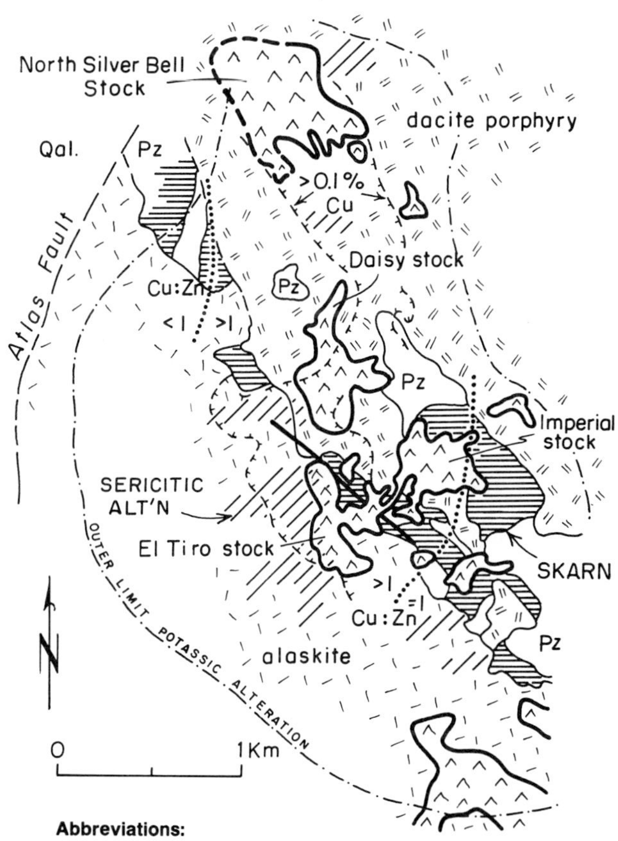

Abbreviations:

Pz = Paleozoic carbonate rocks
Qal = Quaternary alluvium

Figure 7.19. Generalized surface geology of the Silver Bell mining district, Arizona, illustrating distribution of skarn (horizontal ruling) in Paleozoic carbonates relative to the northwest-striking contact of alaskite and the north-trending zone of porphyry stocks, potassium-silicate alteration, and +0.1 percent hypogene Cu mineralization. Cu:Zn ratios in skarn (dotted lines) are broadly related to district-wide alteration patterns and not to individual stocks. El Tiro pit encompasses the southeastern portion of El Tiro and Imperial stocks and related skarn. Based on Richard and Courtright (1966) and Graybeal (1982).

Sericitic alteration generally is weakly developed at Silver Bell. Overall, the porphyry stocks contain 4 percent sericite as a weak, but pervasive, replacement of plagioclase. Locally intense sericitic alteration is restricted to the contact zone between alaskite and porphyry and is superimposed on potassium-silicate alteration as quartz-sericite ± pyrite envelopes on northeast-striking pyrite-quartz veins. In such areas, the pyrite content locally increases to 5 percent (Graybeal, 1982).

Skarn

In the mid-1970s mineralized skarn began to be an important source of copper ore in the eastern half of the El Tiro pit, where skarn and thin, interbedded hornfels extend a minimum of 330 m from the Imperial stock in the Abrigo and overlying Martin formations. The Escabrosa and Horquilla Limestones, exposed southeast of the El Tiro pit, are recrystallized but not extensively converted to skarn. On the basis of refractive index measurements, Buseck (1962) has suggested that garnet, the dominant silicate in calcic skarn, is pure andradite. Paragenetic relations determined by Stewart (1912) indicate the progressive formation of wollastonite, diopside, garnet-quartz, and calcite-quartz. The latter assemblage occurs as open-space fillings. Graybeal (1982) has indicated that chalcopyrite, pyrite, and magnetite occur in skarn as disseminations, replacing garnet, and in cross-cutting veinlets without alteration envelopes. Pyrite:chalcopyrite ratios increase from 2:1 near the stock to 5:1 at the outer marble contact; Zn:Cu ratios are close to 1:1 throughout. Local veins and patches of green garnet and wollastonite, accompanied by bornite-chalcopyrite-sphalerite, occur in marbleized limestone (Einaudi, 1978, personal notes). Garnet is absent from dolomitic members of the Martin Formation, where the dominant skarn association consists of serpentine, magnetite, chalcopyrite, and pyrite (J. L. Galey, 1978, personal communication).

The degree of skarn destruction in the Imperial stock area is relatively minor, in keeping with the dominance of potassium-silicate alteration and general lack of extensive hydrolytic alteration on the eastern side of the stocks. Skarn destruction is limited to veins and breccia dikes (up to 3 m wide), which consist of dense, purplish-black, jasperoidal silica containing garnet relics, finely and uniformly dispersed hematite, and veinlets and patches of chalcopyrite-quartz (Einaudi, 1978, personal notes). Silica-hematite replaces both skarn and marble, and is very similar to lesser occurrences at the Palo Verde mine.

Discussion

On a district scale, garnetite occurs in isolated blocks and patches of Paleozoic carbonate rocks engulfed by quartz monzonite porphyry along the northeast margin of the Alaskite batholith; this trend marks the position of Richard and Courtright's (1966) "major structure," and is located generally within the zone of potassium-silicate alteration as defined by Graybeal (1981). Garnetite occurs in carbonate rocks at contacts with alaskite, dacite porphyry, and quartz-monzonite porphyry, but is not continuous along all such contacts. The apparent lack of a systematic relationship between garnetite and igneous contacts suggests that: (1) some garnetite is metamorphic, dependent only on the presence of argillaceous limestone and a heat source; and (2) metasomatic skarns are related to fluids evolved from some, but not all, quartz monzonite porphyry stocks. The former possibility is supported by one analysis of garnet by Stewart (1912), which yielded grossularite and pyralspite contents (37.4 and 9.1 mole % respectively) not typical of porphyry-related ore skarns (Einaudi, 1982), and by evidence that extensive development of marble, wollastonite, and calc-silicate hornfels is related to the emplacement of dacite porphyry (S. L. Galey, 1978, personal communication; Graybeal, 1982). The latter possibility has been suggested by Graybeal (1982) with respect to the major area of mineralized garnetite, located in the El Tiro-Imperial stock area. In this area the distribution of skarn and of Cu:Zn ratios appears related to the north-striking zone of >0.1 percent copper which passes through the El Tiro, Daisy, and North Silver Bell stocks (see Fig. 7.19). Graybeal has concluded that alteration-mineralization patterns were dominated by district-scale features, rather than by individual intrusive centers. Graybeal (1982) and Galey (1978, personal communication) have suggested that the development of ore-bearing andradite skarn and sulfide-actinolite veinlets in hornfels was broadly contemporaneous with potassium-silicate alteration in igneous rocks.

THE MORENCI DISTRICT

Ore deposits of the Morenci district are exclusively the result of supergene enrichment. The ores mined by underground methods in the years 1872 to 1932 consisted of high grade, exotic, oxide ores in limestone and supergene chalcocite ores in pyritic fissure veins. When open-pit mining commenced in 1942, lower-grade, disseminated, supergene chalcocite in porphyry was the sole source of copper (Moolick and Durek, 1966); it was still the only source in early 1981.

General Setting

Hypogene alteration-mineralization in the district is related to an intrusive complex consisting of a quartz monzonite porphyry stock intruded by a dike swarm of granite porphyry. The complex is exposed along a northeasterly trend for 16 km and varies in width between 1.5 and 6.5 km. Sedimentary strata exposed in the south-central portion of the district consist of a 300-m section of Paleozoic limestone, sandstone, and shale, overlain by sandstone and shale of Cretaceous age. The basal carbonate strata, of Late Cambrian to Late Ordovician age, include sandy limestone and dolomite of the El Paso Limestone and lower Montoya Group, which were included in the now-abandoned "Longfellow Limestone" of Lindgren (1905). These strata resemble the Abrigo in composition and bedding characteristics (Bryant, 1968); even the purest limestone beds contain significant quartz, dolomite, and argillaceous silt. According to Lindgren (1905) and Moolick and Durek (1966), the Longfellow is less susceptible to replacement by garnet skarn than the purer Modoc limestone (Lake Valley Formation), which occurs higher in the section, above an intervening unit of dark shale. The Modoc consists of gray limestone with lesser interbeds of sandstone and dolomite.

Porphyry

At the Morenci pit the quartz monzonite porphyry contains an elliptical enrichment blanket 1.5 km in diameter; Moolick and Durek (1966) have indicated that the protore below the enrichment blanket contains 3.5 to 8 percent pyrite —disseminated and in veinlets—in strongly sericitized porphyry. Minor sulfides include molybdenite, chalcopyrite, and sphalerite. Hypogene copper grade is 0.10 to 0.15 percent and zinc is present in concentrations only slightly less than copper. The pyrite:chalcopyrite ratio decreases to less than 1 at "considerable depth" (Moolick and Durek, 1966).

The description of altered rocks by Lindgren (1905), Reber (1916), and Moolick and Durek (1966) indicate that the Morenci porphyry exhibits moderately intense sericitic alteration at the surface, with pyrite-quartz-sericite largely restricted to envelopes on veinlets and larger pyrite-quartz fissures. The authors listed above all conclude that argillic alteration between sericitic selvages is largely supergene. There is no published evidence for the presence of advanced argillic alteration.

Sedimentary Rocks

In contrast with most porphyry-skarn deposits, the altered sedimentary rocks at Morenci appear to lack any large volumes of greater than 1 percent hypogene copper mineralization. According to Moolick and Durek (1966) high-grade ores mined in the period 1872 to 1932 consisted of two types: (1) irregular tabular bodies of oxide copper minerals in limestone or shale, which were the result of deposition from supergene fluids that leached copper from adjoining non-carbonate rocks (porphyry or skarn-hornfels); and (2) supergene chalcocite ore developed in quartz-sericite-pyrite fissure veins in non-carbonate rocks.

Alteration of calcareous strata at Morenci extends 500 to 600 m from the southern contact of the stock. In this zone abundant porphyry sills and dikes are propylitically altered and lack the strong sericitic alteration exhibited by the main body of the intrusive. Shale is altered to variable mixtures of quartz, kaolinite, amphibole, epidote, and pyrite. Limestone is replaced by salc-silicates up to 30 m from dike contacts. Except for epidote near porphyry, the Modoc skarns are dominated by honey brown to dark brown andradite (Lindgren, 1905). Chemical analyses of two samples from the Modoc horizon indicate a very low grossularite content (0.8 and 1.5% Al_2O_3). Wollastonite has not been reported to occur at garnet-marble contacts. Opaque minerals consist of disseminations and veinlets of magnetite, pyrite, chalcopyrite, and sphalerite; galena is rare. Magnetite locally is concentrated near porphyry or as replacement bodies in limestone. Calc-silicate rocks in the Longfellow Limestone contain more diopside and less garnet than the Modoc skarns (as would be expected, due to its higher dolomite content). Much of the garnet is greenish-brown in color and Moolick and Durek (1966) have suggested that it is aluminous. Calcite-diopside-tremolite hornfels, with disseminations and veinlets of magnetite, pyrite, and chalcopyrite occurs in the lower portion of the Longfellow Limestone in some areas; calcite-pyrite-magnetite veinlets are bordered by tremolite alteration envelopes (Lindgren, 1905). Local, small bodies of magnesian skarn, consisting of serpentine-magnetite, presumably replaced the more dolomitic members of the Longfellow Limestone.

THE ROBINSON MINING DISTRICT

The porphyry copper deposits of the Robinson mining district, also known as the Ruth or Ely district, produced over 255 million tons of 1.1 percent copper ore in the period 1908 to 1963. Some 20 percent of this production was from skarn in carbonate rocks and from hornfels in shale; after 1962, the proportion of skarn ore relative or porphyry ore increased. Thus, in the 1960s and 1970s Ely ranked as one of the major skarn ore districts in North America.

The major sources of geological data on the district include general reviews by Bauer and others (1964, 1966) and detailed studies of altered igneous rocks by Fournier (1967*a*, 1976*b*) and of altered sedimentary rocks by James (1976).

General Setting

According to Bauer and others (1964), a pre-intrusive thrust fault separates the Chainman Shale of Mississippian age from the overlying Ely Limestone of Pennsylvanian age from the Rib Hill Sandstone of Permian age. The fault zone apparently controlled the emplacement of irregular porphyry plugs and sill-like bodies in Mid-Cretaceous time. Post-ore faulting resulted in approximately 50 percent extension and accentuated the east-west trend of the zone of intrusion and mineralization (James, 1976). Faulting also preserved different structural elevations of the original mineralized column (Figs. 7.20 and 7.21); carbonate rocks at Ely display both typical skarn associated with biotite-orthoclase-altered porphyry, and massive silica-pyrite impregnation associated with intensely sericitized porphyry (James, 1976). Thus, Ely forms an important link between the classic porphyry-skarn environment of districts such as Bingham or Mission, and the massive limestone replacement ores at Bisbee.

Base and precious metal replacement deposits occur in a broad belt, 3 km wide, which extends 15 km westward from the town of Ely along the porphyry intrusive trend; production from these peripheral deposits amounted to less than 1 million tons of ore (Bauer et al., 1966).

Porphyry

Alteration-mineralization in igneous rocks is extremely variable, depending in part on level of exposure. Originally deep zones of quartz monzonite, exposed at the surface or intercepted in drill core, reveal fresh magmatic minerals; the adjacent limestone is recrystallized or metasomatically altered over widths of a few centimeters. Major portions of the stocks contain hypogene, ore-grade copper mineralization associated with biotite-orthoclase alteration; pyrite:chalcopyrite ratios average around 4:1 (Bauer et al., 1964) and bornite occurs locally with chalcopyrite. Such high pyrite: chalcopyrite ratios are not characteristic of potassic alteration in porphyry deposits, and at Ely they reflect a sulfidation

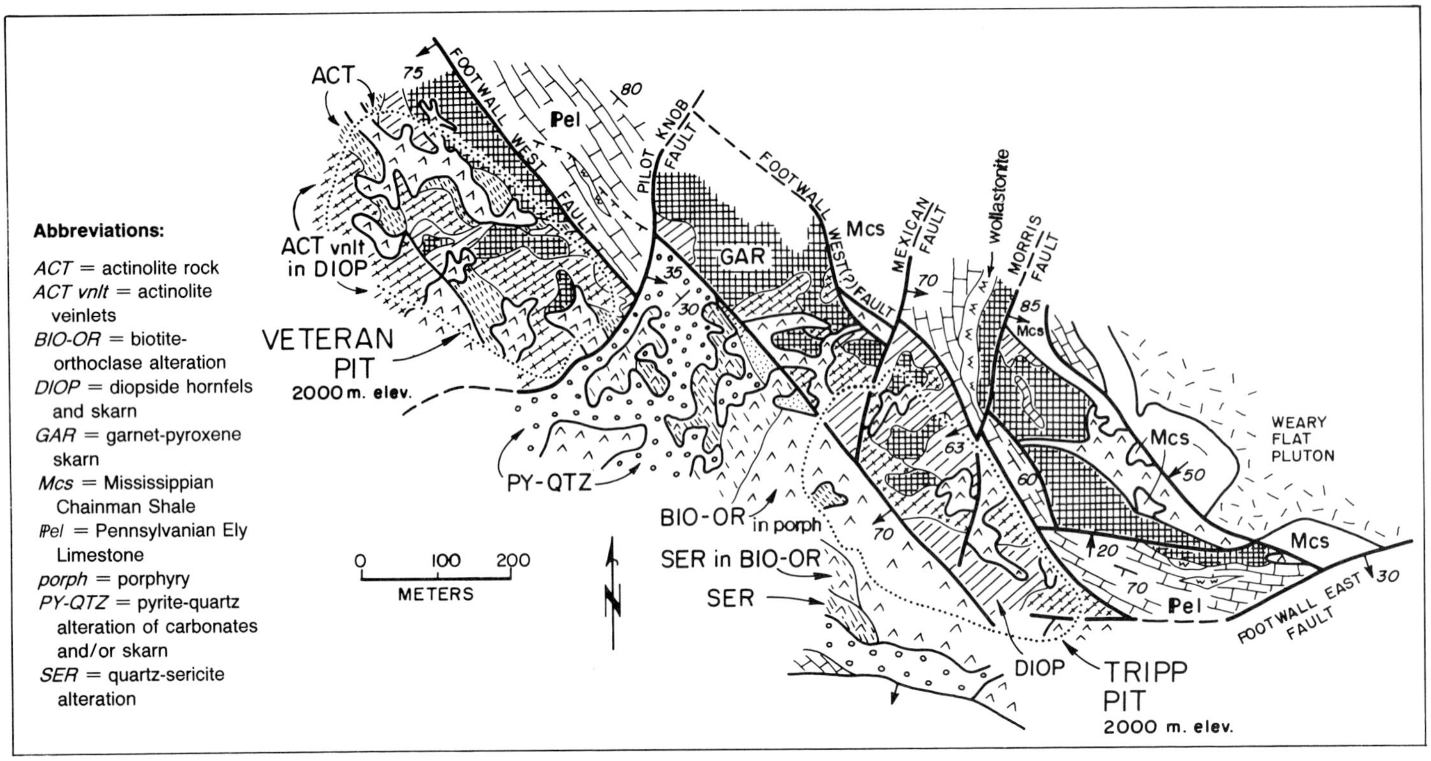

Figure 7.20. Surface geology in the area of the Tripp and Veteran pits in the Robinson (Ely) mining district, Nevada, illustrating the distribution of garnet-pyroxene skarn, diopside, and actinolite veinlet alteration relative to potassium-silicate alteration in porphyry; and the distribution of silica-pyrite alteration of limestone relative to sericitic alteration of porphyry. Redrawn from James (1972).

event accompanying the hydrolytic alteration of plagioclase to montmorillonite-sericite-kaolinite mixtures.

In the uppermost portions of open pits and in fault blocks which can be interpreted to have been originally at a high level relative to biotite-orthoclase alteration, the porphyry is intensely altered to a porous quartz-sericite-pyrite aggregate with subordinate (sub-ore grade) chalcopyrite. Areas of pervasive sericitic alteration grade into biotite-orthoclase alteration cut by quartz-sericite-pyrite veinlets.

Sedimentary Rocks

Two major alteration and mineralization styles occur in sedimentary rocks: calcic skarn and silica-pyrite.

Calcic Skarn. Limestone adjacent to biotite-orthoclase alteration displays a fairly typical skarn assemblage extending outward about 100 m (see Fig. 7.20). According to James (1976), garnet tends to occur near igneous contacts and gives way to garnet-pyroxene as the marble is approached. Red-brown garnet, associated with small amounts of interstitial quartz, calcite, and sulfides, generally contains greater than 90 mole percent andradite (James, 1976; Huang, 1976). A few fluid inclusions in garnet and in quartz-sulfide veinlets cutting garnet without alteration envelopes were studied by Huang (1976); homogenization temperatures ranged from 420 to 575°C. Diopsidic pyroxene, with generally less than 6 mole percent hedenbergite forms light green, fine-grained masses with interstitial quartz and local garnet veinlets.

The contact between skarn and marble locally is marked by a 5- to 10-m-thick zone of wollastonite-quartz with minor diopside, idocrase, and green garnet. Local zones within green garnets associated with wollastonite contain up to 50 mole percent grossularite (James, 1976). In many areas, wollastonite is absent, and skarn gives way to marble with local beds and masses of diopside-saponite-quartz-calcite, garnet-calcite-idocrase with minor fluorite, or pyrrhotite-magnetite-pyrite with local siderite. Small amounts of galena and sphalerite are common in the skarn-marble transition, but do not occur in economic concentrations. Beyond the skarn, bleaching and recrystallization, accompanied by local white clay, occur up to 300 m from known mineralized stocks.

The majority of copper mineralization in skarn is related to quartz-calcite-sulfide-magnetite veinlets concentrated within about 60 m of contacts with mineralization porphyry (Bauer et al., 1964; James, 1976). James (1976) has described the alteration selvages associated with these veinlets, which he has defined as the "clay-sulfide" stage, and has documented their dependence on original skarn mineralogy: in garnet rock, alteration envelopes are largely nontronite-calcite-quartz with lesser magnetite-calcite-quartz and actinolite; in diopside rock, envelopes are largely actinolite-calcite-quartz. The actinolite, which ranges from 17 to 31 mole percent ferroactinolite (James, 1976; Huang, 1976), locally replaces large volumes of diopside rock. In some areas, magnetite veinlets with talc-calcite-quartz alteration envelopes cut actinolite rock. At igneous contacts, actinolite skarn is replaced by phlogopite containing 15 to 33 mole percent annite.

James concludes that the "clay-sulfide" stage of altera-

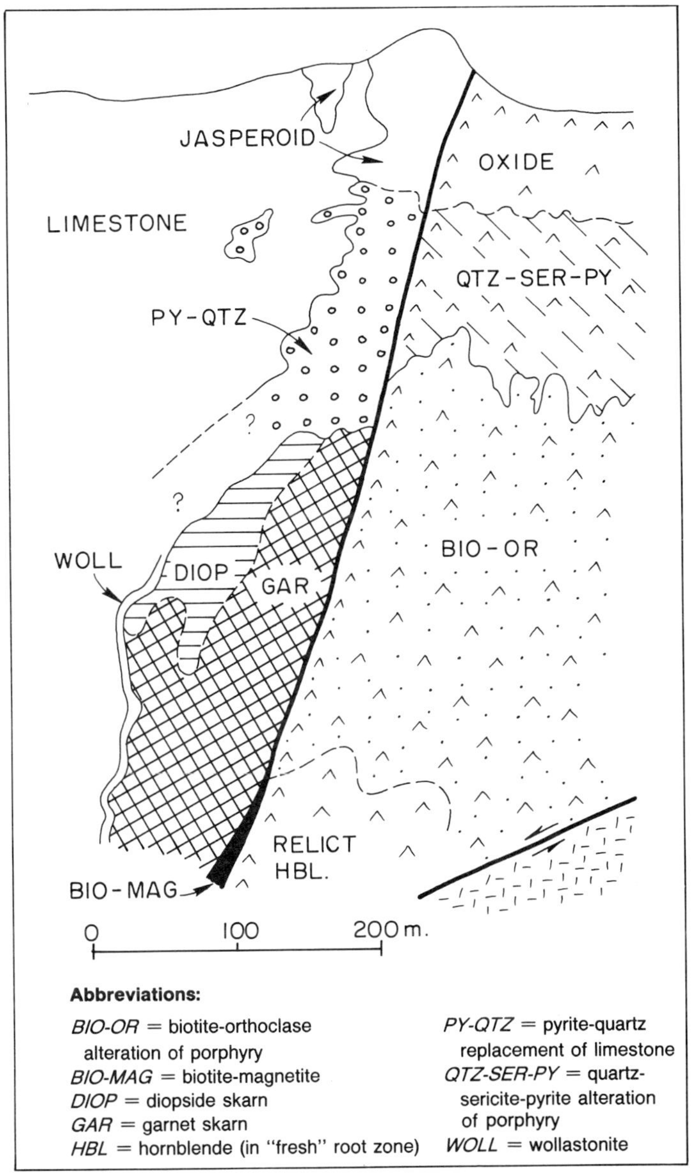

Figure 7.21. Schematic projection of mineral zoning in porphyry and limestone in a reconstructed (unfaulted) vertical cross section of the Robinson (Ely) mining district, Nevada. Redrawn from James (1976).

tion was synchronous with biotite-orthoclase alteration of igneous rocks. However, it is not clear whether actinolite and biotite alteration of diopsidic skarn and calcite-quartz-magnetite alteration of garnetite, which are included in the "clay-sulfide" stage, are synchronous with the formation of nontronite and ferro-saponite. A characteristic feature of many porphyry-related skarns is the presence of dark green actinolite alteration veinlets lacking brown, clay-altered diopside rock. Although this relation could be interpreted as the result of contemporaneous, zoned, actinolite-clay alteration of diopside, the common occurrence of identical actinolite veins in fresh diopside rock suggests that actinolite and clay alteration generally are not age-equivalent. The contemporaneity of actinolite alteration of diopside and biotitic alteration of the stock is convincingly illustrated in a sketch by James (1976, p. 502) of veinlet relations at skarn-stock contracts and is analogous to age relations observed at Bingham and Christmas. Clay alteration of diopside, with actinolite remaining stable, could then have occurred during the trend toward a hydrolytic base-leaching environment at lower temperatures, which resulted in sericitic-argillic alteration of plagioclase in the stock.

The above argument is supported to some extent by the geothermometric studies of Huang (1976). Huang found considerable variation in homogenization temperatures of fluid inclusions in quartz from clay-sulfide stage veinlets (with the majority falling in the range 275 to 475°C), and suggested that either boiling or appreciable temperature changes may have occurred. Ten samples, selected on the basis of internal consistency within a given sample, yielded temperatures of 315 to 445°C. Only 3 of the samples contained clay; the remainder contained quartz-calcite-sulfide-magnetite, with or without actinolite or biotite. Huang also attempted to define the temperature of the clay-sulfide stage by applying oxygen isotope fractionation factors to analyses of quartz-magnetite pairs. Although 9 determinations (355–465°C) fell in the general range of temperatures suggested by fluid inclusions in quartz of the clay-sulfide stage, 12 determinations were considerably higher (487–663°C) and fell in the range of temperatures determined from fluid inclusions of the main skarn stage. The implication is that: (1) veining of garnet-pyroxene skarn by quartz-sulfide-magnetite veinlets occurred over a broad range of temperatures and fluid compositions; (2) a significant amount of this veining occurred in the temperature range typically recorded by fluid inclusion studies of biotite-orthoclase alteration in porphyry systems and may well have been synchronous with such alteration; and (3) alteration of anhydrous calc-silicates along margins of these veinlets to calcite and/or actinolite-bearing quartz-magnetite-pyrite assemblages could have occurred during potassic alteration of the stock.

Silica-Pyrite. James (1976) has documented a close correlation of intense sericitic alteration of porphyry with massive quartz-pyrite replacement of limestone (see Fig. 7.20). One analysis of typical quartz-pyrite alteration yields, in weight percent: 28 percent quartz, 23 percent pyrite, and 48 percent calcite. Nontronite and siderite are present in minor amounts. In some cases, remnant sedimentary textures and patches of limestone indicate that quartz-pyrite replaced limestone; in other cases, it appears that quartz-pyrite replaced skarn. Relict skarn minerals, such as diopside, actinolite, and andradite, were noted near porphyry containing relict biotite-orthoclase alteration; these minerals suggest a transition to deeper skarn, although this transition was not directly observed.

THE MINERALIZED ZONE AT CANANEA

Cananea is located in north-central Sonora, 80 km by road from Bisbee, Arizona. The mineralized zone, 10 km long and 3.5 km wide, follows a northwesterly-striking belt of Laramide quartz porphyry stocks. Within this belt are located the mined-out, high-grade "plums" of the Capote and La Colorada breccia pipes and the immense tonnages of

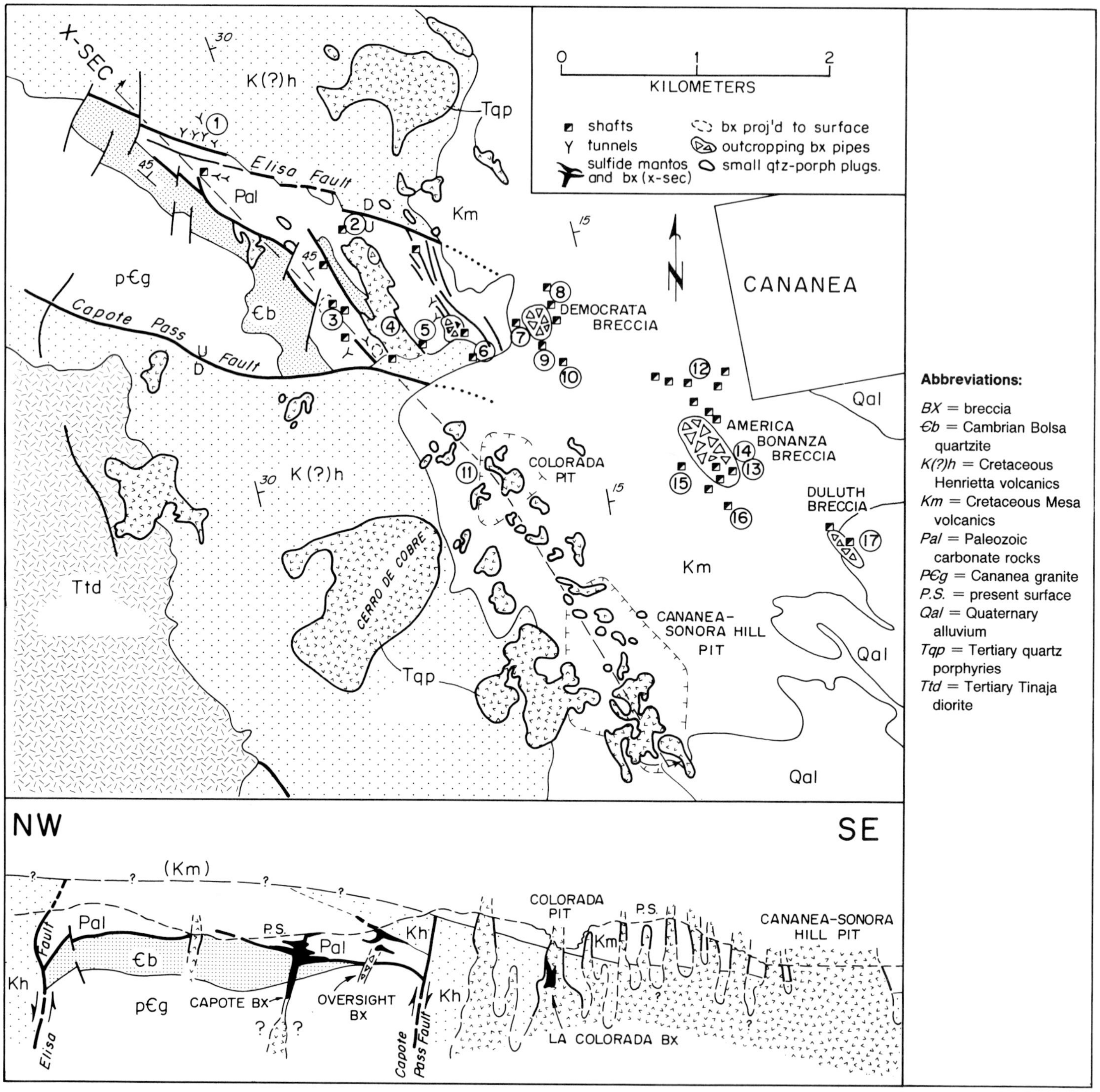

Figure 7.22. Generalized surface geology and cross section (looking northeast) of the Cananea mining district, Sonora, Mexico. The maps illustrate the location of: (1) supergene copper ores associated with the northwest-trending line of quartz porphyry plugs in Mesa volcanics at Colorada-Veta and Cananea-Sonora Hill pits; (2) ore breccia pipes in volcanic terrain at Duluth, America Bonanza, and Democrata; and (3) manto and breccia ores in Paleozoic carbonate rocks of Capote Basin horst. Mine locations: (1) Elisa mine tunnels, (2) Campana shaft, (3) Capote No. 2 shaft, (4) Capote No. 17 tunnel (Oversight), (5) Esperanza No. 1 shaft, (6) Veta Grande No. 5 shaft, (7) Democrata shaft, (8) Cobre Grande No. 5 shaft, (9) Kirk No. 9 shaft, (10) Kirk No. 10 shaft, (11) La Colorada shaft, (12) Cobre Grande shaft, (13) Cananea Central shaft, (14) Bonanza No. 1 shaft, (15) Bonanza No. 2 shaft, (16) Bonanza No. 3 shaft, (17) Cananea Duluth shaft. Based on Emmons (1910), Valentine (1936), and Velasco (1966).

disseminated ores that in 1981 were being mined at the Colorada-Veta and Cananea-Sonora pits. Twenty-year open-pit ore reserves in the latter area, published by Anaconda (Proxy Statement, 1976), were 213 million tons of 0.75 percent Cu; a substantially larger resource of approximately the same grade was estimated to exist beyond the reserves. Later figures indicated reserves of 1,500 million tons of 0.7 percent Cu (Maravilla, 1978).

General Setting

Pre-Laramide rocks exposed at Cananea include Precambrian granite, Paleozoic sedimentary rocks and Mesozoic(?) volcanic rocks. A 1,000-m-thick section of Paleozoic quartzite and limestone (see Fig. 7.2), which has been correlated with the Paleozoic section at Bisbee by Mulchay and Velasco (1954), is exposed in a west-northwest–trending horst, known as Capote Basin (Fig. 7.22). Here, the strata dip moderately to steeply northeast. North and south of the horst, the Paleozoic rocks are unconformably overlain by a minimum of 1,700 m of Mesozoic(?) tuffs and flows of dacitic to latitic composition which dip 30°ENE (Henrietta Formation of Valentine [1936]).

An older set of faults, which pre-dated the outpouring of Henrietta volcanics, are exposed in Capote Basin; they strike N45°W, and repeat the Paleozoic section to the northeast (e.g., Ricketts fault, Fig. 7.23). Younger faults (e.g., Capote Pass and Elisa faults, see Fig. 7.22) strike N20°W and dip vertically; these form the Capote Basin horst, and are post-Henrietta and pre-Laramide in age.

Laramide igneous activity, which extended from approximately 70 to 56 m.y. ago (Damon, 1965; Anderson and Silver, 1977), produced: (1) a complex series of equigranular diorite, granodiorite, and syenite plutons, which are largely exposed in the more deeply eroded terrains in the west-central portion of the range (e.g., Tinaja Diorite; see Fig. 7.22); (2) dominantly andesitic flows and tuffs of the Mesa Formation, which are preserved on the eastern range front, where they dip 15°ENE; and (3) a younger series of small quartz-porphyry stocks, plugs, and breccia pipes which are broadly contemporaneous with hydrothermal alteration-mineralization.

Emplacement of quartz porphyries was controlled on a district scale by the older, N45°W–striking faults, and this trend was especially marked by the belt of porphyry plugs extending through the Cananea–Sonora Hill and Colorado-Veta pits (see Fig. 7.22). On a local scale a set of north- to north-northeast-striking faults, with negligible displacement, and which are presumably of Laramide age, guided the emplacement of porphyries, breccias, and mineralization (Valentine, 1936).

Porphyry

Designation of the porphyries as quartz porphyries reflects their highly altered state; in fact, Schwartz (1947) had indicated that the Cananea porphyries represent the most completely sericitized rocks of the group of southwestern North American porphyry copper deposits he has studied. Work by Ochoa and Echavarri (1978) in the Colorado-Veta pit area suggests that the porphyries consist of at least four separate intrusive phases, ranging in composition from grandiorite to quartz monzonite.

Pervasive hypogene sericitic alteration of porphyry and andesitic wall rocks at the surface is centered on the belt of porphyry plugs. The presence of widespread hypogene alunite (Varela, 1972; Ochoa and Echavarri, 1978) suggests that advanced argillic alteration may be present in significant

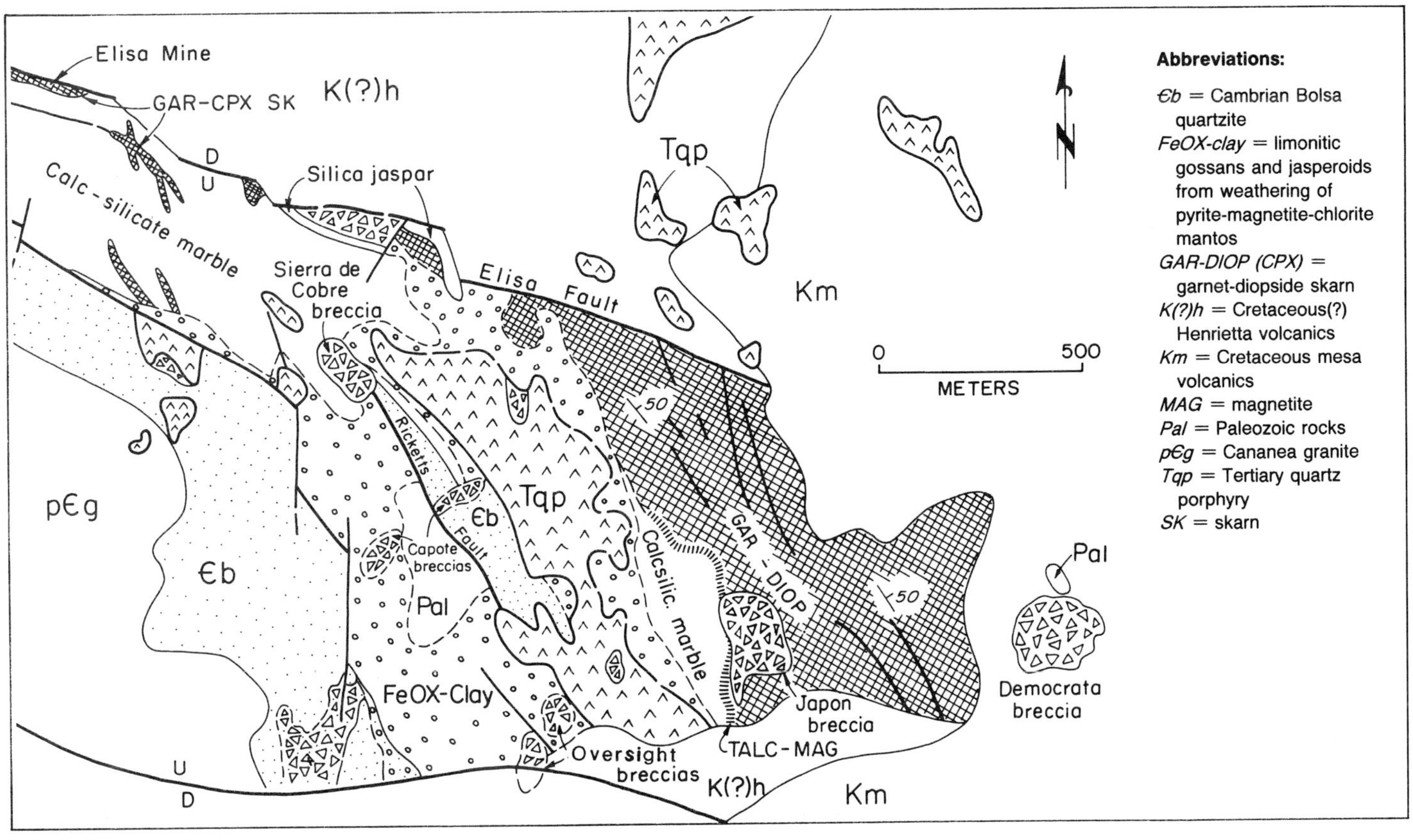

Figure 7.23. Preliminary geologic map of Capote Basin in the Cananea mining district, Sonora, Mexico, illustrating close spatial relation between pervasively sericitized porphyry, mineralized breccia pipes, and pyrite-magnetite-chlorite manto replacement bodies in carbonates. Skarn and calc-silicated marble appear as an earlier event. Based on L. D. Meinert (1977–1978, unpublished).

proportions within the broader sericitic zone, although replacement of sericite by kaolinite or pyrophyllite has not been reported. Quartz-sericite-pyrite alteration at the surface grades outward into propyllitic alteration at distances of approximately 250 m from porphyry contacts and diminishes in intensity with depth, so that at 500 m below the surface, the porphyries contain common fresh K-feldspar, biotite, negligible veining, and less than 1 percent sulfides—largely pyrite (Varela, 1972). Although the intensity of supergene chalcocite replacement renders it difficult to estimate the original content of chalcopyrite, it would appear that the majority of porphyries contained only trace amounts of hypogene copper-iron sulfides. Some porphyries, however, such as the Colorado quartz porphyry types described by Ochoa and Echavarri (1978), appear to have been the main sources of both chalcopyrite and molybdenite, and some deep drill holes have encountered significant intervals of copper-iron sulfide concentrations associated with an early (pre-sericite) generation of quartz veins and quartz breccias (R. Velasco, 1978, personal communication). The evidence suggests, however, that no broad zone of intense potassic alteration associated with disseminated copper mineralization with grades in excess of 0.2 percent Cu was ever formed at Cananea. Rather, copper was concentrated in structural openings —largely breccia pipes.

La Colorada Breccia

In 1926 La Colorada pipe was discovered; this extraordinary hypogene orebody was sacrificed at low copper prices to keep Anaconda in operation during the Great Depression. A series of papers by Perry (1933, 1935, and 1961) have summarized various aspects of La Colorada and other breccia pipe deposits at Cananea; sulfide paragenesis was studied by Kelley (1935). High-grade copper ore at La Colorada was enclosed in a pegmatitic quartz-phlogopite sheath located within a subsidence breccia near the apex of a quartz porphyry plug emplaced in volcanic rocks. During an early stage, a ring of massive molybdenite-chalcopyrite-bornite-chalcocite ore formed inside the quartz shell. Pyrite was concentrated peripherally and in overlying quartz veinlets during this early stage, and low-grade mineralization, consisting of quartz-chalcopyrite-molybdenite veinlets, extended downward at least 500 m below the ore pipe. A late stage is represented by the formation of pyrite-alunite veins containing luzonite, tennantite, covellite, sphalerite, and galena within the massive sulfide ring and by the formation of a brecciated core in the upper levels containing fragments of early sulfides altered to luzonite-tennantite and cemented by alunite and clays. A halo of silicification and sericitization, containing abundant alunite, extends 15 to 60 m outward into quartz porphyry on the bottom levels. Intense alkali-leaching alteration and sulfide mineralization do not extend above the top of the deposit, which was located 200 m below the pre-pit surface; the deposit at La Colorada had little surface expression, other than sporadic areas of slump breccia and quartz veinlets.

Thus, the sequential change from relatively low-sulfur assemblages, chalcopyrite-bornite-chalcocite and molybdenite-chalcopyrite-pyrite, to relatively high sulfur assemblages, containing luzonite and sphalerite, with parallel changes in gangue mineralogy from pegmatitic quartz-phlogopite to quartz-sericite-alunite, is especially well documented at La Colorada. Similar changes can be inferred for the quartz-porphyry belt as a whole.

Ores in Carbonate Rocks

The monumental treatment of Cananea geology by Emmons (1910) remains the best source of published data on the high-grade ores mined in Capote Basin during the turn of the century. The correlation of alteration-mineralization events in the volcanic terrain of the quartz-porphyry belt with events in the carbonate terrain of Capote Basin can be stated only in broad terms on the basis of published information. However, mapping by L. D. Meinert (1977–1978, personal communications) had yielded a sounder framework for such a correlation; some of his preliminary results are incorporated in Figure 7.23 and in the discussion which follows.

Emmons (1910) cast the ores occurring in carbonate rocks of Capote Basin into two general categories: (1) Skarn deposits, such as the Elisa and Puertecitos mines (see Fig. 7.22), in which bornite and chalcopyrite were the dominant copper-bearing sulfides, chalcocite enrichment locally was important, and hypogene grades averaged around 3 percent Cu; and (2) siliceous pyrite bodies in breccias or replacing limestone, such as the Capote, Oversight, Esperanza, and Veta Grande mines (Fig. 7.22), in which sphalerite locally was abundant, chalcopyrite occurred in small amounts, and supergene chalcocite enrichment was necessary to achieve ore grades. Perry (1933) has described the Capote orebody as a vertical breccia pipe cutting Precambrian granite and Cambrian quartzite at depth and grading into massive sulfide replacement bodies in limestone near the surface (see Fig. 7.22, cross section). The breccia, which extends over a known vertical interval of 350 m, contains mineralized angular fragments of porphyry and wall rock cemented by quartz, carbonates, pyrite, chalcopyrite, bornite, and chalcocite. The replacement ore, which occurs within 120 m of the surface, has been described by Emmons (1910) on one level as consisting of a supergene-enriched pyritic body, 100 m long and 50 m wide, containing 20 percent copper. Emmons has estimated that the copper grade of protore in the siliceous pyrite bodies of Capote Basin was less than 2 percent overall. Emmons concluded that these two deposit types represented successive periods of mineralization. He based this conclusion on the presence of transitional types, such as the Democrata, West Cobre Grande, and Kirk mines (see Fig. 7.22) in which early skarn, with minor bornite and sphalterite, was brecciated and cemented by quartz-pyrite, with minor chalcopyrite. In these ores he recognized the successively less important role of skarn formation and the increasing role of low-grade silica-pyrite mineralization.

On the district scale, according to Meinert, calcic skarn (Ad_{65-100}, Hd_{10-30}) was preceded by skarnoid (Ad_{15-50}, Hd_{5-15}), and both calc-silicate–forming events preceded the emplacement of quartz porphyry and breccias at the present level of exposure in Capote Basin. Skarn is restricted to the easternmost portion of the Basin, where it replaces Escabrosa Limestone (Puertecitos Formation of Mulchay and Velasco

[1954]), and does not occur as an envelope on the Capote quartz porphyry (see Fig. 7.23). Carbonate rocks in contact with quartz porphyry are recrystallized to marble and replaced by chlorite. The general area that includes porphyry and breccia pipes is a locus not of skarn, but of manto-type replacement bodies containing largely magnetite and pyrite, a lesser amount of chalcopyrite and specularite, and a gangue of calcite, quartz, and chlorite. Early skarnoid and hornfels are converted to epidote, chlorite, and clays. This type of alteration-mineralization extends in a discontinuous fashion for 3 km in thin-bedded, limestone-skarnoid-hornfels sequences of the Abrigo Formation (Esperanza Limestone of Mulchay and Velasco [1954]) from the deep levels of La Colorada mine on the southeast to the Elisa mine on the northwest (see Fig. 7.22). Weathering at the surface, particularly of the more pyritic zones, yields variable mixtures of iron-oxide, clays, and jasperoidal silica (shown as FeOX-Clay on Fig. 7.23).

The contemporaneity of manto replacement bodies in limestone, the destruction of skarnoid, and the deposition of pyrite-quartz in brecciated skarn with emplacement of quartz porphyry plugs and breccia pipes is suggested by Meinert's data. An intriguing unresolved question is the timing of skarn formation relative to older intrusive events.

THE BISBEE DEPOSIT

Within the group of deposits considered in this chapter, Bisbee fits at the end of the scale toward increasing sulfidation and hydrolytic alteration. The Sacramento stock, a complex of porphyries and intrusive breccias, was emplaced in Cambrian to Premain carbonate rocks (see Fig. 7.2). Hypogene ore containing greater than 3 percent Cu occurs in intrusive breccias and is associated with quartz-pyrite replacement bodies in limestone up to 2 km from the stock contact (Fig. 7.24).

Porphyry-Breccia Complex

Although large tonnages of low-grade, disseminated ore have been mined from intrusive rocks, this ore is exclusively supergene in origin. The primary mineralization-alteration bears little resemblance to the "typical" porphyry copper deposit. According to Bonillas and others (1917) and Bryant (1964, 1968), the primary ore consists largely of massive pyrite-bornite, with minor chalcopyrite, distributed erratically as isolated pods and lenses in highly silicified and sericitized intrusive breccias. The quartz porphyry is pervasively altered to a typical advanced argillic assemblage consisting of quartz-pyrophyllite-sericite with 15 to 18 percent pyrite and

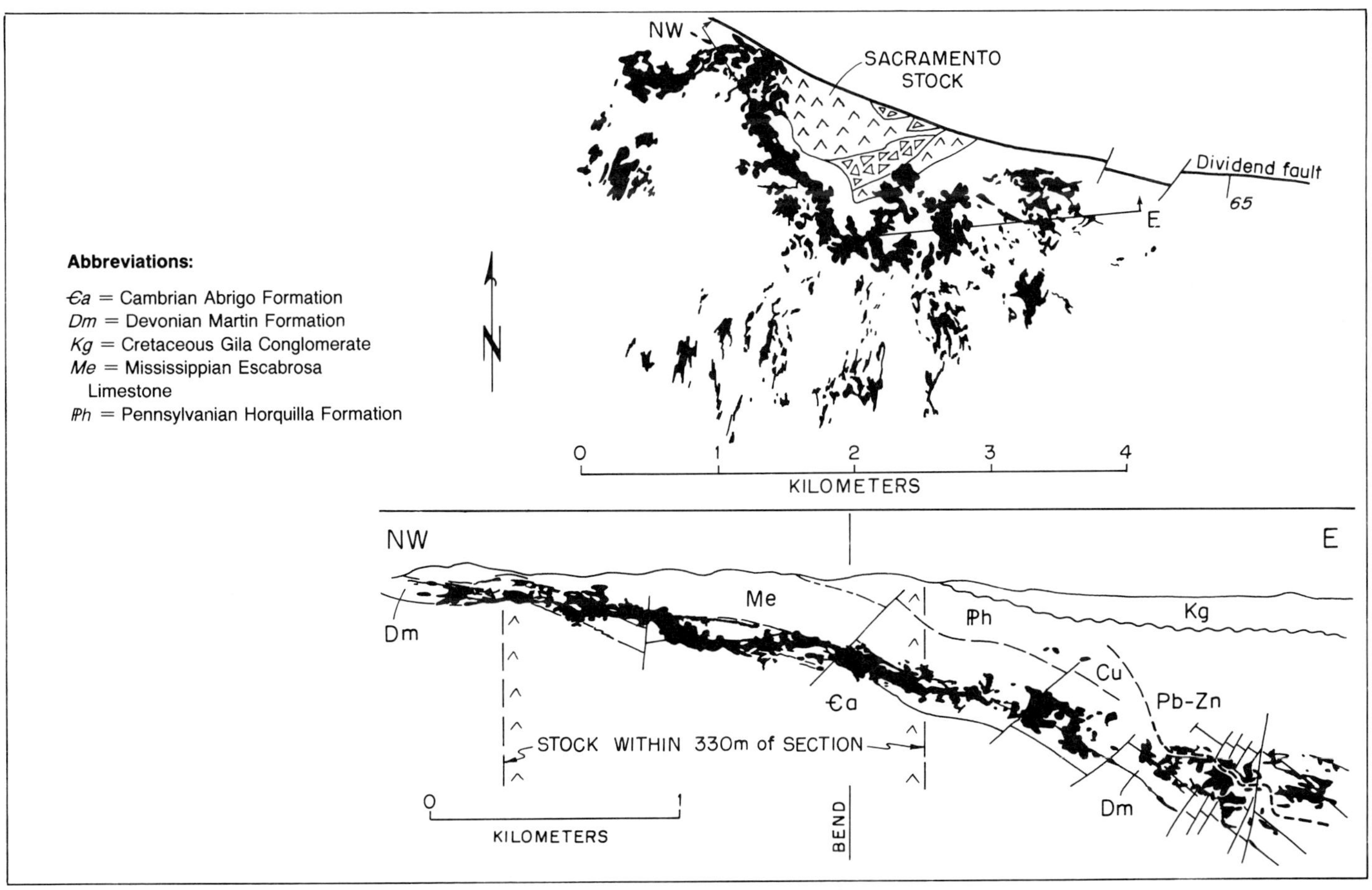

Figure 7.24. Projection of copper and lead-zinc stopes (black) in carbonate rocks to a horizontal plane (*top*) and vertical section (*bottom*) in the area of the Sacramento pit in the Bisbee mining district, Arizona. Only those stopes within 140 m of line of section (*top*) are projected onto vertical section (*bottom*). The figure illustrates the close spatial association of massive sulfide ores of copper in limestone (without skarn) with the porphyry-breccia complex of the Sacramento stock. Based on Bryant (1964).

accessory alunite, dickite, diaspore, and barite (Bryant, 1964). Local occurrences of pyrite-chalcopyrite veinlets with quartz-sericite-chlorite selvages in less-altered quartz-feldspar porphyry are reminiscent of sericitic alteration in the porphyry copper deposits, but there are no published accounts of potassium-silicate alteration.

It is conceivable that advanced argillic alteration destroyed the evidence of an earlier potassic stage. However, if the association of andradite-salite (± magnetite, chalcopyrite) skarn with potassium silicate alteration is accepted as the general case, then the apparent absence of skarn at Bisbee argues against the development of potassic alteration at the present level of exposure.

Sedimentary Rocks

According to Ransome (1904) calc-silicates occur as microscopic grains in greenish marble up to 350 m from the stock; the dominant silicates are tremolite and chlorite, with accessory grossularitic (?) garnet, diopside, and idocrase. These silicates are most prominent in the impure, shaly-sandy limestone of the Abrigo and Martin formations (Bonillas et al., 1917), and it is probable that they are entirely of metamorphic origin. The contact between the porphyry-breccia stock complex and relatively pure Escabrosa Limestone is characterized by only a narrow fringe of calc-silicates developed in marble. Locally up to 60 m from the stock, the marble is replaced by a granular aggregate of quartz-pyrite-calcite. The possibility that this zone represents the destruction of andradite skarn is not suggested by the published descriptions.

According to Trischka (1938) and Bryant (1964), the sulfide replacement bodies in limestone occur as pipe-like and ovoid masses, often associated with dikes and sills of porphyry or intrusive breccia, and are controlled by bedding and cross faults (see Fig. 7.24). The ores extend beyond the zone of contact silicates. The massive sulfide bodies are zoned from quartz-pyrite cores, which average less than 1 percent Cu, to intermediate pyrite-chalcopyrite ± bornite ore, to fringes of pyrite-sphalerite-galena. In some localities, specularite occurs between sulfides and limestone. Analyses of ore (Bonillas et al., 1917) indicate approximately 10–15 percent quartz, 15 percent copper-iron sulfides, and 50 percent pyrite. The ores in limestone at Bisbee, thus, are remarkably similar to the silica-pyrite zones at Ely and the manto ores at Cananea.

CONCLUSIONS

The data on ores in carbonate rocks associated with porphyry plutons indicate that, if the "noise" due to variability in original sedimentary lithologies, multiple intrusions, and early metamorphic events can be filtered out, the changes of alteration-mineralization with time can be correlated directly with events in the associated plutons. Table 7.10 summarizes these correlations.

Given a pluton displaying potassium-silicate alteration, the mineral associations in carbonate rocks can be predicted solely on the basis of original sedimentary lithology. Limestone develops andraditic garnet and diopsidic clinopyroxene with pyrite, chalcopyrite, and magnetite; outer zones may or may not contain wollastonite, but are consistently depleted in pyrite and enriched in bornite (without pyrite), sphalerite, pyrrhotite, and tennantite relative to garnet zones. Dolomite develops forsterite-serpentine-magnetite chalcopyrite skarn. Pyroxene hornfels is altered to actinolite and biotite along pyrite-chalcopyrite ± magnetite veinlets. The conclusion is

TABLE 7.10
Correlation of Generalized Stages of Skarn Evolution in Porphyry Copper Deposits

Temperature Range, °C	Intrusive Rocks	Sedimentary Rocks
900–700	Intrusion of melt	Some reaction with dolomite or, rarely, with limestone; no extensive skarn formed
700–500	Crystallization of pluton margins; emplacement of pre-skarn dikes	Metamorphism: decarbonation-dehydration reactions form light-colored silicates in impure carbonates: diopside forms in dolomitic siltstone; wollastonite (± diopside, grossularite, idocrase) in shaly limestone
600–400	Release of metasomatic fluid in partially solidified & fractured pluton; beginning of potassic alteration and disseminated chalcopyrite	Skarn formation proceeds outward along fissures, pre-skarn dikes, sedimentary contacts, permeable horizons: andradite-salite replaces wollastonite-diopside; magnetite replaces andradite near stock; interstitial sulfides. Actinolite-sulfide veinlets in fractured diopside hornfels
500–300	Continued potassic alteration; transition to sericitic. Disseminated and veinlet chalcopyrite-pyrite, molybdenite-pyrite	Ore deposition occurs before new skarn formation has ceased and continues during early skarn destruction; andradite → magnetite, quartz, pyrite, calcite, (actinolite); diopside → actinolite, calcite, quartz; early chalcopyrite remobilized into veins
350–200	Sericitic alteration accompanies influx of meteoric water; pyrite (± chalcopyrite) in veins. Local advanced argillic alteration	Retrograde alteration of skarn, during and after late stages of ore deposition, forms chlorite, montmorillonite, quartz, calcite, hematite, pyrite; peripheral sphalerite-galena-tennantite veins. Local silica-pyrite replacement bodies

Source: Based on Burt (1972, 1977), James (1976), Atkinson and Einaudi (1978).

NOTE: Emphasis is on calcic skarn.

that the physiochemical characteristics of hydrothermal fluids associated with potassium-silicate alteration in porphyry copper plutons were remarkably similar in the deposits considered.

Variability between porphyry-related skarn deposits largely involves the degree of retrograde alteration and is expressed in porphyry copper deposits in general by the degree of sericitic alteration (e.g., the "variation on a theme" of Gustafson and Hunt [1975]). Early stages of retrograde alteration of anhydrous skarn silicates probably are correlatable with the waning of potassic alteration and the beginning of sericitic; the dominant alteration products are quartz-magnetite (± pyrite, calcite) after andradite, and actinolite after salite. Sulfides are dominantly chalcopyrite with lesser pyrite. Later stages of retrograde alteration, correlated with main sericitic alteration in the pluton, involve increasing amounts of montmorillonoids (nontronite or ferrosaponite), chlorite, siderite, calcite, and hematite, accompanied by increasing pyrite and lesser chalcopyrite, tennantite, and sphalerite. The retrograde vent overprints the early skarn along zones of high permeability, which tend to occur along contacts with the pluton.

Skarns containing high-grade copper mineralization associated with unaltered garnet and pyroxene, such as Christmas and some portions of deep skarn at Carr Fork (Bingham) probably were mineralized prior to any retrograde alteration; in these cases, the better-grade zone tends to occur near the marble contact and a lower-grade garnet zone occurs near the stock. This spatial distribution may be the result of high temperatures near the stock, combined with the tendency for ferrous-clinopyroxene and/or calcite to be more abundant near marble. The latter could control the solubility of sulfides due to a decrease in f_{O_2} or an increase in pH, respectively (e.g., Crerar and Barnes, 1976).

Some deposits contain the highest grade of copper in skarn displaying relatively intense retrograde alteration at contacts with sericitized plutons, while less-altered anhydrous skarn farther out is only weakly mineralized. Examples include Ely and Chino (Santa Rita). These suggest that copper was introduced to the skarn, and not simply remobilized, during the retrograde stage. Possibly, some of this copper originated through leaching of early chalcopyrite in the stock by the relatively low pH fluids of the sericitic stage.

It is proposed that the presence of silica-pyrite bodies replacing limestone at contacts with porphyry plutons is *prima facie* evidence that the pluton never underwent potassium-silicate alteration at that level of exposure. The distribution in a given deposit of andradite skarn, as opposed to silica-pyrite, should enable the definition of the maximum upper extent of original potassium-silicate alteration in areas where this alteration has been overprinted and destroyed by sericitic alteration.

Bisbee and, to some extent, also Cananea differ in many regards from the generally accepted model of porphyry copper deposits. The term "porphyry copper deposit," when applied indiscriminantly to such deposits, masks the differences which are significant clues to variations in ore-forming processes. Table 7.11 and Figures 7.25 and 7.26 present a general classification of porphyry-related deposits; these stress the differences, rather than the obvious similarities, and are intended as a frame of reference with which to compare the deposits discussed in this chapter. The descriptive terms "disseminated" and "lode" are used with reference to the morphology and texture of ore occurrence (see Tables 7.11 and 7.12), but these reflect important differences in geological and geochemical environment, as discussed below. Both styles of sulfide occurrence may be present in a given deposit, but there is a tendency for most of the copper to be restricted to one or the other. Although no true endmember disseminated deposits may be identifiable, some possible endmember lode deposits are shown in Table 7.12 (last group listed under Deposit Examples). The latter, not classed as porphyry copper deposits, commonly are referred to as Cordilleran vein or lode deposits.

Five essential features serve to differentiate between lode mineralization and disseminated mineralization.

The development of major ore zones with intense silicification-sericitization or advanced argillic alteration, associated with pyrite-bornite-chalcocite and enargite, is the dominant feature of the copper zone of lode mineralization. In contrast, the characterizing feature of disseminated mineralization is the development of potassium-silicate alteration at the intermediate sulfidation-oxidation states implied by pyrite-chalcopyrite or chalcopyrite-bornite-magnetite. In both the lode copper and disseminated copper deposits, the trend of physiochemical evolution of the ore fluid with time at a given spot was the same: toward lower temperatures, higher sulfidation-oxidation states, and lower pH. However, the lode deposits reflect the extreme development of this trend, whereas the disseminated deposits show a pronounced development of the earlier stages.

Lateral zoning with distance from an igneous center is well established in the Peruvian lode deposits (see Table 7.12), where the sulfide assemblages record an outward decrease in sulfidation state (Petersen, 1970): enargite gives way to tennantite at approximately the point where pyrite-bornite gives way to pyrite-chalcopyrite and where sphalerite and then galena become abundant. These changes, which, if taken in conjunction with wall-rock alteration, imply an outward increase in pH, are especially pronounced in carbonate wall rocks. However, the same trend occurs in quartzo-feldspathic rocks, such as toward the western extremities of veins in the volcanic vent at Cerro de Pasco (Graton and Bowditch, 1936), near the periphery of the copper zone at Butte (Meyer et al., 1968), and toward the surface in the Magma vein (Hammer and Peterson, 1968). The zoning from core to fringe in the lode deposits is the reverse of the paragenetic sequence: high-sulfur sulfides generally replace low-sulfur sulfides (McKinstry, 1963), and sphalerite pre-dates the copper sulfides in the central copper zone (Meyer et al., 1968; Einaudi, 1977*b*). These data are consistent with outward expanding zones of alteration-mineralization. In contrast, the sulfide zonal pattern in disseminated deposits records an upward and outward increase in sulfidation state; chalcopyrite and chalcopyrite-pyrite give way to pyrite-bornite and minor sphalerite, and the zoning from core to fringe in this case parallels the paragenetic sequence from early to late (e.g., Gustafson and Hunt, 1975). These data are not consis-

TABLE 7.11
Generalized Characteristics of Endmember Types of Porphyry-Related Copper Deposits

LODE TYPE	DISSEMINATED TYPE
Igneous Rocks	
Small, isolated stocks and dikes of quartz monzonite porphry	Small stocks and dikes of quartz monzonite porphyry in many cases associated with multiple, larger, equigranular intrusions
Intrusive breccias common and associated with ore	Pebble dikes and breccias less common and largely post-date ore
Post-ore porphyries absent	Post-ore porphries common
Ore Textures and Grade	
Sulfides occur as massive, open space fillings in veins, breccias; replacement bodies	Sulfides are finely disseminated and in veinlets; peripheral veins
Irregular distribution of sulfides commonly leads to selective mining	Uniform distribution leads to bulk mining
10 million tons of 6% Cu, to 500 million tons of 2% Cu; no large tonnages of 0.5% Cu (except supergene or superimposed on disseminated stage)	100 to 2,000 million tons of 0.35 to 1.0% Cu; higher grades only in skarn
Molybdenum generally absent	Molybdenum generally present, average grade 0.015% Mo
Copper ores with 2 to 4 oz./ton silver; relatively low Cu:Ag	Average around 0.05 oz./ton silver; relatively high Cu:Ag
Contains major lead-zinc-silver ores in peripheral areas of both igneous and sedimentary rocks	Rarely contains major lead-zinc-silver ore; if present, only in limestone
Sulfides, General	
Enargite & bornite major ore minerals	Chalcopyrite major ore mineral
Pyrite abundant and generally early	Pyrite less abundant and generally late
Sphalerite ubiquitous in copper zone and precedes copper mineralization	Sphalerite rare in copper zone and post-dates copper mineralization
Tin-tungsten-bismuth minerals common, trace in central Cu-zone	Molybdenite common in central Cu zone and deeper
Lateral Zoning of Major Opaque Minerals	
Central: pyrite-digenite-enargite, with trace amounts of tin-tungsten-bismuth minerals	*Central:* bornite-chalcopyrite-magnetite, or pyrite-chalcopyrite, with molybdenite
Intermediate: pyrite-bornite-chalcopyrite-tennantite, with minor sphalerite	*Intermediate:* pyrite-chalcopyrite
Peripheral: pyrite-chalcopyrite-tennantite-sphalerite-galena, with minor hematite	*Peripheral:* pyrite, with minor chalcopyrite, tennantite, sphalerite, and galena; hematite or magnetite
Limestone: pyrite, bornite, chalcopyrite, tennantite, sphalerite, galena; minor magnetite or hematite	*Limestone:* pyrite-chalcopyrite-magnetite; minor sphalerite, tennantite, pyrrhotite
Major Gangue Minerals	
Quartz, pyrite, sericite, kaolinite, alunite, barite, carbonates	Feldspars, biotite, quartz, anhydrite, sericite
Lateral Zoning of Alteration Types	
Central: advanced argillic and silicification (pyrophyllite or kaolinite replaces sericite)	*Central:* potassic (biotite replaces hornblende; orthoclase replaces plagioclase)
Intermediate: sericitic (sericite replaces montmorillonite and orthoclase)	*Intermediate:* sericitic (sericite replaces feldspars)
Peripheral: well-developed intermediate argillic grades to propylitic (montmorillonite replaces plagioclase; chlorite replaces mafics)	*Peripheral:* intermediate argillic weak to absent; grades to propylitic
Limestone: massive quartz-pyrite bodies, breccias, mantos; contains siderite, calcite, specularite, magnetite, chlorite, clays	*Limestone:* zoned skarns with andradite-diopside; late actinolite, chlorite, clays, pyrite

NOTE: These characteristics refer to porphyry-related copper deposits which are associated with calc-alkaline magmatism in continental margin mobile belts of Mesozoic and younger age. Possible examples of a continuum between the two endmember types of deposits are listed in Table 7.12.

tent with outward expanding zones of alteration-mineralization; rather, the high-level sericitic zone expands onto the deeper potassic zone. Thus, downward and inward zoning accompanying meteoric water influx in the disseminated deposits mimics the outward zoning of the lode deposits and represents the embryonic development of the lode stage.

Lode deposits in igneous rocks are mined for copper, zinc, and often lead, silver, and manganese. The bulk of the ore minerals in igneous rocks are restricted to through-going vein systems or breccia pipes, are generally massive, and may be erratically distributed in ore shoots or pods. The morphology and texture of ore occurrence suggest that rapid deposition inhibited infiltration or diffusion of metals into wall rocks. These features of ore distribution are reflected in mining grades; selective underground mining in the copper zone of lode deposits characteristically yields ore grades of 2.5 to 5.5 percent Cu, with an average zinc content of nearly 1 percent and a silver content of 2 to 4 oz. per ton; bulk mining methods yield hypogene copper ores that range from 1.2 to 2.0 percent Cu. In contrast, disseminated deposits are mined for copper and molybdenum; silver is a by-product; and peripheral zones rarely contain significant lead-zinc mineralization unless they are rich in carbonate rocks. The ore minerals tend to be uniformly distributed in veinlets or as disseminations in porphyry; late porphyries and breccia pipes commonly are lower in grade. Copper ores rarely achieve grades that would support selective underground mining. The average hypogene copper grade in igneous rocks of 17 North and South American examples (from Lowell and Guilbert, 1970) is 0.44 percent Cu, and it rarely exceeds 1.0 percent.

Minor to trace amounts of bismuth sulfides (bismuthinite, wittichenite), tin sulfides (stannite, colusite), and tungsten minerals (wolframite, scheelite) occur in the copper zone of the lode deposits, but they are not reported from disseminated deposits. In many cases, the tin, tungsten, bismuth minerals are most abundant with enargite in the core of the copper zone: bismuthinite and wolframite occur with

TABLE 7.12
Continuum Between Lode-Type and Disseminated-Type Endmembers in Porphyry-Related Copper Deposits

Degree of Development Disseminated Stage	Degree of Development Lode Stage	Deposit Examples	Alteration in Limestone	Sources
Major, contains all known ore	Unknown (never formed, or removed by erosion)	Christmas, Arizona	Skarn	Koski & Cook, 1982; Perry, 1969
		Twin Buttes, Arizona	Skarn	Barter & Kelly, 1982
		Mission, Arizona	Skarn	Gale, 1965; Einaudi, 1974
		Bingham, Utah	Skarn	Atkinson & Einaudi, 1978
		Silver Bell, Arizona	Skarn	Richard & Courtright, 1966; Graybeal, 1982
		Santa Rita, New Mexico	Skarn	Nielsen, 1968, 1970
Major, highest grade (all of Cu and Mo introduced during this stage?)	Minor, lower grade (Cu leached during this stage?)	Ely, Nevada	Skarn, silica-pyrite	James, 1976
		Red Mountain, Arizona	Limestone absent	Corn, 1975
		El Salvador, Chile	Limestone absent	Gustafson & Hunt, 1975
Major, well-mineralized (all of Mo and most of Cu introduced during this stage?)	Major, highest grade (Cu leached from earlier stage and concentrated?)	Butte, Montana	Limestone absent	Meyer et al., 1968; Brimhall, 1979
		Chuquicamata, Chile	Limestone absent	Lopez, 1939; Perry, 1952
Local, minor, or absent (very minor Cu and Mo introduced?)	Major, highest grade (most of Cu introduced during this stage?)	Cananea, Mexico	Skarn?, silica-pyrite	Emmons, 1910; Kelley, 1935; Perry, 1961
		Morococha, Peru	Skarn, silica-pyrite	Barrentes, 1970; Petersen, 1965
		Bisbee, Arizona	Silica-pyrite	Bryant, 1964
Absent? (no Cu, no Mo)	Major (all of Cu introduced during this stage?)	Magma, Arizona	Silica-pyrite	Hammer & Peterson, 1965
		Cerro de Pasco, Peru	Silica-pyrite	Petersen, 1965; Einaudi, 1977*b*
		Yauricocha, Peru	Silica-pyrite	Petersen, 1965

NOTE: Characteristics of disseminated stage and lode stage are summarized in Table 7.11.

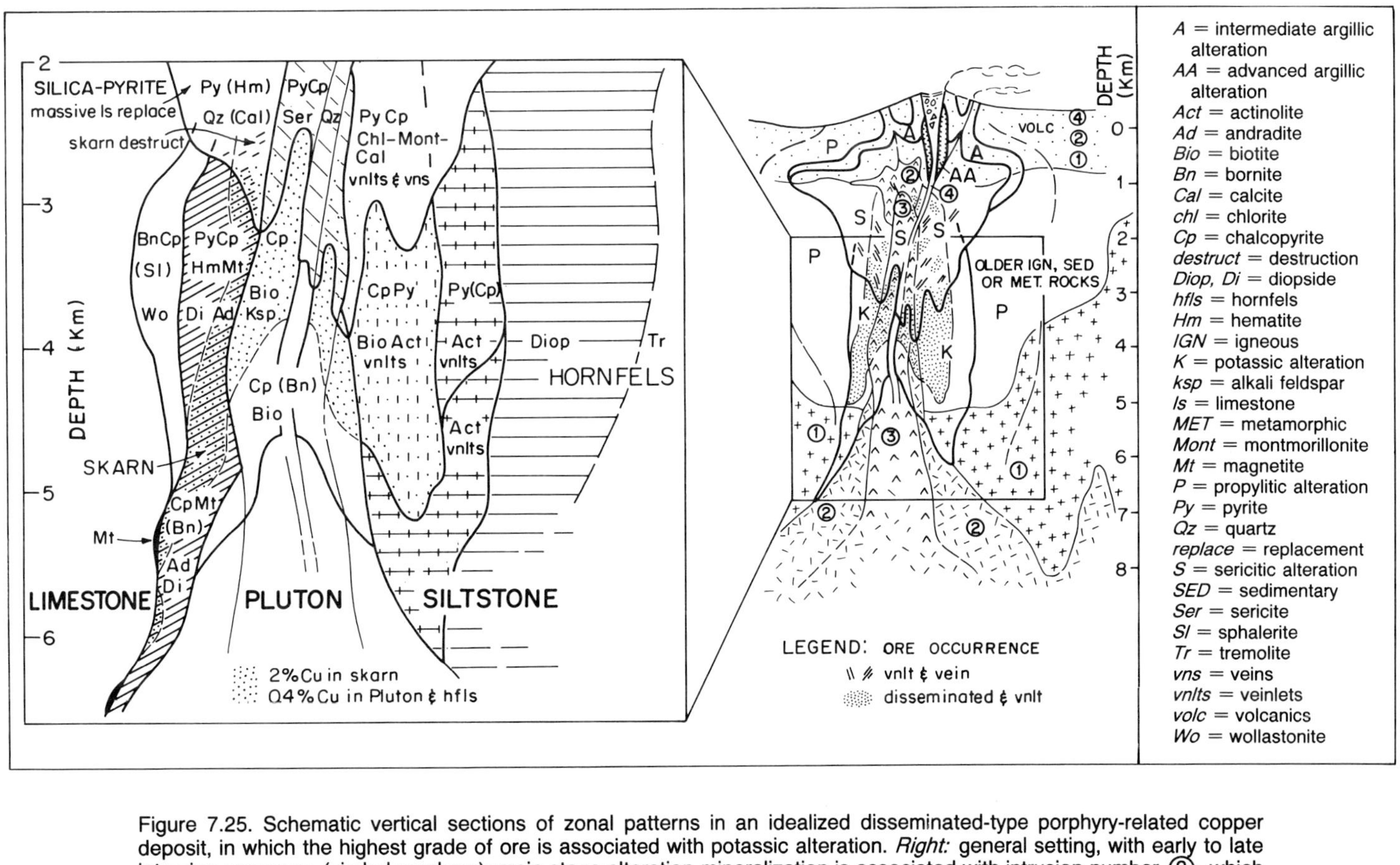

Figure 7.25. Schematic vertical sections of zonal patterns in an idealized disseminated-type porphyry-related copper deposit, in which the highest grade of ore is associated with potassic alteration. *Right:* general setting, with early to late intrusion sequence (circled numbers); main-stage alteration-mineralization is associated with intrusion number ③, which does not vent. Heavy lines enclose dominant alteration types, including a deep and central potassic, peripheral propylitic, and later sericitic. Advanced argillic alteration is restricted to a near-surface vent; argillic and propylitic alteration dominate in the volcanic edifice. Based on Lowell and Guilbert (1970), Sillitoe (1973), Gustafson and Hunt (1975), and Einaudi, Proffett, and others (in preparation). *Left:* equivalent zonal patterns in limestone and calcareous siltstone, mainly based on deposits at Christmas, Arizona, and in the Pima, Bingham, and Robinson mining districts.

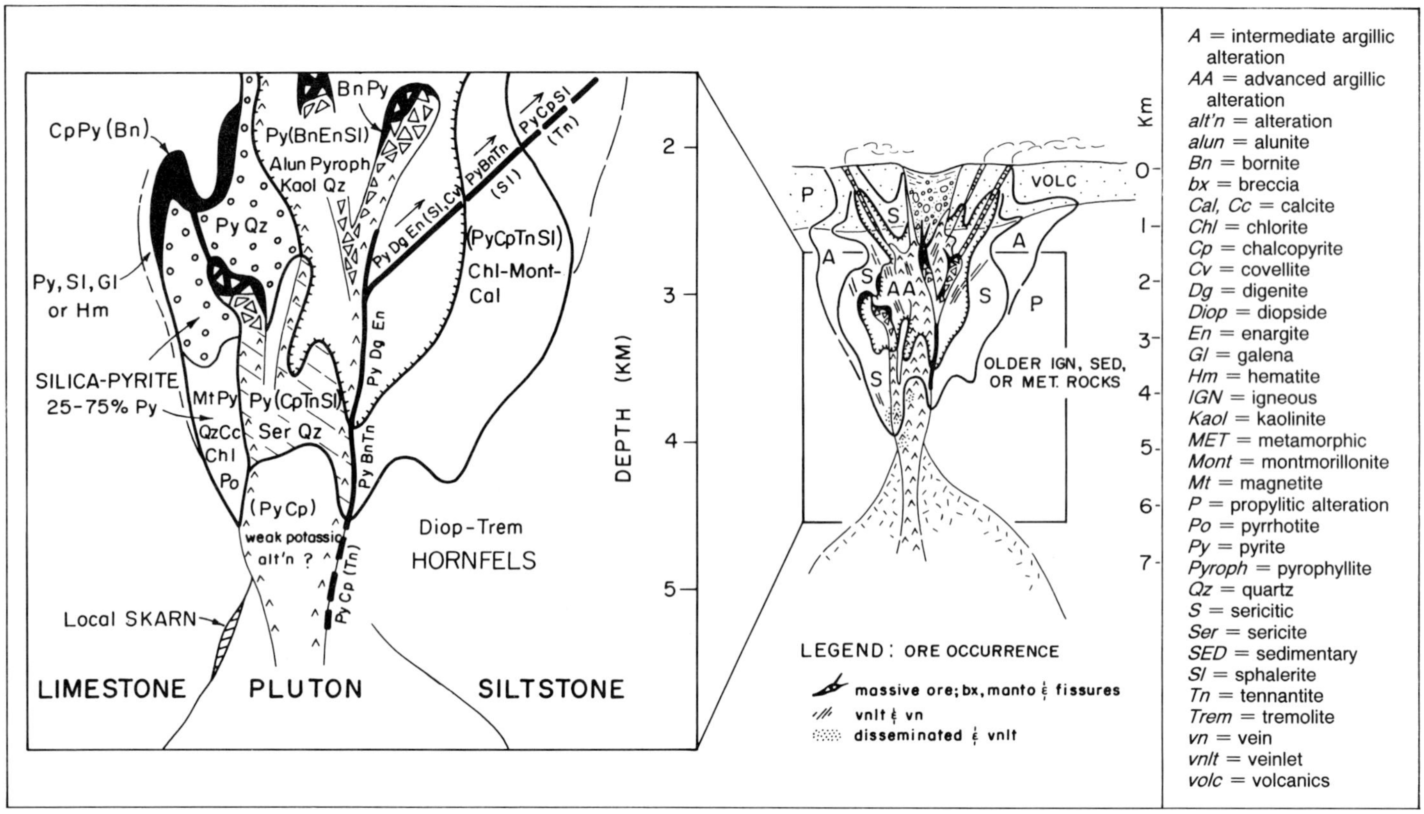

Figure 7.26. Schematic vertical sections of zonal patterns in an idealized lode-type porphyry-related copper deposit, in which the highest grade of ore consists of massive sulfide vein-fillings and mineralized breccias associated with silification and advanced argillic alteration. *Right:* general setting, with heavy lines enclosing dominant alteration types (advanced argillic, with peripheral sericitic and intermediate argillic). Based on Graton and Bowditch (1936) and Meyer and others (1968). *Left:* equivalent zonal patterns in limestone and calcareous siltstone. Based on Hammer and Petersen (1967), Petersen (1965), and Einaudi (1977*b*).

enargite at Yauricocha (Petersen, 1965); stannite, wolframite and scheelite occur in the copper zone at Morococha (Petersen, 1965); colusite and wittichenite are rare constituents of copper ores at Magma (Hammer and Peterson, 1968); colusite and huebnerite are most abundant in the pyrite-covellite-digenite-enargite ores at Butte (John M. Proffett, Jr., 1974, personal communication); and wittichenite and scheelite are also known to occur in the copper zone (Meyer et al., 1968). At Cerro de Pasco, stannite, wolframite, and cassiterite occur in the early, low-sulfur, pyrrhotite stage of mineralization (Einaudi, 1977*b*).

The Limestone wall rocks of the lode deposits characteristically contain copper and lead-zinc ores associated with replacement pipes and mantos of passive pyrite-quartz, with local carbonates and specular hematite; calc-silicates are absent. Sulfide assemblages generally reflect a lower sulfidation state than those in associated igneous wall rocks, with pyrite-chalcopyrite-bornite present, rather than pyrite-bornite-chalcocite, and tennantite present, rather than enargite. Ore pipes and mantos are markedly zoned, with an early, barren pyrite-quartz stage or core zone, surrounded by copper and peripheral lead-zinc ores. In addition to the obvious analogies between Bisbee and Cerro de Pasco (Einaudi, 1977*b*), the zoning in silica-pyrite bodies at Bisbee is a remarkable duplication of zoning in the ore pipes in limestone at Morococha (Petersen, 1965), and also bears some resemblance to ore breccias in limestone at Yauricocha (Thomson, 1960, as summarized by Petersen, 1965) and mantos in limestone near the Magma vein (Hammer and Peterson, 1968).

The lack of ore-bearing skarns in limestone near contacts with leached igneous rocks in lode deposits is one of their most striking features and sets a sharp contrast with the disseminated deposits, where limestone wall rocks characteristically contain ore-bearing andradite-diopside skarns. Metasomatic replacement of limestone in the lode deposits apparently occurred at lower temperatures and/or higher sulfur fugacities than the andradite stability field. The relatively low pH of fluids associated with lode mineralization also effectively suppressed the formation of calc-silicates.

Factors which may control the degree of development of disseminated, as opposed to lode, mineralization in porphyry-related copper deposits have briefly been summarized by Gustafson and Hunt (1975) and Einaudi (1977*b*) and are implicit in the chemical model of Meyer and Hemley (1967). The major variables, as stated by Gustafson and Hunt, include: (1) geometries, time factors, and depth of emplacement of intrusions; (2) abundance of metals and volatiles evolved from the melt; and (3) degree of groundwater availability. The ultimate control may be the timing of groundwater influx.

If the influx is retarded due to deep emplacement, a prolonged period of intrusive activity, large size of intrusions, or relatively dry and impermeable wall rocks, then the mineralizing porphyry system cools slowly, and disseminated ore zones and skarn are favored. As the transition from alkali to hydrogen ion metasomatism occurs, due to decreasing pressure and temperature, accompanied and enhanced by the encroachment of groundwater, a stage of hypogene leaching begins. At Ely and El Savador (Chile) overall depletion of copper may have occurred. At Butte, Brimhall (1979) has suggested that a new hydrothermal system, possibly largely meteoric in origin, was activated by heat supplied by late porphyry plugs. The lode stage, which post-dated the disseminated stage by several million years, initially leached chalcopyrite and resulted in whole-rock copper and iron depletion. This was followed by re-precipitation of copper as pyrite-bornite and pyrite-digenite-covellite in Main Stage veins. Chuquicamata (Chile) also may fit this model. At both Butte and Chuquicamata, the lode stage was superimposed directly onto the earlier stage of disseminated chalcopyrite and potassium-silicate alteration.

If the influx of groundwater occurs early—due to shallow porphyry emplacement, a limited period of intrusive activity, small size of intrusions, or relatively wet and permeable wall rocks—then the mineralizing porphyry cools rapidly, and lode-type deposits in igneous rocks and silica-pyrite replacement ores in limestone are favored. In this case, the lode stage may represent the first introduction of copper into the system. Deposits which may fit this end-member case include Cerro de Pasco (Peru), Yauricocha (Peru), and Magma (see Table 7.12). Bisbee and Cananea may represent deposits intermediate between Butte and Cerro de Pasco.

Alteration and mineralization in carbonate wall rocks of porphyry plutons are intimately tied to the environment of emplacement of the melt, to its subsequent cooling history and volatile evolution, and the geometries of hydrothermal convection. The type of alteration observed in carbonate rocks is an additional clue to unraveling these events. A goal of future research should be to place the above generalizations on a firmer base of field observation, analytical data, experimentation, and thermochemical computation.

ACKNOWLEDGMENTS

The thoughts expressed in this chapter represent the distillation of personal research, publication by authors cited in the text, and discussions with numerous colleagues. The last of these points is the most difficult to acknowledge, yet may be the most productive of ideas. In this regard, the mine geologists acknowledged in the section on individual deposits aided the author in acquiring the local context which could not be acquired by reading the literature. Colleagues who have had a significant influence on the author's thinking on porphyries and skarns include: W. W. Atkinson, Jr., R. C. Baker, D. M. Burt, L. B. Gustafson, and J. P. Hunt. The Anaconda Company, Anamax Mining Company, and U. V. Industries released useful data, and C. F. Barter, D. S. Cook, F. T. Graybeal, J. L. Kelly, R. A. Koski, and D. L. Norton supplied the author with early versions of the manuscripts for the chapters they contributed to this book. An all-day crash drafting session by graduate students at Stanford University saved the author from a great deal of embarassment. Finally, the encouragement and patience of S. R. Titley is gratefully acknowledged.

REFERENCES CITED

Anderson, T. H., and Silver, L. T., 1977, U-Pb isotope ages of granitic plutons near Cananea, Sonora: Econ. Geol., v. 72, p. 827–836.

Atkinson, W. W., Jr., and Einaudi, M. T., 1978, Skarn formation and mineralization in the contact aureole at Carr Fork, Bingham, Utah: Econ. Geol., v. 73, p. 1326–1365.

Barrentes, E. T., 1970, Geología y estructura del yacimiento del proyecto de Morococha, *in* Geología de los yacimientos minerales operados por la Cerro de Pasco Corp., Primer Cong. Latino Americano de Geol., Lima, Peru: La Oroya, Peru, Cerro de Pasco Corp., p. 131–155.

Barter, C. F., and Kelly, J. L., 1982, Geology of the Twin Buttes mineral deposit, Pima Mining District, Pima County, Arizona, *in* Titley, S. R., ed., Advances in Geology of the Porphyry Copper Deposits, Southwestern North America: Tucson, Univ. Ariz. Press, Chapter 20.

Bauer, H. L., Jr.; Breitrich, R. A.; Cooper, J. J.; and Swinderman, J. N., 1964, Origin of the disseminated ore in metamorphosed sedimentary rocks, Robinson mining district, Nevada: AIME Trans., v. 229, p. 131–140.

Bauer, H. L., Jr.; Breitrich, R. A.; Cooper, J. J.; and Anderson, J. A., 1966, Porphyry copper deposits in the Robinson mining district, Nevada, *in* Titley, S. R., and Hicks, C. L., eds., Geology of the Porphyry Copper Deposits, Southwestern North America: Tucson, Univ. Ariz. Press, p. 233–244.

Bonillas, Y. S., Tenney, J. B., and Feuchere, L., 1917, Geology of the Warren mining district: AIME Trans., v. 55, p. 284–355.

Brimhall, G. H., Jr., 1979, Lithologic determination of mass transfer mechanisms of multiple-stage porphyry copper mineralization at Butte, Montana: Vein formation by hypogene leaching and enrichment of potassium-silicate protore: Econ. Geol., v. 74, p. 556–589.

Brant, D. G., 1964, Intrusive breccias and associated ore of Warren (Bisbee) mining district, Cochise County, Arizona: Unpub. Ph.D. thesis, Stanford Univ., 149 p.

———, 1968, Intrusive breccias associated with ore, Warren (Bisbee) mining district, Arizona: Econ. Geol., v. 63, p. 1–12.

Bryant, D. G., and Metz, H. E., 1966, Geology and ore deposits of the Warren mining district, *in* Titley, S. R., and Hicks, C. L., eds., Geology of the Porphyry Copper Deposits, Southwestern North America: Tucson, Univ. Ariz. Press, p. 189–204.

Burt, D. M., 1972, Mineralogy and geochemistry of Ca-Fe-Si skarn deposits: Unpub. Ph.D. Thesis, Harvard Univ., 256 p.

———, 1977, Mineralogy and petrology of skarn deposits: Rendiconti So. Ital. Mineral. Petrol., v. 33, p. 859–873.

Buseck, P. R., 1962, Contact metasomatic deposits at Concepción del Oro, Mexico; Tem Piute, Nevada; and Silver Bell, Arizona: Unpub. Ph.D. Thesis, Columbia Univ., N.Y.

Butler, W. C., 1971, Permian sedimentary environments in southeastern Arizona: Ariz. Geol. Soc. Digest, IX, p. 71–94.

Cooper, J. R., 1960, Some geologic features of the Pima mining district, Pima County, Arizona: U.S. Geol. Survey Bull. 1112-C, p. 63–103.

———, 1971, Mesozoic stratigraphy of the Sierrita Mountains, Pima County, Arizona: U.S. Geol. Survey Prof. Paper 658D, 42 p.

Corn, R. M., 1975, Alteration-mineralization zoning, Red Mountain, Arizona: Econ. Geol., v. 70, p. 1437–1447.

Damon, P. E., compiler, 1965, Correlation and chronology of ore deposits and volcanic rocks: U.S. Atomic Energy Comm. Contract AT(11–1)-689, Ann. Prog. Rept. COO-689-50: Tucson, Geochron. Labs., Univ. Ariz., p. A-II-3.

Eastlick, J. T., 1968, Geology of the Christmas mine and vicinity, Banner mining district, Arizona, *in,* Ridge, J. D., ed., Ore Deposits of the United States, 1933–1967 (Graton-Sales vol.): AIME, New York, p. 1192–1210.

Einaudi, M. T., 1974, Skarn study, Palo Verde mine, Pima County, Arizona: unpublished report, The Anaconda Co., 44 p.

———, 1977*a*, Petrogenesis of copper-bearing skarn at the Mason Valley mine, Yerington district, Nevada: Econ. Geol., v. 72, p. 769–795.
———, 1977*b*. Environment of ore deposition at Cerro de Pasco, Peru: Econ. Geol., v. 72, p. 893–924.
———, 1982, General features and origin of skarns associated with porphyry copper plutons, southwestern North America, *in* Titley, S. R., ed., Advances in Geology of the Porphyry Copper Deposits, Southwestern North America: Tucson, Univ. Ariz. Press, Chapter 8.
Emmons, S. F., 1910, The Cananea mining district of Sonora, Mexico: Econ. Geol., v. 5, p. 312–256.
Forrester, J. D., 1972, Skarn formation and sulfide mineralization at the Continental mine, Fierro, New Mexico: Unpub. Ph.D. Diss., Cornell Univ., 205 p.
Fournier, R. O., 1967*a*, The porphyry copper deposit exposed in the Liberty open pit mine near Ely, Nevada: Part I, Syngenetic formation: Econ. Geol., v. 62, p. 57–81.
———, 1967*b*, The porphyry copper deposit exposed in the Liberty open pit mine near Ely Nevada: Part II, The formation of hydrothermal alteration zones: Econ. Geol., v. 62, p. 207–227.
Gale, R. E., 1965, The geology of the Mission copper mine, Pima mining district, Arizona: Unpub. Ph.D. Thesis, Stanford Univ., 162 p.
Gilluly, J.; Copper, J. R.; and Williams, J. S., 1954, Late Paleozoic stratigraphy of central Cochise county, Arizona: U.S. Geol. Survey Prof. Paper 266, 49 p.
Graton, L. C., and Bowditch, S., 1936, Alkaline and acid solutions in hypogene zoning at Cerro de Pasco: Econ. Geol., v. 31, p. 651–698.
Graybeal, F. T., 1982, Geology of the El Tiro area, Silver Bell mining district, Pima County, Arizona, *in* Titley, S. R., ed., Advances in Geology of the Porphyry Copper Deposits, Southwestern North America: Tucson, Univ. Ariz. Press, Chapter 24.
Greenwood, E.; Kottlowski, F. E.; and Thompson, S. III, 1977, Petroleum potential and stratigraphy of Pedregosa Basin: Comparison with Permian and Orogrande basins: Amer. Assoc. Pet. Geol. Bull., v. 61, p. 1448–1469.
Gustafson, L. B., and Hunt, J. P., 1975, The porphyry copper deposit at El Salvador, Chile: Econ. Geol., v. 70, p. 857–912.
Hallof, P. G., and Winniski, E., 1971, A geophysical case history of the Lakeshore ore body: Geophysics, v. 36, p. 1232–1249.
Hammer, D. F., and Peterson, D. W., 1968, Geology of the Magma mine area, Arizona, *in,* Ridge, J. D, ed., Ore Deposits of the United States, 1933–1967 (Graton-Sales vol.): AIME, New York, v. 2, p. 1282–1310.
Hansen, L. A., 1961, The stratigraphy of the Carr Fork mines, Bingham district, Utah: Utah Geol. Soc., Guidebook to the Geology of Utah, No. 16, p. 71–81.
Hayes, P. T., 1978, Cambrian and Ordovician rocks of southeastern Arizona and southwestern New Mexico: New Mexico Geol. Soc. Guidebook, 29th Field Conf., p. 165–173.
Hernon, R. M., 1949, Geology and ore deposits of Silver City region, New Mexico: West Texas Geol. Soc. Guidebook Field Trip 3.
Hernon, R. M., and Jones, W. R., 1968, Ore deposits of the Central Mining district New Mexico, *in* Ridge, J. D., ed., Ore Deposits of the United States, 1933–1967 (Graton-Sales vol.): AIME, New York, p. 1211–1238.
Himes, M. D., 1973, Mineralization and alteration at Pima mine—a complex porphyry copper deposit: AIME Trans., v. 254, p. 166–174.
Huang, Chi-I, 1976, An isotopic and petrologic study of the contact metamorphism and metasomatism related to copper deposits at Ely, Nevada: Unpub. Ph.D. Thesis, Penn. State Univ., 178 p.
Hunt, J. P., 1957, Rock alteration, mica, and clay minerals in certain areas in the United States and Lark mines, Bingham, Utah: Unpub. Ph.D. Thesis, Univ. Calif., Berkeley, 321 p.
Hunt, R. N., 1924, The ores in limestone at Bingham, Utah: AIME Trans., v. 70, p. 856–883.
Irvin, G. W., 1959, Pyrometasomatic deposits at San Xavier mine: Southern Arizona Guidebook II, Ariz. Geol. Soc. p. 195–197.
James, A. H., 1971, Hypothetical diagrams of several porphyry copper deposits: Econ. Geol., v. 66, p. 43–47.
James, L. P., 1972, Zoned hydrothermal alteration and ore deposits in sedimentary rocks near mineralized intrusions, Ely area, Nevada: Unpub. Ph.D. Thesis, Penn. State Univ., 241 p.
———, 1976, Zoned alteration in limestone at porphyry copper deposits, Ely, Nevada: Econ. Geol., v. 71, p. 488–512.
John, E. C., 1978, Mineral zones in the Utah Copper ore body: Econ. Geol., v. 73, p. 1250–1259.
Jones, W. R.; Hernon, R. M.; and Moore, S. L., 1967, General geology of Santa Rita quadrangle, Grant County, New Mexico: U.S. Geol. Survey Prof. Paper 555, 144 p.
Journeay, J. A., 1959, Pyrometasomatic deposits at Pima mine: Southern Arizona Guidebook II, Ariz. Geol. Soc., p. 198–199.
Kelley, V. C., 1935, Paragenesis of the Colorada copper sulfides, Cananea, Mexico: Econ. Geol., v. 30, p. 663–688.
Kinnison, J. E., 1966, The Mission copper deposit, Arizona, *in* Titley, S. R., and Hicks, C. L., eds., Geology of the Porphyry Copper Deposits, Southwestern North America: Tucson, Univ. Ariz. Press, p. 281–287.
Knopf, A., 1918, Geology and ore deposits of the Yerington district, Nevada: U.S. Geol. Survey Prof. Paper 114, 68 p.
Koski, R. A., 1978, Porphyry-type alteration and mineralization of igneous rocks at Christmas, Arizona: Unpub. Ph.D. Diss., Stanford Univ., 196 p.
Koski, R. A., and Cook, D. S., 1982, Geology of the Christmas porphyry copper deposit, Gila County, Arizona, *in* Titley, S. R., ed., Advances in Geology of the Porphyry Copper Deposits, Southwestern North America: Tucson, Univ. Ariz. Press, Chapter 17.
Lacy, W. C., 1959, Structure and ore deposits of the east side of the Sierrita Mountains, Arizona: Southern Arizona Guidebook II, Ariz. Geol. Soc., p. 185–192.
Langlois, J. D., 1978, Geology of the Cyprus Pima mine, Pima county, Arizona: Ariz. Geol. Soc. Digest, XI, p. 103–113.
Lanier, G.; John, E. C.; Swenson, A. J; and others, 1978, General geology of the Bingham mine, Bingham Canyon, Utah: Econ. Geol., v. 73, p. 1228–1241.
Lanier, G.; Raab, W. J.; Folsom, R. B; and Cone, S., 1978, Alteration of equigranular monzonite, Bingham mining district, Utah: Econ. Geol., v. 32, p. 1270–1286.
Lindgren, W. 1905, The copper deposits of the Clifton-Morenci district, Arizona: U.S. Geol. Survey Prof. Paper 43, 375 p.
Lindgren, W.; Graton, L. C.; and Gordon, C. H., 1910, The ore deposits of New Mexico: U.S. Geol. Survey Prof. Paper 68, 361 p.
Lopez, V. M., 1939, The primary mineralization at Chuquicamata, Chile, S. A.: Econ. Geol., v. 34, p. 674–711.
Lowell, J. D., and Guilbert, J. M., 1970, Lateral and vertical alteration-mineralization zoning in porphyry copper deposits: Econ. Geol., v. 65, p. 373–408.
MacKenzie, F. D., 1959, Pyrometasomatic deposits at the Mineral Hill and Daisy mines: Southern Arizona Guidebook II, Ariz. Geol. Soc., p. 193–194.
———, 1963, Geological interpretation of the Palo Verde Mine based upon diamond drill core: Ariz. Geol. Soc. Digest, VI, p. 41–48.
Maravilla, S., 1978, Minas en producción, minas en preparación y depósitos con reservas o menos conocidas en el Estado de Sonora: 1° Simposio Geol. Potencial Minero, Estado Sonora, Inst. Geol., U.N.A.M., Hermosillo, Sonora, Mexico, p. 85–87.
McKee, E. D., 1951, Sedimentary basins of Arizona and adjoining areas: Geol. Soc. Amer. Bull., v. 62, p. 481–506.
McKinstry, H., 1963, Mineral assemblages in sulfide ores: The system Cu-Fe-As-S: Econ. Geol., v. 58, p. 483–505.

Meyer, C., and Hemley, J. J., 1967, Wall rock alteration, *in* Barnes, H. L., ed., Geochemistry of Hydrothermal Ore Deposits: N.Y., Holt, Rinehart and Winston, p. 166–235.

Meyer, C.; Shea, E. P.; Goddard, C. C., Jr.; and Staff, 1968, Ore deposits at Butte, Montana, *in* Ridge, J. D., ed., Ore Deposits of the United States, 1933–1967 (Graton-Sales vol.): New York, AIME, p. 1373–1416.

Moolick, R. T., and Durek, J. J., 1966, The Morenci district, *in* Titley, S. R., and Hicks, C. L., eds., Geology of the Porphyry Copper Deposits, Southwestern North America: Tucson, Univ. Ariz. Press, p. 221–232.

Moore, W. J., 1978, Chemical characteristics of hydrothermal alteration at Bingham, Utah: Econ. Geol., v. 73, p. 1260–1269.

Moore, W. J., and Nash, J. T., 1974, Alteration and fluid inclusion studies of the porphyry copper ore body at Bingham, Utah: Econ. Geol., v. 69, p. 631–645.

Mulchay, R. B., and Velasco, J. R., 1954, Sedimentary rocks at Cananea, Sonora, Mexico, and tentative correlation with the sections at Bisbee and the Swisshelm Mountains, Arizona: AIME Trans., v. 199, p. 628–632.

Nielsen, R. L., 1968, Hypogene texture and mineral zoning in a copper-bearing granodiorite porphyry stock, Santa Rita, New Mexico: Econ. Geol., v. 63, p. 37–50.

———, 1970, Mineralization and alteration in calcareous rocks near the Santa Rita stock, New Mexico: New Mexico Geol. Soc. Guidebook 21st Field Conf., p. 133–139.

Ochoa, H., and Echavarri, A., 1978, Observaciones preliminares sobre la secuencia de las intrusiones hipabisales en el tajo Colorada-Veta del distrito minero de Cananea: Bol. Dpto. Geol. Uni-Son., v. 1, p. 57–60.

Parkinson, G., 1976, Cyprus develops moly-talc separation float: Eng. Mining Jour., May, 1976, p. 97.

Peirce, H. W., 1976, Elements of Paleozoic tectonics in Arizona: Ariz. Geol. Soc. Digest X, p. 37–57..

Perry, D. V., 1968, Genesis of the contact rocks at the Christmas mine, Gila county, Arizona: Unpub. Ph.D. Thesis, Univ. Ariz., 229 p.

———, 1969, Skarn genesis at the Christmas mine, Gila county, Arizona: Econ. Geol., v. 64, p. 255–270.

Perry, V. D., 1933, Applied geology at Cananea, Sonora, Mexico, *in* Ore deposits of the Western states (Lindgren vol.): New York, AIME, p. 701–709.

———, 1935, Copper deposits of the Cananea district, Sonora, Mexico, *in* Copper Resources of the World: Int. Geol. Cong., 16th, v. 1, p. 413–418.

———, 1952, Geology of the Chuquicamata ore body: Min. Eng. v. 4, p. 1166–1168.

———, 1961, The significance of mineralized breccia pipes: AIME Trans., v. 220, p. 216–226.

Petersen, Ulrich, 1965, Regional geology and major ore deposits of central Peru: Econ. Geol., v. 60, p. 407–476.

———, 1970, Metallogenic provinces in South America: Geol. Rundschau, v. 59, p. 834–897.

Peterson, N. P., and Swanson, R. W., 1956, Geology of the Christmas copper mine, Gila county, Arizona: U.S. Geol. Surv. Bull. 1027-H, p. 351–373.

Proffett, J. M., Jr., 1977, Cenozoic geology of the Yerington district, Nevada, and implications for the nature and origin of basin and range faulting: Bull. Geol. Soc. America, v. 88, p. 247–266.

Proffett, J. M., Jr., and Proffett, B. H., 1976, Stratigraphy of the tertiary ash-flow tuffs in the Yerington district, Nevada: Nev. Bur. Mines Geol., Rpt. 27, 28 p.

Ransome, F. L., 1904, Geology and ore deposits of the Bisbee quadrangle, Arizona: U.S. Geol. Survey, Prof. Paper 21, 168 p.

Reber, L. E., 1916, The mineralization of Clifton-Morenci: Econ. Geol., v. 11, p. 528–573.

Reid, J. E., 1978, Skarn alteration of the Commercial limestone, Carr Fork area, Bingham, Utah: Econ. Geol., v. 73, p. 1315–1325.

Richard, K., and Courtright, J. H., 1959, Some geologic features of the Mission copper deposit: Southern Arizona Guidebook II, Ariz. Geol. Soc., p. 201–204.

———, 1966, Structure and mineralization at Silver Bell, Arizona, *in* Titley, S. R., and Hicks, C. L., eds., Geology of the Porphyry Copper Deposits, Southwestern North America: Tucson, Univ. Ariz. Press, p. 157–164.

Roberts, R. J.; Crittenden, M. D., Jr.; Tooker, E. W.; Morris, H. T.; Hose, R. K.; and Cheney, T. M., 1965, Pennsylvanian and Permian basins in northwestern Utah, northwestern Nevada, and south-central Idaho: Am. Assoc. Pet. Geol. Bull., v. 49, p. 1926–1956.

Rose, A. W., and Baltosser, W. W., 1966, The porphyry copper deposit at Santa Rita, New Mexico, *in* Titley, S. R., and Hicks, C. L., eds., Geology of the Porphyry Copper Deposits, Southwestern North America: Tucson, Univ. Ariz. Press, p. 205–220

Ross, C. A., 1978, Late Pennsylvanian and Early Permian sedimentary rocks and tectonic setting of the Marathon Geosyncline: Permian Basin sec.: Soc. Econ. Paleont. Mineral., Pub. 78–17, p. 181–189.

Ross, C. P., 1925, Ore deposits of the Saddle Mountain and Banner mining districts, Arizona: U.S. Geol. Surv. Bull. 771, 72 p.

Rubright, R. D., and Hart, O. J., 1968, Non-porphyry ores of the Bingham district, Utah, *in* Ridge, J. D., ed., Ore Deposits of the United States, 1933–1967 (Graton-Sales vol.): New York, AIME, p. 886–908.

Schmitt, H. A., 1939, The Pewabic mine, New Mexico: Bull. Geol. Soc. America. v. 50, p. 777–818.

Schwartz, G. M., 1947, Hydrothermal alteration in the "porphyry copper" deposits: Econ. Geol., v. 42, p. 319–352.

Shafiqullah, M., and Langlois, J. D., 1978, The Pima mining district, Arizona—A geochronologic update: New Mex. Geol. Soc. Guidebook, 29th Field Conf., p. 321–327.

Sillitoe, R. H., 1973, Tops and bottoms of porphyry copper deposits: Econ. Geol., v. 68, p. 799–815.

South, D. L., 1972, Sulfide zoning at the Lakeshore copper deposit, Pinal county, Arizona: Unpub. M.S. Thesis, Univ. Ariz., 79 p.

Speed, R. C., 1978, Paleogeographic and plate tectonic evolution of the early Mesozoic marine province of the western Great Basin, *in* Howell, D. G., and McDougall, K. A., eds., Mesozoic paleogeography of the western United States: Pacific Coast Paleogeogr. Symp., Soc. Econ. Paleont. Mineral., v. 2, p. 253–270.

Stewart, C. A., 1912, The geology and ore deposits of the Silver Bell mining district, Arizona: AIME Bull., v. 65, p. 455–506.

Stoddard, Carl, and Carpenter, J. A., 1950, Mineral resources of Storey and Lyon counties, Nevada: Univ. Nev. Bull., Geol. Mining Ser., no. 49, 115 p.

Titley, S. R., 1976, Evidence for a Mesozoic linear tectonic pattern in southeastern Arizona: Ariz. Geol. Soc. Digest, X, p. 71–101.

Trischka, C., 1938, Bisbee district: Ariz. Bur. Mines Bull. 145, p. 32–41.

Valentine, W. G., 1936, Geology of the Cananea Mountains, Sonora, Mexico: Bull. Geol. Soc. America, v. 47, p. 53–86.

Varela, F. E., 1973, Tourmaline in the Cananea mining district, Sonora, Mexico: Unpub. M.S. Thesis, Univ. Calif. Berkeley, 79 p.

Velasco, J. R., 1966, Geology of the Cananea district, *in* Titley, S. R., and Hicks, C. L., eds., Geology of the Porphyry Copper Deposits, Southwestern North America: Tucson, Univ. Ariz. Press, p. 245–250.

Willden, Ronald, 1964, Geology of the Christmas quadrangle, Gila and Pinal counties, Arizona: U.S. Geol. Surv. Bull. 1161-E, p. 1–64.

Wilson, J. R., 1963, Geology of the Yerington mine: Min. Cong. Jour., v. 49, no. 6, p. 30–34.

8

General Features and Origin of Skarns Associated With Porphyry Copper Plutons

SOUTHWESTERN NORTH AMERICA

Marco T. Einaudi

Altered carbonate wall rocks in porphyry copper deposits are sulfide-rich and contain variable mixtures of calc-silicates, various forms of silica, carbonates, clays, and iron oxides. Most commonly, these minerals display a complex zonal and paragenetic distribution which reflects changing structural controls, variations in original composition and permeability of sedimentary rocks, and space-time variations in the physical and chemical properties of the hydrothermal fluid. In spite of these complexities, the following key themes emerge:

1. Within individual deposits, the evolution of alteration mineralization in carbonate rocks can be correlated with hydrothermal events in the pluton: (a) dominantly metamorphic processes accompany the early stages of stock emplacement and crystallization; (b) skarn formation in marbles and biotite-actinolite alteration of hornfelses, accompanied by sulfides, are broadly contemporaneous with potassium-silicate alteration in the stock; and (c) alteration of skarn and hornfels to quartz-clay-carbonate-pyrite accompanies sericitic alteration in the stock. In some deposits, where hypogene leaching evolves to an extreme, silicification and advanced argillic alteration of the stock is accompanied by locally complete skarn destruction and/or formation of massive silica–sulfide–iron-oxide replacement bodies in marble.
2. Variability in alteration styles between deposits in some cases may be a function of level of erosion, but in some extreme cases (e.g., andradite-diopside-chalcopyrite skarn at Christmas versus sulfide-quartz-carbonate replacement pipes at Bisbee) it appears to reflect important differences in the temperature and volatile fugacities of hydrothermal fluids *at the time metasomatic replacement begins.*
3. The distinction between porphyry-related skarns and other copper-dominant skarns largely rests on the degree of development of certain features. Skarns formed in immediate contact with mineralized porphyry plutons are larger, display more massive and fine-grained textures, and contain a higher density of fractures, veins, and retrograde alteration than non-porphyry skarns. Small, copper-bearing skarns associated with barren, phaneritic granodiorite and quartz monzonite stocks may represent either porphyry systems which are deeply eroded or intrusive systems which never generated the hydrothermal fluids and permeabilities required for mineralization of the stocks.
4. The mineralogy of porphyry-related calcic skarns reflects their relatively oxidized, sub-volcanic environment: garnets tend to be andradite (high Fe^{+3}); pyroxenes are diopside-salite (low Fe^{+2}); pyrite rather than pyrrhotite is the dominant iron sulfide; and specular hematite often is abundant, in addition to magnetite.

These and other themes are developed in detail in this chapter. First, the common features of carbonate-hosted ores related to porphyry copper plutons are summarized, based to a large extent on the descriptive data presented in Chapter 7 of this volume. Then, experimental and theoretical data are used to propose a genetic framework.

DEPTHS OF SKARN FORMATION AND CONFIGURATION OF PLUTONS AND CONTACT AUREOLES

Depths of formation of porphyry copper–related skarns have been estimated by various methods, including stratigraphic-structural reconstructions and fluid inclusion studies. Estimates of depths of emplacement at Yerington, Christmas, Bingham, and Ely are summarized in Figure 8.1. The vertical extent of mineralized rocks is on the order of 1 to 2 km, and depths below the volcanic surface range from 1 to 2 km for the shallowest sericitic ore zones to 3 to 5 km for the deepest potassium silicate ore zones. Such depths are compatible with the general depth environment of porphyry

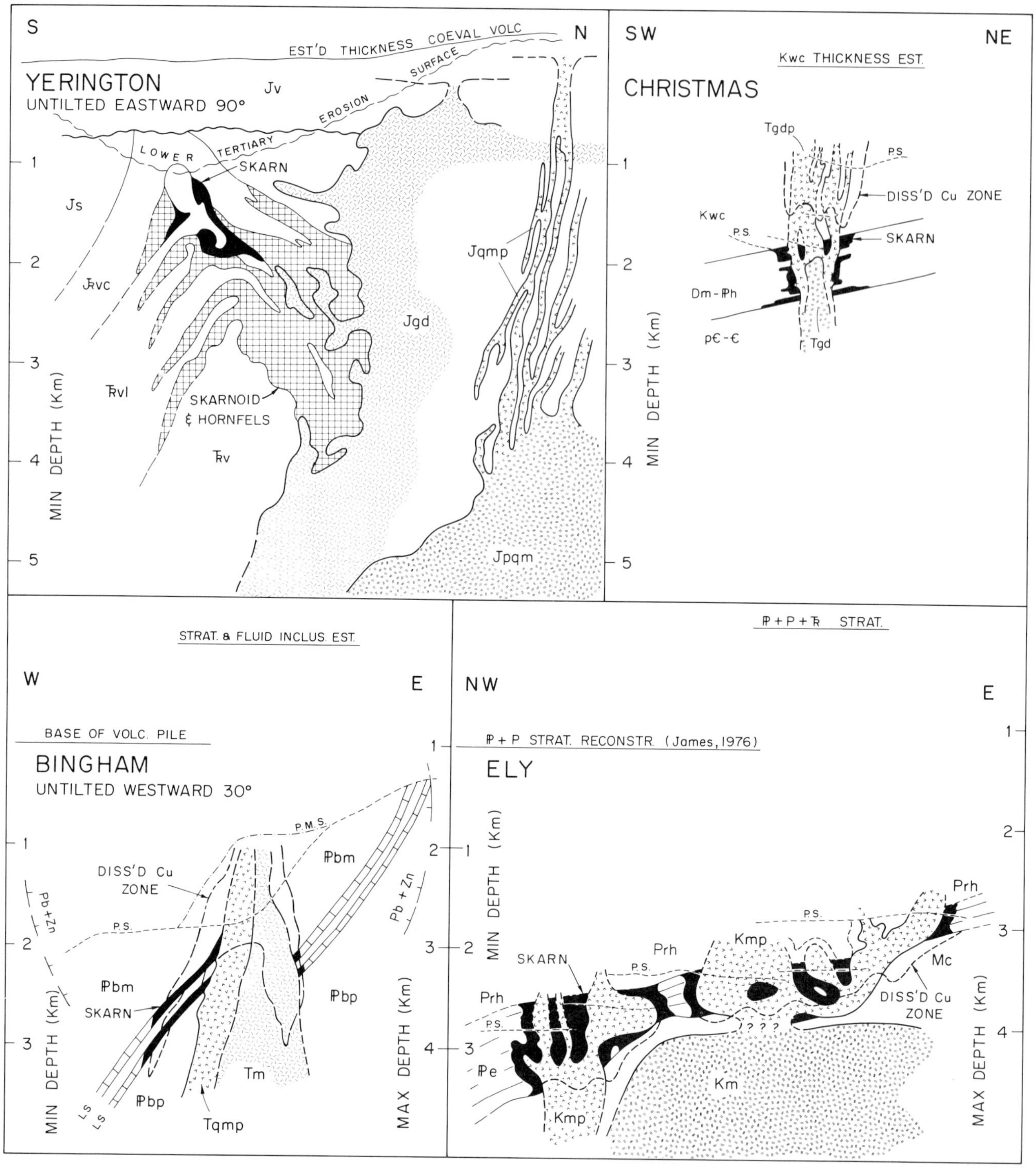

Abbreviations:

pЄ-Є = Cambrian Bolsa quartzite and Precambrian basement
Km = Cretaceous monzonite
Kmp = Cretaceous monzonite porphyry
Kwc = Cretaceous Williamson Creek volcanics
Dm-IPh = Devonian Martin Formation through Pennsylvanian Horquilla Formation
Diss'd = disseminated
Jgd = Jurassic granodiorite
Jpqm = Jurassic porphyritic quartz monzonite porphyry
Jqmp = Jurassic quartz monzonite porphyry
Js = Jurassic sedimentary rocks
JTRvc = Jurassic-Triassic volcanic and clastic sedimentary rocks
Jv = Jurassic volcanic rocks
Ls = Limestone
Mc = Mississippian Chainman Shale
P = Permian
IPbm = Pennsylvanian Bingham Mine Formation
IPbp = Pennsylvanian Butterfield Peaks Formation
IPe = Pennsylvanian Ely Limestone
Prh = Permian Rib Hill Sandstone
P.M.S. = Pre-mine surface
P.S. = Present surface (1974)
Tgd = Tertiary granodiorite
Tgdp = Tertiary grandiorite porphyry
Tm = Tertiary monzonite
Tqmp = Tertiary quartz monzonite porphyry
TRv = Triassic andesite-rhyolite sequence
TRvl = Triassic volcanic-limestone sequence

Figure 8.1. Reconstructed vertical cross sections illustrating depth regimes, pluton morphologies, and spatial relations between disseminated copper zones and skarn, in four porphyry copper deposits. Data for Yerington from J. M. Proffett and M. T. Einaudi, 1972, unpublished data; for Christmas from Perry (1969), Koski (1978); for Bingham from Moore and Nash (1974), Atkinson and Einaudi (1978); for Ely from James (1976).

copper deposits as estimated by numerous workers (e.g., Sillitoe, 1973; Nielsen, 1976) and are equivalent to lithostatic pressures of 220 to 1,100 bars and hydrostatic pressures of 100 to 500 bars.

Approximately one-half of the deposits considered in this chapter are associated with isolated, relatively small, porphyry stock complexes emplaced into a series of sedimentary and volcanic rocks which have not undergone earlier periods of magma-induced metamorphism or hydrothermal alteration. In these cases, the metamorphic and metasomatic rocks can be considered broadly synchronous with porphyry emplacement and in many cases are zoned with respect to the porphyry stock contacts. Local vagaries in zonal patterns may be the result of structural and/or lithological controls or of the possible intrusion by the stock of its own metamorphic/metasomatic envelope. Deposits which fit this general case include Ely, Christmas, Lakeshore, and Bisbee.

At the other end of the scale are districts which show an extended period of plutonic activity pre-dating the emplacement of the porphyry stocks and the formation of their associated ores. The porphyry stocks may intrude earlier batholiths or mixed stock-metamorphic terrain. In these cases, the resulting metamorphic and metasomatic rock distributions bear no simple relation to the porphyry stock. For example, the distribution of hornfels and skarnoid may reflect the earlier plutonic event which, in terms of volume, may have been orders of magnitude larger than the porphyry event (e.g., Yerington, Silver Bell). Also, early skarns formed during emplacement of equigranular, barren stocks of the first stage (such as the skarn magnetite deposits associated with diorite-granodiorite at Yerington, or the skarn zinc deposits associated with the Hanover stock near Santa Rita) may be over-printed by the copper-dominant skarns of the porphyry system. Recognition of these complications is of critical importance not only in exploration but also in establishing field-based models for experimental testing. Deposits which fit this general case include Yerington, Silver Bell, Cananea, Continental, Santa Rita, Twin Buttes and Pima-Mission.

Average horizontal dimensions of plutons range from 600 to 1,500 m. Morphologies include elongate dike swarms (Yerington); single to multiple, upward-branching stocks (Christmas, Ely); and nearly circular, plug-like composite porphyry or porphyry-breccia complexes (Mission, Twin Buttes, Bisbee). In some cases, porphyries are known to extend over vertical depth ranges of 5 km without major changes in size or shape. Configurations at greater depths can be inferred (see Fig. 8.1): at Yerington, the porphyries grade into enlarging stocks of porphyritic quartz monzonite at depths of 4 to 5 km below the co-genetic volcanic surface; at Ely, mutliple porphyry stocks originally overlay a single pluton, at least 3 km in diameter, at depths of 3 to 4 km (James, 1976); aeromagnetic data suggest the presence of batholithic-sized masses at depths below Ely (Carlson and Mabey, 1963) and Bingham (Zietz et al., 1969). These examples suggest that in most cases the mineralized portions of stocks are spatially well removed from their batholithic source, but that in some examples the batholithic connection lies at the relatively shallow depth of about 5 km. This depth is well within the region of possibly high fracture permeabilities; therefore, time-extensive, convective transfer of melt, aqueous fluid, and heat from deeper batholiths to shallow plutons could be an important factor in the mineralization process.

The lateral extent of skarn formation is dependent on the attitude of beds relative to the stock contacts, the thickness of limestone beds, and the presence of permeable zones, such as faults or interbedded sandstone or fractured hornfels beds. Large, well-mineralized skarns rarely extend more than 200 to 400 m from their associated stocks. The low range is represented by deposits formed in thick limestone sections, such as Ely (James, 1976) or Christmas (Perry, 1969); the high range is represented by deposits formed in sedimentary strata containing a large proportion of non-carbonate interbeds, such as Bingham (Atkinson and Einaudi, 1978). In some localities, such as Morenci, Silver Bell, and Mission, skarns are found as far as 500 to 900 m from the central stocks, but these distal skarns tend to be small and are associated with dikes and sills of propylitically altered porphyry. If distances of 200 to 900 m are taken as the general case, then skarn alteration rarely extends into limestone as far as biotitic (potassium-silicate) alteration extends into felsic to intermediate igneous rocks surrounding the porphyry stocks.

In contrast with skarn development, the formation of calc-silicates in sandstone and shale extends 1.5 to 2.0 km from the main stock contacts. Examples include the outermost limit of diopside at 1.5 km and of tremolite at 1.8 km in calcareous quartzite at Bingham (Atkinson and Einaudi, 1978) and comparable outermost limits (1.0–2.0 km) of calc-silicate hornfels in shale beds at Christmas (Perry, 1968, 1969) and Santa Rita (Nielsen, 1970).

Finally, the outermost signs of most large porphyry systems occur beyond the calc-silicate aureole and consist of generally minor lead-zinc-silver veins and replacement bodies with quartz and carbonate gangue. Commonly, such deposits occur up to 2 km from the central stocks; at Bingham, a maximum distance of 2.6 km (Rubright and Hart, 1968) yields an overall bull's-eye of mineralization of about 6 km in diameter.

REPLACEMENT OF SEDIMENTARY STRATA BY ORE-BEARING SKARN

The relative favorability of carbonate units for replacement by ore-bearing skarn appears to be a function of three variables: carbonate content, permeability, and structural configuration. Although skarn tends to be best developed in the purer carbonate beds of a given sequence, the *extent* of skarn formation is dependent on fracture permeability or on the presence of permeable sandy or hornfels interbeds due to the relatively low permeability of pure limestone.

At Bingham and Ely the presence of relatively thin carbonate units within thick sections of non-carbonate clastic rocks resulted in the predictable formation of skarn within the former; metasomatic fluids gained access to the limestone beds by travelling through fractured and relatively non-reactive rocks. In southeastern Arizona and southwestern New Mexico, however, the higher proportion of carbonate strata imposed more subtle controls which varied considerably between districts. Here, no generalizations appear to be valid (with the exception that all carbonate beds, from those in the Cambrian Abrigo to those in the Permian Concha contain skarn in one or another district). For example, at Christmas skarn in the relatively pure, thick-bedded Escabrosa Limestone extends only tens of meters from the stock, whereas skarn in limestone beds of the Horquilla and Martin formations extends up to 120 to 200 m outward (Perry, 1968). Similar relations are described at Silver Bell (Graybeal, 1982), where massive limestone (Escabrosa) is transformed into marble and where carbonate formations containing shaly or silty interbeds (Abrigo, Martin) contain the majority of mineralized skarn. However, the opposite was noted by Lindgren (1905) at Morenci, where the purer Modoc Limestone (Lake Valley Formation) contains the majority of garnetite skarn, in contrast with the apparently less-favorable, impure Longfellow Limestone (El Paso and Montoya Groups). However, the paucity of garnetite skarn in the Longfellow may simply have been due to the inhibiting effect of the dolomitic lithology on garnet formation; a similar contrast is observable in the same formations in the Continental pit, Central mining district, New Mexico.

ALTERATION-MINERALIZATION TYPES IN PORPHYRY COPPER SYSTEMS

Alteration-mineralization styles in porphyry copper skarn deposits may be categorized according to the general processes involved. Early metamorphism and bimetasomatic exchange of components between carbonate and quartzofeldspathic rocks yield a variety of calc-silicate hornfelses and skarnoid. The main period of high-temperature metasomatism yields calcic skarn in limestone and magnesian skarn in dolomite; both of these skarns are altered to various retrograde mineral assemblages as temperatures decline. Low-temperature metasomatism of limestone forms massive silica-pyrite replacement bodies in some deposits.

Hornfels-Skarnoid

Three widespread types of hornfels that are commonly thought to have originated by metamorphic decarbonation and dehydration, without metasomatic addition of components, include wollastonite-bearing rocks developed in cherty and/or sandy limestone, fine-grained diopside hornfelses developed from dolomitic siltstone, and calc-silicate hornfelses developed from calcareous shale. A fourth type is rich in garnet of grossularite or intermediate grossularite-andradite composition; in many cases it is accompanied by diopside and other calc-silicates of low iron content. This type of calc-silicate rock is termed skarnoid, in allusion to its skarn-like aspect.

Wollastonite Rock. The question of origin of wollastonite-bearing rocks is, of course, greatly simplified if there is little or no original quartz in the limestone, in which case metasomatic addition of silica (1.63 grams/cc), accompanied by loss of CO_2 (1.19 grams/cc), transforms the limestone, with insignificant volume change, to pure wollastonite rock. The case for silica-bearing limestone is vastly more complex. Winchell (1924) and Lindgren (1924) have both concluded that the conversion of cherty limestone to wollastonite-bearing rock at Bingham was not accompanied by a volume change and that in most cases the original quartz was not used. If these two constraints are taken together, it becomes impossible to write a reaction which reproduces Lindgren's mineralogical data. For example, in order to convert a calcite$_{70}$ quartz$_{30}$ rock (Yampa limestone, average analyses #1 and #2 [Lindgren, 1924]) to a calcite$_{52}$wollastonite$_{33}$ quartz$_{15}$ rock (analysis 3 w) without reacting quartz, an unlikely volume increase of 100 percent is required. If, however, constant volume is assumed, then producing the same numerical change requires that 26 percent of the calcite and 50 percent of the quartz in the original limestone be consumed, and that 0.19 grams/cc CaO and 0.10 grams/cc SiO_2 be introduced from external sources. Lindgren fully realized the variability of the alteration process from place to place, and he demonstrated in a general way that, whereas the silicates in the Yampa limestone largely were formed from introduced silica, in the Highland Boy limestone most of the detrital quartz was consumed. In the latter case, a possible mechanism to form wollastonite involves the consumption of silica and calcium in the original limestone, with the reaction proceeding to the point at which one of the reactant minerals is consumed; a calcite$_{70}$quartz$_{30}$ rock then produces a calcite$_{30}$wollastonite$_{70}$ rock, which is identical to analysis 5 w of Lindgren (1924). But in this case, the reaction causes a 26 percent volume decrease.

The examples above illustrate the ambiguities involved in attempting to define not only the gains and losses from bulk chemical analyses, but also the possible fluid-rock reactions. Although Lindgren and Winchell have used stratigraphic measurements to rule out volume decreases during formation of calc-silicates at Bingham, other data from the same district indicate that the presence or absence of volume changes cannot be determined, due to variability in original stratigraphic thicknesses. For example, Britt (1976) has documented a stratigraphic thinning of 55 percent for unaltered Highland Boy limestone over a distance of 8 km, and drilling results at Carr Fork indicate as much as 17 percent thinning of garnetized Highland Boy over distances of 200 m.

Diopside Hornfels. Calcareous siltstone lacking significant argillaceous components commonly is converted to diopside-quartz hornfels. Such silty hornfels is abundant in many porphyry copper districts. It is, for example, the most common calc-silicate rock type at Bingham (Atkinson and Einaudi, 1978); it appears in the mid-Scherrer silty-carbonate beds at Pima-Mission (Gale, 1965; Einaudi, 1974) and at Twin Buttes (Barter and Kelly, 1982); and it occurs in quartzite of the Martin Formation at Christmas (Perry, 1969). Diopside and diopside-calcite rocks also are common and appear to form in purer carbonate beds, especially those with an originally significant dolomite content, such as in portions of the Ely Limestone at Ely (James, 1976) and in the upper dolomite beds of the Martin Formation at Christmas (Perry, 1969). Insufficient petrographic and chemical data exist to determine whether these diopside hornfelses are largely metamorphic or metasomatic in nature. However, their highly specialized composition and simple monomineralic or bimineralic nature suggest that most are metasomatic rocks.

At Christmas, Perry (1969) concluded that monomineralic diopside hornfels in the upper Beckers Butte member of the Martin Formation must have resulted from metasomatism; addition of silica is suggested, but whether MgO, CaO and H^+ were added or subtracted during the reaction depends on whether volume changes occurred.

Non-dolomitic calcareous sandstone in the Bingham district was converted to diopsidic quartzite and silty diopside hornfels up to 1.5 km from the stock (Atkinson and Einaudi, 1978). Preservation of finely laminated bedding suggests that no significant volume changes accompanied silication. The fact that detrital quartz grains are only mildly corroded by diopside suggests that only a small fraction (10%?) of the silica originally present was used during silication. With these constraints, a quartz$_{75}$calcite$_{25}$ rock yields a quartz$_{67}$ diopside$_{33}$ rock on addition of 0.39 grams/cc SiO_2 and 0.20 grams/cc MgO; 0.10 grams/cc CaO and 0.30 grams/cc CO_2 are removed. Lack of participation of detrital quartz in silication reactions involving quartzose sedimentary rocks, also noted by Winchell (1924), is not peculiar to Bingham, but is a general phenomenon also at Twin Buttes (Barter and Kelly, 1982). The introduction of silica from an external source may be the general case.

Calc-Silicate Hornfels. Calc-silicate hornfels—consisting of variable proportions of the minerals quartz, tremolite, plagioclase, epidote-clinozoisite, and diopside, generally with little or no garnet—are commonly developed in calcareous shale units in porphyry skarn systems. Examples include portions of the Abrigo, Earp, and Horquilla Formations at Twin Buttes (Barter and Kelly, 1982) and portions of the Syrena Formation in the outer zones at the Chino (Nielsen, 1970) and Continental mines, New Mexico. The rocks are generally light colored, unzoned, and extremely fine-grained, with relic bedding and low Fe : Al ratios; such characteristics are generally sufficient to distinguish these rocks—which are most likely products of simple metamorphic dehydration-decarbonation—from the metasomatic, Fe-rich skarns with which they are commonly associated (or to which they may in some cases be converted.)

Skarnoid. The distinction between metasomatism and metamorphism becomes increasingly difficult if a sequence of impure carbonate and shale beds is replaced on a large scale by coarse-grained, Al-Si–rich garnetite. In porphyry-skarn systems the presence of grossularitic garnetite is suggestive of a dominantly metamorphic or local bimetasomatic process—such as exchange of components between shale and limestone (Vidale, 1969; Thompson, 1975)—because metasomatic skarn garnets typically are andraditic. Such garnet-rich rocks, termed skarnoid, may be difficult to distinguish in the field from true skarn. They generally are not ore-bearing, unless overprinted by metasomatic, skarn-forming fluids.

A probable necessary condition for the development of large volumes of skarnoid is the presence of intimately interbedded carbonate and quartzo-feldspathic rocks, with the latter present in larger amounts than generally is the case in the Paleozoic section of the southwestern U.S. In contrast, the Triassic-Jurassic sedimentary section in the Yerington district of western Nevada was ideally suited for the production of skarnoid.

Approximately 2 km^2 of unmineralized, garnet-rich rocks are exposed at Yerington, formed from a 1,400-m-thick sequence of felsic volcaniclastic rocks, calcareous shale, and limestone. The skarnoid, which contains 50 to 75 percent garnet and 10 to 15 percent pyroxene, displays little or no modal variation as a function of original rock type. A detailed study of bulk mineral and chemical composition of fresh and altered rocks. (Einaudi, 1971, unpub. research) suggests that, although limestone underwent significant metasomatic addition of components during conversion to skarnoid (2 grams/cc), the shales are a reasonable isochemical match (other than volatiles and Fe_2O_3) of the skarnoid, especially if a volume decrease is considered. Furthermore, the components which appear to be added to carbonate rocks are those which are leached from volcaniclastic rocks, and the components added to volcaniclastic rocks are those which are leached from carbonate rocks. Fe_2O_3 is the only component added in moderate amounts (0.3 grams/cc) to all rock types. The above results suggest that exchange of components between different sedimentary rocks was the dominant mechanism of skarnoid formation at Yerington.

Calcic Skarn

The classic association of andradite garnet with chalcopyrite has been established since the early studies of garnetite skarn copper deposits of the western United States (e.g., Lindgren, 1905; Knopf, 1918). Other silicate-sulfide associations are recognized in calcic skarns mined for other metals; this general topic has been reviewed by Zharikov (1970) and Burt (1972, 1977).

Calcic skarn is the dominant skarn type in porphyry copper districts of southwestern North America. Dominant early silicates are garnet, clinopyroxene, and wollastonite. These silicates commonly are zoned relative to intrusive or sedimentary contacts. Some typical patterns are illustrated in Figure 8.2. If Wollastonite is present, it occurs with minor garnet, idocrase, and clinopyroxene in an outer zone near marble. Garnet, accompanied by lesser amounts of clinopyroxene, forms the innermost zone near porphyry or siliceous hornfels beds. Epidote, if present, commonly occurs within a few meters of the porphyry or in endoskarn. The early zonal pattern can be interpreted as the result of activity gradients set up between iron and silica-rich solutions and limestone host rocks (Burt, 1972, 1974; Einaudi, 1977). The zones form simultaneously, with the inner garnet zone replacing (and sometimes over-running) the outer wollastonite zone.

Less obvious calc-silicate zonal and paragenetic features also may be present. Garnet commonly is color-zoned, from reddish brown near the stock to greenish farther out, especially where it replaces wollastonite. In some cases garnet : clinopyroxene ratios decrease away from the stock or vein center; replacement of clinopyroxene by garnet is more common than the reverse, in concert with the general model of simultaneous outward growth of zones.

Garnets in porphyry copper–related skarns belong to the grossularite-andradite ($Ca_3Al_2Si_3O_{12}$-$Ca_3Fe_2Si_3O_{12}$) series; a range in composition from 80 to 100 mole percent andradite is typical (Fig. 8.3). Zoning in individual garnets,

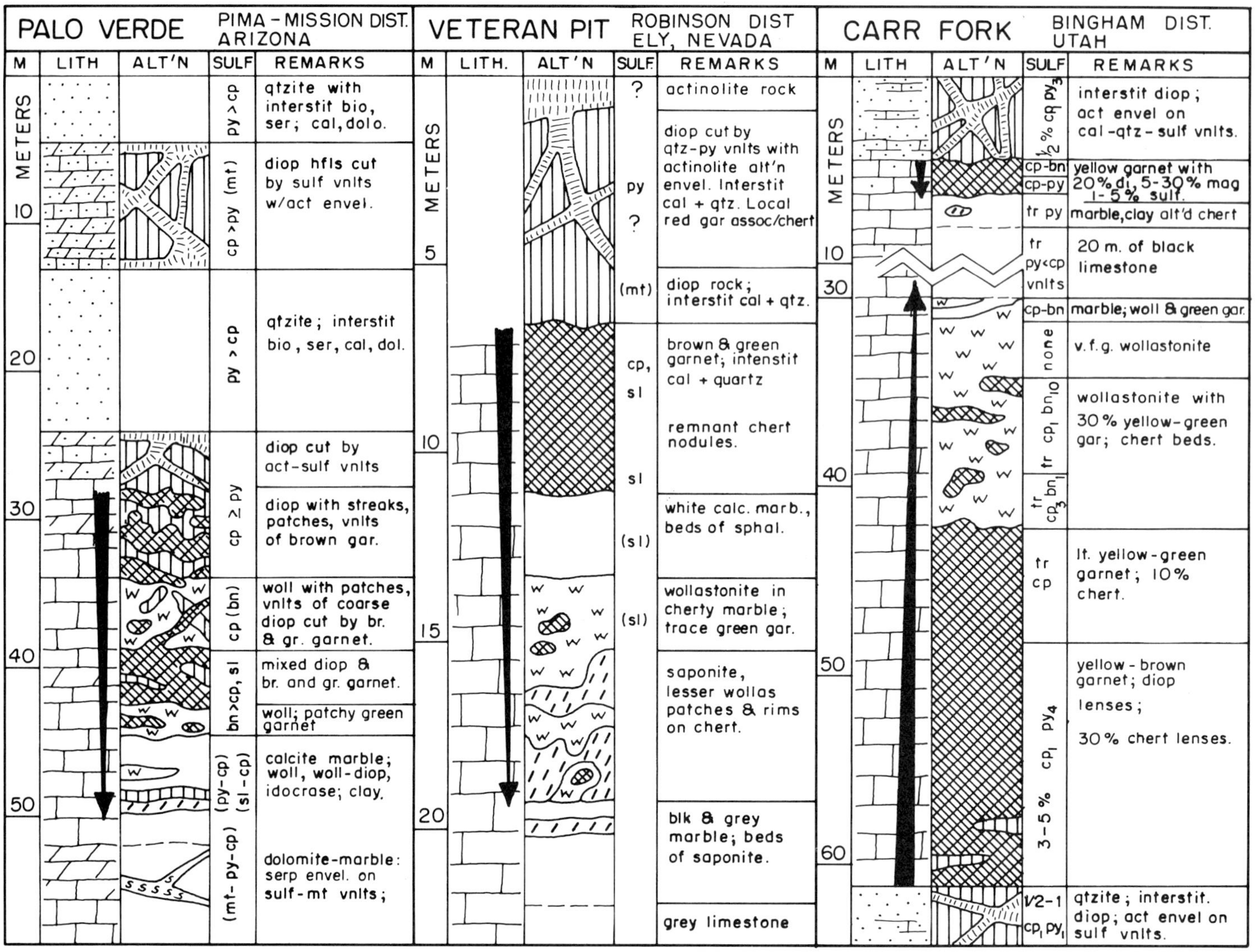

Abbreviations:

Act = actinolite	*cp* = chalcopyrite	*LITH* = original lithology	*ser* = sericite
ALT'N = alteration	*diop* = diopside	*lt.* = light	*serp* = serpentine
bio = biotite	*dolo* = dolomite	*marb* = marble	*tr* = trace
blk = black	*envel* = envelopes	*mt, mag* = magnetite	*v.f.g.* = very fine grained
bn = bornite	*gar* = garnet	*py* = pyrite	*vnlts* = veinlets
br = brown	*gr* = green	*qtz* = quartz	*woll* = wollastonite
cal = calcite	*hfls* = hornfels	*sl, sphal* = sphalerite	

Figure 8.2. Summaries of diamond drill core logs illustrating typical calcic skarn and diopside hornfels mineralogy at Palo Verde (Einaudi, 1974), Ely (James, 1976), and Bingham (Atkinson, unpublished). In all three localities calcic skarn is zoned relative to lithologic contacts (as shown by heavy black arrows) with the sequence: brown andradite-chalcopyrite ±pyrite; green andradite-wollastonite-chalcopyrite ±bornite ±sphalerite; marble with variable wollastonite, clay, idocrase. In all three localities, diopside hornfels is cut by abundant pyrite-chalcopyrite ±magnetite veinlets with actinolite alteration envelopes. Actinolite and andradite may represent the main stage of Fe-metasomatism accompanying sulfide deposition in different lithologies.

overgrowths, and multiple generations of garnet veins are common; where microprobe data are available, the paragenetic data indicate a general increase in iron content with time and toward the stock. Clinopyroxenes belong to the diopside-hedenbergite ($CaMgSi_2O_6$-$CaFeSi_2O_6$) series and typically contain less than a few mole percent of the johannsenite ($CaMnSi_2O_6$) component. A wide range in composition, from 2 to 55 mole percent hedenbergite, is indicated by relatively few analyses (see Fig. 8.3); however, 15 to 35 mole percent hedenbergite is the normal range for typical porphyry-related skarn. Higher iron contents are found in anomalous distant occurences (e.g., Mason Valley mine, Yerington), and many of the low-iron analyses represent clinopyroxene from hornfels of probable metamorphic origin. Actinolite, which is generally associated with salite in skarn, or which replaces early diopside hornfels, contains 20 to 40 mole percent of the iron endmember (see Fig. 8.3). The andradite-salite association of copper-dominant skarns helps to distinguish potential

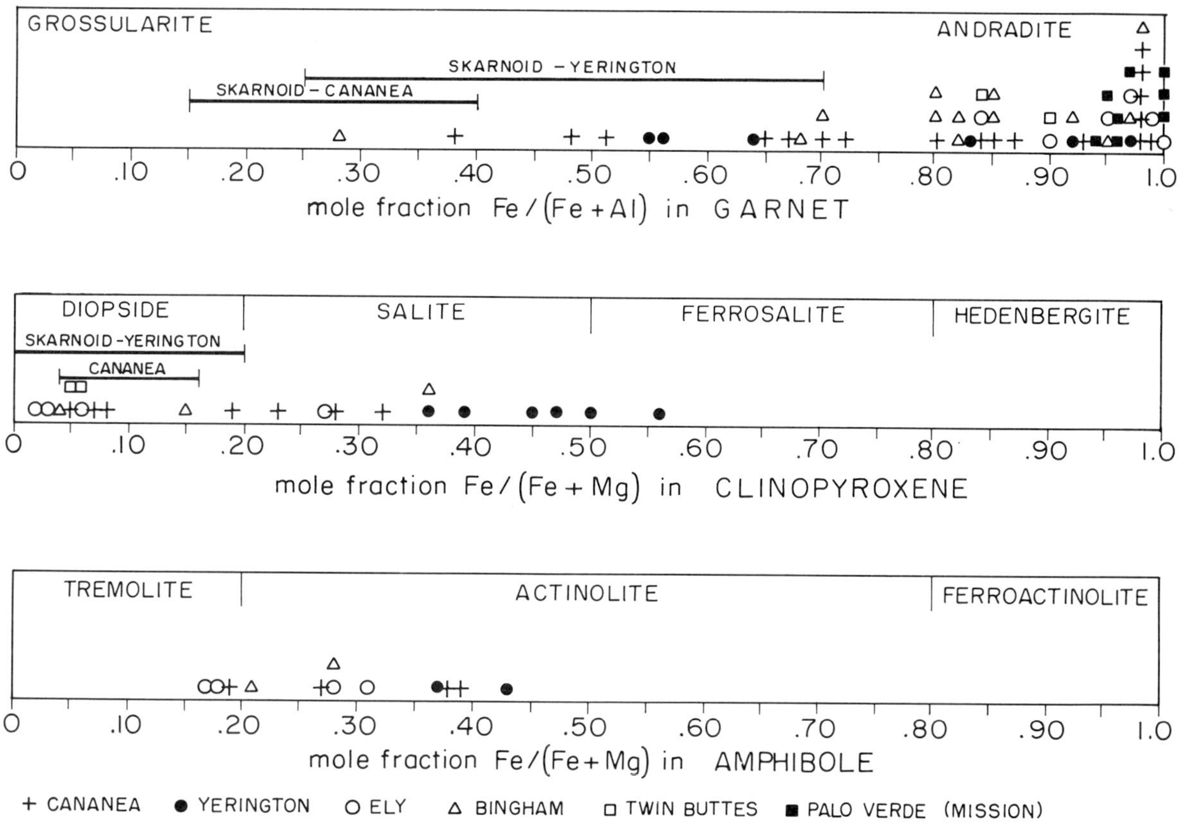

Figure 8.3. Iron-content of grossularite-andradite, diopside-hedenbergite, and tremolite-ferroactinolite solid solutions in porphyry-related skarns. Electron microprobe data on Cananea from L. D. Meinert (1978, personal communication), on Yerington from Einaudi (1977, and unpublished), on Ely from James (1976) and Huang (1976); wet chemical data on Bingham from Atkinson and Einaudi (1978), on Twin Buttes from Einaudi (unpublished); X-ray data on Palo Verde from Einaudi (unpublished).

skarn copper prospects from those of other metals. However, this association may not be specific to porphyry copper-related skarns.

The andradite-salite-chalcopyrite association, which contrasts with the grossularite-hedenbergite-scheelite (molybdenite) association (Zharikov, 1970; Shimazaki, 1974), may be largely a function of the relatively oxidized environments which produce the garnet-chalcopyrite association. The andradite-salite-chalcopyrite association also contrasts with the andradite-manganhedenbergite-sphalerite (galena) association (Zharikov, 1970; Burt, 1972, 1977) and may be largely a function of relatively higher temperature and lesser degree of fluid differentiation in copper-dominant deposits. These concepts are developed in a later section.

Anhydrous calc-silicate minerals of the early zoned skarn stage are replaced by hydrous silicates, sulfides, oxides, and carbonates as temperatures decline and fluid compositions change. In contrast with the early stage, which involves the formation of monomineralic or bimineralic assemblages, late stages lead to complex mineral assemblages of many phases. Common examples include replacement of andradite by quartz, calcite, magnetite and pyrite; of diopside by actinolite, quartz, and calcite; and of wollastonite by calcite and quartz. These relations suggest a shift from dominantly open-system behavior in the early stages to dominantly closed-system behavior in later retrograde stages. The extent of early skarn destruction appears to vary directly with the extent of hydrolytic alteration in the associated stock.

Sulfides and iron oxides occur as disseminations, as massive streaks and veins in skarn, and as massive replacements of marble at the skarn front. Most workers have concluded that the opaque minerals are deposited throughout the sequence of skarn formation and later skarn destruction. The occurrence of most opaque minerals with the silicates and carbonates of the later stage can be interpreted either as the result of late deposition or as remobilization of sulfides deposited during the early stage.

Calcic skarns in porphyry districts typically contain 2 to 15 percent sulfides. Common silicate-sulfide associations are summarized in Table 8.1. The assemblage pyrite-chalcopyrite is characteristic of garnet-rich zones. Pyrite : chalcopyrite ratios reflect those of the adjacent stock and typically range from 1 : 2 to 5 : 1; ratios may be higher near contacts with sericitically altered stocks, due to the late addition of pyrite during retrograde alteration of skarn. Pyrite : chalcopyrite ratios may increase outward through the garnet zone, but commonly drop to 0 near marble, especially if a wollastonite zone is present. In the wollastonite zone, bornite and chalcopyrite and lesser sphalerite, often accompanied by fresh andradite, are the most common sulfides, and pyrite, if present, is not associated with bornite.

Overall, porphyry-related calcic skarns contain up to 10

TABLE 8.1
Generalized Silicate-Sulfide-Oxide Associations in Calcic Skarn Zones Associated With Porphyry Copper Deposits

Zone	Commonly Associated Minerals	Less Commonly Associated Minerals
Garnet	pyrite (chalcopyrite) (magnetite)	—
Garnet-Pyroxene	pyrite chalcopyrite (magnetite)	magnetite after specularite
Garnet-Wollastonite	bornite chalcopyrite (sphalerite)	pyrrhotite (galena) (digenite) (tennantite)
Marble	sphalerite chalcopyrite (magnetite) (pyrite)	pyrrhotite (galena)

NOTE: Parentheses indicate low relative abundance.

percent iron oxides. Magnetite is more common than hematite during the early stages of skarn formation, and it generally precedes or is contemporaneous with sulfides. Magnetite commonly is concentrated at porphyry-skarn contacts, where it replaces andradite or salite, or at garnetite-marble contacts, where it replaces marble; magnetite is sparse in wollastonite zones, where it is rimmed by andradite or calcite + quartz reaction envelopes dependent on T-X_{CO_2} conditions.

The skarn zonal pattern, from pyrite-chalcopyrite-magnetite associated with andradite near pluton contacts to bornite-chalcopyrite associated with wollastonite near marble contacts, presumably reflects the outward trend toward decreasing total iron in the overall skarn, rather than a change in the sulfidation state of fluids. The change from andradite-chalcopyrite to wollastonite-bornite has been explained by Burt (1972) as the result of iron-rich oxidizing solutions that altered wollastonite to andradite. Precipitation of andradite causes a decrease in Fe : Cu ratio in the fluid and could cause the deposition of bornite rather than chalcopyrite; thus, the presence of bornite in skarn is not analogous to the presence of bornite in the plutons in terms of defining a zonal center.

Magnesian Skarn

Skarn dominated by magnesium-rich silicates and containing large amounts of magnetite is a common feature in dolomitic beds of Paleozoic formations of the Southwest, but is absent from deposits in the northern Basin and Range province. Magnesian skarn is developed on a large scale at Christmas in the Martin Formation (Perry, 1968, 1969) and at the Continental mine in the Montoya and El Paso dolomites. Relatively minor occurrences of magnesian skarn are reported from Silver Bell, Pima-Mission, Twin Buttes, and Morenci.

Fosterite, serpentine, and talc are characteristic of silica-deficient environments; talc and tremolite occur in quartz-bearing environments. Forsterite commonly is pervasively altered to serpentine-dominant assemblages; the more pervasive development of retrograde assemblages in Mg skarn relative to Ca skarn reflects the greater ease of alteration of forsterite relative to andradite or diopside in H_2O-rich fluids at temperatures below 400°C.

Relative to calcic skarn, magnesian skarn yields high magnetite contents, low sulfide contents (less than 6%), and low pyrite : chalcopyrite ratios (less than 1 : 2). The high magnetite content is due to the presence of magnesian silicates, such as forsterite, talc, and serpentine, which do not display extensive solid solution toward their ferrous end-members due either to incompatibility of the latter with calcite or to the relatively oxidized state of the skarn-forming environment. Therefore, iron precipitates as iron oxides, in contrast to calcic skarn, where much of the iron is used to form calcium-iron silicates. These contasts are summarized in Figure 8.4, which shows that, for a given iron content, the Ca : Mg ratio determines not only the silicate present, but also the amount of magnetite.

Silica-Pyrite

In addition to the two skarn types discussed above, a common alteration feature associated with sulfide deposition in carbonate rocks of some porphyry copper districts consists of various forms of silica accompanied by abundant pyrite. Silica-pyrite may replace skarn, but more commonly, it replaces limestone as massive irregular bodies, mantos, or

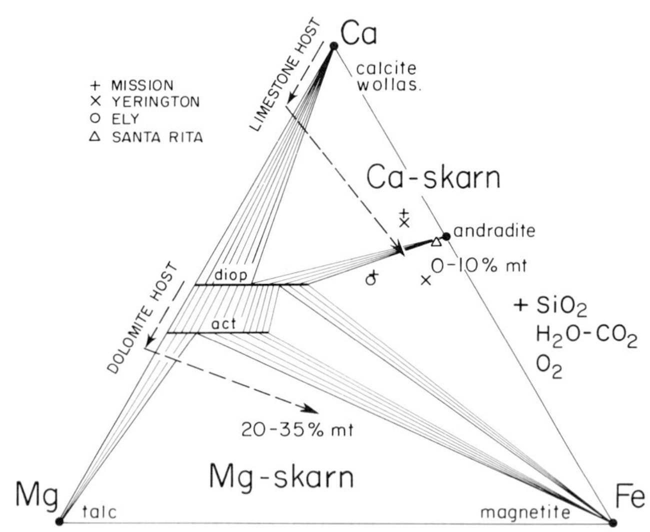

Abbreviations:
act = actinolite
diop = diopside
mt = magnetite
wollas = wollastonite

Figure 8.4. Ca-Mg-Fe diagram (mole proportions) with externally controlled SiO_2, H_2O-CO_2, and O_2, illustrating the most common mineral compositions and compatibilities during porphyry-related skarn formation. General compositional area for calcic skarn based on Gale, 1965 (Mission); Einaudi, 1977 (Yerington); James, 1976 (Ely); and Nielsen, 1970 (Santa Rita). For a comparable degree of Mg and Fe metasomatism (dashed arrows), limestone forms calcic skarn with 0 to 10 percent magnetite, whereas dolomite forms magnesian skarn with 20 to 35 percent magnetite.

steep, structurally controlled breccia pipes. A direct correlation exists between hydrolytic alteration of plutons to sericitic or advanced argillic assemblages and formation of silica-pyrite in carbonate rocks. Of the deposits considered in this chapter, Bisbee, Ely, and Cananea display the greatest degree of development of silica-pyrite. At Bisbee this alteration type is present almost to the exclusion of skarn (Ransome, 1904). At Ely and Cananea large volumes of both skarn and silica-pyrite are present; silica-pyrite is restricted to the upper portions of the Ely system as reconstructed by James (1976) and appears to replace both limestone and earlier skarn at Cananea (Emmons, 1910). In all three districts, jasperoidal silica ledges are distinctive features at the surface; some of these ledges represent oxidized portions of silica-pyrite bodies.

In other porphyry copper districts, silica-pyrite occurs in relatively minor amounts. At Silver Bell and Palo Verde it locally cuts skarn along late veins and breccias and is only weakly developed in marble; at Bingham portions of the Old Highland Boy mine and Yampa footwall vein consisted of pyritic quartz-clay, and the opal-cristobalite zone of the Yampa limestone in the Utah copper pit (Reid, 1978) is a closely related alteration type; at Yerington the Ludwig lode (Knopf, 1918) is representative of silica-pyrite.

At Bisbee and Ely silica in the form of chalcedony, jasper, or massive aphanitic quartz is present in amounts from 10 to 30 percent, and pyrite—present in amounts ranging from 25 to 50 percent (Bryant, 1964; James, 1976), constitutes the dominant mineral. Calcite may be abundant locally, and nontronite, montmorillonite, chlorite, talc, and siderite are common minor phases in most silica-pyrite bodies of porphyry copper districts. In some deposits, notably Silver Bell and Palo Verde, the dominant iron phase is hematite rather than pyrite. At Cananea magnetite and chlorite may be dominant over pyrite and silica (L. D. Meinert, 1978, personal communication).

The hypogene copper grade of silica-pyrite bodies is extremely variable. In districts where copper was deposited at the higher temperatures associated with potassium-silicate alteration and skarn formation—such as Ely—the silica-pyrite stage appears to be largely a product of a late skarn-destructive event which leached copper. In contrast, in districts where most of the copper in the intrusive system appears to have been deposited during a stage transitional to, or characterized by, intense hydrolytic alteration and brecciation—such as Cananea and Bisbee, respectively—the associated silica-pyrite bodies in limestone contain massive, high-grade copper ores which often are accompanied by important sphalerite concentrations.

Silica-pyrite bodies of the porphyry-copper environment are similar in some respects to base and precious metal pyrite-siderite-jasperoid ores in limestone, such as those at Leadville and Gilman, Colorado, and Tintic, Utah. Both are characterized by an abundance of Si, Fe, and Ca, which, for a variety of environmental reasons, did not combine to form calc-silicates. In contrast to porphyry-related silica-pyrite bodies, silica-pyrite ores of the Leadville-type lack a close spatial association with intensely leached plutons; in fact, the spatial-temporal relations with igneous rocks often is ambiguous. These ores also tend to have a greater carbonate content, including mangano-siderite and dolomite, and they contain a different suite of metals (Ag, Pb, Zn, with lesser Cu, Au). Titley (1968, 1973) has suggested that the Leadville-type silica-pyrite alteration is the high-pressure and high-sulfur analogue of the near-surface skarn environment. Within the porphyry copper environment, however, silica-pyrite is the low-temperature and high-sulfur analogue of skarn.

DISTINCTIVE FEATURES OF PORPHYRY-RELATED SKARNS

Although many of the features discussed above are common to non–porphyry-related skarns, some additional features, which appear to be uniquely associated with porphyry-related skarns, may serve to guide exploration and develop genetic models for porphyry copper systems.

Fine-Grained Silicate Textures

Porphyry-related skarns tend to consist of fine-grained to massive aggregates of calc-silicates in which relic bedding may be locally recognizable. Coarsely bladed clinopyroxenes or coarse granular garnet, which are characteristic of zinc-bearing skarns—such as in the Pewabic mine (Schmitt, 1939) or the Linchburg mine (Titley, 1961)—are generally absent, although they can be seen in some distal copper-bearing skarns—such as in the Mason Valley mine (Einaudi, 1977). In porphyry systems characterized by shallow levels of emplacement in highly fractured rocks, relatively high fluid flow rates are conducive to supersaturation, which may result in fine-grained textures due to rapid deposition at numerous nucleation sites. In contrast, non–porphyry-related skarns appear to form in less dynamic magmatic-hydrothermal environments and perhaps at greater depths or greater distances from intrusive margins, where fluid movement is more restricted; in such locations there is less likelihood of supersaturation, and large crystals can grow slowly.

High Veinlet Density

Porphyry-related skarns form during the active structural deformation that accompanies multiple intrusive events; repetitive fracturing of brittle sedimentary rocks, hornfels, and previously-formed skarn is characteristic of this environment and leads to vein densities which are greater than those in non-porphyry skarns.

Actinolite Veins in Diopside Hornfels

One of the most striking and characteristic features of porphyry-related skarns is the density of quartz-sulfide veinlets or sulfide fractures with actinolite alteration envelopes in diopside skarn or hornfels. These veinlets in large part are contemporaneous with biotite-orthoclase alteration of the associated plutons, as illustrated in Figure 8.5. They are absent in skarns formed at considerable distance from potassium-silicate alteration (e.g., Mason Valley mine, Yerington district) and in skarns not associated with potassically altered stocks. The actinolite alteration can be interpreted in terms of equilibria in the system $KAlO_2$-MgO-SiO_2-CaO-CO_2-H_2O

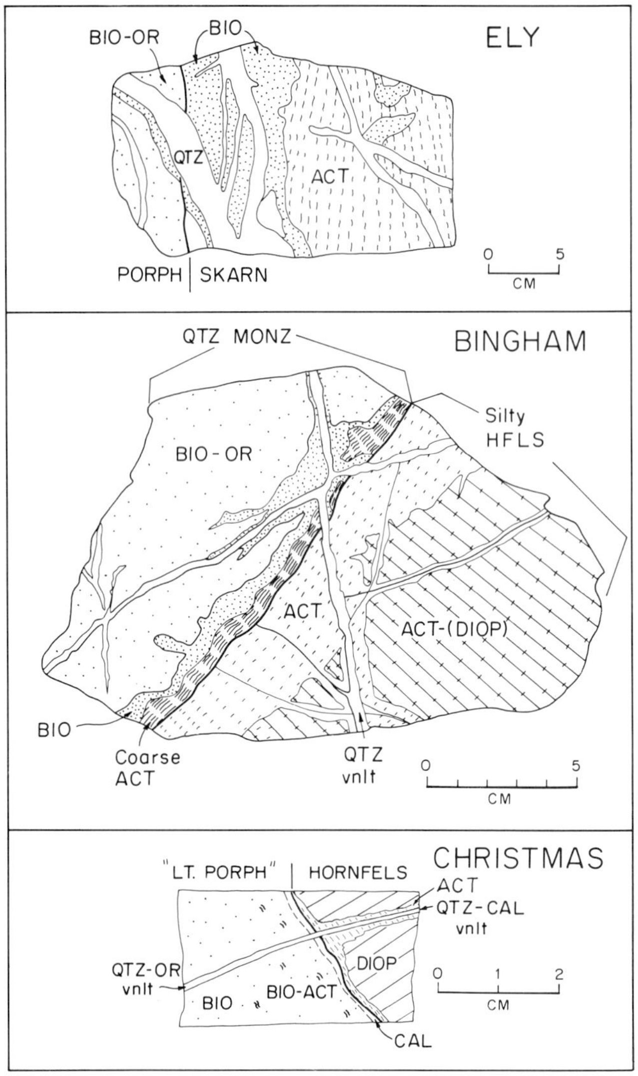

Abbreviations:

ACT = actinolite
BIO = biotite
CAL = calcite
DIOP = diopside
HFLS = hornfels
"LT. PORPH" = "light porphyry"
OR = orthoclase
PORPH = porphyry
QTZ = quartz
QTZ MONZ = quartz monzonite
vnlt = veinlet

Figure 8.5. Veinlet-alteration relations at contacts between intrusions and sedimentary rocks at Ely, Bingham, and Christmas, illustrating contemporaneity between potassium-silicate alteration (quartz-orthoclase-biotite-sulfide veinlets) of porphyry and actinolite alteration (quartz ±calcite ±sulfide veinlets) of diopside hornfels. Ely example redrawn from James (1976).

(Vidale, 1969; Hoschek, 1973) as the reaction between diopside-rich wall rocks and fluids saturated with respect to phlogopite. This alteration is a distinctive feature of the superposition of the early potassium-silicate environment of porphyry copper deposits onto hornfelses of intermediate Ca : Mg ratios.

High Degree of Retrograde Alteration

The quasi-monomineralic nature of skarn zones formed in the early stages of alteration is usually preserved in simple, non-porphyry skarns, but may be largely destroyed in porphyry systems. In the non-porphyry skarns, late-stage assemblages, such as calcite-quartz-chlorite-pyrite, are largely confined to vug fillings in garnetite, minor veins, or immediate skarn-intrusive contacts; low water : rock ratios and low permeabilities presumably block the retrograde process. In contrast, large volumes of porphyry-related skarns are commonly altered to late carbonate–hydrous silicate assemblages, and limestone may be replaced on a large scale by equivalent assemblages (silica-pyrite or clay-chlorite). Presumably, these characteristics reflect the presence of a long-lived, sulfur-rich hydrothermal system operating in a highly fractured, hence permeable, environment. Decrease in temperature below 350°C, oxidation by ground water influx, and low pressure boiling all can contribute to the generation of hydrothermal fluids which are out of equilibrium with plutons and skarns.

TONNAGE AND GRADE OF SKARN-RELATED PORPHYRY COPPER ORE

The tonnage and copper grade of porphyry copper deposits containing skarn are summarized in Table 8.2. A striking feature brought out by this table is the extremely low hypogene copper grades of many of the porphyry stocks associated with large volumes of calcareous sedimentary rocks containing 0.6 to 0.9 percent Cu. The highest grade in stocks at Christmas, Continental, Twin Buttes, Mission, Santa Rita, Silver Bell, and Morenci ranges from 0.05 to 0.3 percent Cu. Although higher grades may have been present in eroded upper portions of the stocks, this possibility is not considered likely as a general case because Mission, Santa Rita, and Morenci can be interpreted as high-level exposures. The interpretation favored here is that low-grade porphyry is symptomatic of porphyry plutons emplaced in carbonate rocks, because copper in the convecting hydrothermal fluid is preferentially abstracted by the carbonates.

Another feature emphasized by the data in Table 8.2 is that porphyry plutons surrounded by major volumes of carbonate rocks (generally those at the top of the table) do not undergo supergene sulfide enrichment; the pH of surface waters is buffered to intermediate values by calcite, so that copper remains insoluble as various carbonate, silicate, or oxide phases. Supergene sulfide enrichment may occur where migrating surface waters in the pluton do not traverse carbonate rocks because of topography (e.g., Bingham, where the pluton is a topographic high) or because of shielding by non-carbonate rocks (e.g., Cananea, where the upper portions of porphyry plugs are emplaced in volcanic rocks overlying carbonate rocks).

Because tonnage and grade in large part are a function of mining method (and, hence, of cut-off grade), the grade data in the table cannot be readily compared between deposits. Open-pit operations, with a cut-off of 0.3 to 0.4 percent Cu, mine a substantial amount of non-skarn rock, including mineralized hornfels and arkose; these rock types commonly are lower grade than skarn. Average hypogene grades for mineralized sedimentary rocks at open-pit mines range from 0.6 to 0.9 percent Cu; the major contribution to this grade comes from skarn, which probably averages near 1 percent Cu. In terms of ore tonnage in sedimentary rocks, Twin

TABLE 8.2

Tonnage and Grade of Skarn-Related Porphyry and Non-Porphyry Copper Ore in Representative Deposits of Southwestern North America

NAME OF DEPOSIT	ENTIRE DEPOSIT		PORPHYRY ORE IN IGNEOUS ROCKS			NON-PORPHYRY ORE IN CALCAREOUS ROCKS			SOURCES
	Ore Tonnage (Millions of Tons)	Overall Grade (% cu)	Percent of Total Ore	Grade of Hypogene Ore (% Cu)	Grade of Supergene Ore[b] (% Cu)	Percent of Total Ore	Grade of Hypogene Ore (% Cu)	Grade of Supergene Ore (% Cu)	
Christmas[a] (Arizona)	~80 p + r	~0.7	0	0.05–0.1	absent	100	~2.0 ug 0.6 op	—	Koski & Cook, 1982; Perry, 1969
Continental (New Mexico)	47 p + r	~1.0	0	0.04	absent	100	~2.0 ug 0.85 op	—	W.T. Worthington, 1978, personal communication
Twin Buttes (Arizona)	500 p + r	0.78	5?	0.1–0.5 ave. <0.3?	absent	80	0.73 op ~1.2 op sk	1.0 ox op	Barter & Kelly, 1982; Anaconda Co., Proxy Statement, 1976
Mission (Arizona)	500 p + r	~0.8	5?	0.1–0.4	absent	80	0.4–2.0 op	—	Gale, 1965; Kinnison, 1966
Bisbee (Arizona)	~150 p	~2.5	35 bx	>3.0 bx ug ~1.0 bx op <0.1 diss	>3.0 bx ug ~1.0 bx op ~0.8 diss	65	~5 ug	~5 ox ug	Bryant, 1964
Lakeshore (Arizona)	265 r	0.8		~0.5?	~1.5 ox		1.7 ug	—	Hallof & Winniski, 1971; South, 1972
Bingham (Utah)	1,350 p	0.9	70	0.62 (1975)	1–2	30[c]	1.5–2.0 ug,r	—	Bray & Wilson, 1975; Einaudi et al., 1978; Anaconda Co., Proxy Statement, 1976
Santa Rita (New Mexico)	~350 p	0.9	80 (supergene)	0.1–0.3	0.9	20	0.9 op	—	Nielsen, 1970; Rose & Baltosser, 1966
Ely (Nevada)	~300 p	1.1	80	0.4–2.0	1.0–2.0	20	—	—	Bauer et al., 1966
Silver Bell (Arizona)	75 p	0.86	85 (supergene)	0.1–0.35	0.81	15	3.5 ug 0.8 op	1.02 ox op	Graybeal, 1982
Cananea (Sonora, Mexico)	~400 p + r	1.0	95 (supergene)	>3.0 bx ug <0.3 diss	0.76 op	5	1–4	3–10 ug	Emmons, 1910; Anaconda Co., Proxy Statement, 1976
Yerington (Nevada)	160 p	~0.75	100	0.75	0.75 ox	distant occur.	2–5 ug	—	Einaudi, unpublished
Morenci (Arizona)	353 p	~1.1	~99 (supergene)	0.1–0.15	2–4 ug 1.00 p	~1	<1	5–20 ox	Moolick & Durek, 1966

NOTE: Deposits are arranged in order of decreasing proportion of non-porphyry to porphyry ore. Blanks in body of table indicate no data.

[a] Mineralization west of Joker Fault

[b] Grade for supergene ore refers to supergene sulfides, unless noted otherwise.

[c] Estimated future potential

KEY:
- bx = breccia
- diss = disseminated
- op = open-pit mining grade
- ox = oxide ore
- p = production
- r = reserves
- sk = skarn
- ug = underground mining grade

Buttes, and Pima-Mission are in the +500-million-ton class; Santa Rita, Ely, and Christmas are at the 100-million-ton mark; and Silver Bell and Continental contain 50 million tons.

Large-scale underground mining of skarn ore by block caving methods has yet to be attempted in southwestern North America. The Lakeshore deposit and a future resource on Anaconda property adjacent to the Carr Fork mine at Bingham yield similar estimates of tonnage and hypogene grade for possible block caving operations in skarn: 150 to 200 million tons of 1.0 to 1.5 percent Cu (Hallof and Winniski, 1971; South, 1972; Proxy Statement, 1976, The Anaconda Co.). More selective underground mining methods can be designed to remove skarn only; such methods, used at Christmas, Continental, and Carr Fork, yield copper grades near 2 percent (at cut-off grades of 0.8–1% Cu) for ore tonnages of 5 to 60 million tons (Koski and Cook, 1982; W. T. Worthington, 1978, personal communication; Proxy Statement, 1976, The Anaconda Co.). The data from smaller underground mines in operation during the early part of the century, when mining was highly selective and cut-off grades were near 1.5 percent Cu, indicate that an upper limit for hypogene copper grade of skarn in blocks of 500,000 tons to a few million tons would be around 2.5 to 3.0 percent Cu.

The presence of 2 to 10 percent calcite in most skarn bodies inhibits the development of supergene sulfide ores, because copper is retained (and slightly enriched) in the oxide zone: oxide ores at Twin Buttes and Christmas average 1.0 percent Cu. High-grade, exotic, copper oxide ores—such as those at Morenci (Moolick and Durek, 1966)—may form in limestone near skarn bodies, in fault zones, or above impermeable shale beds.

Massive sulfide ores associated with silica-pyrite rock have yielded the highest hypogene and supergene copper grades of the porphyry copper environment. Carbonate-free silica-pyrite is ideally suited for supergene enrichment; intense leaching at the surface yields copper-free jasperoidal gossans which may be encased in copper carbonate ores. Oxidized silica-pyrite ores at Bisbee have contained 5 percent Cu (Bryant, 1964), whereas supergene-enriched chalcocite ores in silica-pyrite at Cananea have ranged from 3 to 10 percent Cu (Emmons, 1910). Square-set stopes in the hanging wall of the High Grade fault in the Ruth mine (Robinson district, Nevada) have yielded supergene enriched silica-pyrite ores averaging more than 5 percent Cu (Bauer et al., 1966). Selective underground mining at Cananea and Bisbee has produced tens of millions of tons of primary ore with 2 to 5 percent Cu.

Published data on the content of metals other than copper are sparse; Table 8.3 summarizes available data. Cu:Mo ratios in skarn generally are higher than in the associated plutons. Lead and zinc are present in amounts less than 0.05 weight percent in most skarn deposits; zinc is unusually high in skarn at Silver Bell and Continental, where it reaches 0.5 to 0.8 weight percent overall. Zn:Cu ratios in skarn are higher than in associated plutons, and range from 1:30 at Bingham to 1:1 in the Imperial skarn at Silver Bell. Outlying Pb-zn-Ag fissures in limestone at Bingham display Zn:Cu ratios of 9:1 to 17:1 (Atkinson and Einaudi, 1978); similar fissures in the western portion of the Central mining district, which may or may not be related to the Santa Rita stock, display Zn:Cu ratios which increase westward from 3:1 to 26:1 or 50:1 (Jones et al., 1967). WO_3 commonly occurs in the range 0.02 to 0.04 weight percent in garnetite skarn at Twin Buttes (Barter and Kelly, 1982), and a small Cu-W orebody in shale in contact with the Weary Flat stock at Ely contains an average of 0.50 percent WO_3 (Bauer et al., 1966).

PHYSIOCHEMICAL CHARACTERISTICS OF SKARN-FORMING ENVIRONMENTS

Consideration of the physiochemical conditions of alteration-mineralization in carbonate rocks must take into account not only the *P-T* conditions and the possible ranges of volatile fugacities and pH, but also the activities of nonvolatile components in the hydrothermal fluid. The identification of controlling variables in open systems of many components is virtually impossible; at best, only relative changes in temperature and/or activities of components in solution can be specified as a function of space or time. Consider, for example, the occurrence of andradite versus pyrite-quartz-calcite; both are known to occur as metasomatic replacement of limestone, presumably through the infiltration of a fluid with relatively high activities of silica and iron. The relative stabilities of the two contrasting assemblages can be expressed by:

$$\underset{\text{andradite}}{Ca_3Fe_2Si_3O_{12}} + 3CO_2 + 2S_2 = \underset{\text{pyrite}}{2FeS_2} + \underset{\text{quartz}}{3SiO_2} + \underset{\text{calcite}}{3CaCO_3} + \tfrac{3}{2}O_2 \qquad (1)$$

The reaction is a function of temperature and of f_{O_2}, f_{S_2}, and f_{CO_2} (or the mole fraction $CO_2/CO_2{+}H_2O$, abbreviated as X_{CO_2}). The specification of controlling variables in this case must rely on geological arguments related to the specific case being considered, perhaps enhanced by independent estimates of temperature and X_{CO_2}, based on fluid inclusion or isotopic study.

This section sets a general temperature-fugacity-mole fraction (T-f_{O_2}-f_{S_2}-X_{CO_2}) framework for metamorphism and metasomatism in contact aureoles of porphyry copper plutons. The contrast between the andradite-diopside-chalcopyrite association and other garnet-clinopyroxene ore mineral associations is discussed in order to define general environmental parameters, such as oxidation state and degree of chemical evolution of ore fluids. Within this context, consideration is given to T-X_{CO_2} equilibria involving Ca-Mg silicates, then to equilibria involving Ca-Fe silicates—where f_{O_2} becomes an additional variable—and finally to reactions involving phases of variable Fe:Mg ratios. This discussion sets the stage for consideration of the effects of sulfur and hydrothermal interaction between plutons and carbonate wall rocks.

Contrasts With Other Skarn-Forming Environments

Hedenbergite-Grossularite Skarn. The hedenbergite-grossularite association, typical of the majority of tungsten-bearing skarn deposits (Zharikov, 1970; Shimazaki, 1974, 1977), has not been reported from porphyry-related skarns.

TABLE 8.3
Hypogene Grades and Ratios from Porphyry and Skarn in Representative Porphyry Copper Districts of Southwestern North America

MINING DISTRICT AND DEPOSIT NAME	ORE TYPE	HYPOGENE GRADES				AMOUNT OF SILVER	METAL RATIOS		SOURCES
		%Cu	%Mo	%Pb	%Zn	Ag oz./ton	Cu:Mo	Zn:Cu	
Bingham Mining District, Utah									
Carr Fork	deep calcic skarn, underground	2.2	0.029	—	—	0.4	76	—	Einaudi, 1982; Reid, 1978; James, 1978
Utah Copper	calcic skarn, open pit;	0.65	0.009	0.002	0.02	0.15	72	0.03	
Utah Copper	porphyry, open pit	0.70	0.036	—	—	—	19	—	
Central Mining District, New Mexico									
Continental No. 3	calcic skarn, underground;	~2.0	—	—	~0.5	—	—	0.25	W. T. Worthington, 1978, personal communication;
Continental	calcic skarn, open pit	0.85	—	—	—	—	—	—	
Santa Rita (Chino)	calcic skarn, open pit;	0.9	—	—	—	—	—	—	Rose & Baltosser, 1966; Nielsen, 1970
Santa Rita (Chino)	porphyry, open pit	~0.2	—	—	—	—	—	—	
Morenci District, Arizona									
Morenci	porphyry, open pit	0.12	0.007	—	~0.05	—	17	0.42	Moolick & Durek, 1966; Lowell & Guilbert, 1970
Pima District, Arizona									
Twin Buttes	calcic skarn, open pit;	1.30	0.05	—	—	0.37	27	—	Einaudi, 1982
Twin Buttes	in all types of calc-silicate rocks, open pit	0.73	0.03	—	—	—	24	—	
Mission	skarn + hornfels(?), open pit	0.70	0.009	0.024	—	0.28	78	—	Gale, 1965
Pima	skarn + hornfels, open pit;	0.18	—	—	—	—	—	—	Langlois, 1978
Pima	porphyry, open pit;	0.15	—	—	—	—	—	—	
Pima	overall, open pit	0.47	0.015	—	—	—	31	—	
Silver Bell Mining District, Arizona									
El Tiro	Imperial skarn, open pit;	0.8	—	—	0.8	—	—	1.0	Graybeal, 1982
El Tiro	El Tiro skarn, open pit;	0.8	—	—	<0.8	—	—	<1.0	
El Tiro	Silver Bell porphyry, open pit	~0.2	0.022	—	—	—	9	—	

NOTE: Blanks in body of table indicate no data.

The relative iron contents of co-existing garnet and clinopyroxene could reflect variations in temperature; activities of silica, calcium, and hydrogen ion; as well as oxidation state:

$$\underset{\text{in garnet}}{[Ca_3Fe_2Si_3O_{12}]} + H_4SiO_4 + 2H^+ = \underset{\text{in clinopyroxene}}{2[CaFeSi_2O_6]} + Ca^{++} + 3H_2O + \tfrac{1}{2}O_2 \quad (2)$$

Zharikov (1970), using a relation similar to (2), assumed that temperature, f_{O_2}, and the activities of non-volatile components are relatively constant in deep skarn-forming environments, and concluded that the ratio of the mole fraction of hedenbergite in clinopyroxene to the mole fraction of andradite in garnet (X_{Hd}/X_{Ad}) depends primarily on pH. For these assumptions, skarns with high X_{Hd}/X_{Ad} (tungsten-bearing) reflect relatively lower pH than skarns with lower X_{Hd}/X_{Ad} (copper-bearing).

An alternative view was expressed by Shimazaki (1978) and Einaudi (1977), who concluded that X_{Hd}/X_{Ad} reflects the oxidation state of the skarn-forming environment. In order for X_{Hd}/X_{Ad} to be uniquely a function of the oxidation state, two additional pure solid phases must be present to reduce the variance of the system, as, for example:

$$\underset{\text{in garnet}}{3Ca_3Fe_2Si_3O_{12}} + \underset{\text{quartz}}{9SiO_2} + \underset{\text{magnetite}}{Fe_3O_4} = \underset{\text{in clinopyroxene}}{9[CaFeSi_2O_6]} + 2O_2 \quad (3)$$

Assuming garnet and clinopyroxene are ideal solutions and that quartz and magnetite are pure phases, then the ratio X_{Hd}/X_{Ad} in skarn contining excess quartz and magnetite should be a measure of oxidation state. (Alternately, a similar relation holds for skarns with excess quartz and wollastonite if X_{Hd} is less than about 0.85.)

Figure 8.6 contrasts X_{Hd}/X_{Ad} for North American occurrences of tungsten-bearing skarns and of copper-bearing skarns related to porphyry systems. The diagram is a simplification of complex compositional and space-time relationships and its use in contrasting skarn deposits should be restricted to deposits which (1) lack significant manganese in pyroxene and ferrous iron in garnet and (2) display a limited range in X_{Hd}/X_{Ad}. Although porphyry-related skarns appear to meet the above restrictions, tungsten-bearing skarns in general do not. For this reason, data points for tungsten skarns represent somewhat subjective averages for the main ore-bearing portions of the deposits, in which the pyralspite component of garnet is lower than that in later stages (see, for example, Wright [1973]). With the above caveats in mind, it can be seen that Figure 8.6 illustrates the tendency for tungsten-bearing skarns to display X_{Hd}/X_{Ad} values greater than 0.75 (relatively reduced) and for copper-bearing skarns to display values less than 0.40 (relatively oxidized).

The constant value of X_{Hd}/X_{Ad} displayed by garnet-pyroxene pairs in some skarns suggests that equilibria of type (3) may be operative during skarn formation and that variation in the activity of iron in solution may simply be reflected

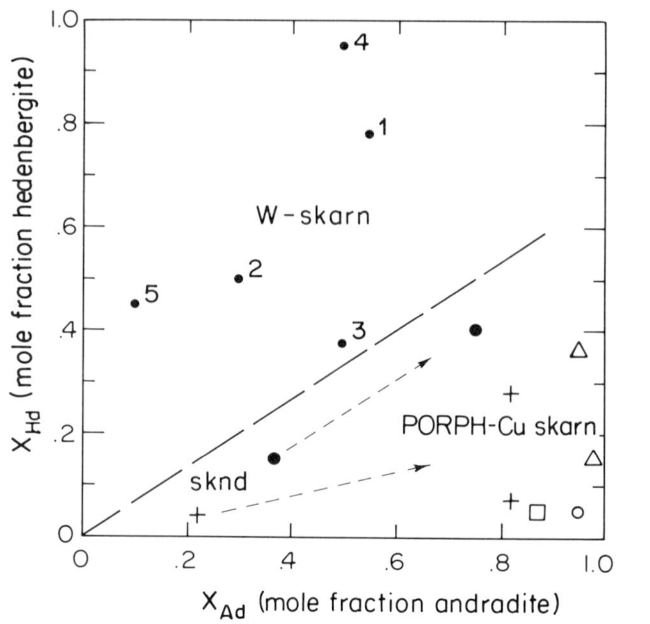

Figure 8.6. Plot of X_{Hd} versus X_{Ad}, illustrating relative oxidation states of North American W-bearing and porphyry-related, Cu-bearing skarns. Data points represent averages of garnet and pyroxene compositions in ore-bearing skarn. Dashed arrows indicate Fe-enrichment trend from early skarnoid *(sknd)* to late skarn at Yerington and Cananea. Key to W deposits: 1 = Granite Creek, Nevada (Taylor, 1976); 2 = Pine Creek, California (Wright, 1973); 3 = Scheelore, 4 = Pappas, 5 = Laurel Lakes (all three in California [Morgan, 1975]). Key to Cu deposits: ● = Yerington, Nevada (Einaudi, 1977), + = Cananea, Mexico (L. D. Meinert, 1978, preliminary data); ○ = Ely, Nevada (James, 1976; Huang, 1976); □ = Twin Buttes, Arizona (Einaudi, unpublished data), and △ = Bingham, Utah (Atkinson and Einaudi, 1978).

by a change in $X_{Hd} + X_{Ad}$ (Einaudi, 1977). The effect of this change could be recognized in the iron enrichment through time at constant X_{Hd}/X_{Ad}, such as from early skarnoid formation to later skarn formation at Yerington and Cananea (see Fig. 8.6, dashed arrows).

The relatively high oxidation state of copper-bearing versus most tungsten-bearing skarns suggested by the calc-silicate compositions is supported by contrasts in geologic settings (high-level stock, as opposed to deeper batholithic environments) and in minor phases (hematite-magnetite-pyrite, as opposed to magnetite-pyrrhotite ±pyrite).

Manganese-Rich Calc-Silicates. Common skarn minerals, which are stable in the relatively oxidized hypabyssal environment of porphyry copper plutons, but which are not known to occur in porphyry-related skarns, include iron- and manganese-rich clinopyroxenes (manganhedenbergite, johannsenite), pyroxenoids (pyroxmangite, bustamite, ferrobustamite, rhodonite), and associated phases, such as ilvaite. As shown earlier, in porphyry-related skarns clinopyroxene is magnesium-rich and actinolite, rather than ilvaite, is stable as a late replacement of clinopyroxene. Burt (1977) has pointed out that, in some skarns, clinopyroxene is enriched in the sequence Mg → Fe^{+2} → Mn as limestone is approached. Enrichment in Fe^{+2} + Mn is especially marked in zinc-bearing skarns, as pointed out by Zharikov (1970) and Burt (1972, 1977) and as exemplified in the United States by skarns in the Magdalena (Titley, 1961) and Central (Schmitt, 1939) mining districts, New Mexico. The early portion of the sequence (Mg → Fe^{+2}) is apparent in the few porphyry-related skarns where data are available: Einaudi (1977) has shown a progressive increase of Fe/(Fe + Mg) in clinopyroxene from 0.36 to 0.56 as marble is approached at the Mason Valley mine, Yerington district; and L. D. Meinert (1978, personal communication) has documented ferrous iron enrichment, accompanied by minor manganese, in late clinopyroxene in skarn at Cananea, Mexico.

Although there is no simple relation between zoning of calc-silicates and time-evolutionary trends in the composition of the hydrothermal fluid in individual deposits, the above data suggest that both the degree of manganese enrichment relative to magnesium and ferrous iron, and a parallel enrichment of the zinc relative to copper, are expressions of the degree of chemical evolution of the ore fluids and may largely be functions of travel distance and temperature, rather than of fundamentally different initial compositions. Thus, the low values of X_{Hd}/X_{Ad}, Mn/(Mg + Fe) and Zn: Cu in porphyry-related skarns may reflect proximity to the source of a primitive, moderately oxidized, hydrothermal fluid associated with mineralized hypabyssal stocks.

Decarbonation-Dehydration Reactions in Skarn Deposits

Considerable experimental data exist on metamorphic reactions involving mixed volatiles and pure endmember minerals in the systems $CaO\text{-}MgO\text{-}SiO_2\text{-}CO_2\text{-}H_2O$ and $CaO\text{-}Al_2O_3\text{-}SiO_2\text{-}CO_2\text{-}H_2O$. Only a few key concepts are considered here; for detailed reviews, the reader is referred to summaries by Kerrick (1974), Greenwood (1976), and Shreyer (1976). A constant total pressure *(P)* of 500 bars, equal to fluid pressure, is assumed in the following discussion. This pressure is based on approximate lithostatic load at the shallow levels of emplacement of porphyry copper plutons. However, because these systems commonly show evidence of a shift with time from $P_{fluid} \geq$ lithostatic to P_{fluid} = hydrostatic, a value of P_{fluid} equal to 500 bars should be considered an approximate upper limit.

At constant pressure, two variables may be used to describe the stabilities of calc-silicates in the above systems: temperature *(T)* and the mole fraction of CO_2 in a $H_2O\text{-}CO_2$ fluid (X_{CO_2}). Reactions which lead to the first appearance of a calc-silicate phase from a carbonate-bearing assemblage have positive slopes on a $T\text{-}X_{CO_2}$ diagram; that is, either an increase in T or a decrease in X_{CO_2} favors formation of the calc-silicate. This characteristic has two important consequences in the interpretation of natural assemblages: (1) in order to specify *T*, the composition of the aqueous phase (X_{CO_2}) must be known; and (2) calc-silicate formation can occur at lower T in H_2O-rich fluids than in CO_2-rich fluids.

X_{CO_2} in Skarn-Forming Environments. Various sources of data indicate that X_{CO_2} in fluids permeating carbonate rocks during metamorphism and metasomatism generally is quite low, probably less than 0.1. Based on oxygen isotope data, Taylor and O'Neil (1977) have estimated X_{CO_2} to be $\leq$0.15 in metamorphic calc-silicate rocks and vein skarns (<3 cm thick), and $\leq$0.035 in massive skarns of the Osgood Mountains, Nevada. Based on fluid inclusion data, Huang (1976) has concluded that X_{CO_2} in fluids that deposited garnet, pyroxene, and quartz in skarn at Ely, Nevada, was less than 0.06. Low values of X_{CO_2} during various stages of alteration also are implied by the presence of certain key minerals: (1) grossularite or clinozoisite formed during early metamorphic stages indicates fluids with X_{CO_2} of $\gtrsim$0.1 at T = <550°C and P = 2kb (Gordon and Greenwood, 1971); and (2) serpentine formed as a retrograde product after olivine or as a metasomatic replacement of marble indicates fluids with X_{CO_2} of <0.05 (Greenwood, 1967*a*) at very low pressures.

In spite of the above arguments, the possibility of significant local variations in X_{CO_2} must not be ignored. These variations may have occurred through time; initial stages of metamorphism in rocks of low permeability (e.g., marbles), before the onset of widespread fracturing and fluid circulation, could have lead to CO_2 enrichment, followed by H_2O enrichment, as fracturing occurred and as CO_2 generated during decarbonation could be more effectively flushed out of the system. This possibility has been suggested by the data of Taylor and O'Neil (1977). Variations in X_{CO_2} also may be expressed as gradients during prograde zoned skarn formation, with X_{CO_2} relatively high near the marble contact and relatively low in the skarn center (Einaudi, 1977), or as gradients between different interstratified lithologies (Atkinson and Einaudi, 1978).

Open-System Versus Closed-System Behavior. The general lack of isobarically univariant assemblages (such as diopside-tremolite-calcite-quartz) in contact metamorphic aureoles associated with porphyry copper plutons implies that the value of X_{CO_2} was controlled by the fluid (system open to H_2O and CO_2); this type of control, in turn, implies high permeabilities and relatively high fluid: rock ratios. In contrast, lower permeabilities and fluid: rock ratios would result in control of X_{CO_2} by the mineral phases present in the rock (system closed to H_2O and CO_2). The low values of X_{CO_2} implied by the arguments given earlier are consistent with open-system behavior, because closed-system behavior can lead to significant enrichment of the fluid phase in CO_2 (see, for example Greenwood [1967*a*, 1975]).

Oxidation-Reduction Reactions in Porphyry-Related Skarns

Because garnet of essentially pure andradite composition is a common phase in porphyry-related skarns, the stability relations in the system Ca-Fe-Si-C-O-H are especially significant. The effect of variable Fe: Mg ratios in clinopyroxene and amphibole can be treated using ideal solution theory and experimental data from the endmember system.

System Ca-Fe-Si-C-O-H. Experimental studies by Liou (1974), Gustafson (1974), and Taylor and Liou (1978) allow the definition of a $T\text{-}f_{O_2}$ grid for anhydrous phases (Fig. 8.7) that confirms the topology predicted by Burt (1972). However, a study by Shimazaki and Bunno (1978) of natural hedenbergite-ferrobustamite assemblages implies that the reaction andradite-quartz = hedenbergite-wollastonite is metastable and that iron-endmember equilibria at low oxidation states will have to be modified. The consequences of such modification are insignificant for the present discussion because, for the relatively high oxidation states of porphyry copper systems, ferrobustamite is not stable relative to

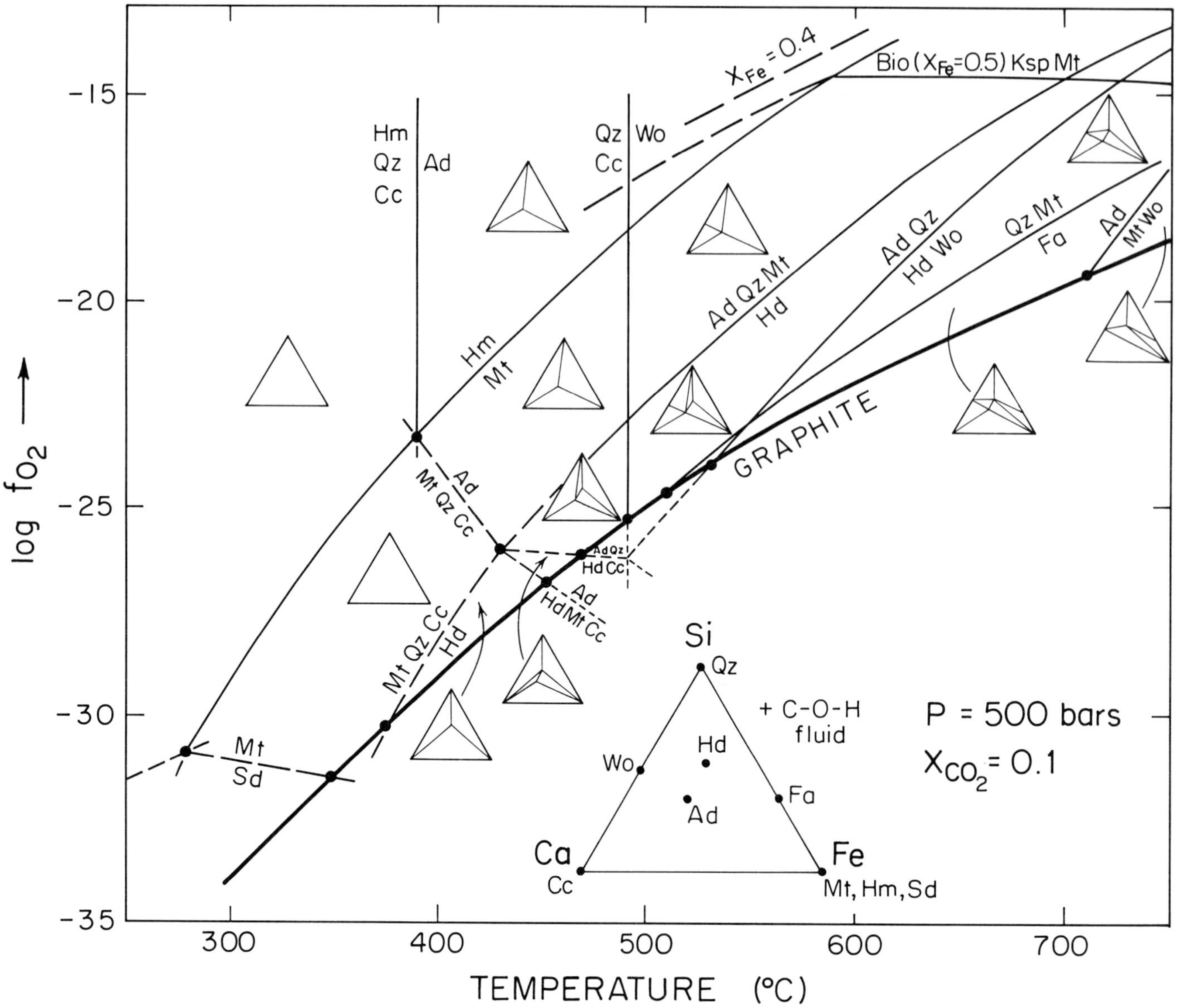

Abbreviations:
Ad = andradite
Cc = calcite
Fa = fayalite
Hd = hedenbergite
Hm = hematite
Ksp = alkali feldspar
Mt = magnetite
Qz = quartz
Sd = siderite
Wo = wollastonite

Figure 8.7. Temperature-log f_{O_2} diagram at 500 bars fluid pressure and $X_{CO_2} = 0.1$ for the system Ca-Fe-Si-C-0-H. Solid line calc-silicate equilibria are based on experimental data from Greenwood (1967*b*), Liou (1974), Gustafson (1974), and Taylor and Liou (1978); dashed lines are approximate locations of equilibria lacking experimental control. Oxide buffers hematite-magnetite, quartz-magnetite-fayalite, and graphite are based on data from French and Eugster (1965) and French (1971). The siderite field is schematic, based on the lack of siderite-hedenbergite and siderite-andradite assemblages in skarns (Burt, 1972). Biotite compositions in mole fraction annite for assemblage biotite–K-feldspar–magnetite(hematite) from Wones and Eugster (1965).

clinopyroxene ($X_{\text{hedenbergite}} < 0.85$) + wollastonite. Key features of Figure 8.7 include the following:

1. Equilibria in the CO_2-free system show that hedenbergite, with iron in the ferrous state, is stable only at relatively low oxidation states, below the magnetite-pyrite-pyrrhotite buffer. The absence of iron-rich clinopyroxene in porphyry-related skarns is due in part to the relatively high oxidation states but more importantly to the relatively high sulfidation states. In contrast, andradite, with iron in the ferric state, has a broad f_{O_2} stability range below 700°C. The stability of andradite, rather than wollastonite-magnetite, below 700°C is an experimental result which is compatible with the absence of the latter assemblage in porphyry-related skarn. Thus, iron-rich solutions, at intermediate to low sulfidation states, deposit andradite rather than magnetite on encountering wollastonite.

2. Only the equilibria involving CO_2 will shift positions as X_{CO_2} is changed from the value of 0.1 used to construct the figure. For example, increasing X_{CO_2} moves the an-

dradite equilibria to higher temperature (the invariant points shift along the CO_2-free equilibria), and thus reduces the size of the andradite stability field. In contrast, the hedenbergite field is significantly less sensitive to variations in X_{CO_2}.

3. It can be predicted that at oxidation states above andradite-quartz-magnetite = hedenbergite an important retrograde reaction at relatively low sulfidation states involving andradite-rich skarn is the magnetite-producing analogue of reaction (1):

$$\underset{\text{andradite}}{Ca_3Fe_2Si_3O_{12}} + 3CO_2 = \tfrac{2}{3}\underset{\text{magnetite}}{Fe_3O_4} + 3\underset{\text{quartz}}{SiO_2} + 3\underset{\text{calcite}}{CaCO_3} + \tfrac{1}{6}O_2 \qquad (5)$$

Effect of Variable Fe : Mg Ratios. One of the limitations inherent in applying Figure 8.7 is the fact that natural assemblages in most cases do not contain phases of endmember composition. Although, as a first approximation, garnets can be treated as pure endmember andradite, the magnesium content of clinopyroxene must be accounted for. Because experimental data are lacking, the shift of endmember reactions on addition of magnesium can be approximated using ideal solution theory. Two examples are given below, based on the approach taken by Mueller (1973).

A common porphyry-related skarn association is andradite, magnetite, and quartz containing clinopyroxene of variable, but low, iron content. The Fe-endmember equivalent of reaction (3),

$$9\underset{\text{hedenbergite}}{CaFeSi_2O_6} + 2O_2 = 3\underset{\text{andradite}}{Ca_3Fe_2Si_3O_{12}} + \underset{\text{magnetite}}{Fe_3O_4} + 9\underset{\text{quartz}}{SiO_2} \qquad (3')$$

determined experimentally by Gustafson (1974), can be used to calculate the oxidation state implied by $X_{Fe}^{clinopyroxene} = 0.15$ to 0.35 in the assemblage clinopyroxene-andradite-quartz-magnetite. Assuming that clinopyroxene behaves as an ideal solution (Mueller, 1961; Saxena, 1971), for which $a_i = X_i^n$ (n = number of equivalent lattice sites per gram formula of exchanging cation, [i]), and that the value of $\Delta V°_r$ (solids) is constant from P_1 to P_2, then

$$\log (f_{O_2})_2 = \frac{\Delta V°_r (P_2-P_1)(0.0239)}{9.152T} + \log (f_{O_2})_1 - \tfrac{9}{2}\log X_{Fe}^{clinopyroxene} \qquad (3'\text{–}1)$$

where subscripts 1 refer to the experimental conditions at P_1 = 2,000 bars, $\log (f_{O_2})_1 = -25.2$ bars, $T = 450 \pm 60$°C, and subscripts 2 refer to conditions of interest here (also at 450°C) at P_2 = 500 bars.

Solving for $X_{Fe}^{clinopyroxene} = 0.15$ to 0.35 at 450°C, $\log f_{O_2}$ ranges from –21.8 to –23.5. This result is consistent with the occurrence of pyrite, rather than pyrrhotite, with andradite-clinopyroxene-magnetite-quartz assemblages (see Table 8.1). It also suggests that in order for hematite to co-exist with andradite-clinopyroxene-quartz, clinopyroxene should contain less than 6 mole percent hedenbergite. Because it may be questioned whether four-phase equilibrium assemblages occur in skarns, the above results must be viewed as general values of oxidation state implied by the associations of porphyry skarns. The agreement of these results with other environmental indicators suggests that the *overall* composition of salite reflects an approach to equilibrium with andradite at oxidation states intermediate between the nickel–nickel oxide and magnetite-hematite buffers at temperatures above 400°C (for $X_{CO_2} = 0.1$, and 500 bars P_{total}).

A second porphyry-related skarn mineral association that can be evaluated in this manner involves actinolite. Ernst (1966) has determined the stability field of endmember ferroactinolite at P_{H_2O} = 3,000 bars to be at temperatures less than 550°C and low oxygen fugacities near, or lower than, the quartz-fayalite-magnetite buffer. Endmember ferroactinolite rarely occurs in nature because of this low f_{O_2} stability, but substitution of magnesium for iron expands the field of the calcic amphibole to higher oxygen fugacities. Actinolite is a common phase in porphyry-related skarns, particularly as an alteration of salite, and is associated with pyrite, magnetite, and chalcopyrite. A relevant reaction, therefore, is reaction *J* of Ernst:

$$\underset{\text{ferroactinolite}}{Ca_2Fe_5Si_8O_{22}(OH)_2} + \tfrac{1}{2}O_2 = 2\underset{\text{hedenbergite}}{CaFeSi_2O_6} + \underset{\text{magnetite}}{Fe_3O_4} + \underset{\text{quartz}}{4SiO_4} + H_2O \qquad (6)$$

A general equation which describes the shift in reaction (6) as a function of Fe : Mg ratio of the phases, assuming that both clinopyroxene and amphibole behave as ideal solutions and that $X_{Fe}^{actinolite} = X_{Fe}^{clinopyroxene}$, can be established in a manner analogous to that for reaction (3'):

$$\log (f_{O_2})_2 = \frac{\Delta V°_r (P_2-P_1)(0.0239)}{2.288} + 2\log (f_{H_2O})_2 - \log (f_{H_2O})_1 - 6\log X_{Fe}^{actinolite} + \log (f_{O_2})_1 \qquad (6\text{–}1)$$

Subscripts 1 indicate Ernst's experimental conditions, at 500°C, whereas subscripts 2 indicate the new conditions (also at 500°C) at P_2 = 500 bars, $X_{CO_2} = 0.1$. In calculating $(f_{H_2O})_2$, it was assumed that H_2O-CO_2 mixtures behave as ideal solutions; fugacity values for pure H_2O were taken from Burnham and others (1969). Equation (6–1) was used to calculate f_{O_2} for a range in $X_{Fe}^{actinolite}$ of 0.15 to 0.40, which corresponds to the composition of actinolite co-existing with salite-quartz-pyrite ±magnetite at Ely, Bingham, and Yerington. Results are a range in $\log f_{O_2}$ (at 500°C) of –20.2 to –22.9, respectively.

The overlap of oxidation state for salite-andradite assemblages (3) and salite-actinolite assemblages (6), implied by these results, was expected on the basis of field evidence discussed earlier; actinolite and andradite represent contemporaneous products resulting from the influx of relatively oxidized metasomatic fluids in equilibrium with potassium-silicate assemblages in the associated plutons.

Effect of Sulfur on Stability of Calc-Silicates

The effect of increasing the sulfidation state to the point at which pyrite or pyrrhotite become stable relative to magnetite is to drastically reduce the stability of calcium-iron silicates. This effect can be computed on the basis of equilibria presented above, in conjunction with sulfidation-oxidation equilibria involving iron sulfides, iron oxides, and anhydrite.

Isothermal Fugacity Diagram, 500°C. Figure 8.8 illustrates the calculated log f_{S_2} – log f_{O_2} diagram for the Fe-Si-Ca-C-O-H-S system at 500°C and $X_{CO_2} = 0.1$. Topologically similar chemical potential diagrams have been presented by Burt (1972); computational methods used to construct fugacity diagrams are reviewed by Garrels and Christ (1965) and Holland (1959).

The limits of andradite stability at 500°C are represented by the following reactions:

$$\underset{\text{andradite}}{2Ca_3Fe_2Si_3O_{12}} + 2S_2 = \underset{\text{wollastonite}}{6CaSiO_3} + \underset{\text{pyrrhotite}}{4FeS} + 3O_2 \quad (7)$$

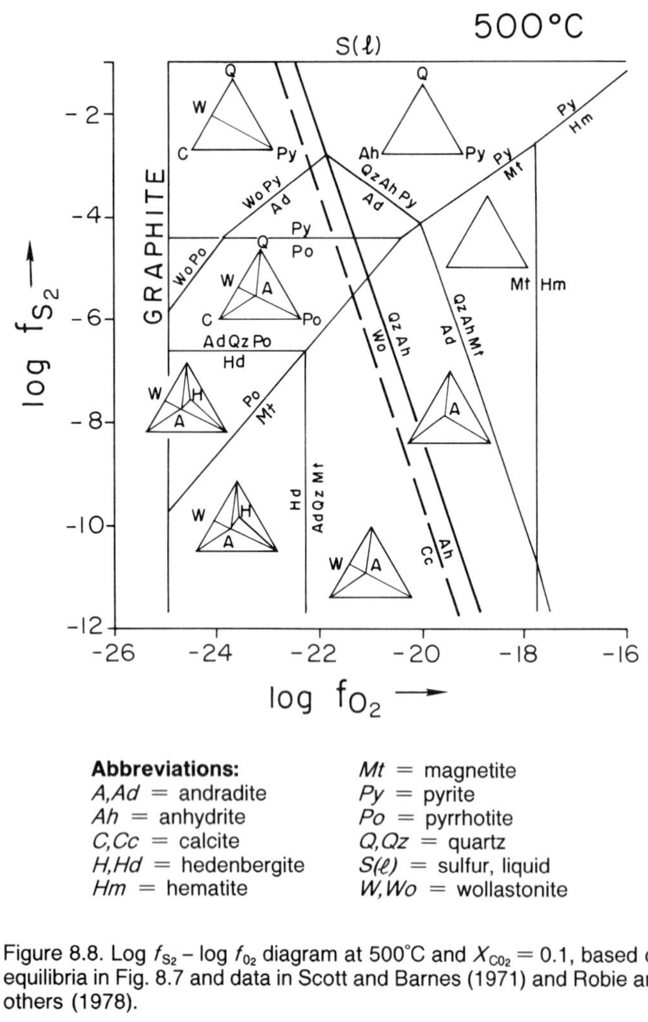

Abbreviations:
A,Ad = andradite
Ah = anhydrite
C,Cc = calcite
H,Hd = hedenbergite
Hm = hematite
Mt = magnetite
Py = pyrite
Po = pyrrhotite
Q,Qz = quartz
S(ℓ) = sulfur, liquid
W,Wo = wollastonite

Figure 8.8. Log f_{S_2} – log f_{O_2} diagram at 500°C and $X_{CO_2} = 0.1$, based on equilibria in Fig. 8.7 and data in Scott and Barnes (1971) and Robie and others (1978).

$$\underset{\text{andradite}}{2Ca_3Fe_2Si_3O_{12}} + 4S_2 = \underset{\text{wollastonite}}{6CaSiO_3} + \underset{\text{pyrite}}{4FeS_2} + 3O_2 \quad (8)$$

$$\underset{\text{andradite}}{2Ca_3Fe_2Si_3O_{12}} + 7S_2 + 6O_2 = \underset{\text{quartz}}{6SiO_2} + \underset{\text{anhydrite}}{6CaSO_4} + \underset{\text{pyrite}}{4FeS_2} \quad (9)$$

$$\underset{\text{andradite}}{6Ca_3Fe_2Si_3O_{12}} + 9S_2 + 26O_2 = \underset{\text{quartz}}{18SiO_2} + \underset{\text{anhydrite}}{18CaSO_4} + \underset{\text{magnetite}}{4Fe_3O_4} \quad (10)$$

Inspection of these reactions and of Figure 8.8 reveals that the stability of anhydrite-quartz relative to wollastonite,

$$\underset{\text{wollastonite}}{2CaSiO_3} + S_2 + 3O_2 = \underset{\text{quartz}}{2SiO_2} + \underset{\text{anhydrite}}{2CaSO_4} \quad (11)$$

has an important effect on the stability of andradite. The topology of Figure 8.8 is valid only if total sulfur (ΣS) and/or $a_{Ca^{++}}$ in the aqueous phase is sufficiently high to stabilize anhydrite relative to its dissolution products at $f_{S_2} - f_{O_2}$ values higher than invariant point (andradite-quartz-anhydrite-magnetite-pyrite). Although the location of the anhydrite dissolution reaction as a function of ΣS and $a_{Ca^{++}}$ cannot be evaluated at the relatively high temperatures of skarn formation, the topology of Figure 8.8 is compatible with the following field data from porphyry systems: (1) the assemblage anhydrite-quartz-magnetite (or pyrite) is relatively common in potassium-silicate-altered stocks associated with andradite skarn; (2) the assemblage andradite-bornite-pyrite is not reported from andradite skarns; (3) the assemblage andradite-anhydrite-pyrite occurs at Christmas and the assemblage andradite-anhydrite-wollastonite occurs at Twin Buttes.

Stability of Andradite, Anhydrite and Sulfides. A series of isothermal log f_{S_2} – log f_{O_2} diagrams, drawn for the andradite bulk composition, are displayed in Figure 8.9, and the univariant T–f_{S_2} curves which define the andradite + Fe-sulfide stability field are projected onto the T–f_{S_2} plane in Figure 8.10. Inspection of these figures leads to the following conclusions:

1. Andradite is stable with iron-sulfides only at low to intermediate oxidation and sulfidation states (and at temperatures above about 400°C for $X_{CO_2} = 0.1$). For these conditions, the opaque mineral assemblages bornite-magnetite, bornite-pyrrhotite, chalcopyrite-pyrrhotite, and chalcopyrite are stable with andradite; they may occur as disseminations in, or replacements of, andradite, but no alteration of andradite would be expected.
2. Andradite is unstable at high sulfidation states irrespective of T or f_{O_2}. Deposition of sulfide assemblages that are stable only at high sulfidation states—such as pyrite-bornite, pyrite-covellite, or pyrite with sphalerite containing less than 1.0 mole percent FeS—should be accompanied by alteration of andradite (see reactions 8 and 9).
3. For the values of X_{CO_2} in Figures 8.9 and 8.10, andradite is not stable with pyrite-hematite. However, under very water-rich conditions, the assemblage andradite-pyrite-hematite becomes stable below about 300 to 350°C because of the following reaction (D.K. Bird and R. P. Gamble, unpublished data):

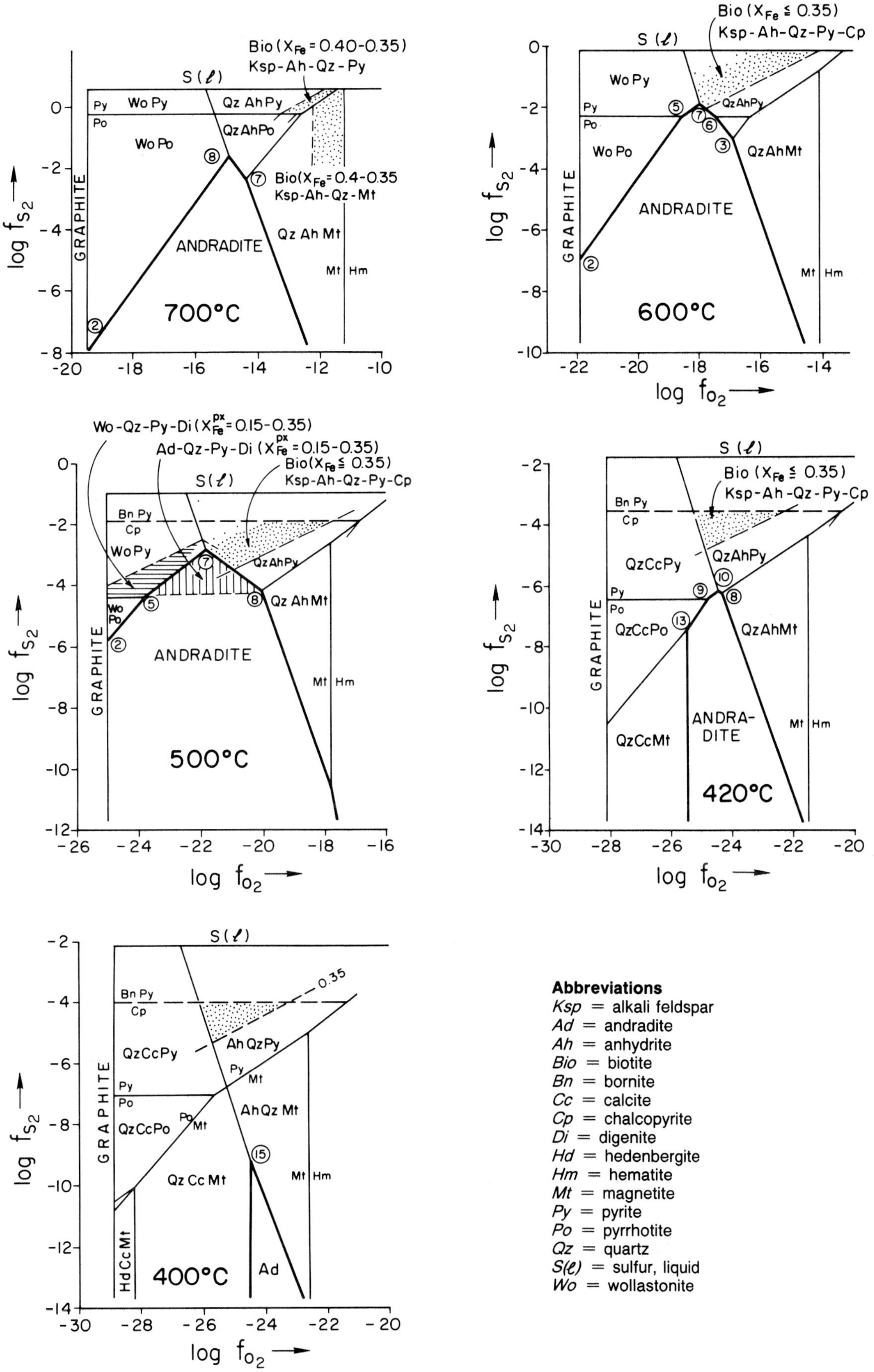

Abbreviations
Ksp = alkali feldspar
Ad = andradite
Ah = anhydrite
Bio = biotite
Bn = bornite
Cc = calcite
Cp = chalcopyrite
Di = digenite
Hd = hedenbergite
Hm = hematite
Mt = magnetite
Py = pyrite
Po = pyrrhotite
Qz = quartz
S(ℓ) = sulfur, liquid
Wo = wollastonite

Figure 8.9. Log f_{S_2} – log f_{O_2} diagrams for andradite bulk composition between 700 and 400°C at $X_{CO_2} = 0.1$. Stippled fields at 700 to 400°C represent estimates of the fugacity environment of K-silicate alteration in the pluton. Ruled areas at 500°C represent the fugacity environment of salite-bearing skarn. Circled numbers represent isobaric univariant assemblages at constant X_{CO_2} shown in Fig. 8.10. Calc-silicate and biotite equilibria based on Liou (1974), Gustafson (1974), Taylor and Liou (1978), and Wones and Eugster (1965). Cu-Fe-S-O-C-H equilibria based on Barton and Skinner (1967), Scott and Barnes (1971), French and Eugster (1965), and Helgeson (1969); anhydrite equilibria based on data in Robie and others (1978).

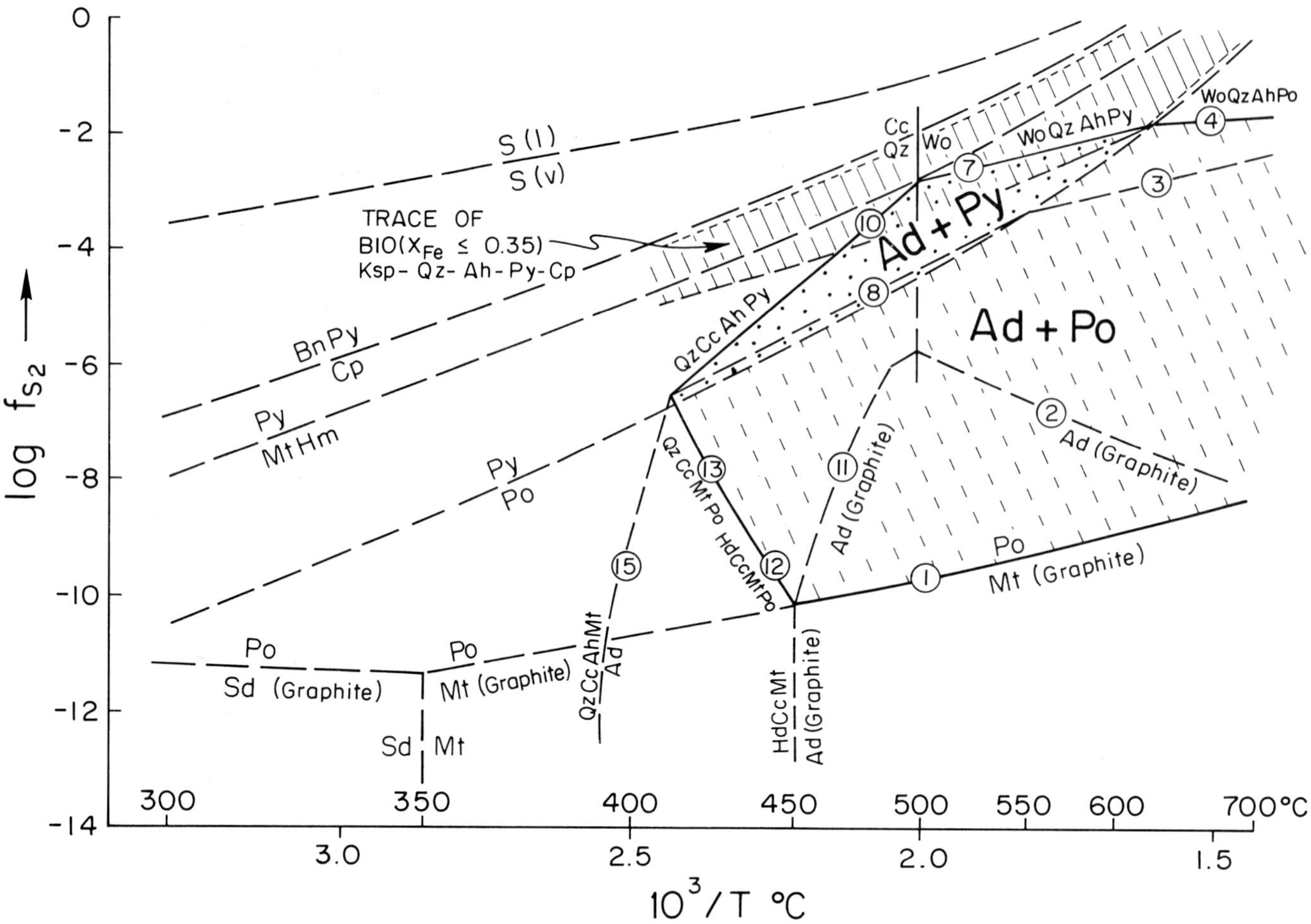

Abbreviations

Ksp = alkali feldspar	*Cp* = chalcopyrite	*Qz* = quartz
Ad = andradite	*Hd* = hedenbergite	*Sd* = siderite
Ah = anhydrite	*Hm* = hematite	*S(l)* = sulfur (liquid)
Bio = biotite	*Mt* = magnetite	*S(v)* = sulfur (vapor)
Bn = bornite	*Py* = pyrite	*Wo* = wollastonite
Cc = calcite	*Po* = pyrrhotite	

Figure 8.10. Log f_{S_2} – temperature diagram illustrating projection of andradite-pyrite and andradite-pyrrhotite stability volume at X_{CO_2} = 0.1; also shown is trace of K-silicate assemblage biotite ($X_{Fe}^{biotite} \leq 0.35$)-orthoclase-quartz-anhydrite-pyrite-chalcopyrite. Based on graphical analysis.

$$\underset{\text{quartz}}{3SiO_2} + \underset{\text{anhydrite}}{6CaSO_4} + \underset{\text{magnetite}}{45Fe_3O_4} = \underset{\text{andradite}}{2Ca_3Fe_2Si_3O_{12}} + \underset{\text{pyrite}}{3FeS_2} + \underset{\text{hematite}}{64Fe_2O_3} \quad (12)$$

Fugacity Environments in Plutons

Specification of the T-f_{O_2}-f_{S_2} environment in plutons, in contrast with that established above for the carbonate environment, yields a basis for discussion of fluid reaction paths during skarn formation and ore deposition.

Potassium-Silicate Alteration. Fugacity ranges for S_2 and O_2 in the late magmatic environment which precedes potassium-silicate alteration can be based on the Fe:Mg ratios of magmatic biotite and on the Fe-S-O opaque mineral assemblages present. Magmatic biotites in porphyry copper plutons commonly display a range of $X_{Fe}^{biotite}$ from 0.35 to 0.40 (Moore and Czamanske, 1973; Roberts, 1973; Koski, 1978); the field of stability of biotite of this composition co-existing with K-feldspar and magnetite or pyrite is shown in Figure 8.9, 700°C, based on experimental data for biotite-sanidine-magnetite equilibria (Wones and Eugster, 1965).

Potassium-silicate alteration typically occurs during initial cooling of the pluton from 600 to 400°C, as deduced from field evidence (Gustafson and Hunt, 1975), fluid inclusion data (Roedder, 1971; Moore and Nash, 1974) and elemental and isotopic partitioning between mineral phases (Sheppard et al., 1971; Brimhall, 1977). Calculated $^{18}O/^{16}O$ ratios indicate that the fluid is "magmatic," although its ultimate origin is unclear (Sheppard et al., 1971; Sheppard and Taylor, 1974). Sulfide assemblages display low S/(Cu + Fe) ratios; typical assemblages are bornite-magnetite, bornite-chalcopyrite, or chalcopyrite with or without minor pyrite.

Fugacity limits for potassium-silicate alteration (traced in Figs. 8.9 and 8.10) may be defined by the composition of hydrothermal biotite in the assemblage biotite-orthoclase-pyrite, based on the experimental data for biotite-sanidine-magnetite. Values of $X_{Fe}^{biotite}$ ranging from 0.35 to 0.15 are taken as representative (Moore and Czamanski, 1973; Beane, 1974). The absence of pyrite-bornite establishes upper limits of F_{S_2} at the reaction chalcopyrite = pyrite-bornite. Lower limits of f_{S_2} and f_{O_2} are established by the reactions anhydrite-quartz = wollastonite and anhydrite-quartz-pyrite = andradite at high temperatures (see Fig. 8.9, 600, 500°C); at lower temperatures, where wollastonite no longer is stable and andradite is not stable at the f_{S_2} of potassic alteration, the lower limits of f_{S_2}-f_{O_2} may approach the graphite boundary, in which case calcite substitutes for anhydrite (see Fig. 8.9, stippled area left of reaction anhydrite = calcite, 420, 400°C).

Sericitic Alteration. The general fluid evolution path over time and toward the peripheries of porphyry copper plutons is toward lower temperature and pressure, higher oxidation-sulfidation states and probably lower alkali : hydrogen ion ratios. This trend is expressed by the appearance of sericitic alteration accompanied by sulfide assemblages such as pyrite-chalcopyrite ±bornite. Temperatures close to 300°C have been suggested on the basis of fluid inclusion data (e.g., Roedder, 1971; Moore and Nash, 1974), and a high meteoric water component has been implied on the basis of oxygen and hydrogen isotope data (Sheppard and Taylor, 1974).

Various mechanisms for the path toward a base-cation leaching environment have been proposed for porphyry copper systems (e.g., Meyer and Hemley, 1967; Rose, 1970). As temperatures decline to 350°C and lower, acids become increasingly dissociated; the shift to lower pH is especially marked in fluids with significant sulfur content and may be enhanced by influx of oxidized meteoric water, especially if some less-ionized H_2S is present to produce more highly ionized H_2SO_4.

Discussion

It can be deduced from Figure 8.9 (700–420°C) that in order for andradite to form in carbonate wall rocks, fluids in equilibrium with potassium-silicate assemblages must shift to lower f_{S_2} and f_{O_2} in addition to having sufficient concentration of silica and iron. In the temperature range 630 to 460°C the pluton and andradite skarn environments overlap (see Fig. 8.10); this temperature interval is the optimum skarn-forming environment for the values of X_{CO_2} and P considered here. Limits on the f_{S_2}-f_{O_2} shift can be placed on the basis of X_{Hd} in clinopyroxene co-existing with andradite-quartz and with an Fe-sulfide or oxide phase, as was done earlier for reaction (3'). One such calculation at 500°C is illustrated in Figure 8.9: clinopyroxene containing less than 35 mole percent hedenbergite is stable with pyrite-chalcopyrite and not with pyrrhotite-chalcopyrite. These results are compatible with field observation (see Table 8.1).

At higher temperatures (Fig. 8.9, ~ 700°C), a significant f_{S_2}-f_{O_2} shift is required if fluids in equilibrium with biotite ($X_{Fe}^{biotite}$ <0.4)–K-feldspar–pyrite are to form andradite; the andradite-equivalent assemblages quartz-anhydrite-pyrrhotite (pyrite) or wollastonite-pyrrhotite may form as precursors to andradite. This possibility is suggested by anhydrite occurrences at Christmas and Twin Buttes.

The path toward lower f_{S_2}-f_{O_2} that has been deduced from the field evidence may be a consequence of several possible reactions. Fluids exiting from the pluton usually are undersaturated with respect to calcite. As the fluid dissolves calcite, the pH increases. A pH increase in sulfate-dominant fluids at constant ΣS is accompanied by a decrease in f_{O_2} and/or f_{S_2}:

$$SO_4^{=} + 2H^+ = H_2O + \tfrac{1}{2}S_2 + \tfrac{2}{3}O_2$$

A pH increase in sulfide-dominant fluids may be accompanied by a decrease in f_{S_2} if the fluid is relatively reduced by reaction with graphite, organic material, or hedenbergitic clinopyroxene present in the wall rocks.

The presence of veins and patches of quartz-calcite-pyrite ±magnetite in some andradite skarns where hydrolytic alteration of the pluton is minor or absent—such as at Christmas (Perry, 1968, 1969) and deep portions of Bingham (Atkinson and Einaudi, 1978)—and temperatures based on fluid inclusions in quartz-calcite-magnetite-sulfide veins at Ely (Huang, 1976) suggest that skarn destruction may begin at relatively high temperature. At temperatures below 460°C (see Fig. 8.9, 420, 400°C), the andradite stability field rapidly shrinks to lower f_{S_2} along the calcite-anhydrite equilibrium line; the f_{S_2} stability limit for andradite (see Fig. 8.9, reaction 15) at 400°C, (X_{CO_2} = 0.1) is 4 log units lower than that indicated for the pluton. Fluids exiting from the pluton at these temperatures may begin to alter previously formed andradite.

As with sericitic alteration of the stocks, destruction of skarn occurs along zones of greatest permeability; such zones are often best developed along the contacts with stocks or dikes. As shown earlier, fluids in equilibrium with pyrite at the low temperatures of sericitic alteration would alter andradite to quartz-pyrite(-hematite)-calcite (or anhydrite) (see Fig. 8.9). Lack of- anhydrite in alteration products of this stage implies that decreasing total sulfur or relatively low values of f_{S_2} and f_{O_2} cause anhydrite to become unstable relative to calcite in carbonate environments below 400°C.

The dominant trend in skarn destruction involves the formation of hydrous silicates which are progressively depleted in calcium as the intensity of alteration increases. Thus, in the earliest (highest temperature) stages epidote (9 mole percent Ca) replaces the grossularite component of garnet (15 mole percent Ca), and tremolite (5 mole percent Ca) replaces diopside (10 mole percent Ca). Later, at lower temperature and under more extreme conditions of calcium-leaching, ferrosaponite (1 mole percent Ca) replaces andradite-salite (10–15 percent Ca), and talc (no Ca) replaces tremolite. Calcium released during this process either is leached from the system or is fixed as calcite.

The path toward decreasing pH may be arrested at the sericitic stage due to a variety of factors. A decrease in ΣS due to earlier deposition of sulfides during potassic alteration reduces the capacity of the fluid to generate hydrogen ion. When this reduced capacity is combined with continued removal of hydrogen ion by exchange with feldspar and with excessive dilution by ground water, the net effect may be a decline in hydrolytic alteration and sulfide deposition in an upward and outward direction from the sericitic zone. This may be the case in porphyry copper deposits which display well-developed, high-grade potassic and skarn zones, such as Christmas, Twin Buttes, and Bingham.

If, however, the evolution of hydrogen ion is unusually high, the fluid path may enter the advanced argillic stage, represented by kaolinite(pyrophyllite)-quartz-pyrite-bornite(digenite). Fluids in plutons displaying advanced argillic alteration interacted with carbonate rocks and formed massive silica-pyrite replacement bodies. At Ely the majority of copper was deposited during an early potassic and skarn-forming event, and zones of pervasive sericitic alteration and silica-pyrite bodies generally are not ore-grade (James, 1976). In contrast, the apparent absence of andradite-salite skarn at Bisbee (Ransome, 1904; Bryant, 1964), and during the quartz-porphyry stage at Cananea (L. D. Meinert 1978, personal communication) implies that conditions conducive to potassic alteration never developed. Suppression of potassic alteration and skarn formation in these cases may have been caused by unusually rapid cooling of the pluton due to shallow emplacement and to early influx of groundwater. The evolution to extremes of sulfidation-oxidation state and low pH occurred while the fluid contained sufficient copper to form well-mineralized breccia pipes and silica-pyrite replacement bodies.

SUMMARY AND CONCLUSIONS

Skarns formed at contacts with mineralized porphyry copper plutons share many of the features of the general class of copper skarn deposits, including a common petrotectonic setting, calc-silicate association and composition, and opaque mineral association. Copper skarn deposits are associated with hypabyssal felsic stocks emplaced in continental margin orogenic belts. Zinc-lead skarn deposits and some magnetite skarn deposits also share this environment, which is distinct from the orogenic batholith environment of tungsten skarn deposits and the post-orogenic granite association of tin skarn deposits. The calc-silicate mineralogy of copper skarns is characterized by andraditic garnet and diopsidic pyroxene, in contrast to the andradite and manganohedenbergite association of zinc-lead skarns and to the grandite, grossularite-spessartine, and hedenbergitic pyroxene association of tungsten skarns and tin skarns. Opaque minerals, dominated by magnetite, chalcopyrite, and pyrite, are relatively abundant in copper skarns; in contrast, magnetite and sulfides, including pyrrhotite and arsenopyrite, are less abundant in tungsten and tin skarns. These features point to a common evolution for copper skarns that differs from that of other classes of skarn deposits—an evolution at relatively high oxidation and sulfidation states that reflects not only a shallow level of formation, but also the specific igneous rock association.

Other features of porphyry copper skarns deviate from the norm of copper skarns. In terms of ore tonnage, porphyry copper skarns are the largest known base-metal sulfide skarn deposits. Also, the relatively high continuity of copper grade appears to violate the rule that skarns display erratic grade distribution. Unusually high fracture and veinlet densities in skarn—in part a function of water-release from magmas of intermediate water contents at shallow depths—contribute to uniform copper distribution by enhancing rock permeability. In addition, the widespread late sericitic alteration event in igneous rocks, which is unique to skarns related to porphyry copper deposits, may act as a hypogene enrichment process; leach solutions from the pluton may infiltrate peripheral and overlying skarn, where they are effectively neutralized. During this process, the sulfide content of the skarn is enhanced as garnet and pyroxene are destroyed.

Unusually high oxidation states of porphyry copper magmas are implied by magmatic biotite compositions, and a continued oxidation trend is recorded by the alteration mineral assemblages in both plutons and skarns. A relatively high oxidation state may be a necessary factor in the generation of porphyry copper deposits, because the sulfur content of magmatic aqueous fluids is dependent not only on the sulfur content of the melt, but also on the oxidation state (Burnham, 1979). High oxidation states favor high sulfur contents in the aqueous phase, which, in turn, favors the development of base metal sulfide concentrations.

Although oxidation state is an important parameter, which controls the partitioning of ferric and ferrous iron between garnet and pyroxene, additional factors must be responsible for the unusual bulk composition of porphyry copper–related skarns. As outlined above, their depletion in manganese and zinc relative to other types of base-metal sulfide skarns is a compositional feature which presumably reflects higher temperatures and proximity to the source of metasomatic fluids. Also, bulk compositional and mineralogical data from skarns formed in limestone free of argillaceous components indicate that porphyry copper-related skarns display the highest Fe : Al ratio of any skarn type. A possible cause is the unusually high chloride content of high temperature hydrothermal solutions in porphyry copper systems; Burnham (1967) and Kilinc (1969) have shown that the Fe : Al molal ratio in aqueous fluids in equilibrium with felsic igneous rocks at high temperatures increases with the cube of the chloride concentration at oxidation states of porphyry copper systems.

Of the general class of skarn deposits, the porphyry copper-related skarns display the clearest and most visible genetic connection to magmatic and post-magmatic processes. They are the only widespread skarn type that clearly forms at the contact with a portion of the intrusive system that generated the ore fluid. In addition, the pervasive and multiple generations of fracture-controlled alteration-mineralization, both in the pluton and in its wall rocks, record in unusual detail the evolution of water-rock relations in both environments.

ACKNOWLEDGMENTS

Many of the ideas expressed in this chapter are the result of discussions with colleagues; particular thanks are extended to D. M. Burt, whose pioneering studies of skarn phase equilibria have had an important influence on the author's thinking. Also, some of the concepts presented are the outgrowth of a graduate seminar at Stanford University; discussions with R. J. Newberry and L. D. Meinert were especially useful. A field workshop and symposium on skarns, sponsored by the National Science Foundation and held in Arizona and New Mexico in April, 1978, helped to clarify differences between skarns in porphyry and non-porphyry environments. Critical reviews of the manuscript by D. M. Burt, L. D. Meinert, and R. J. Newberry improved the presentation; their efforts are gratefully acknowledged.

REFERENCES CITED

Atkinson, W. W. Jr., and Einaudi, M. T., 1978, Skarn formation and mineralization in the contact aureole at Carr Fork, Bingham, Utah: Econ. Geol., v. 73, p. 1326–1365.

Barter, C. F., and Kelly, J. L., 1982, Geology of the Twin Buttes Mineral Deposit, Pima mining district, Pima County, Arizona, *in* Titley, S. R., ed., Advances in Geology of the Porphyry Copper Deposits, Southwestern North America: Tucson, Univ. Ariz. Press, Chapter 20.

Barton, P. B., Jr., and Skinner, B. J., 1967, Sulfide mineral stabilities, in Barnes, H. L., ed. Geochemistry of Hydrothermal Ore Deposits: New York, Holt, Rinehart and Winston, p. 236–333.

Bauer, H. L., Jr.; Breitrich, R. A.; Cooper, J. J.; and Anderson, J. A., 1966, Porphyry copper deposits in the Robinson mining district, Nevada, *in* Titley, S. R., and Hicks, C. L., eds., Geology of the Porphyry Copper Deposits, Southwestern North America: Tucson, Univ. Ariz. Press, p. 233–244.

Beane, R. E., 1974, Biotite stability in the porphyry copper environment: Econ. Geol., 69, p. 241–256.

Bray, R. E., and Wilson, J. C., eds., 1975, Guide Book to the Bingham mining district, Soc. Econ. Geologists, Oct. 23: Kennecott Copper Corp., Bingham Canyon, Utah, 156 p.

Brimhall, G. H., Jr., 1977, Early fracture-controlled disseminated mineralization: Econ. Geol., v. 72, p. 37–59.

Britt, T. L., 1976, Brief discussion of the stratigraphy of the Bingham Mine Formation and structural setting in Middle Canyon: Utah Geol. Assoc., Ann. Field Conf., Pub. 6, p. 22–24.

Bryant, D. G., 1964, Intrusive breccias and associated ore of Warren (Bisbee) mining district, Cochise county, Arizona: Unpub. Ph.D. Diss., Stanford Univ., 149 p.

Burnham, C. W., 1967, Hydrothermal fluids at the magmatic stage, *in* Barnes, H. L., ed., Geochemistry of Hydrothermal Ore Deposits: New York, Holt, Rinehart & Winston, p. 34–76.

———, 1979, Magmas and hydrothermal fluids, *in* Barnes, H. L., ed., Geochemistry of Hydrothermal Ore Deposits, 2nd ed.: New York, John Wiley and Sons, p. 71–136.

Burnham, C. W.; Holloway, J. R.; and Davis, N. F., 1969, Thermodynamic properties of water to 1,000°C and 10,000 bars: Geol. Soc. Amer., Spec. Paper 132, 96 p.

Burt, D. M., 1972, Mineralogy and geochemistry of Ca-Fe-Si skarn deposits: Unpub. Ph.D. Diss., Harvard Univ., 256 p.

———, 1974, Metasomatic zoning in Ca-Fe-Si exoskarns, *in* Hofmann, A. W., and others, eds., Geochemical Transport and Kinetics: Carnegie Inst., Wash. Publ. 634, p. 287–293.

———, 1977, Mineralogy and petrology of skarn deposits: Rendiconti Soc. Ital. Mineral. Petrol., v. 33, p. 859–873.

Carlson, J. E., and Mabey, D. R., 1963, Aeromagnetic and gravity maps of the Ely area, Nevada: U.S. Geol. Survey Map GP 392, 2 p. text.

Einaudi, M. T., 1974, Skarn studies—Palo Verde mine, Pima County, Arizona: Unpub. manuscript, The Anaconda Co., 44 p.

———, 1977, Petrogenesis of copper-bearing skarn at the Mason Valley mine, Yerington district, Nevada: Econ. Geol., v. 72, p. 769–795.

———, 1982, Description of skarns associated with porphyry copper plutons, southwestern North America, *in* Titley, S. R., ed., Advances in Geology of the Porphyry Copper Deposits, Southwestern North America: Tucson, Univ. Ariz. Press, Chapter 7.

Einaudi, M. T.; Moore, W. J.; and Wilson, J. C., 1978, Introduction, Bingham mining district: Econ. Geol., v. 73, p. 1215–1217.

Emmons, S. F., 1910, The Cananea mining district of Sonora, Mexico: Econ. Geol., v. 5, p. 312–356.

Ernst, W. G., 1966, Synthesis and stability relations of ferrotremolite: Amer. Jour. Sci., v. 264, p. 37–65.

French, B. M., 1971, Stability relations of siderite ($FeCO_3$) in the system Fe-C-O: Amer. Jour. Sci., v. 271, p. 37–78.

———, and Eugster, H. P., 1965, Experimental control of oxygen fugacities by graphite-gas equilibriums: Jour. Geophys. Res., v. 70, p. 1529–1539.

Gale, R. E., 1965, The geology of the Mission copper mine, Pima mining district, Arizona: Unpub. Ph.D. Diss., Stanford Univ., 162 p.

Garrels, R. M., and Christ, C. L., 1965, Solutions, Minerals and Equilibria: New York: Harper and Row, 450 p.

Gordon, T. M., and Greenwood, H. J., 1971, The stability of grossularite in H_2O-CO_2 mixtures: Amer. Mineral., v. 56, p. 1674–1688.

Graybeal, F. T., 1982, Geology of the El Tiro Area, Silver Bell mining district, Pima County, Arizona, *in* Titley, S. R., ed., Advances in Geology of the Porphyry Copper Deposits, Southwestern North America: Tucson, Univ. Ariz. Press, Chapter 24.

Greenwood, H. J., 1967*a*, Mineral equilibria in the system MgO-SiO_2-H_2O-CO_2, *in* Abelson, P. H., ed., Researches in Geochemistry, v. 2: New York, John Wiley, p. 542–567.

———, 1967*b*, Wollastonite: stability in H_2O-CO_2 mixtures and occurrence in a contact metamorphic aureole near Salmo, British Columbia, Canada: Amer. Mineral., v. 52, p. 1669–1680.

———, 1975, Buffering of pore fluids by metamorphic reactions: Amer. Jour. Sci., v. 275, p. 573.

———, 1976, Metamorphism at moderate temperatures and pressures, *in* Bailey, D. K., and MacDonald, R., eds., The Evolution of the Crystalline Rocks: London Academic Press, p. 187–259.

Gustafson, L. B., and Hunt, J. P., 1975, The porphyry copper deposit at El Salvador, Chile: Econ. Geol., v. 70, p. 857–912.

Gustafson, W. I., 1974, The stability of andradite, hedenbergite, and related minerals in the system Ca-Fe-Si-O-H: Jour. Petrology, v. 15, p. 455–496.

Hallof, P. G., and Winniski, E., 1971, A geophysical case history of the Lakeshore ore body: Geophysics, v. 36, p. 1232–1249.

Helgeson, H. C., 1969, Thermodynamics of hydrothermal systems at elevated temperatures and pressures: Amer. Jour. Sci., v. 267, p. 729–804.

Holland, H. R., 1959, Some applications of thermochemical data to problems of ore deposits, I: Stability relations among the oxides, sulfides, sulfates, and carbonates of ore and gangue minerals: Econ. Geol., v. 54, p. 184–233.

Hoschek, G. 1973, Die reaktion Phlogopit + Calcit + Quartz = Tremolit + Kalifeldspar + H_2O + CO_2: Contrib. Mineral. Petrol., v. 39, p. 231–237.

Huang, C., 1976, An isotopic and petrologic study of the contact metamorphism and metasomatism related to copper deposits at Ely, Nevada: Unpub. Ph.D. Diss., Penn. State Univ., 178 p.

James, L. P., 1976, Zonal alteration in limestone at porphyry copper deposits, Ely, Nevada: Econ. Geol., v. 71, p. 488–512.

———, 1978, The Bingham copper deposits, Utah, as an exploration target: history and pre-excavation geology: Econ. Geol., v. 73, p. 1218–1227.

Jones, W. R.; Hernon, R. M.; and Moore, S. L., 1967, General geology of Santa Rita quadrangle, Grant County, New Mexico: U.S. Geol. Survey Prof. Paper 555, 144 p.

Kerrick, D. M., 1974, Review of metamorphic mixed volatile (H_2O-CO_2) equilibria: Amer. Mineral., v. 59, p. 729–762.

Kilinc, I. A., 1969, Experimental metamorphism and anatexis of shales and graywackes: Unpub. Ph.D. Diss., Penn. State Univ.

Kinnison, J. E., 1966, The Mission copper deposit, Arizona, *in,* Titley, S. R., and Hicks, C. L., eds., Geology of the Porphyry Copper Deposits, Southwestern North America: Tucson, Univ. Ariz. Press, p. 281–287.

Knopf, Adolph, 1918, Geology and ore deposits of the Yerington district, Nevada: U.S. Geol. Survey Prof. Paper 114, 68 p.

Koski, R. A., 1978, Porphyry-type alteration and mineralization of igneous rocks at Christmas, Arizona: Unpub. Ph.D. Diss., Stanford Univ., 196 p.

Koski, R. A., and Cook, D. S., 1982, Geology of the Christmas Porphyry Copper Deposit, Gila County, Arizona, *in* Titley, S. R., ed., Advances in Geology of the Porphyry Copper Deposits, Southwestern North America: Tucson, Univ. Ariz. Press, Chapter 17.

Langlois, J. D., 1978, Geology of the Cyprus Pima mine, Pima county, Arizona: Ariz. Geol. Soc. Digest XI, p. 103–113.

Lindgren, Waldemar, 1905, The copper deposits of the Clifton-Morenci district, Arizona: U.S. Geol. Survey, Prof. Paper 43, 375 p.

———, 1924, Contact metamorphism at Bingham, Utah: Bull. Geol. Soc. America v. 35, p. 507–534.

Liou, J. G., 1974, Stability relations of andradite-quartz in the system Ca-Fe-Si-O-H: Amer. Mineral. v. 59, p. 1016–1025.

Lowell, J. D., and Guilbert, J. M., 1970, Lateral and vertical alteration-mineralization zoning in porphyry copper deposits: Econ. Geol., v. 65, p. 373–408.

Meyer, Charles, and Hemley, J. J., 1967, Wallrock alteration, *in* Barnes, H. L., ed., Geochemistry of Hydrothermal Ore Deposits; New York, Holt, Rinehart and Winston, p. 166–235.

Moolick, R. T., and Durek, J. J., 1966, The Morenci district, *in* Titley, S. R., and Hicks, C. L., eds., Geology of the Porphyry Copper Deposits, Southwestern North America: Tucson, Univ. Ariz. Press, p. 221–232.

Moore, W. J., and Czamanske, G. K., 1973, Composition of biotites from unaltered and altered monzonitic rocks in the Bingham mining district, Utah: Econ. Geol., v. 68, p. 269–274.

Moore, W. J., and Nash, J. T., 1974, Alteration and fluid inclusion studies of the porphyry copper ore body at Bingham, Utah: Econ. Geol., v. 69, p. 631–645.

Morgan, B. A., 1975, Mineralogy and origin of skarns in the Mount Morrison pendant, Sierra Nevada, California: Amer. Jour. Sci., v. 275, p. 119–142.

Mueller, R. F., 1961, Analysis of relations among Mg, Fe and Mn in certain metamorphic minerals: Geochim. Cosmochim. Acta, v. 25, p. 267–296.

———, 1973, System CaO-MgO-FeO-SiO_2-C-H_2-O_2: some correlations from nature and experiment: Amer. Jour. Sci., v. 273, p. 152–170.

Nielsen, R. L., 1970, Mineralization and alteration in calcareous rocks near the Santa Rita stock, New Mexico: Guidebook, New Mex. Geol. Soc., 21st Field Conf., p. 133–139.

———, 1976, Recent developments in the study of porphyry copper geology—a review, *in* Sutherland Brown, A., ed., Porphyry Deposits of the Canadian Cordillera: CIM, Spec. Vol. 15, p. 487–500.

Perry, D. V., 1968, Genesis of the contact rocks at the Christmas mine, Gila county, Arizona: Unpub. Ph.D. Diss., Univ. Ariz., 229 p.

———, 1969, Skarn genesis at the Christmas mine, Gila county, Arizona: Econ. Geol., v. 64, p. 255–270.

Ransome, F. L., 1904, Geology and ore deposits of the Bisbee quadrangle, Arizona: U.S. Geol. Survey, Prof. Paper 21, 168 p.

Reid, J. E., 1978, Skarn alteration of the commercial limestone, Carr Fork area, Bingham, Utah: Econ. Geol., v. 73, p. 1315–1325.

Roberts, S. A., 1973, Pervasive early alteration in the Butte district, Montana, *in* Miller, R. N., ed., Guidebook for the Butte Field Meeting, Soc. Econ. Geologists: The Anaconda Co., Butte, Montana, p. HH1–HH8.

Robie, R. A.; Hemingway, B. S.; and Fisher, J. R., 1978, Thermodynamic properties of minerals and related substances at 298.15K and 1 bar (10^5 pascals) pressure and at higher temperatures: U.S. Geol. Survey Bull. 1452, 456 p.

Roedder, Edwin, 1971, Fluid inclusion studies on the porphyry-type ore deposits of Bingham, Utah; Butte, Montana; and Climax, Colorado: Econ. Geol., v. 66, p. 98–120.

Rose, A. W., 1970, Zonal relations of wallrock alteration and sulfide distribution at porphyry copper deposits: Econ. Geol., v. 65, p. 920–936.

Rose, A. W., and Baltosser, W. W., 1966, The porphyry copper deposit at Santa Rita, New Mexico, *in* Titley, S. R., and Hicks, C. L., eds., Geology of the Porphyry Copper Deposits, Southwestern North America: Tucson, Univ. Ariz. Press, p. 205–220.

Rubright, R. D., and Hart, O. J., 1968, Non-porphyry ores of the Bingham district, Utah, *in* Ridge, J. D., ed., Ore Deposits of the United States, 1933–1967 (Graton-Sales Vol.): New York, AIME, p. 886–908.

Saxena, S. K., 1971, Mg^{2+}-Fe^{2+} order-disorder in orthopyroxene and the Mg^{2+}-Fe^{2+} distribution between coexisting minerals: Lithos, v. 4, p. 345–354.

Schmitt, H. A., 1939, The Pewabic mine, New Mexico: Bull. Geol. Soc. America, v. 50, p. 777–818.

Schreyer, W., 1976, Experimental metamorphic petrology at low pressures and high temperatures, *in* Bailey, D. K., and MacDonald, R., eds., The Evolution of the Crystalline Rocks: London, Academic Press, p. 261–331.

Scott, S. D., and Barnes, H. L., 1971, Sphalerite geothermometry and geobarometry: Econ. Geol., v. 66, p. 653–669.

Sheppard, S. M. F.; Nielsen, R. L.; and Taylor, H. P. Jr., 1971, Hydrogen and oxygen isotope ratios in minerals from porphyry copper deposits: Econ. Geol., v. 66, p. 515–542.

Sheppard, S. M. F., and Taylor, H. P., Jr., 1974, Hydrogen and oxygen isotope evidence for the origins of water in the Boulder batholith and the Butte ore deposits, Montana: Econ. Geol., v. 69, p. 926–946.

Shimazaki, Hidehiko, 1974, Characteristics of tungsten mineralization in Japanese skarn deposits, *in* Stemprok, M., ed., Metallization Associated With Acid Magmatism: Geol. Surv. Czech., v. 1, p. 312–315.

———, 1977, Grossular-spessartine-almandine garnets from some Japanese scheelite skarns: Can. Mineral. v. 15, p. 74–80.

———, 1978, Main characteristics of non-porphyry skarn deposits in Japan (abs.): Geol. Soc. America, abs. with program, v. 10, p. 147.

Shimazaki, Hidehiko, and Bunno, Michiaki, 1978, Subsolidus skarn equilibria in the system $CaSiO_3$-$CaMgSi_2O_6$-$CaFeSi_2O_6$-$CaMnSi_2O_6$: Can. Mineral., v. 16, p. 539–546.

Sillitoe, R. H., 1973, Tops and bottoms of porphyry copper deposits: Econ. Geol., v. 68, p. 799–815.

South, D. L., 1972, Sulfide zoning at the Lakeshore copper deposit, Pinal County, Arizona: Unpub. M.S. Thesis, Univ. Ariz., 79 p.

Taylor, B. E., 1976, Origin and significance of C-O-H fluids in the formation of Ca-Fe-Si skarn, Osgood Mountains, Humboldt County, Nevada: Unpub. Ph.D. Thesis, Stanford Univ., 285 p.

Taylor, B. E., and Liou, J. G., 1978, The low-temperature stability of andradite in C-O-H fluids: Amer. Mineral. v. 63, p. 378–393.

Taylor, B. E., and O'Neil, J. R., 1977, Stable isotope studies of metasomatic Ca-Fe-Al-Si skarns and associated metamorphic and igneous rocks, Osgood Mountains, Nevada: Contrib. Mineral. Petrol., v. 63, p. 1–49.

Thompson, A. B., 1975, Calc-silicate diffusion zones between marble and pelitic schist: Jour. Petrology, v. 16, p. 314–346.

Titley, S. R., 1961, Genesis and control of the Linchburg ore body, Socorro County, New Mexico: Econ. Geol., v. 56, p. 695–722.

———, 1968, Environment of deposition of the hydrothermal metamorphic (pyrometasomatic) deposits (abs.): Econ. Geol., v. 63, p. 699.

———, 1973, "Pyrometasomatic"—an alteration type: Econ. Geol., v. 68, p. 1326–1329.

Vidale, R. J., 1969, Metasomatism in a chemical gradient and the formation of calc-silicate bands: Amer. Jour. Sci., v. 267, p. 857–874.

Winchell, A. N., 1924, Petrographic studies of limestone alterations at Bingham: AIME Trans., v. 70, p. 884–889.

Wones, D. R., and Eugster, H. P., 1965, Stability of biotite: Experiment, theory and application: Amer. Mineral., v. 50, p. 1228–1272.

Wright, W. A., 1973, Skarn formation at Pine Creek mine, Bishop, California: Unpub. PhD Thesis, Univ. Calif. Berkeley, 135 p.

Zharikov, V. A., 1970, Skarns: Internat. Geol. Rev., v. 12, p. 541–559, 619–647, 760–775.

Zietz, Isidore; Bateman, P. C.; Case, J. E.; Crittenden, M. D. Jr.; Griscom, A.; Kind, E. R.; Roberts, R. J.; and Lorentzen, G. R., 1969, Aeromagnetic investigation of crustal structure for a strip across the western United States: Bull. Geol. Soc. America, v. 80, p. 1703–1714.

9

A Geochemical Study of the Kalamazoo Porphyry Copper Deposit

PINAL COUNTY, ARIZONA

Maurice A. Chaffee

Many investigations have described the mineralization and alteration characteristics of porphyry copper deposits. Most of these studies have taken a mineralogical point of view. In contrast, this chapter describes the application of geochemistry to a porphyry system, with an emphasis on geochemical applications that can be used in the exploration for new mineral deposits.

The region encompassing the southwestern United States and the adjoining sections of northern Mexico contains the highest density of known porphyry copper deposits in the world. It seems likely that most of the exposed porphyry copper deposits that exist in this region have already been found. As a consequence, new techniques or approaches are needed that are capable of detecting mineral deposits that are not exposed at the surface. The search for new approaches has renewed interest in whole-rock geochemistry. The employment of whole-rock sampling, which, until the 1970s, was neglected in geochemical surveys in North America, should be useful in the search for blind porphyry copper deposits occurring at depth within exposed or surficially covered rock bodies.

A number of authors have described element zoning derived from analyses of rock samples collected in porphyry copper districts in the western United States and Canada. These workers include Brabec and White (1971), Cox and others (1975), Creasey (1965), Davis (1974), Eidel and others (1968), Fisher (1972), Gott and others (1966), Gunton and Nichol (1974), Jambor (1974), Krish (1974), Olade and Fletcher (1975, 1976*a*, 1976*b*), Reid (1975), and Theodore and Nash (1973). In addition, Jerome (1966) has summarized the general trace-element zoning around porphyry copper deposits. An earlier report on the Kalamazoo deposit (Chaffee, 1976) has described the distribution of 17 elements relative to the copper ore zone and the alteration-mineralization zones found in the district.

To learn more about the geochemistry of porphyry copper deposits and the potential of rock geochemistry in the exploration for blind porphyry copper deposits, a study has been made of the Kalamazoo deposit, near San Manuel, Pinal County, Arizona (see location map, Fig. 9.1). Zoned copper deposits, such as the Kalamazoo, may contain concentrations of elements occurring in aureoles, or zones, around the copper orebody. The spatial relationship of the aureoles of these pathfinder elements to the known copper ore zone may

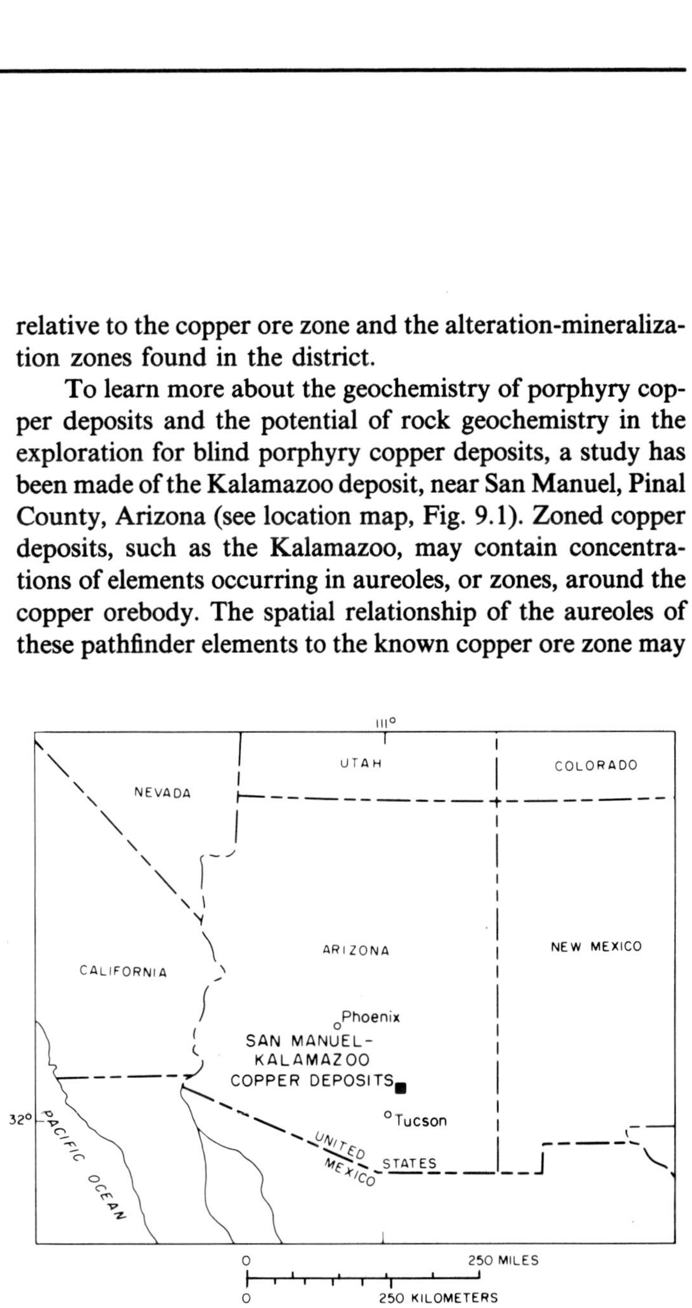

Figure 9.1. Location of the San Manuel and Kalamazoo deposits

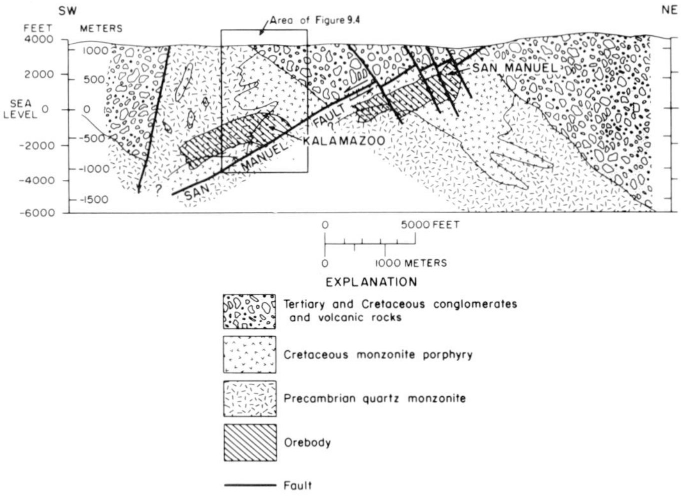

Figure 9.2. Simplified geologic section through the Kalamazoo and San Manuel deposits. Modified from Lowell (1968).

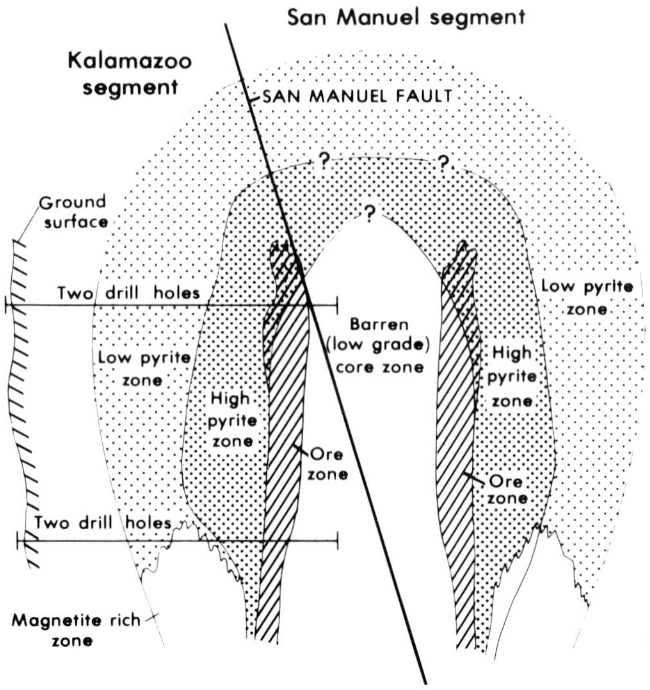

Figure 9.3. Idealized section of Kalamazoo and San Manuel deposits before faulting and rotation. Modifed from Lowell and Guilbert (1970).

provide useful information for understanding the genesis of porphyry deposits and for exploring for additional deposits of this type.

GEOLOGIC SETTING

A description of the geologic setting and spatial relationships of the Kalamazoo deposit and the associated San Manuel deposit has been provided by Lowell (1968). Figure 9.2 is a simplified section through the two deposits that shows three major geologic units (the minor rock units that are known to exist in the area, such as dikes, have been omitted). The oldest of the three units is a large mass of Precambrian quartz monzonite, which is formally known in this area as the Oracle Granite. This widespread unit was intruded in Late Cretaceous time by a zoned stock consisting mostly of monzonite porphyry. (This unit is the granodiorite porphyry of Creasey [1965]. The rock name used in this chapter is the one used in the drill logs.) The Kalamazoo and San Manuel deposits are offset, rotated segments of a single mineral deposit that was formed during the late stages of emplacement of this stock. The deposits are found both within the Cretaceous stock and within the Precambrian wall rocks.

These two older major igneous units are unconformably overlain by a third major unit that consists of a thick sequence of conglomerates, sedimentary breccias, and intercalated volcanic rocks of probable Cretaceous and Tertiary age (Creasey, 1965; Thomas, 1975). This third unit is not subdivided for this report. Erosion to the present surface in the vicinity of the Kalamazoo deposit has locally exposed portions of all three major geologic units.

Figure 9.3, adapted from an illustration by Lowell and Guilbert (1970) shows the probable original orientation and form of the two deposits before they were separated and rotated. Both the approximate orientation of the present surface and the location of the four drill holes whose samples were used in this study are shown on the left. Two of the holes penetrated the upper half of the deposit towards its original top and two holes penetrated the deposit near its roots.

A correctly oriented, somewhat generalized geologic section through the drill holes is shown in Figure 9.4. The two holes on the left were collared in and penetrated mostly the Precambrian wall rock unit, whereas the two holes on the right were drilled mostly through Cretaceous and Tertiary

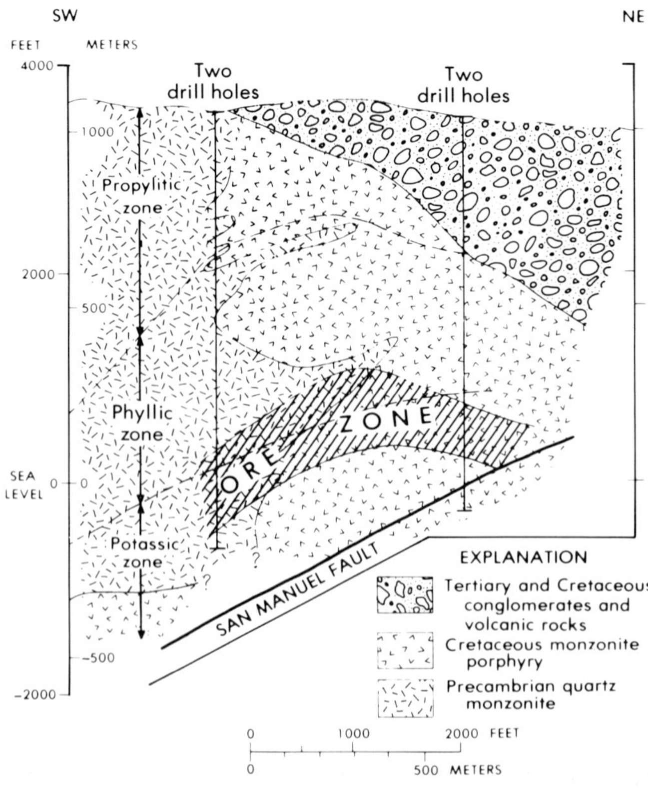

Figure 9.4. Geologic section through the Kalamazoo deposit showing approximate locations of drill holes sampled for this report. Modified from L. A. Thomas (1975).

conglomerates, breccias, and volcanic rocks and the Cretaceous stock. The holes on the left intersected the copper ore zone (defined here as the interval in which copper is equal to or exceeds 0.5 percent), the pyrite zone, and all of the hydrothermal alteration zones found in the area, from the propylitic zone to the potassic zone. In the area penetrated by the holes on the right, most of the propylitic zone had been removed by erosion prior to deposition of the Cretaceous and Tertiary rocks. For the holes studied, the greatest depth from the surface to the top of the ore zone was about 1,130 m (3,700 ft.).

SAMPLING AND ANALYSIS

For this study whole-rock samples were composited from either drill cores or cuttings that were recovered within a specific 3-m (10-ft.) interval. The sampled intervals were spaced approximately 15m (50 ft.) apart along the entire length of each drill hole. The samples from each hole were submitted to the analysts in a random sequence. Analytical data from 311 samples were used in this report. The samples were analyzed for bulk density—using an air pycnometer (McIntyre et al., 1965)—and for 62 different elements. The elements gold, cadmium, mercury, potassium, lithium, sodium, tin, tellurium, thallium, and zinc were determined using atomic absorption spectroscopy (Hubert and Lakin, 1973; Nakagawa and Thompson, 1969; Ward et al., 1969: Welsch and Chao, 1976). The elements aluminum, chlorine, phosphorus, and silicon were determined using X-ray fluorescence (Claisse, 1956). Colorimetry was used to determine arsenic, antimony, selenium, and uranium (Crenshaw and Lakin, 1974; Ward et al., 1963). Sulfur was determined using a titrimetric method described by the Laboratory Equipment Company of St. Joseph, Michigan (no date) and fluorine was determined by specific-ion electrode potentiometry (Ficklin, 1970). Carbon dioxide was determined using a volumetric technique (Watterson et al., 1976). The other 41 elements were determined using a six-step semiquantitative emission spectrographic method (Myers et al., 1961).

A summary of cumulative-frequency percentile values for the 50th (median value), 75th, and 90th percentiles and ranges of values are given for the 62 elements and for bulk density in 178 drill-hole samples of the Precambrian quartz monzonite (Table 9.1) and 133 drill-hole samples of the Cretaceous quartz monzonite porphyry (Table 9.2). The 62 elements shown on these tables were divided into four groups based on geochemical characteristics for the two holes in each rock type. Most of the analyses for Group A elements were reported as being "not detected" at the lower limits of detection for the methods used; as a result, no readily interpretable information was obtained for these elements. More sensitive analytical methods might yet provide meaningful information for some of these elements. Plots of the concentrations of the elements in Group B did not show any changes that could be related in any obvious way to the Kalamazoo deposit. Plots of Group C elements showed zoning patterns, but these patterns were not consistent for the two holes in each rock unit. Plots of Group D elements all produced some type of zoning pattern relative to the Kalamazoo ore zone that was consistent for the two holes in each rock unit. Group D elements are, therefore, the elements that are most useful in a geochemical study of the Kalamazoo deposit.

TABLE 9.1
Statistical Data for Samples Penetrating Mostly Precambrian Quartz Monzonite, Kalamazoo Deposit, Arizona

Element	Percentiles 50	75	90	Ranges of Values
GROUP A				
As	L(10)	15	20	N(10) – 1200
Bi	N(10)	N(10)	N(10)	N(10) – 30
Ce	L(150)	L(150)	L(150)	N(150) – 700
Cl	N(1000)	N(1000)	N(1000)	N(1000) – N(1000)
Eu	N(100)	N(100)	N(100)	N(100) – N(100)
Ge	N(10)	N(10)	N(10)	N(10) – N(10)
Hf	N(100)	N(100)	N(100)	N(100) – N(100)
In	N(10)	N(10)	N(10)	N(10) – N(10)
Nb	15	16	20	L(10) – 30
Nd	70	70	100	N(70) – 300
Pd	N(1)	N(1)	N(1)	N(1) – N(1)
Pr	N(100)	N(100)	N(100)	N(100) – N(100)
Pt	N(30)	N(30)	N(30)	N(30) – N(30)
Re	N(30)	N(30)	N(30)	N(30) – N(30)
Sm	N(100)	N(100)	N(100)	N(100) – N(100)
Ta	N(200)	N(200)	N(200)	N(200) – N(200)
Th	N(200)	N(200)	N(200)	N(200) – N(200)
U	N(4)	N(4)	N(4)	N(4) – N(4)
W	N(100)	N(100)	L(100)	N(100) – 200
GROUP B				
Be	1.9	2.1	3.2	N(1.5) – 7
Cr	140	200	290	5 – 300
Ga	19	21	30	7 – 30
La	58	66	72	N(50) – 300
Sc	14	15	15	L(5) – 30
Y	31	52	60	10 – 150
Yb	5	6	7	1 – 10
Zr	110	150	190	30 – 500
GROUP C				
Al %	6.1	7.3	8.0	3.3 – 11
C (CO_2) %	.73	.96	1.1	.02 – 3.6
Ca %	.5	.7	.8	.15 – 3
Cd	.4	.5	.7	N(.1) – 25
Cs	L(5)	5	7	N(5) – 30
F	310	470	610	140 – 840
Hg	.10	.18	.29	.02 – .8
Mg %	.5	.8	1.0	.1 – 2.0
Na %	.9	1.3	1.9	.1 – 2.4
Ni	8	12	18	L(5) – 150
P	1150	1470	1690	L(440) – 2360
Sb	1.4	3.5	12	N(1) – 1500
Si %	32	33	35	21 – 36
Sn	N(10)	N(10)	10	N(10) – 10
Ti %	.3	.3	.5	.15 – 1
GROUP D				
Ag	N(.5)	.5	1,1	N(.5) – 15
Au	L(.02)	.03	.06	N(.02) – .4
B	L(20)	L(20)	26	N(20) – 200
Ba	720	870	1300	100 – 3000
Co	12	16	24	L(5) – 100
Cu	570	1600	5500	30 – 30,000
Fe %	2.8	3.2	5	.7 – 7
K %	2.8	3.1	3.7	.8 – 4.6
Li	30	40	55	10 – 1100
Mn	170	320	520	30 – 1500
Mo	4	8	35	N(3) – 1000
Pb	19	38	61	N(10) – 1000
Rb	100	110	130	20 – 200
S %	1.5	2.8	4.1	L(.01) – 9.9
Se	1.2	3.4	5.7	L(.1) – 15.8
Sr	120	150	200	30 – 700
Te	L(.1)	.3	1.0	N(.1) – 2.0
Tl	.6	.8	.9	N(.2) – 1.6
V	70	80	100	30 – 300
Zn	34	61	90	5 – 1120
BULK DENSITY	2.73	2.77	2.82	2.63 – 2.91

NOTE: N = Not detected at the lower limit of analytical detection shown in parentheses. L = Detected, but in a concentration less than the lower limit of analytical detection shown in parentheses. All values in ppm unless % shown.

The raw analyses for each element were first plotted on a depth-versus-concentration diagram for each hole (Chaffee, 1976); the curve for magnesium is shown as an example in

TABLE 9.2
Statistical Data for Samples Penetrating Mostly Cretaceous Quartz Monzonite Porphyry, Kalamazoo Deposit, Arizona

Element	Percentiles 50	75	90	Ranges of Values
GROUP A				
As	L(10)	10	10	L(10) - 80
Bi	N(10)	N(10)	N(10)	N(10) - N(10)
Ce	N(150)	L(150)	L(150)	N(150) - L(150)
Cl	N(1000)	N(1000)	N(1000)	N(1000) - N(1000)
Eu	N(100)	N(100)	N(100)	N(100) - N(100)
Ge	N(10)	N(10)	N(10)	N(10) - N(10)
Hf	N(100)	N(100)	N(100)	N(100) - N(100)
In	N(10)	N(10)	N(10)	N(10) - N(10)
Nb	L(10)	L(10)	14	N(10) - 30
Nd	N(70)	L(70)	L(70)	N(70) - 70
Pd	N(1)	N(1)	N(1)	N(1) - N(1)
Pr	N(100)	N(100)	N(100)	N(100) - N(100)
Pt	N(30)	N(30)	N(30)	N(30) - N(30)
Re	N(30)	N(30)	N(30)	N(30) - N(30)
Sm	N(100)	N(100)	N(100)	N(100) - N(100)
Ta	N(200)	N(200)	N(200)	N(200) - N(200)
Th	N(200)	N(200)	N(200)	N(200) - N(200)
U	N(4)	N(4)	N(4)	N(4) - N(4)
W	N(100)	N(100)	N(100)	N(100) - N(100)
GROUP B				
Be	L(1.5)	1.6	2.1	N(1.5) - 3
Cr	26	29	48	5 - 70
Ga	19	20	30	15 - 30
La	L(50)	L(50)	51	N(50) - 70
Sc	7	10	10	N(5) - 15
Y	10	14	15	L(10) - 20
Yb	1.1	1.5	3	N(1) - 3
Zr	74	82	100	30 - 300
GROUP C				
Al %	5.8	7.6	8.1	3.6 - 9.0
C (CO_2) %	.79	1.5	1.8	N(.0003) - 2.7
Ca %	.6	1.1	1.8	.05 - 3
Cd	.2	.4	.5	N(.1) - 2.9
Cs	N(5)	5	7	N(5) - 20
F	420	590	750	100 - 940
Hg	.07	.11	.17	.02 - .26
Mg %	.8	1.0	1.3	.3 - 10
Na %	1.3	2.0	2.3	.1 - 3.2
Ni	18	20	32	N(5) - 50
P	940	1220	1450	L(440) - 1880
Sb	L(1)	L(1)	1.2	N(1) - 5
Si %	30	30	32	20 - 37
Sn	N(10)	N(10)	N(10)	N(10) - 15
Ti %	.2	.3	.3	.03 - .3
GROUP D				
Ag	N(.5)	.6	.9	N(.5) - 7.0
Au	.04	.07	.10	N(.02) - .25
B	L(20)	L(20)	L(20)	N(20) - 100
Ba	570	710	880	70 - 1500
Co	13	17	25	N(5) - 70
Cu	1200	3400	6800	10 - 10,000
Fe %	2.4	5.3	10	.3 - 10
K %	2.1	2.8	3.3	1.0 - 5.0
Li	40	50	60	20 - 270
Mn	140	210	300	7 - 700
Mo	5	25	58	N(3) - 200
Pb	13	19	35	N(10) - 150
Rb	60	100	120	20 - 200
S %	2.0	5.4	8.1	3.6 - 9.0
Se	2.9	4.2	7.1	.1 - 12.8
Sr	150	240	490	30 - 700
Te	N(.1)	L(.1)	.6	N(.1) - 1.0
Tl	.5	.8	1.3	L(.2) - 4.2
V	70	100	150	L(5) - 150
Zn	22	30	46	N(5) - 300
BULK DENSITY	2.72	2.81	2.88	2.60 - 3.20

NOTE: N = Not detected at the lower limit of analytical detection shown in parentheses. L = Detected, but in a concentration less than the lower limit of analytical detection shown in parentheses. All values in ppm unless % shown.

Figure 9.5. Similar plots were made for bulk density values. After the raw data were plotted, a smoothed curve was sketched for each variable. The concentration scales for the element curves illustrated in this report were arbitrarily selected so as to best illustrate the changes in concentration

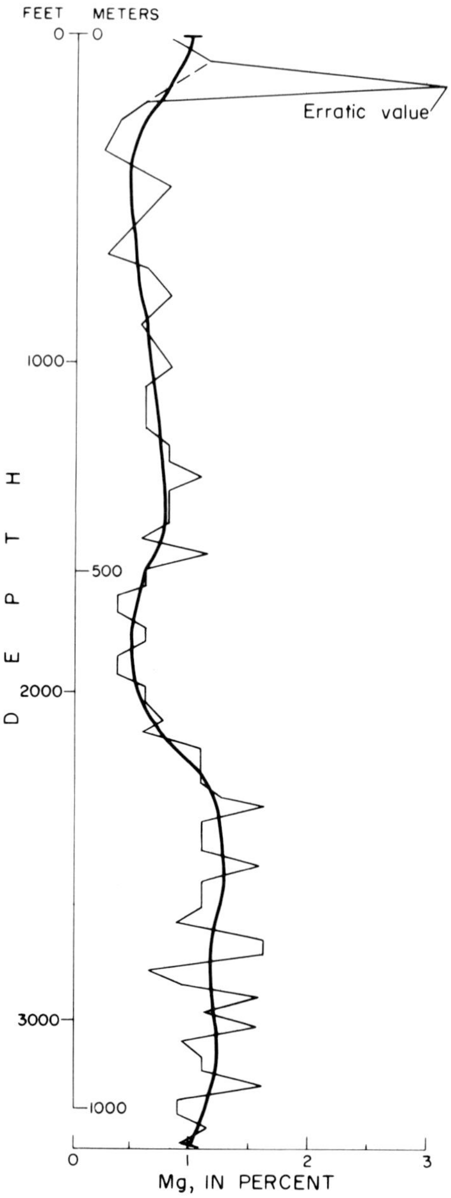

Figure 9.5. Plot of % Mg vs. depth to illustrate raw data plot and resulting smoothed curve. Modified from Chaffee (1976).

for any particular element. The main emphasis in this study has been on determining the broad changes in concentrations; erratic values—such as the one shown at the top of Figure 9.5—have been ignored in constructing the smoothed curves.

DISCUSSION OF RESULTS

Bulk Density

Those elements in Groups B, C, and D were compared, using a U.S. Geological Survey STATPAC correlation analysis program (Sower et al., 1971) with the corresponding values for bulk density. The results indicate that bulk density values correlate best with the concentrations of iron and sulfur. The correlation coefficients for the four holes for density versus sulfur averaged a highly significant value of about 0.90, where a value of 1.00 is a perfect correlation. The

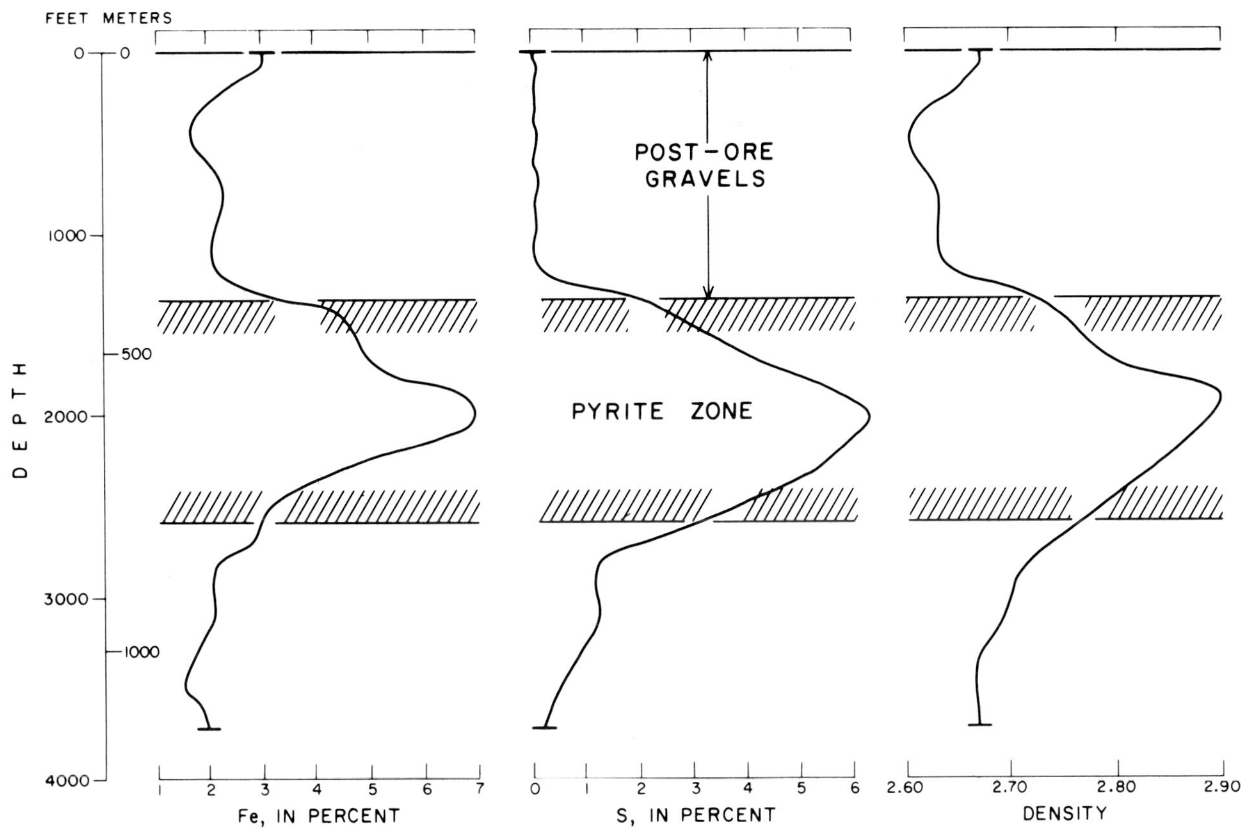

Figure 9.6. Concentration vs. depth curves for iron and sulfur, and value vs. depth curve for density

coefficients for density versus iron were lower, averaging about 0.72; the coefficients for all of the other elements studied were significantly lower.

The smoothed curve for iron, sulfur, and density have similar patterns, as shown for one hole in Figure 9.6. For this particular hole the iron and density curves match quite well. The sulfur curve is similar to the density curve except in the post-ore rock units where sulfur has probably been leached by chemical weathering. The close correlations of iron and sulfur concentrations with values for bulk density and the similarities of the curves in Figure 9.6 suggest, at least for the Kalamazoo deposit, that bulk density is probably more a measure of the pyrite content of the rock than of any other factor.

Mineralogy

A number of characteristically associated minerals are commonly present in most porphyry copper systems. Many of these minerals are readily identifiable in a hand specimen; others can be identified only with a petrographic microscope. Still others are so small that they can be identified only using X-ray or other techniques. The use of chemical analyses of rock samples (element curves) and also the ratios of one element to another (element-ratio curves) may be useful in identifying specific minerals or mineral groups. For example, concentrations of carbon dioxide, which can be determined quantitatively by a simple analytical procedure, can be used to estimate the amount of carbonate minerals—principally calcite—present in the Kalamazoo samples. Correlation analysis of carbon dioxide and the major rock-forming elements determined in this study indicates that the highest correlation values for carbon dioxide are with calcium in three out of the four holes; these values indicate that calcite is probably the most common carbonate mineral present. The correlation value for calcium with carbon dioxide in the fourth hole is lower than for other major elements with carbon dioxide and suggests that carbonate minerals other than calcite may be present in the samples from this hole. Curves showing the close relationship of calcium concentrations to carbon dioxide concentrations are illustrated in Figure 9.7 for samples from one drill hole.

Many curves representing element ratios were examined for this study. In contrast to other studies (Olade and Fletcher, 1976*a*, 1976*b*; Oyarzun M., 1974), few of the curves for Kalamazoo provide information that could not be obtained from a study of curves for individual elements. Most of the useful *trace* elements show enough variation in concentration, so little advantage is gained from a ratio. For the major rock-forming elements, however, ratios may be more useful. For example, ratios of iron to other elements may be helpful in determining the location of the pyrite aureole, or zone, known to be present outside of the copper ore zone.

In an attempt to find any metal ratios that might define the pyrite aureole, the curves for each of the four holes were examined for the ratio of iron to each of the other elements in Groups B, C, and D (see Tables 9.1 and 9.2). Of all the element ratios studied only those of iron to magnesium, calcium, and manganese produced curves that seemed to show

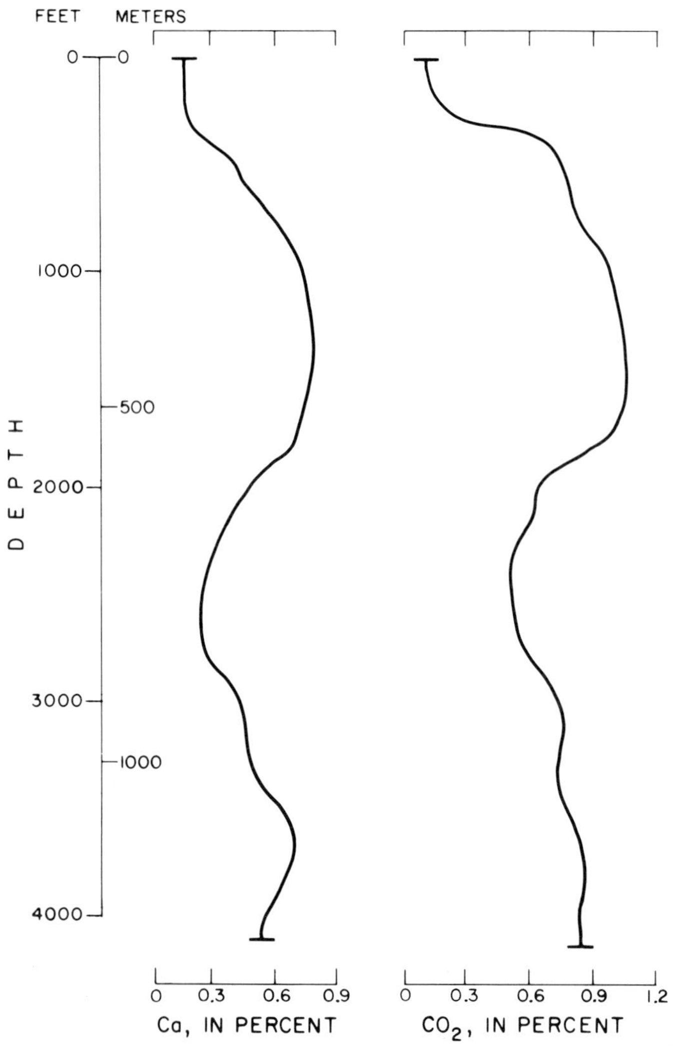

Figure 9.7. Concentration vs. depth curves for Ca and CO_2

any patterns that would define the pyrite aureole. Figure 9.8 shows, for one drill hole, the curve for total iron and several curves for ratios. The curve for iron shows three numbered intervals representing high concentrations, any one of which could represent the pyrite zone. The iron curve alone does not provide information that can be used to separate the interval representing the pyrite zone from the other two intervals, which may represent zones containing concentrations of magnetite or other iron-rich minerals.

The curve for iron-magnesium ratios, just to the right of the iron curve in Figure 9.8, still shows three intervals of high values and is, for this hole, no improvement over the total-iron curve for identifying the pyrite zone. In other holes the iron-magnesium ratio does delineate the pyrite zone. The curve for iron-calcium ratios for this hole is an improvement over the iron-magnesium curve but still shows two intervals with high values, and the interval with the highest values is not the pyrite zone. On the curve for iron-manganese ratios, on the other hand, the most prominent interval of high values is clearly interval 3, the interval containing the pyrite aureole. With the correct interval identified chemically, it was possible to see a close match between the limits of interval number 3 in the iron curve and the limits of the pyrite zone as given in the drill log for this hole. Of the three metal ratios, the iron-manganese ratio was the most successful: it defined the pyrite aureole in all four holes. The iron-calcium ratio was the next best, and the iron-magnesium ratio was the poorest of the three.

These two examples of the use of chemical analyses to interpret mineral abundances pertain to minerals that can be readily identified in hand specimens or thin sections. A chemical analysis of samples, in most cases, is not a substitute for a good mineralogic or petrologic analysis; however, the examples using carbon dioxide analyses and iron-manganese ratios suggest that zones containing high concentrations of less obvious accessory minerals might be defined from a study of curves for other chemical variables, especially where an association between a specific element or elements and a specific mineral has previously been established.

Classification of Anomalies

An examination of the depth-versus-concentration curves suggests that the curves for the 20 selected elements in Group D (see Tables 9.1 and 9.2) can be classified into one or more of four types.

Type 1 Curves. Type 1 curves have the highest concentrations of their respective elements in the lower half of the ore zone or below the ore zone in the barren or low-grade core of the deposit. The curve on the left of Figure 9.9 represents an idealized form of a Type 1 curve. The four elements that have been identified as having Type 1 curves are shown on the right for samples from one hole. In order to emphasize the location of the anomaly for each element—the shaded area along each curve—a background value, represented by the left-hand edge of the shading for each element, has been arbitrarily chosen.

Type 2 Curves. Type 2 curves include those elements that seem to concentrate in the copper ore zone, as shown in Figure 9.10 (*a* and *b*) for samples from one hole. In addition to copper and molybdenum, the elements silver, gold, and probably tellurium and potassium belong in this group. Molybdenum (and in some holes, copper) is also present in anomalous concentrations below the copper ore zone; its presence here suggests that the curve for molybdenum might be characterized as a combination of Type 1 and Type 2 curves.

Type 3 Curves. The Type 3 family of curves includes those elements that have positive anomalies present in aureoles outside the ore zone. Elements having a Type 3 curve include cobalt, vanadium, selenium, iron, sulfur, rubidium, gold, and tellurium. Curves for some of these elements are shown in Figure 9.11 (*a* and *b*) for samples from one hole. Tin, tungsten, and antimony may also belong to this group. Note that gold and tellurium (see Fig. 9.10*b*) seem to have two positive anomalies. These elements exhibit a combination of Type 2 and Type 3 curves. Note that the largest anomaly for gold is in the ore zone and that the smaller anomaly is well outside this zone, whereas for tellurium, the largest anomaly is well outside the ore zone, and only a minor anomaly is associated with the ore zone.

Type 4 Curves. Type 4 curves include those elements that seem to form negative anomalies relative to the ore zone. Elements forming Type 4 curves include manganese, zinc, lead, and thallium, and may also include other elements such

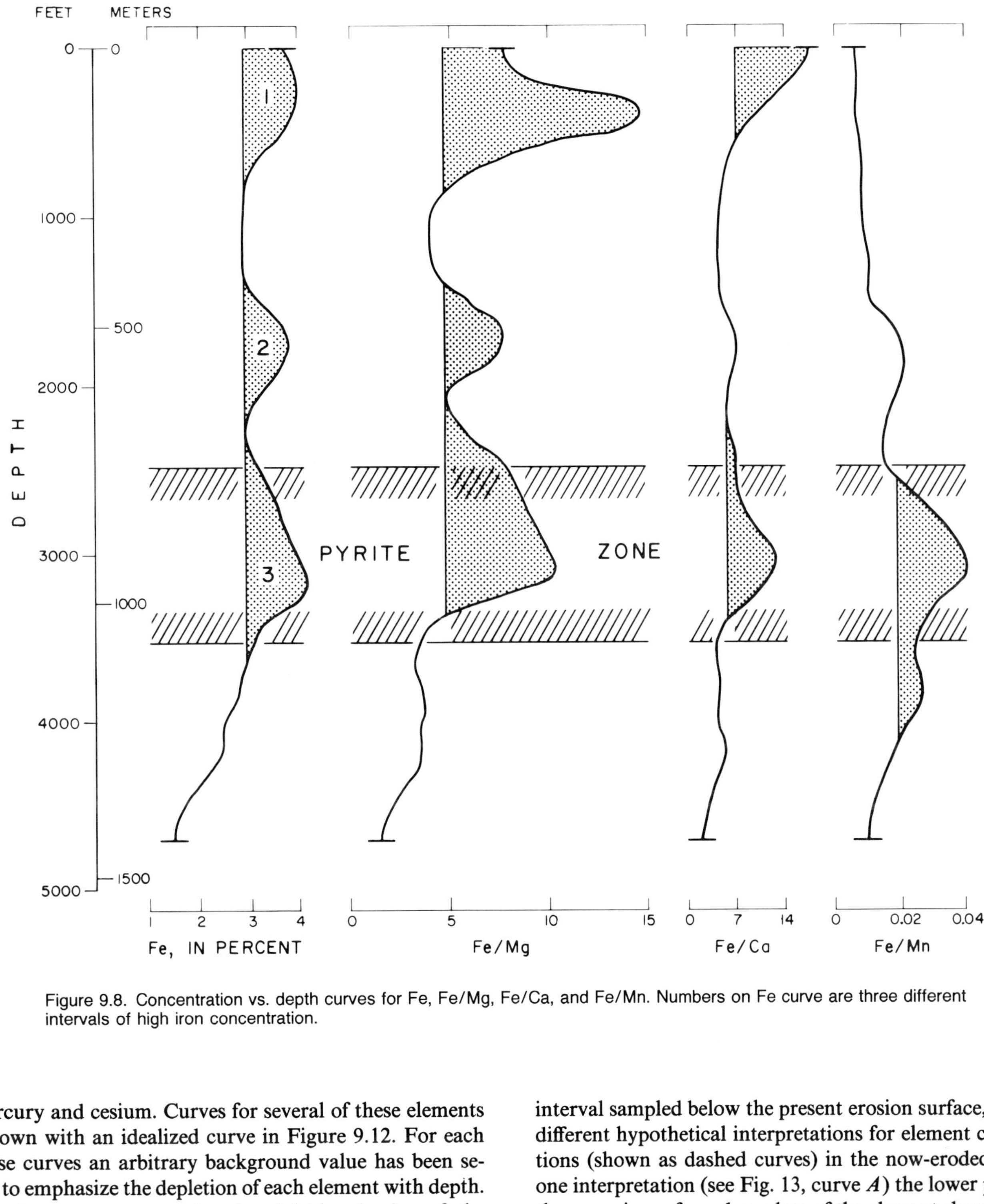

Figure 9.8. Concentration vs. depth curves for Fe, Fe/Mg, Fe/Ca, and Fe/Mn. Numbers on Fe curve are three different intervals of high iron concentration.

as mercury and cesium. Curves for several of these elements are shown with an idealized curve in Figure 9.12. For each of these curves an arbitrary background value has been selected to emphasize the depletion of each element with depth. This value is represented by the right-hand edge of the shaded area. Information in the drill logs indicates that chemical weathering has occurred to varying depths in each hole. Narrow high-concentration peaks near the tops of some curves, such as that for manganese (see Fig. 9.12), are within the interval subjected to chemical weathering and are thought to be the result of weathering processes rather than primary dispersion effects.

Type 4 curves can be interpreted in two different ways; however, correct interpretation for the Kalamazoo deposit is made difficult if not impossible, because the part of the deposit that needs to be sampled has been eroded. Figure 9.13 illustrates two identical, generalized Type 4 curves for the interval sampled below the present erosion surface, with two different hypothetical interpretations for element concentrations (shown as dashed curves) in the now-eroded rock. In one interpretation (see Fig. 13, curve *A*) the lower portion of the curve is confirmed as a loss of the element shown relative to a given background level established some distance away from the copper deposit. In this case, a Type 4 curve represents a true negative anomaly.

A second interpretation of Type 4 curves (see Fig. 9.13, curve *B*) shows that the hypothetical curve peaks out and then drops off with increasing distance from the ore zone. In this interpretation, Type 4 curves become, in effect, Type 3 curves with positive anomalies in aureoles that are located well beyond the anomalies for the Type 3 elements. This second interpretation seems more compatible with what is generally known about the zoning for elements such as manganese, zinc, and lead in many porphyry copper districts. At

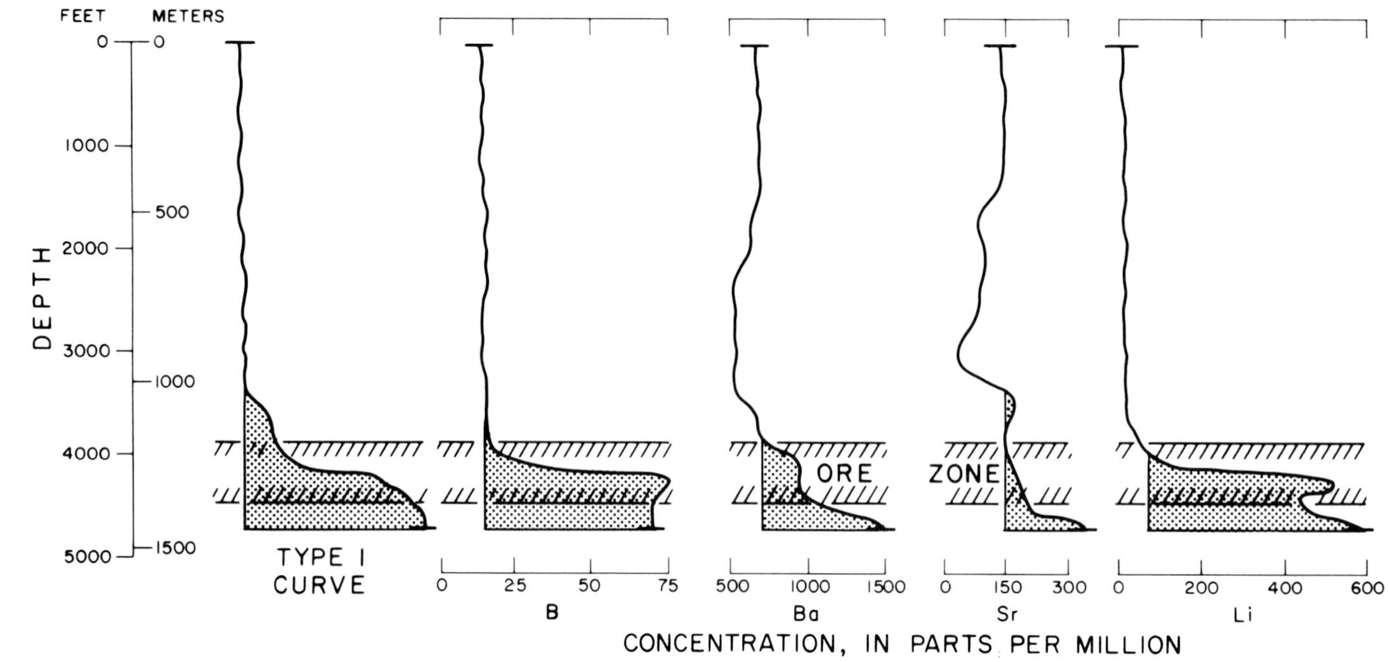

Figure 9.9. Concentration vs. depth curves for Type 1 elements, including B, Ba, Sr, and Li. Shaded areas represent anomalies.

least one study describing the distribution of mercury in the vicinity of a porphyry copper deposit (Gott and McCarthy, 1966) and one describing the distribution of thallium (Cox et al., 1975) suggest that these two elements are concentrated in aureoles outside their respective copper ore zones. No other published information is available to confirm or deny the Type 4 curves also seen for cesium in the present study.

GEOCHEMICAL MODEL OF THE KALAMAZOO DEPOSIT

Besides having distinct zones, or intervals, of high or low concentrations, nearly all the 20 elements in the D group on Tables 9.1 and 9.2 have distinct concentration peaks within their intervals of high concentration (Fig. 9.14, curve *A*), rather than just a broad zone of high but similar concentrations (Fig. 9.14, curve *B*). The distance of the concentration peak or peaks from the outer edge of the copper ore zone was determined for each of the 20 elements in each of the four drill holes. This distance was nearly the same for each element in samples from the two holes drilled near the top of the deposit and was also consistent for each element in samples from the two holes drilled near the roots of the deposit. For most elements, the locations of the concentration peaks are more consistent from hole to hole than are the locations of the intervals of high (or low) concentrations.

Based on the locations of intervals with high concentrations and the locations of concentration peaks, a three-dimensional geochemical model of the Kalamazoo-San Manuel deposit has been synthesized (Fig. 9.15). The framework used for the geochemical model is based on the configuration for the copper ore zone at San Manuel (Creasey, 1965). This configuration shows a slight tapering from top to bottom of a roughly cylindrical ore zone. Because information is limited to the analyses of samples from only four holes, the model should be considered as somewhat speculative. The tentative geochemical model presented in Figure 9.15. shows solid lines representing the approximate location of each zone based on the coincidence of concentration peaks for the elements shown. The changes in concentrations for each element are gradational away from this line in both directions (see Fig. 9.14, curve *A*). In the center of the deposit is the barren or low-grade core, containing boron, barium, strontium, and lithium. The inward extent of the anomalies of these four elements is not known, as indicated by the queries.

The ore-zone elements, including copper, molybdenum, silver, gold, and probably tellurium and potassium, have coincident peaks in a zone that surrounds the core elements. Just outside of the ore zone is an aureole that includes the elements cobalt, vanadium, and selenium. Outside of this zone is the most significant part of the pyrite zone, represented by an aureole that includes the coincident peaks for iron and sulfur. The samples from the two holes penetrating the deep part of the deposit show a rubidium aureole outside the pyrite zone. This rubidium aureole is not present in the samples from the two holes penetrating the upper part of the deposit, probably because the rock has been removed by erosion to a depth below where the aureole should occur.

Outside of the iron-sulfur and rubidium aureoles occurs one more aureole representing a second coincidence of peaks for tellurium and gold. This aureole does not have the same configuration as the others; rather, it appears to expand outward rapidly with depth. Further, the lower part of this tellurium-gold aureole also contains a coincident peak for iron. This enrichment of iron deep in the deposit seems to correlate with the deep magnetite zone in Lowell and Guilbert's (1970) generalized mineralogical model for porphyry deposits (see Fig. 9.3). There is no immediate explanation

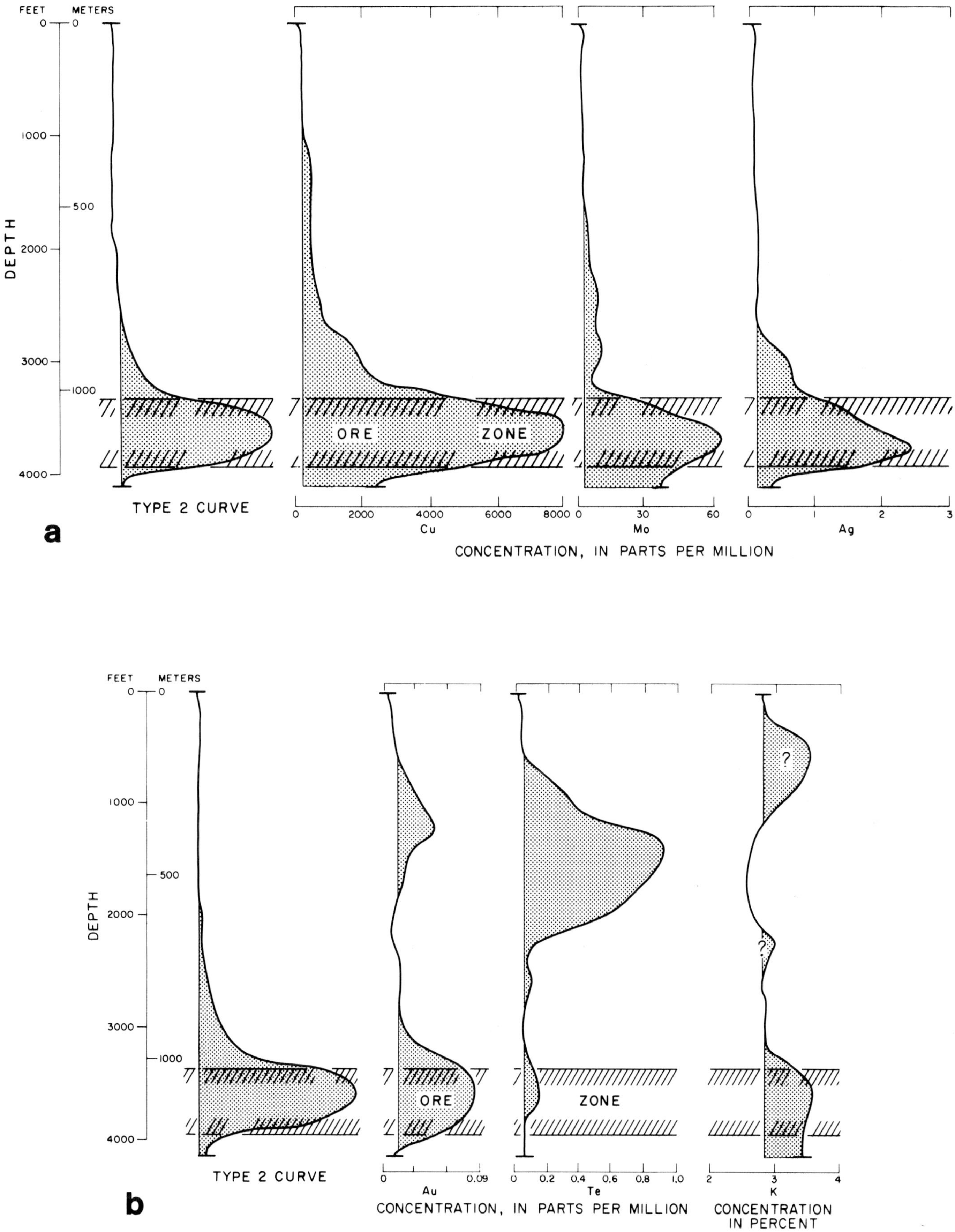

Figure 9.10. Concentration vs. depth curves for Type 2 elements: (*a*) Cu, Mo, and Ag; (*b*) Au, Te, and K. Shaded areas represent anomalies.

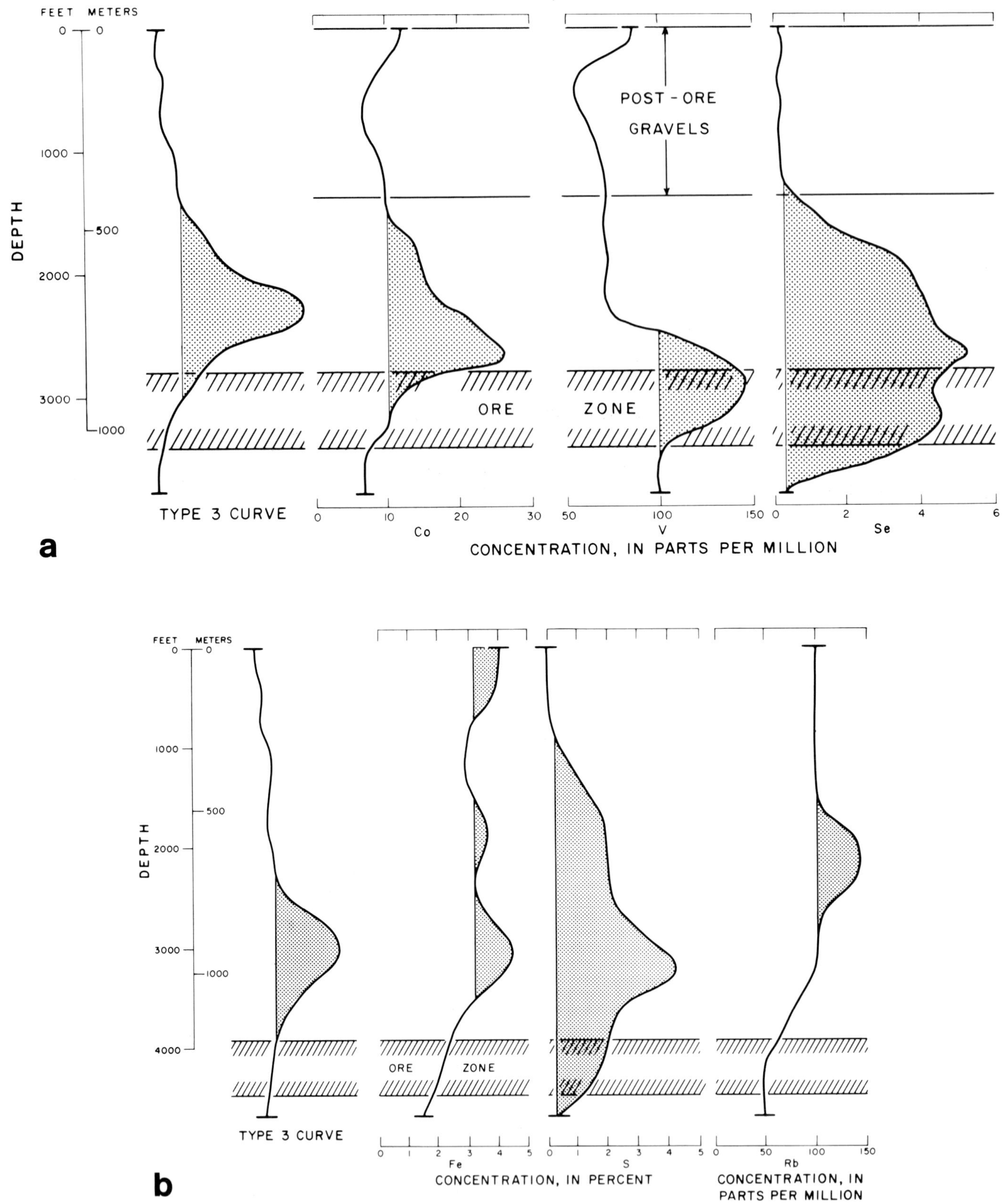

Figure 9.11. Concentration vs. depth curves for Type 3 elements: (*a*) Co, V, and Se; (*b*) Fe, S, and Rb. Shaded areas represent anomalies.

as to why this outer gold-tellurium aureole does not have the same configuration as the other metal aureoles; more information is needed to solve this problem.

The study by Jerome (1966) and general field observations in many porphyry copper districts suggest that additional aureoles should be present at Kalamazoo outside of those described here. Sampling farther from the ore zone in future studies may reveal distinct aureoles for elements such as lead, zinc, and manganese.

The approximate locations of the boundaries between the potassic, phyllic, and propylitic alteration zones have been added to the geochemical model in Figure 9.15, based

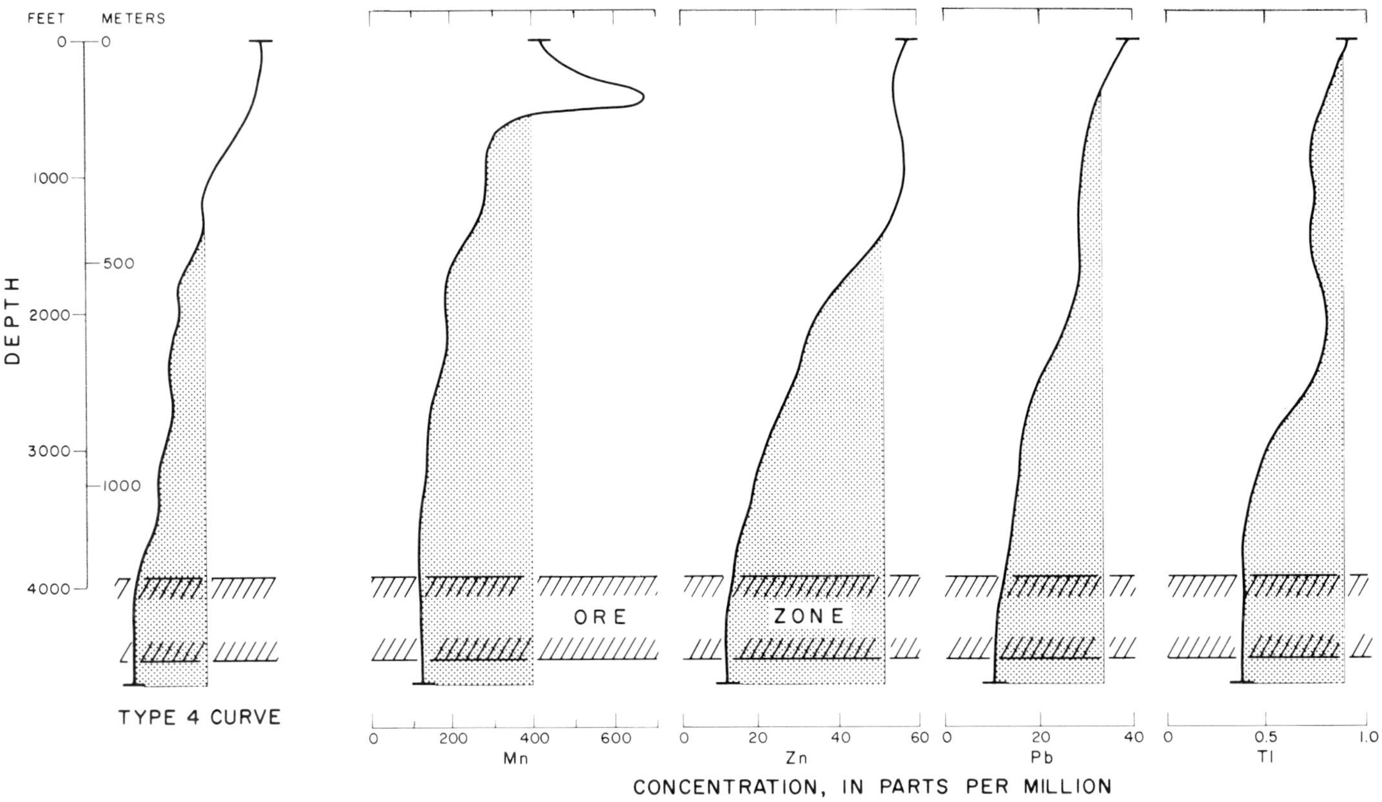

Figure 9.12. Concentration vs. depth curves for Type 4 elements, including Mn, Zn, Pb, and Tl. Shaded areas represent anomalies.

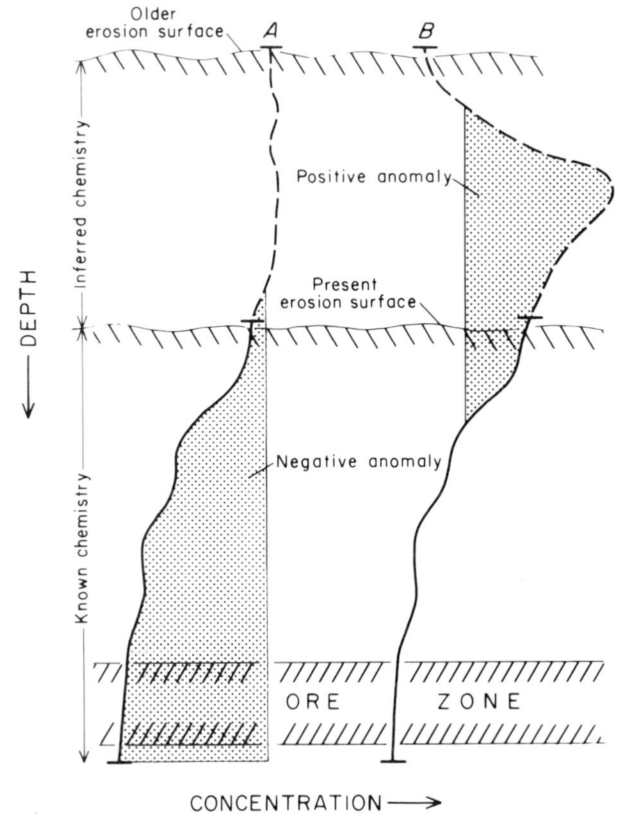

Figure 9.13. Concentration vs. depth curves for Type 4 elements, showing two interpretations based on hypothetical chemical analyses in now-eroded rock. Shaded areas represent anomalies.

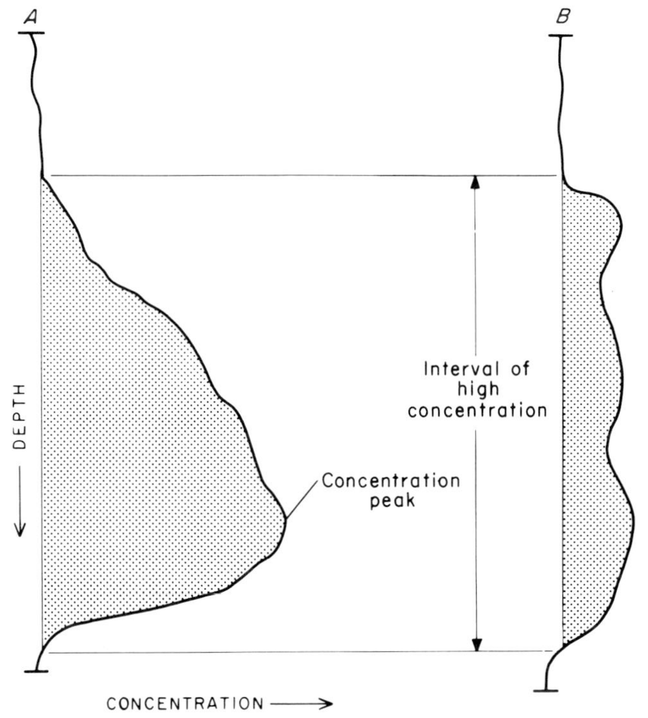

Figure 9.14. Schematic concentration vs. depth curves, showing relation between intervals of high concentration of an element and the concentration peak. Shaded areas represent anomalies. Curve *A* shows distinct concentration peak; curve *B* does not.

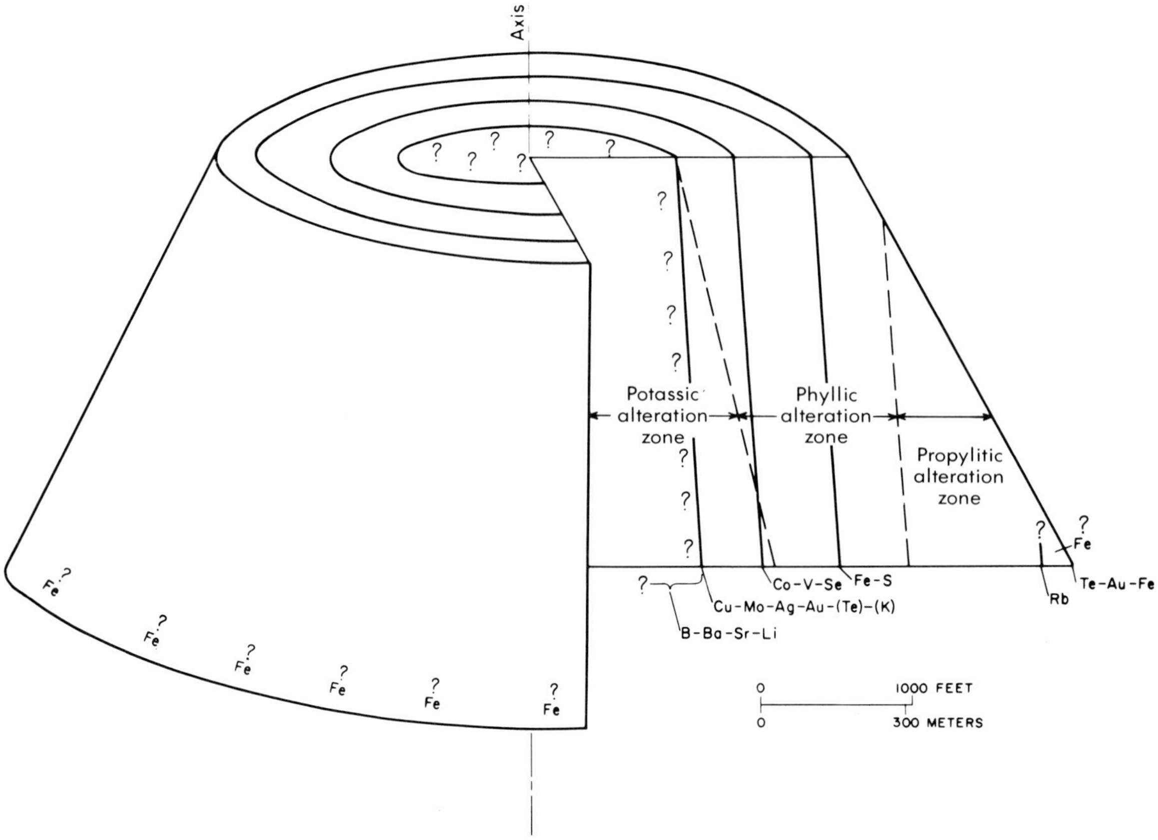

Figure 9.15. Geochemical model of the San Manuel-Kalamazoo porphyry copper system. Alteration zone boundaries (dashed lines) are from data given in drill logs.

on information given in the drill logs. The boundary between the phyllic and propylitic alteration zones appears to be roughly similar in configuration to most of the metal zoning. In contrast, the boundary between the potassic and phyllic zones seems to cross the metal aureoles.

EFFECTS OF WEATHERING

From a practical standpoint, most geochemical sampling is done using weathered material that is readily accessible at the surface. Rock outcrops, except in areas of rapid erosion, are usually altered as a result of chemical weathering. If geochemical surveys using outcrop material are to be successful in the search for blind porphyry copper deposits, then geochemists will need to learn more about the effects of chemical weathering on the primary concentrations of many elements, including those described in this study. The two drill holes that were collared in the Precambrian quartz monzonite at Kalamazoo exhibit the effects of chemical weathering to depths of as much as 180 m (about 600 ft.). Concentrations of various elements in the zone of weathering were compared to their respective concentrations in unweathered rock immediately underlying the weathered rock. The assumption was made that any significant differences in concentration in these two areas were predominantly the result of weathering processes. Unfortunately, only a limited number of the ore-related elements provided information that was consistent for both holes.

The effect of weathering at Kalamazoo is best illustrated by curves for sulfur (Fig. 9.16). For both holes a sharp break in the curves can be seen at the base of the zone of weathering. Clearly, sulfur has been rather thoroughly leached as a part of the weathering process; consequently, this element will probably not provide much useful information in weathered samples.

Some other ore-related elements seem to have been little affected (or to have actually been enriched) in the zone of weathering. Figure 9.17 shows that copper, for example, seems to have been enriched in this zone; zinc and rubidium, on the other hand, do not seem to have been either enriched or depleted. Copper at Kalamazoo is present in anomalous concentrations well beyond the actual copper ore zone; rubidium and, probably, zinc occur in aureoles that are also distant from the ore zone. Thus, analyses of rocks for these three elements in combination should be especially useful in the search for blind porphyry copper deposits. Other somewhat immobile ore-related elements—such as gold, silver, lead, tellurium, and selenium—may also be useful in evaluating samples of weathered rock; however, the effects of weathering on these and other elements were not consistent for the two holes, or the levels of concentrations were too low to be detected in the upper parts of the holes. Further studies of many of the elements discussed in this report are needed before analyses of these elements in weathered rock samples can be used in routine geochemical surveys.

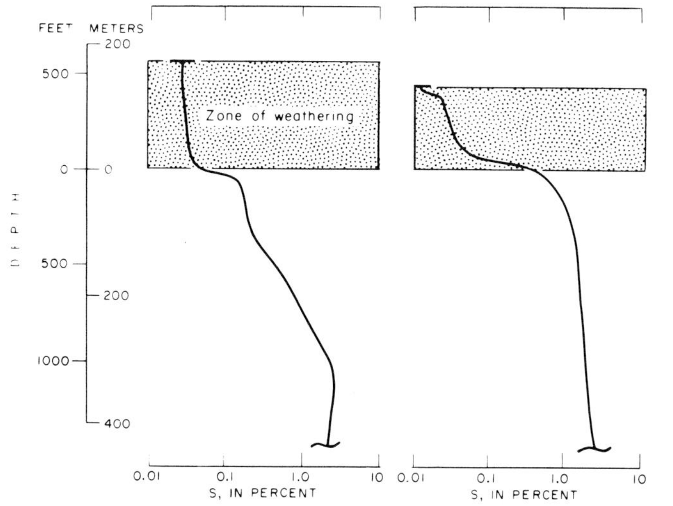

Figure 9.16. Concentration vs. depth curves for sulfur, illustrating the effects of weathering. Only the upper parts of two drill holes are shown. Zero on the depth scales represents the base of the zone of weathering.

APPLICATIONS TO EXPLORATION

An understanding of geochemical zoning in a porphyry copper deposit should be useful in prospecting for deposits similar to the Kalamazoo. Some of the results obtained at the Kalamazoo deposit suggest the value of using element zoning, especially with a combination of elements, to locate the position of a sample relative to a possible copper ore zone.

First, samples containing low copper and molybdenum values but high concentrations of boron, barium, strontium, or lithium may indicate that the samples are from the barren core of a deposit. In contrast, low copper and molybdenum concentrations combined with low boron, barium, strontium, or lithium values should indicate a different, perhaps more favorable, location beyond any ore zone.

Second, the presence of high tellurium concentrations in magnetite-rich samples may indicate that the samples are from locations near the outer root zone of a porphyry deposit. Samples with high tellurium but low iron concentrations may be from locations near the top of a porphyry system.

Third, for a systematic series of samples, such as core samples collected periodically along the length of a drill hole, the order in which concentration peaks for various elements are encountered—especially when combined with alteration information—may be an important criterion in determining where a given sample is located spatially within a porphyry system and, therefore, whether to continue drilling. For example, if core samples from a hole being drilled define a tellurium anomaly near the top of the hole, followed by a sulfur peak lower down, and then a selenium peak even lower down—in addition to slight increases in copper and molybdenum values—then drilling should be continued.

The Kalamazoo system has been examined in detail, but this study is only a beginning, and many problems remain to be solved. For example, it is not yet known if the same suite of elements is present around other deposits in similar concentrations and locations relative to a copper ore zone. And it is not known if there are predictable relationships between the grade and tonnage of a blind porphyry copper deposit and the spatial positions and relative concentrations of surrounding aureoles for various pathfinder elements. Limited geochemical information from other deposits plus the similar alteration-mineralization zoning patterns present around many other porphyry copper deposits suggest that the same

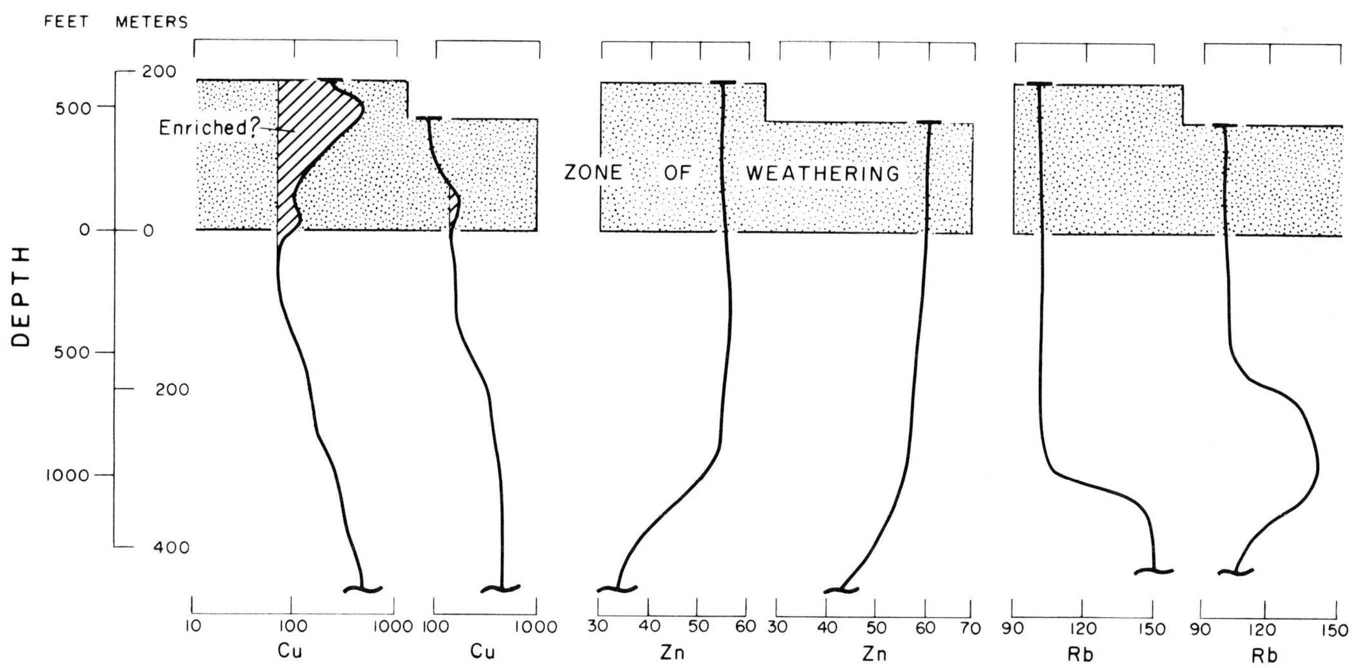

Figure 9.17. Concentration vs. depth curves for Cu, Zn, and Rb, illustrating the effects of weathering. Only the upper parts of two drill holes are shown. Zero on the depth scales represents the base of the zone of weathering.

pathfinder elements may be present in many of these deposits. As a consequence, the evaluation of element zoning may be useful in the search for new porphyry copper deposits that are present at depth within exposed or surficially covered rock bodies.

ACKNOWLEDGMENTS

A project the size of this one could not have been completed without the help of many individuals. I would like to express my appreciation to the staff of Magma Copper Company, and especially to Lloyd Thomas, Chief Geological and Planning Engineer, for providing the sample material and much valuable assistance. I am also grateful to a large number of chemists in the U.S. Geological Survey for their help in providing the analyses used in this chapter. These analysts include: J. W. Baker, L. A. Bradley, G. L. Crenshaw, C. A. Curtis, L. D. Forshey, J. G. Frisken, J. D. Hoffman, D. M. Hopkins, J. B. McHugh, R. L. Miller, E. L. Mosier, J. C. Negri, R. M. O'Leary, J. D. Sharkey, Z. C. Stephenson, S. J. Sutley, J. H. Turner, R. L. Turner, J. G. Viets, J. S. Wahlberg, E. P. Welsch, and R. J. Young.

REFERENCES CITED

Brabec, D., and White, W. H., 1971, Distribution of copper and zinc in rocks of the Guichon Creek batholith, British Columbia, *in* Boyle, R. W., and McGerrigle, J. I., eds., Geochemical Exploration: Canadian Inst. Mining, Metall., Spec. Vol. 11, p. 291–297.

Chaffee, M. A., 1976, The zonal distribution of selected elements above the Kalamazoo porphyry copper deposit, Pinal County, Arizona: Jour. Geochem. Explor., v. 5, no. 2, p. 145–165.

Claisse, Fernand, 1956, Accurate X-ray fluorescence analysis without internal standard: Que. Dep. Mines. Prelim. Rept., no. 327, 24 p.

Cox, D. P.; Gonzalez, I. P.; and Nash, J. T., 1975, Geology, geochemistry, and fluid-inclusion petrography of the Sapo Alegre porphyry copper prospect and its metavolcanic wallrocks, west-central Puerto Rico: U.S. Geol. Survey Jour. Research, v. 3, no. 3, p. 313–327.

Creasey, S. C., 1965, Geology of the San Manuel area, Pinal County, Arizona: U.S. Geol. Survey Prof. Paper 471, 64 p.

Crenshaw, G. L., and Lakin, H. W., 1974, A sensitive and rapid method for the determination of trace amounts of selenium in geologic materials: U.S. Geol. Survey Jour. Research, v. 2, no. 4, p. 483–487.

Davis, J. D., 1974, Geothermometry, geochemistry, and alteration of the San Manuel porphyry copper orebody, San Manuel, Arizona: Unpub. Ph.D. Diss., Univ. Arizona, 269 p.

Eidel, J. J.; Frost, J. E.; and Clippinger, D. M., 1968, Copper-molybdenum mineralization at Mineral Park, Mohave County, Arizona, *in* Ridge, J. D., ed., Ore Deposits of the United States, 1933–1967: New York, American Inst. Mining, Metall., p. 1258–1281.

Ficklin, W. H., 1970, A rapid method for the determination of fluoride in rocks and soils using an ion-selective electrode, *in* Geological Survey research 1970: U.S. Geol. Survey Prof. Paper 700-C, p. C186–C188.

Fisher, F. S., 1972, Tertiary mineralization and hydrothermal alteration in the Stinkingwater mining region, Park County, Wyoming: U.S. Geol. Survey Bull. 1332-C, p. C1–C33.

Gott, G. B., and McCarthy, J. H., Jr., 1966, Distribution of gold, silver, tellurium, and mercury in the Ely Mining District, White Pine County, Nevada: U.S. Geol. Survey Circ. 535, 5 p.

Gott, G. B.; McCarthy, J. H., Jr.; Oda, Uteana; Lakin, H. W.; and Thompson, C. E., 1966, Preliminary report comparing geochemical halos around an exposed and a concealed copper deposit, *in* CENTO Seminar on field techniques for mineral investigations, Iran, 1965: Ankara, Turkey, Office U.S. Econ. Coordinator CENTO Affairs, p. 133–144.

Gunton, J. E., and Nichol, Ian, 1974, Chemical zoning associated with the Ingerbelle-Copper Mountain mineralization, Princeton, British Columbia, *in* Elliott, I. L., and Fletcher, W. K., eds., Geochemical Exploration 1974: Amsterdam, Elsevier Scientific Publishing Co., Inc., p. 297–312.

Hubert, A. E., and Lakin, H. W., 1973, Atomic absorption determination of thallium and indium in geologic materials, *in* Jones, M. J., ed., Geochemical exploration 1972: Internat. Geochem. Explor. Symposium, 4th, London 1972, Proc., London, The Inst. Mining and Metallurgy, p. 383–388.

Jambor, J. L., 1974, Trace element variations in porphyry copper deposits, Babine Lake area, B.C.: Canada Geol. Survey Paper 74-9, 30 p.

Jerome, S. E., 1966, Some features pertinent in exploration of porphyry copper deposits, *in* Titley, S. R., and Hicks, C. L., eds., Geology of the Porphyry Copper Deposits, southwestern North America: Tucson, Univ. Ariz. Press, p. 75–85.

Krish, E. J., 1974, Relationship of trace element distribution to level of erosion in some porphyry copper deposits and prospects, southwestern United States and northwestern Mexico: Unpub. M.S. Thesis, Colorado School of Mines, 156 p.

Laboratory Equipment Company, no date, LECO automatic sulfur determinator: Laboratory Equipment Company, 1415 Hilltop Road, St. Joseph, Michigan 49085, 6 p.

Lowell, J. D., 1968, Geology of the Kalamazoo orebody, San Manuel district, Arizona: Econ. Geol., v. 63, no. 6, p. 645–654.

Lowell, J. D., and Guilbert, J. M., 1970, Lateral and vertical alteration-mineralization zoning in porphyry ore deposits: Econ. Geol., v. 65, no. 4, p. 373–408.

McIntyre, D. B.; Welday, E. E.; and Baird, A. K., 1965, Geologic application of the air pycnometer: A study of the precision of measurement: Geol. Soc. America Bull., v. 76, no. 9, p. 1055–1060.

Myers, A., T.; Havens, R. G.; and Dunton, P. J., 1961, A spectrochemical method for the semi-quantitative analysis of rocks, minerals, and ores: U.S. Geol. Survey Bull. 1084-I, p. 207–229.

Nakagawa, H. M., and Thompson, C. E., 1969, Atomic absorption determination of tellurium, *in* Geological Survey research 1968: U.S. Geol. Survey Prof. Paper 600-B, p. B123–B125.

Olade, M. A., and Fletcher, W. K., 1975, Primary dispersion of rubidium and strontium around porphyry copper deposits, Highland Valley, British Columbia: Econ. Geol., v. 70, no. 1, p. 15–21.

——— 1976*a*. Distribution of sulphur, and sulphide-iron and copper in bedrock associated with porphyry copper deposits, Highland Valley, British Columbia: Jour. Geochem. Explor., v. 5, no. 1, p. 21–30.

——— 1976*b*, Trace element geochemistry of the Highland Valley and Guichon Creek Batholith in relation to porphyry copper mineralization: Econ. Geol., v. 71, no. 4, p. 733–748.

Oyarzun, M., Jorge, 1974, Rubidium and strontium as guides to copper mineralization emplaced in some Chilean andesitic rocks, *in* Elliott, I. L., and Fletcher, W. K., eds., Geochemical Exploration 1974: Amsterdam, Elsevier Scientific Publishing Co., Inc., p. 333–338.

Reid, J., 1975, Skarn alteration of the Commercial Limestone in the Carr Fork area, *in* Bray, R. E., and Wilson, J. C., eds., Guidebook to the Bingham Mining District: Soc. Econ. Geologists Guidebook, p. 105–118.

Sower, F. B.; Eicher, R. N.; and Selner, G. I., 1971, the STATPAC system: U.S. Geol. Survey computer contribution no. 11, 36 p.

Theodore, T. G., and Nash, J. T., 1973, Geochemical and fluid zonation at Copper Canyon, Lander County, Nevada: Econ. Geol., v. 68, no. 4, p. 565–570.

Thomas, L. A., 1975, written communication.

Ward, F. N.; Lakin, H. W.; Canney, F. C.; and others, 1963, Analytical methods used in geochemical exploration by the U.S. Geological Survey: U.S. Geol. Survey Bull. 1152, 100 p.

Ward, F. N.; Nakagawa, H. M.; Harms, T. F.; and VanSickle, G. H., 1969, Atomic-absorption methods of analysis useful in geochemical exploration: U.S. Geol. Survey Bull. 1289, 45 p.

Watterson, J. R.; Ficklin, W. H.; and Turner, J. H., 1976, A modification of Shapiro's technique for CO_2: U.S. Geol. Survey Open-File Rept. 76-530, 5 p.

Welsch, E. P., and Chao, T. T., 1976, Determination of trace amounts of tin in geological materials by atomic absorption spectrometry: Anal. Chim. Acta, v. 82, p. 337–342.

10

Sulfur and Copper in Magma and Rocks

RAY PORPHYRY COPPER DEPOSIT, PINAL COUNTY, ARIZONA

Norman G. Banks

The study reported in this chapter was initiated to trace the development of S, Cu, H_2O, and Cl in the suite of Laramide igneous rocks near the Ray porphyry copper deposit, Arizona, and to evaluate the data with respect to the pluton causative models of porphyry copper genesis that assume causal relations, in one or more ways, between porphyry deposits and igneous rocks associated in time and space with them. Although many variations and combinations exist, the two endmember models are (1) the classical magmatic or orthomagmatic model, which assumes that magma in an exposed or nearby hidden pluton carried the metals, fluids, and sulfur from a deeper source into or near the deposits, and (2) the meteoric water model, which postulates that Cu and S were leached, transported, and deposited by groundwaters whose circulation was induced by magmatic heat.

Both the meteroic water and orthomagmatic models are based on the well-documented space-time association of porphyry-type deposits and calc-alkaline plutons, and both have accumulated a large volume of circumstantial support. However, neither one has produced unambiguous data that establish a direct causative connection between ore generation and upper crustal plutons. In fact, surprisingly few direct data testing the models have been gathered, and much of the appropriate but indirect data that have been published, rather than demonstrating proof, have required amendment of the two basic models.

Earlier studies at Ray found it unlikely that Cl-rich waters were evolved from the Laramide plutons associated with the deposit in the amounts and at the times required to support the orthomagmatic model (Banks, 1976). Additionally, it became evident that although propylitic alteration of basement igneous rocks (of Precambrian through Laramide age) might have introduced sulfur to circulating meteoric waters (Banks, 1973), it could have provided only a fraction of the sulfur in the deposit (Banks, 1973, 1974*a*); at the same time, this alteration produced a mineralogy that would have removed, rather than introduced, copper from the water in the outer reaches of a circulation cell (Banks, 1974*b*).

This chapter provides data on magmatic sulfides and concentrations of S and Cu in rock samples and their component minerals in the intrusive bodies associated in time and space with the Ray porphyry copper deposit, Arizona. They include petrologic descriptions of magmatic sulfide minerals; emission spectrochemical, electron microprobe, and ion microprobe analyses of Cu and S in the major and minor minerals of the rocks; and petrologic descriptions and analyses of the whole-rock samples for S and Cu. These data allow interpretation of the magmatic behavior of S and Cu and evaluation of the application of both the orthomagmatic and meteoric water models of porphyry copper generation to the Ray deposit.

This evaluation proves critical of both models, because, when viewed in a context which includes all the petrochemical data for the rocks, the S and Cu data seem best explained if the ore-age magmas contained little S and Cu and if most of both elements was utilized by the igneous minerals during crystallization of the magmas. Furthermore, the petrochemical data from Ray are not unique when compared to equivalent information from other calc-alkaline igneous suites, including those in provinces barren of porphyry copper mineralization. This commonality of petrochemical data suggests that the explanation of the space-time relation of porphyry-type deposits and calc-alkaline plutons might be consistent with the petrochemical findings and interpretations at Ray, but alternative to the ore-genesis models described above.

BACKGROUND GEOLOGY AND PETROLOGY OF LARAMIDE IGNEOUS ROCKS

The concerns of this report are the distribution and magmatic behavior of S and Cu in the Laramide rocks at Ray, but these data cannot be interpreted properly without a basic geologic and petrologic framework of the samples used in the study. The pertinent background information can be obtained in detail from Cornwall and others (1971), Banks and others (1972), Banks and Stuckless (1973), Banks (1973, 1974*a*, 1974*b*, 1976), Cornwall and Banks (1977), Banks and Page (1980) and Cornwall (1982) and is described briefly in this section.

Ray is a major porphyry copper deposit, located about 110 km north of Tucson and 120 km east of Phoenix, Arizona. The main hosts of the hypogene sulfides (mainly pyrite, chalcopyrite, molybdenite) are schist, Ruin Granite (a quartz nonzonite), quartzite, and diabase; all are of Precambrian age. As seen in Figure 10.1, the center of mineralization occurs near the west-central edge of the Sonora quadrangle near the junction of major northwest-trending and northeast-trending fault systems at the end of an elongate zone of stocks and chronolithic masses of one of the Laramide rock types in the area, the Granite Mountain porphyry. Thus, neither the deposit nor intense deposit-associated alteration coincides with the densest dike swarms and largest plutons of ore age exposed near the commercial mineralization. This relation makes Ray an attractive place to investigate igneous processes that occurred in magma associated in time and space with a major porphyry copper deposit.

The Laramide rocks near Ray were intruded over a period of 10–11 m.y. that—for convenience of description, without necessarily implying episodic magmatism—has been described by Banks and others (1972) in terms of 5 intrusive periods (see Fig. 10.1). These intrusive periods include at least 12 rock types that are cut by sulfide veinlets, and at least 11 of them were emplaced prior to deposition of ore in the deposit 60 m.y. ago (Banks et al., 1972; Banks and Stuckless, 1973). Whole-rock chemical and petrologic data have been collected for one or more samples of each of the 12 rock types, and a summary of these data is presented by Cornwall in Chapter 11 of this volume. The samples used in this study were collected at the sites indicated in Figure 10.1; they include 8 of the 12 rock types and, in addition, one sample (78/79–4) of intrusive andesite of a still earlier period (70–85 m.y. ago) of basaltic and andesitic magmatism (Banks and Krieger, 1977; Cornwall, 1982; Koski and Cook, 1982). This older intrusive type is represented in the study area by only a few sills and dikes.

One or more stocks representing 5 rock types were emplaced in each of the first 4 intrusive periods. Four of these rock types (Tortilla Quartz Diorite, Rattler Granodiorite, Granite Mountain Porphyry, and Teapot Mountain Porphyry) were included in this study (Fig. 10.1, Table 10.1). The excepted rock type represents a granodiorite of intrusive period II, which crops out extensively outside of the immediate study area in the Grayback quadrangle (see Cornwall, Chapter 11 of this volume). Andesitic to quartz latitic dikes were emplaced in intrusive periods II, IV, and V. Samples of these dikes chosen for this study came from three rock types of intrusive period II (samples 61–4, 17–16, and GM100, Table 10.1) and one rock type of period V (sample 61–2F, Table 10.1).

Bulk compositions of the major Laramide plutons are progressively more felsic (increasing differentiation index) with decreasing age of the intrusive type; these ages (see Table 10.1) were determined by geologic relations (Cornwall et al., 1971) and by K-Ar and fission-track ages (Creasey and Kistler, 1962; Damon and Mauger, 1966; Damon et al., 1970; Banks et al., 1972; Banks and Stuckless, 1973). Compositions of the dike rocks are not always intermediate between those of rock types that they crosscut and that crosscut them. However, standard petrochemical plots of whole-rock normative minerals, major elements, and trace elements indicate that the magmas of both the dikes and the stocks of Laramide age near Ray developed along smooth chemical trends (Banks et al., 1972; Cornwall and Banks, 1977; Cornwall, 1982). The results are compatible with, but do not distinguish between, either consanguinity or a common-source partial melting origin of the igneous suite. The various facies of one pluton, the Rattler Granodiorite, almost duplicate in one intrusive mass the chemical, textural, and mineralogical variations that occur in the entire sample suited studied (see Table 10.1). This duplication allows comparison of the S and Cu content in one stock with that in a series of dikes and stocks intruded in the 10-m.y. period at different levels of emplacement—ranging from 1.5 km or less to 3 km or more (but less than 5 km, Banks and Stuckless, 1973).

Some knowledge of the paragenesis of the igneous minerals (details in Banks, 1976, and Cornwall, 1982) is required for proper interpretation of the magmatic behavior of S and Cu; particularly important is the paragenesis of apatite, biotite, and hornblende, which contain most of the Cl, H_2O and S in the rocks, and of magnetite, which is associated with the bulk of the magmatic sulfide minerals. Plagioclase and, where present, pyroxene were the first minerals formed in the melts of all rock types. In the Tortilla Quartz Diorite and mafic facies of the Rattler Granodiorite, hornblende followed crystallization of plagioclase and pyroxene, and biotite, quartz, and K-feldspar are interstitial to and also replace these early minerals. In the progressively more felsic facies of the Rattler Granodiorite and in all facies of the Granite Mountain Porphyry, part of the quartz and K-feldspar, in addition to the bulk of the plagioclase, crystallized before biotite began forming, and hornblende either is not present or is present as a trace mineral. In all of the holocrystalline rocks, the bulk of the apatite and magnetite occurs with the biotite, although both accessory minerals, particularly in the more mafic samples, occur as small inclusions in the early silicates. Most of these early, but modally less significant and physically smaller, occurrences of magnetite and apatite are considered to have resulted from local saturation of the melt with the accessory minerals. The saturation resulted from rejection of their component elements by growth of the including and adjacent major silicate phases, rather than from melt-wide saturation. The above paragenesis applies to the bulk of igneous rock exposed, but variations are displayed in the Teapot Mountain Porphyry, porphyritic facies of the

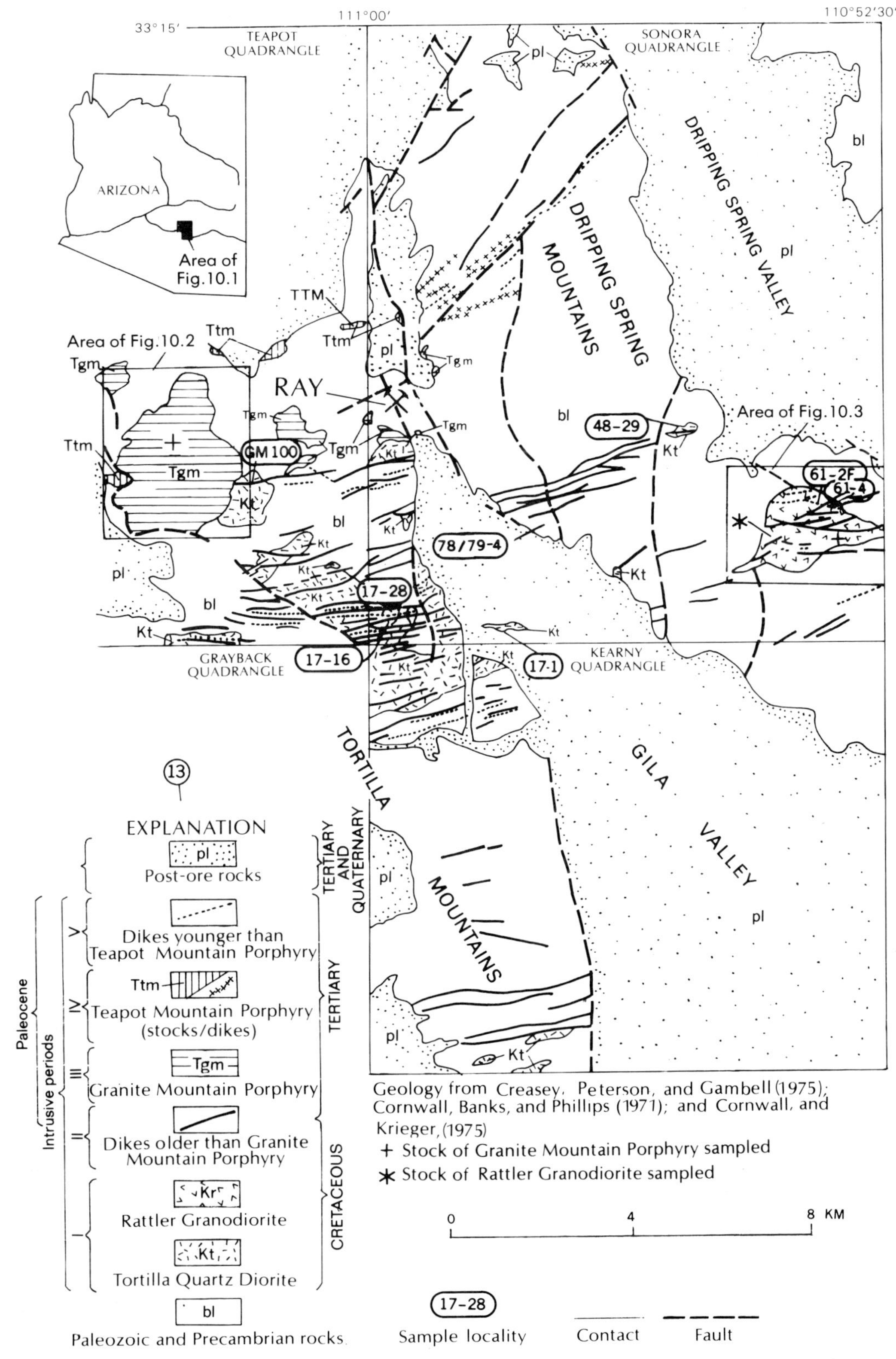

Figure 10.1. General geology and samples locations, Ray area

Rattler Granodiorite and in the porphyritic dike rocks in which phenocrystic magnetite, biotite, and apatite suggest an earlier separation from the melt than in the holocrystalline plutons.

Although the samples were collected as much as several kilometers from commercial ground and were specifically chosen to minimize alteration, occasional hairline- to millimeter-thick sulfide veinlets were observed at or near almost every sample site. The veinlets are most abundant near or along strike of the larger plutons or dike swarms, and they show strong preferred orientation in contrast to fractures (radial, concentric, sheeting joints) related to solidification

TABLE 10.1
Differentiation Index, Texture, and Mafic Silicates in Laramide Rocks Near Ray

Rock Sample[1]	Rock Differentiation Index[2]	Texture	Mafic Silicates Present: Pyroxene	Hornblende	Biotite
Tortilla Quartz Diorite (71–70 m.y.)[3]					
17–28	51.4	Intersertal	X	X	X
17–1	51.9	Intersertal	X	([4])	X
48–29	53.2	Intersertal	X	X	—
Rattler Granodiorite (70 m.y.)					
46–99B	48.4	Hypidiomorphic-seriate	X	X	X
60–113D†	64.7	Porphyritic	—	X	X
60–114†*	72.2	Porphyritic	—	X	X
60–108	72.3	Hypidiomorphic-seriate	Trace	X	—
61–25†	72.4	Porphyritic	—	X	X
60–91	72.5	Seriate porphyritic	—	X	X
60–111	72.7	Chilled	—	—	X
60–124*	72.8	Hypidiomorphic-seriate	—	X	X
60–98	75.2	Hypidiomorphic-seriate	—	X	X
46–11G	75.4	Hypidiomorphic-seriate	—	X	X
60–131	76.4	Seriate porphyritic	—	—	X
60–130	76.9	Hypidiomorphic-seriate	—	—	X
60–132*	77.7	Hypidiomorphic-seriate	—	—	X
60–96A	87.3	Aplitic	—	—	X
46–11A	93.3	Aplitic	—	—	X
Granite Mountain Porphyry (61–60 m.y.)					
RB5	79.7	Granitoid	—	—	X
GM14	80.5	Seriate porphyritic	—	—	X
GM12	81.8	Porphyritic	—	—	X
GM18	81.9	Granitoid	—	Trace	X
GM6G	83.5	Seriate porphyritic	—	Trace	X
GM1A	[5]94.7	Aplitic	—	—	X
GM2A	94.7	Aplitic	—	—	X
Teapot Mountain Porphyry (61–60 m.y.)					
Ttm†	83.6	Porphyritic	—	X	X
Andesite and Rhyodacite Dikes[6]					
78/79–4†*	51.6	Porphyritic	X	X	—
61–4†*	54.7	Porphyritic	—	X	Trace
17–16†	—	Porphyritic	—	X	X
GM100†	[7]80.0	Porphyritic	—	X	X
61–2F†	81.0	Porphyritic	—	X	X

NOTE: Table includes only samples with whole rock chemistry and mineral analyses, omits samples with emission spectrochemical data only.

† Samples with phenocrystic magnetite and hydrous phases.

* No mineral analyses in the following tables.

[1] A numeral 2 preceding the sample numbers in the following tables indicates that the probe mount is a duplicate probe sample.

[2] Modified from Thornton and Tuttle (1960): uses quartz plus albite plus K-feldspar from molecular catanorm rather than the CIPW norm.

[3] Ages from Banks and Stuckless (1973); Banks and others (1972).

[4] Fibrous amphibole reaction rims on pyroxene.

[5] Aplite assumed to have approximately same differentiation index as sample GM24.

[6] Ages as follows: Sample 78/79-4 (<85, >70 m.y.); samples 61-4 and 17-16 (<69, >63 m.y.); sample GM100 (63 m.y.); sample 61-2F (questionable, either 70 m.y. or <60 m.y.).

[7] Rock analysis from the same dike type but not the same dike used for the mineral analyses.

of the plutons. (Compare attitudes of the veinlets and dikes that are nearby which crosscut the plutons with the attitudes of the aplite dikes in the plutons, Figs. 10.2, 10.3.) Strong preferred orientation of dikes and sulfide veinlets in and near porphyry copper deposits has been noted elsewhere in Arizona (Rehrig and Heidrick, 1972, 1976) as well as in other crustal areas (for example, Goossens and Hollister, 1973; Hollister, 1974; Hollister et al., 1975). The age of the veinlets has not been determined for all areas near Ray, but in the deposit they are about 60 m.y. old, and the veinlets crosscutting the Rattler Granodiorite (70 m.y.) were emplaced at least 7 m.y. after solidification of the stock, because they crosscut dikes of intrusive period II which are 63 m.y. old (Fig. 10.4*A*, Table 10.1). These relations indicate a regional tectonic control on development of the sulfide veinlets rather than a control related to the crystallization of the immediate host sampled. Therefore, considerable efforts were made to eliminate the sulfide veinlets from the samples analyzed by whole-rock methods (see Appendix II).

NATURE AND DISTRIBUTION OF IGNEOUS SULFIDE MINERALS

Sulfide minerals with textural relations indicating their direct magmatic heritage are present in most igneous rocks (Newhouse, 1936), and they have been found to occur in the Laramide intrusive rocks near Ray. Presumably, they also occur in rocks associated with other porphyry copper deposits.

Knowledge of the abundance, textures, paragenesis, and compositions of demonstrably magmatic sulfides and an understanding of how these petrologic parameters change with the changing age and chemistry of rocks associated with porphyry-type ore deposits would aid greatly in interpreting the content and behavior of magmatic S and Cu in the plutons and in evaluating models of porphyry copper generation. Surprisingly, such knowledge is almost nonexistent and is limited to the classic but broad and unquantified study of Newhouse (1936), a few notations in petrologic studies unrelated to porphyry deposits, and inferences from the more detailed but largely unrelated studies of sulfide minerals in mafic and ultramafic rock. This paucity of applicable data is probably in part due to the common superposition of porphyry copper mineralization and alteration on magmatic textures of the plutons, a superposition from which the Laramide intrusive rocks near Ray happily are largely exempt. Other inhibiting factors may be the necessarily considerable investment in time and expense and the need for microanalytical instruments to measure and observe the pertinent petrologic parameters.

Details of the analytical techniques used here are available in Appendix I. Briefly, modal and textural data (Table 10.2) were gathered using polished thin sections (ca 4–5 cm^2) and a combination of microscope and electron microprobe observations and measurements. The polished thin sections came from samples that were carefully screened in outcrop, sawed slab, and thin section and for which detailed chemistry and petrology were already available (Cornwall et al., 1971; Banks et al., 1972; Banks, 1976; Cornwall and Banks, 1977; Banks and Page, 1980; Cornwall, 1982). The screening was meant to eliminate biasing of the data by

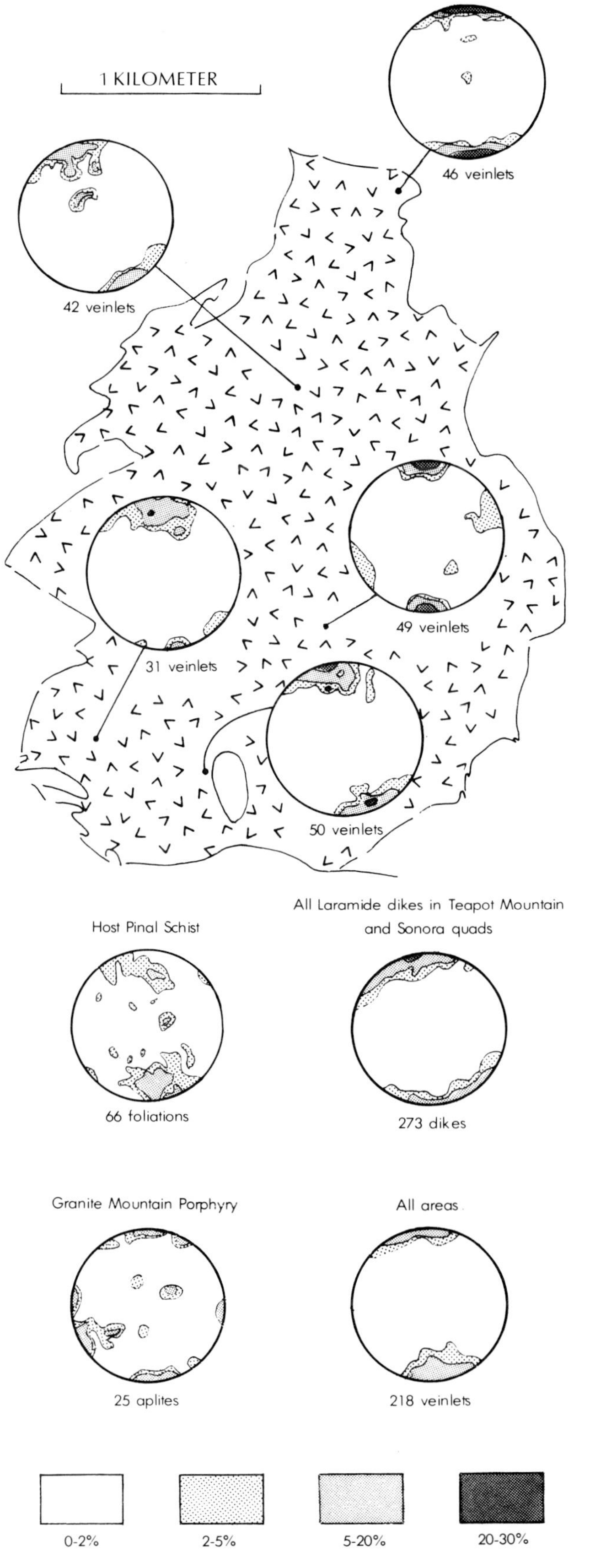

Figure 10.2. Orientation of sulfide veinlets and aplites cutting the Granite Mountain Porphyry, Laramide dikes in the district, and foliation of Pinal Schist intruded by Granite Mountain Porphyry. Data are poles to the planar features plotted on the lower hemisphere, equal area projection. Geology and schist foliations from Creasey and others (1975). Dike orientation data from Cornwall and others (1971).

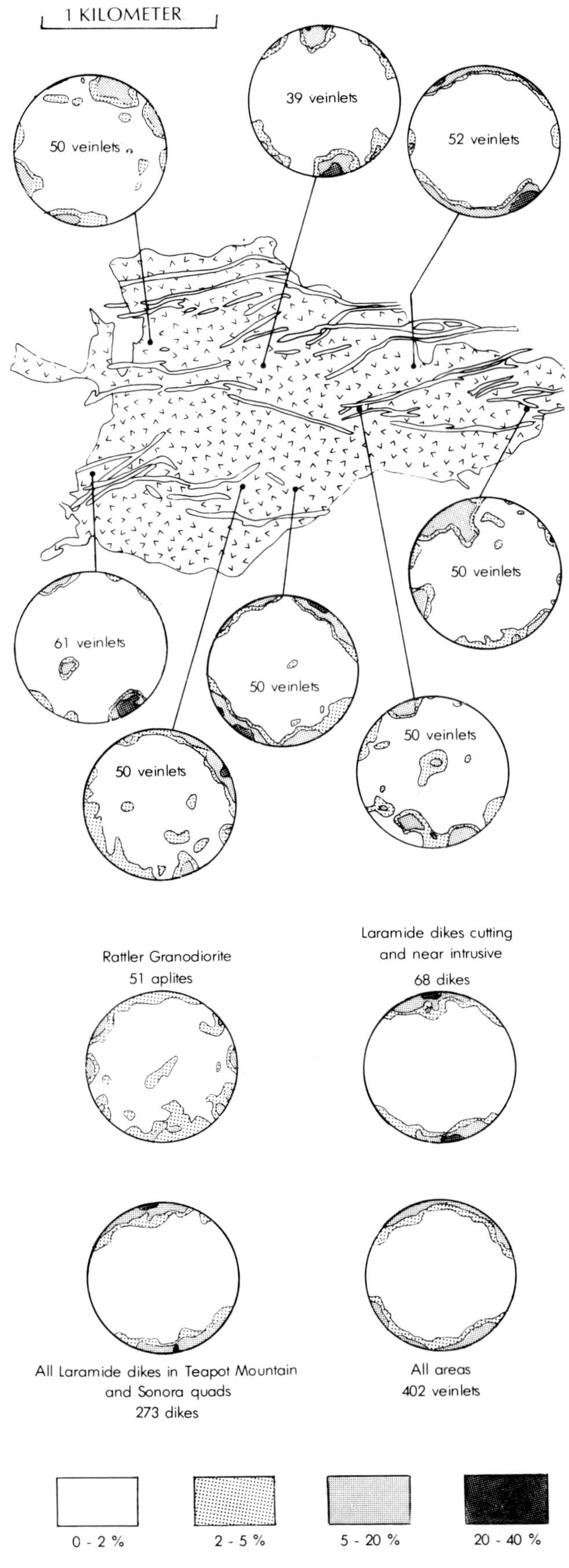

Figure 10.3. Orientation of sulfide veinlets, aplites, and Laramide dikes cutting the Rattler Granodiorite and orientation of all the Laramide dikes in the district. Data are poles to the planar features plotted on the lower hemisphere, equal area projection. Geology and dike orientation data from Cornwall and others (1971).

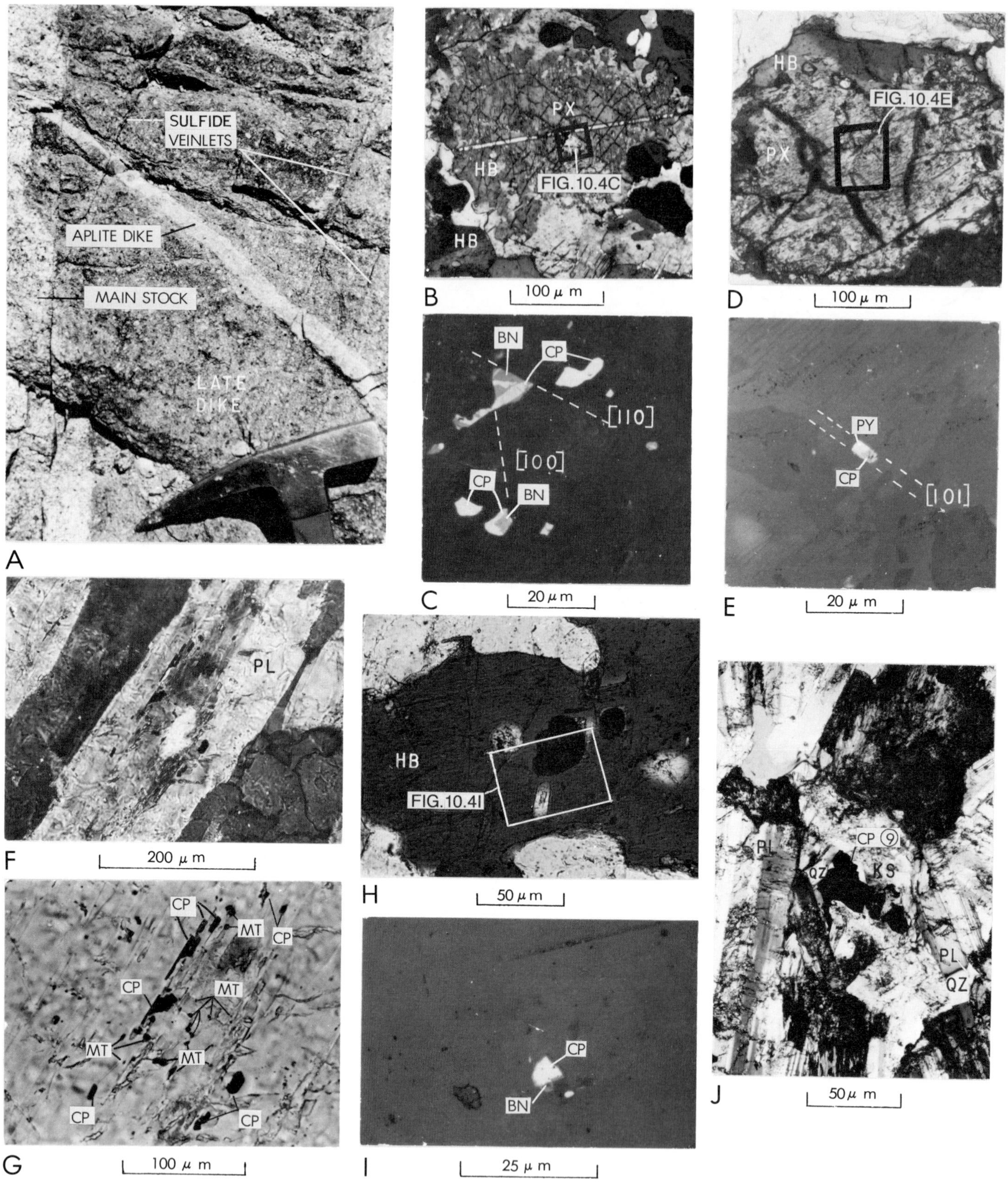

Figure 10.4. Textural relations of sulfide minerals in Laramide igneous rocks near Ray. *A,* sulfide veinlets (<63 m.y.) cutting the late dike facies and an aplitic differentiate located on a sheeting joint in the Rattler Granodiorite (70 m.y.). *B,* sample 17–28, two-phase bornite-chalcopyrite inclusions surrounding optical core of pyroxene twin, partially crossed nicols. *C,* enlargement of area shown in *B,* reflected light. Dotted lines indicate crystallographic orientation of host pyroxene. *D,* sample 17–28, two-phase pyrite-chalcopyrite filling of negative crystal in core of pyroxene grain, reflected light. *E,* enlargement of area shown in *D,* reflected light. Dotted lines indicate [101] crystallographic orientation of host pyroxene. *F,* sample 17–1, chalcopyrite filling negative crystals around optical core of plagioclase twin, partially crossed nicols. *G,* enlargement showing forms of grains in core area shown in *F,* uncrossed nicols. *H,* sample 48–29, large two-phase bleb of bornite-chalcopyrite in hornblende, uncrossed nicols. *I,* enlargement of area shown in *H*, reflected light. *J,* sample 217–1, anhedral chalcopyrite occurring with interstitial quartz and potassium feldspar, partially crossed nicols. Number refers to analysis in Table 10.3. Key: BN = bornite; CP = chalcopyrite; HB = hornblende; KS = potassium feldspar; μm = micrometers; MT = magnetite; PL = plagioclase; PY = pyrite; PX = pyroxene; QZ = quartz.

TABLE 10.2
Modal Data for Sulfides in Samples of Igneous Rocks Associated With the Ray Porphyry Copper Deposit

Rock Type	Sample Number[1]	Modal Abundance in ppm[2] PY	CP	BN	Number of Grains Counted[3]	Number of Two-Phase Grains	Average Size of Grain[4] (μm^2)	Relative Host Mineral[5] Occurrence in Volume Percent PX	PL	HB	SP	BI	MT	QZ	KS	GB	Volume Percent[6] Occurrence With Alteration	Occurrence With Fractures	Relative Percent by Volume of Grain Form[7] Bleb	Negative Crystal	Subhedral and Euhederal
Tortilla	17–28	0.01 —	2.1 (0.06)	0.35	58 (1)	6	16 (25)	71	16	12	—	—	1	—	—	—	15CP	3CP	95	5	—
Quartz	17–1	5.5 —	68 (1.5)	—	158 (6)	14	141 (77)	tr	17	1	—	2	39	1	—	32	20CP	9CP	23	66	12
Diorite	248–29	0.06 —	0.87 —	[8]1.4	33 —	5	29 —	28	25	19	—	—	10	—	—	18	3CP,11BN	1CP,2BN	91	9	—
Rattler	246–99B	7.3 (0.41)	— —	—	30 (3)	0	93 (57)	—	25	2	46	—	21	6	—	tr	22PY	5PY	73	—	27
Granodiorite	60–113D	— —	1.2 —	1.0	37 —	15	26 —	—	—	6	—	—	94	—	—	—	—	—	99	1	—
	60–108	— —	— —	—	— —	—	— —	—	—	—	—	—	—	—	—	—	—	—	—	—	—
	61–25	0.05 —	1.3 —	—	12 —	0	43 —	—	—	—	—	—	100	—	—	—	—	—	77	23	—
	60–91	0.03 (0.03)	1.1 (0.03)	—	7 (2)	0	69 (15)	—	15	14	—	—	68	—	—	3	6PY,5CP	3PY,3CP	32	68	—
	60–111	0.24 (0.01)	0.22 —	—	8 (3)	1	19 (1.5)	—	7	—	—	—	86	7	—	—	3PY	3PY	59	33	8
	60–98	— —	0.69 (1.6)	—	14 (1)	0	19 (600)	—	5	—	—	—	95	—	—	—	70CP	70CP	22	78	—
	46–11G	— —	0.99 —	—	14 —	0	29 —	—	—	—	—	—	100	—	—	—	—	—	71	29	—
	60–131	0.76 —	0.33 —	—	9 —	5	47 —	—	25	—	—	—	75	—	—	—	2CP	—	74	9	17
	60–130	0.23 —	0.97 (0.02)	—	17 (1)	3	27 (9)	—	13	—	—	—	81	—	—	6	2CP	2CP	75	18	7
	60–96A	0.34 (14.2)	0.29 —	—	10 (11)	1	20 (390)	—	47	—	—	—	47	6	—	—	96PY	96PY	17	17	83
	46–11A	0.10 (0.81)	0.05 (0.28)	—	4 (10)	—	16 (44)	—	100	—	—	—	—	—	—	—	98PY,97CP	95PY,96CP	—	—	100
Granite	RB–5	— —	0.39 (0.09)	—	10 (1)	0	16 (39)	—	34	—	—	—	61	5	—	—	43CP	35CP	60	9	31
Mountain	GM14	— —	0.22 —	—	3 —	0	33 —	—	100	—	—	—	—	—	—	—	—	—	100	—	—
Porphyry	GM12	— —	— —	—	— —	—	— —	—	—	—	—	—	—	—	—	—	—	—	—	—	—
	GM18	0.11 —	0.03 —	—	2 —	0	30 —	—	—	—	—	—	100	—	—	—	—	—	50	50	—
	GM6G	— —	— (0.04)	—	0 (1)	0	— (15)	—	—	—	—	—	—	—	—	—	100CP	100CP	—	—	—
	GM2A	0.08 (0.02)	— (0.01)	—	1 (2)	0	34 (6)	—	—	—	—	—	—	—	100	—	15PY,10CP	100PY,100CP	—	—	100
Teapot Mountain Porphyry	2TTM	— —	— —	—	— —	—	— —	—	—	—	—	—	—	—	—	—	—	—	—	—	—

[1] Arranged in order of increasing differentiation index for each rock type.

[2] Calculated from area of slide and area of mineral grains. Numbers in parentheses indicate modal abundance of secondary sulfide mineral grains in the slide located on fractures with alteration halos. *PY* = pyrite, *CP* = chalcopyrite, *BN* = bornite.

[3] Numbers in parentheses indicate number of secondary sulfide grains as defined in footnote 2.

[4] Numbers in parentheses indicate average size of secondary sulfide grains as defined in footnote 2.

[5] *PX* = pyroxene, *PL* = plagioclase, *HB* = hornblende, *SP* = sphene, *BI* = biotite, *MT* = magnetite, *QZ* = quartz, *KS* = potassium-feldspar, *GB* = grain boundary.

[6] Includes secondary sulfides located on fractures with alteration halos. *CP* = chalcopyrite, *PY* = pyrite, *BN* = bornite.

[7] Subhedral and euhedral may include some occurrences of negative crystals where the crystallographic orientation of the host mineral could not be determined.

[8] Includes digenite occurring with bornite.

sulfide grains associated with the tectonically controlled fractures, but despite the care, approximately half of the samples had hairline fractures visible on the polished surface, and some of these had microscopically visible alteration halos and sulfide minerals distributed along them. These fracture-controlled sulfide grains in altered mineral hosts are not considered indigenous to the samples and were not included in construction of the figures. However, for completeness, the data for these secondary sulfide grains are included in parentheses in Table 10.2. Grains occurring near a fracture in an unaltered mineral host or in an altered host not accompanied by a fracture were considered to be magmatic; thus, the data for the magmatic grains are probably biased toward inclusion rather than exclusion of secondary grains. Corrections for the secondary sulfides were small, except in two samples of aplite (60–96A and 46–11A, Table 10.2). The sulfides considered to be secondary in these samples were much larger than the magmatic sulfides in the rocks and were located on only one or two clearly crosscutting fractures with alteration halos.

Occurrence, Modal Abundance, Form, and Variations of the Magmatic Sulfide Minerals

Microscopic sulfide minerals whose textural features strongly suggest that they were present in the rocks prior to solidification and that therefore, they are magmatic, occur in most of the least-altered Laramide igneous rocks near Ray. They occur largely as inclusions in igneous minerals and are dominantly bornite, chalcopyrite, and pyrite. Digenite and covellite occur with some of the bornite grains, but the data do not distinguish whether they exsolved with bornite from a high-temperature bornite solid-solution phase or are low-temperature alteration products of bornite.

The features that suggest the magmatic origin of the sulfide occurrences are location, abundance, size, morphology, and the fact that some of these parameters change regularly with changes in age and chemistry of the host rock. On the other hand, these parameters do not measurably respond to alteration imposed upon the samples since their solidification.

The sulfides in the more mafic older rocks are more abundant, began forming paragenetically earlier, and had a long crystallization history. In the older and less differentiated samples (Tortilla Quartz Diorite and more mafic samples of Rattler Granodiorite), magmatic sulfides occur most commonly in zones in or around the cores of the early formed silicates (see Table 10.2), pyroxene (see Fig. 10.4*B–E*), plagioclase (see Fig. 10.4*F–G*), and hornblende that at least in part replaces pyroxene (see Fig. 10.4*H–I*). They fairly commonly are associated with the interstitial minerals (see Fig. 10.4*J;* Table 10.2) and included in magnetite (Fig. 10.5*A–B;* Table 10.2). In the younger more felsic samples (most of Rattler Granodiorite and Granite Mountain Porphyry), the dominant host for the sulfides is paragenetically late magnetite (see Table 10.2; Fig. 10.5*C–G*) although some grains are found in plagioclase (see Table 10.2). They occur only rarely in all samples in the paragenetically later formed silicates, K-feldspar, quartz, and biotite, and most of these occurrences are in the more mafic samples (Table 10.2). The correlation between rock chemistry and age and the occurrence of inclusions is shown graphically in Figure 10.6*A*. The large scatter in Figure 10.6*A* for the Granite Mountain Porphyry is caused by its small number of sulfide grains compared to the other rock types (see Table 10.2), and no sulfide minerals were observed in the sample of Teapot Mountain Porphyry studied. Because of greater likelihood of xenoliths and the stronger alteration and fracturing compared to the stocks, no sulfide studies were attempted for the dike rocks.

Another parameter indicative of magmatic origin of the sulfide inclusions is their morphology. They are dominantly bleb shaped (see Table 10.2; Figs. 10.4*C, H–J;* 10.5*A–E, G;* 10.6*B*), but a considerable number are two phase, and most of those with planar boundaries have these boundaries parallel to the principal crystal forms of the host mineral. Most of the tabular grains, therefore, appear to occupy negative crystals of the host mineral; they do not display the crystal form characteristic of the sulfide mineral, although it was not possible in all cases to rule out the possibility that a subhedral grain was included in an oriented manner in the host mineral. These morphologies suggest that the sulfide grains were liquid when included and thus were formed at magmatic temperatures. Examples of probable negative crystals are seen in Figure 10.4*C, E–G, I;* and in Figure 10.5*A–B, D–G.* In Figure 10.4*C, E* the geometric shapes are attained at the edges of two-phase sulfide occurrences and clearly cannot represent the crystal forms of either sulfide; in addition, the sides of the forms are parallel to one, or to more than one, of the major crystallographic directions of the host pyroxenes. In Figure 10.4*I,* the sulfide outcrop has some linear sides, but the grain is two phase and, in overall form, bleb shaped (Fig. 10.4*H*). In Figure 10.5*E,* both tabular (larger grains) and blebby (smaller grains) forms are found in the same host mineral grain. In Figure 10.5*A–C, E–G,* one or more linear edges of the sulfide grains are parallel or sub-parallel to those of the host grain; in Figure 10.5*A–B, D, G,* it is only with coexisting silicate inclusions that blebby, one- or two-phase sulfide grains fill the tabular or regular void in the host mineral.

The magmatic sulfides are both small and modally insignificant components of the rocks; they average <5 ppm by volume (see Table 10.2). Thus, they provide little S and Cu to the whole rock. As shown in Figure 10.7, most of the grains are from 1 to 200 μm^2 (square micrometers) in area (average, 30 μm^2), but some are as large as 4,000 μm^2 (in the more mafic samples). The size distributions of the magmatic sulfides in the three main rock types studied are approximately the same (see Fig. 10.7); however, the distribution is very slighly skewed toward the finer grain sizes, particularly in the Granite Mountain Porphyry. More importantly, the modal abundance of the sulfide grains decreases with an increasing differentiation index (Fig. 10.8*A*) in the entire sample suite, in the Granite Mountain Porphyry and, more strongly, in the Rattler Granodiorite (which has, as noted earlier, a range in composition similar to the entire rock suite). There also is a marked decrease in average abundance of sulfide grains in the main stocks with decreasing age of the samples. These are additional responses of the

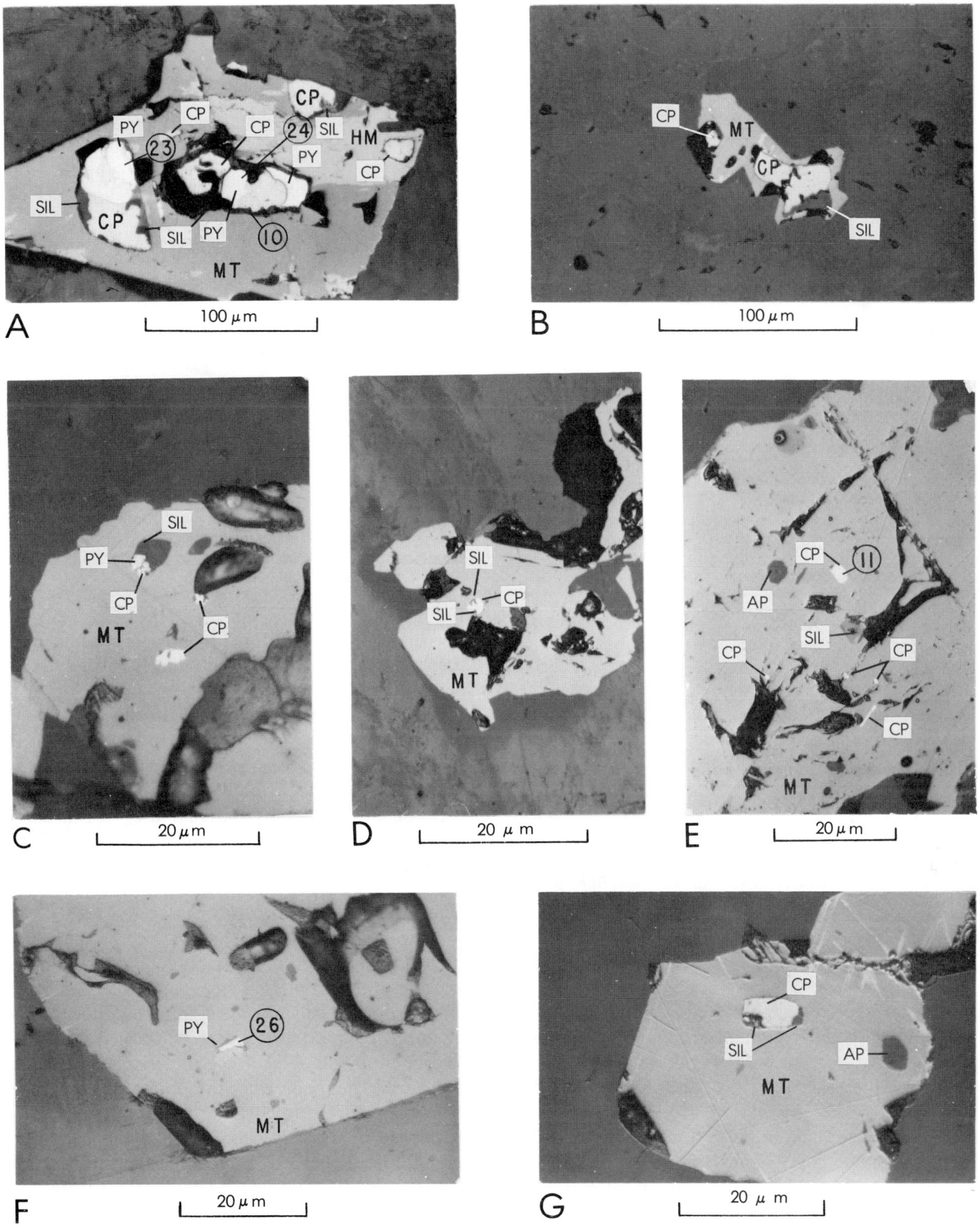

Figure 10.5 Textural relations of magmatic sulfide inclusions in magnetite in Laramide igneous rocks near Ray. *A,* sample 17–1, two-phase sulfide blebs included with silicate phases in magnetite, reflected light. Hematite, probably of post-magmatic origin, replaces part of the magnetite. Numbers refer to analyses in Table 10.3. *B,* sample 217–1, bleb- and geometric-shaped chalcopyrite grains co-existing with silicate as fillings of negative crystals in magnetite, reflected light. *C,* sample 60–113D, chalcopyrite blebs and three-phase chalcopyrite-pyrite-silicate inclusion in magnetite, reflected light. *D,* sample 246-11G, chalcopyrite bleb with silicate filling a negative crystal in magnetite, reflected light. *E,* sample 261–25, chalcopyrite blebs (smaller grains) and tabular forms (larger grains) in magnetite, reflected light. Number refers to analysis in Table 10.3. *F,* sample 60–131, pyrite either euhedral or filling negative crystal in magnetite, reflected light. Number refers to analysis in Table 10.3. *G,* sample 60–91, chalcopyrite bleb filling negative crystal with silicate in magnetite, reflected light. Key: AP = apatite; CP = chalcopyrite; HM = hematite; μm = micrometers; MT = magnetite; PY = pyrite; SIL = silicate.

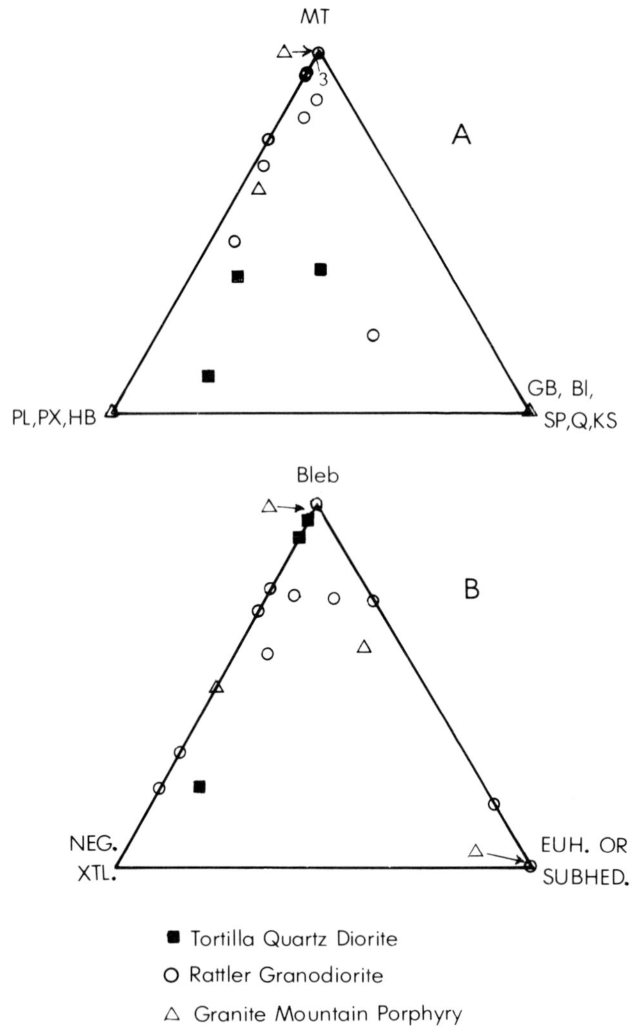

Figure 10.6. Host mineral occurrence (*A*) and crystal form (*B*) of magmatic sulfides in Laramide igneous rocks near Ray. Key: BI = biotite; GB = grain boundary; HB = hornblende; KS = K-feldspar; MT = magnetite; PL = plagioclase; PX = pyroxene; Q = quartz; SP = sphene; Neg. Xtl. = negative crystal; Euh. = euhedral; Subhed. = subhedral.

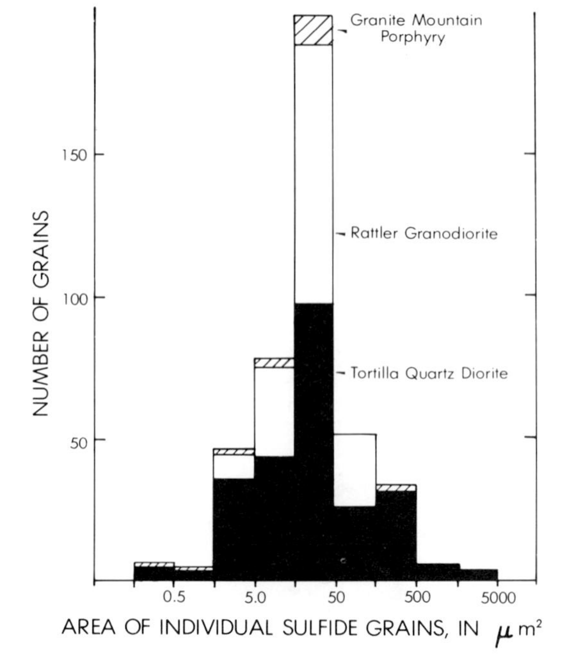

Figure 10.7. Size distribution of individual magmatic sulfide grains in Laramide rocks associated with the Ray porphyry copper deposit. Note that the abscissa is nonlinear.

magmatic sulfides to petrologic parameters of the host rock. However, although the largest grains are found in the most mafic samples, the average size of the grains does not correlate statistically with either the age or the chemistry of the sample.

Also apparent in the data gathered (see Table 10.2) is the overall decrease in the copper sulfide:pyrite ratio with an increasing differentiation index in the suite of samples as a whole, in the Granite Mountain Porphyry, and (excepting the mafic endmember) in the Rattler Granodiorite. This trend is also considered to be magmatic and is similar to that noted for the Skaergaard intrusion by Wager and others (1957) and Wager and Brown (1967).

In contrast to the several parameters that suggest magmatic affiliation of the sulfide inclusions, there is no correlation between their modal abundance and the degree of alteration of either biotite or plagioclase in the samples (Fig. 10.9); this fact indicates that the abundance of the sulfide inclusions was not detectably changed when the samples were partially altered. Further, there is a lack of corrosion of the sulfide grains in magnetite that is partially converted to hematite along fractures and at the grain margins (see Fig. 10.5*A–B*) and a lack of alteration of silicate grains enclosing most of the sulfide grains (see Fig. 10.4*B, D, F, G, H;* Table 10.2). These observations strengthen the premise that the sulfide grains are magmatic in origin (not deuteric, hydrothermal, or supergene) and that their form, amount, and distribution has been little changed since their crystallization from the magma that formed the samples studied.

Chemistry of the Sulfides

Twenty-four of the larger magmatic sulfide grains yielded analyses with acceptable totals. These are presented in Table 10.3 and plotted on Figure 10.10 along with values for appropriate stoichiometric minerals and two analyses of fracture-localized pyrite grains. The analyses shown in Table 10.3 confirm the optical determinations and semi-quantitative probe analyses that the microscopic-size magmatic sulfides are bornite (analysis 5), chalcopyrite (analyses 9–21), and pyrite (analyses 22–28). They also confirm that the dominant Cu-Fe-S phase is stoichiometric or near-stoichiometric chalcopyrite rather than the phases stable at lower temperatures (cubanite, talnakhite, mooihockite, and haycockite; Cabri, 1973). The small deviations from stoichiometry toward the Fe corner of Figure 10.10 of analyses 11–20 are satisfactorily explained by the small size of the grains and the resulting gain of iron intensity data from the host magnetite, and the relatively low total (see Table 10.3) and shift away from the Fe corner of Figure 10.10 for analysis 21 can be attributed to a corresponding loss in iron intensity data from the host plagioclase. The shift of analysis 5 away from stoichiometric bornite might also be attributed to a gain in copper intensity data from the co-existing digenite. However, it is possible

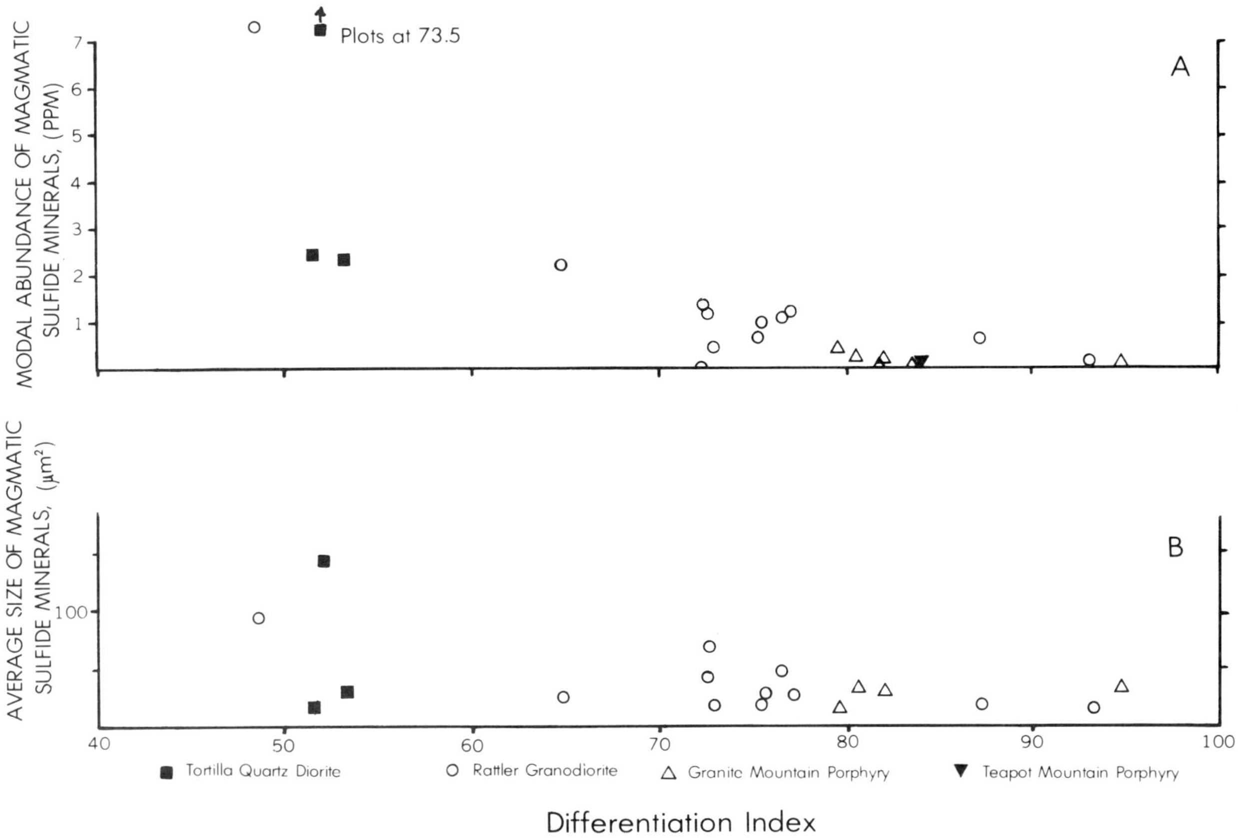

Figure 10.8. Variations of modal abundance (*A*) and average size (*B*) of magmatic sulfide grains with differentiation index of Laramide host rocks near Ray

that at least part of the iron shift of the chalcopyrite and copper shift of the bornite may be real and may indicate incomplete exsolution of the high-temperature phases.

The origin of the pale-blue isotropic digenite (analyses 6 to 8, Table 10.3; Fig. 10.10) is uncertain. The mineral occurs with several bornite grains in sample 248–29 and with one grain in sample 17–28 (see Table 10.2) and contains in addition to wisps of bornite, rare, very small, golden areas that may be chalcopyrite. Several grains also contain pleochroic vermicular (exsolution?) domains of anistropic (indigo blue) covellite. The digenite and covellite may represent exsolution products of the high-temperature bornite solid-solution phase or may be alteration products of bornite. If they are the latter, however, there is a problem in the lack of a source in the rocks for the additional copper.

Comparison of analyses 22 to 28 with 29 and 30 in Table 10.3 suggests that hydrothermal pyrite grains are not distinguishable from magmatic pyrite on the basis of copper content and major-element composition. A similar lack of distinction has been observed in major-element composition of hydrothermal chalcopyrite (not listed in Table 10.3 because of low totals) and of magmatic chalcopyrite occurring in the same sample. The possibility that Co, Ni, or other trace elements might distinguish the magmatic from secondary sulfides in the rocks has not been investigated.

Attempts to analyze by electron microprobe the largest silicate phases co-existing with the sulfide blebs in magnetite hosts resulted in highly variable and non-reproducible values and, for the most part, in low totals. The low totals are a result of the small size of the grains, and the variable results probably indicate the presence of multiple mineral species in the areas analyzed; for example, see 4 or more domains with different reflectivities in the silicate co-existing with the sulfide blebs in Fig. 10.5*A*.

Interpretation of the Origin of Magmatic Sulfides

Experimental data (Yund and Kullerud, 1966; Kullerud et al., 1969; Cabri, 1973) indicate that stoichiometric bornite, chalcopyrite, and particularly, pyrite are not stable at magmatic temperatures, in apparent conflict with the textural and modal data discussed above. Thus, composition of the grains observed must have resulted from their re-equilibration with the melt or host mineral. On the basis of chemistry, the blebby, two-phase bornite-digenite and chalcopyrite-bornite grains in the more mafic samples are compatible with the interpretation that they were trapped as liquid or liquid plus solid-solution phases (bornite solid solution and intermediate solid solution [Iss]) at magmatic temperatures of 800°C or more (Yund and Kullerud, 1966; Kullerud et al., 1969; MacLean, 1969; Cabri, 1973) and that they attained their present near-stoichiometric compositions by sub-solidus exsolution without chemical exchange with the magma or host mineral. Likewise, a few of the chalcopyrite grains might have resulted from cooling of magmatic Iss of fortuitous composition. However, there are too many chalcopyrite

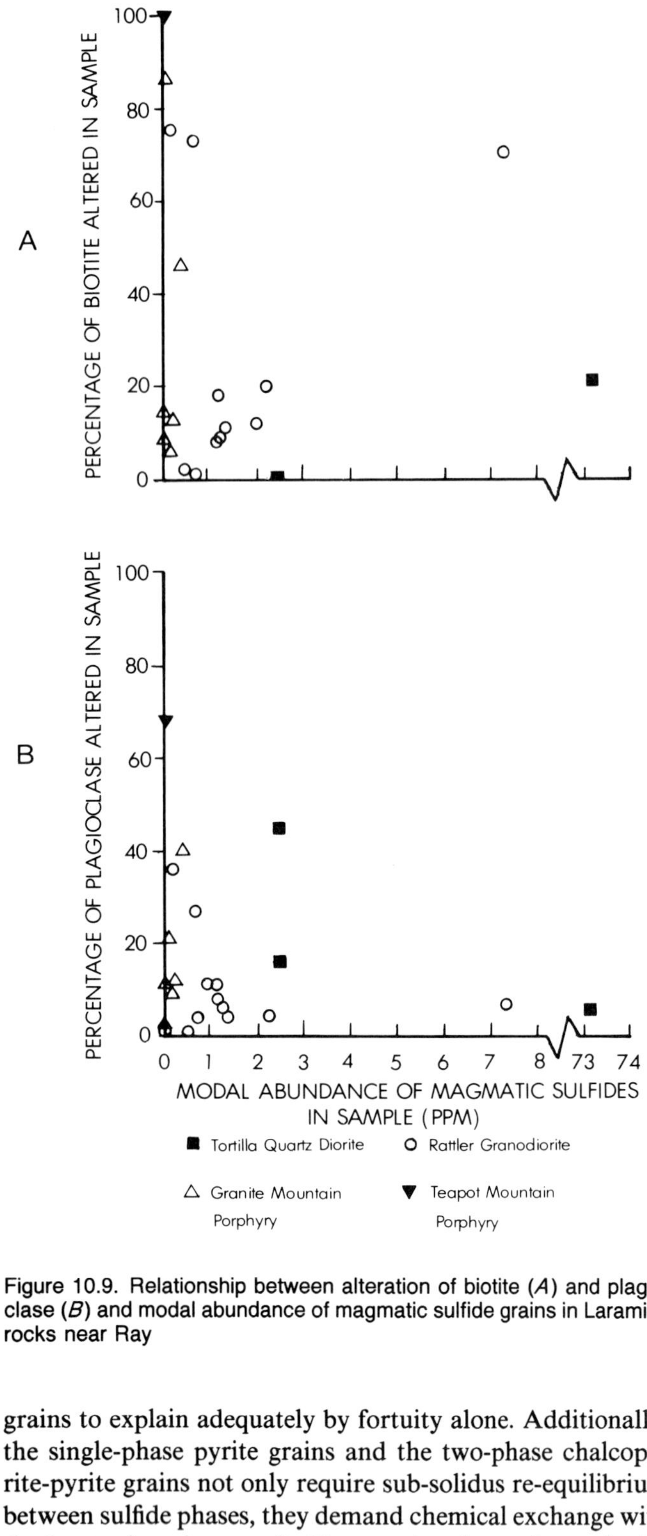

Figure 10.9. Relationship between alteration of biotite (*A*) and plagioclase (*B*) and modal abundance of magmatic sulfide grains in Laramide rocks near Ray

grains to explain adequately by fortuity alone. Additionally, the single-phase pyrite grains and the two-phase chalcopyrite-pyrite grains not only require sub-solidus re-equilibrium between sulfide phases, they demand chemical exchange with the host minerals or melt. Thus, estimations of meaningful temperatures of formation for the sulfides from experimental data seem precluded, even if the seemingly insurmountable problem of determining accurate modal ratios of two-phase blebs from two-dimensional outcrops of the sparse tiny grains could be resolved.

To elaborate, stoichiometric chalcopyrite and pyrite form respectively at 547°C and 742°C at 1 atmosphere (atm) (Kullerud and Yoder, 1959; Toulmin and Barton 1964; Yund and Kullerud, 1966), temperatures well below the solidus of the magmas, particularly the more mafic ones. Pressures up to a few kilobars raise these temperatures a few tens of degrees, but they remain well below the interpreted silicate solidus. Chalcopyrite and pyrite mixtures do not lie on tie lines of solid phases (Iss or Iss + pyrrhotite solid solution) that are stable and that coexist with sulfide liquids at magmatic temperatures (Kullerud and Yoder, 1959; Yund and Kullerud, 1966; Kullerud et al., 1969; Cabri, 1973). Therefore, the single-phase pyrite, the two-phase chalcopyrite-pyrite, and the majority of the single-phase chalcopyrite grains must have exchanged copper, sulfur, or iron with their hosts in order to explain the shift in composition toward the tie line between chalcopyrite and pyrite (the stable phases at sub-solidus temperatures of the magmas. This chemical exchange could have involved either diffusion of S from the host or magma into the sulfide liquid and solid sulfide phases, or the diffusion of Fe out of the sulfide grains, with or without diffusion of Cu into or out of the grains. The calculations described below suggest that the second of these processes is more likely.

The amount of each element diffused into and out of the co-existing magnetite, silicate, and sulfide grains depends on the size of each sulfide grain and on its original and present (equilibrated) composition. The case requiring the largest addition or subtraction of material is conversion of pyrrhotite solid solution to pyrite (conversion of Iss or Iss + pyrrhotite to chalcopyrite or chalcopyrite + pyrite requires less mass transfer). The pyrrhotite conversion requires that about 7 X 10^{-11} gm of S had to be added to the average high-temperature pyrrhotite grain (3 μm radius) to convert it to pyrite. If the host was magnetite, about 0.13 weight percent S had to be supplied to the sulfide grain from the magnetite in a spherical volume with a radius of 30 μm. If the host was a silicate or melt, a slightly larger radius would be required. If the radius of the contributing material was 40 μm, about 500 ppm had to be supplied by the host silicate, oxide, or melt. However, sulfur occurs below the 50 ppm detection level of the microprobe in magnetite, plagioclase, and pyroxene (whether or not they contain sulfide inclusions), and the required amount of S is probably much too high for silicate melts of the composition of the Ray magmas (Haughton et al., 1974). Additionally, introduction of post-magmatic, sulfur-bearing gas or water (at temperatures of about 550°C or less) does not offer a likely alternative for the apparent lack of adequate sulfur sources within the magma to convert the high-temperature sulfide phases to pyrite and chalcopyrite because: (1) the grains for the most part are well armored by large oxide or silicate grains; (2) the apparently total conversion of pyrrhotite to pyrite in all the samples seems unlikely by such a process, unless very large amounts of this fluid passed through each of the rocks studied in amounts are not very consistent with the degree of their alteration; and (3) the lower temperature forms of Cu-Fe sulfide described by Cabri (1973), expected to have formed by reaction of the sulfides with a cooling fluid phase, were not observed in the samples. Thus, either S diffused to the grains from the surrounding silicates, oxides, and magma, from distances of at least 100 μm away, depleting that volume by less than 40 ppm, or,

TABLE 10.3
Analyses of Sulfide Grains in Igneous Host Rocks Near Ray
(In Weight Percent)

	Text and figure reference number*														
Element	1	2	3	4	5	6	7	8	9	10	11	12	13	14	15
Cu	—	34.6	63.3	79.9	64.3	76.5	76.8	78.0	34.7	34.5	33.5	33.7	33.1	32.8	33.4
Fe	46.6	30.4	11.1	—	9.3	1.3	1.1	.8	30.2	30.0	32.3	31.9	31.6	32.1	32.0
S	53.4	35.0	25.6	20.1	25.2	22.2	22.1	20.4	35.0	34.8	34.5	34.8	35.0	35.0	34.4
Σ	100.0	100.0	100.0	100.0	98.8	100.0	100.0	99.2	99.9	99.3	100.3	100.4	99.7	99.9	99.8
Host†					HB	HB	HB	PL	INT	MT	MT	MT	MT	MT	MT
	Text and figure reference number*														
	16	17	18	19	20	21	22	23	24	25	26	27	28	29	30
Cu	32.7	32.3	32.7	32.4	32.9	34.0	.50	.29	.12	ND	.61	ND	.54	ND	ND
Fe	32.5	32.8	33.1	33.3	32.3	28.6	46.2	46.1	46.6	46.0	46.2	45.5	46.1	46.4	46.0
S	35.0	34.3	34.4	34.0	34.3	34.5	53.8	53.0	53.6	53.7	53.2	52.3	52.4	53.6	53.6
Σ	100.2	99.4	100.2	99.7	99.5	97.1	100.5	99.4	100.3	99.7	100.0	97.8	99.0	100.0	99.6
Host†	MT	MT	MT	MT	MT	PL	MT	MT	MT	QZ	MT	MT	MT	FRAC	FRAC

*1–4, stoichiometric mineral compositions; 5, magmatic bornite; 6–8, digenite occuring with magmatic bornite; 9–21, magmatic chalcopyrite; 22–28, magmatic pyrite; 29–30, fracture localized pyrite. Identification of analysis, sulfide minerals in parentheses in footnotes co-exist with the analyzed phase.

†*HB* = hornblende, *INT* = interstitial, *MT* = magnetite, *PL* = plagioclase, *QZ* = quartz, *FRAC* = fracture.

1. Stoichiometric pyrite
2. Stoichiometric chalcopyrite
3. Stoichiometric bornite
4. Stoichiometric chalcocite
5. 248–29 S1BN (digenite, covellite)
6. 248–29 S1D (bornite, covellite)
7. 248–29 S1D2 (bornite, covellite)
8. 48–29 S1D (bornite, covellite)
9. 217–1 S3CP (none, see Fig. 10.4J)
10. 17–1 S3CP (pyrite, see Fig. 10.5A)
11. 61–25 S3CP (none, see Fig. 10.5E)
12. 61–25 S3CP1 (none)
13. 60–98 S1CP (none)
14. 60–98 S2CP (none)
15. 246–11G S1CP1 (none)
16. 246–11G S2CP (none)
17. 60–111 S1CP (none)
18. 60–130 S3CP1 (none)
19. 260–96A S1CP (none)
20. 60–96A S5CP (none)
21. GM14–T3CP (none)
22. 217–1 S1PY (chalcopyrite)
23. 17–1 S3PY (chalcopyrite, see Fig. 10.5A)
24. 17–1 S3PY2 (chalcopyrite, see Fig. 10.5A)
25. 46–99B S1PY (none)
26. 60–131 S3PY (none, see Fig. 10.5F)
27. 60–131 S2PY1 (chalcopyrite)
28. 60–131 S2PY2 (chalcopyrite)
29. 246–11A S3PY2 (none)
30. GM1A S4PY2 (none)

more likely, Fe diffused out of the sulfide liquid + solid solution into and, perhaps, through the host minerals. Pyrite could have formed from pyrrhotite by diffusion of about 13 weight percent iron or about 17 weight percent iron oxides from a sulfide liquid + pyrrhotite solid-solution mixture. Iron oxide exsolves directly from the sulfide melt and precipated as magnetite (MacLean, 1969; Naldrett, 1969; Shimazaki and Clark, 1973) could account for some of the iron depletion; because of the small size of the sulfide grains, the small amount of iron exsolved from a solid high-temperature sulfide phase could have been incorporated without too much difficulty in pyroxene, magnetite, and even plagioclase hosts (Armbrusmacher and Banks, 1974) or combined with hematite exsolved from the same hosts to precipitate more magnetite on the walls of the enclosing crystal or as nearby individual magnetite crystals in a silicate host (for example, see Fig. 10.4*G*). The process would have been aided by, but does not require diffusion of, some S and perhaps Cu into the sulfide grains from adjacent or nearly melt, silicate, or oxide phases.

Magmatic Behavior of Sulfur Indicated by the Sulfide Minerals

The presence of the magmatic sulfides in the Laramide igneous rocks near Ray indicates that the melts were saturated at least locally with sulfide, and their morphology suggests that separation was largely as immiscible liquid. Beyond this, the data do not provide a unique interpretation of how the saturation and distribution of sulfide were obtained. However, local controls, attained on a scale comparable to the grain size of the rocks and dominated by enrichment of S and reduction of sulfide solubility in melt immediately adjacent to growing larger minerals, seem to fit the data better than controls operating throughout the magmas. Local saturation from an initially unsaturated state, rather than melt-wide saturation, is suggested by the occurrence of the sulfides in specific locations and only a very few of the many such locations available, rather than random occurrences in all mineral phases in the rocks. To review, the sulfide minerals are rare, and in the more mafic (older) samples, they occur for the most part in and around the cores of early-formed pyroxene, hornblende, hornblende after pyroxene, and plagioclase. They occur also in the more mafic samples as inclusions in magnetite and, compared to the younger rocks, more commonly near grain boundaries or between grains of the interstitial quartz and potassium feldspar. In the more felsic samples, the dominant host of the sulfides is late-formed magnetite.

To elaborate, the occurrence of the sulfides near the centers of early-formed plagioclase and pyroxene crystals is adequately explained as the result of local concentration and saturation of the sulfide in the melt owing to cooling of the

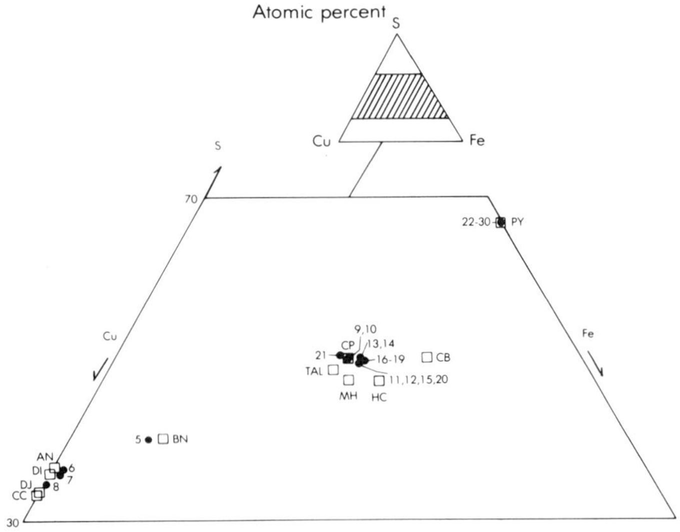

Figure 10.10. Mineral compositions in atomic percent of magmatic minerals in Laramide igneous rocks near Ray. Numbers refer to data in Table 10.3. Symbol size approximates 1 standard deviation in microprobe data. Key to stoichiometric minerals: AN = anilite; BN = bornite; CB = cubanite; CC = chalcocite; CP = chalcopyrite; DI = digenite; DJ = djurleite; HC = haycockite; MH = mooihoekite; PY = pyrite; TAL = talnakhite.

melt (Fincham and Richardson, 1954; MacLean, 1969; Shimazaki and Clark, 1973; Haughton et al., 1974), combined with local enrichment of sulfide components adjacent to the growing sulfur-poor host minerals. The relatively fewer occurrences of sulfide minerals in paragenetically later (Banks, 1976) biotite, quartz, and potassium feldspar and outer rims of hornblende, pyroxene, and plagioclase, can be attributed to fewer instances of saturation of sulfides. This reduction of saturation may be due in part to local enrichment of the melt in FeO (Haughton et al., 1974) during precipitation of plagioclase, but probably is due in larger part to removal of sulfur from the melt by the apatite, biotite, and hornblende (data presented in a later section). The few exceptions may be attributed to continued cooling of the magma and to an inadequate rate of diffusion of S to the nearest biotite, apatite, and hornblende grain to avert some instances of saturation. Likewise, the relatively abundant occurrence of sulfide inclusions in magnetite (which formed predominantly at above the same time as the hornblende, biotite, and apatite) can be attributed to inadequate diffusion rate and a strong local reduction of the sulfide-carrying capacity of the melt (Fincham and Richardson, 1954; MacLean, 1969; Page, 1971; Haughton and Roeder, 1971; Haughton and Skinner, 1972; Nagashima and Katsura, 1973; Katsura and Nagashima, 1974; Haughton et al., 1974) caused by depletion of iron in the melt adjacent to the growing magnetite. Presence of the interstitial sulfide grains in the more mafic samples can be explained by a sufficient initial sulfur content, continued decrease in magma temperature, and confirmed crystallization of the sulfur-poor quartz and potassium feldspar, possibly with proportionally lesser amounts of co-precipitated sulfur-bearing biotite and apatite.

The sulfide occurrences in the more felsic samples can be explained in the same manner as those in the more mafic samples, but several observations suggest that the younger, more felsic magmas contained less S than the older more mafic magmas. These are:

1. lesser abundance and more delayed crystallization history of the sulfides in the more felsic samples
2. the extreme rarity of interstitial sulfides in the more felsic samples
3. greater abundance of sulfur-poor silicates (plagioclase, K-feldspar, and quartz) in the felsic rocks, coupled with fewer sulfur-bearing major minerals (biotite, hornblende, and apatite); Banks, 1976
4. probable lower emplacement temperatures of the more differentiated magmas
5. experimental data of MacLean (1969), Haughton and Roeder (1971), Haughton and Skinner (1972), Shimazaki and Clark (1973), Haughton and others (1974), and Katsura and Nagashima (1974) on basaltic melts, suggesting that S should have been less soluble in the younger, more felsic melts than in the more mafic melts by virtue of their lower FeO, MgO, MnO, TiO^2, and CaO contents and higher silica content and
6. the much greater proportions of sulfide occurrences in magnetite in the more felsic samples.

In other words, the younger, more silicic magmas were more capable of achieving sulfide saturation at an earlier stage of crystallization or at a lower concentration of S than the more mafic magmas, yet they not only achieved saturation later and much less frequently, they required almost everywhere the local removal of FeO from the melt to induce saturation.

There are several explanations possible for the real decrease in modal abundance of the sulfide mineral occurrences (Fig. 10.8*A*) and the apparent decrease in S content of the melts with development of the Rattler Granodiorite, Granite Mountain Porphyry, and entire magmatic series. The simplest is that less S was incorporated or soluble in sequentially later partial melts at the source area and that, once they began forming, the hydrous minerals were efficient enough in removing sulfur from the melt to avert most instances of sulfide saturation. This interpretation explains the data adequately but precludes the stocks and any related upper crustal batholith as sources of the Cu and S in the deposit. A less likely explanation, because it implies extraordinary diffusion rates, is that, once formed, the sulfides themselves were extremely efficient in scavenging S from melt. Another unlikely alternative is that, rather than reflecting depletion of S in the melt, the decreased sulfide occurrences in the more felsic magma resulted from settling of sulfides from the magma in a presumed batholithic parent or by flow differentiation in the batholith or along conduits. What makes this alternative unlikely is (1) the removal of the sulfides by settling would be strongly hampered by their inclusion in the larger major and minor mineral phases of the magmas, and (2) their removal by flow differentiation should result in a skew to the larger grain sizes in the remaining sulfide grains (Newhouse, 1936; Komar, 1972*a*, 1971*b*; Barrie, 1976), rather than in the observed slight skew toward smaller grains (Fig. 10.7). However, neither alternative is compatible with an increase of sulfide content in the melt with development of the magmas, because, given the cooling and increased differentiation of the magma, a greater, rather than a more restricted, occurrence of sulfide inclusions would then be expected.

Another interpretation of the data postulates that a magmatic vapor phase was causitive in inducing or averting saturation of the melts with sulfides or in modifying their form and distribution afterwards. However, this interpretation finds no supporting evidence in the S contents of the other sulfur-bearing crystalline phases that formed at the same time as the sulfide grains (data later in this report), unless the S in the magmatic vapor involved an inconsequential amount of the S in the magma-vapor system. Furthermore, it does not seem possible, at present, to predict what effect the evolution of water would have on the formation of sulfides in the magmas. For examples, even a small amount of S removed with the vapor phase might tend to avert sulfide saturation, as would the exothermic crystallization of silicates induced by vapor withdrawal. On the other hand, evolution and expansion of the vapor phase would cool and oxidize the magma and induce sulfide precipitation. Which of these factors would prevail with respect to sulfide solubility in the magma depends on a great number of unknowns, such as: composition of gas phase and magma, depth at time of sulfide and vapor formation, vapor overpressure required to induce evolution of vapor, original and subsequent sulfur species in the magma and vapor, partitioning coefficients of sulfur species in the vapor and magma, temperature of the magma, chemical effect on the sulfide-carrying capacity of the magma caused by the induced precipitation of major silicate and oxide phases, and knowledge of what part of these phases formed prior to evolution of the vapor phase.

Thus, evolution of magmatic vapor is not necessary to explain the sulfide data, and there is no evidence for predicting that the sulfide petrology has been modified by exposure to magmatic water. Moreover, a large body of other physical and chemical data for the rocks (Banks, 1976) suggests that little if any vapor phase evolved from the stocks. Such data include the following:

1. The volume of pegmatite and aplite dikes is very low.
2. Thermal aureoles are restricted or absent even in impure carbonate hosts rocks.
3. Miarolitic features are lacking in the stocks.
4. Fluid inclusions are sparse, relatively dilute, and homogenize at temperatures below 450°C.
5. Ferromagnesian mineral grains, although zoned, do not show patterns of Mg enrichment at their rims.
6. The Fe/Mg ratios of the ferromagnesian minerals are higher rather than lower in the younger more felsic rocks than in the older more mafic rocks.
7. The bulk of the magnetite in the rocks formed paragenetically late, and the more felsic rocks contain less, rather than more, magnetite.
8. Adjacent biotite grains still maintain measurably different F contents and the F contents of the grains become higher, rather than lower, in progressively younger more differentiated samples.
9. Hydrous minerals formed paragenetically late in most of the rocks, particularly in the more felsic rocks.
10. Experimental data indicate that at the depths of emplacement, formation of the hydrous minerals would have tended to avert saturation of the magmas with water, and
11. Calculations and paragenetic relations of the hydrous minerals indicate that they were likely to have used most of the water present in the magmas.

There is one sample, 17–1 on Table 10.2, still requiring explanation. Sulfide grains in this sample are twice as abundant (10 times in modal abundance) as in each of the other samples, and their average size is two or more times that of each of the others. Another difference in this sample, compared to others from the same rock type, is the replacement of pyroxene by a fibrous magnesian amphibole and fine-grained magnetite rather than hornblende. In bulk chemistry, grain size, and texture, however, sample 17–1 is very similar to samples from the other stocks of Tortilla Quartz Diorite. Furthermore, each of the seven or more intrusive bodies of Tortilla Quartz Diorite in the area, although containing about the same amount of plagioclase, potassium feldspar, quartz, and mafic minerals, contains very different proportions of the three mafic minerals, pyroxene, hornblende, and biotite. The variations in mafic mineral ratios in the different stocks of Tortilla Quartz Diorite have been explained by slightly different water contents or conditions of crystallization (Banks, 1976). Because the sulfide content of sample 17–1 is so small (only 40 ppm more Cu and 30 ppm more S, compared to the other samples) and the magmas appear to be undersaturated, except locally, with sulfide and thus capable of assimilating more sulfide, a similar hyphothesis can be applied here. Better access to Cu, S, and H_2O could be obtained at the point of origin by longer residence time in a zone of partial melting or by slightly different starting materials. At the site of emplacement, better access to Cu and S could be obtained by access to meteoric or hydrothermal fluids or by incorporation of sulfide-rich xenoliths.

SULFUR AND COPPER CONTENT OF THE IGNEOUS MINERALS

The sulfide petrology indicates that the Laramide magmas at Ray were saturated only locally and rarely with sulfides and strongly suggests that the more felsic rocks were progressively less able to precipitate sulfides; however, there remains the possibility that appreciable amounts of S and Cu were in the magmas but were stored or complexed in the melt and other crystalline phases. This possibility was investigated mainly by use of the electron microprobe, because the areas of microprobe analysis are essentially pinpoint-size and can be selected optically at will; such characteristics allow non-magmatic effects on the igneous minerals to be minimized, as well as identified and investigated. Analyses of mineral separates and whole-rock samples were also made (see Appendix II for the description of analytical methods used in this section), but they serve mainly as checks on the microprobe study, because of the probable presence of non-magmatic sulfide minerals on undetected hairline fractures and the slight but ubiquitous alteration of some of the igneous minerals (since incipient propyllitic alteration of biotite can cause loss of S and gain of Cu in igneous rocks and their mineral separates (Banks, 1973, 1974*b*). The disadvantage of the electron microprobe is its relatively high detection level for S (50 ppm) and Cu (90–100 ppm). This disadvantage was somewhat minimized by a sparse but representative set of mineral analyses with an ion microprobe, which has a detection level of about 1 ppm for Cu under ideal conditions, and by analyses of mineral separates (also with 1 ppm detection levels), which indicate the maximum amount of Cu in the minerals. Likewise, the whole-rock S and Cu analyses of the freshest samples were useful, when compared with calculated whole-rock values, in determining whether or not most of the S and Cu in the rocks could be accounted for by the amounts detected by microprobe analysis.

Sulfur occurs at 50 to 1,000 ppm levels in the hydrous igneous minerals in the Laramide plutons but was not detected in the other major, minor, and trace igneous minerals analyzed in the samples. All the biotite, apatite, and some of the hornblende and igneous(?) epidote contain S at or considerably above the dectection level (50 ppm). Sulfur is more abundant in apatite than in biotite, which, in turn, contains more S than either hornblende or epidote. Copper was detected by electron microprobe in about 15 percent of the biotite grains analyzed but was not observed at a detection level of 100 ppm in any other major or minor non-sulfide igneous minerals. Almost every occurrence of detectable Cu in the biotite can be attributed to alteration products of biotite (Banks, 1974*B*), and, excepting magnetite and biotite, nil or very low ppm amounts of Cu were detected by ion microprobe and emission spectrochemical analysis of the major and minor non-sulfide igneous minerals. The abundances of S and Cu found agree well with the range of values in the literature for rocks and minerals occurring with other deposits and in ore-barren provinces (Banks and Page, 1980). These results and comparisons are summarized below.

Biotite

Sulfur occurs at an average abundance of 200 ppm in all grains of igneous biotite analyzed in the Laramide rocks at Ray (Table 10.4; see also Banks, 1973, 1974*b*). Sulfur analyses of biotite are rare in the literature, but those found indicate similar values for biotites occurring near other porphyry deposits (Banks, 1973) and in plutons not associated with ore provinces (200–300 ppm; Foster, 1960).

Copper was detected in 17 of 123 electron microprobe analyses of igneous biotite in the Ray rocks (Table 10.4; see also Banks, 1974*b*), and the values indicate a very erratic distribution of Cu. The spectrochemical and ion probe data (Table 10.5) for Cu in biotite are as erratic as the data from the electron microprobe. Copper was detected in 73 percent of the biotite areas or separates analyzed by these more sensitive means; it averaged less than 58 ppm (calculated assuming the maximum allowable level for D and ND analyses in Table 10.5), and ranged from more than 280 ppm to less than 3 ppm.

Almost every occurrence of Cu in biotite (see Tables 10.4, 10.5) can be attributed to (although not proven to be) Cu in vermiculite(?) and chlorite alteration products of the biotite; the occurrence may result either directly, by excitation of the Cu in an alteration mineral near or below the analyzed spot, or indirectly by Cu smeared from the alteration mineral onto the surface of the biotite (Banks, 1974*b*).

TABLE 10.4
Sulfur and Copper Content of Igneous Biotite From Intrusive Rocks Near Ray
(By Electron Microprobe)

Rock Type	Probe Sample	Analysis Number[1]	Contents (ppm) [2]S	[2]Cu
Tortilla Quartz Diorite	217–28	2BIC	200 ± 10	ND
		2BIE	200 ± 20	ND
		4BIC	240 ± 20	ND
		4BIE	220 ± 10	ND
	217–1	5BIC	190 ± 20	ND
		5BIE	170 ± 30	ND
		6BIC	150 ± 30	ND
		6BIE	180 ± 20	ND
Rattler Granodiorite	60–91	1BIC	370 ± 20	ND
		1BIE	150 ± 10	ND
		4BIC	190 ± 10	ND
		4BIE	150 ± 10	ND
	60–111	2BIC	210 ± 10	ND
		2BIE	190 ± 10	ND
		2BI2C	210 ± 10	ND
		2BI2E	220 ± 10	ND
	60–98	1BIC	180 ± 10	ND
		1BIE	90 ± 10	ND
		3BIC	100 ± 10	ND
		3BIE	150 ± 40	ND
	60–131	1BIC	190 ± 20	ND
		1BIE	130 ± 10	ND
		2BIC	110 ± 10	ND
		2BIE	130 ± 10	ND
		3BIC	210 ± 10	ND
		3BIE	130 ± 10	ND
	60–130	2BIC	180 ± 10	ND
		2BIE	190 ± 10	ND
		4BIC	220 ± 20	ND
		4BIE	140 ± 20	ND
		M2BIC	420 ± 20	ND
	246–11A	MBIC	170 ± 20	580 ± 40
		MBIE	160 ± 10	690 ± 500
		M1BIC	140 ± 10	ND
		M1BIE	190 ± 50	ND
Granite Mountain Porphyry	RB5	6BIC	220 ± 10	ND
		6BIE	250 ± 10	ND
		7BIC	200 ± 10	ND
		7BIE	180 ± 30	ND
	GM18	MBIC	170 ± 10	ND
		MBIE	210 ± 10	ND
		M1BIC	120 ± 10	ND
		M1BIE	80 ± 10	ND
		M2BIC	380 ± 10	ND
	GM2A	1BIC	130 ± 10	ND
		1BIE	130 ± 20	ND
Rhyodacite Dike	61–2F	1BI	230 ± 20	ND
		9BI	180 ± 10	ND
		MBI	290 ± 20	ND

NOTE: Additional published analyses used in the construction of figures are found in Banks (1973, 1974*b*).

[1] Analysis numbers ending in *C* or *E* indicate data points located at grain center or edge, respectively.

[2] Microprobe analyses; background counts taken above and below peaks for each analysis. Precision calculated from standard counting error of the mean of 4 to 6 data points. *ND*, not detected at 50 ppm S or 100 ppm Cu.

Rehrig and McKinney (1976) also report Cu-rich vermiculite associated with biotite, and Dodge (1973) likewise notes that chlorite separates contain excess Cu over separates of their biotite precursors. The vermiculite(?) contains as much as

TABLE 10.5
Copper Content of Minerals From Laramide Igneous Rocks Near Ray
(By Spectrochemistry and Ion Microprobe Analysis)

Rock Type	Sample Number	Analysis or Separate Number	Mineral	Content of Cu (ppm): Emission Spectrochemistry[1]	Ion Microprobe[2]
Tortilla Quartz Diorite	217–28	4MT	Magnetite		[3]D20
		4HB	Hornblende		[4]ND9
		4PX	Pyroxene		ND6
		4BI	Biotite		ND3
Rattler Granodiorite	246–99B	1MT	Magnetite		D6
		3HB	Hornblende		ND3
		1PX	Pyroxene		D6
		3BI	Biotite		[5]280 ± 12
	61–25	PL	Plagioclase	ND2	
		PL2	Plagioclase	6	
		HB	Hornblende	13	
		BI1	Biotite	40	
		BI2	Biotite	50	
		KS	K-feldspar	5	
	246–11G	4MT	Magnetite		D1
		3HB	Hornblende		13 ± 3
		3BIC	Biotite		ND6
	260–96A	5BIC	Biotite		ND8
	246–11A	6MT	Magnetite		34 ± 13
		1BIC	Biotite		59 ± 14
		2BI	Biotite		[6]163
		6BID1	Biotite		40 ± 8
		6BID2	Biotite		44 ± 16
		6BID3	Biotite		47 ± 12
		1CLA	Chlorite		[5]950 ± 4
Granite Mountain Porphyry	RB5	MMT	Magnetite		41 ± 1
		BIE1	Biotite		23 ± 16
		7BIC	Biotite		34 ± 30
		BI	Biotite	50	
		PL	Plagioclase	ND2	
		KS	K-feldspar	8	
		QZ	Quartz	ND2	
	GM18	M2MT	Magnetite		3 ± 2
		T1HBC	Hornblende		ND9
		MBIC	Biotite		ND18
		MPG	Plagioclase		ND3
		MKS	K-feldspar		ND1
		MQZ	Quartz		ND1

[1] Analysis of mineral separate. Analyst R. E. Mays, values accurate to ±15 percent of amount present.
[2] Analysis of mineral grain. Analyst J. R. Hinthorne, Applied Research Laboratories. Error bar is 1σ of counting statistics. Values considered accurate to ±10 percent of amount present (J. R. Hinthorne, 1977, oral communication).
[3] D20, detected at or below level indicated.
[4] ND9, not detected at level indicated.
[5] Minimum value, probe beam larger than grain analyzed.
[6] One determination, no statistics.

105,000 ppm Cu and the chlorite contains as much as several thousand ppm Cu (Banks, 1974*b*); thus, Cu in alteration products of biotite can explain not only the bulk of Cu in whole-rock analyses of biotite-bearing rocks, but also the universally erratic distribution of Cu in separates of biotite from both ore-related and ore-barren plutons (Parry and Nockowski, 1963; Putman and Burnham, 1963; Dodge and Moore, 1968; Dodge et al., 1969; Lovering, 1969; Putman and Alfors, 1969; Al-Hashimi and Brownlow, 1970; Lovering et al., 1970; Dodge and Ross, 1971; Lovering, 1972; Graybeal, 1973; Kesler et al., 1975).

Apatite

Sulfur occurs in the igneous apatite grains analyzed (Table 10.6) at an average concentration of 640 ppm, and the occurrence of S is not surprising because sulfate apatites have been successfully synthesized (Kreidler and Hammel, 1970). The amount found in the Ray apatites is similar to that found in igneous apatite in the Iron Hill Complex and in the Shonkin Sag laccolith, two igneous suites unassociated with porphyry deposits (200–1,200 ppm; Nash, 1972*a*, 1972*b*).

Copper was not detected (<100 ppm) in the apatites studied by electron microprobe (Table 10.6), and the apatites were not analyzed by ion probe or spectrochemistry because apatite would account for less than 1 ppm of Cu in the rock even if present at 100-ppm levels in the mineral. However, search of the literature suggests low copper content for apatite. Lee and others (1973) have reported Cu at 2–12 ppm in separates of igneous apatite from rocks in the Snake Range in Nevada, and Nockolds and Mitchell (1946) have reported

TABLE 10.6
Sulfur and Copper Content of Igneous Apatite From Laramide Intrusive Rocks Near Ray

(By Electron Microprobe)

Rock Type	Probe Sample	Analysis Number[1]	Grain Occurrence[2]	Contents (ppm) [3]S	[3]Cu
Tortilla Quartz Diorite	217–28	1A	H	620 ± 80	ND
		5A	P	470 ± 60	ND
		5AA	P	400 ± 100	ND
	217–1	1A	P	240 ± 140	ND
		5A[4]	P	240 ± 70	ND
		7A	M	270 ± 30	ND
	248–29	1A	P	790 ± 120	ND
		2A	P	1130 ± 290	ND
		3A	P	740 ± 60	ND
Rattler Granodiorite	246–99B	1A	H	1420 ± 210	ND
		2A	I	450 ± 260	ND
		3A	H	1950 ± 50	ND
	60–113D	T21A[5]	P	610 ± 270	ND
		T22AC	P	1100 ± 230	ND
		T22AE	P	450 ± 30	ND
	60–108	1AC	P	500 ± 110	ND
		1AE	P	650 ± 100	ND
		3A[6]	P	840 ± 340	ND
		6AC	P	440 ± 80	ND
		6AE	P	570 ± 60	ND
	61–25	T14A	P	530 ± 30	ND
		T15A	GM	590 ± 130	ND
	60–91	1A	P	530 ± 70	ND
		2A	B	450 ± 70	ND
		6A[6]	P	620 ± 60	ND
	60–111	1AC	P	560 ± 60	ND
		1AE	P	1530 ± 120	ND
		2A[4]	P	650 ± 50	ND
	60–98	1A	M	800 ± 30	ND
		3A	B	520 ± 40	ND
		6AC	P	970 ± 30	ND
		6AE	P	560 ± 50	ND
	246–11G	6A	P	440 ± 60	ND
		6AA	P	420 ± 70	ND
		7A	B	620 ± 60	ND
	60–131	MAC	PL	510 ± 30	ND
		MAE	PL	580 ± 40	ND
		M1AC	P	530 ± 80	ND
		M1AM	P	460 ± 20	ND
		M1AE	P	520 ± 20	ND
		M2A[4]	GM	1750 ± 470	ND
	60–130	2AC	PL	1860 ± 40	ND
		2AE	PL	1070 ± 40	ND
		3A[4]	B	1110 ± 580	ND
		M2AC	I	650 ± 60	ND
		M2AE	I	740 ± 60	ND
Rattler Granodiorite (*cont'd.*)	260–96A	2A[4]	B	520 ± 40	ND
		3A[6]	B	600 ± 60	ND
		3AA[6]	B	570 ± 40	ND
	246–11A	1A	P	640 ± 130	ND
		3A[5]	B	740 ± 200	ND
		4A	P	350 ± 30	ND
Rhyodacite Dike	17–16	1AC	P	200 ± 10	ND
		1AE	P	150 ± 20	ND
		M1AC	P	330 ± 30	ND
		M1AE	P	630 ± 50	ND
		M2A	P	1530 ± 60	ND
	GM100	3AC	P	440 ± 30	ND
		3AE	P	130 ± 20	ND
		M5AC	P	170 ± 30	ND
		M5AE	P	140 ± 30	ND
		XA	P	450 ± 50	ND
Granite Mountain Porphyry	RB5	2AC	B	440 ± 130	ND
		2AM	B	460 ± 150	ND
		2AE	B	670 ± 90	ND
		3A	B	580 ± 90	ND
		3AA	B	440 ± 190	ND
	GM14	T33AA[4]	B	520 ± 70	ND
		T33BA[6]	B	630 ± 190	ND
	GM12	2AC	B	530 ± 50	ND
		2AE	B	660 ± 30	ND
		3A[6]	B	400 ± 40	ND
		4A	B	1110 ± 240	ND
	GM18	7AC	P	700 ± 30	ND
		7AE	P	570 ± 120	ND
		8A[5]	P	440 ± 60	ND
	2GM6G	1MA[6]	P	790 ± 290	ND
		2MA[6]	B	640 ± 60	ND
		5AC	P	610 ± 40	ND
	2GM1A	1A	P	570 ± 90	ND
		1AA	P	480 ± 110	ND
		2A	P	510 ± 140	ND
	2GM2A	5A	PL	870 ± 70	ND
		5AA	PL	820 ± 80	ND
Teapot Mountain Porphyry	2TTM	1A[7]	B	1730 ± 90	ND
		2A	GM	490 ± 50	ND
		5A[4]	B	530 ± 350	ND
		5AA	GM	570 ± 80	ND
Rhyodacite Dike	61–2F	T10A[5]	P	440 ± 130	ND
		T18A[7]	GM	350 ± 70	ND
		MAC	P	450 ± 20	ND
		MAE	P	460 ± 20	ND

[1] Analysis numbers ending in *A* indicate 3 to 12 data points distributed randomly over grain; analysis numbers ending in *C, E,* or *M* indicate 3 to 5 data points at grain center, edge, or median point between grain center and edge; footnoted analysis numbers indicate data points gathered along traverses described in footnote.

[2] Grain occurrence: *P* = phenocryst or large grain, *H* = inclusion in hornblende, *B* = inclusion in biotite, *M* = inclusion in magnetite, *PL* = inclusion in plagioclase, *I* = interstitial; and *GM* = groundmass.

[3] Microprobe analysis. Precision calculated from standard counting error of the mean of data points described in footnotes 1 and 4 to 7. *ND* = not detected at 50 ppm S or 100 ppm Cu.

[4] Four to six data points on traverse from center to edge of grain along *a* axis.

[5] Four to twelve data points on traverse from edge to edge of grain along *a* axis.

[6] Four to eleven data points on traverse from center to edge of grain along *c* axis.

[7] Four to nine data points on traverse from edge to edge of grain along *c* axis.

the copper content of separates of igneous apatite from Caledonian rocks to be 10 ppm or less; but these values must be considered maximum because of the possibility of contamination of the separates or inclusions of sulfide grains.

Hornblende, Sphene, and Epidote

Sulfur occurs at or above detection level in about 30 percent of the igneous hornblende analyzed in the Ray rocks (Table 10.7), and most of the other hornblende grains give counts at the S wavelength that suggest that S occurs in them in amounts just below detection at the 3 σ level (50 ppm). Sulfur was not detected in 15 analyses of igneous sphene, but it was detected at 70–100 ppm levels in 3 of 5 analyses of interstitial igneous(?) epidote (Table 10.7). Analyses of S in these minerals were not found in the literature.

As was the case with apatite, Cu was not detected in the hornblende, sphene, or epidote by electron microprobe analysis (see Table 10.7), and analyses by ion microprobe and emission spectroscopy indicate nil or very low ppm Cu content for the igneous hornblende in the Ray plutons (see Table 10.5). Analyses of hornblende separates from rocks not associated with ore deposits also indicate low ppm content of Cu (Nockholds and Mitchell, 1946; Dodge et al., 1968; Putman and Alfors, 1969; Dodge and Ross, 1971). Those separated from rocks near other porphyry deposits indicate very low to high (as much as 700 ppm) and erratic Cu content (Graybeal, 1973) which may be attributed to chlorite and vermiculite that remained in the mineral separates. Sphene and igneous epidote can account for less than 1 ppm of Cu in the whole rock and were not analyzed by more sensitive methods. Sphene separates are rarely analyzed for Cu but those reported in the literature usually have nil or low ppm Cu content (Nockholds and Mitchell, 1946).

Magnetite, Pyroxene, Feldspars, Quartz, and Zircon

Neither S nor Cu was detected by electron microprobe analyses of 10 or more grains each of the rest of the major and accessory minerals in the Laramide plutons (magnetite,

TABLE 10.7
Sulfur and Copper Content of Igneous Hornblende, Sphene, and Epidote From Laramide Intrusive Rocks Near Ray
(By Electron Microprobe)

Rock Type	Probe Sample	Analysis Number[1]	Contents (ppm)	
			[2]S	[2]Cu
Tortilla Quartz Diorite	217–28	4HC	ND	ND
		4HE	ND	ND
		5HC	ND	ND
		5HE	ND	ND
	17–1	[3]T18FH1	ND	ND
		[3]T18FH2	ND	ND
	217–1	6PSC	ND	ND
		6PSE	ND	ND
		6PEPC	ND	ND
		6PEPE	ND	ND
	248–29	1HC	60 ± 10	ND
		2HC	50 ± 20	ND
		2HE	60 ± 10	ND
		1PEP	80 ± 20	ND
Rattler Granodiorite	246–99B	3HC	70 ± 20	ND
		3HE	50 ± 20	ND
		4HC	ND	ND
		4HE	ND	ND
		MPS	ND	ND
		4PS	ND	ND
		MPEP	100 ± 30	ND
	60–108	1H	60 ± 10	ND
		4HC	ND	ND
		4HE	ND	ND
		6HC	ND	ND
		6HE	ND	ND
		1PS	ND	ND
	261–25	MHC	ND	ND
		MHE	ND	ND
		M1HC	60 ± 10	ND
		M1HE	70 ± 10	ND
	60–91	4HC	ND	ND
		4HE	ND	ND
		M2HC	ND	ND
		M2HE	ND	ND
	60–98	NHC	ND	ND
		MHE	ND	ND
		M1HC	ND	ND
	246–11G	3HC	ND	ND
Rattler Granodiorite *(cont'd)*		3HE	ND	ND
		4HC	ND	ND
		4HE	ND	ND
		MH	ND	ND
		MPS	ND	ND
Rhyodacite Dike	17–16	2HC	ND	ND
		2HE	ND	ND
		MHC	ND	ND
		MHE	ND	ND
		M1HC	ND	ND
		M1HE	ND	ND
Rhyodacite Dike	GM100	HMIC	ND	ND
		HMIE	50 ± 10	ND
		M3HC	ND	ND
		M3HE	ND	ND
		M4HC	ND	ND
		M4HE	ND	ND
Granite Mountain Porphyry	RB5	5PSC	ND	ND
	2GM14	4PS	ND	ND
	GM14	T1PS	ND	ND
		T4PEP	70 ± 10	ND
	GM12	M1PSC	ND	ND
		M2PSE	ND	ND
	GM18	T1HC	50 ± 10	ND
		T1HE	70 ± 20	ND
		9PSC	ND	ND
		10 PSC	ND	ND
	2GM6G	M3PSC	ND	ND
		M3PSE	ND	ND

NOTE: Additional published analyses in Banks (1973).

[1] The letters *H, PS,* and *PEP* in the analysis numbers identify the analyses as hornblende, sphene, and epidote, respectively. Analysis numbers ending in *C* or *E* indicate data points located at grain center or edge, respectively.

[2] Microprobe analysis; background counts taken above and below peaks for each analysis; peak confirmed by stepping over peak wavelength. Precision calculated from standard counting error of the mean of 4 to 6 data points. *ND*, not detected at 50 ppm S or 100 ppm Cu.

[3] Fibrous magnesian amphibole of deuteric or hydrothermal origin.

pyroxene, plagioclase, K-feldspar, quartz, and zircon.) Copper was detected by ion probe in all magnetite grains analyzed, averaging less than 10 ppm and ranging from 41 ppm to less than 1 ppm; except for the alteration products of biotite magnetite, and the magmatic sulfide minerals, all other mineral grains and separates analyzed by more sensitive means than the electron microprobe contain low or nil ppm amounts of Cu (Table 10.5). Copper was detected at less than 6 ppm in one of the two pyroxenes analyzed and occurs in plagioclase at an average of less than 3 ppm. It was not detected in plagioclase by ion probe analyses. Copper abundance is slightly higher in the mineral separates of K-feldspar than in those of placioclase, but Cu was not detected in the feldspars by the ion microprobe (<1 ppm). Copper was not detected in the quartz mineral separate or in the grain analyzed by ion microprobe. Nil or low ppm content of Cu for magnetite, pyroxene, feldspars, and quartz are common in the literature (Nockolds and Mitchell, 1946; Putman and Alfors, 1969). Cu values for zircon were not found in the literature, and because only trace amounts of Cu could be contributed to the samples by zircon and rarer accessory minerals, these minerals were not analyzed here by the more sensitive but time-consuming and expensive methods. Analyses of S in igneous magnetite, pyroxene, plagioclase, K-feldspar, quartz, and zircon are almost nonexistent in the literature.

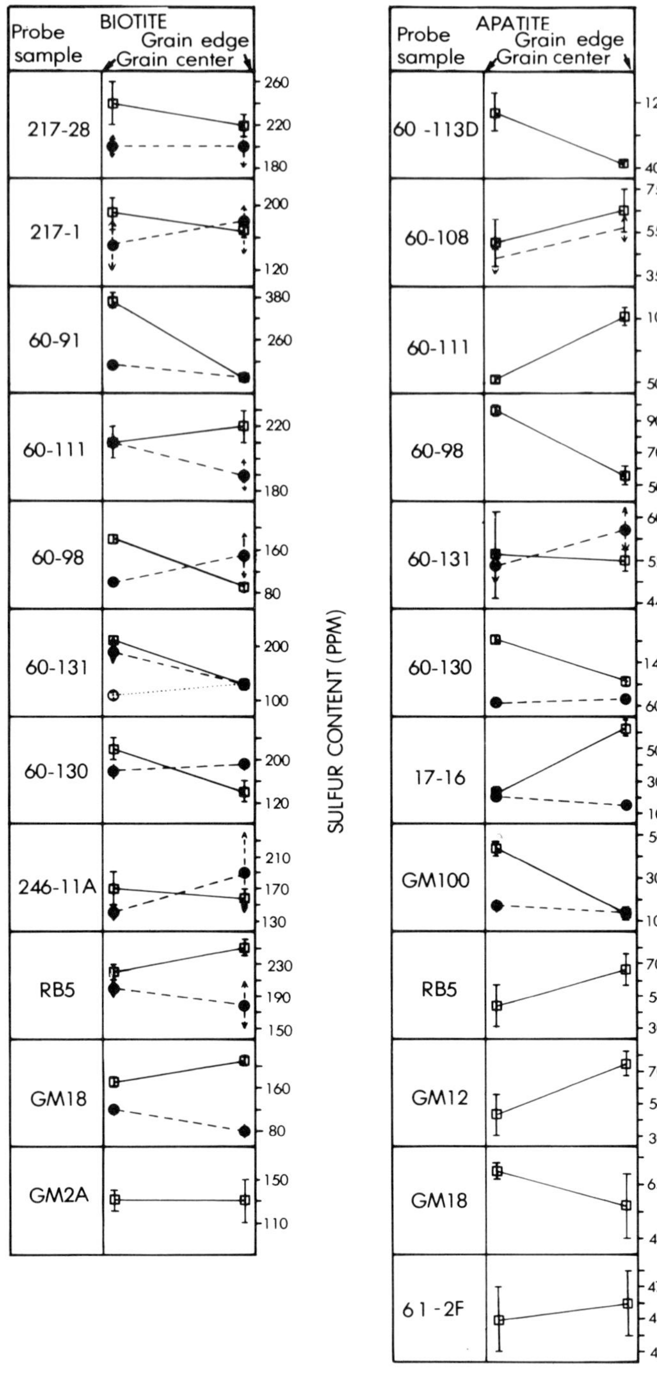

Figure 10.11. Zoning of sulfur in igneous biotite and apatite as indicated by analyses of grain centers and edges. Symbol or bar indicates limits of counting error plus sample inhomogeneity at the area of analysis.

VARIATIONS IN SULFUR AND COPPER ABUNDANCE

Analyses have shown that S and Cu are not abundant in the non-sulfide igneous minerals comprising the plutons associated with Ray, and the data are similar to those from other igneous suites, both associated with and barren of porphyry-type mineralization. Sulfur occurs ubiquitously at ppm levels in the hydrous igneous minerals but was not detected in other minerals. Likewise, Cu occurs at low ppm levels in magnetite and in erratic (but still ppm) amounts in some biotite grains, but was essentially absent in all other minerals. The ubiquitous occurrence of sulfur in the hydrous minerals suggests that it occurs in the structure of the minerals, but most of the Cu detected can be attributed to contamination of grain surfaces and mineral separates by Cu present in post-magmatic alteration products and to undetected sub-micron sulfide blebs in the minerals. Several petrologic parameters can be used to compare the S and Cu content of the minerals at Ray in order to further define the petrology of the S and Cu.

Intrasample Variations and Zoning of Sulfur

Several observations indicate that the igneous minerals studied have not been homogenized with respect to S (or other constituents [Banks, 1976]) by exchange with magma, magmatic fluid, or post-magmatic fluid. Measurably different abundances of S occur between similar mineral grains in the same sample, between different areas in the same grain, and between like mineral grains in the same rock type or stock (see Tables 10.4, 10.6, 10.7). Additionally, analytically distinguishable zoning of S occurs in 36 percent of the biotite grains studied for zoning (Table 10.4, Fig. 10.11) and in 53 percent of the apatite grains studied for zoning (Table 10.6, Figs. 10.11, 10.12). However, there is not a pattern of zoning within like mineral grains (Figs. 10.11, 10.12) or between different minerals in the same sample. Zoning was not detected in the few grains of hornblende and epidote with detectable S that were studied for zoning, but measurably different amounts of S occur between like mineral grains in the same sample or rock type (see Table 10.7).

The abundance of S in the igneous minerals does not appear related to the amount of alteration in the sample (Fig. 10.13), to proximity of a visibly unaltered analyzed spot to an area of alteration in the slide, or to potential susceptibility of the area analyzed to gain or loss of S by virtue of proximity

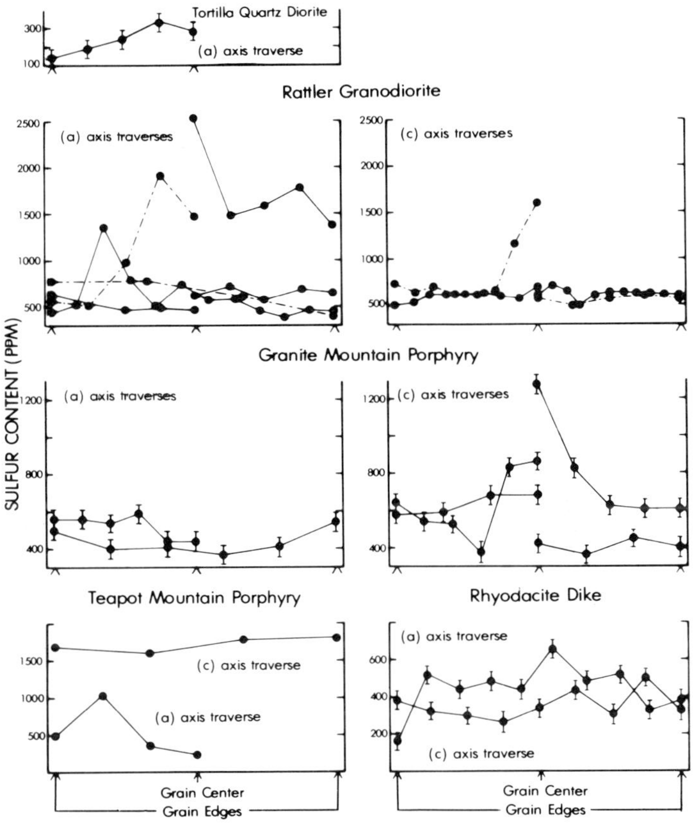

Figure 10.12. Zoning of sulfur in igneous apatite as indicated by traverses across grains. Symbol or bar indicates estimated limit of error of the data point; (*a*) and (*c*) refer to traverse directions parallel respectively to the *a* and *c* axes of the mineral.

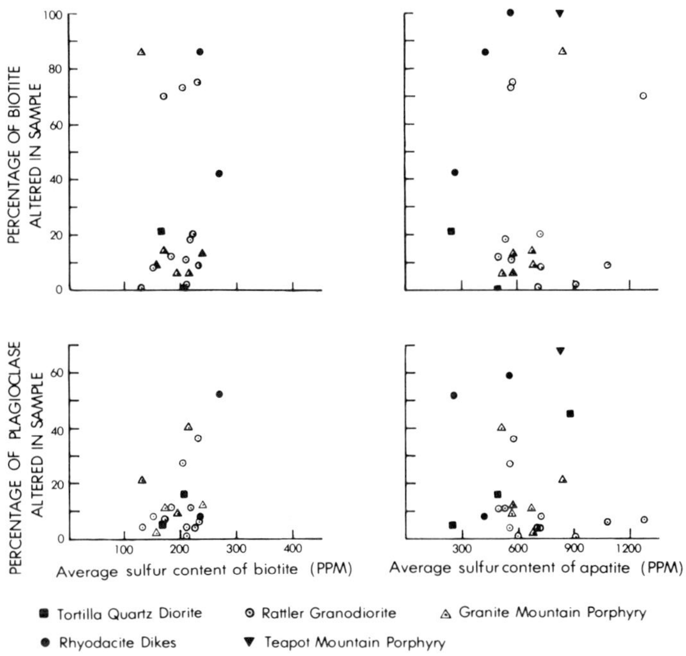

Figure 10.13. Relations between average sulfur content in igneous biotite and apatite and the percentage of biotite and plagioclase altered in the rock

of the area to the edge of the grain (Figs. 10.11, 10.12, 10.14), by virtue of inclusion of a grain in other minerals (see mineral occurrence data in Table 10.6), or by virtue of the size of a grain. This lack of correlation suggests that the observed abundances are likely the result of variations either in amounts of S in the melt or in conditions that affected incorporation of S in the minerals. Because these variations are relatively large and were operative over very short distances (millimeter scale or less), it seems more likely that they were caused by local variations in abundance of S in the melts (as favored by the sulfide petrology) or by coupled substitution of S with other elements in the minerals (improbable, as demonstrated later), rather than by complex variations in other conditions throughout the magmas.

Correlation of Intersample Variations in Igneous Minerals With Host Rock Chemistry, Age, Texture, and Modal Abundance

No correlations were found between S and Cu content of the minerals and variations in other petrologic parameters. The abundances of S in biotite and in apatite do not vary detectably with variations in whole-rock chemistry (as indicated by the differentiation index of the host samples, Fig. 10.15), in agreement with the works of Nash (1972*a*, 1972 *b*). Likewise, trends are not observed in the S content of the minerals with changing age of the host rock (compare data for different rock types, Fig. 10.15 or Tables 10.1, 10.4, 10.6), or changes in texture of the rock (Fig. 10.16). In addition, there is no apparent correlation with changes in modal abundance of the major sulfur-bearing minerals in the rocks, because all samples decrease in modal abundance with increasing differentiation (see Fig. 10.8), while the abundance of S in the minerals does not measurably change with the differentiation index of the sample (Fig. 10.15). Moreover, there is no consistent intersample pattern of high or low abundance of S when comparing the sulfur-bearing minerals in one sample with those in other samples of the same rock type or stock. Data for the abundance of S in hornblende and igneous(?) epidote are too scanty for conclusions regarding variations with respect to changing petrologic parameters.

The highly erratic distribution of Cu in biotite in the Ray rocks and the demonstrated association of Cu with Fe-Mg alteration minerals precludes useful comparison of Cu in biotite with indicators of magmatic development, and attempts at this comparison by other workers have resulted in highly conflicting conclusions. A decrease in the Cu content of hornblende with decreasing age of the samples has been noted in one study (Dodge et al., 1968) but not in another (Dodge and Ross, 1971). Graybeal (1973) has noted a correlation of Cu in both biotite and hornblende with rock texture. Lovering (1972) and Graybeal (1973) have suggested that the abundance of Cu in biotite increases with differentiation of rock series. Nockolds and Mitchell (1946) have suggested the opposite, and Dodge and Moore (1968), Dodge and others (1969), and Dodge and Ross (1971) have found no trends for three other rock suites. Parry and Nackowski (1963), Lovering and others (1970), Lovering (1972), and Parry (1972) have suggested that high Cu content indicates a potential mineralizing stock, but Tan (1973) and Kesler and others (1975) suggest the opposite, and Bradshaw (1967) finds no such correlation. These conflicting results appear adequately

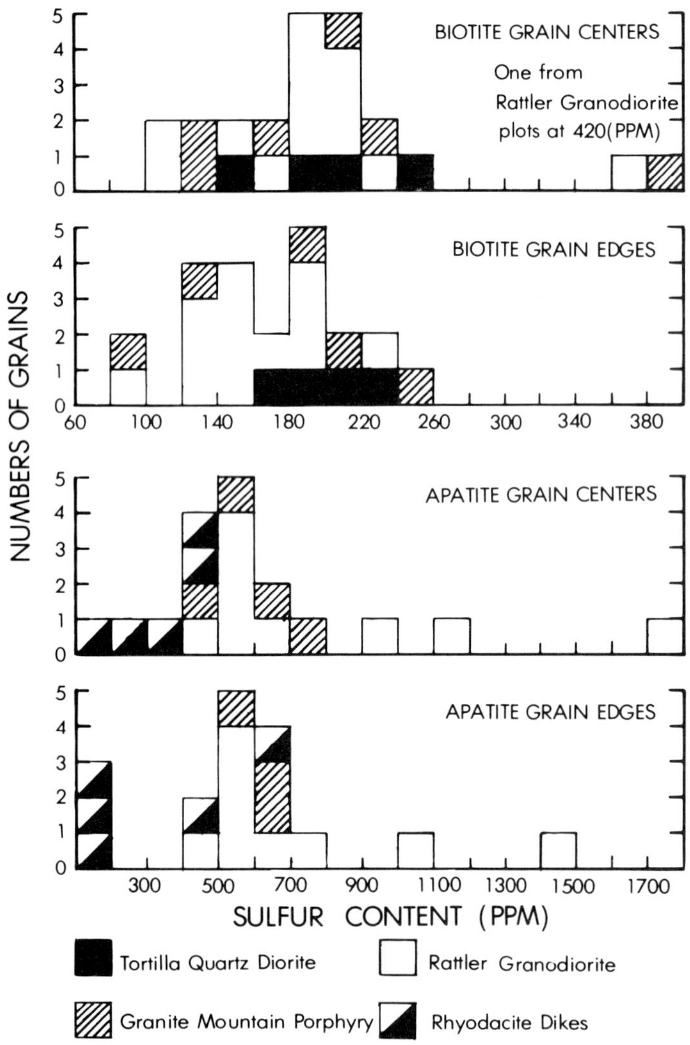

Figure 10.14. Frequency distribution of sulfur content in the centers and edges of igneous biotite and apatite, Laramide rocks near Ray

explained by the presence of Cu-bearing Fe-Mg alteration products in the mineral separates used in these studies.

There are a few intersample correlations between Cu contents of the various minerals; however, these appear to be random and are inconsistent when compared to primary petrologic parameters of the rocks. Appreciable Cu in magnetite occurs in two samples (see 246-11A and RB5, Table 10.5) but not in the third (see 246–99B, Table 10.5), for which appreciable Cu was detected in the coexisting biotite. The Cu content of biotite in one sample (246–11A, Table 10.5) of aplite of the Rattler Granodiorite is higher than two samples (61–25 and 246–11G) of the main stock, but the Cu content of biotite of the other aplite sample (260–96A) is not. Similarly, high (relatively) Cu content for magnetite is found in the more differentiated samples of Rattler Granodiorite and the opposite is true of the Granite Mountain Porphyry. The high Cu content of the biotite is at least suspect of being of secondary origin, but it is unknown whether the relatively high Cu content of magnetite is derived from the magma, results directly or indirectly from secondary processes, or represents coincidence of primary and secondary contributions of Cu. The high Cu values in magnetite might also reflect the presence of sub-optical or sub-surface copper sulfides, because of the propensity of magmatic sulfides to occur in magnetite (see Table 10.2). At any rate, as is the case with S, there does not appear to be consistent depletion or enrichment of Cu in any igneous mineral from progressively younger or more differentiated rocks, nor consistent correlation of the Cu content of any mineral with other primary petrologic parameters for the rocks.

Variations of Sulfur Content in Minerals With Changes in Mineral Composition

The possibility remains that the uptake of S from the melt by the minerals might be the result of coupled substitution of other elements in the minerals; this substitution could obscure slight but real trends in the S content of the minerals with magma differentiation. This possibility was investigated by comparing variations of S content of the minerals with variations of abundances of the other components in the minerals, using (1) individual grains and (2) like minerals grains (a) from the individual stocks or rock types and (b) from all rock types. For the first comparison, the number and type of correlation (positive, negative, or none) were tabulated for all grains of biotite and apatite studied for zoning. No trends emerged from these comparisons (Table 10.8). For the second comparison, correlation matrices were constructed to check for coupled substitution of S with other elements in the minerals; but in these data also, the correlations were either not significant or not consistent (Tables 10.9, 10.10); such results indicate that variations of S content of the minerals are not likely to be the result of coupled substitution.

Sulfur and Copper Content of Rocks

The data for S and Cu in the igneous minerals, when combined with the modal abundance and appropriate densities of the minerals, suggest that the Laramide intrusive rocks near Ray contain about 20 ppm and no more than 80 ppm S and about 10 ppm and no more than 50 ppm Cu (Table 10.11). The measured S content of a few selected samples agrees (with two exceptions) with these values, and there is a remarkably good correlation between measured and calculated Cu contents in the samples with very low measured Cu contents. The two exceptions for S (samples RB5 and 61–2F, Table 10.11) are easily explained by the presence of a few sulfide grains on unobserved hairline fractures in the samples submitted for analysis.

There appears to be no correlation between the measured Cu content of the sample and either the occurrence of sulfides in the sample prior to cleaning or the amount of cleaning done on replicate samples (see Table 10.11, footnote 3). Furthermore, the measured Cu content of the whole-rock samples is very erratic and does not appear responsive to changes in rock chemistry (Fig. 10.17*A*) or to alteration of minerals in the samples (Fig. 10.18). These findings are similar to those of other workers (Putman and Burnham, 1963; Putman, 1975) and are consistent with an interpretation that Cu is present in whole-rock samples in sometimes significant, but highly variable, amounts associated with the alteration products of biotite (Banks, 1974*b*).

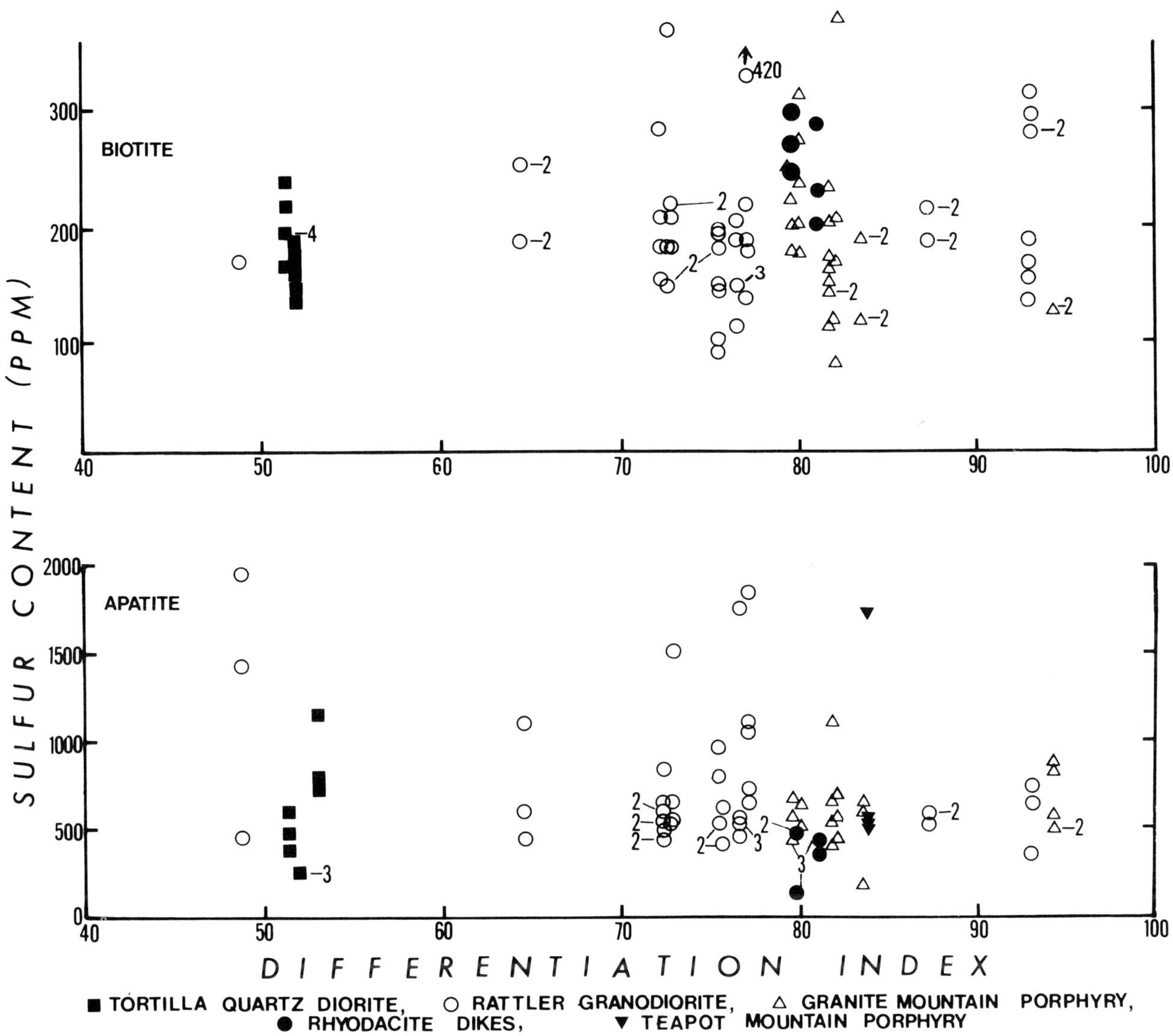

Figure 10.15. Variations of sulfur content of igneous biotite and apatite with rock differentiation index. The large scatter in the data results from heterogeneity of sulfur in and between grains rather than analytical error. The symbols in most cases cover the range of analytical uncertainty of the data points. Numbers with leaders indicate the number of analyses plotted on the symbol.

A plot of the calculated content of Cu (see Fig. 10.17*B*) shows no correlation with chemistry or age of the sample, while the abundance of S decreases slightly with increasing differentiation index of the samples (see Fig. 10.17*C*). The lack of correlation of Cu is the result of low and very erratic Cu contents of the major igneous minerals (a plot of Cu contributed to the samples by the sulfide minerals shows only a negative correlation with rock differentiation). The negative correlation shown by S (Fig. 10.17*C*) is due primarily to the decreasing modal abundance of the major sulfur-bearing minerals—sulfide minerals (see Fig. 10.8) and biotite, apatite, and hornblende (Banks, 1976).

SUMMARY AND DISCUSSION OF THE DISTRIBUTION AND MAGMATIC BEHAVIOR OF SULFUR AND COPPER

The preceding data indicate that sulfide separated, at least partly as immiscible liquid, from the melts of the major plutons associated with the Ray porphyry copper deposit; that this separation, rather than being the result of saturation of sulfide throughout the melts, was probably controlled by cooling of the magmas, coupled with local processes of concentration of S adjacent to other crystalline phases and a decrease in sulfide-carrying capacity of melt induced by growth of Fe-bearing minerals. The magmatic sulfides are rare (<5 ppm average); their modal abundance and, in general, their copper sulfide:pyrite ratio decreases with development of the entire igneous series and individual stocks; and their occurrence and distribution suggest that not much S was available for sulfide formation in magmas and that the younger rocks contained less S than the older rocks. Furthermore, when combined with the observations of Newhouse (1936) and Ramdohr (1940) and the predictions of Ringwood (1955), Curtis (1969), and Nockolds (1966)—which indicate that most of the Cu in unaltered igneous rocks should occur in sulfide minerals rather than in silicates—the data suggest that little Cu was present and that it too became less

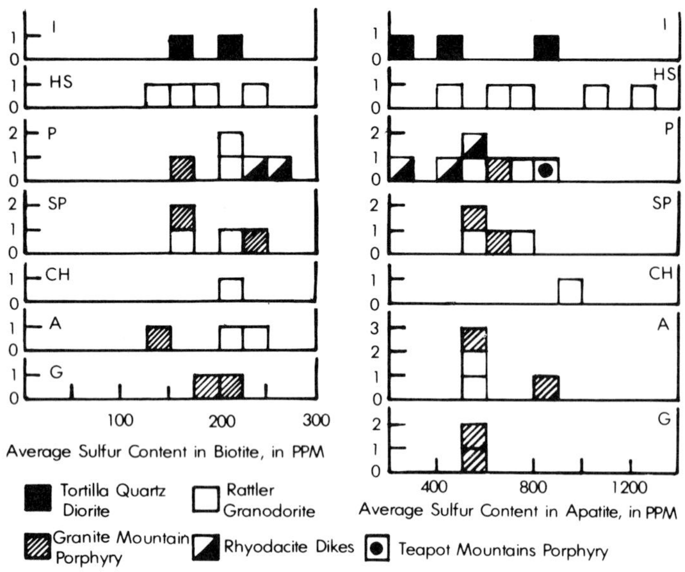

Figure 10.16. Frequency distribution of the average abundance of sulfur in igneous biotite and apatite in samples with differing textures. Key: I = intersertal; HS = hypidiomorphic seriate; P = porphyritic; SP = seriate porphyritic; CH = chilled; A = aplitic; G = granitoid.

abundant in the progressively younger, more differentiated magmas. The sulfide data, like data for the Cl, F, and H_2O in the igneous minerals (Banks, 1976), do not require—and, in fact, are possibly incompatible with—the presence of appreciable magmatic vapor in the magma system.

The data for the non-sulfide igneous minerals in the rocks are compatible with those for the sulfide minerals.

TABLE 10.8
Comparative Zoning of Sulfur in Igneous Biotite and Apatite From Laramide Rocks Near Ray

	Sulfur Detectably and Sympathetically Zoned	Sulfur Detectably and Antipathetically Zoned	Sulfur Only or Oxide-Element Only Detectably Zoned	Sulfur or Oxide-Element Not Detectably Zoned
Biotite				
SiO_2	0	0	6	5
Al_2O_3	0	2	6	3
FeO*	1	0	6	4
MgO	2	1	6	2
MnO	0	0	7	4
TiO_2	0	2	5	4
K_2O	0	0	7	4
Cl	0	0	4	7
F	0	1	4	6
H_2O†	0	0	4	7
Apatite				
SiO_2	1	1	3	3
CaO	0	0	5	3
Na_2O	0	0	5	3
P_2O_5	0	0	5	3
Cl	1	0	4	3
F	1	2	2	3
H_2O†	0	0	5	3

NOTE: Data are number of correlations tabulated for all grains studied for zoning of both sulfur and other elements.

* All Fe calculated as FeO.

† Calculated.

Sulfur is present, but at variable ppm levels (50–1,000) in all igneous biotite, apatite, and probably also in most of the igneous hornblende and igneous epidote analyzed; it was not detected in other igneous minerals. Thus the rocks contain less than 80 ppm S; they average about 20 ppm S, and show less S in progressively more differentiated samples. Variations in abundance of S in the igneous hydrous minerals are large and are not responsive to changes in mineral chemistry; sample age, texture, mineralogy, or chemistry; mild alteration of the sample; or potential susceptibility of the analyzed area of a mineral grain to exchange with a melt or an aqueous fluid. These data suggest that the S content of the igneous minerals analyzed was not measurably influenced by coupled substitution, by exchange with a pervasive magmatic or post-crystallization vapor, or by magmatic processes occurring throughout the melt. Although other unknown factors might also apply, the lack of response of variations in S abundance to variations in melt-wide igneous parameters appears best explained (like the petrology of the magmatic sulfides) as the result of local variations in the content of S in the melts caused by the simultaneous use and rejection of S during the growth of adjacent sulfur-bearing and sulfur-poor minerals. The lack of correlation between the S content of the minerals and the suggested lower S content of the younger, more differentiated magmas is explained by the compensating lesser amount of igneous minerals present (sulfides, apatite, biotite, and hornblende) to remove S from the melts (modal hydrous mineral data from Banks, 1976).

Copper occurs in nil or very low ppm amounts in all non-sulfide igneous minerals in the rocks except magnetite and biotite. It occurs in magnetite in low ppm amounts (40 ppm maximum, <20 average, <1 minimum) and in biotite in amounts ranging from <3 to several hundred ppm. Variations of Cu abundance in biotite and magnetite are large and erratic both within and between mineral grains, rock samples, and stocks and rock types, and they do not correlate consistently with any primary igneous parameter. Most of the Cu in the biotite and in the whole-rock samples is from Cu in alteration products of biotite, and the Cu in magnetite may be in part from magmatic sulfides or non-magmatic sources. The Cu content of the rocks, calculated to avoid the Cu in the alteration products of biotite and occasional sulfide grains of non-igneous origin on hairline fractures, indicates very low Cu content in the Laramide plutons and the basement rocks (<10 ppm average), and samples with low measured Cu content agree well with the calculated values.

INTERPRETATION OF PORPHYRY COPPER GENESIS

The data presented here appear best explained if the exposed stocks and, by analogy, any parental pluton contained little S and Cu and if the present amounts of magmatic S and Cu in the stocks represent their approximate amounts in the parental magmas of the rocks. Thus, the Laramide magmas and solidified plutons were unlikely sources of the sulfides in the Ray deposit and in its satellitic sulfide mineral occurrences. Furthermore, the data presented here and in

TABLE 10.9
Partial Pearson Correlation Matrix for the Chemistry of Igneous Biotite, Sulfur Content of Biotite, and Rock Differentiation Index (D.I.) in Laramide Rocks Near Ray

	SiO_2	Al_2O_3	FeO*	MgO	MnO	TiO_2	K_2O	Cl	F	H_2O†	D.I.
Tortilla Quartz Diorite (N, 3)											
S	*-0.50*	*0.94*	*0.77*	*-0.50*	*0.96*	*-0.96*	*-0.50*	*-0.97*	0.99	*-0.87*	-1.00
D.I.	*.50*	*-.94*	*-.77*	*.50*	*-.96*	*.96*	*.50*	*.97*	-.99	*.87*	1.00
Rattler Granodiorite (N, 22)											
S	*-0.37*	-0.53	*0.12*	*0.26*	*0.33*	*0.07*	*-0.03*	*0.06*	0.46	-0.52	*0.16*
D.I.	*.08*	*.15*	*-.01*	*-.23*	*-.18*	.63	*-.34*	*-.36*	.66	*-.24*	1.00
Granite Mountain Porphyry (N, 17)											
S	*-0.13*	*-0.12*	*0.46*	*-0.39*	*0.08*	*0.19*	*0.03*	*0.26*	-0.58	0.57	*-0.30*
D.I.	*.47*	.59	-.81	*.10*	*-42*	*-.47*	-.83	*-.39*	*.37*	*-.47*	1.00
All Rock Types (N, 44)											
S	-0.32	*-0.27*	0.30	*-0.03*	*0.12*	*0.00*	*0.00*	*0.16*	*-0.19*	*0.05*	*0.03*
D.I.	*-.24*	.47	*.23*	-.53	.43	*-.27*	-.38	-.57	.66	-.63	1.00

NOTE: Italic figures represent correlation at less than 95 percent confidence level; *N* = number of observations in a population.

* All Fe calculated as FeO.

† Calculated.

TABLE 10.10
Partial Pearson Correlation Matrix for the Chemistry of Igneous Apatite, Sulfur Content of Apatite, and Rock Differentiation Index (D.I.) in Laramide Rocks Near Ray

	SiO_2	CaO	Na_2O	Cl	F	P_2O_5	H_2O†	D.I.
Tortilla Quartz Diorite (N, 9)								
S	*-0.47*	*-0.50*	*-0.08*	-0.82	*-0.45*	*-0.22*	*0.55*	0.74
D.I.	*-.52*	-.79	*-.79*	*-.57*	-.73	*-.27*	0.74	1.00
Rattler Granodiorite (N, 25)								
S	*0.03*	*-0.32*	0.54	*0.28*	*0.03*	*-0.17*	*-0.20*	*-0.15*
D.I.	*-.10*	*-.09*	*.37*	*-.29*	*0.00*	*-.14*	*.11*	1.00
Granite Mountain Porphyry (N, 16)								
S	*0.07*	*-0.07*	*0.17*	*0.35*	*0.24*	*-0.28*	*-0.29*	*0.34*
D.I.	*.69*	*-.04*	.64	*.28*	*.05*	*-.37*	*-.07*	1.00
Teapot Mountain Porphyry (N, 4)								
S	*-0.02*	*-0.93*	0.97	*0.70*	*-0.49*	*-0.29*	*-0.45*	—
D.I.	—	—	—	—	—	—	—	—
All Rock Types (N, 60*)								
S	*-0.04*	*-0.22*	*0.28*	*-0.11*	*0.11*	*-0.16*	*-0.12*	*0.09*
D.I.	*-.10*	-.31	*.21*	-.65	.61	*.19*	-.55	1.00

NOTE: Italic figures represent correlation at less than 95 percent confidence level; *N* = number of observations in a population.

† Calculated.

* Includes 6 apatites from dike rocks.

Banks (1976) and Banks and Page (1980) do not require the presence of a magmatic vapor phase; in fact, they conflict with a model whereby the rocks and minerals were in contact with appreciable amounts of magmatic water. In other words, because the orthomagmatic model of porphyry copper genesis requires copious amounts of magmatic water that has access to adequate amounts of magmatic S and Cu, the data from the Ray rocks raise serious questions about the applicability of the orthomagmatic model of porphyry copper genesis to Ray. Likewise, the data for the Ray rocks challenge whether circulating meteoric water can be postulated as causative of the deposit (without removing the possibility of involvement). This challenge results from the low abundance of Cu and particularly of S (non-sedimentary S is required because of the "magmatic" isotopic character of ore sulfides; for example, Jensen, 1967, 1971) in the Laramide

TABLE 10.11
Whole-Rock Sulfur and Copper Abundance Data From the Least-Altered Laramide Igneous Rocks Near Ray

Rock Type	Sample Number[1]	Percentage of Biotite in Rock Altered	Percentage of Plagioclase in Rock Altered	Vein Sulfides Detected in Sample Prior	Measured Content of S in ppm[2]	Measured Content of Cu in ppm[3]	Calculated Content of S in ppm[4]	Calculated Content of Cu in ppm[5]
Tortilla Quartz Diorite	17–28 I	tr	16	Yes	<80	140–80	31 (38)	<7 (<8)
	17–1	21	5	Yes	<80	130–75	57 (72)	<38 (<47)
	48–29	—	45	No		55	36 (36)	<5 (<11)
Rattler Granodiorite	46–99B I	70	7	Rare		50, 180	21 (25)	<3 (<4)
	60–113D	20	4	No		8	27 (28)	<4 (<11)
	60–114	4	3	No		11		
	60–108	—	1	No		5	3 (6)	<2 (<5)
	61–25 S	11	4	Yes	<80	12	18 (19)	<7 (<8)
	60–91	18	11	Yes		95, 130	16 (16)	<3 (<9)
	60–111	2	1	No		8	28 (28)	<2 (<11)
	60–124	11	10	Yes		230, 500		
	60–98	1	4	No		3	12 (12)	<3 (<9)
	46–11G I	12	11	Yes	<80	150, 10	18 (19)	<3 (<4)
	60–131	8	8	No		22	14 (14)	<2 (<8)
	60–130	9	6	No		24	23 (23)	<3 (<9)
	60–132	18	7	Yes		28		
	60–96A I	73	27	Yes		60, 70	17 (17)	<2 (<4)
	46–11A I	75	36	Yes	<80	90, 50, 100	10 (10)	<4 (<7)
	60–105	22	8	No		70		
	60–106	9	6	Yes		160		
	60–115	11	4	Yes		20		
	60–117	5	7	Yes		10		
	60–119	7	9	Yes		100		
	60–129	13	4	Yes		95		
	60–136	12	6	Yes		120		
	60–137	21	12	Yes		130		
Granite Mountain Porphyry	RB5 IS	6	40	Yes	280	50	24 (24)	<7 (<7)
	GM14	13	12	Yes		23	22 (22)	<3 (<8)
	GM12	14	11	No		60	15 (15)	<2 (<8)
	GM18 I	6	9	No		55	23 (23)	<4 (<4)
	GM6G	9	2	Yes		70	14 (14)	<3 (<8)
	GM2A	86	21	Yes		8	1 (1)	<2 (<5)
	GM1A	100	41	Yes		44		
	GM3	41	8	Yes		70		
	GM4V	17	3	Yes		55		
	GM5	14	6	No		65		
	GM10	15	2	Yes		480, 340		
	GM11	34	9	Yes		60		
	GM13	19	11	No		110		
	GM15	10	12	Yes		110		
	GM16	28	7	No		60		
Teapot Mountain Porphyry	TTM	100	68	Yes	<80	75		
Rhyodacite and Andesite Dikes	78/79–4	—	72	No	<80	40		
	61–4	100	22	Yes	<80	20		
	GM100	42	52	No		35		
	61–2F	86	8	Yes	680	50		

[1] Includes all samples with spectrochemical data; an *I* or *S* after the sample number indicates, respectively, that ion probe (*I*) or spectrographic (*S*) data is available for minerals in the sample (see Table 10.5).

[2] Wet chemical analyses in the Analysis Laboratory under Leonard Shapiro (see Shapiro, 1975). Analysts P. Elmore, G. Chloe, J. Glen, H. Smith.

[3] Emission spectrochemical analysis. Analysts R. E. Mays and Chris Heropoulos. In cases with two or three values, the first value is for 1 cm slabs, the second is for 2 mm slabs, and the third is for 1 mm slabs as defined in Appendix II.

[4] Values calculated using modal abundances of igneous biotite, hornblende, epidote, and sulfides; normative abundances of apatite; measured rock densities; assumed mineral densities; average measured abundance of S in biotite, hornblende, epidote, and apatite (assuming 0 ppm for quartz, pyroxene, magnetite, feldspars and mineral analyses resulting in *ND* in Table 10.7); and ideal sulfur contents of the sulfides. Values enclosed in parentheses indicate maximum amount of igneous S in sample calculated as above but assuming 40 ppm for the analyses resulting in *ND* (for the minerals in Table 10.7.

[5] Values calculated using modal abundances of sulfides and major rock-forming minerals, measured rock densities, assumed mineral densities, and either the average measured copper abundances of the major rock-forming minerals or, where not measured, the minimum copper value measured by ion probe for each mineral species present in the rock. Values enclosed in parentheses indicate the probable maximum amount of igneous copper in the sample calculated as above, but assuming instead the average value of copper (measured plus detection levels) by ion probe and emission spectroscopy for the unanalyzed minerals in each sample.

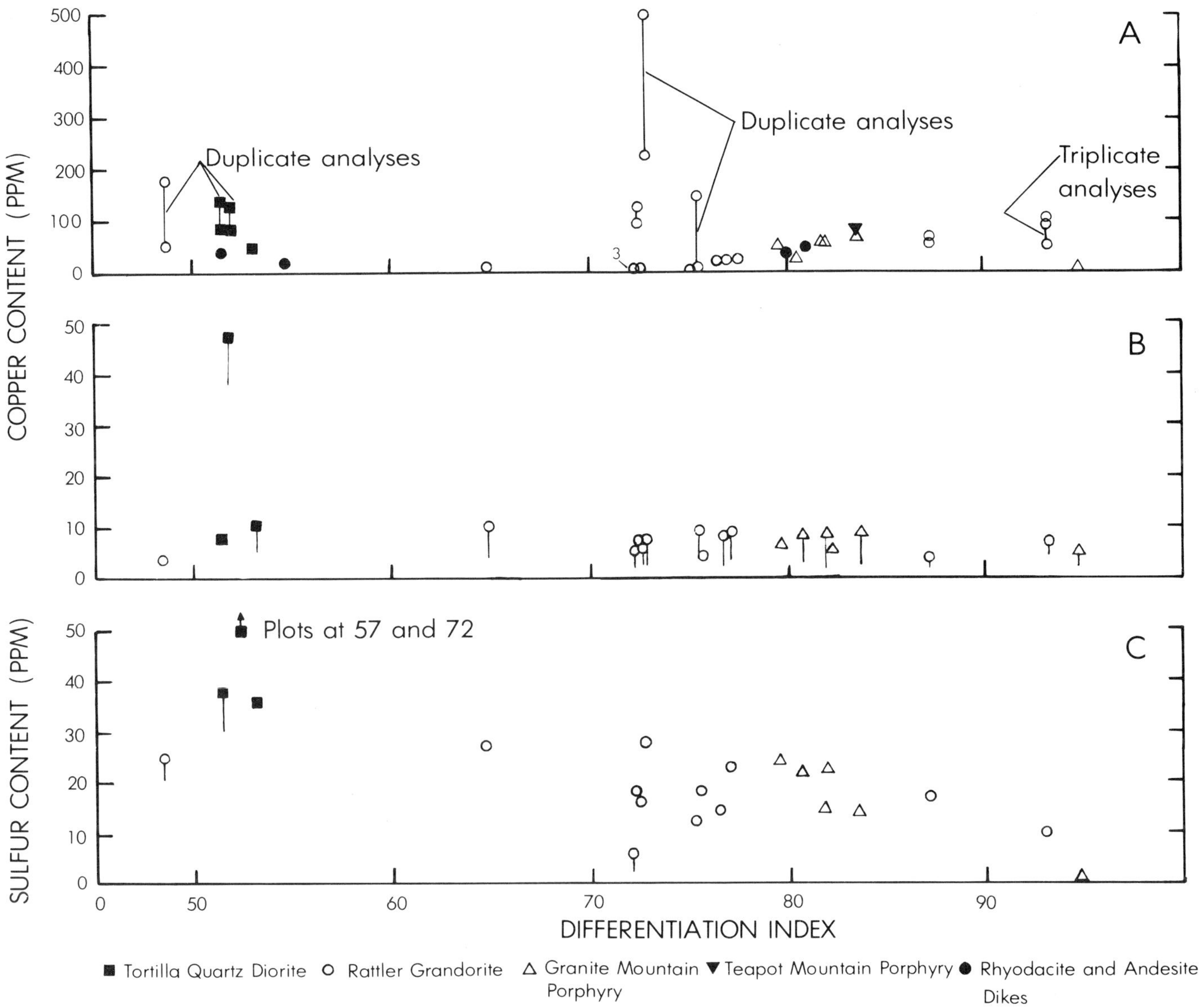

Figure 10.17. Variation of copper and sulfur contents of Laramide rocks with rock differentiation index. Numbers with leaders indicate the number of analyses plotted on the symbol. *A,* copper content measured by emission spectroscopy. *B,* probable maximum copper content of unaltered samples calculated from rock and mineral densities, mineral modal abundances, and copper content of the sample's component minerals, measured by ion microprobe and emission spectroscopy. The average of all analyses of each mineral species was used when no analysis was available for a component mineral in a given sample. Tails on the symbols point to the values calculated assuming the minimum ion probe value, rather than the average value for all unanalyzed mineral species in a given sample. *C,* probable maximum sulfur content of unaltered sample calculated from rock and mineral densities, mineral modal abundances, and average sulfur contents of biotite, apatite, sulfide minerals, epidote, and hornblende in the rocks assuming no sulfur in pyroxene, quartz, feldspar minerals, or magnetite and assuming 40 ppm for sulfur in the analyses of the hornblende, epidote, and sphene that resulted in ND in Table 10.7. Tails on some of the symbols point to values calculated assuming 0 ppm for the analyses that resulted in ND in Table 10.7.

and basement rocks revealed in this study and in Banks (1973), coupled with the likelihood that Cu is more likely scavenged from, rather than added to, water during low-grade alteration in the outer reaches of a circulation cell (Banks, 1974*b*). Furthermore, postulation of a hidden special magma or igneous source rock does not easily solve the problems in the Ray data for the orthomagmatic or meteoric water models, because the Ray data were not unique compared to data for other porphyry copper systems and for igneous systems in ore-barren provinces, with respect to major- and minor-element chemistry and rock petrology (Cornwall and Banks, 1977; Banks and Page, 1980; Cornwall, 1982) and with respect to ore-fluid components of the rocks and their constituent minerals (data from this study and from Banks, 1973, 1974*b,* 1976).

The basic time-space association of magmatism and the deposits and a need for supply of S from depth seem documented beyond question. However, problems and inconsistencies in application of the orthomagmatic and meteoric water models to porphyry copper genesis have been noted by past workers (for a review see Banks and Page, 1977), and direct data on ore-fluid elements in the Ray rocks and component minerals, which monitored the behavior of H_2O, C1, Cu, and S in the magmas, are not satisfactorily explained by

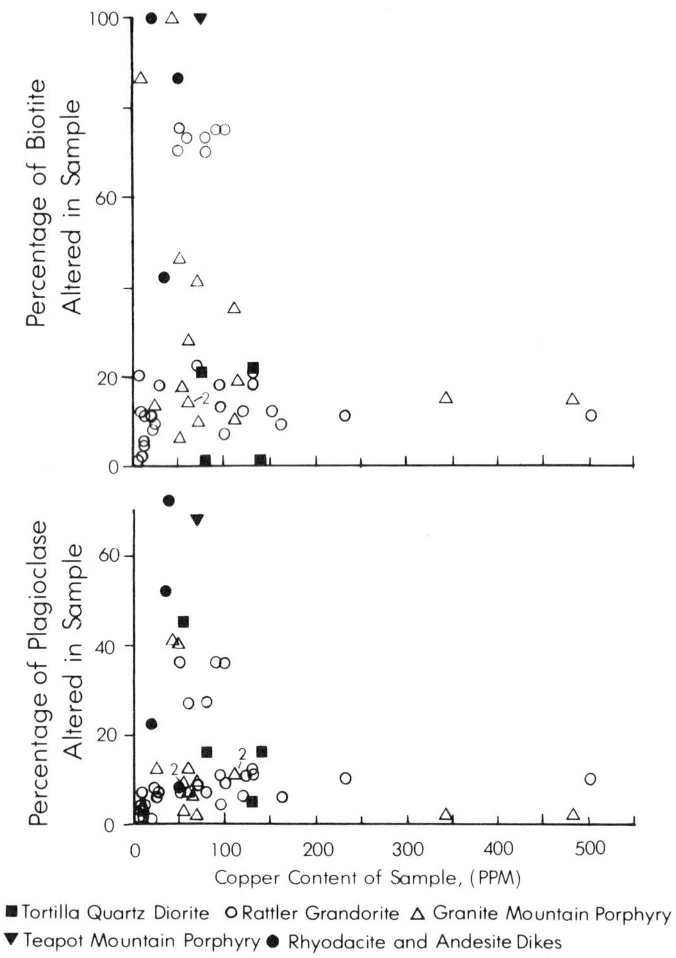

Figure 10.18. Variation of measured copper abundance with alteration of biotite and plagioclase in whole-rock samples

either of these two models. Thus, a re-evaluation of the mechanism that can produce both ore fluids and magmatism seems warranted, and if the re-evaluation is not based on the data available for the Ray rocks (see Banks and Page, 1977), it should at least be consistent with it.

APPENDIX I
Analytical Methods Used in Modal and Chemical Analyses of Igneous Sulfide Minerals

Modal abundance of igneous sulfide minerals was calculated from the area (ca 4–5 cm^2) of polished thin sections of the least-altered samples of the stocks in relation to the area of sulfide grains exposed at the surface of the thin sections. The polished areas of the thin sections were determined with the aid of photographic enlargements (ca 250 cm^2) of the slides. The location of the sulfide grains was observed by slowly moving the slide on the X axis under a microscope with both reflected and transmitted light capabilities at $\geq 160X$ magnification on a grid spacing on the Y axis of one-half the field of view. Sulfide grains and other areas of reflectivity that possibly were sulfide grains were plotted on the photographic enlargement of the slide and notes were taken on their shape, when distinguishable, and mode of occurrence. The slide was then observed visually at $280X$ magnification in an ARL EMX microprobe by slowly moving the slide (depending on the number of sulfide grains present, complete coverage of the slide took about 5–12 hours) on the X axis on a grid spacing on the Y axis of one-half the field of view. All areas of the slide were thus visually observed four times, twice with a microscope and twice in the probe. Each of the real and possible sulfide occurrences plotted on the photographic map of the slide was checked off as it was observed in the probe. After half of the samples had been observed in this fashion, the preliminary examination with the microscope was discontinued owing to a higher degree of success in finding and identifying sulfides in the microprobe. However, in the second half of the study, the sample was moved more slowly in the microprobe, and the beam was left scanning in a line 10- to 20-μm long along the Y axis as the slide was moved. Any increase in the X-ray intensity of sulfur was indicated by a buzzer, and the area checked. Only four grains (of the several hundred observed) were discovered in this manner, and, because of their small size, they represented a modally insignificant fraction of the grains observed. The sulfide minerals were identified and their areas measured with the aid of the analytical and beam scanning and oscilloscope projection capabilities of the microprobe. The shape and mode of occurrence of grains discovered in the probe were recorded and, if necessary, checked under the petrographic microscope. Remeasurement of one of the slides a year later resulted in essentially the same modal data for all the sulfide species in the slide. The polished thin sections were of exceptional quality with less than 10 to 15 percent of the measured surface marred by plucking and scratches.

Chemical analyses of some of the larger sulfide grains were done with the microprobe, using the following: a LIF crystal for Cu and Fe and an ADP crystal for S, counting times of about 20 seconds terminated on fixed beam current, an excitation voltage of 15 kv, sample current of 1.5×10^{-8} A, and a fully focused beam that was centered on and moved about the grains by magnetic deflectors. Several (4–10) observation points were used for each analysis, and the X-ray intensity data were corrected by computer (Beeson, 1967; Beaman and Isasi, 1970) or by the on-line FRAME program (Yakowitz et al., 1973). The standards—synthetic bornite and pyrite and stoichiometric Ookiep chalcopyrite—were furnished by Gerald K. Czamanske. Data for the same grain when reduced by the two different programs gave values that were analytically indistinguishable.

APPENDIX II
Analytical Methods Used to Determine Sulfur and Copper Content of Igneous Minerals and Rocks

Major and minor elements (including S for a few samples) of whole-rock samples and mineral separates were analyzed by the rapid-rock methods of Shapiro and Brannock (1962) and Shapiro (1975); Cu was analyzed by the quantitative emission spectrochemical methods of Bastron and others (1960). Several hundred mineral grains were analyzed for S, Cu, and major elements with electron and ion microprobe analyzers. The sample sites were chosen to optimize rock variation and minimize alteration. The samples ranged in size from 5 to 30 kg and were cleaned with unpainted hammers in the field. To further reduce contamination by hydrothermal minerals, each sample was subsequently sawed to ±1 cm-thick slabs and cleaned by sawing out all planar alteration features noted on the wet surfaces (in most cases, very few). Each sample was then divided into two groups using alternate slabs, one for mineral separation and the other for chemical analyses. Except for a few of the larger samples, the slabs used for chemical analyses were re-slabbed to ±2 mm to check for and remove any remaining planar zones of alteration. The slabs of the excepted larger samples were subdivided again into two or three subgroups, one of 1-cm-thick slabs and one or two others that were cut to ±2 mm and ± 1 mm slabs and cleaned as above. These subgroups were submitted as replica samples to check whether the cleaning process affected the analytical results (see Table 10.11). All sawed surfaces were lapped with corundum on steel plates (to remove brass smeared from the saw on the slabs and chips) and, finally, washed in distilled water. The clean chips (a minimum of 1000*X* the volume of the largest phenocryst) were crushed and milled with ceramic-faced machinery prior to analysis. After selection of suitable material for petrologic and microprobe studies, the slabs used for mineral separations were crushed to –30 to +60 mesh and selected component minerals were concentrated, using standard heavy-liquid, electromagnetic, electrostatic, and handpicking methods. These concentrates were then carefully recrushed with repeated screenings, generally to –100 to +150 mesh, and again purified using centrifuge heavy-liquid methods, electrostatic and electromagnetic separators, and handpicking. The resulting separates were thus clean of almost all binary and non-desired mineral species. The main contaminates (less than 1%) were microscopic mineral inclusions and trace amounts of alteration products of the inclusions and host mineral.

The sample preparation, standards, run parameters, and methods of data reduction for the mineral analyses with the electron microprobe for S and Cu in the igneous minerals have been described in detail elsewhere (Banks, 1973, 1974*b,* 1976). In brief, the samples were polished thin sections, carefully prepared to eliminate external contamination by copper of the analytical surface. The analytical instrument was an ARL EMX electron microprobe analyzer with both energy dispersive and wave-length dispersive analyzers, and detection limits (at the run conditions) for Cu of 90–100 ppm and for S of 50 ppm. The average S content determined for biotite in sample 61–25 by electron microprobe was 210 ppm (Banks, 1974*b;* see also Table 10.1), which compared well with the 200 ppm determined by H. N. Elsheimer by X-ray fluorescence analyses of a biotite mineral separate of the same sample. The S content of Wilburforce apatite analyzed by S. T. Neil by gravimetric separation as $BaSO_4$ was 2,360 ppm, which compared well with an average of 2,300 ppm (range of 3,100–1,500 ppm) determined with the electron microprobe. Repeated analysis of a synthetic glass (NBS 610) containing 444 ±4 ppm Cu yielded 400 ±40 ppm by electron microprobe analysis (Banks, 1974*b*).

The same polished sections used for the electron microprobe were used for analyses by an ion microprobe mass analyzer at the ARL-Hasler Research Center. Run parameters included silicon as the internal standard, a negatively charged monatomic oxygen ($^{16}O^-$) as the primary beam, operating voltage of 18.5 kv, variable counting times, and an elliptical beam 150 μm in length. The local thermal equilibrium (LTE) model was used to calculate the ionization correction factors for reducing the raw intensity data (Anderson and Hinthorn, 1973).

The ion microprobe has the advantage over the electron microprobe in that as a mass analyzer, it ideally has a detection level of about 1 ppm for Cu. In practice, because the mass of complex ions of some elements interferes, the statistical error bar on the raw data might increase the effective detection level to as high as 20 ppm; this level, however, is still substantially lower than that of the electron microprobe. In analyzing the same spots, Cu was detected by both the ion and electron microprobe in a biotite and a chlorite (see Table 10.5, grains 246–99B 3BI and 246–11A 1CLA; see also Banks, 1974*b,* Table 1). The values obtained by the ion probe were respectively 60 and 30 percent lower than the amount previously detected by electron microprobe (see Banks, 1974*b,* Table 1). The lower values were expected because the grains analyzed were smaller than the ion beams (in the case of the biotite grain, about half the area of the ion beam).

ACKNOWLEDGMENTS

The manuscript was improved by fruitful discussion with N. J. Page and the helpful reviews of N. J. Page, P. B. Barton, H. R. Cornwall, and S. R. Titley. Emission spectrochemical analyses were done by R. E. Mays and Chris Heropoulus; rapid-rock analyses for S were done by G. Chloe, P. Elmore, J. Glenn, and H. Smith; ion probe analyses were done with J. R. Hinthorne. Mineral separations were aided by R. J. McLaughlin, and measurement of some of the sulfide minerals was done by R. D. Dockter, who also aided in drafting some of the figures. J. M. Schmidt and P. E. Venuti also aided in preparation and drafting of some of the figures.

REFERENCES CITED

Al-Hashimi, A. R. K., and Brownlow, A. H., 1970, Copper content of biotites from the Boulder batholith, Montana: Econ. Geol. v. 65, p. 985–992.

Andersen, C. A., and Hinthorne, J. R. 1973, Thermodynamic approach to the quantitative interpretation of spattered ion mass spectra: Anal. Chemistry, v. 45, p. 1421–1438.

Armbrusmacher, T. J., and Banks, N. G., 1974, Clouded plagioclase in metadolerite dikes, southeastern Bighorn Mountains, Wyoming: Am. Mineral., v. 59, no. 7–8, p. 656–665.

Banks, N. G., 1973, Biotite as a source of some of the sulfur in porphyry copper deposits: Econ. Geol., v. 68, p. 697–703.

———, 1974*a,* Biotite as a source of some of the sulfur in porphyry copper deposits—A reply: Econ. Geol., v. 69, p. 705.

———, 1974*b* Distribution of copper in biotite and biotite alteration products in intrusive rocks near two Arizona porphyry copper deposits: U.S. Geol. Survey Jour. Research, v. 2, no. 2, p. 195–211.

———, 1976, Halogen contents of igneous minerals as indicators of magmatic evolution of rocks associated with the Ray porphyry copper deposit, Arizona: U.S. Geol. Survey Jour. Research, v. 4, p. 91–117.

Banks, N. G.; Cornwall, H. R.; Silberman, M. L.; Creasey, S. C.; and Marvin, R. F., 1972. Chronology of intrusion and ore deposition at Ray, Arizona—Part 1, K-Ar ages: Econ. Geol., v. 67, p. 864–878.

Banks, N. G., and Stuckless, J. S., 1973, Chronology of intrusion and ore deposition at Ray, Arizona—Part 2, Fission-track ages: Econ. Geol., v. 68, p. 657–664.

Banks, N. G., and Krieger, M. H., 1977, Geologic map of the Hayden Quadrangle, Pinal and Gila Counties, Arizona: U.S. Geol. Survey Geol. Quad. Map GQ 1391, scale 1:24000, text 15 p.

Banks, N. G., and Page, N. J. 1977, Some observations that bear on the origin of porphyry copper deposits: U.S. Geol. Survey open-file rept. 77–127, 14 p.

———, 1980, Some observations that bear on the origin of porphyry copper deposits: Proc. 5th Quad. IAGOD Symp. v. 1, Stuttgart, E. Schweiiz, Verlags., p. 49–73.

Barrie, Michel, 1976, Flow differentiation, limitation of the Bagnold effect to narrow intrusions: Contr. Mineralogy and Petrology, v. 55, p. 139–145.

Bastron, Harry; Barnett, P. R.; and Murata, K. J., 1960, Method for the quantitative spectrochemical analysis of rocks, minerals, ores, and other materials by a powder d-c arc technique: U.S. Geol. Survey Bull. 1084-G, p. G165–G182.

Beaman, D. R., and Isasi, J. A., 1970, A critical examination of computer programs used in quantitative electron microprobe analysis: Anal. Chemistry, v. 42, p. 1540–1568.

Beeson, M. H., 1967, A computer program for processing electron microprobe data: U.S. Geol. Survey open-file report, 40 p.

Bradshaw, P. M. D., 1967, Distribution of selected elements in feldspar, biotite, and muscovite from British granites in relation to mineralization: Inst. Mining and Metallurgy Trans., v. 76, sec. b, p. 137–148.

Cabri, L. J., 1973, New data on phase relations in the Cu-Fe-S system: Econ. Geol., v. 68, p. 443–545.

Cornwall, H. R., 1982, Petrology and chemistry of igneous rocks, Ray porphyry copper district, Pinal County, Arizona, *in* Titley, S. R., ed., Advances in Geology of the Porphyry Copper Deposits, Southwestern North America: Tucson, Univ. Ariz. Press, Chapter 11.

Cornwall, H. R.; Banks, N. G.; and Philips, C. H., 1971, Geologic map of the Sonora quadrangle, Pinal and Gila Counties, Arizona: U.S. Geol. Survey Geol. Quad. Map GQ-1021.

Cornwall, H. R., and Krieger, M. H., 1975, Geologic map of the Kearny quadrangle, Pinal County, Arizona: U.S. Geol. Survey Geol. Quad. Map GQ–1188.

Cornwall, H. R., and Banks, N. G., 1977, Igneous rocks and copper mineralization in the Ray porphyry copper district, Arizona: U.S. Geol. Survey open-file rept. 77–255, 10 p.

Creasey, S. C., and Kistler, R. W., 1962, Age of some copper-bearing porphyries and other igneous rocks in southeastern Arizona, *in* Geological Survey Research, 1962: U.S. Geol. Survey Prof. Paper 450-D, p. D1–D5.

Creasey, S. C.; Peterson, D. W.; and Gambell, N. A., 1975, Geologic map of the Teapot Mountain quadrangle, Pinal County, Arizona: U.S. Geol. Survey open-file map 75–314.

Curtis, C. D., 1969, Applications of the crystal-field theory to the inclusion of trace transitional elements in minerals during magmatic differentiation: Geochim. et Cosmochim. Acta, v. 28, p. 389–403.

Damon, P. E., and Mauger, R. L., 1966, Epeirogeny-orogeny viewed from the Basin and Range province: Soc. Mining Engineers Trans., v. 235, p. 99–112.

Damon, P. E. (compiler), and others, 1970, New K-Ar dates for the southern Basin and Range province, *in* Ann. Reports to the Research Division: U.S. Atomic Energy Comm., June 1970, p. 38.

Dodge, F. W. C., 1973, Chlorites from granitic rocks of the central Sierra Nevada batholith, California: Am. Mineralogist, v. 39, p. 58–64.

Dodge, F. C. W., and Moore, J. G., 1968, Occurrence and composition of biotites from the Cartridge Pass pluton of the Sierra Nevada batholith, California, *in* Geological Survey Research, 1968: U.S. Geol. Survey Prof. Paper 600-B, p. B6–B10.

Dodge, F. C. W.; Papike, J. J.; and Mays, R. E., 1968, Hornblendes from granitic rocks of the central Sierra Nevada batholith, California: Jour. Petrology, v. 9, no. 3, p. 378–410.

Dodge, F. C. W.; Smith, V. C.; and Mays, R. E., 1969, Biotites from granitic rocks of the central Sierra Nevada batholith, California: Jour. Petrology, v. 10, p. 250–271.

Dodge, F. C. W., and Ross, D. C., 1971, Coexisting hornblendes and biotites from granitic rocks near the San Andreas fault, California: Jour. Geology, v. 79, 2, p. 158–172.

Fincham, C. J. B., and Richardson, F. D., 1954, The behavior of sulfur in silicate and aluminate melts: Royal Soc. [London] Proc., series A, v. 223, p. 40–62.

Foster, M. D., 1960, Interpretation of the composition of trioctahedram micas: U.S. Geol. Survey Prof. Paper 354-B, p. B11–B49.

Goossens, P. J., and Hollister, V. F., 1973, Structural control and hydrothermal alteration pattern of Chaucha porphyry copper, Ecuador: Mineralium Deposita, v. 8, no. 4, p. 321–331.

Graybeal, F. T., 1973, Copper, manganese, and zinc in coexisting mafic minerals from Laramide intrusive rocks in Arizona: Econ. Geol., v. 68, p. 785–798.

Haughton, D. R., and Roeder, P. L., 1971, Iron and sulphur in basaltic liquids: Geol. Assoc. Canada-Mineralog. Assoc. Canada, Joint Ann. Mtg, May 13–15, Abs. of Papers. p. 31–32.

Haughton, D. R., and Skinner, B. J., 1972, Chemistry of sulfur in melts: Internat. Geol. Cong., 24th, Montreal, Canada, Resumes, abs., p. 420.

Haughton, D. R.; Roeder, P. L.; and Skinner, B. J., 1974, Solubility of sulfur in mafic magmas: Econ. Geol., v. 69, p. 451–467.

Hollister, V. F., 1974, Regional characteristics of porphyry copper deposits of South America: Soc. Mining Engineers Trans., v. 255, p. 45–54.

Hollister, V. F.; Allen, J. M.; Anzalone, S. A.; and Seraphim, R. H., 1975, Structural evolution of porphyry mineralization at Highland Valley, British Columbia: Canadian Jour. Earth Sci., v. 12, no. 5, p. 807–820.

Jensen, M. L., 1967, Sulfur isotopes and mineral genesis, *in* Barnes, H. L., ed., Geochemistry of Hydrothermal Ore Deposits: New York, Holt, Rinehart and Winston, p. 143–165.

———, 1971, Provenance of Cordilleran intrusives and associated metals: Econ. Geol., v. 63, p. 34–42.

Katsura, Takashi, and Nagashima, Shigeru, 1974, Solubility of sulfur in some magmas at 1 atmosphere: Geochim. et Cosmochim. Acta, v. 38, p. 517–531.

Kesler, S. E.; Issigonis, M. J.; Brownlow, A. H.; Damon, P. E.; Moore, W. J.; Northcote, K. E.; and Preto, V. A., 1975, Geochemistry of biotites from mineralized and barren intrusive systems: Econ. Geol., v. 70, p. 559–567.

Komar, P.D., 1972*a,* Mechanical interactions of phenocrysts and flow differentiation of igneous dikes and sills: Geol. Soc. America Bull. v. 83, p. 973–988.

———, 1972*b,* Flow differentiation in igneous dikes and sills, profiles of velocity and phenocryst concentration: Geol. Soc. American Bull. v. 83, p. 3443–3448.

Koski, R. A., and Cook, D. S., 1982, Geology of the Christmas porphyry copper deposit, Gila County, Arizona, *in* Titley, S. R., ed., Advances in Geology of the Porphyry Copper Deposits, Southwestern North America: Tucson, Univ. Ariz. Press, Chapter 17.

Kreidler, E. R., and Hammel, F. A., 1970, The crystal chemistry of apatite-structural fields of fluor- and chlorapatite: Am. Mineralogist, v. 55, p. 170–184.

Kullerud, Gunnar, and Yoder, H. S., 1959, Pyrite stability relations in the Fe-S system: Econ. Geol., v. 54, p. 533–572.

Kullerud, Gunnar; Yund, R. A.; and Moh, G. H., 1969, Phase relations in the Cu-Fe-S, Cu-Ni-S, and Fe-Ni-S systems, *in* Magmatic Ore Deposits, A Symposium: Econ. Geol. Monog. 4, p. 323–343.

Lee, D. E.; Brandt, E. L. M.; Van Loenen, R. E.; Rose, H. J., Jr., 1973, The chemistry of five accessory rock-forming apatites: U.S. Geol. Survey Jour. Research, v. 1, no. 3, p. 267–272.

Lovering, T. G., 1969, Distribution of minor elements in samples of biotite from igneous rocks, *in* Geological Survey Research, 1969: U.S. Geol. Survey Prof. Paper 650–B, p. B101–B106.

———, 1972, Distribution of minor elements in biotite samples from felsic intrusive rocks as a tool for correlation: U.S. Geol. Survey Bull. 1314–D, 29 p.

Lovering, T. G.; Cooper, J. R.; Drewes, Herald, and Cone, G. G., 1970, Copper in biotite from igneous rocks in southern Arizona as an ore indicator, *in* Geological Survey Research, 1970: Geol. Survey Prof. Paper 700–B, p. B1–B8.

MacLean, W. H., 1969, Liquidus phase relations in the FeS-FeO-Fe_3O_4-SiO_2 system and their application in geology: Econ. Geol., v. 64, p. 865–884.

Nagashima, Shigeru, and Katsura, Takashi, 1973, The solubility of sulfur in Na_2O-SiO_2 melts under various partial pressures: Chem. Soc. Japan Bull, v. 46, p. 3099–3103.

Naldrett, A. J., 1969, A portion of the system Fe-S-O between 900 and 1080°C and its application to sulfide ore magmas: Jour. Petrology, v. 10, p. 171–201.

Nash, W. P., 1972*a,* Apatite-calcite equilibria in carbonatite-chemistry of apatite from Iron Hill, Colorado: Geochim. et Cosmochim. Acta, v. 36, p. 1313–1319.

———, 1972*b,* Apatite chemistry and phosphorous fugacity in a differentiated igneous intrusion: Am. Mineralogist, v. 57, p. 877–886.

Newhouse, W. H., 1936, Opaque oxides and sulfides in common igneous rocks: Geol. Soc. America Bull., v. 47, p. 1–52.

Nockolds, S. R., 1966, The behavior of some elements during fractional crystallization of magma: Goechim. et Cosmochim. Acta, v. 30, p. 267–278.

Nockolds, S. R., and Mitchell, R. L., 1946, The geochemistry of some Caledonian plutonic rocks, A study in the relationship between the major and trace elements in igneous rocks and their minerals: Royal Soc. Edinburgh Trans., v. 61, p. 533–575.

Page, N. J., 1971, Sulfide minerals in the G and H chromite zones of the Stillwater Complex, Montana: U.S. Geol. Survey Prof. Paper 694, 20 p.

Parry, W. T., 1972, Chlorine in biotites from Basin and Range plutons: Econ. Geol., v. 67, p. 972–975.

Parry, W. T., and Nackowski, M. P., 1963, Copper, lead, and zinc in biotites from Basin and Range quartz monzonite: Econ. Geol., v. 58, p. 1126–1144.

Putman, G. W., 1975, Base metal distribution in granitic rocks, II —Three dimensional variation in the Lights Creek stock: Econ. Geol., v. 70, 1225–1241.

Putman, G. W., and Burnham, C. W., 1963, Trace elements in igneous rocks, northwestern and central Arizona: Geochim. et Cosmochim. Acta, v. 27, p. 53–106.

Putman, G. W., and Alfors, J. T., 1969, Geochemistry and petrology of the Rocky Hill stock, Tulare County, California: Geol. Soc. America Spec. Paper 120, 109 p.

Ramdohr, Paul, 1940, Die erzminalien in gewöhnlichen magmatishen gestein: Preuss Acad. Wiss. Abh., nr. 2, 43 p.

Rehrig, W. A., and Heidrick, T. L., 1972, Regional fracturing in Laramide stocks of Arizona and its relationship to porphyry copper mineralization: Econ. Geol. v. 67, p. 198–213.

———, Regional tectonic stress during the Laramide and Late Tertiary intrusive periods, Basin and Range Province, Arizona: Arizona Geol. Soc. Digest, v. 10, p. 205–228.

Rehrig, W. A., and McKinney, C. N., 1976, The distribution and origin of anomalous copper in biotite: SME-AIME Preprint 76-L-64, 34 p.

Ringwood, A. E., 1955, The principles governing trace element distribution during magmatic crystallization, Part 1—the influence of electronegativity: Geochim. at Cosmochim. Acta, v. 7, p. 189–202.

Shapiro, Leonard, 1975, Rapid analysis of silicate, carbonate, and phosphate rocks—Revised edition: U.S. Geol. Survey Bull. 1401, 76 p.

Shapiro, Leonard, and Brannock, W. W., 1962, Rapid analysis of silicate, carbonate, and phosphate rocks: U.S. Geol. Survey Bull. 1144–A, 56 p.

Shimazaki, Hidehiko, and Clark, L. A., 1973, Liquidus relations in the FeS-FeO-SiO_2-Na_2O system and geological implications: Econ. Geol., v. 68, p. 79–96.

Tan, Li-Ping, 1973, Copper content of biotites from the andesitic rocks in northern Taiwan: Acta Geol. Taiwanica, no. 16, p. 47–55.

Thornton, C. P., and Tuttle, O. F., 1960, Chemistry of igneous rocks—[Pt.] 1, Differentiation index: Am. Jour. Sci., v. 258, p. 664–684.

Toulmin, Priestley III, and Barton, P. B., Jr., 1964, A thermodynamic study of pyrite and pyrrhotite: Geochim. et Cosmochim. Acta, v. 28, p. 641–671.

Wager, L. R.; Vincent, E. A.; and Smales, A. A., 1957, Sulfides in the Skaergaard intrusion: Econ. Geol., v. 52, p. 855–903.

Wager, L. R., and Brown, G. M., 1967, Layered Igneous Rocks: San Francisco, W. H. Freeman and Co., 588 p.

Yakowitz, H.; Myklebust, R. L.; and Heinrich, K. F. J., 1973, FRAME, an on-line correction procedure for quantitative electron probe analysis: Natl. Bur Standards Tech. Note 796, 46 p.

Yund, R. A., and Kullerud, Gunnar, 1966, Thermal stability of assemblages in the Cu-Fe S system: Jour. Petrology, v. 7, p. 454–488.

11

Petrology and Chemistry of Igneous Rocks

RAY PORPHYRY COPPER DISTRICT, PINAL COUNTY, ARIZONA

Henry R. Cornwall

The Ray porphyry copper deposit has many of the geologic characteristics common to most major porphyry copper deposits in the North America Cordillera (Lowell and Guilbert, 1970; Phillips et al., 1974). Its most striking difference is that the bulk of the hypogene and supergene ore occurs in host rocks to the ore-age intrusive rocks rather than in the intrusive rocks themselves. This relation is not unique to Ray, and many major deposits have one or more characteristics that deviate from the typical or average copper deposit (Lowell and Guilbert, 1970). The large proportion of relatively unaltered intrusive rock around the Ray deposit makes this area igneous attractive for gathering detailed petrochemical data that identify igneous processes occurring in magma associated in time and space with a major porphyry copper deposit.

The Ray porphyry copper district is approximately 110 km north of Tucson and 120 km east-southeast of Phoenix in southeastern Arizona. The major disseminated deposit at Ray has estimated reserves of 650 million tons (590 metric tons), 0.8 percent copper (N. A. Gambell, 1976, oral communication); three-fourths of the reserves is primary sulfide ore in which chalcopyrite is the main ore mineral, and the rest is secondary silicate ore in which chrysocolla is the main ore mineral. The ore at Ray occurs mostly in Precambrian Y diabase; other mineralized rocks are small intrusive bodies of early Tertiary granodiorite, the Granite Mountain Porphyry, and a few plugs and dikes of similar composition and age. Before the early 1970s, production was mostly from an irregular zone of chalcocite, a few to a hundred or more meters thick, in Precambrian X schist west of the diabase orebody. Major production from this deposit, reported to have contained 2.7 million tons of copper (N. A. Gambell, 1977, written communication), started in 1911; the Kennecott Copper Corporation has operated the mine since 1933.

GENERAL GEOLOGY OF THE REGION

The geology of the deposit and surrounding area (Fig. 11.1) has been described by a number of geologists (Ransome, 1919, 1923; Metz and Rose, 1966; Metz et al., 1968; Cornwall et al., 1971; Phillips et al., 1974; and Creasey et al., 1975), and various details of the associated igneous rocks have been discussed by Banks and other geologists (Banks et al., 1972; Banks and Stuckless, 1973; and Banks, 1973, 1974, 1976). The ore-age and older rocks are locally overlain unconformably by middle Tertiary and younger conglomerate and tuff (Fig. 11.2). Major high-angle, northwest-trending normal faults extend through the deposit area, intersected by major northeast-trending faults at the north end of the deposit (Fig. 11.1). Movement on some of these faults began in late Precambrian, near the time of diabase intrusion, but major deformation along these faults occurred before, after, and perhaps during intrusion of ore-age dikes and stocks. One or more slightly domed, low-angle faults occur in the area of the secondary chalcocite deposit but do not extend east of the easternmost major northwest-trending normal fault zone.

Laramide intrusive bodies representing at least 12 different rock types were emplaced near Ray during a 10-m.y. period, 70 to 60 m.y. ago. For convenience of discussion, but not necessarily implying distinct magma pulses, these rock types are grouped into five intrusive periods (Banks et al., 1972; Banks and Stuckless, 1973; Banks, 1976). All rock types are cut by sulfide veinlets, although not all occur in the ore deposit. Major plutons, together representing five rock types, were emplaced during each of the first four periods: I, Tortilla Quartz Diorite and Rattler Granodiorite; II, Tea Cup Granodiorite; III, Granite Mountain Porphyry; IV, Teapot Mountain Porphyry (see Figs. 11.1 and 11.2).

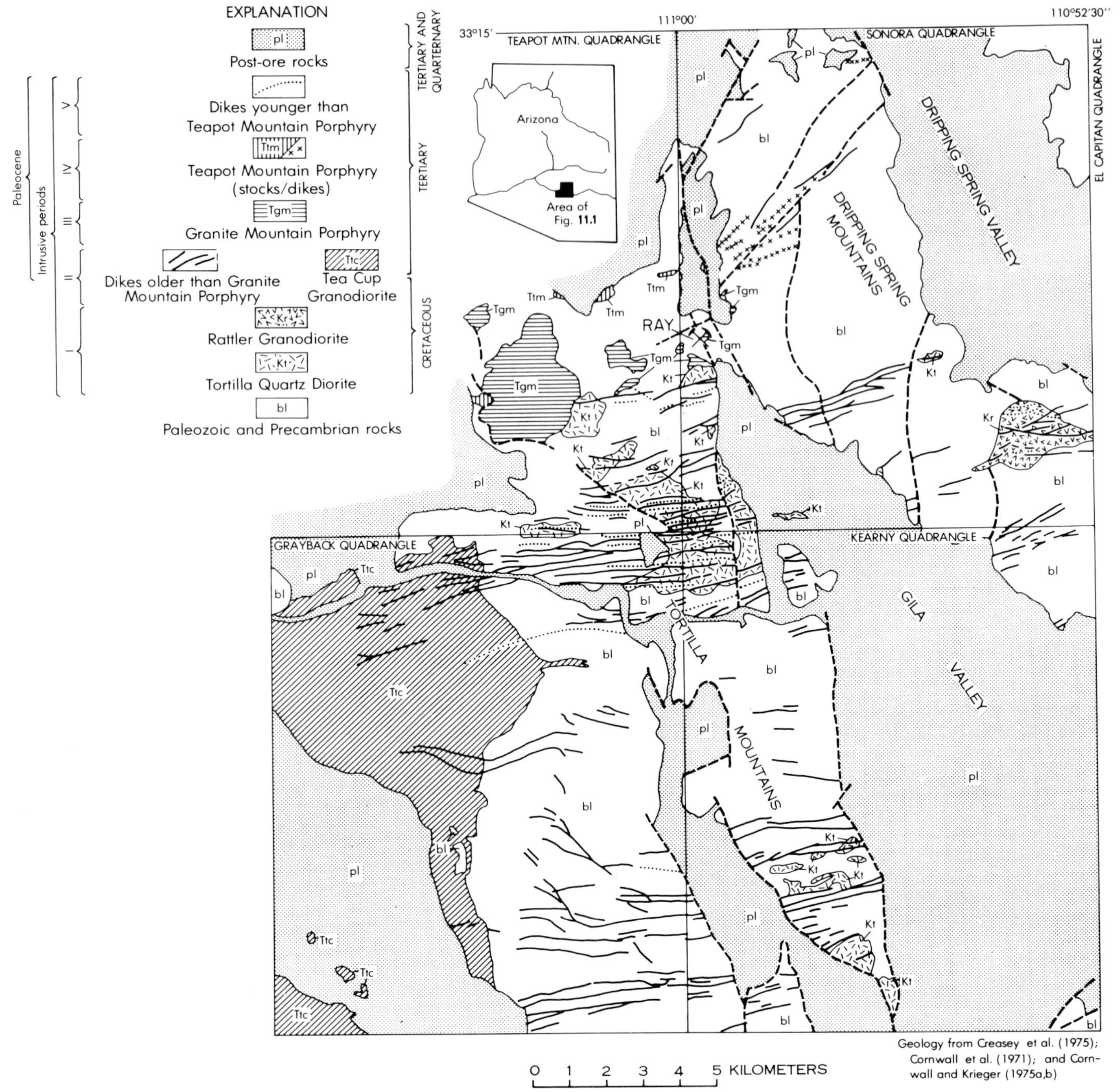

Figure 11.1. General geology of the Ray district and vicinity, Arizona. Faults shown as heavy dashed lines.

Andesitic to quartz latitic dikes were emplaced in periods II, IV, and V. A few basalt and andesite dikes emplaced west and south of the deposit prior to intrusive period I are thought to be correlative with the 70- to 85-m.y.-old volcanic rock and crosscutting diorite sills in the Hayden and Christmas quadrangles south of the study area (Banks, 1976; Banks and Krieger, 1977; Koski and Cook, 1982). Bulk compositions of the major Laramide plutons are progressively more felsic (increasing differentiation index) with decreasing age of the intrusive type—as determined by geologic relations (Cornwall et al., 1971) and by K-Ar and fission-track ages (Creasey and Kistler, 1962; Damon and Mauger, 1966; Damon, 1970; Banks et al., 1972; Banks and Stuckless, 1973).

Standard petrochemical plots of whole-rock normative minerals, major elements, and trace elements indicate that the magmas of both the dikes and the stocks of Laramide age near Ray developed along smooth chemical trends; the results are compatible with, though not proof of, either consanguinity or a common-source partial melting origin of the igneous suite. Compositions of the dike rocks are not always intermediate between those of rock types that they crosscut and that crosscut them.

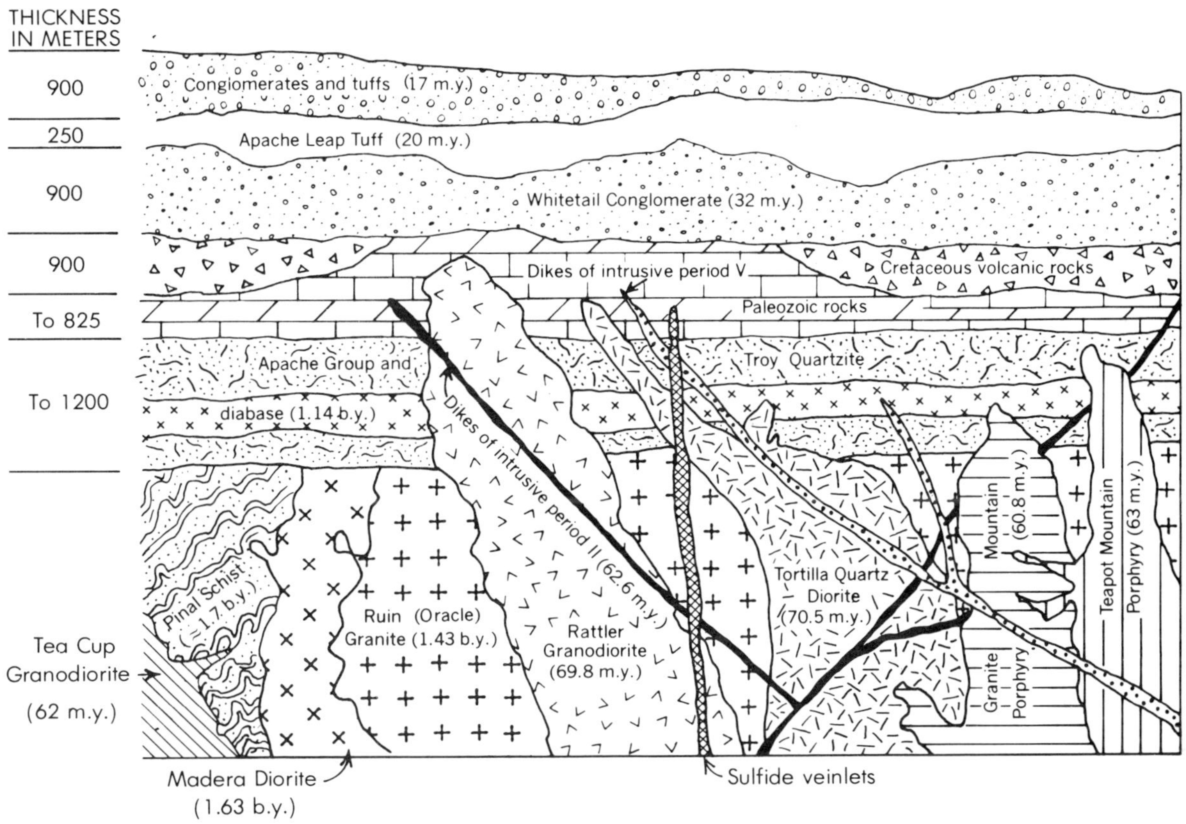

Figure 11.2. Schematic geologic section at Ray and vicinity, Arizona

Stratigraphic reconstructions indicate that the depth of cover in the Ray district at the time of the Laramide pluton intrusions was between 1 and 3 km. This depth range is similar to that estimated for the Bingham stock in the Bingham mining district, Utah, by Gilluly (1932, 1946) and Moore (1973). The maximum depth of the upper parts of the Rattler Granodiorite and some of the Tortilla Quartz Diorite is estimated to have been 1.5 km., and that of the Granite Mountain and Teapot Mountain porphyries, 2.5 km. Concordance of apatite fission-track ages with other mineral ages indicates a maximum allowable depth of 5 km for these plutons and for the Ray copper deposit during and since Laramide time (Banks and Stuckless, 1973). Stratigraphic reconstruction of the depth of intrusion of the Tea Cup Granodiorite is not possible, for it was intruded into older Precambrian granite of unknown thickness.

PETROGRAPHY

Modal data for petrographic studies were gathered using a combination of stained and unstained rock slabs and thin sections of samples determined to be typical of the 12 rock types identified during the mapping of the Sonora (Cornwall et al., 1971), Teapot Mountain (Creasey et al., 1975), and Grayback (Cornwall and Krieger, 1975*b*) quadrangles. Mineral abundance was determined by point counts (typically 500–2,000 points) of stained rock slabs with areas a minimum of 100 times the area of the largest mineral grain in the sample. These data were modified with point counts (typically 1,000–2,000 points) of stained thin sections to correct for mafic mineral ratios, minor and accessory mineral content, and ratios of groundmass minerals. Modal data for some samples of the finer-grained nonporphyritic rocks were determined with thin section counts only.

Tortilla Quartz Diorite (Intrusive Period I)

The Tortilla Quartz Diorite occurs 5 km south of the Ray mine (see Fig. 11.1) in an irregular, somewhat discontinuous mass, 5 km long and 3 km wide. It also crops out as small stocks in this area—northward into the deposit area, in the southern part of the Kearny quadrangle and eastern part of the Sonora quadrangle, and in the central El Capitan Mountain quadrangle, east of the area shown in Figure 11.1. The average age of the stocks—based on four K-Ar ages on biotite and four fission-track ages on apatite and zircon from four localities—is 70.4 ± 1.3 m.y. (Banks et al., 1972; Banks and Stuckless, 1973). This diorite intrudes Precambrian intrusive and sedimentary rocks and Paleozoic sedimentary rocks. Where intrusive into Paleozoic limestone at Elder Gulch in the southern part of the Sonora quadrangle, it is partly surrounded by breccia masses containing fragments of Pennsylvanian limestone and older rocks in a comminuted rock matrix. The Tortilla Quartz Diorite, though generally similar from stock to stock, is variable in details of composition and appearance, ranging from pyroxene-hornblende diorite to the more common biotite-hornblende-pyroxene quartz diorite and granodiorite (Figs. 11.3 and 11.4). It is fine- to medium-grained, typically with hypidiomorphic-intersertal texture, partly porphyritic, with andesine, hornblende, pyroxene (mostly augite), biotite, and magnetite-ilmenite in an interstitial matrix of quartz and potash feldspar. Locally, hornblende megacrysts occur in pods and fracture-controlled arrays (Banks et al., 1972) suggestive of late magmatic or metasomatic growth. Accessory minerals are sphene, zircon, apatite, epidote, pyrite, chalcopyrite, and bornite.

Rattler Granodiorite (Intrusive Period I)

The Rattler Granodiorite crops out as a pear-shaped body in the southeastern Sonora quadrangle. The average age in this pluton, based on three K-Ar dates on biotite and two fission-track dates on sphene and apatite from three localities, is 69.2 ± 1.2 m.y. (Banks et al., 1972; Banks and Stuckless, 1973). The granodiorite body is 2.7 km long, east to west, and 0.3 to 1.8 km wide with two apophyses to 0.9 km long extending westward from the main body (see Fig. 11.1). A second pluton of Rattler Granodiorite, 0.6 km wide and 0.9 km long, crops out 0.8 km to the east in the El Capitan Mountain quadrangle. It is overlapped on the east and north by Tertiary and Quaternary gravels. The granodiorite intrudes Precambrian sedimentary rocks and Paleozoic sedimentary rocks as young as Devonian. The main pluton ranges in composition from quartz diorite to quartz monzonite but is dominantly a granodiorite (Figs. 11.4 and 11.5) and is cut by dikes of aplitic leucocratic quartz monzonite that occupy a few of the many radial, concentric, and sheeting joints cutting the pluton.

Texturally, the Rattler Granodiorite grades from fine- to medium-grained hypidiomorphic-seriate to porphyritic rocks. Where porphyritic (Fig. 11.5*D*), the phenocrysts are most commonly plagioclase (predominantly andesine) but

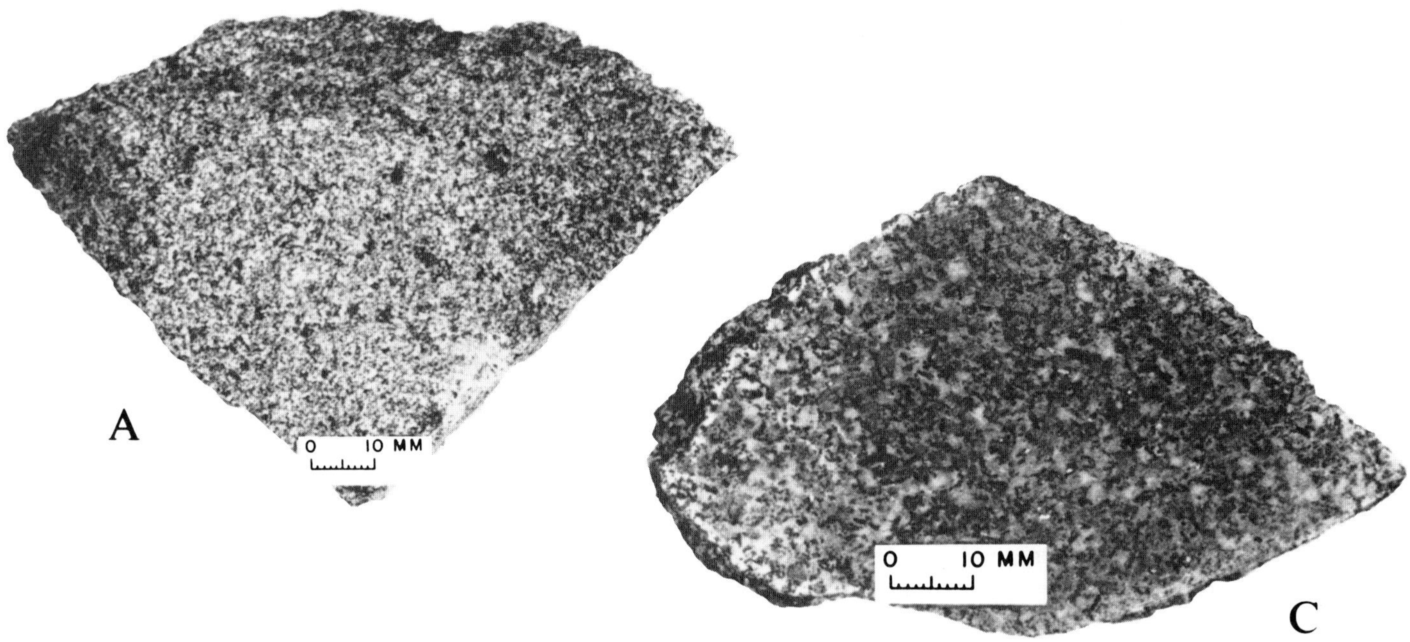

B

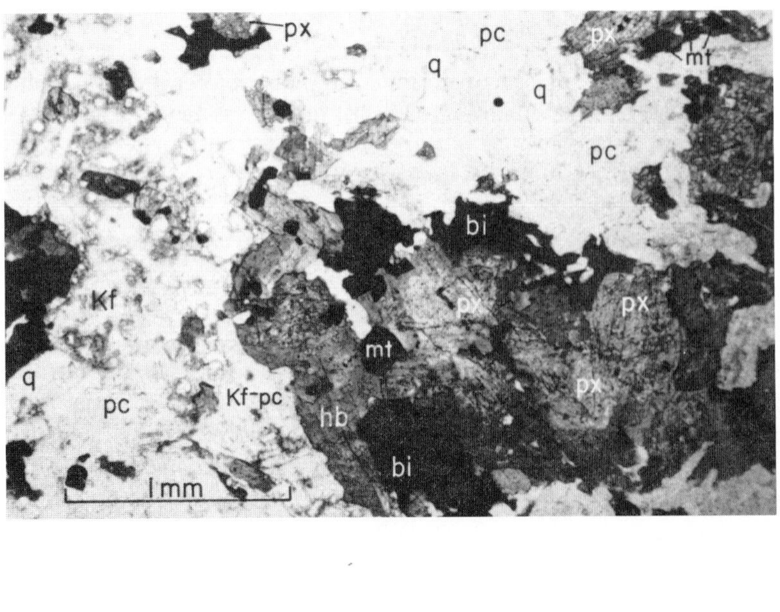

Figure 11.3. Two varieties of Tortilla Quartz Diorite: *A*, fine-grained, biotite-hornblende-pyroxene, quartz diorite; *B*, photomicrograph of intersertal texture of sample *A*; *C*, pyroxene-hornblende diorite. Key: *bi* = biotite, *hb* = hornblende, *Kf* = K-feldspar, *mt* = magnetite, *pc* = plagioclase, *px* = pyroxene, *q* = quartz.

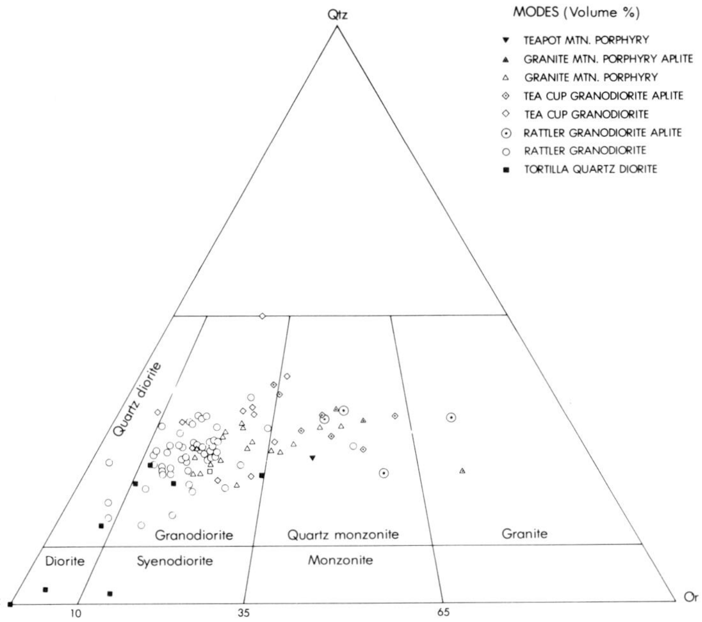

Figure 11.4. Modal proportions of K-feldspar (*Or*), quartz (*Qtz*), and plagioclase (*Pc*) of Laramide plutons in the Ray area

also include quartz, biotite, hornblende, magnetite, and apatite, 1 to 4 mm long. The groundmass and smaller grains in the seriate rocks consist of the same minerals plus magnetite, interstitial K-feldspar and quartz, and accessory minerals: apatite, sphene, zircon, sulfides, and locally primary epidote and allanite. The magmatic sulfides present here are pyrite and chalcopyrite.

Tea Cup Granodiorite (Intrusive Period II)

The Tea Cup Granodiorite occupies much of the western part of the Grayback quadrangle about 10 km southwest of the Ray copper deposit and extends south of the quadrangle for possibly 35 km and west for about 8 km (see Fig. 11.1). It is overlapped on the west and partly on the south by Tertiary and Quaternary gravels. The granodiorite has a biotite K-Ar age of 62.9 ± 1.3 m.y. (Damon, 1970) and a garnet fission-track age of 61.4 ± 3.2 m.y. (Banks and Stuckless, 1973). The pluton cuts Precambrian granite, diabase, and schist. Local apophyses of the granodiorite and its aplitic facies extend into the host rock for as much as 1,200 m. The Tea Cup Granodiorite ranges in composition from granodiorite to quartz monzonite (Figs. 11.4 and 11.6). It is medium grained and locally contains aplitic dikes and pegmatitic segregations. In some areas the pegmatitic rocks and adjacent granodiorite or quartz monzonite contain two micas, phengite and biotite, and traces to 1 percent of almandine garnet (see Fig. 11.6 *D*). Elsewhere the granodiorite and aplite contain only biotite. The texture is hypidiomorphic-seriate, porphyritic, and granitic (see Fig. 11.6). Phenocrysts, where present, are plagioclase (oligoclase-andesine), quartz, and locally hornblende up to 12 mm long. The groundmass and smaller grains in the granitic and seriate-textured rocks are of these same minerals plus K-feldspar, biotite, magnetite, and accessory minerals.

Granite Mountain Porphyry (Intrusive Period III)

The Granite Mountain Porphyry crops out in eight areas of mappable size and six smaller areas, mostly in Precambrian X schist in the southeastern Teapot Mountain quadrangle and southwestern Sonora quadrangle (see Fig. 11.1). The outcrops occupy a zone elongate in an east-northeast direction for 8 km. At the west end of the zone the outcrop width is 4 km; at the east end, 0.6 km. The Ray porphyry copper deposit is in the eastern part of this zone.

The Granite Mountain Porphyry is mostly granodiorite, but in part quartz monzonite (see Fig. 11.4). Textures grade from granitic to porphyritic (Fig. 11.7). Phenocrysts are plagioclase (oligoclase and andesine), quartz, and K-feldspar. In addition, the rock contains biotite, magnetite, and the accessory minerals sphene, apatite, zircon, allanite, monazite, hornblende, and sparse magmatic sulfides. The average of four K-Ar ages on biotite and one sphene fission-track age for four samples of the main pluton is 60.6 ± 1.5 m.y. (Banks et al., 1972; Banks and Stuckless, 1973).

Teapot Mountain Porphyry (Intrusive Period IV)

The Teapot Mountain Porphyry is one of the youngest Laramide intrusive rocks in the area. The most concentrated occurrence of small plugs and dikes of this porphyry is in the Teapot Mountain and Sonora quadrangles in a zone just north of the zone of Granite Mountain Porphyry plugs (see Fig. 11.1). The rock is quartz monzonitic in composition (see Fig. 11.4) and similar in appearance to some varieties of the rhyodacite porphyry dikes. It is distinguishable by the presence of large phenocrysts of pink K-feldspar that have yielded an anomalously old K-Ar age, 63.0 ± 0.7 m.y. (Banks et al., 1972). It also contains phenocrysts of quartz, plagioclase, and biotite in an aphanitic groundmass (Fig. 11.8).

Dikes (Intrusive Periods: Pre-I, II, IV, and V)

Laramide dikes and small plugs, ranging in composition from andesite to quartz latite, are closely related temporally and spatially to the larger plutons described. The oldest (pre-intrusive period I) are basaltic and andesitic (Fig. 11.8*B*), with K-Ar ages of 70 to 85 m.y. (Koski and Cook, 1982; unpublished fission-track ages in Hayden quadrangle, C. W. Naeser, 1977, written communication); the youngest (from intrusive period V) are rhyodacitic and quartz latitic, with a probable age of about 60 m.y. (Fig. 11.9*C*, *D*); the most numerous are andesitic and rhyodacitic dikes of intrusive period II—ca. 62 m.y. (Figs. 11.8*C*-*E*, 11.9*A*, *B*). The Laramide dikes thus range from older to somewhat younger than the larger intrusive bodies. The dikes are steep to vertical and trend mainly east-west to N70°E, locally northwest or northeast. They are generally less than 30 m thick, most commonly 1 to 5 m thick.

The andesite dikes contain phenocrysts of pyroxene, hornblende, and labradorite in a groundmass of these minerals plus a little quartz, K-feldspar, ilmenite-magnetite, and accessory minerals. The rhyodacite porphyries contain phenocrysts up to 15 mm long of andesine, hornblende, quartz, biotite, and magnetite in a groundmass of the same

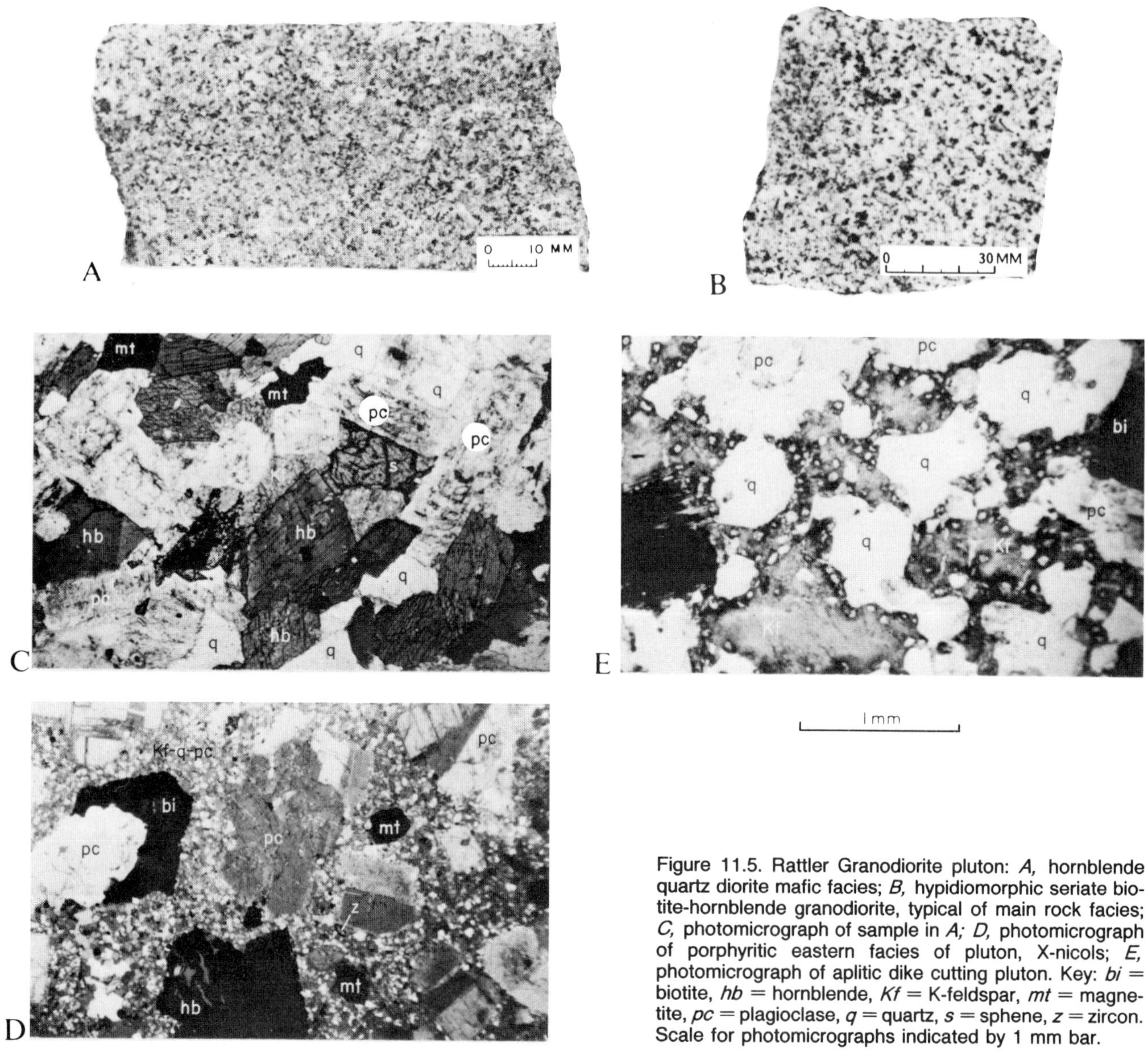

Figure 11.5. Rattler Granodiorite pluton: *A,* hornblende quartz diorite mafic facies; *B,* hypidiomorphic seriate biotite-hornblende granodiorite, typical of main rock facies; *C,* photomicrograph of sample in *A; D,* photomicrograph of porphyritic eastern facies of pluton, X-nicols; *E,* photomicrograph of aplitic dike cutting pluton. Key: *bi* = biotite, *hb* = hornblende, *Kf* = K-feldspar, *mt* = magnetite, *pc* = plagioclase, *q* = quartz, *s* = sphene, *z* = zircon. Scale for photomicrographs indicated by 1 mm bar.

minerals plus K-feldspar and accessories. The quartz latite porphyry dikes are similar to the rhyodacite dikes, but contain more K-feldspar in the groundmass and generally fewer phenocrysts. Both the rhyodacite and quartz latite are similar to facies of Teapot Mountain Porphyry that have few or sparse K-feldspar phenocrysts.

A modal ternary plot of the dikes and small plugs on K-feldspar–quartz–plagioclase (Fig. 11.10) shows a compositional field similar to that of the major plutons (see Fig. 11.4), but with less modal quartz. This composition probably reflects greater uncertainty in resolving groundmass minerals in the dikes than in the plutons because the dikes do not fall into a separate field with respect to normative and other chemical plots.

MINERAL PARAGENESIS

The paragenesis of the minerals in igneous intrusive rocks can generally be determined by microscopic examination of the textural relations. For example, phenocrysts are considered to be older than the enclosing groundmass, euhedral crystals are older than interstitial subhedral to anhedral minerals, and euhedral crystals in larger euhedral crystals are older than the enclosing crystals. These relations can be misleading, however. Euhedral crystals of one species may develop early, at the expense of displaced silicate magma, whereas formation of euhedral faces on another species may occur later, at the expense of anhedral crystal development of adjacent but contemporaneous silicate minerals. Early inclusion of one mineral in another might also result from local concentration of the required components caused by their rejection during growth of the larger host prior to saturation of the included mineral throughout the magma. A valid paragenetic sequence is still determinable when the same pattern of relations is repeatedly observed. Under these criteria, the following general paragenetic sequence for the main facies of the major Laramide intrusives at Ray is obtained (see also Banks, 1976).

Among the major minerals, plagioclase and pyroxene, where present, formed first and are commonly euhedral.

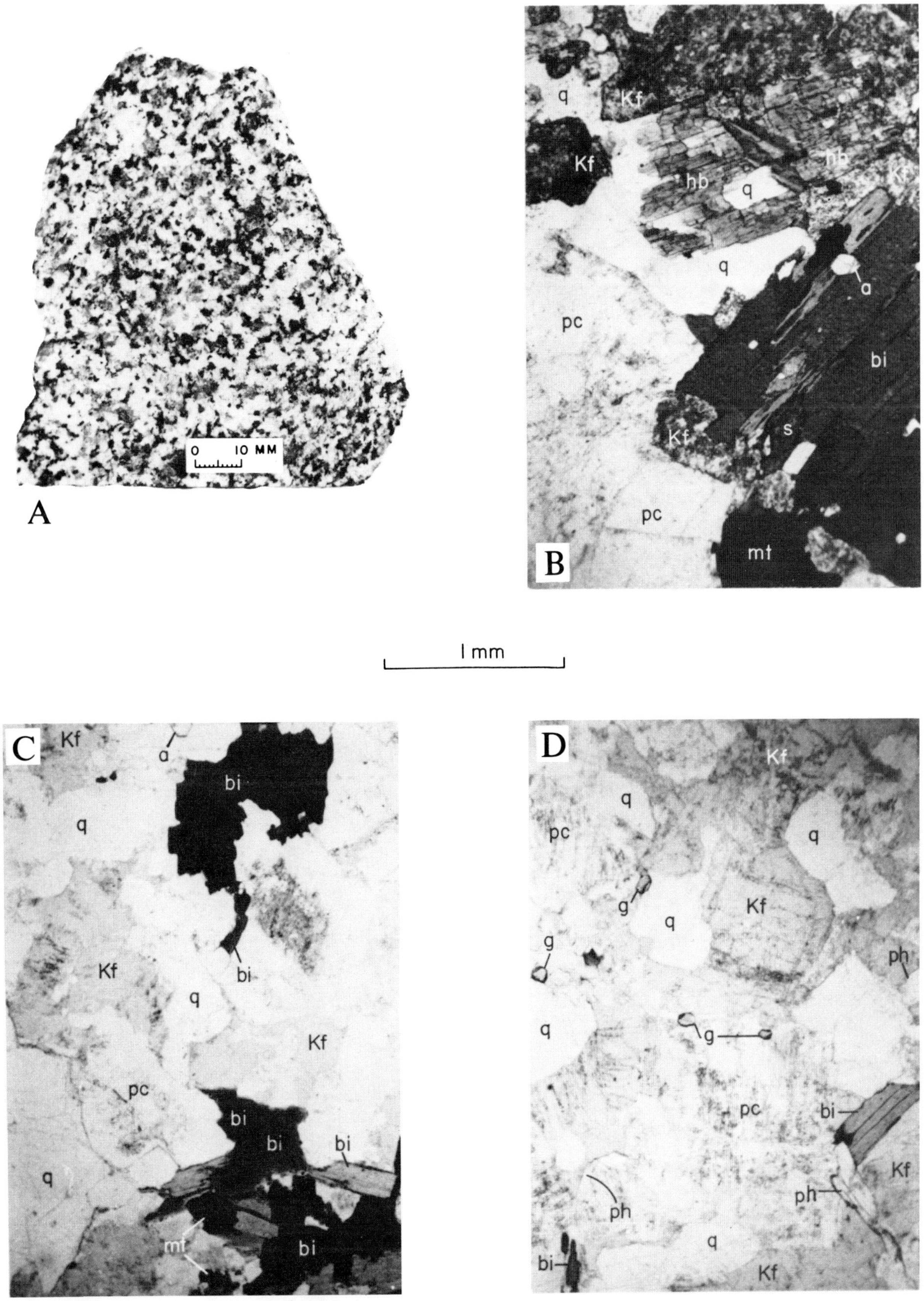

Figure 11.6. Tea Cup Granodiorite: *A,* Hypidiomorphic-seriate, hornblende-biotite granodiorite; *B,* photomicrograph of hypidiomorphic seriate, hornblende-biotite granodiorite; *C,* photomicrograph of granitoid biotite quartz monzonite; *D,* photomicrograph of two-mica, garnet-bearing aplitic facies. Key: *a* = apatite, *bi* = biotite, *g* = garnet, *hb* = hornblende, *Kf* = K-feldspar, *mt* = magnetite, *pc* = plagioclase, *ph* = phengite, *q* = quartz, *s* = sphene. Scale for photomicrographs (*B, C, D*) indicated by 1 mm bar.

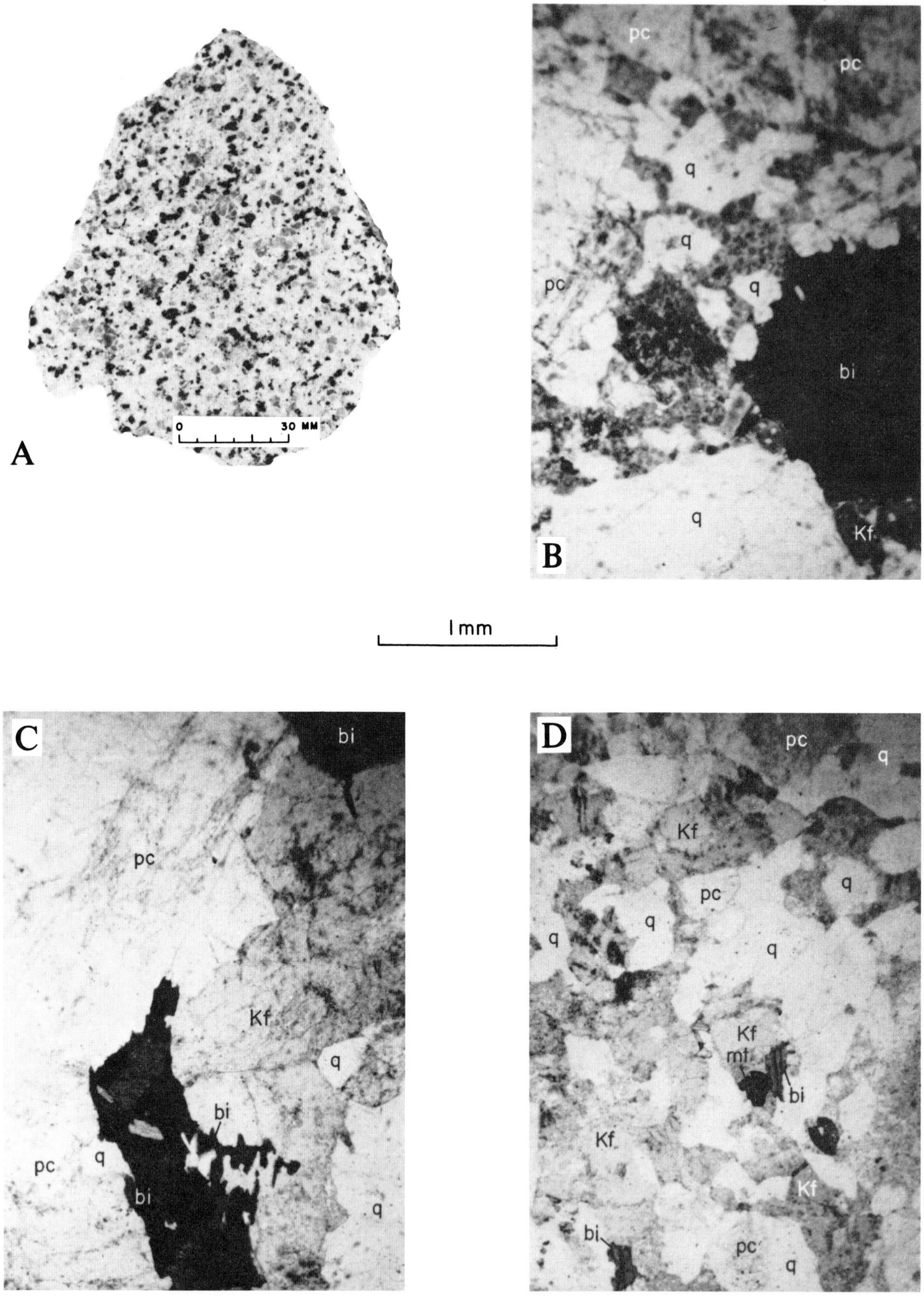

Figure 11.7. Granite Mountain Porphyry: *A,* porphyritic granodiorite facies of main pluton; *B,* photomicrograph of sample in *A; C,* photomicrograph of granitoid facies of Granite Mountain Porphyry; *D,* photomicrograph of aplitic dike. Key: *bi* = biotite, *Kf* = K-feldspar, *mt* = magnetite, *pc* = plagioclase, *q* = quartz. Scale for photomicrographs (*B, C, D*) indicated by 1 mm bar.

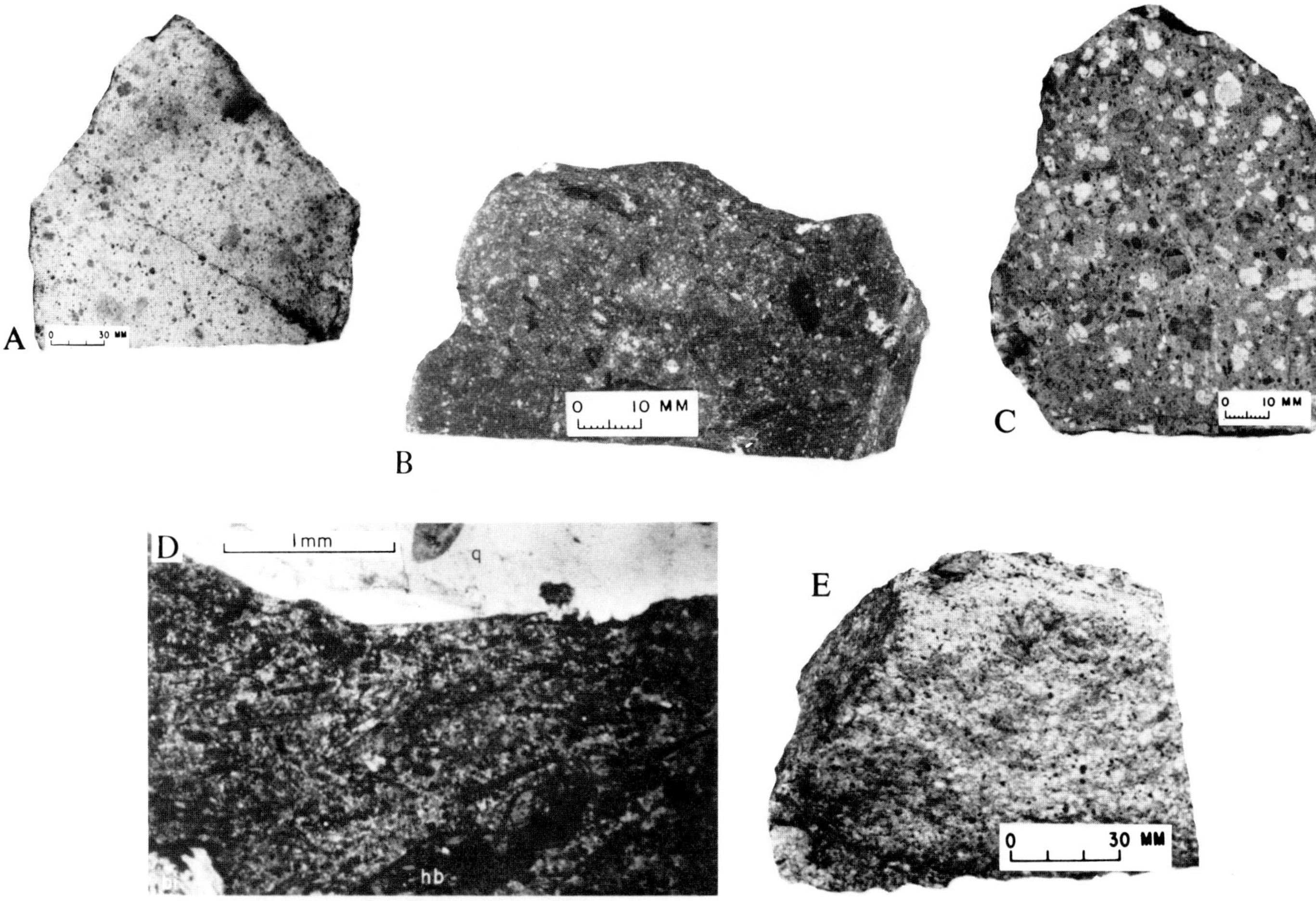

Figure 11.8. Teapot Mountain Porphyry and representative rock types in dikes near Ray: *A,* large phenocrysts (K-feldspar) and smaller phenocrysts (plagioclase, quartz, and biotite) in stained specimen of Teapot Mountain Porphyry; *B,* pre-intrusive period I, hornblende-pyroxene andesite dike; *C,* early melanocratic rhyodacite dike of intrusive period II; *D,* photomicrograph of sample in *C; E,* rhyodacite dike with quartz phenocrysts. Key: *bi* = biotite, *hb* = hornblende, *q* = quartz.

Hornblende, where present, is an early mineral but in part formed by reaction between the melt and pyroxene. Accessory zircon and apatite grains also are commonly euhedral and occur to some extent in the early-formed minerals. However, they are larger and occur most commonly in or with late- and intermediate-stage minerals; these characteristics suggest that their occurrence with the early-formed minerals is the result of local processes of concentrations of the required chemical components. Sphene appears to be late in the more mafic rocks and intermediate in the more felsic. Igneous epidote and allanite, where present, appear to be late interstitial minerals. Paragenesis of the sulfide minerals is treated by Banks in Chapter 10 of this volume.

In the intermediate stage of crystallation, plagioclase formed along with quartz, biotite, and magnetite. Pyroxene and hornblende ceased to form during this stage. The late stage was characterized by the same minerals as those formed in the intermediate stage plus K-feldspar. In the more felsic rocks, K-feldspar and quartz crystallization began earlier relative to biotite and magnetite than in the more mafic rocks.

The paragenetic sequence described was observed, with moderate local variations, in all the major Laramide plutons at Ray. In the dikes and small plugs early-formed minerals occur as phenocrysts in fine-grained to aphanitic groundmasses of quartz, K-feldspar, and plagioclase, together with biotite, hornblende, and opaque minerals. The andesites contain phenocrysts of pyroxene, hornblende, and plagioclase. Some of the rhyodacite and quartz latite dikes contain phenocrysts of quartz, biotite, and magnetite, as well as of plagioclase and hornblende. The Teapot Mountain Porphyry contains these same phenocrysts but has prominent large K-feldspar crysts in place of hornblende.

CHEMICAL DATA

The normative ternary plot of K-feldspar–quartz–plagioclase (Ab + An), shown in Figure 11.11, illustrates a similar but more orderly trend relative to the correlative modal plots (see Figs. 11.4 and 11.10). This similarity probably results from a combination of fewer data and more averaged data because of the large size of the individual samples analyzed. There is a shift of the mafic end of the normative plot toward the K-feldspar corner produced by the substantial amount of K_2O in biotite, which is quite abundant in the quartz diorite and mafic granodiorite and is calculated as K-feldspar in this diagram. The normative K-feldspar, anorthite, and albite

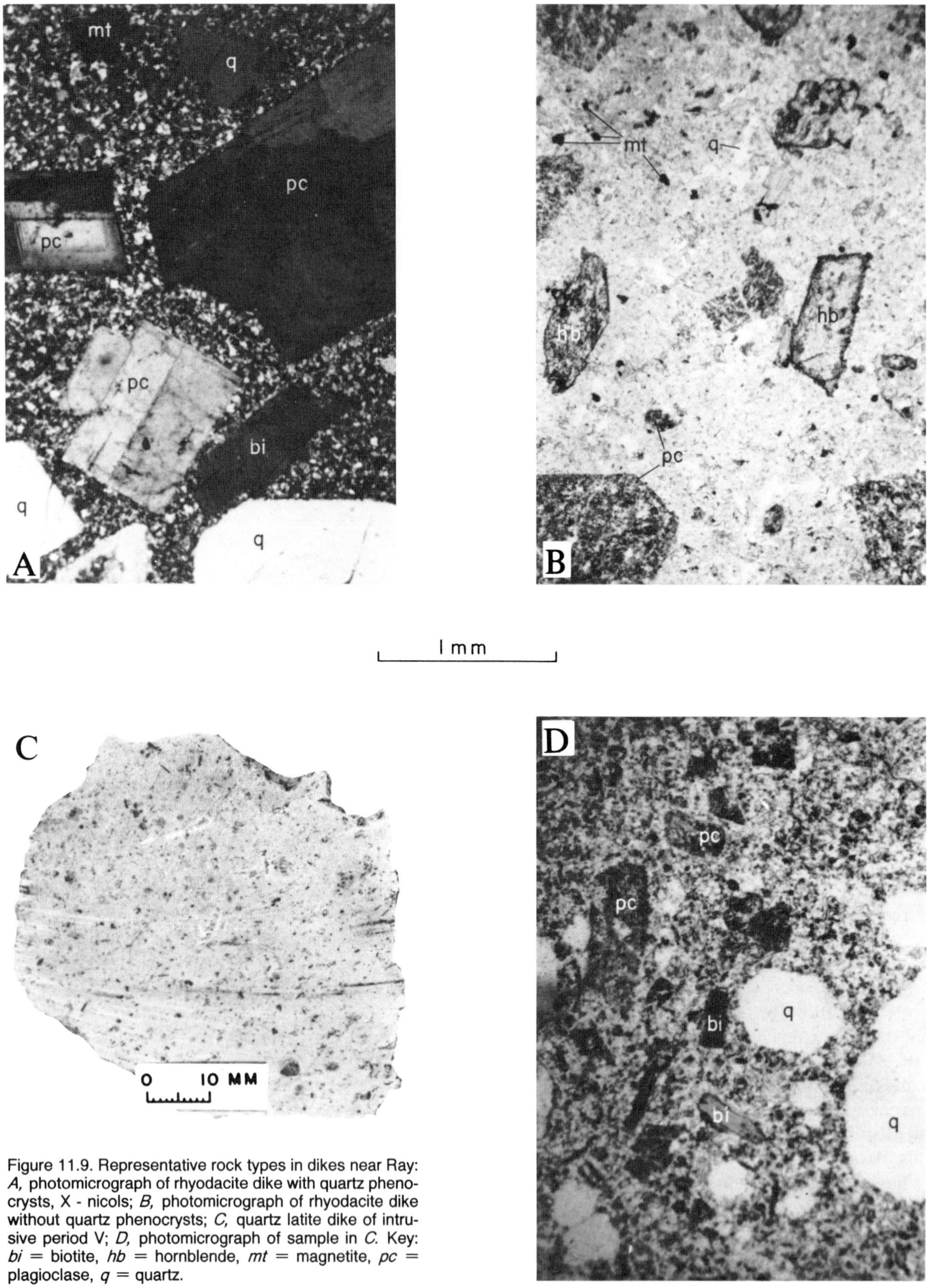

Figure 11.9. Representative rock types in dikes near Ray: *A,* photomicrograph of rhyodacite dike with quartz phenocrysts, X - nicols; *B,* photomicrograph of rhyodacite dike without quartz phenocrysts; *C,* quartz latite dike of intrusive period V; *D,* photomicrograph of sample in *C.* Key: *bi* = biotite, *hb* = hornblende, *mt* = magnetite, *pc* = plagioclase, *q* = quartz.

and K-feldspar, quartz, and albite ternaries (Figs. 11.12 and 11.13) show, as expected, a trend from anorthite and albite to quartz and K-feldspar in progressively younger rocks, both within individual plutons and between progressively younger, more differentiated plutons and dikes. The rocks lowest in anorthite and albite and richest in quartz and K-feldspar are the Teapot Mountain Porphyry and the aplitic facies of the older plutons.

The oxides of the major cations plotted relative to differentiation index (Thornton and Tuttle, 1960) in Figure 11.14

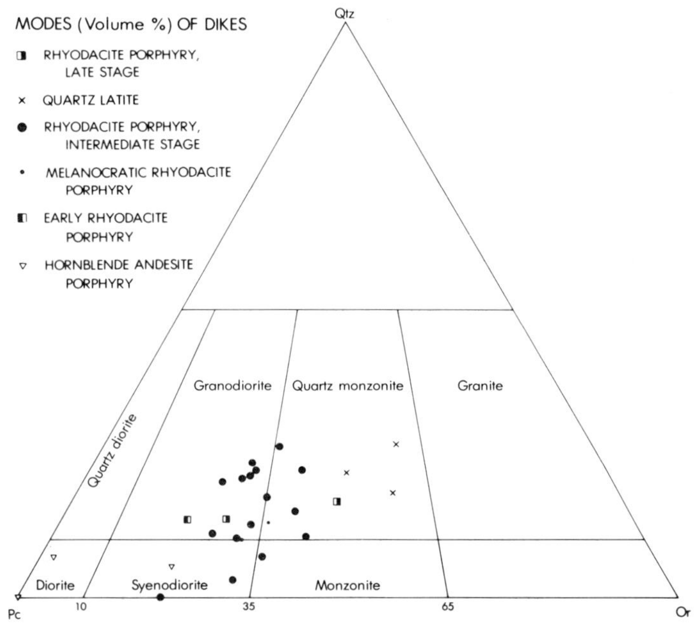

Figure 11.10. Modal proportions (volume %) of K-feldspar (*Or*), quartz (*Qtz*), and plagioclase (*Pc*) of dikes in the Ray area

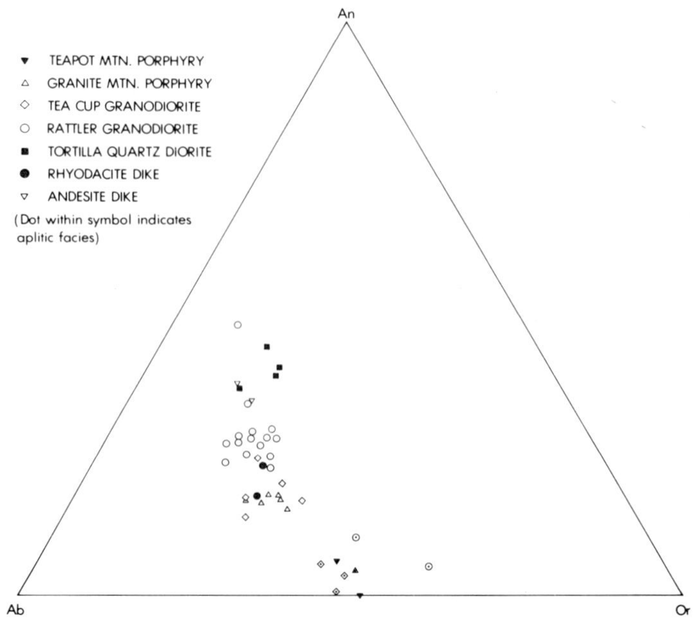

Figure 11.12. Normative proportions (weight %) of K-feldspar (*Or*), anorthite (*An*), and albite (*Ab*)

show a range in D.I. from 48 for the most mafic to 96 for the most silicic rocks. The andesites, Tortilla Quartz Diorite, and mafic facies of the Rattler Granodiorite are the most mafic, ranging in D.I. from 48 to 58. The main body of the Rattler Granodiorite is intermediate in composition, ranging in D.I. from 65 to 78. The Granite Mountain Porphyry and Tea Cup Granodiorite are the most silicic of the major plutons, ranging in D.I. from 79 to 87. Dikes and small stocks of rhyodacite and Teapot Mountain Porphyry overlap the Rattler Granodiorite and Granite Mountain Porphyry in D. I. Aplites of the Rattler Granodiorite, Granite Mountain Porphyry, and Tea Cup Granodiorite range in D.I. from 93 to 96 except for one of 87 from the Rattler Granodiorite.

SiO_2 and K_2O show an orderly increase with increasing D.I.: the SiO_2 from 55 to 76 percent, the K_2O from 1.5 to 6 percent. Al_2O_3, total Fe as FeO, MgO, and CaO decrease with increasing D.I.: Al_2O_3, 19 to 13 percent; ΣFe, 9 to 0.5 percent; MgO, 4 to 0 percent; CaO, 8 to 0.3 percent. For all of these constituents the trends are reasonably orderly, except for MgO in an andesite with a D.I. of 55 that has a high MgO content of 5.3 percent. Na_2O ranges from 2.7 to 4.2

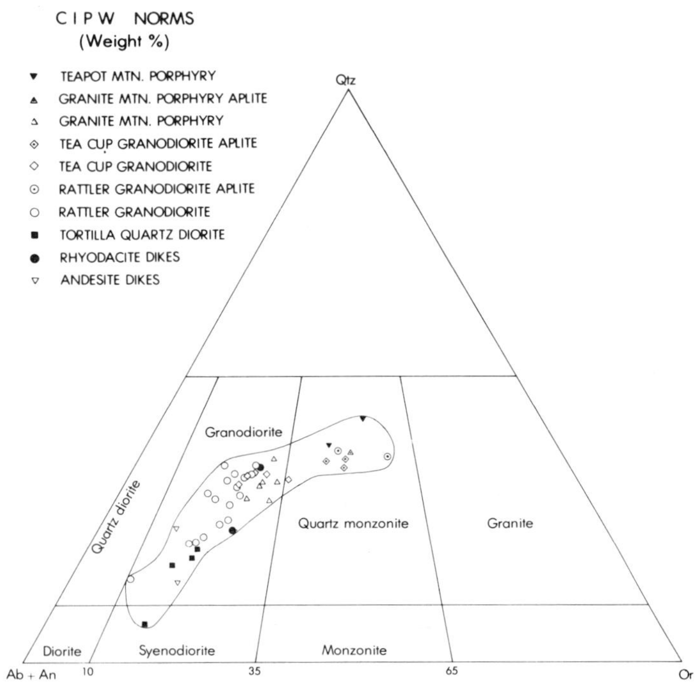

Figure 11.11. Normative proportions (weight %) of K-feldspar (*Or*), quartz (*Qtz*), and plagioclase (*Ab* + *An*)

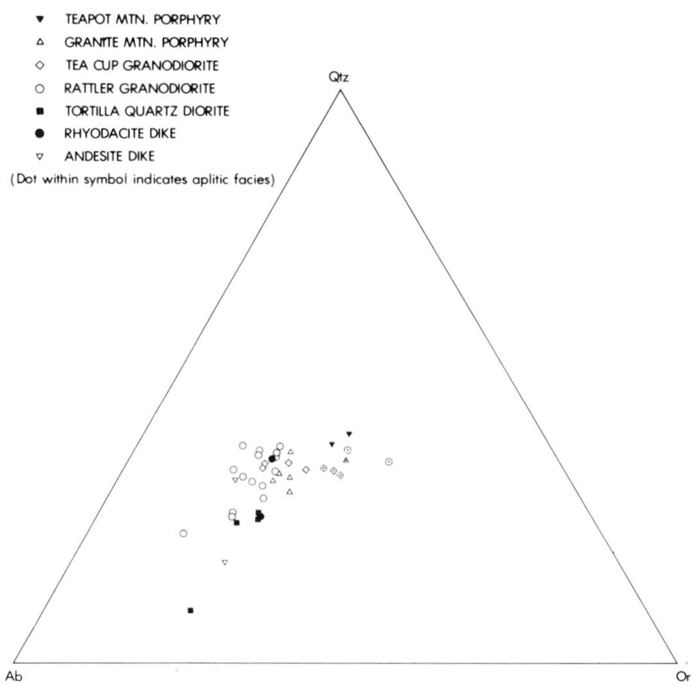

Figure 11.13. Normative proportions (weight %) of K-feldspar (*Or*), quartz (*Qtz*), and albite (*Ab*)

percent in these rocks but does not show an appreciable trend with increasing D.I.

In considering the trends of the oxides, it should be kept in mind that because the sum of the oxides in an analysis is constant, a large increase in one oxide (commonly SiO_2) causes a proportionate decrease in the sum of the remaining oxides. The true trends of individual oxides, though modified by this effect, still convey a general impression of relative increases and decreases, especially where marked. This problem has been discussed by Chayes (1967), Krauskopf (1967), and other workers.

The minor elements show similar tight grouping of data along differentiation trends within and between the individual plutons. The associations between minor elements and between minor elements and major elements and D.I. are indicated in Table 11.1 by the Spearman non-parametric rank correlation coefficients for all the chemical data from the individual plutons and all the plutons. Strong positive correlations have been found between manganese (Mn), cobalt (Co), scandium (Sc), and vanadium (V) and between these elements and the major elements A1, Ti, Fe, Mg, Ca, P. (The Mn-P correlation, 0.54, is not strong and is below the cutoff of 0.59 for this table). Strontium shows a similar strong correlation for all the elements except Mn. Except for Sr-Si, these elements show a strong negative correlation with D.I., Si, and K (Sr-Si coefficient –0.56).

Yttrium (Y) correlates positively with Ti, Fe, Mg, Ca, P, and Yb (Ytterbium), and negatively with D.I. Gallium correlates positively with Fe and P and negatively with Si. Lead correlates positively with D.I. and negatively with Fe, Mg, and Ca. Copper has poor correlation with other elements, the highest with Ti, Fe, Mg, P (coefficient 0.37–0.42).

TABLE 11.1
Correlation of Minor Elements With Other Minor and Major Elements and Differentiation Index (D.I.)

Positive Correlations				
Mn-Al	Co-Al	Sc-Al	Sr-Al	V-Al
Mn-Ti	Co-Ti	Sc-Ti	Sr-Ti	V-Ti
Mn-ΣFe	Co-ΣFe	Sc-ΣFe	Sr-ΣFe	V-ΣFe
Mn-Mg	Co-Mg	Sc-Mg		V-Mg
Mn-Ca	Co-Ca	Sc-Ca	Sr-Ca	V-Ca
	Co-P	Sc-P	Sr-P	V-P
Mn-Co	Co-Mn			V-Mn
Mn-Sc	Co-V	Sc-Mn		V-Co
	Co-Sc	Sc-Co	Sr-Ba	V-Sc
Mn-V		Sc-V	Sr-V	V-Sr
	Y-Ti	D.I.-Pb		
Ga-ΣFe	Y-ΣFe			
	Y-Mg			
	Y-Ca			
Ga-P	Y-P			
	Y-Yb			

Negative Correlations					
D.I.-Mn	Mn-Si	Co-Si	Ga-Si	Sc-Si	V-Si
D.I.-Co	Mn-K	Co-K	Sr-K	Sc-K	V-K
D.I.-Sc	Pb-ΣFe				
D.I.-Sr	Pb-Mg				
D.I.-V	Pb-Ca				
D.I.-Y					

NOTE: Correlations are indicated by ± Spearman rank correlation coefficients greater than 0.59, significant at 99 percent confidence level, and based on 76 minor vs. minor element pairs, 37 minor vs. major element pairs, and 37 minor vs. D.I. pairs.

The correlations between elements within individual plutons, where there are sufficient element pairs to be significant, are similar to those shown in Table 11.1 and discussed for the combined data, except that in the Rattler Granodiorite there are no negative correlations between Pb and Fe, Mg, or Ca. These data suggest a common source for the magmas but do not distinguish between common-source partial melting in the upper mantle or lower crust and upper crustal batholithic differentiation.

COMPARISON WITH OTHER IGNEOUS SUITES

Chemistry

Laramide igneous rocks in the Ray porphyry copper district do not appear to be unique among other calc-alkaline suites. Using the criterion of Peacock (1931), the trend line of $Na_2O + K_2O$ crosses the trend line of CaO at about D.I. 60, where the SiO_2 line is at 60 percent (see Fig. 11.14). This is in the calc-alkalic (calc-alkaline) range. These rocks also fall in the calc-alkaline field using the criteria of Irvine and Baragar (1971). The similarity of the Laramide igneous rocks at Ray to other calc-alkalic suites is probably best illustrated by the ternary plot of normative Or-Qtz-Ab + An (Fig. 11.15) for the rocks in the Ray district and by the trend lines for all available analyses of Laramide intrusives in southern Arizona (S. C. Creasey, 1977, written communication), for the eastern and western Sierra Nevada batholith (Ross, 1972), and for five analyses of granodiorite related to a porphyry copper deposit at Battle Mountain, Nevada (Theodore et al., 1973). The similarity of these diverse suites, some related to porphyry copper deposits and some barren of copper mineralization, is very striking and significant, though not a new observation.

The trends of the percentages of various oxides plotted against D.I. of the Laramide igneous rocks at Ray are similar to igneous suites in general, as evident, for example, in the 5,000 igneous-rock analyses compiled by Washington (1917) and contoured by Thornton and Tuttle (1960); the igneous rocks of the Coast and Transverse Ranges, California (Ross, 1972); and the igneous rocks at Bingham, Utah (Moore, 1973).

Volatile Content of the Magmas

As has been pointed out by Banks (1976), several petrochemical features of the Laramide plutons in the Ray area suggest that they did not saturate early during their crystallization nor evolve much water. The MgO content of the biotite decreases slightly with increasing D.I. but markedly with decreasing age of the intrusives. Wones and Eugster (1965) have suggested that such a trend indicates undersaturation of water in the melt. Low content of volatiles in the magmas is indicated by the following characteristics: scarcity of aplites and pegmatites in the plutons, only minor metamorphic aureoles around all of the intrusive bodies, absence of miarolitic cavities, sparsity of fluid inclusions in quartz, and the fact that these inclusions are dilute, two-phase, and homogenious below 450°C (J. T. Nash, 1971, 1972, written communications; M. J. Logsdon, 1973, oral communication).

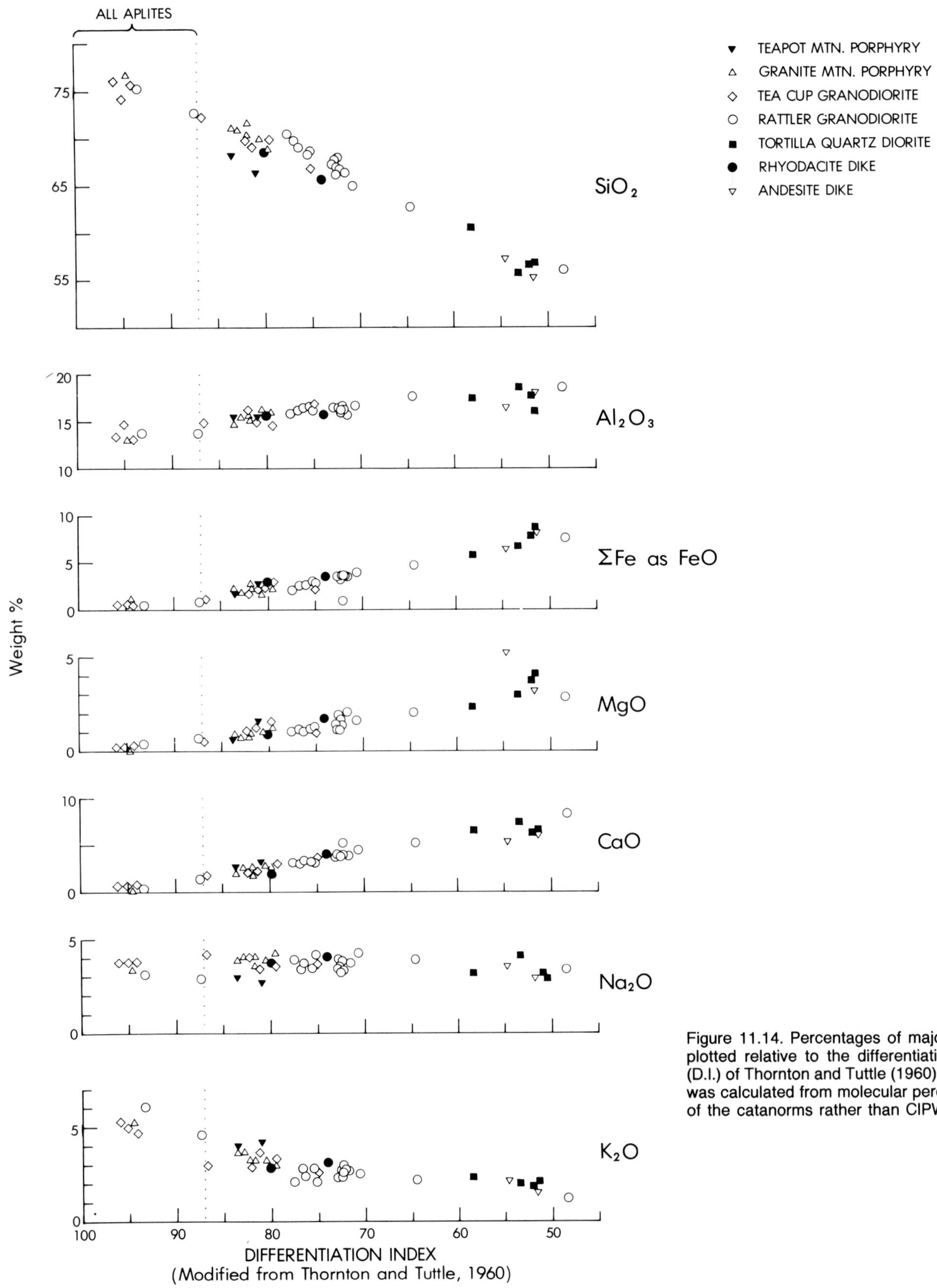

Figure 11.14. Percentages of major oxides plotted relative to the differentiation index (D.I.) of Thornton and Tuttle (1960). The D.I. was calculated from molecular percentages of the catanorms rather than CIPW norms.

The water content of the magmas at their emplacement is indicated by the point during crystallization at which hydrous minerals first formed. In the rhyodacite dikes, Teapot Mountain Porphyry, and a restricted porphyritic facies of the Rattler Granodiorite, phenocrysts of biotite and hornblende occur in a fine-grained groundmass that makes up 30 to 50 percent of the rock; this composition indicates that the hydrous minerals started to form before the midpoint of crystallization. However, in the Granite Mountain Porphyry, Tea Cup Granodiorite, Tortilla Quartz Diorite, and the main

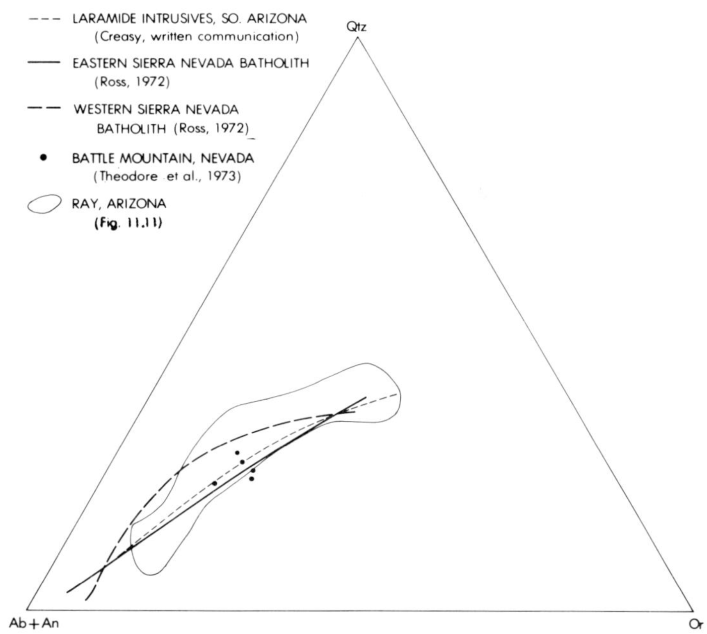

Figure 11.15. Comparison of normative (weight %) K-feldspar (*Or*), quartz (*Qtz*), and plagioclase (*Ab* + *An*) of Ray intrusives with other Laramide intrusives in southern Arizona (54 analyses), with the Sierra Nevada Batholith, and with intrusives in the Battle Mountain mining district, Nevada.

facies of the Rattler Granodiorite the hydrous minerals are intergrown with quartz and K-feldspar and are interstitial to plagioclase, which makes up about 50 percent of the rocks. In these rocks—which largely constitute the intrusive bodies at Ray—biotite and hornblende probably did not start to form before the midpoint of solidification.

At their depths of emplacement, the intrusive rocks at Ray should have contained 2.5 to 3.0 weight percent H_2O before biotite started to form (D. R. Wones, 1973, oral communication; Wones and Dodge, 1966). If, as indicated, biotite first formed after the plutons were 50-percent crystallized, then the initial water content of the more mafic magma must have been less than 1.5 percent and even less in the more felsic magma. These amounts approximate those now locked in the rocks in primary hydrous minerals and are less than the amounts required to saturate the magmas at the depth of intrusion with water; this fact suggests that little water escaped the magmas. Textural studies show that the hydrous minerals have crosscutting, interstitial, and coeval relations with the late-forming anhydrous minerals (mainly quartz, K-feldspar, and plagioclase) and that they occur in late-stage aplitic differentiates of all the plutons. Therefore, the hydrous phases would have continued to maintain the amount of water present in the silicate melt at 2 to 3 percent, until only a small amount—if any—liquid remained.

Banks (1976), in a study of the halogen contents of igneous minerals in Laramide intrusive rocks at Ray, has found no indication that Cl or H_2O build up in individual melts or with development of the igneous suite as a whole, as required for the generation of magmatic ore solutions. He has revealed that the rocks in the Ray district cannot be distinguished from other calc-alkaline suites with respect to rock or mineral contents of Cl, F, and H_2O or with respect to the trends of these contents with indicators of rock differentiation. The results of his study can be summarized as follows (Banks, 1976, p. 91):

1. Apatite and biotite in younger, more silicic rocks contain more F but less Cl and H_2O+ than apatite and biotite in older, more mafic rock; the same relations hold for F and H_2O+ in sphene.
2. The contents of Cl, F, and H_2O+ in whole-rock samples decrease with increasing differentiation index and decreasing age.
3. The data are satisfactorily although not exclusively explained by postulating that the melts each contained progressively less Cl, F, and H_2O and that the hydrous minerals consumed most of the Cl, F, and H_2O in the magmas.
4. The data are similar to those for plutons that are not associated with porphyry copper deposits.

SOURCE OF COPPER IN THE RAY DEPOSIT

In speculating on the source of the copper and the mineralizing solutions that formed the Ray deposit, several factors should be considered. The age of mineralization has been determined by K-Ar dating of hydrothermal biotite intergrown with ore minerals at 65 m.y. (Banks et al., 1972). This date is close to but anomalously older than the K-Ar age of 61 m.y. for the Granite Mountain Porphyry, which was mineralized by the ore solutions at the deposit. The K-Ar age of the hydrothermal biotite is also close to but slightly older than the age of 63 m.y. (Banks et al., 1972) for the Teapot Mountain Porphyry, which crops out as a northeast-trending zone of small stocks and dikes 0.8 km north of the Ray deposit. The Tortilla Quartz Diorite, dated at 70 m.y. (Banks et al., 1972), crops out in a small stock 0.8 km south of the deposit and in a large pluton 3 km to the southwest.

These intrusives plus east-trending rhyodacite dikes in the area are the intrusive rocks that are spatially, and possibly genetically, closely related to the Ray copper deposit. Ore solutions may have emanated directly from one of these igneous bodies or from a common source beneath the area at shallow or great depth. The ore deposit and two of the intrusive bodies (Granite Mountain Porphyry and Teapot Mountain Porphyry) occur near the intersection of major northwest- and northeast-trending fault zones. These intersecting shear zones provided access to the surface from great depth for both magmas and hydrothermal solutions.

I favor a model of magmas and copper-bearing hydrothermal solutions ascending from considerable depth, probably from the upper mantle. Derivation of the copper-bearing solutions directly from one of the nearby plutons does not appear likely, in view of the probable small amounts of volatiles that could have evolved from these intrusives. If a local source directly from a pluton is postulated, the Granite Mountain Porphyry is the most likely one. The small stocks in the area of the copper deposit should be underlain at shallow depth by a larger body from which the solutions could have emanated.

ACKNOWLEDGMENTS

I am grateful to Norman G. Banks for his support in this study and for his suggestions concerning the significance of the data obtained. Critical review of this chapter by Norman G. Banks and Arthur S. Radtke is also acknowledged. Chemical data presented here are based on rapid rock analyses by P. L. D. Elmore, Gillison Chloe, J. L. Glenn, Lowell Artis, John Kelsey, and Hezekiah Smith and on quantitative and semi-quantitative spectrographic analyses by R. E. Mays and Chris Heropoulos.

REFERENCES CITED

Banks, N. G., 1973, Biotite as a source of some of the sulfur in porphyry copper deposits: Econ. Geol., v. 68, p. 697–703.

———1974, Distribution of copper in biotite and biotite alteration products in intrusive rocks near two Arizona porphyry copper deposits: U.S. Geol. Survey Jour. Research, v. 2, no. 2, p. 195–211.

———1976, Halogen contents of igneous minerals as indicators of magmatic evolution of rocks associated with the Ray porphyry copper deposit, Arizona: U.S. Geol. Survey Jour. Research, v. 4, no. 1, p. 91–117.

Banks, N. G.; Cornwall, H. R.; Silberman, M. L.; Creasey, S. C.; and Marvin, R. F., 1972, Chronology of intrusion and ore deposition at Ray, Arizona—Part I, K-Ar ages: Econ. Geol., v. 67, p. 864–878.

Banks, N. G., and Krieger, M. H., 1977, Geologic map of the Hayden quadrangle, Pinal and Gila Counties, Arizona: U.S. Geol. Survey Geologic Quad. Map GQ-1391, 1:24,000, 15 p. text.

Banks, N. G., and Stuckless, J. S., 1973, Chronology of intrusion and ore deposition at Ray, Arizona—Part II, Fission-track ages: Econ. Geol., v. 68, p. 657–664.

Chayes, Felix, 1967, On the graphical appraisal of the strength of associations in petrographic variation diagrams, *in* Abelson, P. H., ed., Researches in Geochemistry, v. 2: New York, John Wiley and Sons, p. 322–339.

Cornwall, H. R.; Banks, N. G.; and Phillips, C. H., 1971, Geologic map of the Sonora quadrangle, Pinal and Gila Counties, Arizona: U.S. Geol. Survey Quad. Map GQ-1021, 1:24,000.

Cornwall, H. R., and Krieger, M. H., 1975*a*, Geologic map of the Kearny quadrangle, Pinal County, Arizona: U.S. Geol. Survey Geol. Quad. Map GQ-1188, 1:24,000.

—1975*b*, Geologic map of the Grayback quadrangle, Pinal County, Arizona: U.S. Geol. Survey Geol. Quad. Map GQ-1206, 1:24,000.

Creasey, S. C., and Kistler, R. W., 1962, Age of some copper-bearing porphyries and other igneous rocks in southeastern Arizona, *in* Geological Survey Research, 1962: U.S. Geol. Survey Prof. Paper 450-D, p. D1–D5.

Creasey, S. C.; Peterson, D. W.; and Gambell, N. A., 1975, Preliminary geologic map of the Teapot Mountain quadrangle, Pinal County, Arizona: U.S. Geol. Survey Open-file Rept. 75–314, 1:24,000.

Damon, P. E., 1970, New K-Ar dates for the southern Basin and Range province, *in* Annual Progress Reports to Research Division: U.S. Atomic Energy Comm., June, p. 38.

Damon, P. E., and Mauger, P. E., 1966, Epeirogeny-orogeny viewed from the Basin and Range province: Soc. Mining Engineers Trans., v. 235, p. 99–111.

Gilluly, James, 1932. Geology and ore deposits of the Stockton and Fairfield quadrangles, Utah: U.S. Geol. Survey Prof. Paper 173, 171 p.

———1946, The Ajo mining district, Arizona: U.S. Geol. Survey Prof. Paper 209, 112 p.

Irvine, T. N., and Baragar, W. R. A., 1971, A guide to the chemical classification of the common volcanic rocks: Canadian Jour. Earth Sci., v. 6, p. 523–548.

Koski, R. A., and Cook, D. S., 1982, Geology of the Christmas porphyry copper deposit, Gila County, Arizona, *in* Titley, S. R., ed., Advances in Geology of the Porphyry Copper Deposits, Southwestern North America: Tucson, Univ. Ariz. Press, Chapter 17.

Krauskopf, K. B., 1967. Introduction to Geochemistry: New York, McGraw-Hill Book Co., 721 p.

Lowell, J. D., and Guilbert, J. M., 1970, Lateral and vertical alteration-mineralization zoning in porphyry ore deposits: Econ. Geol., v. 65, p. 373–408.

Metz, R. A.; Phillips, C. H.; and Caviness, C. R., 1968, Recent developments in the geology of the Ray area, *in* Southern Arizona Guidebook 3: Ariz. Geol. Soc., p. 137–146.

Metz, R. A., and Rose, A. W., 1966, Geology of the Ray copper deposit, Ray, Arizona, *in* Titley, S. R., and Hicks, C. L., eds., Geology of the Porphyry Copper Deposits, Southwestern North America: Tucson, Univ. Arizona Press, p. 176–188.

Moore, W. J., 1973, Igneous rocks in the Bingham mining district, Utah: U.S. Geol. Survey Prof. Paper 629-B, 42 p.

Peacock, M. A., 1931, Classification of igneous rock series: Jour. Geology, v. 39, p. 54–67.

Phillips, C. H.; Gambell, N. A.; and Fountain, D. S., 1974, Hydrothermal alteration, mineralization, and zoning in the Ray deposit: Econ. Geol., v. 69, p. 1237–1250.

Ransome, F. L., 1919, The copper deposits of Ray and Miami, Arizona: U.S. Geol. Survey Prof. Paper 115, 192 p.

———1923, Description of the Ray quadrangle, Arizona: U.S. Geol. Survey Geol. Atlas, Ray Folio, No. 217, 24 p.

Ross, D. C., 1972, Petrographic and chemical reconnaissance study of some granitic and gneissic rocks near the San Andrea fault from Bodega Head to Cajon Press, California: U.S. Geol. Survey Prof. Paper 698, 92 p.

Theodore, T. G.; Silberman, M. L.; and Blake, D. W., 1973, Geochemistry and potassium-argon ages of plutonic rocks in the Battle Mountain mining district, Lander County, Nevada: U.S. Geol. Survey Prof. Paper 798-A, 24 p.

Thornton, C. P., and Tuttle, O. F., 1960, Chemistry of igneous rocks—I, Differentiation index: Am. Jour. Sci., v. 258, p. 664–684.

Washington, H. S., 1917, Chemical analyses of igneous rocks published from 1884–1913 inclusive, with a critical discussion of the character and use of analyses: U.S. Geol. Survey Prof. Paper 99, 1201 p.

Wones, D. R., and Dodge, F. C. W., 1966, On the stability of phlogopite: Geol. Soc. America, Ann. Mtg., Program, with Abstracts, p. 243 (abs.).

Wones, D. R., and Eugster, H. P., 1965, Stability of biotite—experiment, theory, and application: Am. Mineralogist, v. 50, p. 1228–1272.

12

Characteristics of Leached Capping and Techniques of Appraisal

James A. Anderson

In detailing the characteristics of leached capping, this chapter examines the nature of mineralogical and chemical changes produced during the oxidation and enrichment of sulfide deposits. The research has been directed toward developing an understanding of the nature and origin of various products of weathering, particularly as they may be related to the nature of former sulfide assemblages, to host rocks, and to variations in physiography and climate. As a result of these studies, it has become possible to assess the probable history and implications of secondary mineral assemblages present in the zone of supergene effects as they may relate both to enriched copper grades and to the nature of primary sulfide assemblages. The results are broadly applicable and can be used in the study of porphyry copper systems with different host rocks and with widely different sulfide contents and ratios.

Interpretations of published experimental studies reveal that variations in the pH of waters, produced by acids derived from oxidation of primary and secondary sulfide minerals, exert a strong and predictable control on the resulting secondary mineral assemblage. The characteristics of this secondary assemblage can, therefore, be used as one basis for interpretation of the nature of the primary mineral suite. This concept has focused research on quantitative mineralogical and chemical studies of limonite and other oxide minerals, of sulfide mineralogy, and of silicate alteration assemblages, as well as of copper content and distribution in the zones of capping, sulfide and oxide enrichment, and primary sulfides.

The data presented here consist primarily of theoretical, empirical, and practical bases for the interpretation of secondary mineral assemblages. Interpretation of various assemblages of limonite minerals is particularly important because these minerals, taken together with other criteria—such as rock and alteration mineralogy, rock copper geochemistry, ore textures, and geologic inferences—may be used to predict the copper grade and sulfide mineralogy of subjacent sulfide zones. These criteria, which have been tested in field studies in the western hemisphere, are illustrated in the chapter by charts, nomographs, and compositional diagrams which relate mineral stabilities to limonite-copper correlations.

FUNDAMENTALS OF OXIDATION AND ENRICHMENT OF SULFIDES

The oxidation and enrichment of sulfide minerals is dependent on the oxidation potential of the chemical environment. This potential is a function of the availability of free oxygen and can be expressed in terms of the partial pressure of oxygen (pO_2), as shown in Figure 12.1.

Role of Oxygen

The highest pO_2 obtained in nature is that of air, i.e., atmospheric pO_2. Oxidation potentials approaching this value are found in air-saturated porous rocks in the zone of capillary water above the ground-water table. This zone periodically becomes saturated for short durations by oxygenated meteoric recharge waters derived from surface runoff. Because air does not readily gain access to rocks where the pore space is saturated with water, the pO_2 decreases rapidly at the groundwater table.

The decrease in pO_2 below the groundwater table marks the transition between oxidizing and reducing environments for copper and iron minerals (see Fig. 12.1). Local oxidizing conditions prevail along structures that conduct oxygenated recharge waters below the groundwater table. Also, reducing conditions may persist locally in the zone of capillary water above the groundwater table.

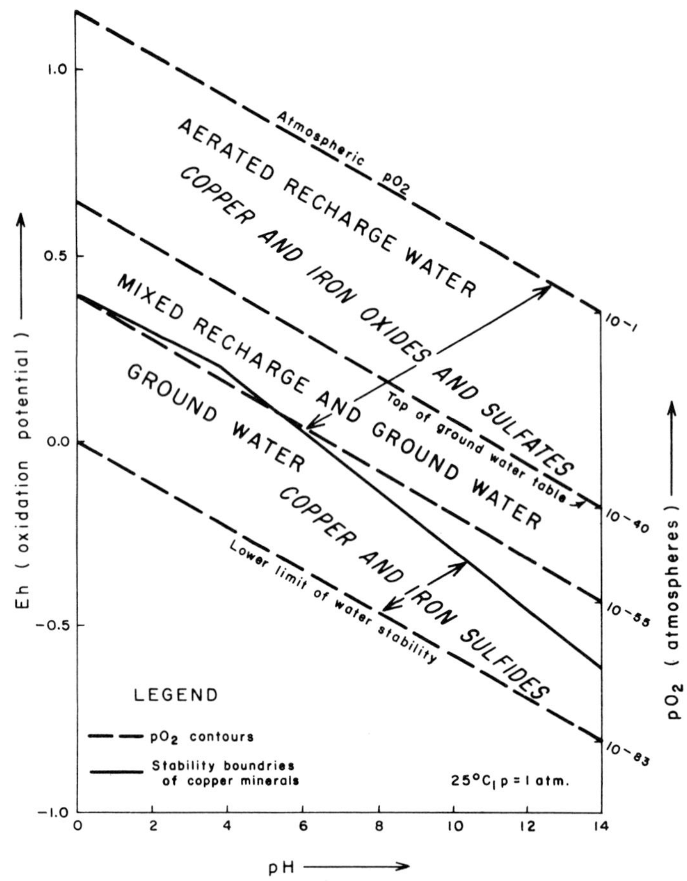

Figure 12.1. Diagram showing stability ranges of copper and iron compounds with respect to oxidation potential and pH.

Stability of Sulfide Minerals

Changes in the oxidation potential (pO_2) of a system are accompanied by changes in the stability of sulfide minerals (see Fig. 12.1). Sulfides are stable in reducing environments, but they liberate metal and sulfate ions in oxidizing environments. Figure 12.2 shows the effects of oxidation in high- and low-sulfide environments. Most of the metal ions released by oxidation of deposits containing a high total sulfide content (Fig. 12.2*A*) are carried away in solution from the site of oxidation during periodic flushing by meteoric recharge water (Fig. 12.2*B*). Most of the metal ions liberated by oxidation of deposits containing a low total sulfide content (Fig. 12.2*E*) are precipitated as hydroxides, oxides, carbonates, sulfates, or silicates at the site of oxidation (Fig. 12.2*F*).

Metal ions (particularly copper) that migrate to reducing environments precipitate by reaction with hypogene sulfides to form a zone of supergene sulfide enrichment. Most supergene copper sulfides (chalcocite and covellite) form in the zone of reduction below the groundwater table (see Figs. 12.1, 12.2*B*), but they also form in local reducing environments that persist in the zone of capillary water above the water table (Fig. 12.2*C*).

Influence of Climate

Climatic conditions influence the oxidation of sulfide deposits by controlling chemical weathering, which is dependent on temperature and amount of precipitation. Temperature influences the rate of chemical reactions: tropical climates promote rapid chemical reactions, temperate climates produce moderate reaction rates, and polar climates prevent significant chemical reaction.

Precipitation influences the rate of leaching of metal ions from the oxide zone. It also determines the depth of oxidation by controlling the level of the groundwater table. Humid climates have high water tables that prevent deep oxidation. Semiarid climates are favorable for deep oxidation, leaching, and enrichment because low water tables allow periodic recharge water to remove capillary solutions from the oxide zone. Extreme arid conditions are favorable for deep oxidation but do not promote rapid leaching and enrichment because of the deficiency of recharge water.

Oxidation of sulfide minerals occurs to some extent in all but polar climates, but the chemical weathering that produces deep oxidation, leaching, and enrichment of sulfide deposits is most strongly promoted by tropical, semiarid climates. The duration of the favorable climate is an important factor in the effectiveness of enrichment by chemical weathering.

Oxidation Cycles

Oxidation of sulfide deposits proceeds in cycles that are controlled by fluctuations in the groundwater table. These fluctuations are produced by changes in the base level or climate of the area. First-cycle oxidation with leaching and enrichment (see Fig. 12.2*B*) or first-cycle oxidation without leaching and enrichment (see Fig. 12.2*F*) continues until the primary sulfides exposed to oxidizing environments above an established water table are completely oxidized.

Second-cycle oxidation (see Figs. 12.2*C*, 12.2*G*) is initiated by a relative lowering of the groundwater table, which exposes additional sulfides to oxidizing environments. However, this process can be terminated at any stage by a rise in the groundwater table to levels above the sulfide zone. Second-cycle oxidation attacks primary sulfides and first-cycle supergene chalcocite. A large drop in the water table (usually caused by regional uplift) may produce a large gap between first- and second-cycle supergene enrichment zones, as shown by the arrow in Figure 12.2*C*. Minor drops in the water table commonly produce a zone of overlap between the first- and second-cycle chalcocite blankets. Second-cycle oxidation stops when oxidation of sulfides is complete above the new groundwater table.

Repeated cycles of oxidation, leaching, and enrichment in porphyry copper deposits (related to repeated adjustments in the water table) produce increases in the copper content of successive enrichment zones (compare Figs. 12.2*B,C*). This increase in grade culminates in complete replacement of hypogene sulfides by chalcocite (depicted by 2–3% copper values in Figs. 12.2*B,C*). Subsequent oxidation of this chalcocite blanket produces *in situ* oxide ore (crosshatch pattern in Figs. 12.2*C,D*). This type of oxide ore commonly overlies

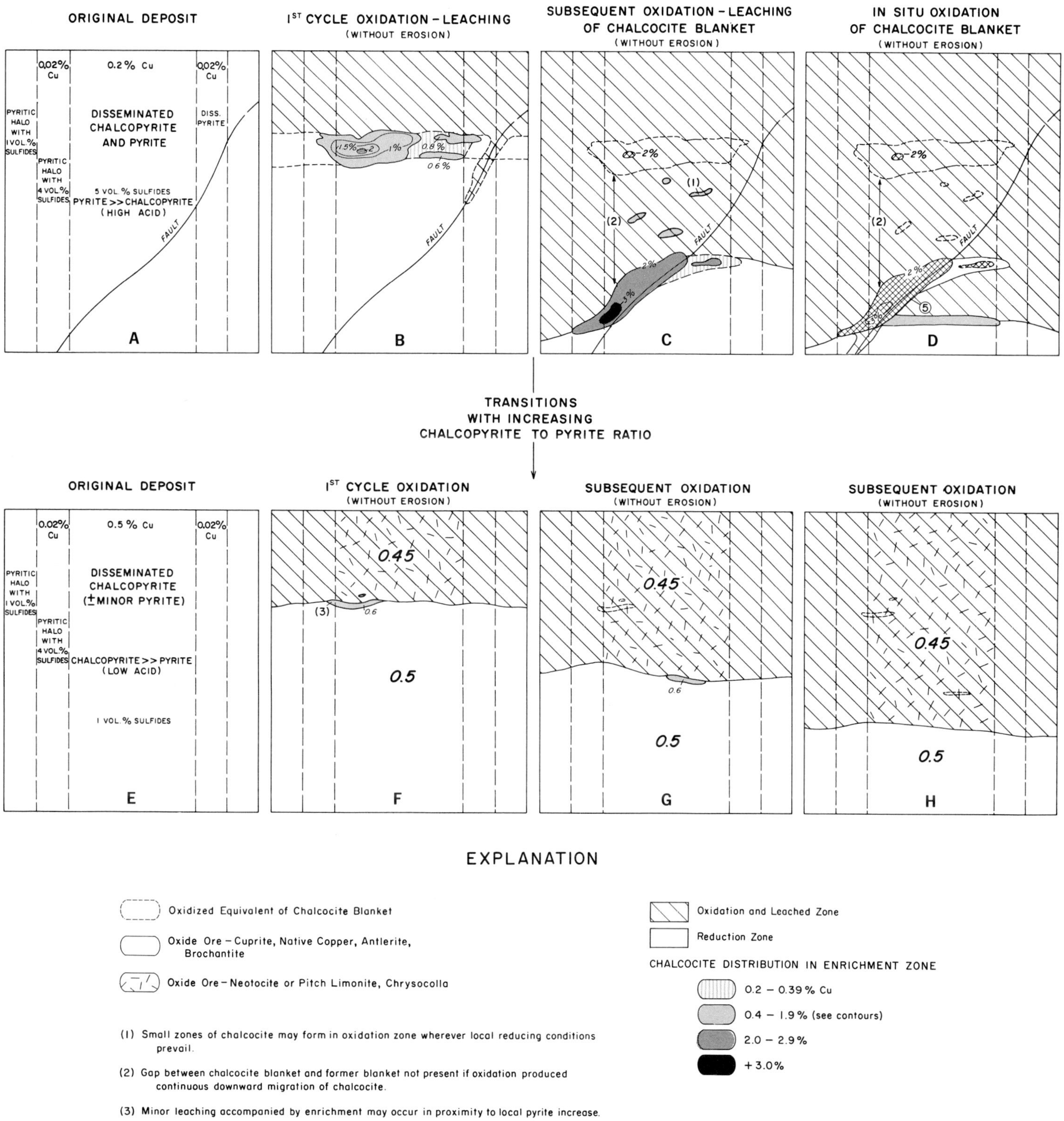

Figure 12.2. Idealized cross sections through typical porphyry copper deposits showing the evolution of oxidation, leaching, and enrichment in a mineralized system containing 0.2 percent copper and a 5 volume percent total sulfide *(A-D)* and in a mineralized system contain 0.5 percent copper and 1 volume percent total sulfide *(E-H)*.

zones of leaching and enrichment formed by oxidation of deeper primary sulfides.

The pH of Capillary Water

Oxidation of copper and iron sulfides in the zone of oxidation above the groundwater table affects the pH balance of water by releasing copper sulfate, iron sulfate, and sulfuric acid into capillary solutions. The amount of these compounds available to the solution is a function of: (1) the total sulfide content, (2) the copper sulfide to iron sulfide ratio, and (3) the mineralogy of the copper sulfides.

Effect of Sulfide Oxidation. Oxidation of rocks with a

high total sulfide content produces abundant sulfuric acid. An increase in the copper sulfide to iron sulfide ratio or in the copper content of copper minerals lowers the amount of available sulfur and thus decreases the amount of sulfuric acid produced during oxidation. The factors controlling sulfuric acid generation are illustrated by the following possible reactions:

$$4FeS_2 + 7H_2O + 14\tfrac{1}{2}O_2 = 2HFeO_2 + 6H_2SO_4 + 2FeSO_4 \quad (1)$$

$$6CuFeS_2 + 12H_2O + 25O_2 = 4HFeO_2 + Cu_4(OH)_6SO_4 + 7H_2SO_4 + 2CuSO_4 + 2FeSO_4 \quad (2)$$

A lowering of the total sulfide content of the rock also decreases the amount of sulfuric acid generated by oxidation.

Some of the acid generated by oxidation of sulfides is consumed by reactive gangue—such as calcite, feldspar, and mafic minerals—in the host rock. The pH of the oxidizing capillary solution is a measure of the equilibrium attained between acid production and acid consumption; it is, therefore, a "built-in" system of accounting for the variables that control oxidation and leaching.

Effect on Leaching of Copper and Iron. Experimental and thermodynamic data on equilibrium stability fields of cupric ion (Fig. 12.3) and ferrous ion (Fig. 12.4) demonstrate that the solubility of copper and iron is determined by the pH and pO_2 of the solution. These data indicate that a decrease in the pH of capillary solutions leads to greater solubility of copper and iron from the oxide zone; on the other hand, an increase in the pH of a saturated solution results in the precipitation of copper and iron. Copper and iron minerals are also precipitated from saturated capillary solutions by increasing the pO_2 of the system.

The pH control over the solubility of copper and iron indicates that the amount of leaching from the zone of oxidation is related to the sulfide content and to the reactive mineral composition of the host rock. Oxidation of unreactive rocks with a high total sulfide content produces low pH capillary solutions which accomplish nearly complete leaching of copper and iron from the zone of oxidation. An increase in the reactivity of the rock or an increase in the copper sulfide to iron sulfide ratio raises the pH balance of the capillary water. This change reduces solubility and, therefore, lowers the amount of leaching of copper and iron. Oxidation of rocks with low total sulfide content produces high pH capillary solutions, which result in *in situ* precipitation of copper and iron compounds in the zone of oxidation. Because copper is more soluble than iron (see Figs. 12.3, 12.4), oxidation results in the preferential leaching of copper in comparison to iron.

Effect on Supergene Copper Mineralogy. Experimental, thermodynamic, and geologic data suggest that the pH value of capillary solutions controls the mineralogy of supergene copper, iron, and silica compounds formed during oxidation and enrichment. The pH control of supergene copper minerals is illustrated in the stability field boundaries shown in Figure 12.3. Low pH supergene solutions are required for

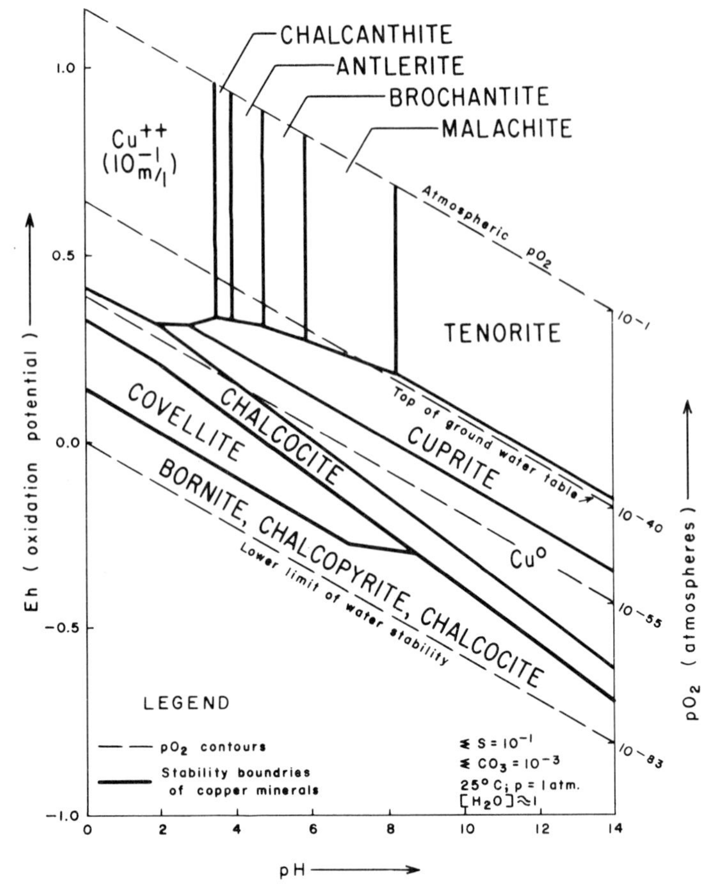

Figure 12.3. Eh-pH diagram showing the stability fields of copper minerals in the system Cu-S-H_2O.

thorough leaching and enrichment of copper. The stability fields of cupric ion (Cu^{++}), chalcanthite ($CuSO_4 \cdot 5H_2O$), chalcocite (Cu_2S), and covellite (CuS) dominate this environment. Since water soluble chalcanthite that precipitates from low pH capillary solutions is redissolved by dilute recharge waters that periodically flush the oxide zone, the residual copper in most thoroughly leached cappings is present in some form other than stable copper minerals. Analytical data show that the residual copper in this type of capping is camouflaged (included) in co-precipitating limonite minerals and in copper-iron mineraloids, including pitch limonite [$H(Fe,Cu)O_2$], neotocite [$(Cu,Fe,Mn)SiO_2$], and, more rarely, turquoise ($CuO \cdot 3Al_2O_3 \cdot 2P_2O_5 \cdot 9H_2O$).

Moderate pH solutions produce partial leaching of copper from the capping. The stability fields of antlerite [$Cu_3(OH)_4SO_4$], brochantite [$Cu_4(OH)_6SO_4$], cuprite (Cu_2O), native copper (Cu^0), and chalcocite (Cu_2S) dominate this environment. Co-precipitating limonite minerals are saturated with camouflaged residual copper. Geologic associations indicate that chrysocolla ($CuSiO_3 \cdot 2H_2O$) forms instead of brochantite when capillary solutions are high in dissolved silica; malachite [$Cu_2(OH)_2CO_3$] forms instead of brochantite in cappings containing highly reactive carbonate gangue minerals.

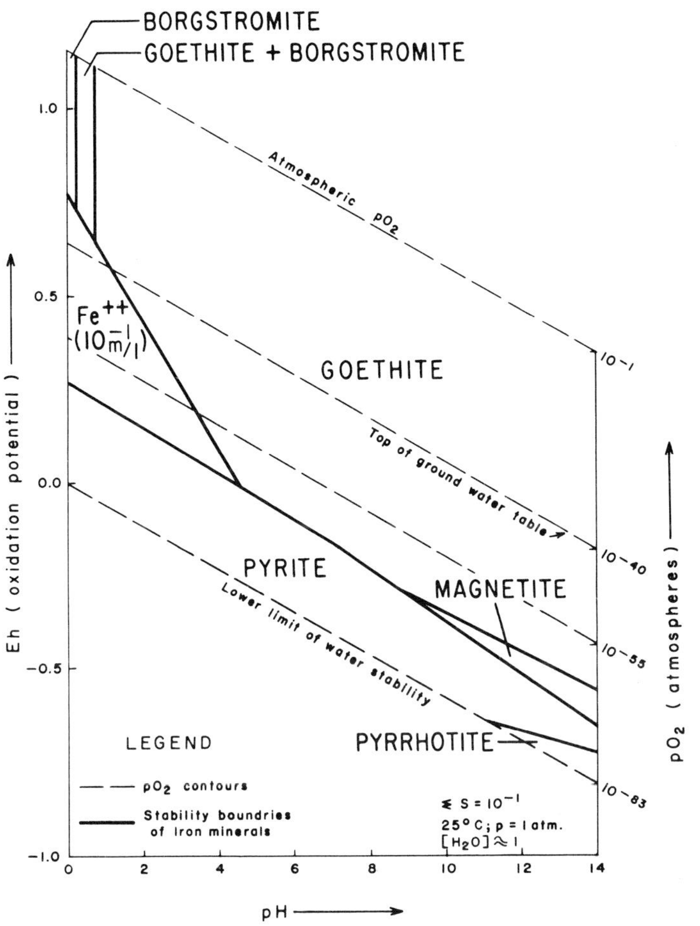

Figure 12.4. Eh-pH diagram showing the stability fields of some iron minerals in the system Fe-S-$H_2$0.

Neutral to alkaline (high pH) solutions do not produce significant leaching of copper from the oxide zone. The presence of tenorite (CuO) and abundant malachite or azurite are diagnostic of this environment.

Effect on Supergene Iron Mineralogy. The pH control over formation of supergene iron minerals is shown by the goethite ($HFeO_2$) and borgstromite-jarosite [$(K,H)Fe_3(SO_4)_2(OH)_6$] stability boundaries in Figure 12.4. Experimental data indicate that hematite does not precipitate from Fe-S-H_2O solutions at temperatures below ~125°C—the dehydration temperature of goethite to hematite. The stability relations of borgstromite, goethite, and hematite have important implications in leached capping interpretations. The pH dependence of the borgstromite-goethite boundaries indicates that the ratio of these minerals is related to the nature and amount of sulfides that produce sulfuric acid during oxidation. The pH control over the solubility of copper and iron provides a correlation between the borgstromite-goethite ratio and the amount of leaching of these metals from the zone of oxidation. The occurrence of hematite in oxidized, low temperature, sulfur-rich systems is anomalous from the standpoint of present experimental evidence. The abundance of this mineral in oxide zones formed by oxidation of a sulfide zone containing chalcocite suggests that the oxidation mechanism of chalcocite stabilizes the hematite structure at low temperatures.

The presence of borgstromite or jarosite implies that oxygenated capillary water has a pH lower than 2.2, the lowest value recorded for recharge runoff waters. This anomalous condition suggests that most sulfide oxidation is accomplished by capillary waters. The recharge water, it appears, merely serves to flush the saturated acidic capillary water from the system and to replenish the system with new capillary water which rejuvenates oxidation. Oxidation halts when oxygenated solutions reach equilibrium with sulfides and reactive minerals.

Influence on Supergene Silicate and Silica Alteration. Some of the variables controlling the stability of supergene silicate and silica minerals are summarized in Figures 12.5 and 12.6. The pH of the solution is an important control on mineral stability, and the concentration of elements essential in silicate minerals exerts similar controls on mineral stabilities. For example, a decrease in either the pH or the potassium ion concentration of capillary solutions attacking orthoclase may produce identical alteration sequences (see Fig. 12.6). As shown in Figure 12.5, the concentration of silica in the solution also appears to control the presence or absence of sericite and quartz in alteration assemblages.

Supergene silicate alteration is independent of the oxidation potential of the system because free oxygen is not required in silicate alteration reactions:

$$2KAlSi_3O_8 + H_2SO_4 + H_2O = Al_2Si_2O_5(OH)_4 + 4SiO_2 + 2K^+ + SO_4^{=} \quad (3)$$

This condition implies that supergene alteration is not confined to the oxide and supergene chalcocite enrichment zones of an oxidizing sulfide deposit. Supergene silicate alteration commonly extends for considerable depths into the primary sulfide zones. The mineralogy of supergene silicate alteration gradually changes with increasing depth in the hypogene sulfide zone. This change is attributed to reactive mineral acid consumption, which produces a downward increase in the pH of acid solutions originating in the oxide zone. Chlorite and biotite (magmatic or hypogene) serve as a measure of the extent of supergene acid attack because they are only stable under neutral to alkaline conditions at low temperatures and pressure (see Fig. 12.6). The upper limit of chlorite, biotite, and possibly gypsum in the hypogene sulfide zone may, therefore, mark the depth of supergene acid alteration. Supergene gypsum precipitates from calcium-bearing sulfate solutions under neutral to alkaline conditions and may, therefore, occur with the chlorite or biotite.

X-ray studies of leached capping samples have shown that kaolinite is present in most leached cappings located over chalcocite enrichment ore. This observation of "unreactive clay" can be readily explained by considering the kaolinite to be the product of supergene acid attack on reactive gangue, including calcite, plagioclase, and mafic minerals. Such an explanation is supported by experimental, thermodynamic, empirical data (see Fig. 12.5) and by field observa-

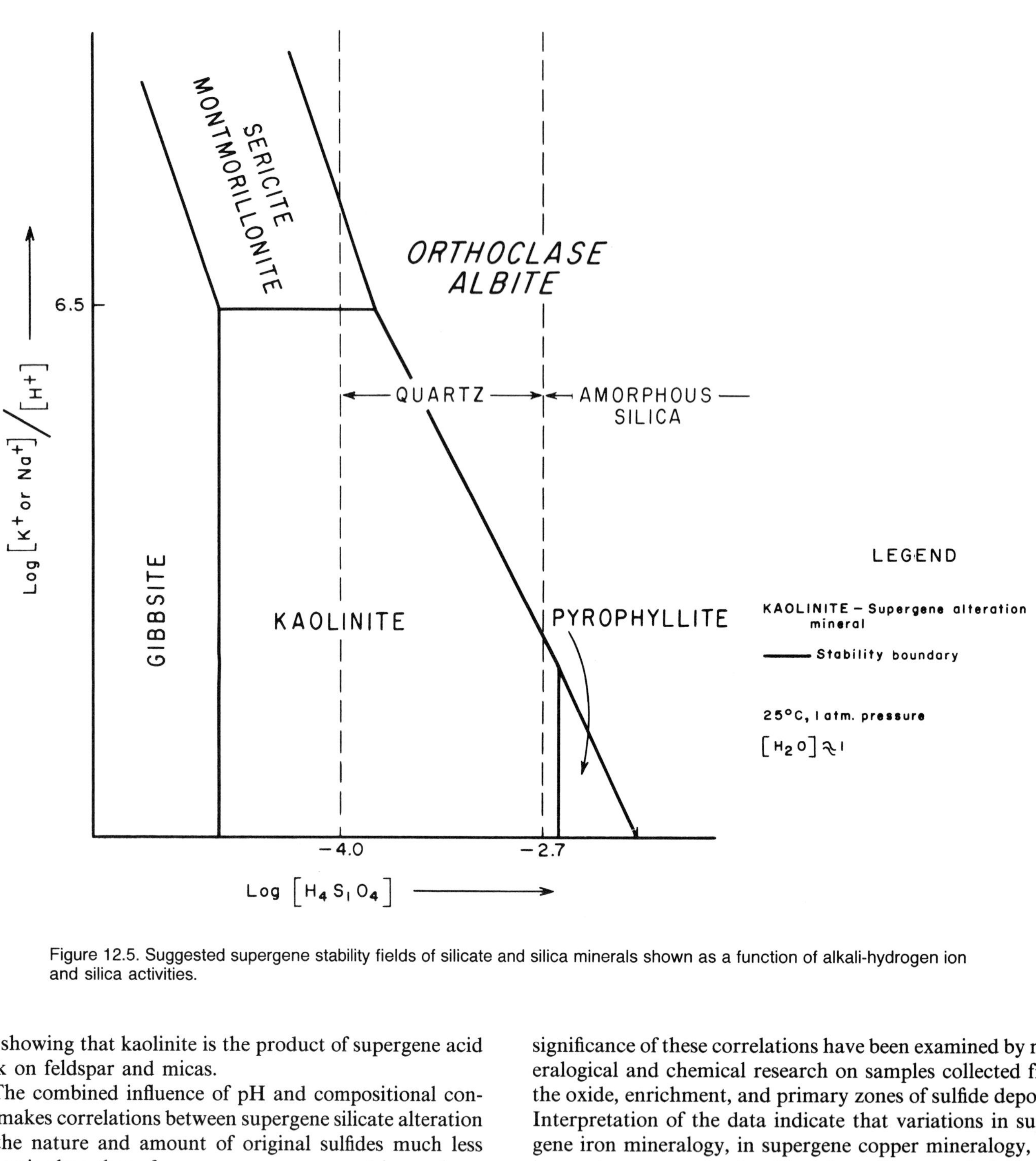

Figure 12.5. Suggested supergene stability fields of silicate and silica minerals shown as a function of alkali-hydrogen ion and silica activities.

tions showing that kaolinite is the product of supergene acid attack on feldspar and micas.

The combined influence of pH and compositional controls makes correlations between supergene silicate alteration and the nature and amount of original sulfides much less diagnostic than those for supergene copper and iron minerals. The sensitivity of the correlation is further complicated by the presence of hypogene sericite and clay minerals in some deposits.

CHARACTERISTICS OF SUPERGENE MINERALIZATION IN LEACHED CAPPINGS AND CORRELATIONS WITH FORMER SULFIDE MINERALIZATION

Experimental, thermodynamic, empirical, and theoretical data reviewed in the preceding sections suggest that some quantitative correlations exist between supergene mineralization and the former sulfide mineralization. The nature and significance of these correlations have been examined by mineralogical and chemical research on samples collected from the oxide, enrichment, and primary zones of sulfide deposits. Interpretation of the data indicate that variations in supergene iron mineralogy, in supergene copper mineralogy, and in capping copper geochemistry show close correlations with significant differences in the former sulfide mineralization. These relationships are summarized in the following sections.

Sulfide Oxidation Control of Supergene Mineralization

Oxidation of copper and iron sulfides in the zone of capillary water above the groundwater table produces copper sulfate, iron sulfate, and sulfuric acid. The pH (net acidity) of the capillary water is controlled by: (1) the total sulfide content of the rock, (2) the copper sulfide:iron sulfide ratio, (3) copper sulfide mineralogy, and (4) the reactivity of the host rock. The pH of the capillary water in turn regulates the amount of leaching of copper and iron from the zone of

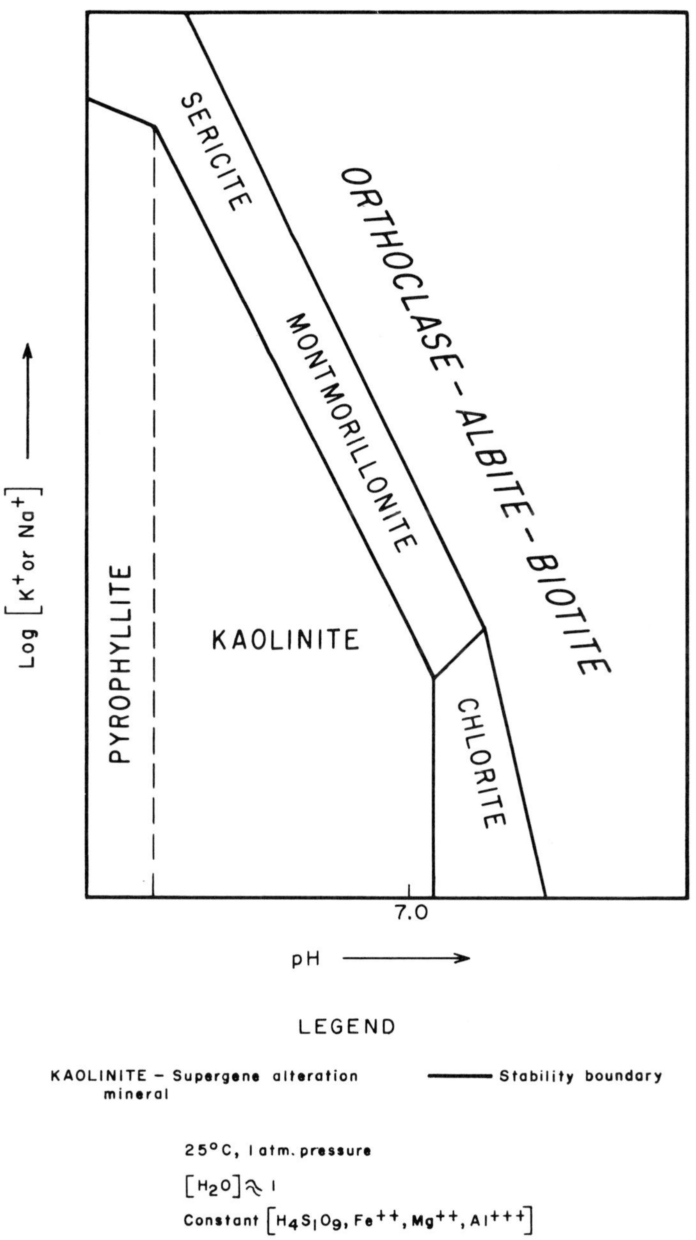

Figure 12.6. Suggested supergene stability fields of silicate minerals shown as a function of pH and activity of alkalis.

oxidation. The pH of the solution also determines the mineralogy of the supergene compounds of copper, iron, and silica that are precipitated from saturated capillary waters in the oxide zone.

Supergene Iron and Copper Mineralogy

Supergene ferric iron minerals, broadly referred to as "limonites," and supergene copper minerals are listed in Figure 12.7. Mineralogic analyses of samples from cappings over sulfide deposits demonstrate that the common limonite and oxidized copper minerals include goethite, jarosite-borgstromite, hematite, neotocite, pitch limonite, chrysocolla, turquoise, antlerite, brochantite, cuprite, and native copper. Significant quantities of copper are also camouflaged in coprecipitating limonite minerals.

Tenorite is rare in cappings over sulfide deposits. This situation is explained by the neutral to alkaline conditions required for its stability field (see Fig. 12.3). Tenorite does, however, commonly accompany malachite (or, locally, azurite) which occurs in cappings that contain abundant carbonates, because the carbonates neutralize most of the sulfuric acid generated by sulfide oxidation.

Chalcanthite is common in the mixed oxide-sulfide zone of most copper deposits. This mineral is rarely encountered in oxide cappings, since it is water soluble and is readily dissolved by dilute recharge waters that periodically flush the zone of oxidation.

The hydrated ferric sulfates shown by solid triangles in Figure 12.7 are rarely found in cappings because of the extreme arid conditions required for their formation. They are, however, reported in the oxide zone of sulfide deposits in the Atacama Desert of northern Chile. Lepidocrocite is a common limonite mineral in sulfur deficient, weathered zones, e.g., most soils. Martite, the octahedral hematite pseudomorph after magnetite, has not been observed in capping samples. As shown in Figure 12.7, a number of hydrous iron oxide minerals described in the literature have been discredited by X-ray studies by Posnjak and Merwin (1922).

Alunite is common in certain types of cappings. It is included with the limonite minerals because of the solid solution series it forms with jarosite. Jarosite may also form a solid solution series with the mineral borgstromite (compare formulas in Fig. 12.7).

Correlation of Limonite and Copper Oxide Mineralogy With Former Sulfide Content and Mineralogy

Quantitative data on the limonite and oxide copper mineralogy of cappings and on the underlying sulfide mineralization have been obtained on approximately 4,500 surface and drill core samples from 85 properties. Empirical correlations of limonite and copper mineralogy with the former sulfide mineralization, made in areas where vertical zoning in the upper part of the primary sulfide zone is negligible are summarized in the three-dimensional diagram shown in Figure 12.8.

The empirical relationships illustrated in Figure 12.8 and, in more detail, in the sections in Figures 12.9 and 12.10 demonstrate that the limonite and copper mineralogy of a capping are sensitive indicators of the total sulfide content and sulfide mineralogy of the former sulfide zone. The percent of goethite in limonite, i.e., $100 \times G/G + H + J$, ($G =$ goethite, $H =$ hematite, and $J =$ jarosite), is diagnostic of the total sulfide content of the former sulfide zone (curved planes in Fig. 12.8 or contours of goethite composition in Figs. 12.9 and 12.10). The percent hematite in limonite is related to the amount and relative proportions of chalcocite in the former sulfide zone (dashed contours in Fig. 12.10). Jarosite does not form with copper sulfates in the capping (see Fig. 12.8). Supergene copper minerals form in a capping when the mole ratios of chalcopyrite:pyrite and chalcocite:pyrite are greater than 0.5 in the sulfide zone (see Figs. 12.8, 12.9, and 12.10). The mineralogy of the copper precipitates is controlled by the

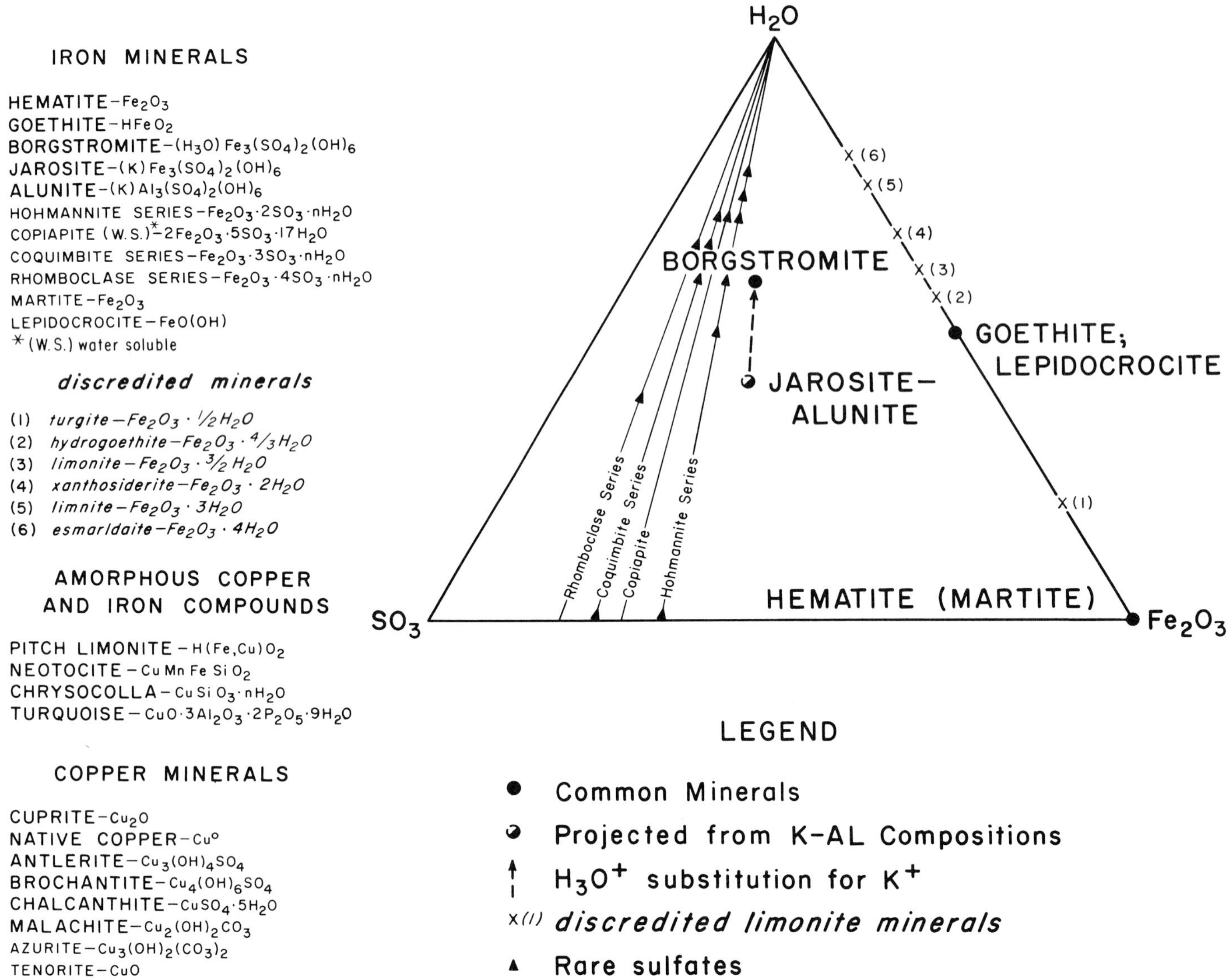

Figure 12.7. Compositions of supergene ferric iron and copper minerals shown as functions of H_2O-SO_3-Fe_2O_3.

abundance and mineralogy of iron and copper sulfides. The intensity of iron staining in a goethite capping (100% goethite in limonite) is proportional to the sulfide-iron content of the former sulfide zone, because significant leaching of iron from a capping does not occur until solutions have sufficient acidity to form jarosite or hematite.

The empirical correlations summarized in Figures 12.8, 12.9, and 12.10 demonstrate that the limonite and copper mineralogy of a capping provide sufficient evidence to make field estimates of the approximate sulfide mineralogy and total sulfide content of the former sulfide zone at each outcrop examined. The maximum and minimum limits of copper grade of the former sulfide zone can be calculated from these estimates by the use of the nomograph shown in Figure 12.11. This method of reconstructing the grade of the former sulfide zones results in low estimates in the case of cappings in limestone, dolomite, or other reactive host rocks. This condition is explained by carbonate neutralization of sulfuric acid, which increases the goethite content of limonite and results in lower total sulfide estimates.

Limonite Compositions, Copper Geochemistry, and Copper Leaching

Empirical correlations of limonite mineralogy and capping copper geochemistry with copper leaching are summarized on the primary-grade prediction chart in Figure 12.12. The primary-grade contours in this chart demonstrate that the percent of goethite in limonite is equal to the percent of the original copper that is retained in the capping. Thus, for example, 50 percent of the copper originally present in sulfides is retained in a capping that contains 50 percent goethite in limonite. This correlation of the percent of goethite in limonite with the residual copper content of the capping is valid for all degrees of rock reactivity, because the pH of the capillary solutions influences the ratios of limonite

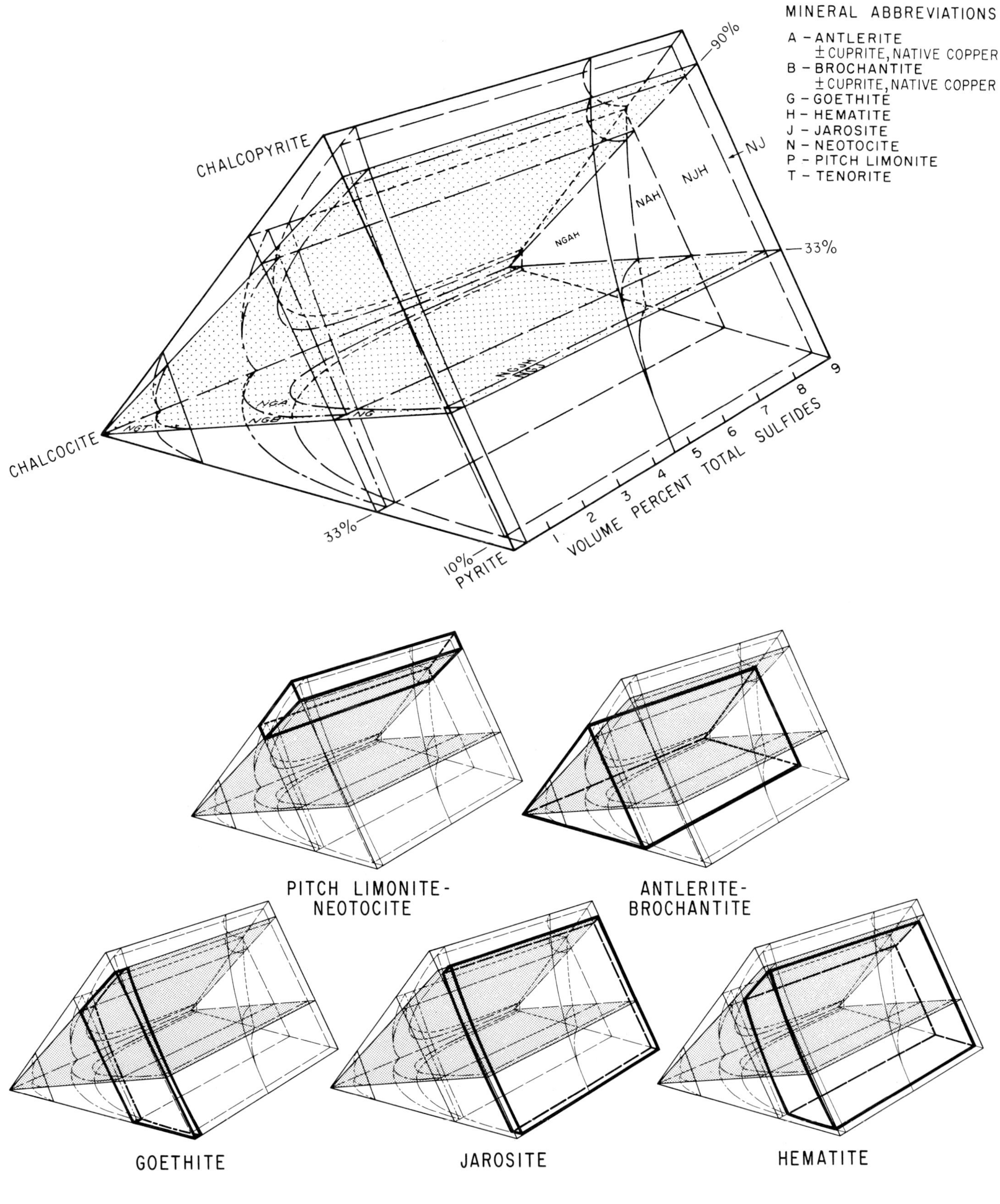

Figure 12.8. Correlation of limonite and copper mineralogy with former sulfide mineralization.

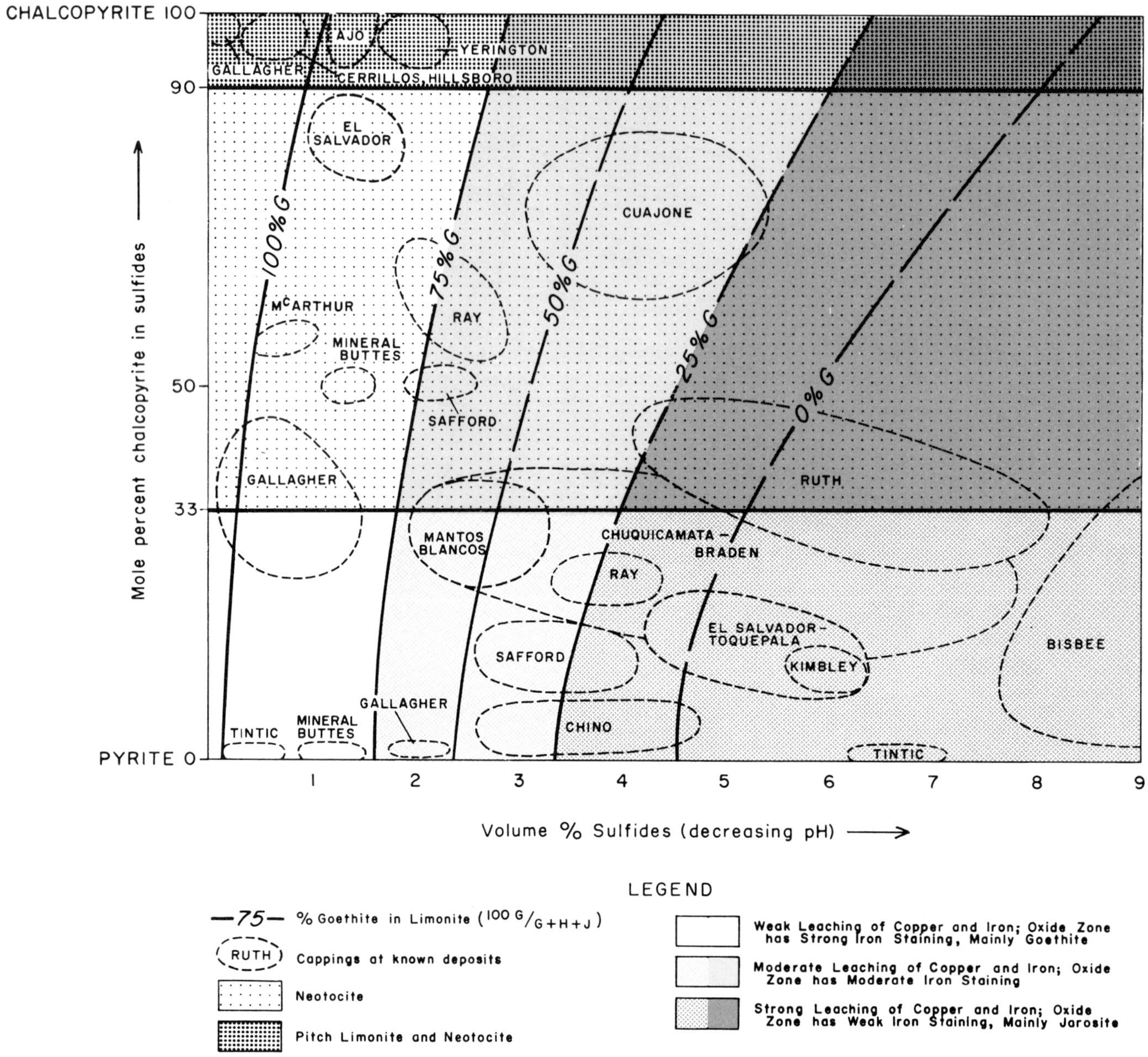

Figure 12.9. Correlation diagram of limonite and copper mineralogy with former pyrite and chalcopyrite in various copper deposits.

precipitates (see Fig 12.4) and, therefore, automatically accounts for differences in the reactivity of rock.

The above correlations demonstrate that solutions derived from the oxidation of sulfide deposits with a low total sulfide content or high proportion of chalcocite (see white area in Fig. 12.10) are not capable of leaching significant copper or iron. The oxide zone is, therefore, characterized by moderate to strong iron staining, predominantly goethite. Conversely, highly acid solutions derived from the oxidation of sulfide deposits with a high total sulfide content or low proportion of chalcocite (area with dark shading in Fig. 12.10) are capable of leaching most of the copper and iron from the oxide zone. These cappings are characterized by weak iron oxide staining, predominantly jarosite or hematite. In both examples, most of the copper in the capping is camouflaged in the limonite minerals when the chalcopyrite: pyrite ratio (see Fig. 12.9) or the chalcocite:pyrite ratio (see Fig. 12.10) is less than 0.5 (i.e., less than 33 mole %). In these figures it may be seen that diagnostic copper minerals—e.g., antlerite, brochantite, pitch limonite, neotocite—occur in cappings over deposits with chalcopyrite:pyrite or chalcocite:pyrite ratios greater than 0.5 (i.e., greater than 33 mole %).

The grade predictions obtained from the chart in Figure 12.12 represent the grade of the primary sulfide assemblages which have been oxidized for most deposits. If, however, either antlerite, brochantite, cuprite, native copper, or residual chalcocite occurs in the capping, the values obtained from the chart represent the grade of the former chalcocite enrichment zone at the point of observation. This correlation of limonite composition and rock copper geochemistry with the grade of the former enrichment zone for this type of capping is explained by the marked reduction in acidity, and, thus, in copper leaching produced by oxidation of chalcocite:pyrite or chalcocite:chalcopyrite ratios greater than 0.5 (refer to the marked inflection in percent goethite contours shown in Fig. 12.10).

Limonite Compositions, Copper Geochemistry, and Copper Enrichment

Empricial data summarized in Figures 12.8, 12.9, and 12.10 demonstrate that the percent of hematite in limonite in cappings over sulfide deposits shows a direct correlation with the percent of chalcocite in the former sulfide zone. Additional empirical correlations demonstrate that the percent of hematite in limonite and the residual copper content of the capping are related to the amount of copper enrichment at depth; the relationship between these parameters is shown on the chalcocite-enrichment prediction chart in Figure 12.13. The contour lines on this chart represent values of feet–percent copper enrichment in the sulfide zone—i.e., the amount of secondary enrichment copper added to the primary grade. Methods of evaluating the amount of chalcocite enrichment included plotting: (1) the average grade of the chalcocite enrichment zone, (2) the enrichment factor (ratio of enrichment grade to primary grade), and (3) the feet–percent copper enrichment. This third method was the only one yielding satisfactory results. The values obtained (V) correspond to the equation V (in ft. % Cu) = $(EG - PG)T$, where EG is the average grade of the enrichment zone, PG is the average grade of the primary zone (the average grade of the upper part of the primary sulfide zone is used if vertical sulfide zoning occurs), and T is the thickness of the enrichment zone. The average grade of the chalcocite enrichment

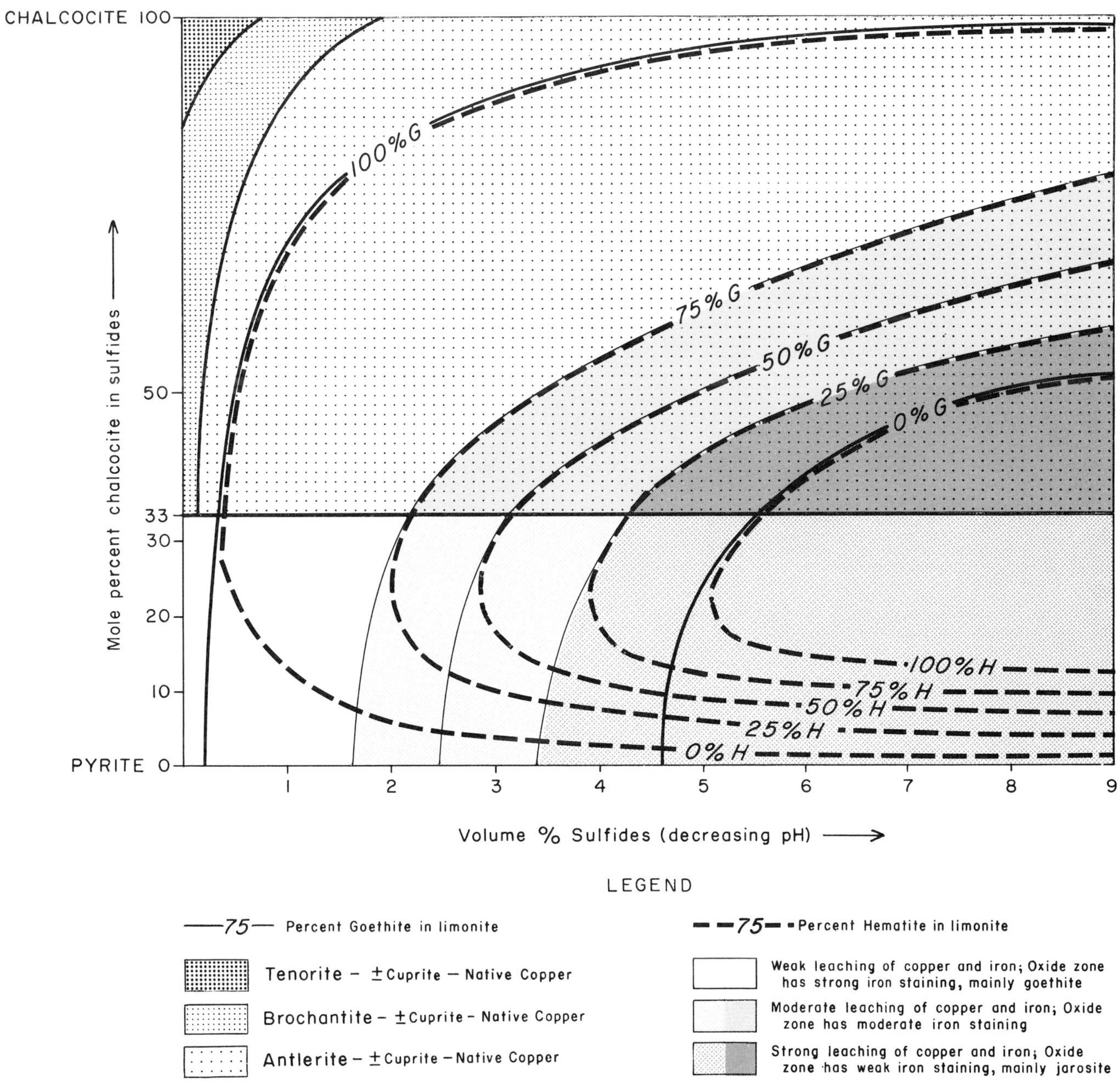

Figure 12.10. Correlation of limonite and copper mineralogy with former pyrite, chalcocite, and chalcopyrite mineralization.

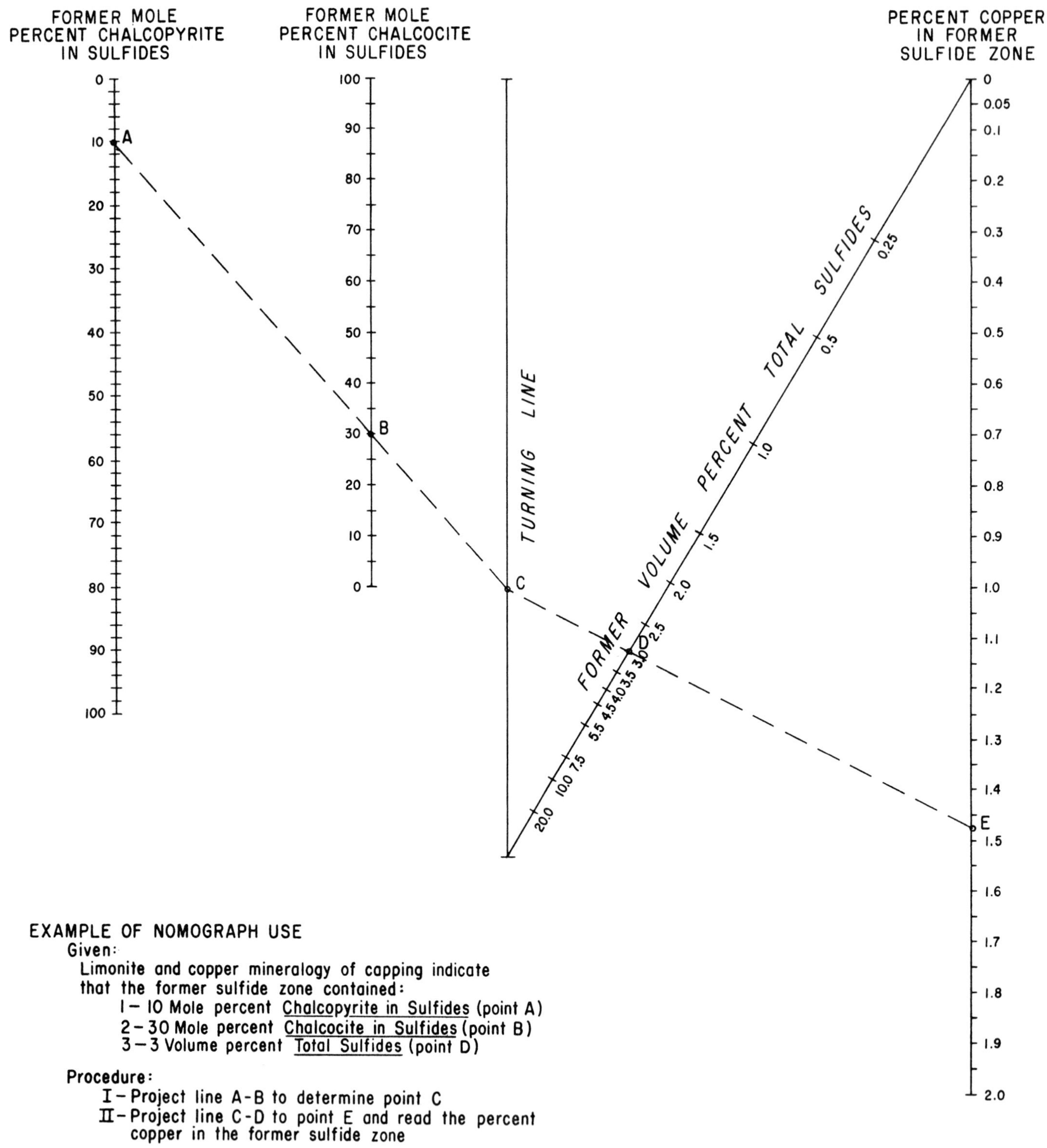

Figure 12.11. Nomograph for converting volume percent sulfide to weight percent copper in rock.

zone can be predicted from calculations using the primary grade and feet-percent copper enrichment predictions if the thickness of the enrichment zone is known, can be estimated, or can be assigned a set of possible limits. These methods of estimating the amount of chalcocite enrichment are valid for all degrees of rock reactivity because of the pH (net acidity) control on limonite mineralogy.

The chalcocite-enrichment grade predictions obtained from the chart in Figure 12.13 represent the amount of enrichment expected in the chalcocite zone below the capping of most deposits. Chalcocite enrichment predictions for cappings containing either cuprite, native copper, antlerite, brochantite, or residual chalcocite represent the enrichment value of the former blanket at the point of observation, since

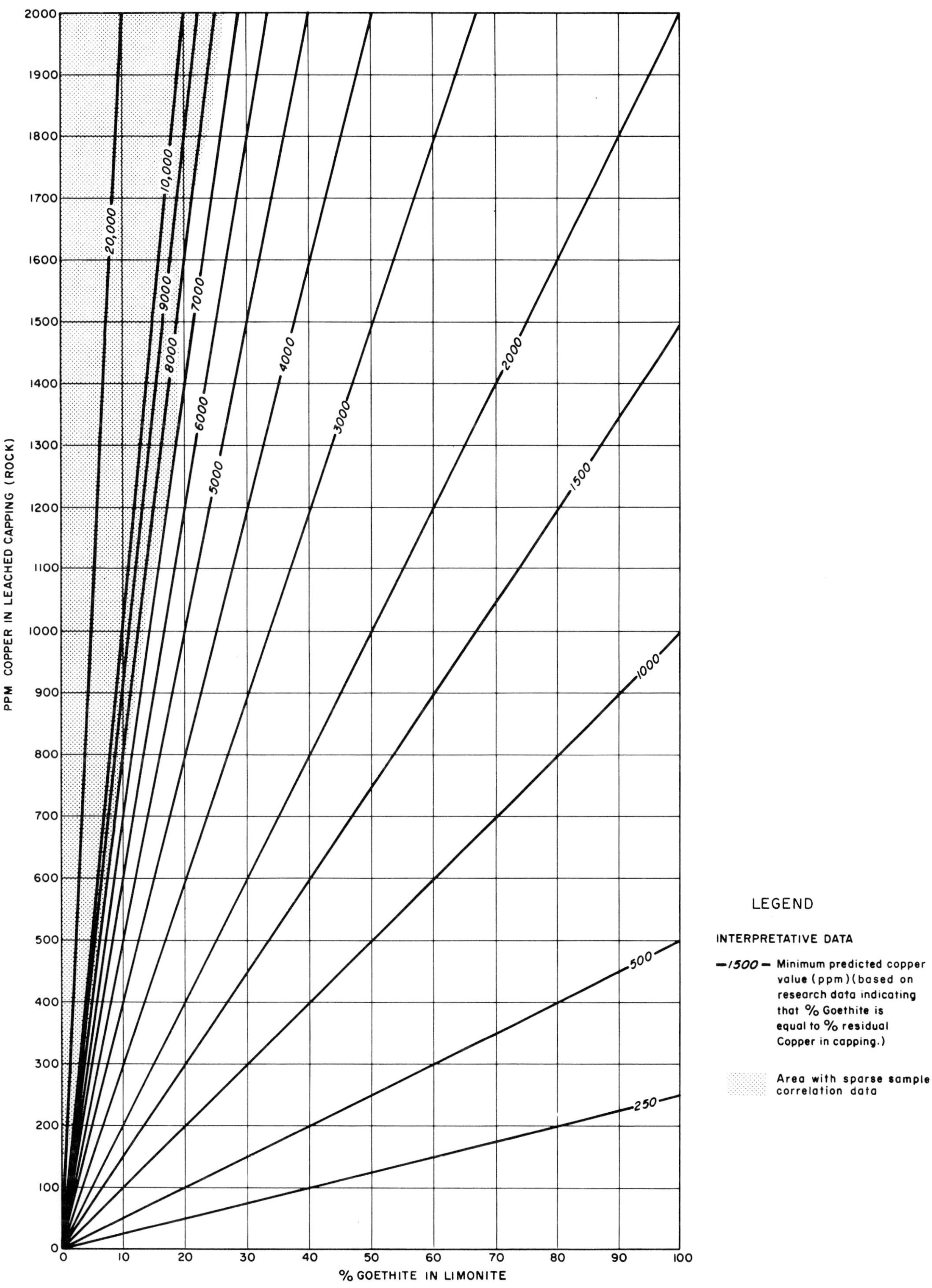

Figure 12.12. Grade prediction chart shows original grade of primary mineralization or, if either antlerite, brochantite, cuprite, native copper, or residual chalcocite is present, the grade of secondary sulfide enrichment originally present at the point of observation.

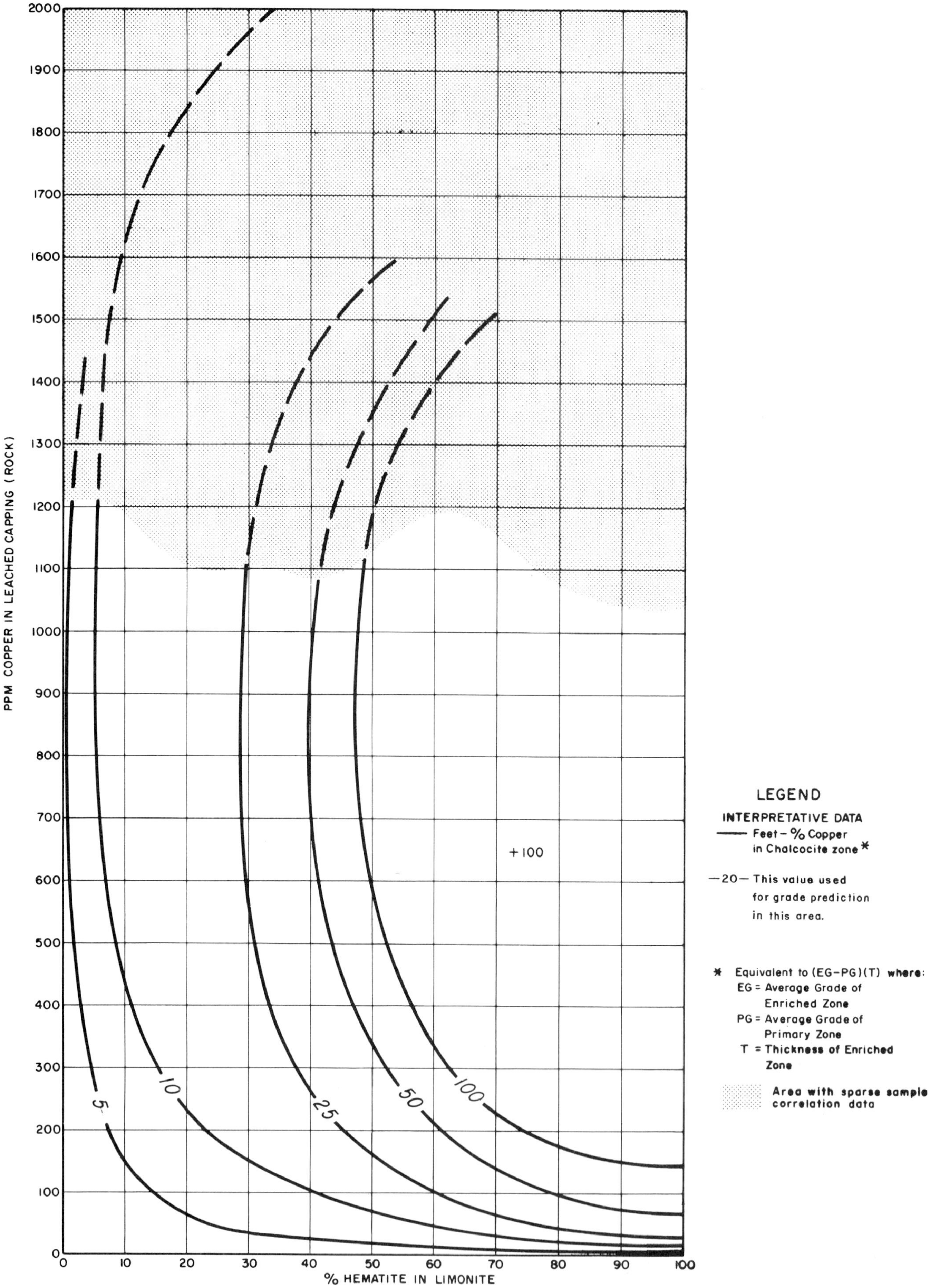

Figure 12.13. Chalcocite-enrichment prediction chart based upon hematite and copper contents of capping. If antlerite, brochantite, cuprite, native copper, or residual chalcocite is present in the sample, the chart gives the grade of the sulfide enrichment blanket originally present at the point of observation.

most of the copper is retained in this type of capping and is not available to produce further enrichment. The small amount of leaching from cappings of this type is explained by the marked reduction in acidity and, thus, in copper leaching, produced by oxidation of chalcocite:pyrite or chalcocite:chalcopyrite ratios greater than 0.5 (refer to goethite contours in Fig. 12.10).

Enrichment possibilities below cappings derived from the oxidation of sulfide zones containing pyrite and chalcopyrite, but not chalcocite, cannot be evaluated by the above methods because of the lack of hematite, so more indirect qualitative methods—such as applying commonly observed enrichment ratios to estimated primary grades or evaluating the enrichment indications of local isolated "pods" of hematite formed by second-cycle oxidation of local zones of prior chalcocite enrichment—are the only techniques available.

APPLICATION OF CONCEPTS OF CAPPING APPRAISAL

The data and interpretations concerning supergene mineralization and former sulfide mineralization summarized in the preceding sections were developed for the purpose of applying the results to the exploration evaluation of leached capping. The basic purpose of such evaluation is to predict the copper grade and the nature of sulfide mineralization that may lie beneath the surface. The field evaluation procedures necessary to accomplish these objectives are summarized in the following sections. These procedures utilize capping classification, limonite mineralogy, supergene copper mineralogy, and residual copper content of the capping in predicting primary copper grade, chalcocite enrichment grade, and characteristics and intensity of the underlying sulfide mineralization. Vertical primary sulfide zoning, lateral downward migration of supergene solutions, and changes in rock type or structure must be anticipated by geologic interpretations.

Classification of Capping

Capping classification is based on limonite mineralogy, copper mineralogy, and oxidation cycles. Six types of cappings are recognized: (1) goethite, (2) jarosite, (3) hematite, (4) pitch limonite-neotocite, (5) antlerite-brochantite, and (6) malachite. A summary of the distribution and characteristics of each type of capping is depicted in the idealized cross sections through typical porphyry copper deposits shown in Figure 12.14. Field verifications of some of these examples are shown in the color photographs in Figures 12.15, 12.16, and 12.17. Grade predictions for each type of capping utilize empirical correlations of the primary grade and chalcocite enrichment grade of the sulfide zone with the (a) percent goethite in limonite, (b) percent hematite in limonite, (c) percent jarosite in limonite, (d) diagnostic copper mineralogy, and (e) residual copper content of the capping.

Recognition and Interpretation of Cappings

First-cycle oxidation-leaching of the pyrite-chalcopyrite deposit in Figure 12.14*A* produces a chalcocite enrichment blanket overlain by an oxide capping containing goethite and jarosite (see Fig. 12.14*B*). The capping formed over the pyritic halo containing 0.5 volume percent pyrite contains goethite and may, therefore, be classified as a goethitic capping (represented by classification type 1 in Fig. 12.14). No copper or iron is leached from this type of capping.

Limonite in the capping formed over the pyritic halo containing 4 volume percent pyrite consists of jarosite with minor goethite, while limonite in the capping over the ore zone containing 5 volume percent total sulfides consists of pure jarosite. Both of these cappings are classified as the jarositic type (see the upper jarosite capping at Toquepala shown in Fig. 12.15; represented by classification type 2 in Fig. 12.14.). Most of the copper and iron has been leached from these cappings. The primary grade of the sulfide zone beneath each of these cappings may be reconstructed by the use of the prediction chart in Fig. 12.12. The amount of chalcocite enrichment in the sulfide zone below these jarositic cappings must be evaluated by qualitative indirect methods, such as applying a range of probable enrichment factors to the primary-grade prediction values. Enrichment factors observed in similar deposits range from 1.5x to >10x. The most common range is 2x to 6x.

Oxidation of sulfides in the limestone inclusion shown in Figure 12.14 *A–D* is not accompanied by leaching of copper or iron, because the acid is consumed by the reactive carbonate minerals. A goethitic capping is formed in the limestone inclusion in the pyritic halo. Trace amounts of malachite may be observed in the capping over a pyritic halo that contains 0.02 percent copper. A malachite capping (represented by classification type 3 in Fig. 12.14), which consists of malachite (local azurite) and goethite, is formed in the limestone inclusion over the copper zone.

Successive cycles of oxidation-leaching of the pyrite-chalcopyrite deposit in Figure 12.14*A–D* produce progressively higher-grade chalcocite enrichment blankets (compare Figs. 12.14*B* and 12.14*C*) that are overlain by one or more of the following cappings:

1. original jarositic capping formed by oxidation of a pyrite-chalcopyrite zone (see upper jarosite capping in Fig. 12.15; represented by classification type 2 in Fig. 12.14);
2. hematitic capping, containing hematite, jarosite, and goethite, formed by oxidation of the former chalcocite enrichment blanket (see hematite capping at Chino in Fig. 12.16 and hematite layer in capping at Toquepala in Fig. 12.15; represented by classification type 4 in Fig. 12.14);
3. lower jarositic capping, containing small zones of chalcocite enrichment or subsequent small zones of hematitic capping, formed by oxidation of a pyrite-chalcopyrite zone occupying a gap between two enrichment zones (see lower jarosite capping at Toquepala in Fig. 12.15 and jarosite capping at Butte in Fig. 12.17; represented by classification type 2A in Fig. 12.14.
4. antlerite-brochantite capping, containing antlerite or brochantite with hematite, goethite, and occasionally cuprite, native copper, or residual chalcocite, formed by the *in situ* oxidation of multi-cycle, high-grade, chalcocite enrichment blankets in which chalcocite:pyrite or chalcocite:chalcopyrite mole ratios are greater than 0.5 (represented by classification type 5 capping shown as the crosshatch pattern in Fig. 12.14*C,D*).

Gaps are commonly present between successive chalcocite blankets. These gaps form as a result of large, rapid, downward adjustments of the groundwater table produced by sudden uplift or lowering of the base level. Subsequent oxidation of these deposits produces layered jarosite and hematite cappings, such as those at Toquepala, Peru (see Fig. 12.15). Minor downward adjustments in the groundwater table that take place over prolonged periods of time commonly produce a zone of overlap between downward migrating enrichment zones. Subsequent oxidation of these deposits produces a hematite capping such as that at Chino, New Mexico (see Fig. 12.16).

The primary grade of the sulfide zone underlying jarositic and hematitic cappings may be estimated by using the prediction chart shown in Figure 12.12. Chalcocite enrichment grades for the sulfide zone below jarositic cappings must be estimated by indirect methods, such as applying probable enrichment factors to primary-grade estimates or by evaluating the enrichment indications of local isolated pods of hematitic cappings formed by oxidation of local zones of chalcocite enrichment (see Figs. 12.14*C,D* and 12.17). Estimates of chalcocite enrichment indicated by hematitic cappings may be obtained from the prediction chart in Figure 12.13. Note that the irregular nature of the grade in the chalcocite enrichment zone in Figure 12.14*B* is preserved by the distribution of hematite in the capping shown in Figure 12.14*C*. This relationship may also be observed in the photograph of the layered hematite capping in Figure 12.15.

Only minor leaching of copper occurs from *in situ* oxidation of antlerite-brochantite capping (classification type 5 in Fig. 12.14). The limonite and copper mineralogy and the residual copper content of this capping can be used to reconstruct the grade and the feet–percent copper enrichment value of the former enrichment zone by referring to the grade prediction charts in Figures 12.12 and 12.13. The grade of the primary sulfide zone below this sulfate capping can then be calculated by the formula $V = (EG - PG)\ T$, where $V =$ feet–percent enrichment copper from Figure 12.13, $EG =$ average grade of enrichment zone from Figure 12.12, $PG =$ the average primary grade that is being sought, and $T =$ thickness of the zone, known or reasonably estimated.

All transitions from primary pyrite-chalcopyrite mineralization (see Fig. 12.14*A*) to primary mineralization consisting only of chalcopyrite (see Fig. 12.14*E*) are found in nature. A common occurrence of the chalcopyrite type is depicted in Figure 12.14*E*, wherein the sulfide mineralization consists of approximately 1 volume percent chalcopyrite. First-cycle oxidation of this chalcopyrite deposit produces a pitch limonite-neotocite capping (classification type 6 in Fig. 12.14*E–H*) consisting of oxide ore containing pitch limonite, neotocite, chrysocolla, goethite, and occasionally residual chalcopyrite. No copper or iron is leached from this capping except in local areas of higher sulfide content. Successive cycles of oxidation produce similar cappings (see Fig. 12.14 *G,H*). Neotocite cappings form over deposits with chalcopyrite:pyrite ratios ranging from 9.0 to 0.5 (see Figs. 12.8 and 12.9).

Oxidation of chalcopyrite deposits with higher total sulfide content produces oxidation-leaching-enrichment zones equivalent to those portrayed in Figure 12.14*A–D*, with the exception that pitch limonite or neotocite is present in each type of capping over the ore zone. Primary-grade and chalcocite-grade prediction techniques outlined above for the cappings shown in Figure 12.14*E–H* also apply for these cappings. Field observations at Chuquicamata, Chile, and Cuajone, Peru, have confirmed that antlerite-brochantite, neotocite, and neotocite-antlerite-bronchantite cappings overlie zones of enrichment formed by oxidation and leaching of deeper primary sulfides (refer to chalcocite enrichment zone shown in Figure 12.14*D*). This relationship in oxide ore zones has important exploration implications.

The indiscriminate use of hematite as indication of the presence of chalcocite should be avoided because of the occurrence of hematite as thin layers of "desert varnish" resulting from dehydration of limonite minerals by high surface temperatures caused by forest fires or by sun action. (This phenomenon has been observed in northern climates, e.g., British Columbia, as well as in desert areas.) Other common occurrences of hematite that are unrelated to chalcocite include solfataric alteration, compacted "red bed" sediments, hot spring deposits, iron formations, lateritic and desert soils, etc. Deposits of this type are normally low in copper. Grade predictions from the chart in Figure 12.12 do not indicate chalcocite enrichment. Note also that oxide copper values (rather than totals) must be used for the residual copper values to determine the amount of copper leaching from cappings containing visible sulfide minerals.

Field Applications and Techniques

Field estimates of the limonite and copper mineralogy of a capping provide sufficient evidence for capping classification and for estimates of the maximum and minimun copper grades of the former sulfide zone. Semi-quantitative predictions of the primary grade and chalcocite enrichment grade of the sulfide zone below the capping require geochemical analyses for copper in rock and detailed mapping of the limonite and copper mineralogy.

The empiricial correlations summarized in Figures 12.8, 12.9, and 12.10 demonstrate that field estimates of the percent goethite in limonite ($100 \times G/G + H + J$), of the percent hematite in limonite, of the percent jarosite in limonite, and of the copper mineralogy of a capping can be used to make semi-quantitative estimates of the approximate sulfide mineralogy and the total sulfide content of the former sulfide zone. This information can be used in conjunction with the nomograph in Figure 12.11 to calculate the maximum and minimum limits of copper grade in the former sulfide zone for each outcrop examined.

The limonite and copper mineralogy of areas deemed worthy of further interest should be mapped in detail. Zones with 0, 0 to 10, 10 to 25, 25 to 50, 50 to 75, 75 to 100, and 100 percent goethite, hematite, and jarosite in limonite, as well as areas of specific copper minerals, should each be outlined. Generally, these zones are easily recognized and mapped at a rapid rate (much faster than alteration zones, for

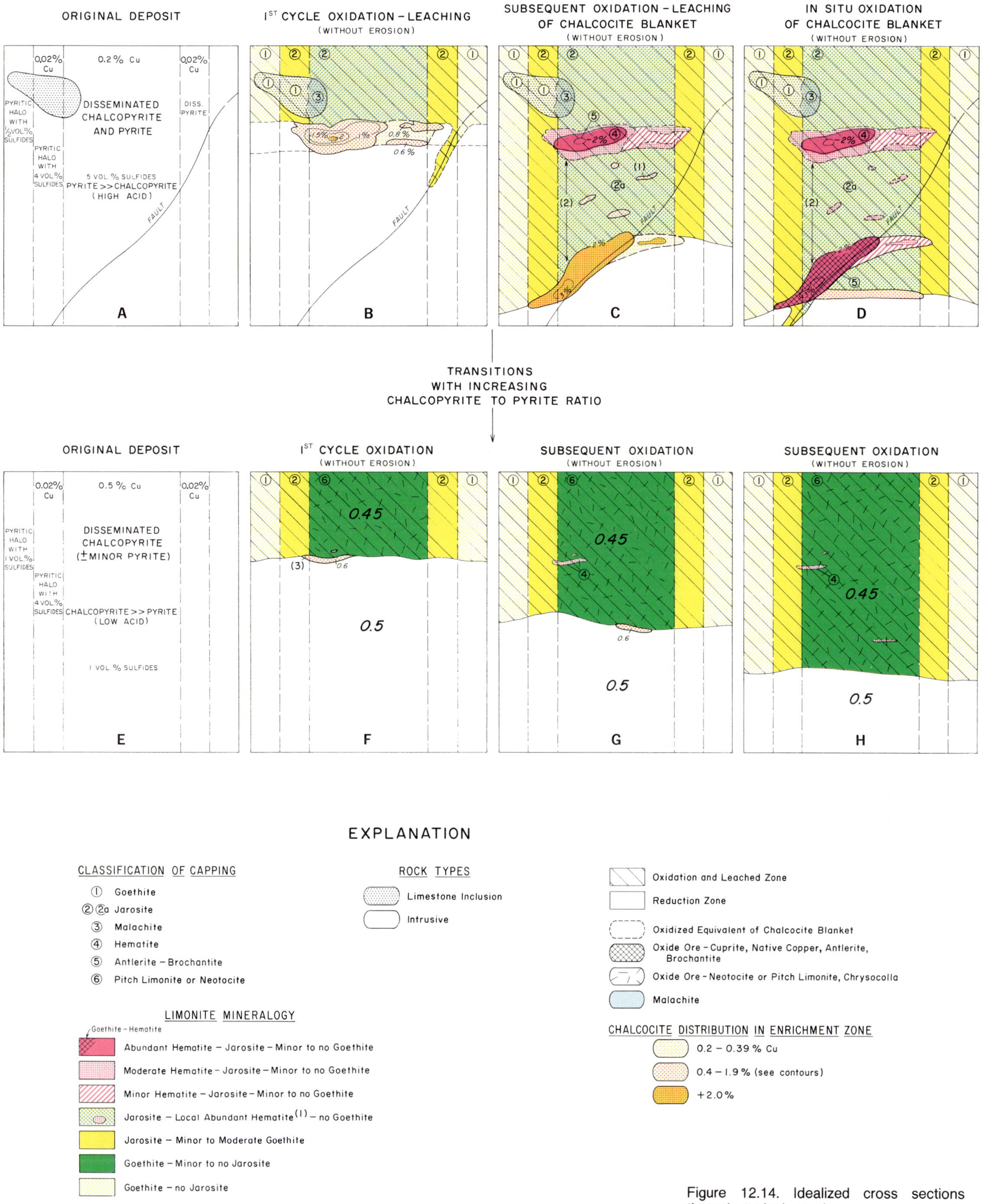

(1) Small zones of chalcocite may form in oxidation zone wherever local reducing conditions prevail.

(2) Gap between chalcocite blanket and former blanket not present if oxidation produced continuous downward migration of chalcocite.

(3) Minor leaching accompanied by enrichment may occur in proximity to local pyrite increase.

Figure 12.14. Idealized cross sections through typical porphyry copper deposits showing oxidation cycles, capping classification, and limonite characteristics. Interpretations shown for a system with 0.2 percent primary copper and 5 volume percent total sulfides *(A-D)* and for a system with 0.5 percent primary copper and 1 volume percent total sulfides *(E-H)*.

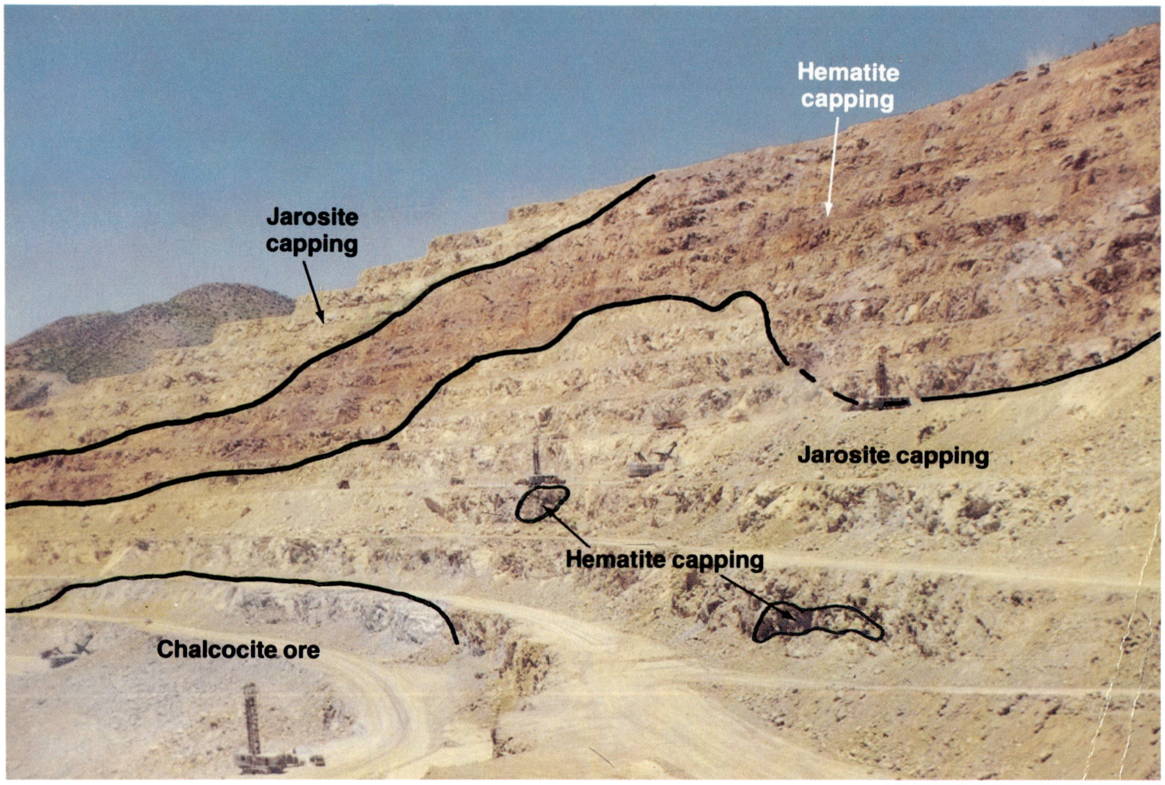

Figure 12.15. Layered jarosite and hematite capping overlying chalcocite ore at Toquepala, Peru. Upper jarosite capping formed by oxidation of pyrite-chalcopyrite. Hematite capping formed by oxidation of a chalcocite enrichment blanket (layer). Lower jarosite capping formed by oxidation of a pyrite-chalcopyrite zone between two chalcocite enrichment blankets. The gap between the former and present chalcocite enrichment blankets is the result of a marked drop in the groundwater table produced by sudden uplift and tilting.

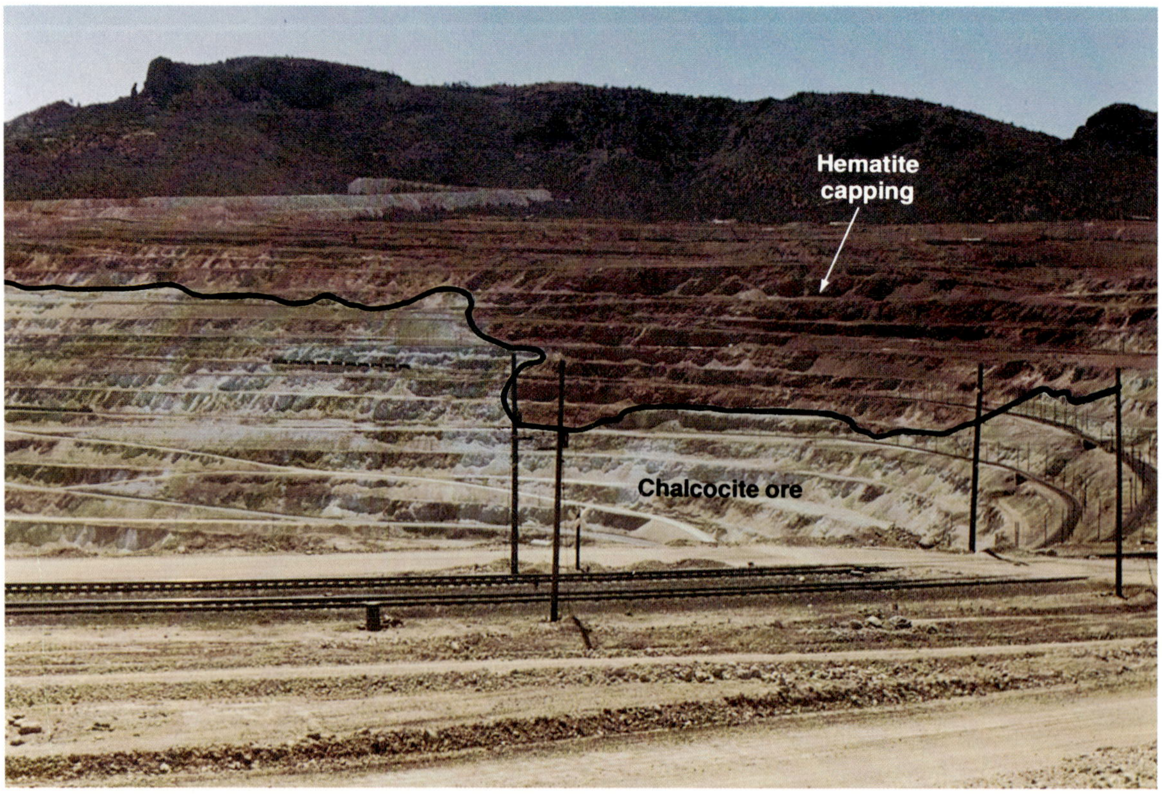

Figure 12.16. Hematite capping overlying chalcocite ore at Chino (Santa Rita), New Mexico. The hematite capping formed by oxidation of a chalcocite enrichment blanket. Continuous lowering of the groundwater table produced vertical continuity of chalcocite enrichment zones with subsequent continuous development of a hematite capping.

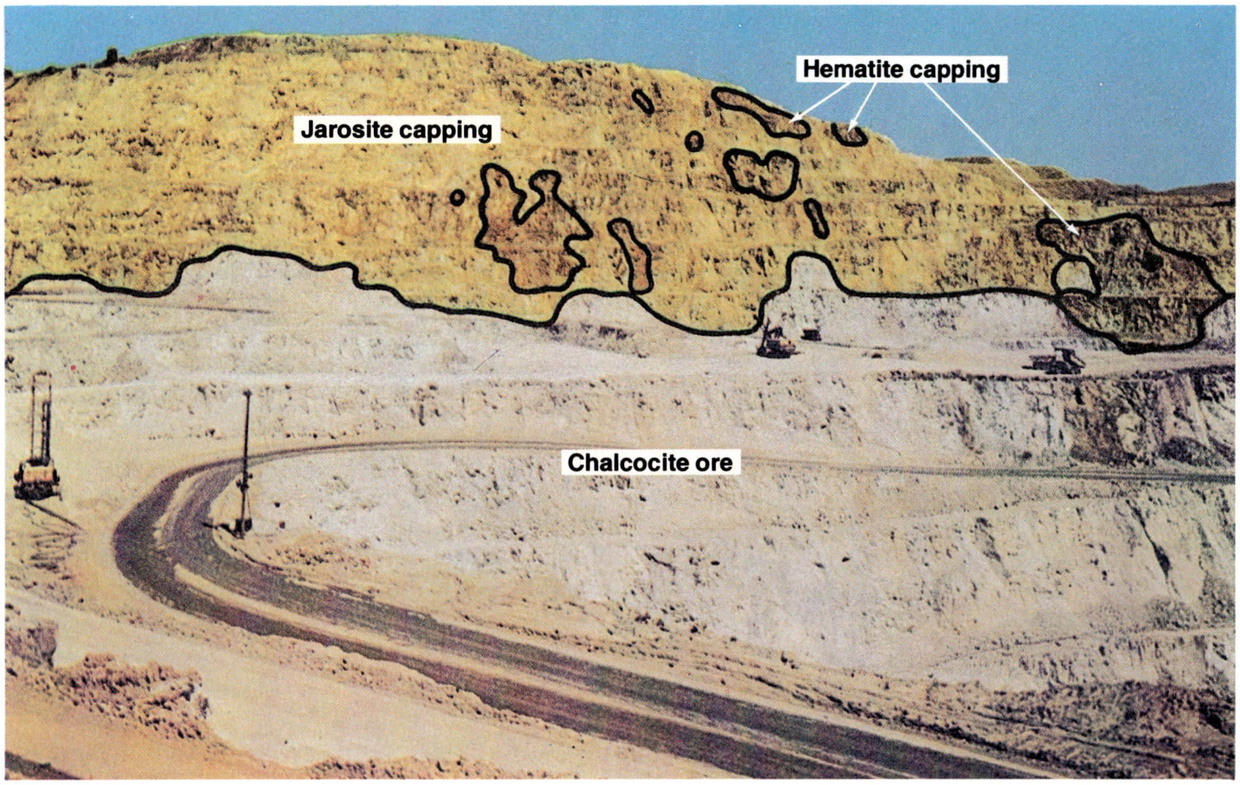

Figure 12.17. Jarosite capping with local zones of hematite capping over chalcocite ore at Butte, Montana. Jarosite capping formed by oxidation of pyrite-chalcopyrite. Hematite capping formed from destruction of local zones of chalcocite enrichment.

example). The size, shape, and control of these limonite map units provide the measure for the distribution of former sulfide mineralization. Brief experience with this type of mapping soon shows, in some areas, the inadequacy of grid sampling for capping appraisal purposes in porphyry copper prospects.

Representative rock samples from each type of capping and each mappable unit should be collected during the mapping program. Visual estimates of the limonite and copper mineralogy should be completed and recorded at the time of sample collection. The rock samples should then be submitted for geochemical copper analyses. Grade predictions for each sample site can then be obtained from the empirical correlations summarized in Figures 12.12 and 12.13. Verifications of visual limonite mapping should be obtained by X-ray on limonite concentrates prepared from a few of the more critical samples. The lowest detection limit of goethite in limonite by X-ray techniques is approximately 4 percent. This value corresponds to the visual detection limit for the writer, but visual limits are not consistent for all observers.

The above-described procedure of capping appraisal provides a method of predicting primary and chalcocite enrichment grades that is suitable for reconnaissance, examination, and project decisions.

Identification of Limonite Mixtures and Copper Minerals. The observed colors of limonite mineral mixtures are influenced by grain size, surface weathering ("desert varnish"), nature of illumination, impurities, and the color sensitivity of the viewer. Most of these variables can be compensated for by scratching the limonite in the rock sample and comparing the color of the resulting powder (streak) with standard powders. A limonite color chart, containing standard mixtures of actual mineral powders, is a useful aid in the field identification of mixtures of goethite, jarosite, and hematite.

Neotocite [$(Cu,Mn,Fe)SiO_2$] and pitch limonite [$H(Fe,Cu)O_2$] (?) may sometimes be confused with manganese oxide and goethite, respectively. Neotocite is distinguished from manganese oxide by its vitreous black to drab black appearance and by a black to dark olive, waxy streak when scratched; fine-grained mixtures of goethite in a sample commonly impart a brownish tint to the streak. Neotocite, which may contain up to 21 percent copper, can also be distinguished by a simple field test for copper. This test consists of applying 10 percent sulfuric acid to the mineral surface; rubbing the acid-wetted surface with metallic iron, such as a knife blade; and examining the blade for an obvious coating of metallic copper.

Pitch limonite may be distinguished from goethite in the field by its brown resinous appearance and shining black conchoidal fractures, which commonly show red internal reflection when viewed with a hand lens. It can also be identified by the field test for copper described above; this test is particularly useful for fine-grained occurrences, since the color of the powder (streak) is identical to that of goethite. This similarity to goethite is explained by X-ray studies, which indicate that pitch limonite is a copper-bearing hydrous iron oxide mineraloid that occasionally gives weak X-ray reflections similar to those of goethite.

Limitations of Capping Interpretations

The grade prediction techniques summarized in this chapter are by no means a panacea for porphyry copper outcrop evaluation. On the contrary, the validity of this approach to capping appraisal (outcrops or sub-outcrops) relies heavily on correct interpretations of structure and petrology. Supergene solutions, for example, may show lateral downward migration because of shallow dipping contacts, fracture systems, or faults, such as those illustrated in Figure 12.14 *A–D.* Pre-ore or post-ore structures may control or produce offsets in sulfide mineralization. Rock types commonly have a marked influence on the distribution of primary sulfides. Highly reactive carbonate rocks below the outcrop may inhibit copper migration, as shown in Figure 12.14*A–D.* The possibility of vertical sulfide zoning must be evaluated by geological concepts and tested by geophysical techniques or drilling. The above considerations, and many more, must be used in conjunction with the grade prediction techniques in order to properly evaluate the potential of a capping. These factors must also be considered when evaluating the grade predictions in light of subsequent drilling results.

SUMMARY

The characteristics of leached capping can be used to predict copper grades and the nature of sulfide mineralization that may lie beneath the surface. The procedures involved include the use of capping classifications, limonite mineralogy, supergene copper mineralogy, and the residual copper content of the capping. Capping classifications are based upon limonite mineralogy, copper mineralogy, and oxidation cycles. Six types of cappings are recognized: (1) goethite, (2) jarosite, (3) hematite, (4) pitch limonite-neotocite, (5) antlerite-bronchantite, and (6) malachite. Grade predictions for each type of capping utilize empirical correlations of the primary grade and chalcocite enrichment grade of the sulfide zone with (a) percent goethite in limonite, (b) percent hematite in limonite, (c) percent jarosite in limonite, (d) diagnostic copper mineralogy, and (e) and the residual copper content of the capping.

Visual estimates of the limonite and copper mineralogy of the capping provide sufficient data for capping classifications and for semi-quantitative field estimates of the maximum and minimum copper grades of the former sulfide zone at each outcrop examined. Quantitative predictions of the primary grade and chalcocite enrichment grade of the sulfide zone below capping require geochemical analyses for copper in rock and detailed mapping of limonite and copper mineralogy.

As a part of the study reported here, copper grade predictions were completed at 9 properties prior to drilling and post-mortem capping appraisals were made at 9 other properties. Drilling results available demonstrate that over 75 percent of the primary-grade predictions (in % Cu) agreed within 30 percent of the actual values encountered in drilling. Over 80 percent of the chalcocite enrichment predictions (in ft. % Cu) agreed within 20 percent of the values obtained by drilling.

ACKNOWLEDGMENTS

The author wishes to acknowledge the assistance and cooperation of Kennecott Copper Corporation, particularly personnel at Bear Creek Mining Company. The writer is especially indebted to D. R. Cook, P. A. Bailly, T. W. Mitcham, D. L. Norton, F. F. Clark, Annan Cook, R. E. Gilbert, J. A. Gower, A. H. James, R. E. Lehner, J. D. Mancuso, G. J. Stathis, T. N. Walthier, Alfred Weiss, J. C. Wilson, and J. R. Woodcock for their interest and support, ideas, suggestions, and aid in data interpretation and presentation; to R. J. Broadhead, D. B. Roberts, W. M. Tuddenham, and J. D. Stephens for their contributions to the development of new analytical techniques and for carrying out the work; and to D. H. Adair, G. Aguilar, W. W. Baltosser, H. E. Bauer, A. R. Grant, R. A. Metz, T. A. Netelbeek, G. C. Reed, M. D. Regan, W. M. Shepard, David Snyder, R. R. Weaver, and J. E. Worthington for their assistance in collection, interpretation, field application, and evaluation of research data.

SELECTED REFERENCES

Baas Becking, L. G. M.; Kaplan, I. R.; and Moore, D., 1960, Limits of the natural environments in terms of pH and oxidation-reduction potentials: Jour. Geol., v. 68, p. 243–284.

Bladh, K. W., 1978, The weathering of sulfide-bearing rocks associated with porphyry-type copper deposits: Unpub. Ph.D. Diss., Univ. Ariz., 98 p.

Blanchard, Roland, 1968, Interpretation of leached outcrops: Nevada Bur. Mines Bull. 66, 196 p.

Brown, J. B., 1971. Jarosite-goethite stabilities at 25°C, 1 atm: Mineral Deposita, v. 6, p. 245–252.

Emmons, W. H., 1917, The enrichment of ore deposits: U.S. Geol. Survey Bull. 625, 530 p.

Garrels, R. M., and Christ, C. L., 1965, Solutions, Minerals and Equilibria: San Francisco, Freeman, Copper and Co., 450 p.

Garrels, R. M., and MacKenzie, F. T., 1971, Evolution of Sedimentary Rocks: New York, W. W. Norton and Co., 397 p.

Garrels, R. M., and Thompson, M. E., 1960, Oxidation of pyrite by iron sulfate solutions: Amer. Jour. Sci., v. 258A, p. 57–67.

Hodge, E. T., 1915, The compositions of water in mines of sulphide ores: Econ. Geol., v. 10, p. 123–139.

Latimer, W. M., 1952, The Oxidation States of the Elements and Their Potentials in Aqueous Solutions, 2nd ed.: Englewood Cliffs, N.J., Prentice-Hall, Inc., 392 p.

Locke, Augustus, 1926, Leached Outcrops As Guides to Copper Ores: Baltimore, Williams and Wilkins Co., 166 p.

Lovering, T. S., 1948, Geothermal gradients, recent climatic changes, and rate of sulfide oxidation in the San Manuel district, Arizona: Econ. Geol., v. 43, p. 1–20.

Merwin, H. E., and Posnjak, E., 1937, Sulphate incrustations in the Copper Queen Mine, Bisbee, Arizona: Am. Mineral. v. 22, p. 567–571.

Posnjak, E., and Merwin, H. E., 1922, the system Fe_2O_3-SO_3-H_2O: Jour. Amer. Chem. Soc., v. 44, p. 1965–1994.

Posnjak, E., and Tunell, G., 1929, The system cupric oxide-sulphur trioxide-water: Amer. Jour. Sci., Fifth Ser., v. 18, no. 103, p. 1–34.

Ransome, F. L., 1919, The copper deposits of Ray and Miami, Arizona: U. S. Geol. Survey Prof. Paper 115, 192 p.

Sato, M., 1960, Oxidation of sulfide ore bodies: 1, Geochemical environments in terms of Eh and pH: Econ. Geol., v. 55, p. 928–961.

Sillman, J. F. B., 1958, The stabilities of some oxidized copper minerals in aqueous solutions at 25°C and 1 atm total pressures: Unpub. Ph.D. Diss., Harvard Univ., 98 p.

Tunell, George, 1930, The oxidation of disseminated copper ores in altered porphyry: Unpub. Ph.D. Diss., Harvard Univ., 105 p.

Tunell, George, and Posnjak, E., 1931, A portion of the system, ferric oxide-cupric oxide-sulphur trioxide-water: Jour. Phys. Chem., v. 35, p. 929–946.

White, D. E.; Hem, J. D.; and Waring, G. A., 1963, Chemical composition of sub-surface water: U.S. Geol. Survey Prof. Paper 440-F, 67 p.

13

Geochemical Prospecting Techniques for Porphyry Copper Deposits

SOUTHWESTERN UNITED STATES AND NORTHERN MEXICO

Maurice A. Chaffee

The porphyry copper province of the southwestern United States and northern Mexico contains the highest density of known major copper deposits of any area in the world. Because this region has been so well endowed, exploration activity, especially during the years 1960 to 1980, was quite intense, and most of the exposed deposits have probably now been found. The region may still contain undiscovered copper deposits that are present beneath a thin layer of post-mineralization pediment gravels or volcanic rocks or that are present at depth within rock bodies that are exposed at the surface. Finding such blind deposits requires the use of indirect exploration techniques. To this end, geophysical techniques have been successful in finding several deposits buried under post-mineralization pediment gravels.

Geochemical prospecting techniques should also be useful in finding new blind porphyry copper deposits. A review of geochemical exploration techniques applicable in the search for copper deposits (Chaffee, 1975) described both proved and untried geochemical prospecting techniques. Some of these techniques are particularly well suited to geochemical prospecting in the semi-arid climate of the southwestern United States and northern Mexico. This chapter discusses some of the more useful sampling techniques for this region and describes the results of several investigations undertaken to learn more about how geochemical prospecting can be used.

ROCK SAMPLING

The possible levels of erosion for porphyry copper systems vary from those that expose the deepest root level of an actual copper deposit, or deeper (Fig. 13.1, level A), to those that expose the pyrite halo level (Fig. 13.1, level B), to those that expose only hypogene altered rock or apparently unaltered rock (Fig. 13.1, levels C and D). (A porphyry copper system includes the copper deposit as well as the surrounding rock that has been affected by the mineralizing processes.) Alteration-mineralization zoning, which has long been recognized around porphyry deposits, has been very useful in the discovery of a number of copper deposits, including many whose copper-rich zone was not exposed at the surface. Element zoning, based on analysis of whole-rock and (or) soil samples, should also be useful in locating copper deposits that are present deep within exposed rock bodies—perhaps even those buried so deep that no alteration is apparent (Fig. 13.1, level D).

Element zoning has been investigated using analyses of whole-rock samples from the deeply buried and zoned Kalamazoo porphyry copper deposit near San Manuel, Arizona (see location map in Fig. 13.2). The orebody is found within both a Precambrian quartz monzonite batholith and a Cretaceous quartz monzonite porphyry stock that intruded the Precambrian unit (Lowell, 1968). The top of the ore zone ($\geq$ 0.5% Cu) occurs as deep as 1,130 m (3,700 ft). Results of the investigation are shown in Figure 13.3. They indicate that intervals of high or low concentrations of at least 21 elements are spatially related to the known ore zone (Chaffee, 1976*a*, 1982). The elements boron, barium, strontium, and lithium are most concentrated in the lower part of the copper ore zone and below the ore zone in the barren, or low-grade, core of the deposit. Surrounding the zone containing these four elements is the ore zone, in which copper, molybdenum, silver, and gold are concentrated. Outside of the ore zone are, successively, aureoles of (1) cobalt, vanadium, and selenium; (2) iron (pyrite-related) and sulfur; (3) rubidium; and (4) tellurium, gold, and iron (in the root zone only). The aureoles for rubidium and for tellurium, gold, and root-zone iron are

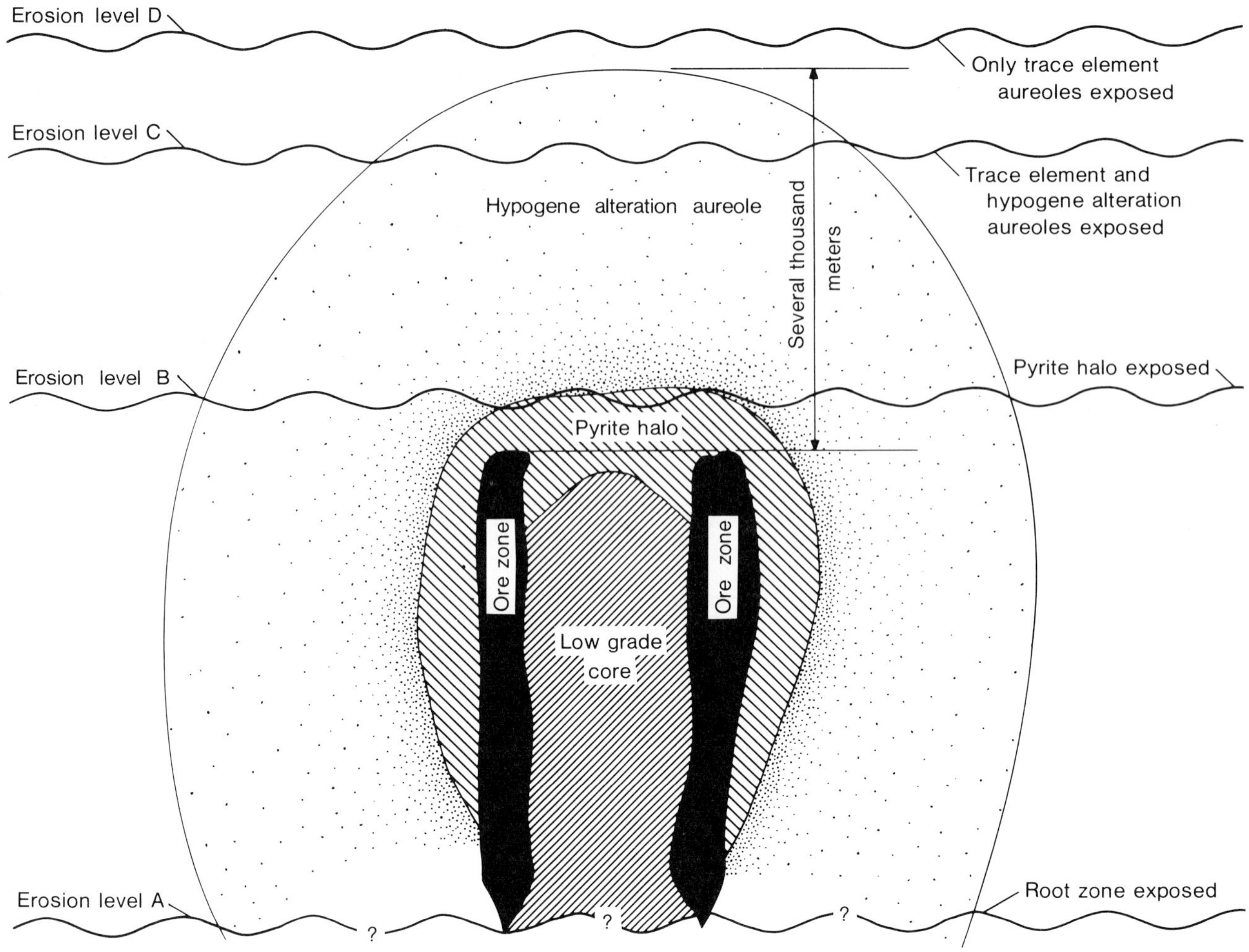

Figure 13.1. Schematic diagram of a porphyry copper system, showing hypothetical levels of erosion. Modified after Lowell and Guilbert (1970).

present well out into the propylitic zone; the aureoles for cobalt, vanadium, and selenium and for sulfur and pyrite-related iron also occur well outside the ore zone. Information presently available suggests that some additional elements (manganese, zinc, lead, thallium, and possibly some others) may be concentrated in aureoles that are even farther from the ore zone than those shown in Figure 13.3.

Element suites need to be determined in rock samples from other known deposits to determine whether common suites of elements exist for most porphyry copper deposits. The results of the study at Kalamazoo suggest that analysis of suites of ore-related elements in rock samples should be a useful method for evaluating exposed rock bodies for buried copper deposits.

The Kalamazoo study utilized whole-rock samples. Many specialized samples derived from rock samples may also be useful in geochemical exploration for porphyry copper deposits. Mineral separates, which tend to concentrate certain elements, may further enhance the widths and element concentrations of aureoles of various elements present in the outer zones of a porphyry system. The element contents of biotite, magnetite, pyrite, and other minerals have been discussed in a number of studies cited in Chaffee (1975). An investigation by Williams (1976) suggests that physical parameters, as well as the trace-element content, of accessory minerals such as apatite and rutile may be important in evaluating exposed rock bodies for their possible relation to

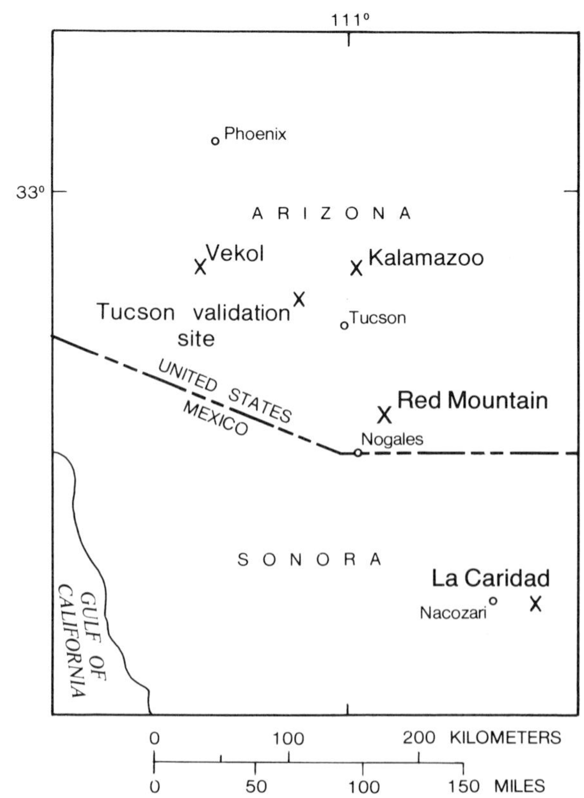

Figure 13.2. Map showing locations of areas discussed in chapter

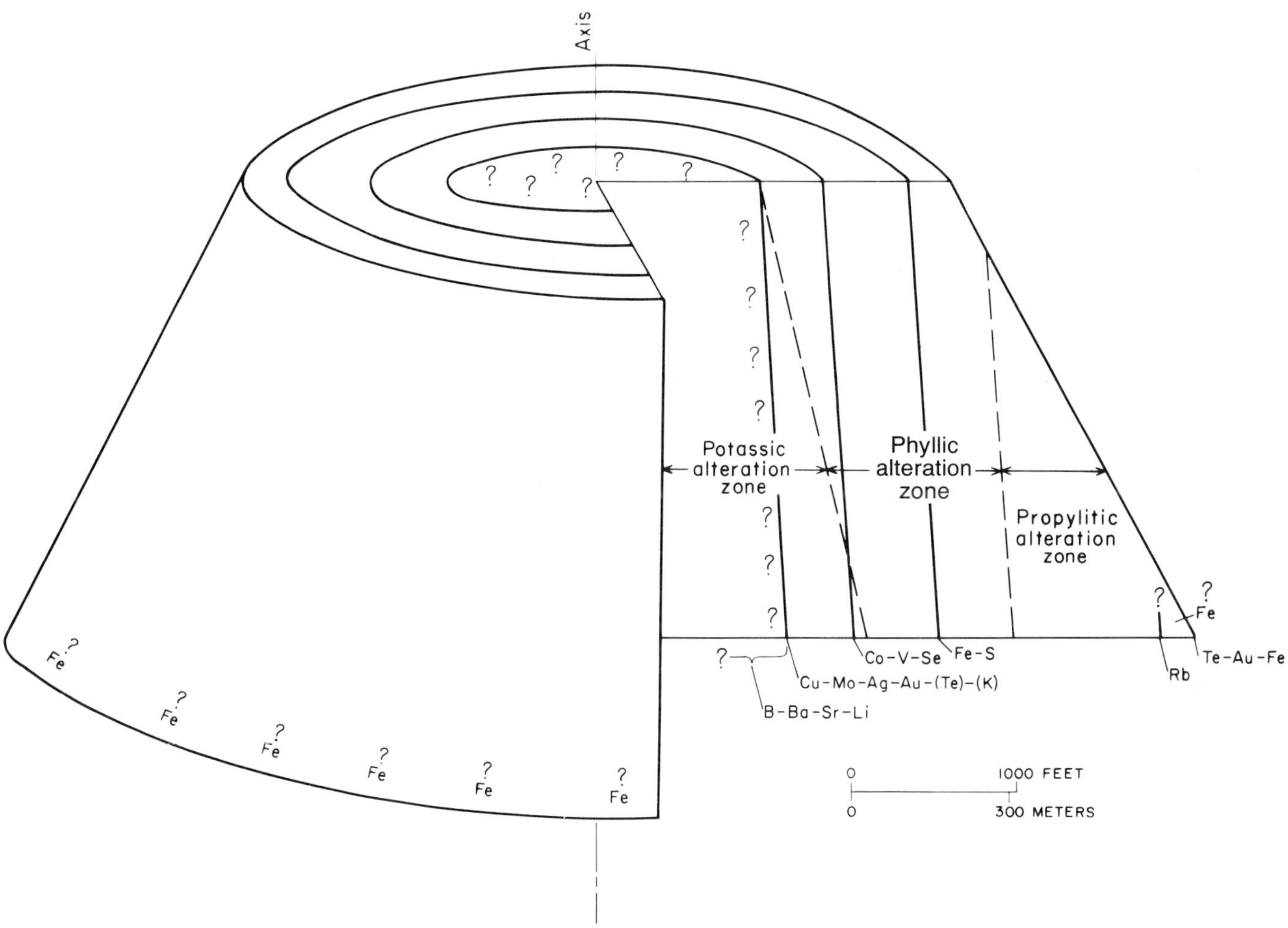

Figure 13.3. Geochemical model of the Kalamazoo-San Manuel porphyry copper deposits. Heavy lines for each element suite represent approximate location of coincident concentration peaks for elements in that suite. Alteration zone boundaries (dashed lines) are based on information given in drill logs.

blind orebodies. Other types of specialized rock samples such as iron- or manganese-oxide coatings, gossans, leached cappings, and fluid inclusions, may also be useful in prospecting for blind porphyry copper deposits (Chaffee, 1975).

SOIL SAMPLING

Soil is a sample medium commonly used in geochemical prospecting. The chemical analyses of samples of residual soil may indicate the presence of one or more pathfinder elements that can define the outer aureoles in the upper or outer parts of a porphyry copper system. Soil sampling techniques were used in a geochemical survey conducted in the vicinity of the Vekol porphyry copper deposit near Casa Grande, Arizona (see location map, Fig. 13.2). The geology and geochemistry of this deposit have been described in several reports (Chaffee and Hessin, 1971; Steele, 1976; Chaffee, 1977). The deposit is genetically associated with a Cretaceous stock that intruded a thick, layered sequence of Precambrian, Paleozoic, and Mesozoic rock units. The copper is concentrated in the host-rock units rather than in the stock. Some outcrops in the vicinity of the deposit are weakly mineralized and altered. Only a small part of the actual deposit crops out; most of the deposit is covered by post-mineralization pediment gravels (Chaffee and Hessin, 1971).

A residual-soil sample was collected at each site shown in Figure 13.4. An evaluation of the analyses of these soil samples indicates that the Vekol porphyry copper system is chemically zoned. Samples of soil collected on the small exposure of the central part of the deposit predictably contain the highest concentrations of copper and molybdenum; in contrast, samples of soil collected from the surrounding area, which is mainly composed of carbonate-rich rock units, contain the highest concentrations of zinc, manganese, silver, lead, cadmium, and bismuth (Fig. 13.5). This pattern of distribution and abundance suggests that a crude aureole of concentrations of these pathfinder elements is present around the copper and molybdenum anomaly. Furthermore, the increase in copper concentrations toward the small outcrop in the center of the deposit and the metal zoning of the system suggest that a soil survey would probably have selected the site of the actual copper deposit as the most favorable location for such a deposit even if the small exposure containing the highest concentrations of copper and molybdenum did not crop out. Thus, soil sampling should be a useful geochemical prospecting technique to use in the search for copper deposits even where only the outer aureoles of pathfinder elements can be detected at the surface.

Several specialized types of soil-related materials have also been used in geochemical surveys (Chaffee, 1975). Of

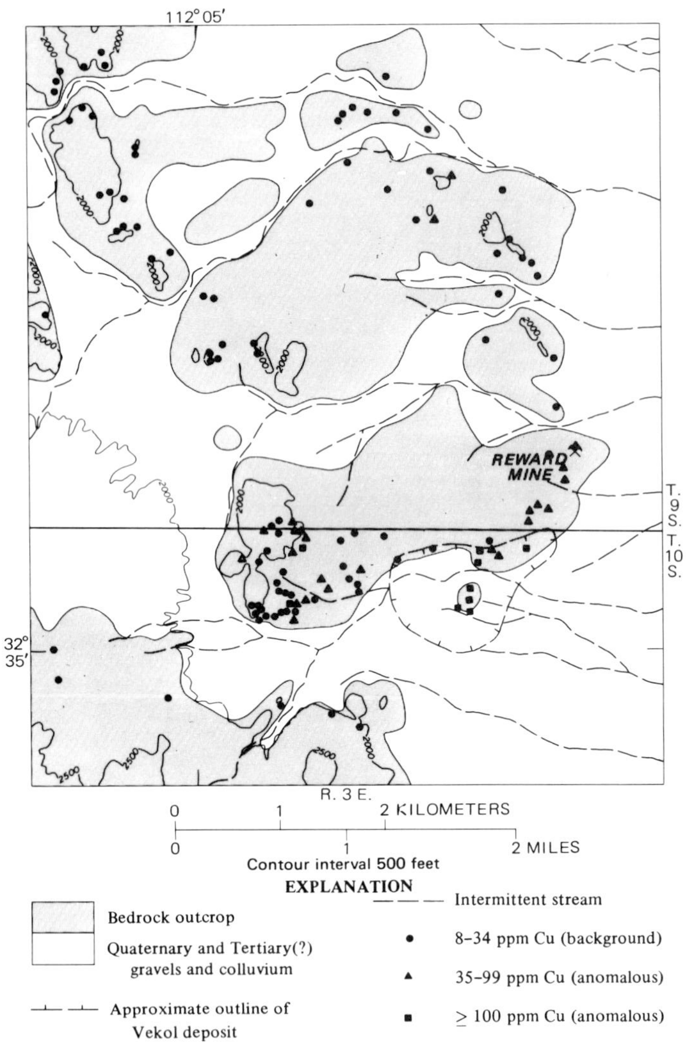

Figure 13.4. Distribution and abundance of copper in samples of residual soil collected in the vicinity of the Vekol copper deposit. The distributions of molybdenum anomalies are similar to those for copper (≥ 100 ppm). Modified after Chaffee (1977).

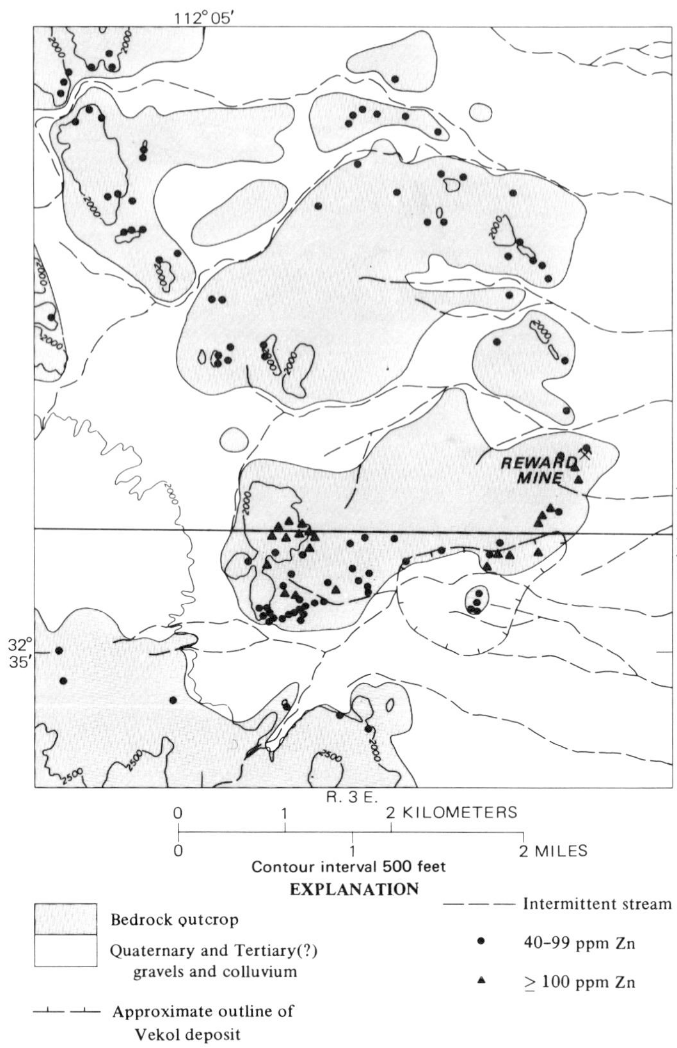

Figure 13.5. Distribution of zinc in samples of residual soil collected in the vicinity of the Vekol copper deposit. The distributions of manganese, silver, lead, cadmium, and bismuth anomalies are similar to those of zinc. Modified after Chaffee (1977).

these, probably only two are of interest in geochemical prospecting for copper in the semi-arid environment: caliche and desert varnish. Caliche is a calcium-carbonate-rich material that is developed as part of the soil-forming process in many arid regions. For geochemical prospecting purposes, caliche that forms in layers deposited directly on bedrock surfaces, or in the overburden immediately above them, is suitable as a sampling medium (Chaffee, 1975). If copper were present in an exposure of bedrock that was later covered with caliche or caliche-cemented overburden, then this superjacent caliche may concentrate any mobilized copper (Huff, 1970). However, for most geochemical surveys, caliche is probably not a very useful sampling medium. Exposures containing caliche are not always present throughout an area; consequently, one may not be able to achieve an effective sample density in an area.

Desert varnish is an iron- or manganese-rich oxide coating that forms on the exposed surfaces of rocks in the arid environment. Desert varnish is known to concentrate various elements (Chaffee, 1975); however, as may be the case for caliche, desert varnish is usually found only in restricted areas. Thus, the use of this type of sample material is limited to those areas where it is widely distributed.

STREAM SEDIMENT SAMPLING

Sediment collected in active stream channels has been used successfully throughout the world as a geochemical sampling medium. Because of the relatively high percentage of rock exposure and the generally good access to most field areas in the southwestern United States, this sampling medium has not been as widely used here as it has in other climatic and geologic environments and in less accessible regions. In addition, some complications exist that may affect the value of stream sediment as a sampling medium in the arid environment. In desert areas, material is eroded from outcrops and transported as sediment in stream channels only during relatively infrequent periods of heavy rainfall. Thus, sediment that remains in place in a channel during dry periods may be contaminated by streambank material or even by wind-borne material. Stream sediment may also be contaminated easily by material from old mine dumps or other man-made sources.

Reconnaissance geochemical surveys using stream sediment have been successfully employed in arid regions. Such a program in northern Mexico located the La Caridad porphyry copper deposit (see location map, Fig. 13.2), which occurs in association with a Tertiary quartz monzonite porphyry stock that intruded older plutonic and volcanic rocks (Saegart et al., 1974). Compared to that around many other porphyry copper deposits, the relief in the immediate vicinity of La Caridad is unusually high—about 1,000 m (about 3,300 ft.). This fact, together with the large size and high grade of the deposit and the well-integrated drainage system, made the La Caridad area an unusually good place to study element migration in stream sediments in the vicinity of a porphyry copper deposit. As a consequence, a detailed stream-sediment survey was conducted in the vicinity of this deposit to learn more about the surface geochemistry of the area before it was greatly disturbed by mining activity. Samples of stream sediment were collected in the vicinity of, and downstream from, the deposit and were analyzed for as many as 37 elements. Of these 37, the analyses for total copper, cold-extractable copper, molybdenum, zinc, silver, and tungsten produced anomalies that could be related to the known deposit (Chaffee et al., 1976*a*). Molybdenum produced the anomaly that extended the farthest downstream—a distance of at least 32 kilometers (about 20 miles). The distribution of molybdenum is shown in Figure 13.6.

In another study regional stream-sediment sampling was conducted in the Patagonia Mountains of southern Arizona (see Fig. 13.2) to learn more about the regional geochemical features of a portion of the Arizona copper province and to determine which elements best define the known large, deeply buried porphyry copper system at Red Mountain. The results of this investigation (Chaffee et al., in press) indicate that samples containing a combination of high concentrations of molybdenum, lead, and tellurium and low concentrations of manganese best define the location of the Red Mountain system. The results also indicate that, relative to other parts of southern Arizona, much of the entire Patagonia Mountain area contains high concentrations of lead, copper, and tellurium; such high concentrations suggest that these elements may be especially useful in defining the limits of areas that may contain undiscovered porphyry copper deposits in southern Arizona or elsewhere.

Concentrates panned from raw stream sediment have also been widely used in reconnaissance geochemical surveys; however, little published information has been available concerning their use in prospecting for porphyry copper deposits in arid regions. In order to provide such information

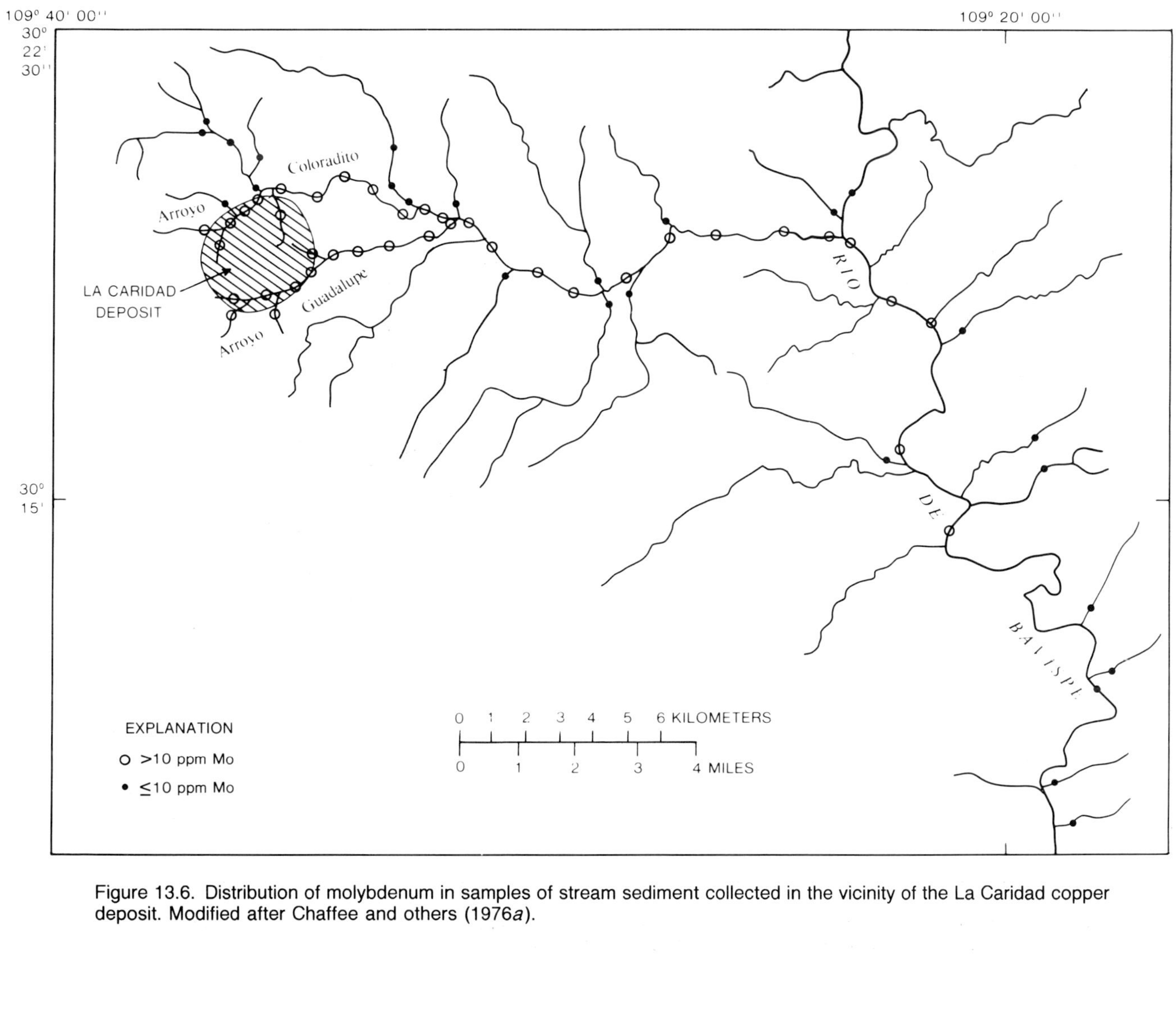

Figure 13.6. Distribution of molybdenum in samples of stream sediment collected in the vicinity of the La Caridad copper deposit. Modified after Chaffee and others (1976*a*).

panned concentrates were prepared from splits of the stream-sediment samples collected for the geochemical survey of the La Caridad deposit. Evaluation of the chemical analyses of these concentrates indicated that only copper, molybdenum, and tungsten produced anomalies related to the deposit (Chaffee et al., 1976*a*).

Figure 13.7 shows the distribution of tungsten anomalies revealed by analyses of the panned concentrates. The anomaly related to the La Caridad deposit continues for about 11 kilometers (about 7 miles) below outcrops of the deposit—an impressive distance for an element not commonly studied in connection with porphyry copper deposits. Because of the relatively high (100 ppm) lower limit of detection for tungsten in the concentrates, the actual content of this element could not be determined in many of the samples collected downstream from the deposit. If a more sensitive lower limit could have been used, the tungsten anomaly related to the deposit would probably have extended much farther downstream. The anomaly for molybdenum in panned concentrates extends about as far as that determined for molybdenum in the samples of stream sediment (see Fig. 13.6),and a more sensitive measurement of tungsten in panned con-centrates might reveal that the tungsten anomaly is equally extensive. Thus, the results of this study at La Caridad indicate that surveys using either stream sediments or panned concentrates would have readily discovered the deposit.

Copper anomalies can be found in sediments collected in many stream channels in the southwestern United States and northern Mexico. Most of these anomalies, however, are probably not associated with porphyry copper deposits. The study at La Caridad found significant anomalies of molybdenum, zinc, silver, and tungsten in addition to anomalies of copper. These results suggest that the determination of elements in addition to copper shou'd help in evaluating other areas for their potential for porphyry copper deposits. If one assumes that most of the exposed porphyry copper deposits in this part of the United States and Mexico have already been discovered, then most stream-sediment surveys probably should emphasize such elements as gold, lead, zinc, tellurium, selenium, and rubidium, which may be concentrated in aureoles outside of the copper-rich zone of a porphyry system. The presence of anomalies of some of these pathfinder elements in stream sediments may help to identify areas with exposed rock bodies containing blind porphyry copper deposits.

VEGETATION SAMPLING

Both geobotanical and biogeochemical prospecting techniques have been used in the search for new porphyry copper

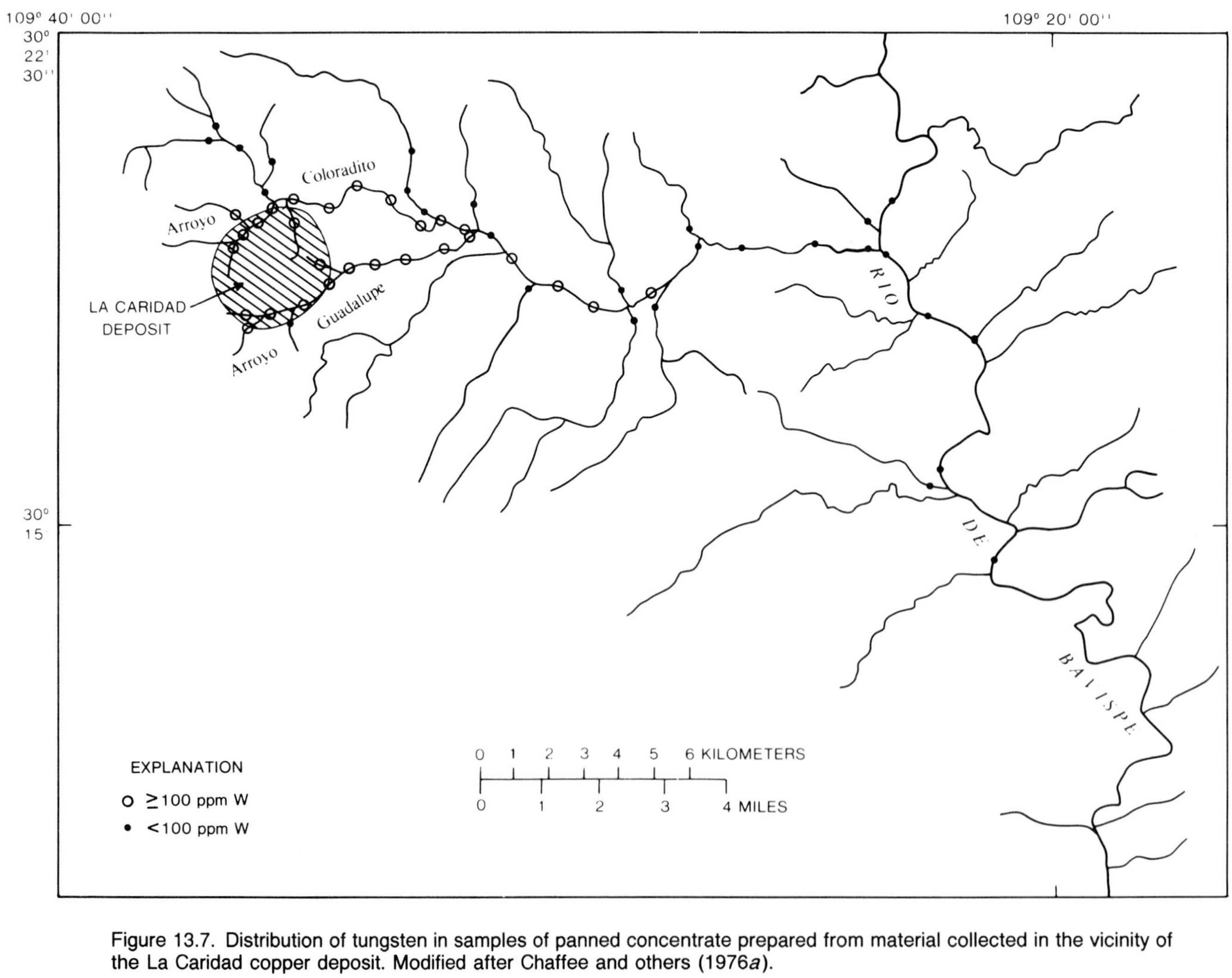

Figure 13.7. Distribution of tungsten in samples of panned concentrate prepared from material collected in the vicinity of the La Caridad copper deposit. Modified after Chaffee and others (1976*a*).

deposits; however, only a few reports dealing with applications of these techniques in the southwestern United States or northern Mexico have been published.

Geobotanical Sampling

Geobotanical surveys applied to the search for porphyry copper deposits in the southwestern United States have not been very successful. To date only one copper-indicator plant species has been found that demonstrates any relationship to concentrations of copper in surficial materials. This species, the California poppy (*Eschscholtzia mexicana*), has been recognized growing in copper-rich soils near many porphyry deposits (Lovering et al., 1950; Warren et al., 1951; Cannon, 1960; and Chaffee and Gale, 1976). One deposit where this species has been recognized is at Mineral Butte, Arizona (see location map, Fig. 13.2). A generalized geologic map (Fig. 13.8*A*) shows a small copper deposit associated with a biotite-quartz monzonite stock of Cretaceous age that has intruded Precambrian granite (Chaffee, 1976*b*). Concentrations of copper were determined for rock and soil samples collected over and around this deposit. The abundance of poppy plants was also mapped in this area (Fig. 13.8*B*). Mapping revealed a close relationship between the area of high copper content in soil samples and the area containing the highest density of poppy plants (Chaffee and Gale, 1976).

In spite of the apparent success of the geobotanical method at Mineral Butte, the technique probably has only limited value for exploration in the southwestern United States and northern Mexico. Many areas of copper-rich soil in this region do not seem to support poppy plants. Also, wild poppy populations have been observed growing in areas where only a normal concentration of copper is present in the soil. Residual soil is usually available for sampling in desert areas where geobotanical surveys would be effective, so that geobotanical prospecting, which requires someone trained in botany to be effective, might not be justified. In addition, the method is not very practical in arid regions because during years of low rainfall, many species of desert plants simply do not germinate, do not flower, or are stunted; such conditions make identification of a given species difficult or impossible.

In spite of these drawbacks, a geobotanical survey can be a rapid, inexpensive, and effective prospecting technique. Such surveys may prove useful in locating blind porphyry

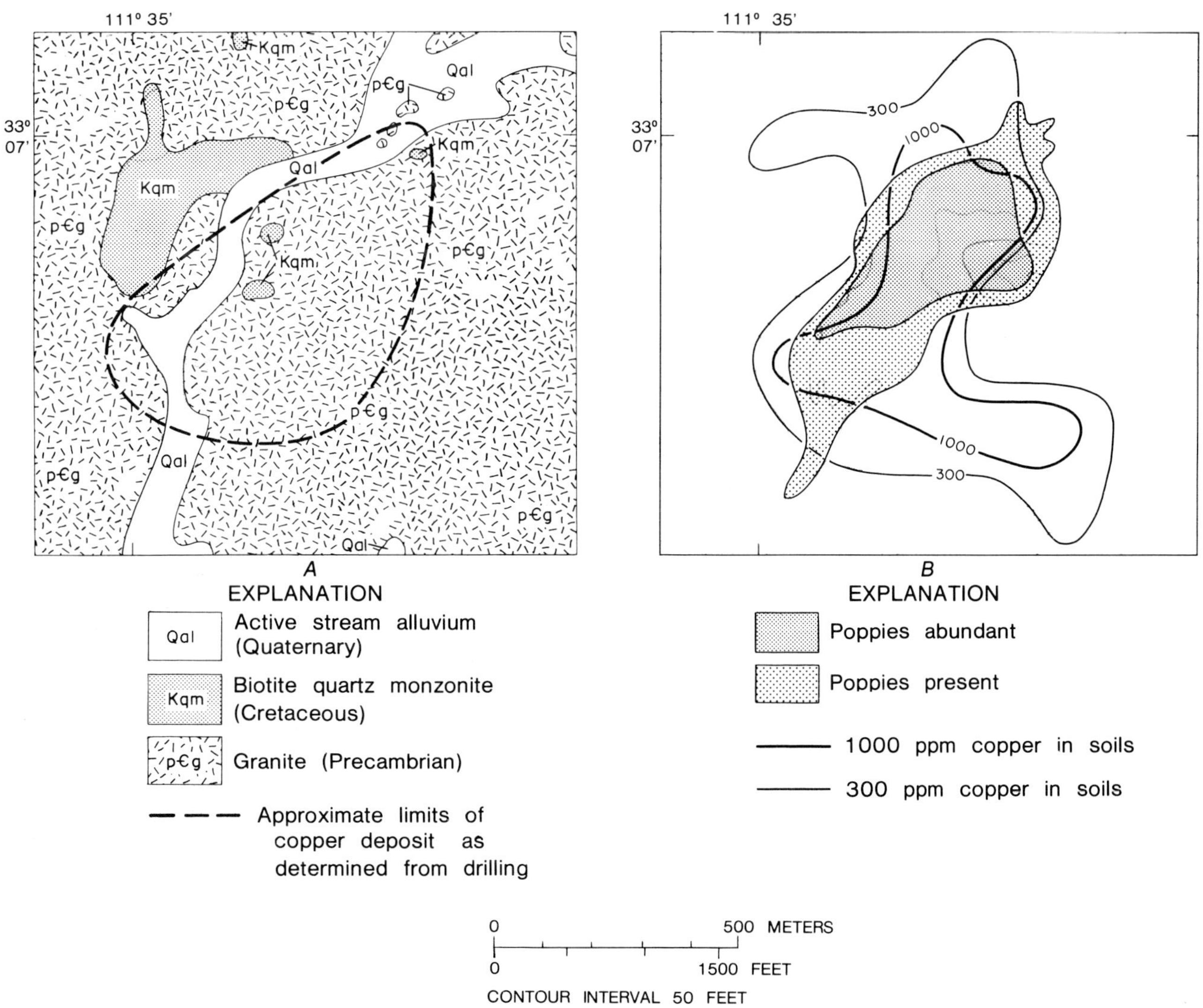

Figure 13.8. The Mineral Butte copper deposit. *A*, generalized geologic map and approximate location of the deposit; *B*, distribution of copper in samples of residual soil as compared to the distribution of California poppy plants in the vicinity of the Mineral Butte deposit. Modified after Chaffee (1976*b*) and Chaffee and Gale (1976).

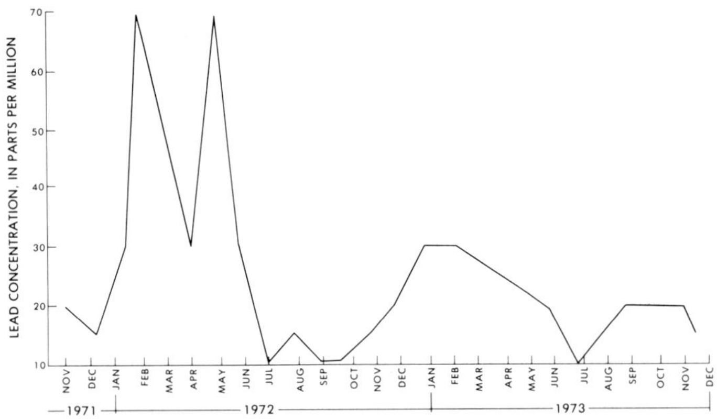

Figure 13.9. Distribution of lead in the ash of mesquite leaves over time. The samples were collected at the International Biological Program Tucson Validation Site. Element variation is both annual and longer-term, and similar variations occur for other plant parts and elements.

copper deposits if indicator plants can be identified for some of the common pathfinder elements known to be associated with this type of deposit, especially those elements that seem to occur in aureoles well outside of the copper-rich zone. The geochemical study at Kalamazoo described in Chapter 9 of this volume suggests that plant species that are specific indicators for elements such as manganese, zinc, gold, sulfur (or sulfate), selenium, and tellurium, might be successful in locating favorable areas. Unfortunately, no studies have as yet been made around porphyry copper deposits in the Southwest to identify species that might be indicative of any of these elements.

Biogeochemical Sampling

Biogeochemical surveys have more proven potential than geobotanical surveys in the search for new porphyry copper deposits. As with other prospecting methods, there are some drawbacks to the biogeochemical method. Perhaps the most serious problem relates to the time required for a sampling program. Analyses from samples collected over a period of more than two years at the International Biological Program Tucson Validation Site, north of Tucson, Arizona (see location map, Fig. 13.2), indicate that the element contents of plant parts often vary with time (Chaffee et al., 1976*b*). Figure 13.9 illustrates one example of this phenomenon. Because of such natural variations, it is impossible to be sure that analytical data from plants collected during one field season will be comparable with data from plants collected at some later time.

Another disadvantage to biogeochemical prospecting can be the limited distribution of some desirable plant species. In a sampling program that covers a large region (perhaps tens of square kilometers, or greater), it may not be possible to find the desired species at all required sample sites. This problem can often be overcome by sampling two or more species concurrently throughout the area being studied. Lastly, for surveys covering a large region, natural variations may be encountered in background values, caused by local variations in climate rather than variations in substrate chemistry. Orientation surveys are therefore recommended for every new area sampled.

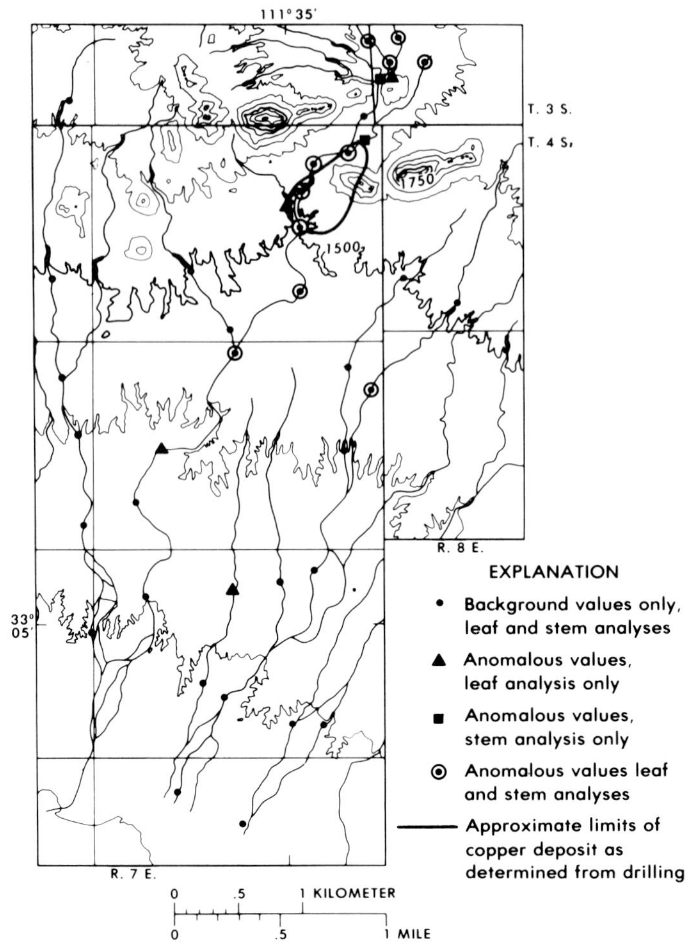

Figure 13.10. Distribution of copper in the ash of mesquite leaves and stems collected in the vicinity of the Mineral Butte deposit. The most significant anomalies are those at sites where both plant parts are anomalous. Modified after Chaffee (1976*b*).

In spite of these drawbacks, biogeochemical prospecting should be an important technique to use in the arid environment. Biogeochemical studies near the Mineral Butte, Vekol, and La Caridad deposits (Chaffee, 1976*b*, 1977; Chaffee et al., 1976*a*) clearly indicate that all three of these deposits could have been located using analyses of plant samples collected downstream from each deposit. At the Mineral Butte deposit the most effective biogeochemical sampling was achieved using the copper content in the ash of the leaves and stems of mesquite (*Prosopis juliflora*) and catclaw acacia (*Acacia greggii*) (Chaffee, 1976*b*). Of the two species, mesquite (Fig. 13.10) seems to give a slightly better indication of the location of the known deposit. This plant-element combination yielded anomalies at least 2 kilometers (about 1.2 miles) downstream from any mineralized outcrops.

At the Vekol deposit a number of elements (copper, molybdenum, manganese, zinc, lead, silver, cadmium, and bismuth) were found to be anomalous in the soils and rocks (Chaffee, 1977). Copper, molybdenum, zinc, and silver were also found to be strongly anomalous in the ash of several plant species—including mesquite, catclaw acacia, blue paloverde (*Cercidium floridum*), and ironwood (*Olneya tesota*)—collected downstream in the channels draining away from the immediate area of the deposit. Samples collected in other channels yielded only background concentration levels. As one example, Figure 13.11 shows the distribution of zinc in the ash of leaves and stems of ironwood—a fairly common desert tree of the region. Of all the plant-element combinations studied, this combination identified the Vekol deposit at the greatest distance downstream from any mineralized outcrops, a distance of over 2 kilometers (about 1.2 miles).

At the La Caridad deposit anomalous concentrations of copper, molybdenum, zinc, and silver were found in ashed samples of mesquite and oak (*Quercus* sp.) (Chaffee et al., 1976*a*). Anomalies of the first three elements extended at least 15 kilometers (about 9 miles) downstream from the deposit; the silver anomaly did not extend quite as far. Figure 13.12 shows the anomalies for copper in samples of the two plant species.

The findings at Mineral Butte, Vekol, and La Caridad indicate that biogeochemical surveys can effectively locate exposed copper deposits at considerable distances downstream from any mineralized outcrop, a distinct advantage in reconnaissance surveys. This sampling method also offers some unique advantages for reconnaissance surveys that might be undertaken to locate copper deposits buried beneath a thin veneer of pediment gravels. Most biogeochemical surveys in arid lands utilize plant species called phreatophytes, which have deep roots that tap the permanent groundwater table. The metal concentrations measured in the ash of these species is probably directly related to the element content of the groundwater that is nourishing the plants. Phreatophytes growing on permeable pediment gravels may have tap roots extending to depths of 15 m (about 50 ft.) or more. Many of the more recently discovered porphyry copper deposits in Arizona, such as the Vekol, Lakeshore, Sacaton, and Poston Butte deposits, do not crop out much more than about 15 m above the surrounding pediment gravels. From a statistical standpoint, then, one should expect that a like number of yet undiscovered deposits may be present beneath 15 m or less of post-mineralization overburden. Clearly, biogeochemical prospecting should be especially useful in locating such copper deposits.

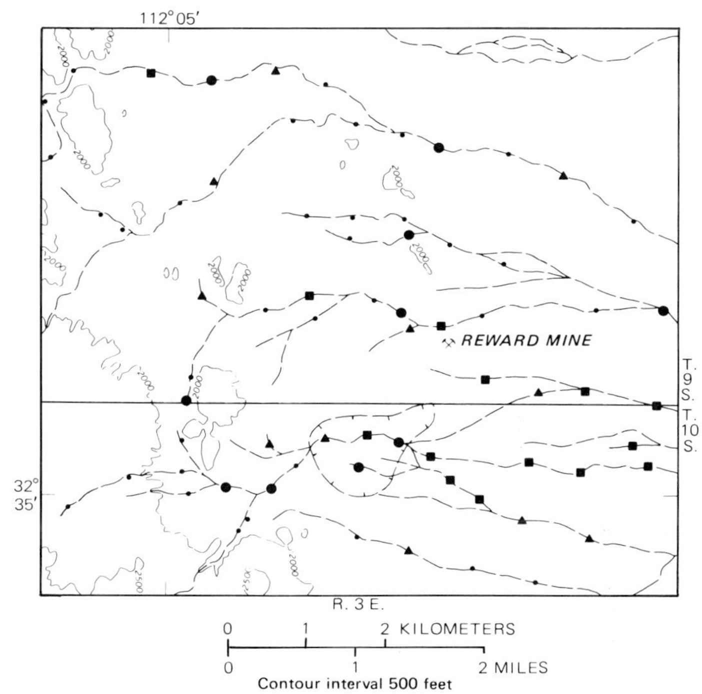

EXPLANATION

- Intermittent stream
- Approximate outline of Vekol deposit
- • Neither plant part anomalous for Zn
- ● Only leaves anomalous (>260 ppm Zn)
- ▲ Only stems anomalous (≥500 ppm Zn)
- ■ Both plant parts anomalous

Figure 13.11. Distribution of zinc in the ash of ironwood leaves and stems collected in the vicinity of the Vekol deposit. The most significant anomalies are those at sites where both plant parts are anomalous. Modified after Chaffee (1977).

GROUNDWATER SAMPLING

In the past geochemical surveys using water as the sample medium have not been popular, mainly because the extremely low concentrations of most elements in natural waters could only be detected by relatively involved analytical methods. Techniques developed in the last few years now make analysis of water for its trace elements much easier; consequently, geochemical surveys using water should become more widely used in the future.

In the arid southwestern United States and northern Mexico, surface water commonly is not present; analysis of well waters, however, may be useful in the search for buried porphyry copper deposits. One of the few geochemical studies of well waters in the southwestern United States that has been published was conducted by Trost and Trautwein (1975). These researchers collected water samples at a number of localities in Arizona and concluded that the concentrations of molybdenum ions, sulfate ions, and total dissolved solids were the three most useful parameters to measure in a well-water survey. Major drawbacks to this method can include the lack of a sufficient number of wells in a given area and also the fact that the pump for a deep well must be running when a sample is needed. Because the chemistry of plants that tap the groundwater table probably reflects the chemistry of the water itself, the disadvantages to well-water sampling might be overcome by using a combination of well-water samples and phreatophyte samples in a prospecting program.

SOIL GAS SAMPLING

Another geochemical technique that may prove useful in the search for buried porphyry copper deposits is the measurement of concentrations of various gases that may be present in the overburden. The many volatile elements and compounds that have been shown to be associated with mineral deposits are cited by Chaffee (1975). Gases such as sulfur dioxide, hydrogen sulfide, or mercury may be formed near an oxidizing sulfide deposit. If the material overlying a buried deposit, whether pre-mineralization or post-mineralization rock or unconsolidated overburden, is permeable, then any gases formed may migrate upward to the surface, where they can be measured.

At the close of the 1970s the use of soil gas in geochemical prospecting had not succeeded in locating any new buried

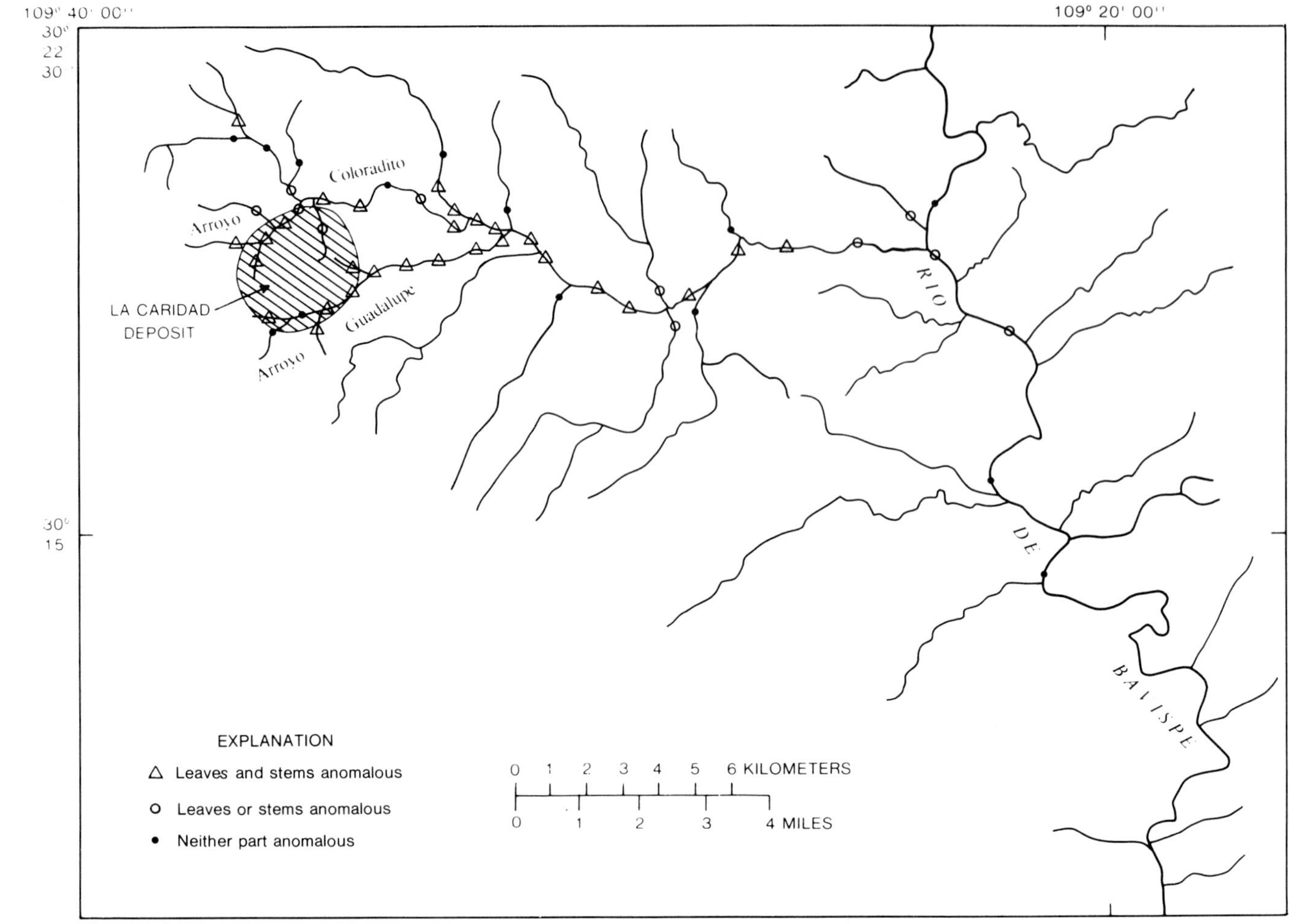

Figure 13.12. Distribution of copper in the ash of mesquite and oak leaves and stems collected in the vicinity of the La Caridad copper deposit. The most significant anomalies are those at sites where both plant parts are anomalous. Modified after Chaffee and others (1976*a*).

copper deposits. However, because of the great depths (or the absence) of groundwater tables in many arid regions, any gases formed over mineral deposits in such an environment have a better chance to migrate upwards than they would have in a more humid region. Thus, if perfected, this technique could be especially useful in the search for blind porphyry copper deposits in the southwestern United States or northern Mexico.

REFERENCES CITED

Cannon, H. L., 1960, Botanical prospecting for ore deposits: Science, v. 132, no. 3427, p. 591–598.

Chaffee, M. A., 1975, Geochemical exploration techniques applicable in the search for copper deposits: U.S. Geol. Survey Prof. Paper 907-B, 26 p.

———, 1976*a*, The zonal distribution of selected elements above the Kalamazoo porphyry copper deposit, San Manuel district, Pinal County, Arizona: Jour. Geochem. Explor., v. 5, no. 2, p. 145–165.

———, 1976*b*, Geochemical exploration techniques based on distribution of selected elements in rocks, soils, and plants, Mineral Butte copper deposit, Pinal County, Arizona: U.S. Geol. Survey Bull. 1278-D, 55 p.

———, 1977, Geochemical exploration techniques based on distribution of selected elements in rocks, soils, and plants, Vekol porphyry copper deposit, Pinal County, Arizona: U.S. Geol. Survey Bull. 1278-E, 78 p.

———, 1982, A geochemical study of the Kalamazoo porphyry copper deposit, Pinal County, Arizona, *in* Titley, S. R., ed., Advances in Geology of the Porphyry Copper Deposits, Southwestern North America: Tucson, Univ. Ariz. Press, Chapter 9.

Chaffee, M. A., and Gale, C. W. III, 1976, The California poppy (*Eschscholtzia mexicana*) as a copper indicator plant—a new example: Jour. Geochem. Explor., v. 5, no. 1, p. 59–63.

Chaffee, M. A., and Hessin, T. D., 1971, An evaluation of geochemical sampling in the search for concealed "porphyry" copper-molybdenum deposits on pediments in southern Arizona, *in* Geochemical Exploration (Internat. Geochemical Explor. Symposium, 3d, Proc.): Canadian Inst. Mining and Metallurgy Spec. Vol. 11, p. 401–409.

Chaffee, M. A.; Hill, R. H.; Sutley, S. J.; and Watterson, J. R., in press, Regional Geochemical Studies in the Patagonia Mountains, Santa Cruz County, Arizona: Jour. Geochem. Explor.

Chaffee, M. A.; Lee-Moreno, J. L.; Caire, L. F.; Mosier, E. L.; and Frisken, J. G., 1976*a*, Results of geochemical investigations comparing samples of stream sediment, panned concentrates, and vegetation in the vicinity of the Caridad porphyry copper deposit, northern Sonora, Mexico: U.S. Geol. Survey Open-file Report 76-559, 34 p.

Chaffee, M. A.; Mosier, E. L.; Nishi, J. M.; VanTrump, George; and Faust, W. F., 1976*b*, Charts showing rainfall and temperature data and chemical analyses for 7 common desert plant species collected between October, 1971 and October, 1974 at the International Biological Program Tucson Validation Site, Pima County, Arizona: U.S. Geol. Survey Open-file Report 76-616, 337 p.

Huff, L. C., 1970, A geochemical study of alluvium-covered copper deposits in Pima County, Arizona: U.S. Geol. Survey Bull. 1312-C, 31 p.

Lovering, T. S.; Huff, L. C.; and Almond, Hy, 1950, Dispersion of copper from the San Manuel copper deposit, Pinal County, Arizona: Geol. Soc. America Bull., v. 45, no. 6, p. 493–514.

Lowell, J. D., 1968, Geology of the Kalamazoo ore body, San Manuel district, Arizona: Econ. Geol., v. 63, no. 6, p. 645–654.

Lowell, J. D., and Guilbert, J. M. 1970, Lateral and vertical alteration-mineralization zoning in porphyry ore deposits: Econ. Geol., v. 65, no. 4, p. 373–408.

Saegart, W. E.; Sell, J. D.; and Kilpatrick, B. E., 1974, Geology and mineralization of La Caridad porphyry copper deposit, Sonora, Mexico: Econ. Geol., v. 69, no. 7, p. 1060–1077.

Steele, H. J., 1976, Vekol Hills copper deposit [abs.]: Program with abstracts, Porphyry Copper Symposium, March 18–20, Tucson, Arizona Geol. Soc.; p. 5–6.

Trost, P. B., and Trautwein, Charles, 1975, Interpretation of molybdenum content in groundwater utilizing Eh, pH, and conductivity, *in* Elliott, I. L., and Fletcher, W. K., eds., Geochemical Exploration 1974: New York, Elsevier Scientific Publishing Co., p. 531–545.

Warren, H. V.; Delavault, R. E.; and Irish, R. I., 1951, Further biogeochemical data from the San Manuel copper deposit, Pinal County, Arizona: Geol. Soc. America Bull., v. 62, no. 8, p. 919–930.

Williams, S. A., 1976, Petrographic criteria unique to porphyry copper deposits [abs.]: Abstracts, 25th Internat. Geol. Cong., Sydney, v. 1, p. 67–68.

PART II

Deposit Descriptions

Introduction

Descriptions of twelve deposits and one district are presented in Part II. The basis for geologic description ranges from that of the broad platform of information developed from continuous study during mining operations to the information developed from drill-hole and underground exploration of deposits still awaiting development.

In the study of the nature and habits of porphyry copper deposits—not only those considered here, but also those in other regions—individual geologists often perceive many similarities or differences among deposits of the genetic type. However, from a very basic point of view, porphyry copper deposits share only the commonality of an association with an intrusion of a felsic porphyry pluton, usually of small (ca. 1–2 km) diameter. The porphyry is usually strongly shattered and either flanks or is central to prominently zoned alteration and copper-iron sulfide mineralization. The diversity of other features, especially the geometry of mineralization, is great and is important to a proper understanding of the deposits, not only to geologists concerned with ore genesis, but also to geologists concerned with discovery and exploitation.

Variations in the characteristics of these deposits are the result of many different factors, including the influences of regional or tectonic settings, which affect how and where porphyry plutons are emplaced. These variations in characteristics are also due, in great part, to differences in composition of both the porphyries and the wall rocks in which they are emplaced, and differences between deposits are certainly results of post-mineralization histories that involve different styles of weathering and, in many regions, a variety of styles of post-mineralization faulting. The chapters in Part II, which review geology in detail, reveal marked differences among deposits in southwestern North America. To the exploration geologist, an appreciation of the ways in which these systems differ is probably fully as important as the knowledge of features of commonality.

In the first volume concerned with deposits of this region (*Geology of the Porphyry Copper Deposits, Southwestern North America,* S. R. Titley and C. L. Hicks, eds.: Tucson, University of Arizona Press, 1966) descriptions of the deposits were arranged in an order that reflected progressively more important involvement of wall rock in the mineralizing process as it was interpreted at the time. The advances in understanding of the deposits and the ore-forming process have led to an increased awareness of the genetic and economic importance of those wall rocks. It is probably valid to say that by 1980, "wall-rock ore" had become vastly more important economically than ore in the porphyries with only a few significant exceptions (e.g., Morenci and Bingham). The order of presentation in this volume is geographical, letting the importance of wall rock fall where it may. The descriptions commence in the east with deposits in New Mexico, move more-or-less westerly across Arizona and finish with Battle Mountain in Nevada.

Since 1955, new discoveries or "rediscoveries" through economic reassessment have resulted in the addition of some nineteen occurrences to the inventory of major porphyry copper deposits in southwestern North America. Descriptions of eight of these deposits are presented in Part II: Copper Canyon (Chapter 27, by T. G. Theodore, D. W. Blake, and E. L. Kretschmer); Copper Flat ([Hillsboro] Chapter 14, by P. G. Dunn); Dos Pobres (Chapter 16, by J. M. Langton and Sidney A. Williams); Poston Butte ([Florence] Chapter 18, by P. W. Nason, A. V. Shaw, and K. D. Aveson); Sacaton (Chapter 25, by R. B. Cummings); Sierrita (Chapter 21, by R. J. West and D. M. Aiken), San Xavier North (Chapter 23, by J. R. King); and Twin Buttes (Chapter

20, by C. F. Barter and J. L. Kelly). Descriptions of Copper Basin, Kalamazoo, La Caridad, and Red Mountain have been published elsewhere, and information on the remaining ones—Casa Grande, Copper Creek, Al Arco, Lake Shore, Nacozari, Rosemont-Helvetia, and Vekol—was not available for inclusion in this volume.

As mining has advanced, continuing and meaningful study of the ores in many porphyry copper deposits has led to increased understanding of the nature and evolution of these systems. Such advances in knowledge have led to new descriptions in Part II that summarize or augment previously reported features of the following deposits: Christmas (Chapter 17, by R. A. Koski and D. S. Cook); Copper Canyon (Chapter 27, by T. G. Theodore, D. W. Blake, and E. L. Kretschmer); El Tiro ([Silver Bell]), Chapter 24, by F. T. Graybeal); Mineral Park (Chapter 26, by W. H. Wilkinson, Jr., L. A. Vega, and S. R. Titley); Mission (Chapter 22, by L. J. Jansen); and Tyrone (Chapter 15, by Joseph Kolessar). In addition, the descriptions of Sierrita-Esperanza (Chapter 21, by R. J. West and D. M. Aiken) and Twin Buttes (Chapter 20, by C. F. Barter and J. L. Kelly) present a considerable volume of important new information and interpretations concerning two completely different and contrasting styles of porphyry copper mineralization of the same age and in the same district.

As more detail is worked out in deposits and is augmented by heightened understanding of the place of these deposits in a regional geologic framework, it may become possible to develop important geological tools and concepts that will increase the efficiency of exploration. Many aspects of regional geology and district geology still remain enigmatic in the early 1980s, and many summaries of the geology of districts are either old (but still useful) or incomplete. In order to provide newer information, a summary of the geology of the Pima mining district (Chapter 19, by S. R. Titley) is presented in Part II. This chapter outlines some important aspects of geologic history and establishes a geologic framework in which chapters that discuss deposits in the district may be considered.

S.R.T.

14

Geology of the Copper Flat Porphyry Copper Deposit

HILLSBORO, SIERRA COUNTY, NEW MEXICO

Peter G. Dunn

The Copper Flat porphyry copper deposit is in Sierra County in south-central New Mexico about 35 miles east-northeast of the Santa Rita deposit near Silver City and about 100 miles northwest of El Paso. It lies in Sections 26 and 35, T.15 S., R.7 W. in the Hillsboro, or Las Animas, mining district about 3½ miles north-northeast of the town of Hillsboro and about 15 miles west of the Rio Grande. The deposit is in a topographic low, Copper Flat, at the western foot of Animas Peak, which is a distinctive conical peak with an elevation of 6,170 ft. Copper Flat is approximately 700 ft. lower and is drained by Grayback Wash, an intermittent tributary to the Rio Grande.

Ore was first discovered in the Hillsboro district in April, 1877 (Jones, 1904), along one of the veins that extend southwest from the quartz monzonite stock in Copper Flat. Placer gold was discovered later in the same year. Production up to 1931 from the district was about $7 million using the prices at the time of production—nearly two-thirds of that amount from gold-silver-copper underground mines along the various veins (Harley, 1934). The deepest of these mines was about 500 ft., and most of the production occurred before 1893, although minor periods of activity continued until a few years prior to World War II (Lindgren et al., 1910).

The rest of the production from the district came from gold placers. Most of this gold was also produced early in the history of the area, but an additional 15,000 oz. of gold were produced between 1935 and 1942 (Segerstrom and Antweiler, 1975). The tailings from that operation were visible in the district, and a few small operators were still producing placer gold from gravels in the existing drainages in 1981.

Although about 200 tons of oxide copper ore were produced from the Sternberg mine in Copper Flat from 1911 to 1931 (Harley, 1934), no exploration of the Copper Flat stock for a potential porphyry copper deposit was made until 1952. Newmont Mining Company drilled 6 angle holes in Copper Flat in that year for a total of 3,369 ft. (Kuellmer, 1955), but the results were not encouraging. In 1958 and 1959 Bear Creek Mining Company drilled 20 holes in Copper Flat for a total of 9,346 ft. Their results indicated that a porphyry copper deposit, including a mineralized breccia pipe, existed in the Copper Flat stock but that no large supergene deposit was present.

Inspiration Consolidated Copper began work at Copper Flat in 1967, and by 1973 had drilled an additional 28 holes in the porphyry deposit for a total of 23,046 ft. They also did some deep drilling in the surrounding andesite, drilled two shallow water wells, and made a preliminary feasibility study and mine plan for a possible open-pit mine.

Quintana Minerals Corporation leased the property from Inspiration in 1974. Between August, 1974, and June, 1976, Quintana drilled 127 holes within the deposit for a total of 94,097 ft. This drilling was supplemented by 2,241 ft. of underground development (approximately 150 ft. below the surface) to provide bulk samples for pilot plant metallurgical testing and to provide a check on the reliability of ore reserve calculations made from vertical drill holes. Additional drilling was also done on potential mill sites, and an adequate water supply was established. The immediate area of the porphyry deposit was mapped at a scale of 1:2,400, and approximately 100 thin sections were examined.

A feasibility study on the Copper Flat deposit was completed in 1976, but the project was temporarily shelved at that time because of low copper prices. It was re-evaluated in 1979, and construction began in 1980. Starting in 1982, the concentrator was scheduled to produce both a copper concentrate with recoverable amounts of gold and silver and a molybdenum concentrate.

REGIONAL GEOLOGY OF THE HILLSBORO DISTRICT

The Hillsboro mining district is in the Animas Hills, a low range formed by a horst at the western edge of the Rio Grande rift, and is separated from the Black Range by a graben in which the town of Hillsboro lies (Woodward et al., 1975). The faults that formed the Animas Hills horst are presumably related to the tectonic activity of the Rio Grande rift, which did not begin until early Miocene (Chapin and Seager, 1975), and were therefore not involved in the localization of the Cretaceous ore deposit.

The central part of the Animas Hills is underlain by a nearly circular block of andesite about 4 miles in diameter; it is shown on Figure 14.1, which has been simplified from the map of Hedlund (1975). The eastern edge of the andesite block coincides with the eastern edge of the horst, where the andesite is in fault contact with the Santa Fe group sediments. A hole drilled for water in the southwestern corner of T.15 S., R.6 W. immediately east of the highway was still in the sediments at a total depth of 2,000 ft.

The rest of the periphery of the volcanic terrain is marked by nearly vertical faults along which the andesite has been down-dropped against Paleozoic sedimentary rocks. The vertical displacement along these faults is not known; deep drill holes in the andesite block were still in andesite at total depths of over 3,000 ft. Some isolated blocks of older rocks have been found in the andesite, and one drill hole has encountered Paleozoic sedimentary rocks underlying the andesite. The thickness of the andesite and the circular fault pattern suggest that the andesite, with related intrusive rocks and mineralization, represents a deeply eroded Cretaceous caldera.

The andesite has been intruded by the Copper Flat quartz monzonite in the center of the caldera, the Warm Springs quartz monzonite along the southern contact, and numerous latite dikes that radiate from the Copper Flat stock. The mineralization of the Hillsboro mining district is found in the Copper Flat stock and the associated dikes; the Warm Springs stock is fresh, with no related mineralization. The entire porphyry copper deposit is contained within the Copper Flat quartz monzonite stock.

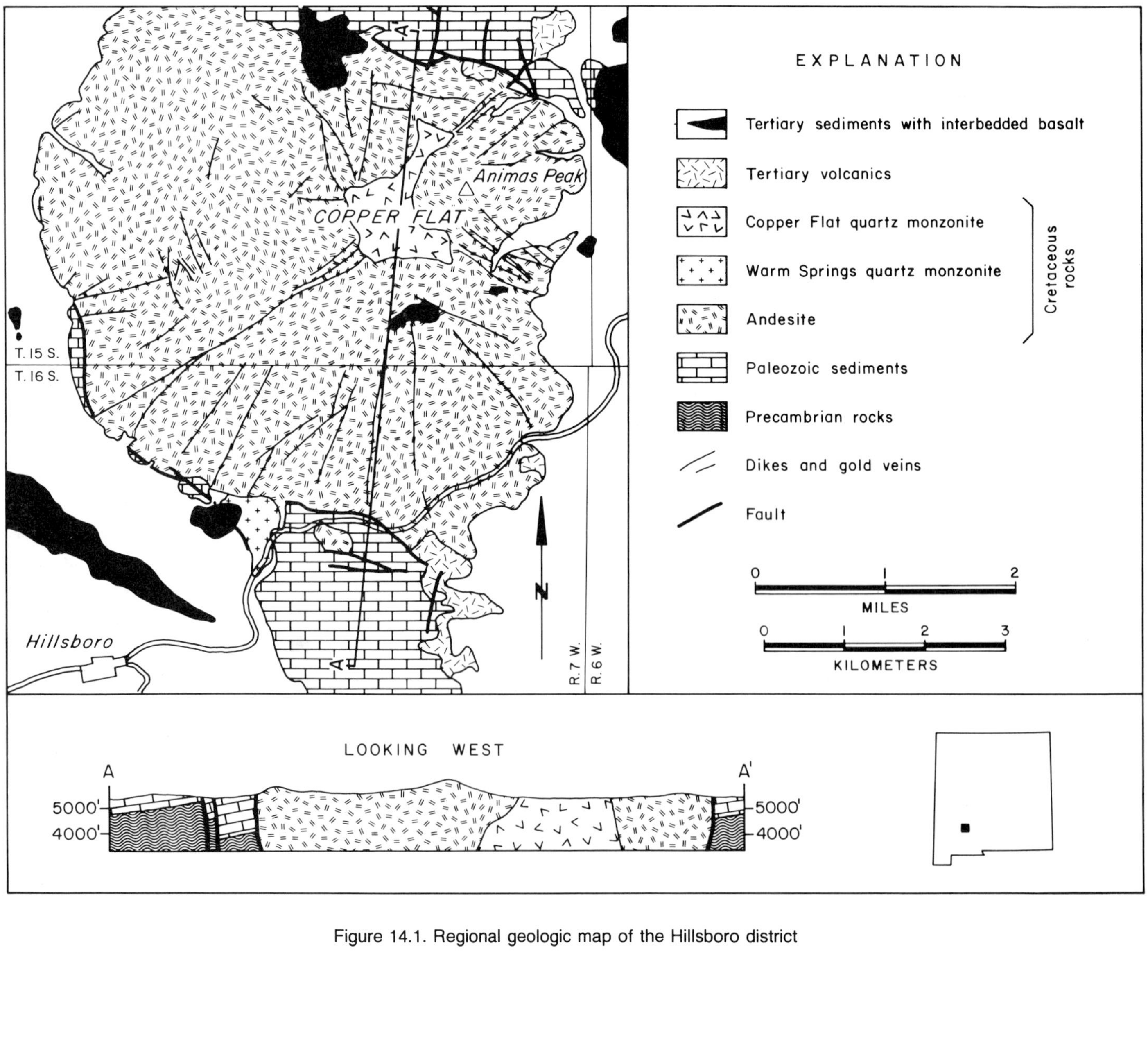

Figure 14.1. Regional geologic map of the Hillsboro district

The latite dikes cut both the andesite and the Copper Flat quartz monzonite, but do not cut the Warm Springs quartz monzonite. Most of the vein mineralization that has provided the production from the Hillsboro district occurs along the contacts of the latite dikes with the andesite (Harley, 1934). The productive veins range from 2 to 8 ft. wide and consist primarily of quartz with calcite, pyrite, chalcopyrite, and minor bornite; gold and silver production has come from the zone of oxidation, where enrichment took place (Reeves, 1963).

The Copper Flat quartz monzonite, the latite dikes, and probably the andesite are thought to be comagmatic. The mineralization of both the porphyry copper deposit and surrounding veins is also probably part of the same igneous sequence. The barren Warm Springs quartz monzonite appears to have been emplaced after the period of mineralization, but is still probably related to the other igneous rocks. Hedlund (1974) reported a K-Ar age date of 73.4 million years from biotite concentrate taken from Inspiration drill core. Secondary biotite is locally abundant from that portion of the Copper Flat stock, and the age date may indicate the age of mineralization.

Post-mineral rocks in the area include Tertiary siliceous pyroclastics (southeast of the andesite outcrop) and basalt flows. Rare dikes related to both of these post-mineral extrusive rocks cut the andesite and the Copper Flat stock. The basalt flows are interbedded with the Santa Fe group sediments in the Palomas Basin east of the Animas Hills and are therefore of Miocene or Pliocene age (Hawley et al., 1969). Both the pyroclastic rocks and the basalt are younger than the faults that bound the caldera. The gold placer deposits of the district occur in recent gravels that overlie the Santa Fe group sediments.

GEOLOGY OF COPPER FLAT

The geologic map of Copper Flat, Figure 14.2, has been simplified from Quintana mapping originally done at a scale of 1 in. to 200 ft. The mineable portion of the porphyry copper deposit is the shaded area of the map. It occurs entirely within the quartz monzonite and includes a central mineralized breccia pipe. Much of the deposit and almost all the breccia lie beneath 5 to 35 ft. of alluvial cover in Copper Flat; the outline of the breccia and the numerous faults shown in the covered area were determined from close-spaced drilling and underground development.

Lithology

The andesite is generally a fine-grained porphyritic rock with phenocrysts of plagioclase (originally andesine) and amphibole in a groundmass of plagioclase and potash feldspar with rare quartz. Agglomerates or flow breccias are locally present, but the andesite is generally massive and attitudes are difficult to determine. The andesite immediately south of the quartz monzonite is coarse-grained and may represent a shallow intrusive phase. Magnetite is commonly associated with the mafic phenocrysts, and accessory apatite is found in nearly every thin section.

An irregular mass of andesite breccia is shown along the northwestern contact of the quartz monzonite. It contains potash feldspar phenocrysts and andesitic rock fragments in a matrix of sericite with minor quartz; it is probably a pyroclastic unit. Similar tuff breccias have been encountered in drill holes and also occur in a few other outcrops in the map area that are too small to be mapped separately. Magnetite, chlorite, epidote, and accessory apatite are also present in the andesite breccia.

The Copper Flat quartz monzonite occupies the central portion of the map; the narrow neck shown in Figure 14.1 extends an additional 2,500 ft. to the northeast beyond the edge of the map in Figure 14.2. The stock contains a few mappable xenoliths or roof pendants of andesite, and a few isolated outcrops of quartz monzonite occur within the andesite. The andesite at the contact shows no obvious contact metamorphism, and the quartz monzonite rarely shows visible evidence of chilling at the contact.

Most of the quartz monzonite is porphyritic, with large orthoclase phenocrysts up to 5 cm long. It consists of about equal amounts of plagioclase (andesine) and orthoclase, although in places either feldspar may comprise more than 50 percent of the rock. Plagioclase usually occurs as smaller phenocrysts, less than 1 cm long; orthoclase comprises much of the groundmass. Quartz makes up 15 percent of the rock, and occurs as small phenocrysts and as part of the groundmass. Both hornblende and biotite occur as primary minerals. Magnetite is common, associated with the mafic minerals, and apatite is a ubiquitous accessory. Rare sphene crystals are present.

Several textural and compositional variants of the quartz monzonite have been observed, but have not been mapped separately. The rock is locally a nearly equigranular rock, and elsewhere is porphyritic but with only the small plagioclase phenocrysts. Quartz is absent in some parts of the stock. Some of the textural variations appear to be the result of later hydrothermal alteration. Although more detailed mapping may indicate that some of the variations represent separate intrusive phases, all the rock types of the stock are older than the later fine-grained dikes and older than the mineralization and alteration.

The latite dikes and plugs shown on the geologic map cut both the andesite and the quartz monzonite. Three different types of dikes can be distinguished in hand specimens, but they are not distinguished on this map. Many of the smaller dikes have also been omitted. Most of the dikes are fine-grained latite containing 5 to 10 percent euhedral plagioclase phenocrysts ranging up to 5 mm long in a groundmass of plagioclase, potash feldspar, and minor quartz. Apatite is again present. The other two types are similar; one contains 1 to 2 percent rounded quartz phenocrysts up to 2 mm, and the other contains no quartz but does contain abundant large orthoclase phenocrysts up to 25 mm long. Cross-cutting relationships indicate that the dikes with the quartz eyes are older than the latite, and that the dikes with the large phenocrysts are younger. The dikes are generally 5 to 30 ft. wide.

The two plugs on the map in Figure 14.2 consist of the fine-grained latite. The larger irregular plug to the north is not well exposed except for its contact with the quartz monzonite. Several small outcrops of both andesite and quartz monzonite occur within the plug, which may actually be a

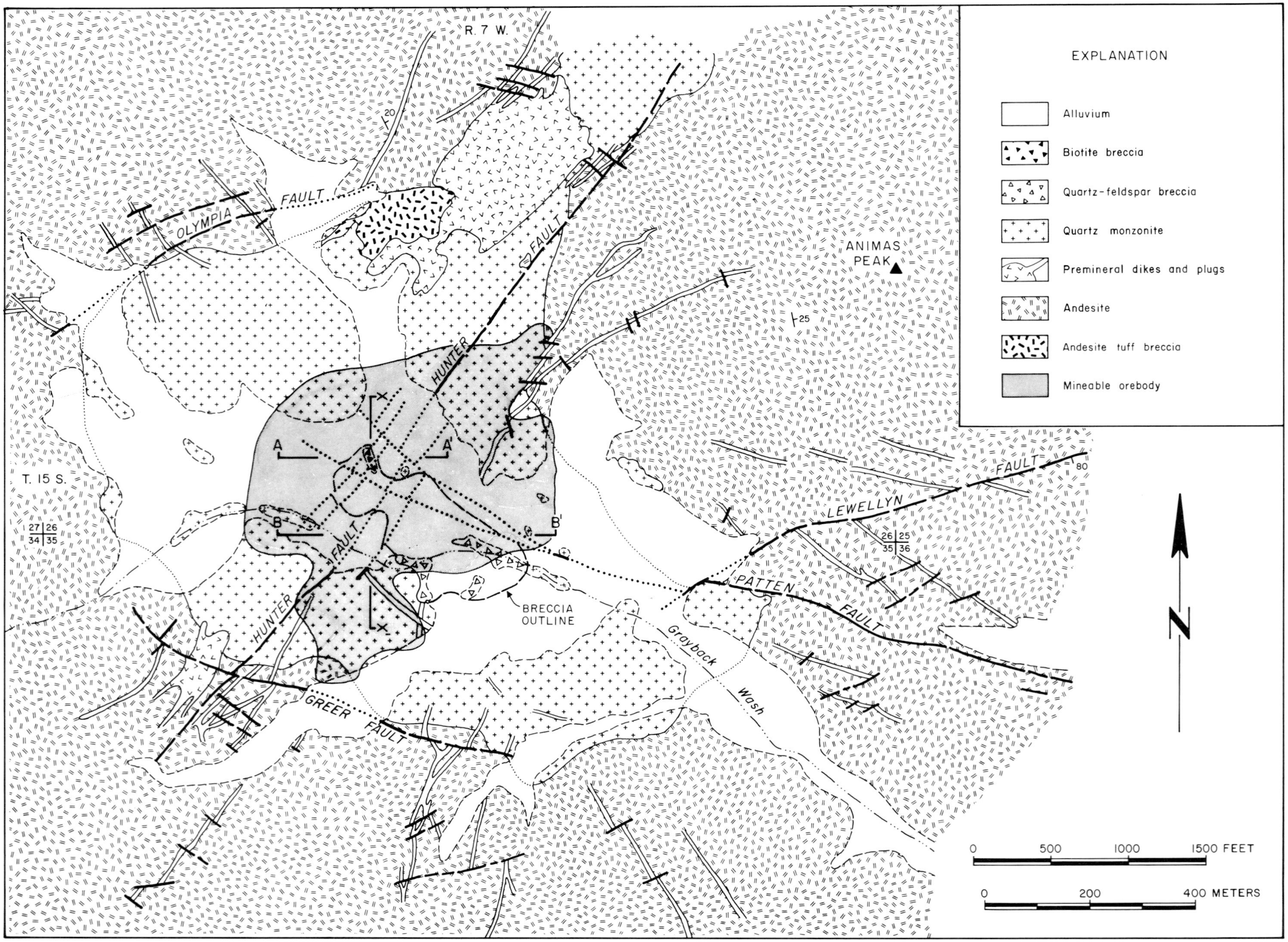

Figure 14.2. Geologic map of the Copper Flat mineralized area

complex dike swarm. The smaller plug to the south is better exposed and is a single body of latite.

Postmineral rocks have been omitted from the geologic map. The only postmineral rocks in the area are a single feldspar porphyry dike that cuts the andesite northwest of the larger latite plug, and a few narrow basalt dikes that cut both the andesite and the quartz monzonite.

Structure

The structural elements in Copper Flat were established prior to the emplacement of the quartz monzonite stock and were controlling factors in the later igneous events and subsequent mineralization. The same structures were still active after the mineralization process; the alluvial covered area, Copper Flat, is due to more active erosion at the intersection of the numerous faults that have had post-mineral movement resulting in wide, strongly brecciated fault zones. Some of the post-mineral dikes have been emplaced within these fault zones.

Three principal structural directions are present in the area. The most prominent of these is northeast—a direction that includes the Hunter fault and the other parallel faults in Copper Flat. The other two structural directions are west-northwest, marked by the Patten and Greer faults, and east-northeast, marked by the Olympia and Lewellyn faults. All these structures are nearly vertical; the Hunter fault system dips 80° to the west, and both the other fault systems dip between 80° to the south and 90°.

The outline of the Copper Flat stock generally parallels one of these structural directions, although nowhere has the stock been emplaced by faulting. The southern contact nearly parallels the Greer fault, although the contact is cut by the fault, and the southeastern and northwestern contacts are roughly parallel to the Olympia and Lewellyn faults. The elongate neck of the stock is parallel to the Hunter fault system. It has not been possible to determine whether there was movement on the fault systems prior to the emplacement of the stock or whether these were simply well-defined fracture systems.

Most of the latite dikes strike in one or another of the three principal fracture directions; the majority, including those related to the most productive vein mines in the district, strike northeast. A narrow zone of fault gouge commonly occurs along the contact between a dike and the andesite, with the mineralization younger than the faulting (Harley, 1934). There is evidence at the extreme west of the map of fault movement during the period of emplacement of the dikes. A younger porphyritic dike was emplaced in a fault (possibly an extension of the Patten fault) that had previously offset an early latite dike.

Sulfide mineralization within the quartz monzonite has been controlled by the fractures following the same principal directions. The attitudes of 162 mineralized fractures in the quartz monzonite surrounding the breccia pipe have been plotted and contoured on an equal-area net and are shown on Figure 14.3. Three of the maxima shown on the diagram correspond very closely to the main structural directions as indicated by the faults and dikes. A fourth concentration indicates a set of fractures that strike N4°W. Although no faults with that orientation were noted in the surface mapping, some of the basalt dikes trend in that direction, and they are thought to have been emplaced along fault zones.

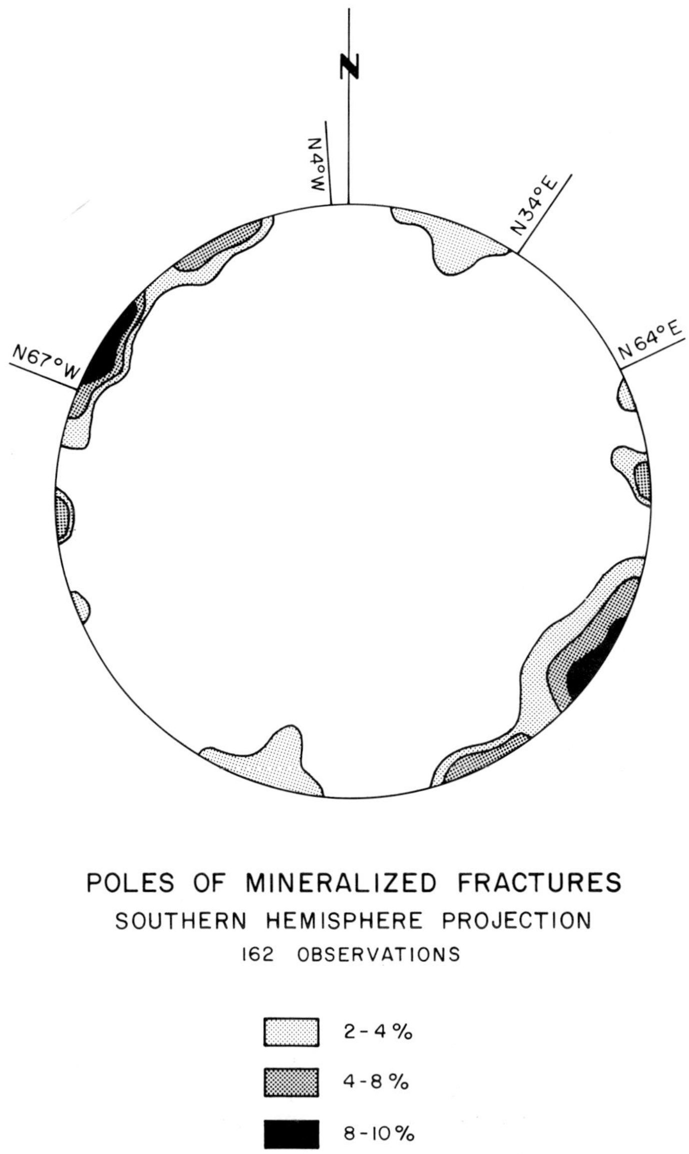

Figure 14.3. Orientation of mineralized fractures in quartz monzonite

The three principal structural directions have been marked by post-dike movement, and both the Hunter fault and the Patten fault systems have had definite post-mineral movement. They are both marked by smeared-out sulfides, and both offset the breccia pipe and the zones within it. Both in drill core and in the underground workings the fault surfaces are marked by nearly horizontal slickensides. This apparent strike-slip movement is usually compatible with the displacement of the dikes mapped on the surface. The Greer fault, however, shows both right-lateral and left-lateral displacement of different offset features; such evidence indicates that there has been some vertical displacement.

Limited information on the fault zones (from drill hole intersections and from the underground workings) suggests that the material within the fault zones is different in the differently oriented faults. The material in the northeast fault zones contains a high proportion of wet gouge, often with no recognizable rock fragments. Where the Hunter fault zone has been encountered underground, material in it has had the same consistency as wet concrete and has actually flowed. The material in the east-northeast fault zones, however, contains only highly broken rock and little obvious gouge. The fault zones in both systems range in width from less than a foot to nearly 25 ft. along the Patten fault east of Copper Flat. The width of the fault zones varies along strike. Despite the intense brecciation within the fault zones, the total displacement along the faults does not appear to exceed a few tens of feet.

Breccia Pipe

The central high-grade portion of the deposit is contained in a mineralized breccia pipe that is almost completely covered by the alluvium in Copper Flat. The shape of the body (beneath the alluvium) is shown on the geologic map in Figure 14.2. The eastern portion of the breccia is outside the outline of mineable ore; the rest of the breccia, however, has a higher grade than the surrounding quartz monzonite. The result of this mineralization is that the breccia will produce nearly one-half of the copper from the mineable deposit although it comprises only about one-third of the total ore that will be mined.

The breccia pipe is a zone within the quartz monzonite that has been cut by numerous, randomly oriented, irregular veins that are thicker and coarser-grained than the narrow fracture-controlled veinlets in the surrounding stock. Part of the northwestern section of the pipe contains angular, rotated fragments cemented by the same hydrothermal matrix. The extent of breccia with rotated fragments can be determined only roughly, because most of the data have come from drill core samples. The entire breccia pipe in Copper Flat, therefore, corresponds to both Zone 2 (crackle breccia) and Zone 3 (breccia pipes) in Copper Basin, Arizona, as described by Johnston and Lowell (1961).

The pipe is 1,300 ft. long and approximately 600 ft. wide at the surface with the long axis perpendicular to the predominant northeast fracture direction. The breccia is exposed in only a few places. It has a vertical extent of over 1,000 ft., with veins of coarse pegmatitic material occurring almost 1,700 ft. deep in one drill hole. Close-spaced drill holes, approximately 100 ft. apart within the center of the deposit, show that the breccia pipe occurs as a single, continuous body. Only two drill holes outside the breccia encountered short intervals of stockwork veining similar to that in the main breccia pipe.

The shape of the main body is shown in detail on the geologic map of Copper Flat at the 5,300 ft. level (the elevation of the underground workings) in Figure 14.4. This map and two vertical cross sections (Fig. 14.5*a*, *c*) also show the approximate extent of the zone containing rotated fragments; cross section *B-B'* (Fig. 14.5*b*) is south of that zone. Although the breccia does reach the surface beneath the alluvium, much of the body is covered by overlying quartz monzonite. This upper contact with the quartz monzonite is relatively sharp, and is shown on the cross sections to have a gentle south dip, suggesting that the top of the pipe has barely been uncovered by erosion.

The pipe has a steep plunge to the southwest, which may be the result of post-mineral rotation. A few attitudes taken in the andesite show 20° dips to the east; if these do represent later movement, the breccia would have originally been vertical. Drill holes at the eastern edge of the pipe drill back into quartz monzonite with a relatively sharp contact. If rotation has taken place, these holes actually drill out the side of the breccia pipe. Drill holes along the western edge drill from breccia into quartz monzonite but with a long gradational contact; this probably represents the true bottom of the pipe.

Most of the fragments in the breccia consist of mineralized quartz monzonite. Fragments of mineralized latite are locally abundant; these are usually found where dikes exposed in the quartz monzonite can be projected into the brecciated zone. Andesite fragments in the breccia pipe occur only as mixed fragments partially in contact with intrusive quartz monzonite; these fragments are clustered within short intervals in only a few drill holes. These observations indicate that the andesite fragments represent only the brecciation of original andesite xenoliths in the quartz monzonite. No other rock types have been recognized as fragments in the breccia.

The matrix of the breccia consists primarily of varying proportions of quartz, biotite (phlogopite), potash feldspar, pyrite and chalcopyrite. Magnetite, molybdenite, fluorite, and calcite are locally common, and apatite is again a common accessory mineral. No tourmaline has been found in the breccia matrix or in the surrounding veins. Minerals in the matrix are commonly quite large, with biotite books up to 5 cm across, and much of the quartz-feldspar matrix has a pegmatitic texture. Either biotite or potash feldspar has formed along the edge of the breccia fragments, and the quartz and sulfide minerals have generally formed in the center of the matrix. Large biotite crystals have generally grown nearly perpendicular to the matrix-fragment contact, which in these instances is very sharp. Magnetite is common in the matrix and is the principal matrix mineral in one drill hole near the center of the body. The primary magnetite, however, has been destroyed in the quartz monzonite immediately surrounding the breccia pipe and in the fragments. Some open cavities lined with euhedral crystals, generally quartz and sulfides, have been found but are not common. Fluorite, calcite, and apatite also occur in open cavities. Apatite also forms as euhedral crystals up to 10 mm across in the center of large sulfide or magnetite crystals. It appears to be concentrated near the center of the breccia pipe associated with magnetite.

Although the matrix is in sharp contact with the fragments in many instances, other fragments are quite diffuse as a result of the formation of a broad alteration envelope of

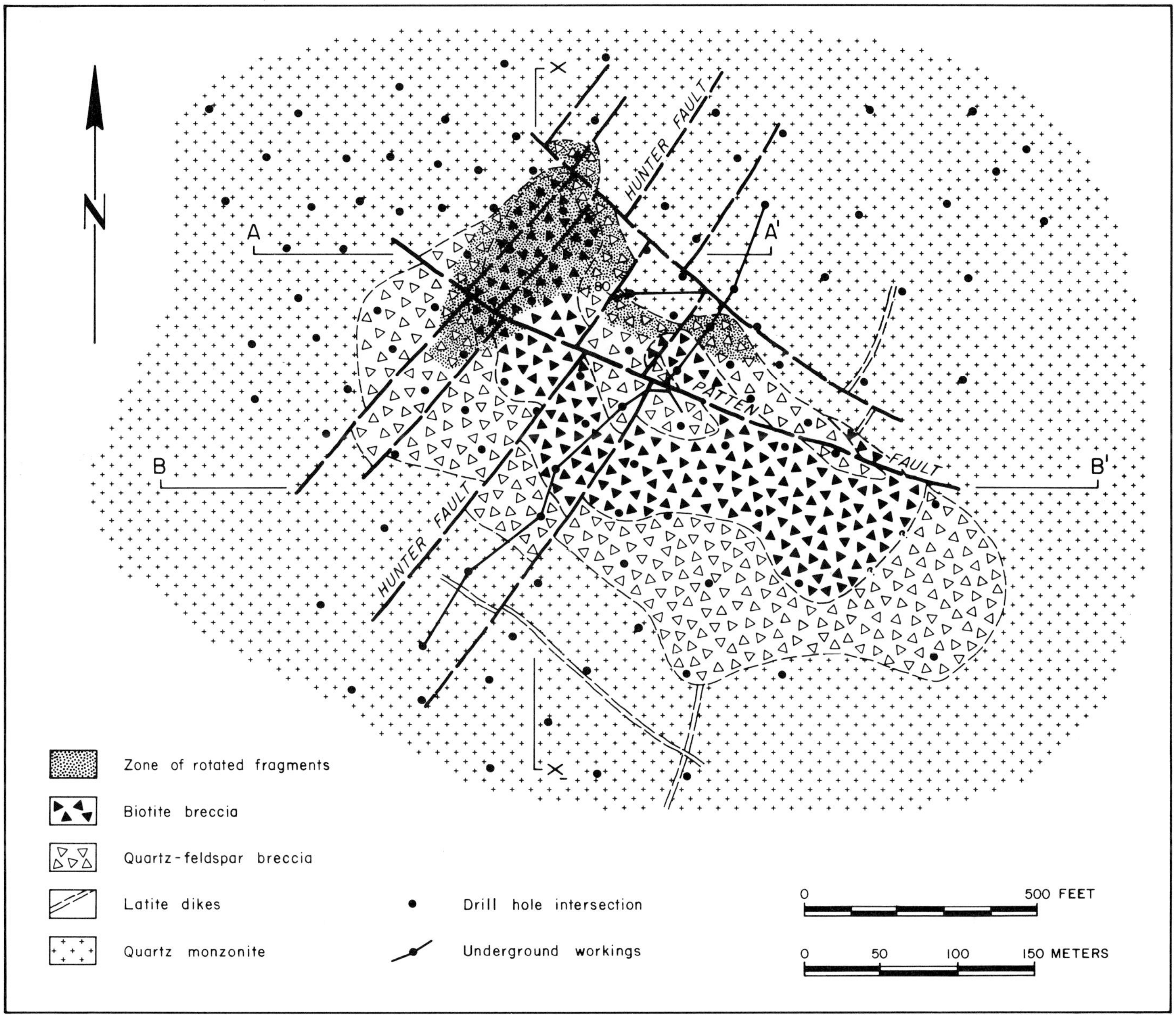

Figure 14.4. Geologic map of Copper Flat at the 5,300-ft. level

very fine grained secondary biotite surrounding the matrix. Other fragments are deeply embayed, and appear to have been corroded by the hydrothermal fluid that formed the matrix.

The proportions of the major hydrothermal minerals vary in different parts of the breccia, and the pipe has been divided—on the basis of the principal gangue minerals in the matrix—into biotite breccia and quartz-feldspar breccia. These sub-divisions do not correspond to the division between breccia with or without rotated fragments. The distribution of biotite breccia is important because it almost always forms high-grade chalcopyrite ore. The grade in the quartz-feldspar breccia is considerably more variable; in general the chalcopyrite content varies with the quartz content. The matrix in the eastern waste portion of the breccia consists primarily of pegmatitic potash feldspar with subordinate amounts of quartz and pyrite and only rare chalcopyrite.

This elliptical body of breccia that forms the center of the Copper Flat porphyry deposit is very similar to the high-grade core of the Ajo orebody that Gilluly (1946) ascribed to pegmatitic replacement. Much of the high-grade core has been mined out at Ajo, but some large boulders are still present in the pit. These contain definite rotated angular fragments of quartz monzonite in a matrix of very coarse grained chlorite, quartz, and chalcopyrite.

MINERALIZATION AND ALTERATION

The mineralization and alteration at Copper Flat are similar to most of the porphyry copper deposits in the South-

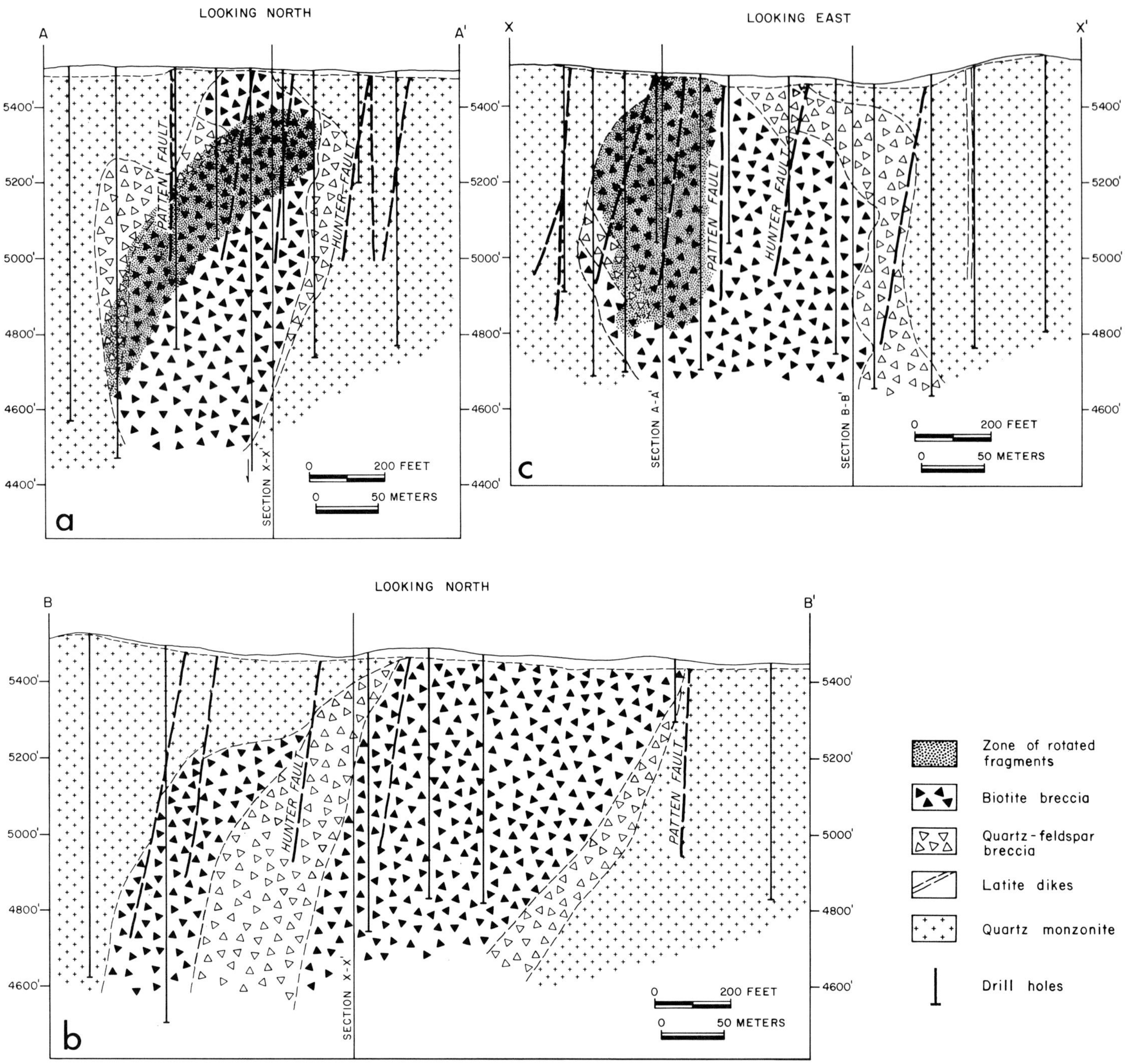

Figure 14.5. Geologic cross sections at Copper Flat: *a,* cross section *A-A'*; *b,* cross section *B-B'*; *c,* cross section *X-X'*.

west, differing in that much of the economic mineralization occurs in the breccia pipe and that few supergene effects are present.

Primary Mineralization

The Copper Flat porphyry deposit is almost entirely a hypogene sulfide deposit with nearly all the copper occurring as chalcopyrite. Pyrite is the other main sulfide mineral; subordinate amounts of molybdenite, galena, and sphalerite are present. Rare bornite has been recognized but, surprisingly, most of it occurs outside the orebody. A few small tetrahedrite crystals have been found in drill core samples. The total sulfide content is generally low compared to most of the porphyry copper deposits in the Southwest; it ranges from approximately 1 percent (by volume) in the eastern portion of the breccia pipe and the surrounding quartz monzonite to 5 percent in the quartz monzonite surrounding the mineable orebody to the south and west. Sulfide content is highly variable within the breccia, with small areas containing as much as 20 percent sulfides. Sulfide mineralization is restricted almost entirely to the quartz monzonite, with an abrupt drop in the sulfide content at the andesite contact. Minor pyrite mineralization extends into the andesite along the pre-mineral dikes.

Mineralization within the quartz monzonite consists of pyrite, which occurs as disseminations or along discontinuous, fracture-controlled veinlets, and chalcopyrite, which occurs principally as disseminations associated with the original mafic minerals. Pyrite is more abundant than chalcopyrite in the quartz monzonite except in two separate areas: (1) a narrow zone immediately surrounding and overlying the western end of the breccia pipe containing abundant chalcopyrite in quartz-sulfide veinlets, and (2) the outcrops southeast of the breccia and south of Grayback Wash, where disseminated chalcopyrite is present with no associated pyrite. The first area contains the highest-grade quartz monzonite ore. Changes in the copper grade in the quartz monzonite, due to changes in the total sulfide content and in the ratio of pyrite to chalcopyrite, are gradational both laterally and vertically.

Molybdenite is not abundant in the quartz monzonite. Where it is present, it occurs either in quartz veins or as thin coatings on fractures. Minor sphalerite and galena are present in both carbonate and quartz veinlets in the stock.

Sulfide mineralization in the pre-mineral dikes is similar to that in the surrounding quartz monzonite. Both pyrite and chalcopyrite generally occur as disseminations. In some areas the copper grade in the dikes is lower than that in the adjacent stock, but in most places there is no marked change in grade between the two rock types.

Mineralization within the breccia pipe is characterized by large, irregular masses of pyrite and chalcopyrite as part of the breccia matrix, and is associated with large crystals of quartz, biotite, and potash feldspar. Some of the larger sulfide masses encountered in the underground workings have measured up to 2 ft. across. Molybdenite occurs in the matrix as coarse crystals up to 2 in. across. Minor amounts of pyrite and molybdenite, with rare sphalerite and galena, occur in narrow quartz and carbonate veinlets that cut both the fragments and the breccia matrix.

Chalcopyrite is most abundant within the biotite breccia, which is almost invariably ore-grade material. The chalcopyrite occurs both as large, irregular masses and as fine disseminations within the large biotite books. A definite horizontal mineral zoning occurs within the quartz-feldspar breccia. In general the highest copper content is at the western end of the breccia and is associated with abundant quartz and only subordinate amounts of potash feldspar. The highest molybdenum content occurs in this area. Pyrite and potash feldspar both become increasingly abundant to the east at the expense of chalcopyrite, molybdenite, and quartz, and even pyrite becomes scarce at the extreme eastern edge of the breccia.

The breccia outside the mineable orebody shown on the map in Figure 14.2 has a matrix comprised almost entirely of pegmatitic potash feldspar and a copper grade of less than 0.1 percent. This matrix mineralization has been superimposed on the existing disseminated mineralization within the fragments of quartz monzonite. The form of the resulting mineralization within the breccia pipe has caused abrupt changes in the copper content over very short distances. Copper assays of adjacent intervals in the same drill hole sample within the breccia may differ by more than 1 percent copper.

Supergene Mineralization

Very little oxidation and supergene enrichment have occurred at Copper Flat, presumably because erosion has been able to keep pace with the rate of oxidation, which, in turn, may have been slower than elsewhere in the Southwest due to the low total sulfide content. Fresh pyrite and chalcopyrite can be found in outcrops along Grayback Wash within the orebody.

A small chalcocite zone occurs in the quartz monzonite adjacent to and overlying the breccia pipe. It also extends to the northeast for about 200 ft. along the N35°E fracture direction. Chalcocite has been found as deep as 200 ft. in some drill holes, but in most places it occurs only within a few tens of feet of the surface. The chalcocite occurs as film on chalcopyrite and rarely comprises any significant amount of the copper within the zone of enrichment. Almost no chalcocite has been recognized within the breccia pipe.

No sizeable tonnage of oxidized copper mineralization is present, although some oxidized copper minerals are present overlying the area of chalcocite enrichment. The base of oxidation is abrupt and is nowhere deeper than 50 ft., in most places it is less than 30 ft., even within fault zones. Malachite and chrysocolla are the main oxidized minerals; small aggregates of euhedral malachite and azurite are found in the post-mineral basalt dikes within the zone of oxidation.

The copper and molybdenum assays in some of the drill hole samples that intersected visible chalcocite mineralization show a remarkable correlation between high-grade enriched copper and high-grade molybdenum within the same assay intervals. The assay results of samples from the top of one of these drill holes are shown graphically on Figure 14.6. These data give at least empirical support for molybdenum enrichment.

The form of the molybdenum in these higher-grade samples is not known. No visible ferrimolybdite or other oxide minerals have been identified, and visible molybdenite is almost completely absent in these samples. Quartz veins are also rare or absent. Below the zone of enrichment at Copper Flat, molybdenite is easily recognized with a hand lens in samples containing as little as 0.010 percent molybdenum, and samples with a high molybdenum grade—comparable to those in the zone of enrichment—usually contain obvious coarse-grained molybdenite in quartz veins.

Several other drill holes also encountered minor chalcocite enrichment, but with no apparent enrichment in the molybdenum. The difference between these core samples and those that do show molybdenum enrichment is in the original total sulfide content and the ratio of pyrite:chalcopyrite. Molybdenum enrichment occurs in areas of low total sulfides (1 to 2 volume %) and approximately equal amounts of pyrite and chalcopyrite; samples that have chalcocite but no molybdenum enrichment are in areas where total sulfides are 3 to 5 volume percent and where pyrite is several times more abundant than chalcopyrite.

This field relationship is in agreement with chemical data on the behavior of molybdenum under oxidizing conditions (Titley and Anthony, 1961; Hansuld, 1966). In an acid

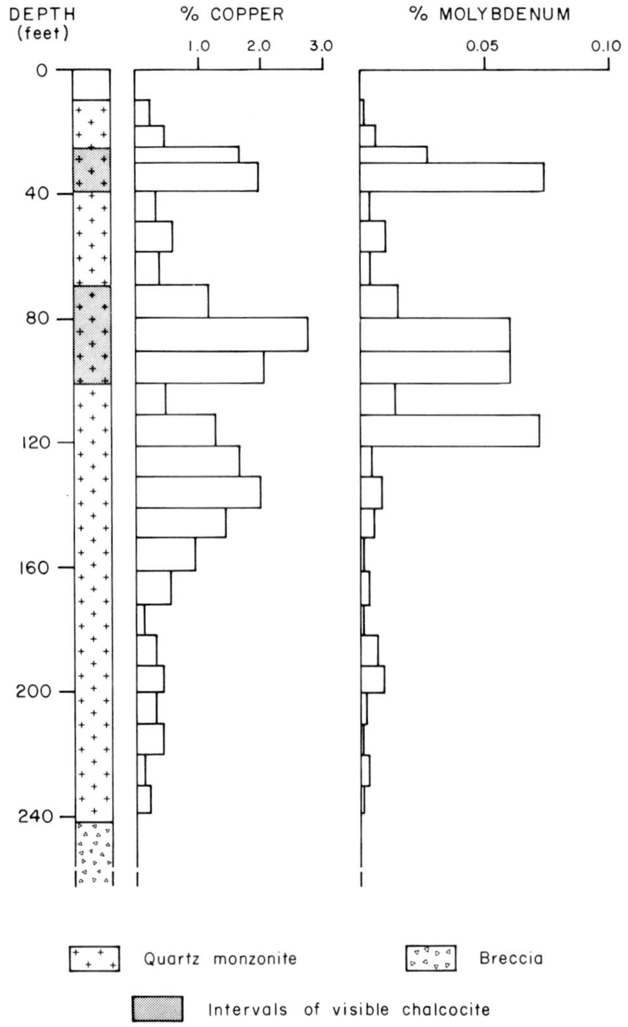

Figure 14.6. Drill hole assays for copper and molybdenum

environment (high pyrite) oxidized molybdenum is fixed; it would remain in the oxidized zone and eventually would be removed by erosion. A more alkaline environment (pH of 6 or greater) causes molybdenum to be mobile and allows it to travel downward into the zone of enrichment. This more alkaline environment, however, is one in which copper is less mobile, so the range of pH under which both copper and molybdenum could form supergene mineralization is quite small.

Alteration

The Copper Flat deposit does not show the symmetrical zoning of alteration types that is considered typical of porphyry copper deposits in the Southwest, although the same alteration minerals are present. A central zone of potassic alteration extends from the breccia pipe almost to the southeastern contact of the quartz monzonite stock and includes the area of chalcopyrite mineralization with no associated pyrite.

The strong potassic alteration within and immediately surrounding the breccia pipe is the most prominent alteration feature of the deposit. Secondary biotite and potash feldspar occur in the breccia matrix as large crystals and also replace the rock fragments. The biotite that forms as replacement occurs as finely shredded aggregates; euhedral primary biotite books in the quartz monzonite are apparently stable, although they have locally been partially altered to chlorite. The secondary potash feldspar occurs as narrow veinlets or alteration envelopes along quartz veins and as almost complete replacement of the original rock, with only vague outlines remaining to indicate the original texture. Quartz occurs as veinlets and in the breccia matrix; it apparently formed together with biotite and potash feldspar during the period of potassic alteration. Chlorite is locally associated with secondary biotite but may have formed later at the expense of biotite. Anhydrite is absent, although rare gypsum occurs as thin coatings on fractures.

Sericite alteration has affected almost the entire quartz monzonite stock and the related dikes; it has also affected the fragments in the breccia. Sericite has replaced the plagioclase and also occurs in the groundmass of the rocks; both sericite and chlorite have replaced original mafic minerials. Quartz and carbonate veins and minor kaolinite are associated with the sericite alteration. Rare zeolites have also been tentatively identified.

Sericite alteration is strongly developed in one near-surface zone south and west from the breccia pipe. Both the quartz monzonite and the dikes in this area have been completely altered to sericite and quartz to the extent that the original texture has been obliterated and it is difficult to distinguish the stock from the dikes on the surface. This intense alteration, however, extends only a few tens of feet from the surface and is clearly a supergene effect that was controlled by the original high pyrite:chalcopyrite ratio in this area. The zone of supergene alteration extends for about 500 ft. south of Grayback Wash and to within about 500 ft. of the western margin of the stock.

Two separate periods of hypogene sericite alteration occurred at Copper Flat—one prior to the formation of the breccia and the potassic alteration, and a later one that postdates the potassic alteration. The sericite in the stock and in the fragments in the breccia surrounding it has been replaced by both secondary biotite and secondary potash feldspar. Areas of pervasive secondary feldspar and the breccia matrix have been subsequently cut by quartz veinlets with only minor sulfides but with well-developed sericite envelopes. The two periods of sericite alteration are associated with a different assemblage of sulfide minerals—pyrite with minor chalcopyrite in the early period, and pyrite, galena, and sphalerite in the later period.

Propylitic alteration is common in the andesite and the andesite breccia, but it is rarely developed in the quartz monzonite or in the latite dikes. Dikes containing weak quartz-sericite alteration with minor pyrite have been observed cutting unmineralized andesite, which shows only chlorite and epidote alteration.

Paragenesis

The sequence of mineralizing events that formed the Copper Flat deposit is depicted schematically on Figure 14.7. Three stages of hypogene mineralization have been recorded, although it is likely that these were not three separate periods but rather a continuous change during time. The three stages

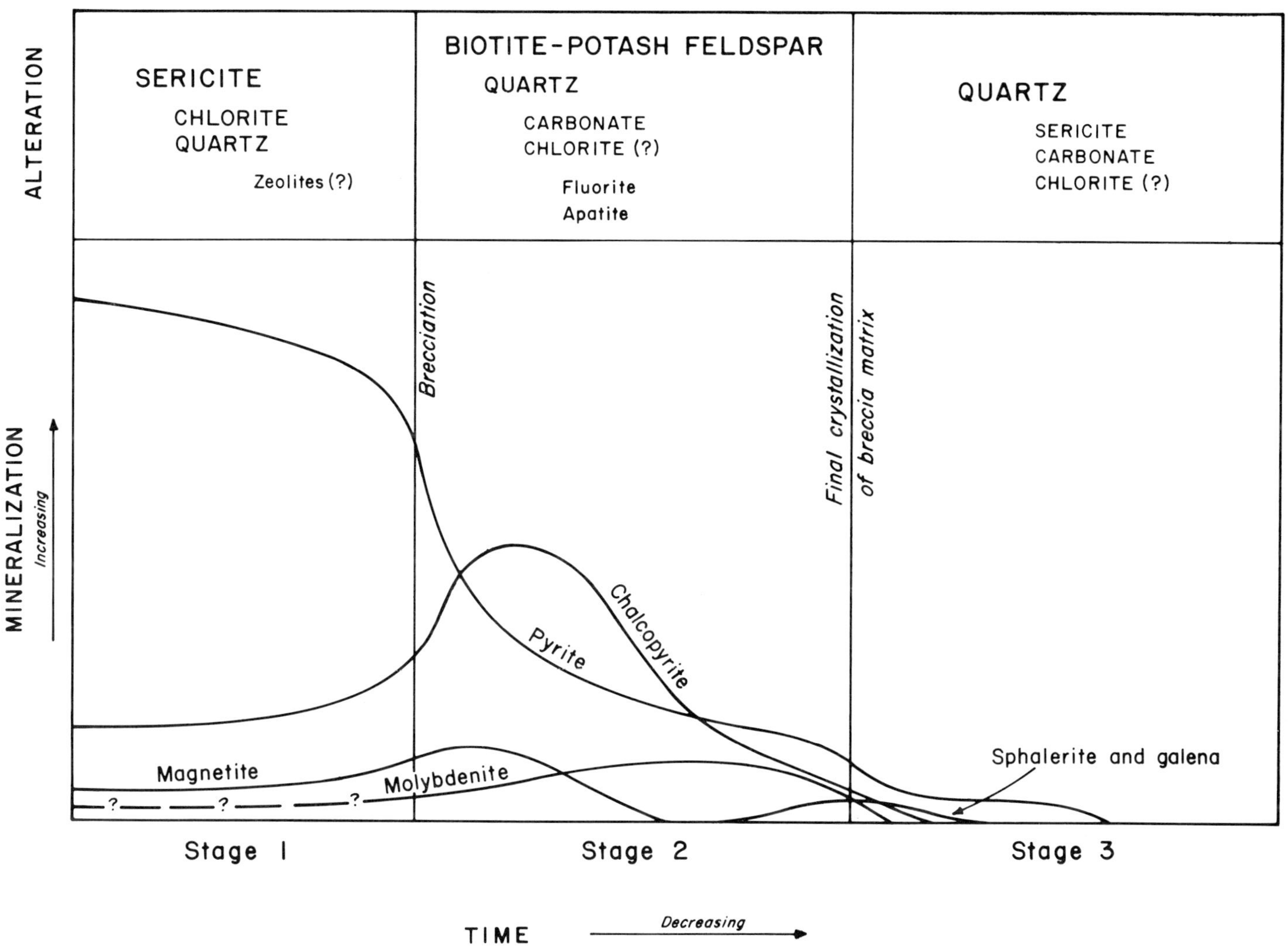

Figure 14.7. Schematic paragenetic sequence for the Copper Flat deposit

are associated with different sulfide and alteration assemblages. No absolute figures are available for the temperature, pressure, or time for the mineralization.

The first stage of mineralization—the introduction of pyrite with subordinate amounts of chalcopyrite—affected nearly the entire stock. This stage occurred after the formation of the latite dikes but prior to the formation of the breccia pipe. The chalcopyrite generally formed as disseminations and the pyrite as coatings along fractures and as discrete veins. No definite first stage molybdenite can be identified. Magnetite formed during this stage as replacements of original mafic minerals. This mineralization was associated with the first stage of sericite and chlorite alteration with subordinate quartz and minor carbonates. It probably formed no ore-grade material.

The second stage began with the formation of the breccia and continued through the crystallization of the breccia matrix. Pyrite and chalcopyrite were both deposited with subordinate amounts of molybdenite and magnetite and trace amounts of sphalerite and galena. This stage affected the breccia pipe and the surrounding and overlying quartz monzonite. Most of the mineralization formed as open space filling between the fragments and as veins in the stock, although some second stage mineralization formed as replacement—particularly of the fragments within the breccia. Higher-grade veins of quartz, chalcopyrite, and molybdenite have been emplaced along the N35°E fracture system for several hundred feet away from the breccia and are thought to have formed during the second stage of mineralization. The gold-silver-copper veins surrounding the Copper Flat quartz monzonite stock are also thought to be related to the second stage. Second stage mineralization was associated with the strong potassic alteration minerals that were forming gangue minerals in the breccia matrix. There is no clear evidence of the age relationship between the biotite breccia and the quartz-feldspar breccia, although the pegmatitic potash feldspar matrix at the extreme eastern edge of the breccia pipe is thought to have been the last material to crystallize.

The first-stage mineralization may have been only peripheral disseminated mineralization that formed contemporaneously with the breccia mineralization. Careful examination of the fragments in the breccia, however, has led to the conclusion that two stages were involved. A few fragments contain narrow quartz-pyrite veinlets or narrow chlorite veinlets that are restricted to the fragment; such veining indicates pre-breccia mineralization. Many of the fragments show only disseminated pyrite and minor chalcopyrite mineralization with sericite alteration, but they are cemented by a matrix of chalcopyrite, magnetite, and molybdenite, with secondary biotite and potash feldspar. This difference between the mineralization in the fragments and that in the matrix suggests that the mineralizing periods were separated in time.

The third stage of mineralization is clearly separate from the second stage: it occurs as narrow quartz, pyrite, and chalcopyrite veinlets that cut both the fragments and the matrix of the breccia. Molybdenite in quartz veins and sphalerite and galena in carbonate veins are also related to third-stage mineralization. These veins have alteration envelopes of late sericite. Third-stage mineralization contributes a very minor amount of sulfide minerals to the Copper Flat deposit compared to the first two stages.

ORIGIN OF THE BRECCIA PIPE

Any hypothesis concerning the origin of the breccia pipe that forms the high-grade center of the Copper Flat porphyry copper deposit must account for the following observations:

1. The matrix cementing the breccia fragments consists entirely of hydrothermal minerals—the same minerals which formed the second stage veins that cut the surrounding stock. No rock flour nor any igneous rock material occurs as part of the matrix.
2. The quartz monzonite and latite fragments within the breccia were mineralized prior to the formation of the breccia.
3. Only a small proportion of the breccia pipe contains definite rotated fragments. The most intense brecciation occurs near the top of the breccia body along the northern and western margin. The zone containing rotated fragments plunges to the west and shows a gradual decrease in the amount of separation and rotation with depth.
4. The bottom of the breccia pipe is marked by a gradual decrease in the number of stockwork veins within the quartz monzonite.
5. The amount of displacement between rotated fragments appears to be very slight. Much of the movement between fragments was no more than a few inches—the width of the intervening matrix. First stage veins can often be traced from one fragment to an adjacent one, even though these veins have been cut by the breccia matrix.
6. Latite fragments within the pipe are concentrated along the projection of the dikes that intrude the stock, and andesite fragments are found together (apparently the brecciation of andesite xenoliths).
7. The long axis of the breccia pipe is perpendicular to the principal fracture direction (northeast) in the stock—parallel to the least-stress direction.

The lack of any rock flour or gouge in the matrix indicates that brecciation was not the result of tectonic movement. The apparent lack of appreciable movement between the fragments and the gradational contact between true breccia and the zone of stockwork veining preclude any explosive mechanism for the brecciation. The process of mineralization-stoping (Locke, 1926) would result in appreciable downward movement and mixing of the fragments; it is therefore precluded at Copper Flat by the same observations.

The mechanism for the formation of the Copper Flat mineralized breccia pipe that appears most compatible with the above observations is that of autobrecciation caused by retrograde boiling when the pressure of the mineralizing fluid exceeded the confining pressure (Phillips, 1973). Expansion and brecciation caused by retrograde boiling within consolidated rock form breccia with the following characteristics that are observed at Copper Flat:

1. The breccia consists of zones of rotated fragments with no appreciable displacement. The zones of true breccia are enclosed within a body of stockwork or crackle breccia where no movement of the rock has occurred.
2. The most intense brecciation occurs near the top of the body, where the difference between the vapor pressure of the hydrothermal fluid and the confining pressure was greatest. The amount of brecciation decreases with depth due to increased confining pressure.
3. Horizontal expansion is greatest parallel to the least-stress direction resulting in an elongate body oriented in the same direction.
4. Retrograde boiling and subsequent expansion and fracturing initially had to occur beneath a cover of unfractured rock; when the fracturing reached the surface, the vapor pressure was released and brecciation ceased.

Unbrecciated quartz monzonite still overlies much of the breccia at Copper Flat, and the dip of the upper contact suggests that the breccia has only been unroofed by later erosion. Small, high-grade breccia bodies within the quartz diorite at El Teniente (Camus, 1975) and elsewhere in Chile (Kents, 1964) are very similar to the Copper Flat breccia pipe. These are still covered by unfractured rock and are thought to have formed through autobrecciation. Camus suggests that those at El Teniente formed at a depth of about 2,000 m; the depth of formation of the Copper Flat breccia pipe may be of the same magnitude.

The open spaces in the breccia at Copper Flat provided by the expansion were filled by hydrothermal minerals forming the matrix of the breccia and the irregular veins in the surrounding crackle breccia. Some part of the second stage mineralization occurred as replacement, which modified the original breccia texture.

The geology of Copper Flat indicates that the hypogene mineralization, including the formation of the breccia pipe, was the result of the final crystallization of the igneous melt that formed the quartz monzonite stock and related dikes. The mineralization was the culminating event of an igneous sequence that probably began with the extrusion of the andesite that forms the caldera.

ACKNOWLEDGMENTS

I thank Corbin J. Robertson, Jr., President of Quintana Minerals, for permission to publish the results of the study and acknowledge the support of W. E. Saegart, who directed the overall Copper Flat project. Bill Saegart also critically reviewed this chapter.

I am particularly pleased to acknowledge the help of B. Y. Kim, who was resident geologist at Copper Flat during the two-year period of exploration and development. His work provided much of the data for this study, and our many discussions were helpful in reaching an understanding of the geology.

REFERENCES CITED

Camus, Francisco, 1975, Geology of the El Teniente orebody with emphasis on wall-rock alteration: Econ. Geol., v. 70, p. 1341–1372.

Chapin, C. E., and Seager, W. R., 1975, Evolution of the Rio Grande rift in the Socorro and Las Cruces areas: New Mex. Geol. Soc. Guidebook, 26th Field Conf. p. 297–321.

Gilluly, James, 1946, The Ajo mining district, Arizona: U.S. Geol. Survey Prof. Paper 209, 112 p.

Hansuld, J. A., 1966, Eh and pH in geochemical exploration: CIM Bull., v. 59, p. 315–322.

Harley, G. T., 1934, The geology and ore deposits of Sierra County, New Mexico: New Mex. Bur. Mines Bull. 10, 220 p.

Hawley, John; Kottlowski, F. E.; Straw, W.S.; Seagar, W. R.; King, W. E.; and Le Mone, D. V., 1969, The Santa Fe group in the south-central New Mexico border region: New Mex. Bur. Mines Circular 104, p. 52–76.

Hedlund, D. C., 1974, Age and structural setting of base-metal mineralization in the Hillsboro-San Lorenzo area, southwestern New Mexico (abs.): New Mex. Geol. Soc. Guidebook, 25th Field Conf., p. 378–379.

———, 1975, Geologic map of the Hillsboro quadrangle, Sierra and Grant Counties, New Mexico: U.S. Geol. Survey open-file report 75–108, 19 p.

Johnston, W. P., and Lowell, J. D., 1961, Geology and origin of mineralized breccia pipes in Copper Basin, Arizona: Econ. Geol., v. 56, p. 916–940.

Jones, F. A., 1904, New Mexico Mines and Minerals: Santa Fe, New Mexico Printing Company, 349 p.

Kents, Paul, 1964, Special breccias associated with hydrothermal developments in the Andes: Econ. Geol., v. 59, p. 1551–1563.

Kuellmer, F. J., 1955, Geology of a disseminated copper deposit near Hillsboro, Sierra County, New Mexico: New Mex. Bur. Mines Circ. 34, 46 p.

Lindgren, Waldemar; Graton, L. C.; and Gordon, C. H., 1910, The ore deposits of New Mexico: U.S. Geol. Survey Prof. Paper 68, 361 p.

Locke, Augustus, 1926, The formation of certain ore bodies by mineralization stoping: Econ. Geol., v. 21, p. 431–453.

Phillips, W. J., 1973, Mechanical effects of retrograde boiling and its probable importance in the formation of some porphyry ore deposits: Instn. Mining and Metall. Trans., v. 82, Sec. B, p. B90–B98.

Reeves, C. C., 1963, Economic geology of a part of the Hillsboro, New Mexico, mining district: Econ. Geol., v. 58, p. 1278–1286.

Segerstrom, Kenneth, and Antweiler J. C. III, 1975, Placer-gold deposits of the Las Animas district, Sierra County, New Mexico: U.S. Geol. Survey open-file report, 39 p.

Titley, S. R., and Anthony, J. W., 1961, Some preliminary observations on the theoretical geochemistry of molybdenum under supergene conditions: Ariz. Geol. Soc. Digest, IV, p. 103–116.

Woodward, L. A.; Callender, J. F.; Gries, J.; Seagar, W. R.; Chapin, C. E.; Zelinski, R. E.; and Shaffer, W. L., 1975, Tectonic map of Rio Grande region from New Mexico-Colorado border to Presidio, Texas: New Mex. Geol. Soc. Guidebook, 26th Field Conf.

15

The Tyrone Copper Deposit

GRANT COUNTY, NEW MEXICO

Joseph Kolessar

The Tyrone copper deposit, a property of Phelps Dodge Corporation, is in the Burro Mountains mining district, Grant County, New Mexico, 10 miles southwest of Silver City, the county seat. The town of Tyrone is 4½ miles south of Silver City on New Mexico State Route 90 at an elevation of 5,700 ft. (Two previous townsites called Tyrone, the first in Niagara Canyon north of the mine and the second in the vicinity of the plant area, have ceased to exist.) The mine and concentrator are 6 miles southeast of the town at an average elevation of approximately 6,000 ft. A flash smelter designed to process Tyrone concentrates was completed in 1976; it is situated at the south end of Playas Lake in Hidalgo County, 64 air miles south of the mine.

HISTORY OF DEVELOPMENT AND PRODUCTION

Robert and John Metcalf made the first recorded discovery of copper and turquoise in the district in 1871, but hostile Indian activity in the area prevented development of their find at that time. In 1875 John E. Coleman rediscovered turquoise and staked the first claim. James Bullard, John Swisshelm, and J. W. Fleming discovered and developed the St. Louis Mine in 1879; two years later, operation of that mine was taken over by the Valverde Mining Company, which had been organized by Paschal R. Smith. A smelter was erected in Deadman Canyon by the Denver Reduction Works Company, and the town of Paschal was built south and west of the smelter. When the Denver Reduction Works venture failed in 1882, Smith organized the Queen City Mining and Smelting Company, which built a smelter immediately east of the Oak Grove Ranch. This enterprise lasted less than a year.

A number of other mining companies were active in the district in the years that followed, the most important being the Alessandro Mining Company and the Southwestern Mining Company. The Leopold brothers of Chicago acquired the properties of the latter company in 1904 and organized the Burro Mountain Copper Company the same year. By 1905 the Burro Mountain Copper Company's mine at the townsite of Leopold was the principal mine in the district. It consisted of an inclined shaft 500 ft. deep and a vertical shaft 220 ft. deep. Four levels comprising several thousand feet of workings were developed from the vertical shaft. The 125-ton-per-day mill included a crusher, rolls, Huntington mills, Wilfley tables, and Frue vanners. Mill capacity was increased to 250 tons per day in 1909.

During 1905 the Comanche Mining and Smelting Company, controlled by Silver City interests, and the Copper Gulf Development Company began development of their respective properties. These two firms later merged as the Savanna Copper Company. In 1906 Briggs Oliver Development Company (later called the Tyrone Development Company and finally the Chemung Copper Company) began developing the Burro Chief group of claims.

Phelps Dodge entered the Burro Mountains mining activity by purchasing the Burro Mountain Copper Company in 1909. Included in the purchase were the Sampson, St. Louis, and Boston mines and the concentrator. In 1912 the Chemung Group, including the Niagara Tunnel and the Nos. 1, 2, and 3 Niagara shafts, was purchased from the Chemung Copper Company, and shortly thereafter Phelps Dodge moved its local headquarters from Leopold to the original town of Tyrone in Niagara Canyon. Acquisition of additional claims and other lands to fill out Phelps Dodge's holdings continued into 1916.

The Leopold concentrator was shut down and dismantled in 1913. A 50-ton-per-day pilot concentrator was built in 1914 and was operated until March, 1915. Construction of a 1,400-ton-per-day concentrator east of the Continental Divide near Brick Kiln Gulch was commenced in June, 1914, and completed in August, 1916. Phelps Dodge's operations were conducted under the name "Burro Mountain Branch."

The Burro Mountain Branch mines and concentrator operated at the rate of 1,400 tons of ore per day until May, 1919, at which time the concentrator was shut down for remodeling and expansion. Production resumed in August, 1920, at the rate of 2,000 tons of ore per day, but low copper prices and declining ore grade resulted in suspension of underground operations at the Burro Mountain Branch in April, 1921. Production figures for the underground mine are shown in Table 15.1.

From 1949 to 1958 a continuous drilling program involving 720 holes blocked out an orebody measuring 1¾ miles by 1¼ miles in dimensions. Plans for reopening Tyrone as an open-pit mine were announced on September 1, 1966, and removal of overburden began May 1, 1967. By September, 1969, 95 million tons of overburden had been removed and a concentrator had been constructed having a daily capacity of 29,000 tons of ore. An expansion of concentrator capacity to 50,000 tons per day was begun early in 1971 and was completed in July, 1972. Additional drilling expanded the limits of the orebody to 1¾ miles by 2 miles. Daily mine output in 1976, including ore, leach, and waste material, totaled 250,000 tons. Between 1972 and 1979 the Tyrone mine produced about 100,000 tons of copper contained in concentrates annually. Production figures for the open-pit mine are shown in Table 15.2.

GEOLOGICAL SETTING

The Burro Mountains are separated into two distinct areas known as the Little Burro Mountains and the Big Burro Mountains. The Little Burros attain an elevation of 6,625 ft. above sea level and the Big Burros reach 8,035 ft.; the surrounding country averages about 6,000 ft. in elevation.

TABLE 15.1
Burro Mountain Branch Mine Production, 1914–1921
(In Tons)

Year*	Ore Treated by Concentrator	Copper Produced
1914	9,804	114
1915	16,255	609
1916	253,782	3,674
1917	473,443	6,749
1918	585,083	7,906
1919	184,946	2,820
1920	231,152	3,384
1921†	169,413	888
Total	1,923,878	26,144

* Production records are incomplete, but less than 100,000 tons of ore of variable grade were estimated to have been treated by the Burro Mountain Copper Company concentrator prior to Phelps Dodge acquisition.

† Mining operations suspended after 1921 until 1967, when the area was reopened as an open-pit mine.

TABLE 15.2
Tyrone Open-Pit Mine Production, 1967–1979
(In Tons)

Year	Total Material Removed	Ore Treated by Concentrator	Copper Produced
1967	17,592,840	145,549	—
1968	46,127,000	2,739,057	—
1969	51,610,000	2,849,370	17,653
1970	43,030,318	9,147,522	60,743
1971	46,487,441	8,797,558	61,563
1972	56,851,312	11,425,236	78,417
1973	72,620,031	15,407,249	103,151
1974	69,124,839	15,230,458	98,387
1975	53,361,922	12,386,795	76,009
1976	70,930,958	15,586,995	91,614
1977	71,666,753	15,073,537	84,734
1978	68,607,043	14,981,372	82,215
1979	80,118,281	17,770,783	100,651
Total	748,128,738	141,541,481	855,137

The Continental Divide traverses the orebody and the southeastern end of the mountains as well as the summit of the Big Burros. The mountains are separated by the Mangas Valley, which contains Gila conglomerate of Middle Miocene to Pleistocene Age and bolson deposits of Upper Pleistocene to Holocene Age and Recent alluvium.

The main mass of the Little Burro Mountains in which the Tyrone deposit occurs is located on the northeast side of the Mangas Valley, north and east of the Tyrone Mine site. The mountains trend northwest-southeast along a northeasterly tilted fault block. The west side of the Little Burro Mountains is faulted against bolson fill by the northwest-southeast trending Mangas fault, which forms a faceted scarp northeast of the Tyrone copper deposit. The Little Burro range consists of Precambrian granite and Cretaceous sedimentary rocks, intruded by andesite and rhyolitic rocks, all of which are overlain by Tertiary volcanic flows.

The Big Burro Mountains are located southwest of the Mangas Valley. Precambrian granite is the principal rock type in these mountains and is widely exposed except to the northeast in the area occupied by the Tyrone laccolith. The exposed part of the laccolith is elliptical in shape, 6 miles long and 4 miles wide. Potassium-argon dating of the biotite in the laccolith was reported at 56.2 ±1.7 million years by the New Mexico Bureau of Mines (August, 1971).

Drilling in the initial pit outline during the period 1949 to 1958 was patterned on a 200-ft. grid. Quartz monzonite porphyry is the predominant rock type in the south half of the orebody. Many holes drilled in this area bottomed in granite. Early literature on Tyrone described the quartz monzonite intrusion as an elliptical stock, but drilling results have indicated that the granite is overlain by quartz monsonite porphyry. The only plausible conclusion from the drilling results is that the intrusion is a laccolith.

Figure 15.1 shows the geologic setting of the Tyrone area. The Tyrone copper deposit is confined to a triangular area bounded on the northwest by the Burro Chief fault, limited to the south by a hinge-line fault extending eastward from the Candlestick fault area (Fig. 15.1). The deposit is covered to the northeast by bolson fill. The orebody is located in a horst

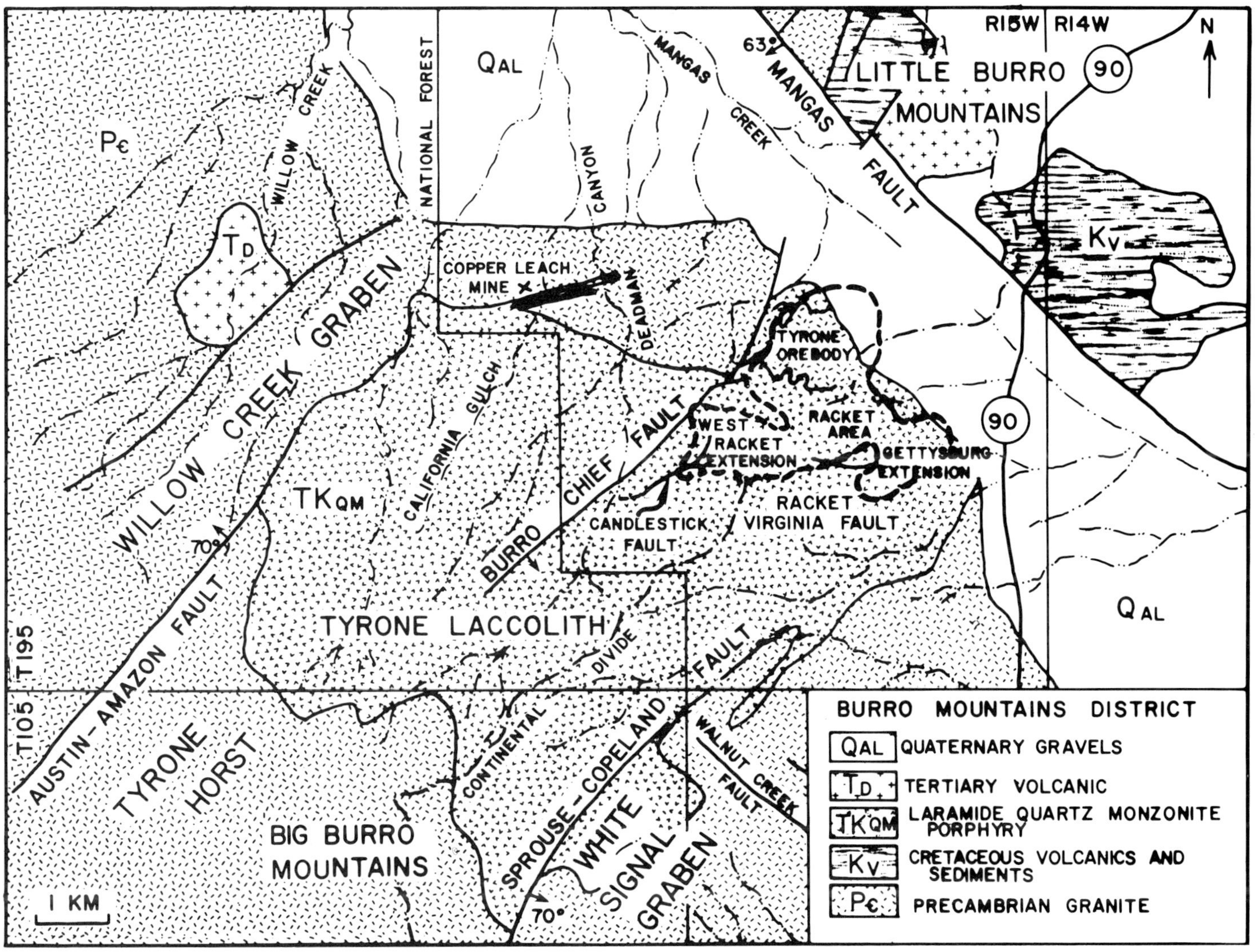

Figure 15.1. Geologic setting of the porphyry copper deposit and surrounding area at Tyrone

which is defined on the northwest by the Austin-Amazon fault and on the southwest by the Sprouse-Copeland fault. The resulting structures have been designated by Gillerman (1964) as the White Signal graben, Tyrone horst, and Willow Creek graben. The Burro Chief fault bisects the horst and tilts the Tyrone copper deposit along an east-west axis in a northerly direction.

Rock Types

Precambrian Rocks. Precambrian granites are the oldest exposed rock in the vicinity and within the Tyrone mine area. The granites are medium- to coarse-grained rocks containing rather large grains of pink orthoclase or plagioclase when fresh and abundant irregularly shaped grains of quartz. Biotite occurs, but not commonly, and some hornblende has been noted. Accessory minerals are sphene, zircon, tourmaline, apatite, magnetite, rutile, and ilmenite. The granite can be recognized megascopically by its abundant irregularly shaped quartz grains, which are evident even when intensely altered.

All plutonic igneous rocks of Precambrian age are included as part of the Burro Mountain batholith complex. Burro Mountain granite constitutes the major exposed part of the batholith, but small, separate, isolated masses of anorthosite, metadiabase, diorite, syenite, shrine granite, and larger masses of quartz diorite gneiss are included. These minor rock types are older than the Burro Mountain granite and are intruded by it. The older series does not appear in the vicinity of the copper deposit.

The granite in the vicinity of the mine is intruded by mineralized diabase dikes. These dikes have not been noted intersecting quartz monzonite porphyry. Granitic areas surrounding the mine site have also been intruded by dikes and plugs of mineralized diabase. This pattern of intrusions suggests an era of mineralization of the diabase younger than the granite but older than the mineralization at the Tyrone copper deposit.

The effects of hydrothermal alteration and weathering are widespread in the granite. Feldspars are argillized, although near mineralized areas they are more commonly sericitized or silicified. Biotite is altered to chlorite, hornblende to chlorite. Limonite, geothite, and supergene hematite veins and stains are common. Silicification is most common along any contact with the quartz monzonite porphyry.

Laramide Rocks. Quartz monzonite porphyry appears in the Burro Mountain granite as a series of intrusions forming the Tyrone laccolith. The porphyries invade the zone between the granite and the overlying sediments and volcanics (now removed by erosion) as dikes and plugs which differ in texture, composition, and sequence of intrusion. Fresh quartz monzonite porphyry outside of the mineralized area consists of moderate quartz, oligoclase, orthoclase, and sporadic occurrences of chloritized biotite.

Textural differences in the intrusion have been reported by Somers (1915) and by Paige (1922). The structural relationship of these varied quartz monzonite porphyries can be observed in areas excavated for open-pit mining. At least five porphyry types have been noted. The oldest, most common porphyry in the mineralized sequence is the intensely altered, fine-grained quartz monzonite porphyry which serves as the host rock for most of the ore mined at Tyrone. Coarser-textured rocks and intrusive breccia intrude the abundant finer-textured porphyry.

One of the more unusual younger course-textured intrusions is the quartz monzonite porphyry with poikilitic orthoclase phenocrysts. Some of these phenocrysts measure 3 in. long and may contain inclusions of quartz, oligoclase, biotite, magnetite, apatite, and sphene. This courser-grained porphyry is seldom, if ever, as thoroughly altered and mineralized as the older, ore-bearing variety which it intrudes. Occurrences of diorite are rare: only one dike has been mapped (east of the Burro Chief shaft).

Intrusive Breccia. Mining activity has exposed several intrusive breccias, two of which were noted prior to open-pit mining. The "breccia orebody" above the 5,669-ft. level cannot be associated with any known fault system. Some fragments are rounded and consist of granite and quartz monzonite porphyry. The matrix contains smaller fragments and is, in turn, fractured (Paige, 1922). The largest intrusive breccia exposed is an elongated body in the southwestern part of the Gettysburg extension (Fig. 15.2) Part of the breccia is uneconomic, but the northwesterly and southeasterly extremities constitute some of the higher-grade ore in the Gettysburg extension. Fragments in the elongated breccia are relatively rounded and are not as tightly welded as the fragments in the breccia across the canyon to the northeast.

In the northwest Gettysburg area a highly mineralized outcrop—indicative of excellent supergene enrichment—displays graphic quartz veining, copious supergene hematite in the form of veins, hydrous iron oxide coatings, and pyrite casts filled and crusted with dark maroon supergene hematite. Fragmentation in this area is difficult to discern; in some breccia outcrops, intensive mineralization obliterates fragmentation to some degree, especially in tightly welded breccias.

With the exception of the breccia orebody which is located near the north-central portion of the Tyrone orebody outline, almost all intrusive breccias noted have been located in the Gettysburg extension and near the eastern limit of the orebody (see Fig. 15.2). Some intrusive breccias at Tyrone have a fragmented pyrite matrix which is coated with supergene chalcocite. Since breccias usually contain a larger sulfide volume than porphyry and granite, the ore grade in these enriched intrusive breccias is usually higher than in the surrounding rocks. The interstices in breccias permit a degree of permeability not displayed in the relatively homogenous rock types. The protore grade in most breccias at Tyrone is similar to the protore grade in the porphyry and granite.

The youngest porphyry at Tyrone is the least important economically. The medium-grained textured porphyries occur as plugs and dikes and contain as an ordinary constituent chloritized biotite and not the secondary biotites that are so characteristic of potassic alteration zones.

In the Racket area of the mine, which is located northwest of the Gettysburg extension (see Fig. 15.2), these young porphyries are mineralized by pyrite. Feldspars are altered to montmorillonite and generally are relatively fresh in appearance as compared with the highly sericitic and pyritic surrounding rocks. In the Gettysburg area, pyrite mineralization in young porphyries is meager.

Drilling located slightly east of the central eastern orebody outline has intersected a sill of relatively fresh, barren pyritic porphyry within thoroughly leached maroon cap rock that is ordinarily indicative of excellent enrichment. A barren porphyry dike has also been noted intersecting Gila conglomerate in a railroad cut of the old El Paso and Southwestern Railroad less than 2 miles east of the ore deposit. These rocks may post-date enrichment.

Cretaceous Rocks. Cretaceous sediments and volcanics are largely confined to the Little Burro Mountains. Beartooth Quartzite (a thin-bedded to massive, vitreous, fine- to very fine-grained sandstone containing thin shale partings) rests unconformably on Precambrian granite. The Colorado Formation (an olive green and brown, calcareous and sandy shale) overlies the Beartooth Quartzite. Cretaceous andesites and dacites complete the Cretaceous section in the Little Burro Mountains.

Tertiary and Quaternary Rocks. Tertiary rhyolites and andesites overlie Cretaceous andesites and dacites in the Little Burro Mountains. In the immediate vicinity of the mine, the only Tertiary deposit is the Gila Conglomerate, of late Tertiary and early Quaternary age. Bolson deposits of Upper Pleistocene and Holocene age are the youngest sediments.

Local Structures

The Mangas fault, dipping 63°SW, forms a prominent scarp with the Little Burro Mountains; Gila Conglomerate and bolson deposits were displaced along this fault and positioned against older rocks of the Little Burro Mountains.

The Burro Chief fault, striking northeast and dipping southeast, is located in the central northern part of the horst (see Fig. 15.1). This fault places Precambrian granite against bolson fill in the area northwest of the orebody. The Burro Chief fault is also the western limit of the Tyrone copper deposit. Fluorite veins were deposited along the fault during middle to late Tertiary time. Many small fluorite deposits

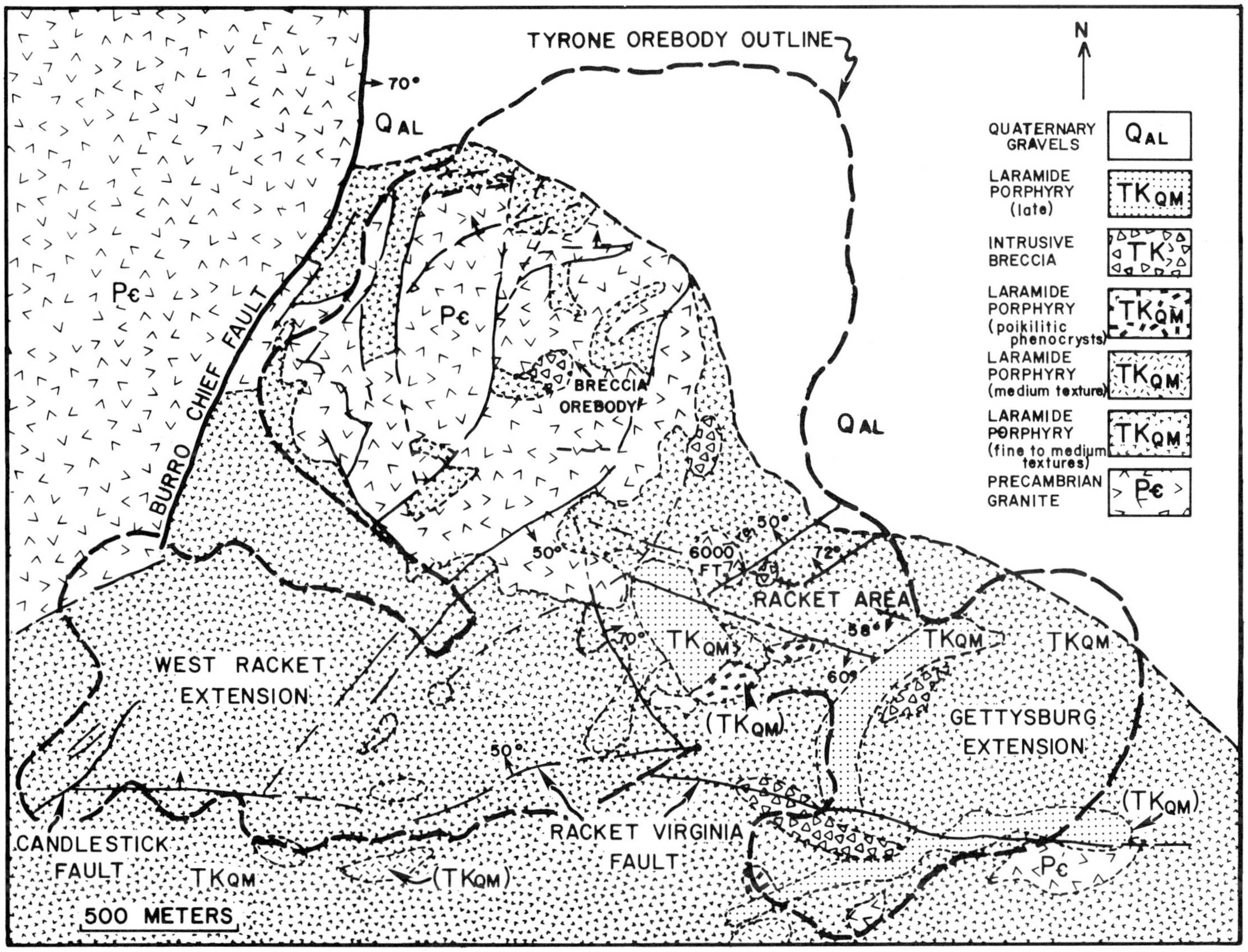

Figure 15.2. Geologic map of the Tyrone deposit

surrounding the quartz monzonite laccolith are associated with faults that cut middle to late Tertiary volcanic rocks. Fluorite in the district has also been noted in fractures within the Gila Conglomerate. A hinge-type movement for the entire block southeast of the fault is plausible. The latest movement on the fault tilted the ore deposit 5 to 8° northwesterly. The area of major displacement is located at or near the intersection of the Burro Chief and Mangas faults.

The Racket-Virginia hinge-line fault zone extends eastward from the Candlestick fault near Deadman Canyon and can be traced for almost two miles.

Major copper mineralization occurs within the area circumscribed by the structures mentioned above; however, there are three notable occurrences of oxide copper outside these limits. Several occurrences of copper oxides are found west of the Burro Chief fault. The most prominent is the copper oxide mineralization at the Copper Leach property (formerly the Ohio mine area). In this area, a mineralized dike of quartz monzonite porphyry intrudes into Precambrian granite and strikes northeasterly through California Gulch and Deadman Canyon. Less prominent oxide copper mineralization occurs in areas south of the Racket-Virginia fault zone and less than ½ mile west of New Mexico Highway 90 and ¾ mile south of the Gettysburg extension.

ECONOMIC GEOLOGY

Description of Orebody

The Tyrone orebody occurs within the Tyrone quartz monzonite laccolith and the underlying Precambrian granite. The quartz monzonite porphyry is a deeply eroded remnant of the original intrusion. The major portion of the laccolith was removed by erosion, and only the many dikes and plugs which invade the Precambrian basement were left (see Fig. 15.2). The orebody consists of a supergene blanket of erratic chalcocite coating on pyrite mineralization. The blanket varies from a few feet to over 300 ft. in thickness. The orebody slopes northeasterly and tilts 8° northwesterly toward the Burro Chief fault. The top of the enrichment blanket is very irregular, with sporadic remnants of sulfide ore in the oxidized capping.

More copper ore occurs in the granite at Tyrone than in the porphyry. The granitic rocks, intruded by dikes and plugs of quartz monzonite porphyry, are exposed prevalently in the north half of the pit. Molybdenum content is also greater in the granite. Within the mine area, there are at least 20 partially mined-out high-grade areas of chalcocite ore averaging 2 to 3 percent copper. These deposits were the principal mining areas at the time underground operations closed down in 1921; they trend roughly northeasterly along the larger fractures, most of which parallel the Burro Chief fault. Aside from minute amounts of gold and silver recovered from the ore, copper is the only product resulting from the mining.

An old water table, evident at the top of the sulfide zone, sharply differs from the location of the 1980 water level. Ore is found above the 1980 water table in the southern sector of the pit boundary and below it (from the 5,700-ft. elevation) in the northern part of the orebody. The outline of the top of the orebody corresponds reasonably with the topography. Ore occurs within a few feet of the surface in the West Racket extension near the St. Louis shaft and at 500 to 600 ft. below the surface in the northeast sector of the orebody. The bottom of the orebody is also irregular and grades into protore averaging approximately 0.10 percent copper. Ultimately, the pit may reach a depth of 1,300 ft., with lateral dimensions of approximately 2 miles along the north-south axis and about 2 miles along the east-west axis.

Mineralization

Although erratic and limited in distribution, chrysocolla is the most abundant copper mineral in the oxidized zone. Tenorite, malachite, and azurite, together with rare cuprite, native copper, brochantite, and chalcanthite, are present in capping and near the Burro Chief fault zone. The ore minerals occur in fractures, as disseminations in the country rock adjacent to fractures, and as matrix in breccias. Most of these fractures are less than an inch wide and only rarely range up to a foot in width.

Chalcocite, the most important ore mineral, and covellite are the supergene sulfide minerals that replace pyrite, chalcopyrite, and sphalerite. Chalcocite occurs most often as a thin coating on pyrite grains, although in some siliceous breccias it occurs as almost pure blebs, possibly as a replacement of chalcopyrite or sphalerite. The pyrite:chalcocite ratio is approximately 6:1.

The primary sulfide minerals are pyrite, chalcopyrite, and sphalerite, with occurrences of molybdenite and trace quantities of bornite in the granitic (northern) part of the orebody. Pyrite, which contains small inclusions of quartz and chalcopyrite, is the most abundant sulfide mineral and commonly is partially replaced by chalcocite at its margins or along veinlets. Chalcopyrite is generally observed as particles in quartz and is also present as small inclusions in pyrite and sphalerite. Sphalerite is commonly associated with pyrite and has replaced it in part.

Molybdenite, which appears as curved shreds unassociated with other sulfide minerals, occurs as a thin coating on joints and fractures in the porphyry and as veins (with quartz) in the granite. Of very minor significance, bornite occurs as sparse remnants of crystals largely replaced by chalcocite. Sulfide content in the protore is less than 6 percent by weight. Of the six species of copper phosphates found in porphyry copper deposits, at least four occur at Tyrone: libethenite, torbernite, pseudomalachite, and turquoise. Lead meta-autunite has been identified in the West Racket vicinity.

Hydrothermal Alteration

Hydrothermal alteration and associated processes may contribute to preparation of the rock for enrichment by development of porosity and permeability in addition to introducing the necessary primary sulfides. In some areas the porous, earthy, altered porphyries serve as host rocks for the supergene enrichment process, but there are enriched areas that do not conform to this description. Sericite is the most abundant hydrothermal alteration product. Hypogene clay minerals occur in the younger porphyries and in the area below the bottom of enrichment.

Argillic alteration occurs erratically, but quartz-sericite is the dominant form of alteration. Propylitic alteration occurs peripherally to the northeast on the edge of the Gettysburg extension, along the Burro Chief fault zone in the northwest part of the West Racket extension, and near the geographic center of the orebody between the original pit and the West Racket extension at the 1,600-ft. level. The younger porphyries exhibit chloritization of biotite, with feldspar altering to montmorillonite, and development of pyrite in the Racket area; only biotite, chloritization, and meager pyritization occur in the Gettysburg area.

The poikilitic orthoclase feldspars for the most part appear relatively fresh, occasionally exhibiting a thin alteration zone on the periphery of the phenocrysts, although in some areas the phenocrysts are completely altered. Some of the most important chemical changes in the porphyry at Tyrone can be noted by the free quartz content, which may range from less than 15 percent in the fresh rocks to 40 to 70 percent in the altered varieties. The Na_2O content, which may vary from 2 to 5 percent in fresh rocks, is invariably reduced to less than 1 percent in the orebody with the destruction of the plagioclase feldspars.

The fact that enormous amounts of water have been added to hydrothermally altered rocks is evident in ignition loss, which is measurably significant because of the abundance of sericite. There has not been any significant change in the K_2O content in the altered and fresh varieties. The chemical comparisons are based on analyses of fresh rocks from the surrounding barren porphyries and on altered rocks sampled from within the orebody.

Silicification is prevalent in the Precambrian granite-quartz monzonite contact zone, a phenomenon repeated in at least one other southwestern porphyry copper deposit. The zone of silicification meanders midway across the narrower expanse of the main orebody outline and then moves along the extreme northeastern pit limits. Silicification also prevails around granite apophyses in the lower levels of the southeast sector of the main orebody (the Racket area).

Nontronite occurs in the transition zone between the bottom of the capping and the top of sulfides. Alunite occurs in localized veins in the granite-porphyry contact zone and has been observed as matrix in a breccia in the area between the Gettysburg extension and the main orebody. In the protore, the preponderance of a yellowish brown montmorillonite immediately below the chalcocite zone suggests that the normal hypogene alteration is obscured by supergene effects; the bleached appearance of enriched sulfide zones is absent.

Leached Capping

The appearance of conditions in the supergene cap rock at Tyrone does not vary significantly with rock type; granites display the same general appearance as porphyries and breccias. The cap rock over the Tyrone copper deposit is a classic example of all stages, from extremely immature to well-defined, mature, supergene capping. The most important constituent—and certainly one of the most abundant minerals in capping over Tyrone and other disseminated copper deposits—is supergene hematite.

Supergene hematite is present as the principal mineral filling the cavities vacated by the sulfides. As a filling, it has a finely fibrous appearance, while as a crust, the surface is made up of tiny spherules. Supergene hematite, which is generally of a porous nature, also forms narrow seams and veinlets, and stains the surrounding rock a prominent maroon. To be of economic significance at Tyrone the area must exhibit supergene hematite in both veins and disseminations; rarely does a preponderance of one form or the other indicate ore-grade, enriched sulfides.

In the northwest area of the mine site, the fissure outcrops exhibit considerable hematite, and chalcedony is stained deep maroon with hematite. In the southwest sector of the main orebody—designated as the Racket-Virginia area—fissure outcrops consist of hematite, granular quartz, and irregular deposits of chrysocolla. Tenorite has been noted in outcrops above areas of thorough oxidation, and neotocite occurs around the periphery of economically important areas.

GEOLOGIC HISTORY

The geologic environment prior to Laramide intrusion consisted of Precambrian granite overlain by Cretaceous volcanics and sediments. During the Laramide Revolution, the Tyrone laccolith intruded the area as a multiple intrusion north of the Big Burro range. In early Tertiary time following Laramide intrusion, an uplift then tilted this area to the northeast, and at approximately the same time the Burro Chief fault bisected the laccolith. Displacement of the area east of the fault limited mineralization to the northwest. The uplift accelerated erosion and removed the Cretacous cover over the laccolith, exposing the porphyry. During uplift, the entire vicinity north of the Mangas fault scarp was essentially an area of moderate relief, with flat-lying Cretaceous and Tertiary flows. If any barren Tertiary volcanics were deposited above the site of the Tyrone orebody, their removal by erosion probably contributed to an intensified supergene process in the area.

Several movements occured along the Burro Chief fault; the last occurred during Pleistocene time and tilted the deposit into its present position. The same era of faulting resulted in tilting of the entire Little Burro mountain range northeasterly, creating the present land forms.

SUMMARY

The Burro Mountains District has progressed from a minor turquoise and copper producer in the 1870s to a major United States copper producer a century later. Mining prior to and during World War I concentrated on developing enriched sulfide veins and breccias. The orebody is a classical example of supergene enrichment of a disseminated pyrite-chalcopyrite protore in a host rock of quartz monzonite porphyry and granite. The protore, averaging about 0.10 percent copper, has been enriched to a grade averaging less than 1 percent copper. The thickness of the enriched ore varies from a few feet to over 300 ft. Leached capping varies from several feet to 500 ft. in thickness. The laccolith of quartz monzonite porphyry was intruded between Precambrian granite and overlying volcanics and sediments. Most of the volcanics have been removed by erosion. The laccolith was invaded by many scattered dikes and plugs of various textured porphyries intruded at several times; usually finer-grained rocks were followed by varieties which cooled slowly and resulted in coarser textures. Uplift and deep erosion of the laccolith then resulted in an enriched orebody with a large volume of leached cap rock.

REFERENCES CITED

Gillerman, Elliot, 1964, Mineral deposits of western Grant County, New Mexico: N. Mex. Bur. Mines Bull. 33, p. 41–48.

Paige, Sidney, 1922, Copper deposits of the Tyrone district, New Mexico: U.S. Geol. Survey Prof. Paper 122, 53 p.

Somers, R. E., 1915, Geology of the Burro Mountains copper district, New Mexico: AIME Trans., v. 52, p. 604–656.

16

Structural, Petrological and Mineralogical Controls for the Dos Pobres Orebody

LONE STAR MINING DISTRICT, GRAHAM COUNTY, ARIZONA

Jackson M. Langton and Sidney A. Williams

The Dos Pobres orebody is one of the four known porphyry copper deposits discovered in the Lone Star mining district, situated on the southwest slope of the Gila Mountains in Graham County, Arizona. This ore deposit is located approximately nine miles north of Safford, the county seat (Fig. 16.1). Surface elevations over the orebody range between 3,900 and 4,200 ft.

Phelps Dodge Corporation optioned the property in the fall of 1957 and commenced drilling on November 21, 1957. By early 1960 sufficient economic mineralization had been delineated to warrant purchase of the optioned claims (Richard Moolick, 1968, personal communication). Exploratory drilling continued intermittently after 1959 and the first exploration and development shaft was begun in November, 1968. As of July 1, 1979, approximately 189,000 feet of rotary drilling and diamond coring had been completed in the immediate vicinity of the orebody and more than 79,100 feet of shaft sinking, crosscutting and drifting had also been accomplished (K. C. Bennett, 1979, personal communication). All exploratory drilling and development work has confirmed reserves of approximately 400 million tons of 0.72 percent copper sulfide ore.

The early phase of exploratory drilling indicated that the ore geometry resembled an inverted funnel, with the minable copper values draped over a relatively barren granodiorite stock at depth. The second phase of delineation, which consisted of diamond coring on a 400-ft. grid and underground development work, provided sufficient information to meliorate previous concepts and to ascertain several facts that were pertinent to localizing the orebody. Extensive petrographic studies correlated with computerized whole-rock chemical analyses and geologic mapping were an integral part of the research conducted on the Phelps Dodge orebody.

DISTRICT GEOLOGY

The Dos Pobres orebody occurs in folded, consanguineous metavolcanics and metavolcaniclastics that are genetically related to Laramide diorite, tonalite, quartz monzonite, granodiorite, and andesite intrusives. The Cretaceous-Tertiary kindred locally crops out from beneath upper Tertiary volcanics and Pliocene to Recent pediment gravels along a regional, northwest-trending structural belt (Fig. 16.2). Hornblende and pyroxene andesite flows and agglomerates dominate the kindred, but are often intercalated with latites, glassy dacites, dacite tuffs, and volcanic conglomerates, wackes, and breccias. The volcaniclastic members generally dip and thicken away from the central belt of principally volcanic rocks.

This enormous thickness of older andesites was derived from an underlying parental tonalite-granodiorite pluton(s), interpreted as Late Cretaceous to Paleocene in age (Table 16.1). Two outcrops of the pluton(s) have been observed by the authors and a third one has been described by Robinson and Cook (1966); Figure 16.2 shows the location of these outcrops. Several localities where apophyses of the pluton(s) are relatively close to the surface have been observed. One hole actually penetrated the Laramide metavolcanics and intrusives and encountered an amphibolite derived from sediments of probable Precambrian age.

Xenoliths of Precambrian gneiss, schist, quartzite, and granite in the metavolcanics, quartz diorite pluton(s), and, occasionally, in the quartz monzonite porphyries have been recognized on the surface and in numerous drill hole samples. The nearest outcrops of Precambrian gneisses and schists, however, are south of Safford on Graham Mountain at elevations up to 10,700 ft. Since more than 5,000 ft. are allowed for Miocene uplift, it appears that the narrow belt of

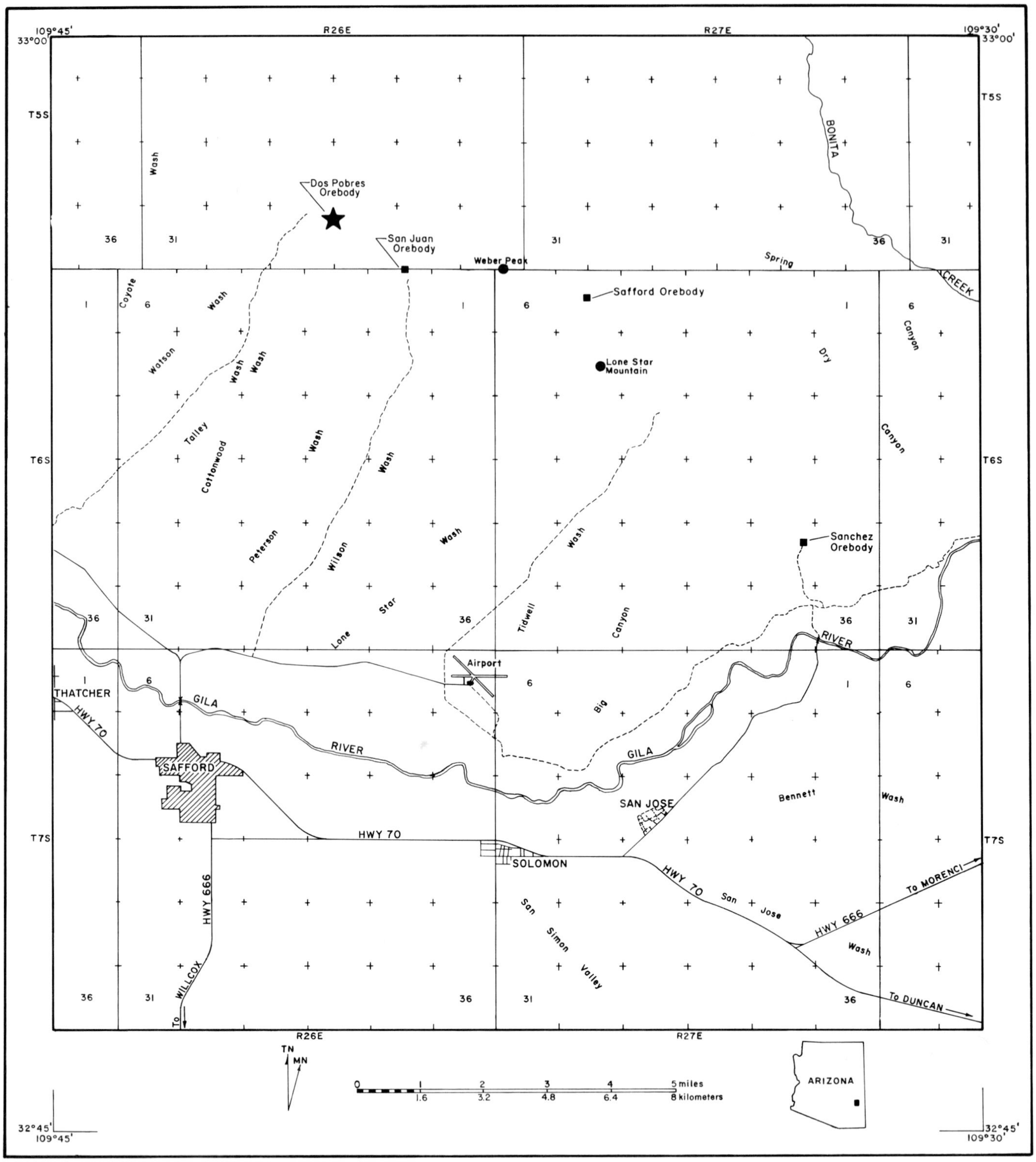

Figure 16.1. Index map of the Lone Star mining district

Laramide andesites were extruded in a structural trough with more than 10,000 ft. of topographic relief. The andesites that have been drilled are sub-aerial in character, and deep exploration throughout the district has failed to find volcanics of spilitic affinity.

The Dos Pobres orebody is remarkably similar to some of the porphyry copper deposits in British Columbia (Carson and Jambor, 1974), the Philippines (Saegart and Lewis, 1976), the Solomon Islands (Fountain, 1972), and the Andes (Hollister, 1973; Camus, 1975; Gustafson and Hunt, 1975).

A rather subtle unconformity exists between the Tertiary-Cretaceous Safford andesites and Tertiary Baboon agglomerates (see Table 16.1). The agglomerates are intruded by non-productive hornblende andesite dikes, sills, and plugs,

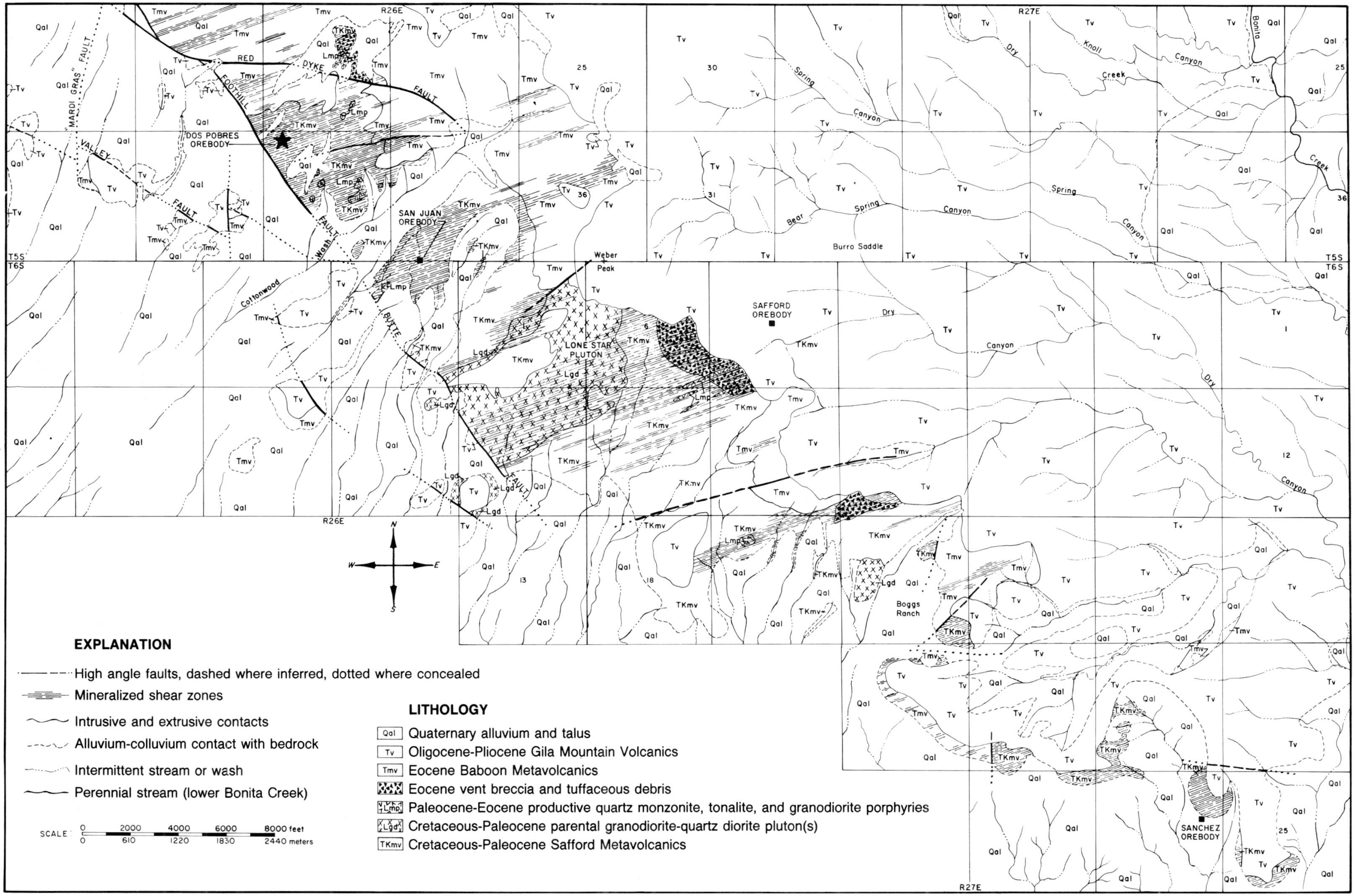

Figure 16.2. Geologic map of the Lone Star mining district.
Mapped and collated by R. Geer and others, Phelps Dodge Corp., 1972.

TABLE 16.1
The Geologic Column at the Dos Pobres Orebody

Rock Type	Composition	Thickness (in ft.)	Age	Symbol
Alluvium, Terrace Gravels, Basin Fill	Sands, claybeds, gravels, siltstones, conglomerates	0–2,000+	Pleistocene-Recent	*Qal*
	Unconformity			
Gila Mountain Volcanics	Basalt & rhyolite dikes, sills, plugs; basalt flows, tuffs, rhyolites, agglomerates, vent debris, basal conglomerate	0–3,000+	Miocene-Pliocene	*Tv*
	Unconformity			
Baboon Metavolcanics-Metavolcaniclastics	Hornblende andesite dikes, sills, plugs	—	Eocene	*Tha*
	Propylitized andesite agglomerates, flow breccias, mud flows, lithic tuffs, conglomerates	0–1,500+	Eocene	*Tmv*
	Unconformity			
Productive Porphyries	Tonalite-quartz monzonite-monzonite-granodiorite porphyry stock(s), dikes, and sills	—	Paleocene-Eocene	*Lmp*
Lone Star Pluton(s)	Quartz diorite-granodiorite batholith	—	Upper Cretaceous-Paleocene	*Lgd*
Safford Metavolcanics-Metavolcaniclastics	Metamorphosed hornblende and pyroxene andesite flows, breccias, agglomerates, wackes, & mud flows	3,500+	Upper Cretaceous-Pleocene	*TKmv*
	Unconformity			
	Amphibolite, gneiss, granite, quartzite, schist	—	Precambrian	*P€s*

most of which are clearly younger than the productive porphyries and appear to be genetically related to the flows. The productive quartz monzonite porphyries do not intrude the Tertiary Baboon sequence, but the agglomerates are often well mineralized along the hornblende andesite dikes and shear zones. These agglomerates crop out northwest, north, and northeast of the Dos Pobres orebody (Fig. 16.3).

Analogous to the large Morenci-Metcalf district, 20 miles to the northeast, the major fault zones of the Lone Star district strike north-south, east-northeast–west-southwest, and northwest-southeast. The north-south faults are poorly defined and appear to have had older left-lateral movement; they may possibly have offset the pluton(s) and Precambrian basement for thousands of feet in some cases. The northwest-southeast *en echelon* faults are the most pronounced features in the district. Although they were conceivably part of an older, regional, right-lateral system, gravity movement since Miocene time characterized the displacements along most of these structures. Hinge- and scissor-type slippage has been delineated along several of the faults.

Basalts, tuffs, rhyolite, and agglomerates of Miocene to Late Pliocene age cap the Gila Mountains and attain thicknesses of more than 3,000 ft. (see Table 16.1). Preceding and contemporaneous with this volcanism, a pediment was developing along the southwest flanks of the Tertiary-Cretaceous volcanic belt. This pediment is principally composed of eroded propylitized volcanic debris cemented with clays and pyroclastic debris; it is covered with clay beds that thicken to the southwest and that crop out locally near the Gila River north of Safford. A younger pediment, developed on the clays and younger volcanics, is, in turn, locally covered with recent basin fill, terrace gravels, and alluvium.

OREBODY GEOLOGY

The surface geologic map in Figure 16.3 portrays the principal rock types, structure, and hydrothermal alteration associated with the ore and may be compared to the geologic map of the 2,500-ft. level (Fig. 16.4), which is approximately 1,500 ft. below the surface. Below the surface to a depth of 800 ft. the ore is pipe-like in shape, partially leached and thoroughly oxidized. The ore pipe persists to a depth of 1,200 ft., but oxidation is accompanied by moderately enriched sulfide mineralization. Below the 2,900-ft. elevation the hypogene ore expands rapidly, achieving a diameter of approximately 3,000 ft. in a northwest-southeast direction.

Rock Types

Safford Metavolcanics. More than 75 percent of the ore at Dos Pobres occurs in the Safford metavolcanics, a metamorphosed Cretaceous-Tertiary sequence. The bulk of the volcanic pile is andesitic in composition, but dacites, dacite tuffs, and latites have been recognized. Specifically, the majority of the flows and breccias are hornblende or pyroxene

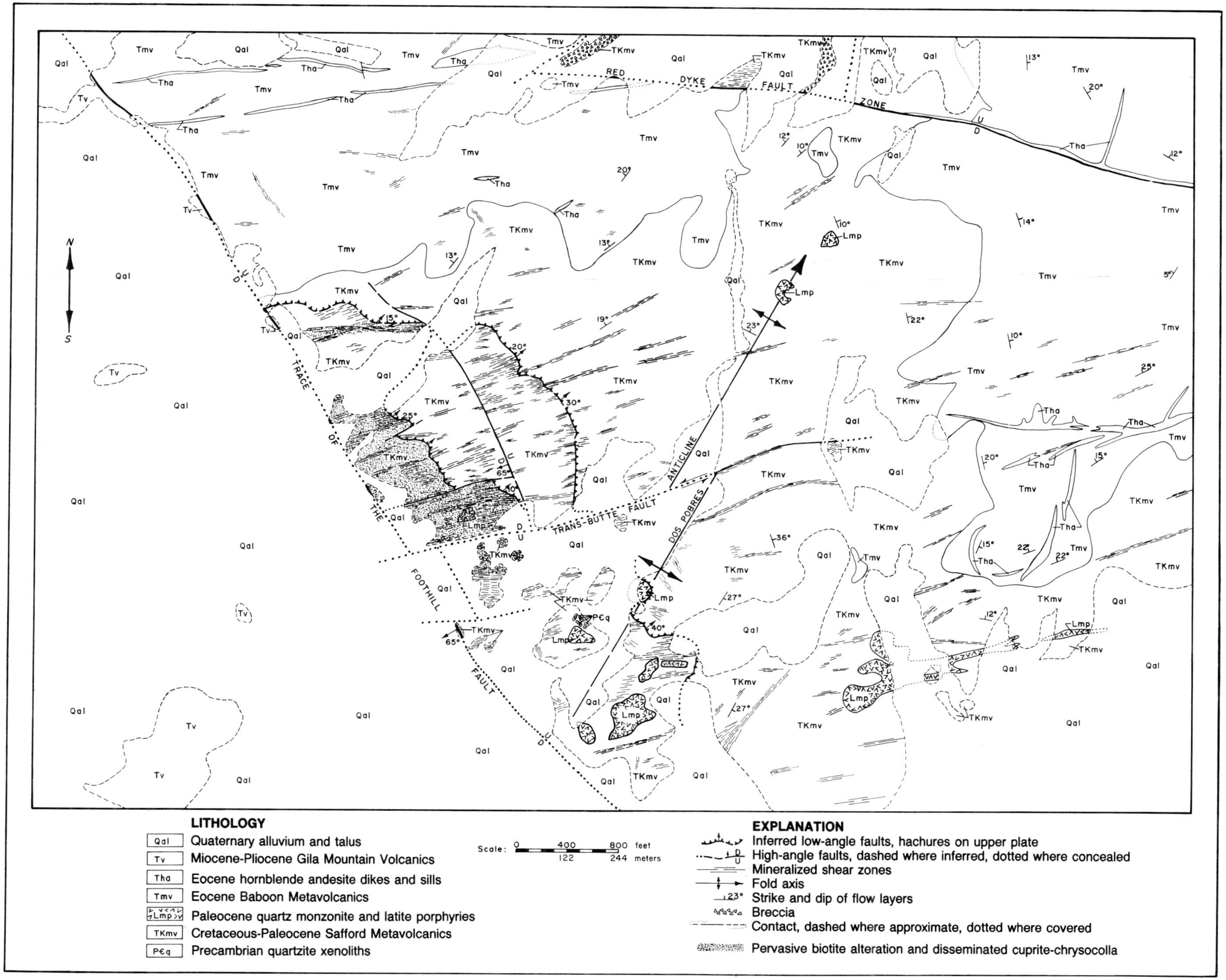

Figure 16.3. Geologic map of the surface of the Dos Pobres orebody and vicinity

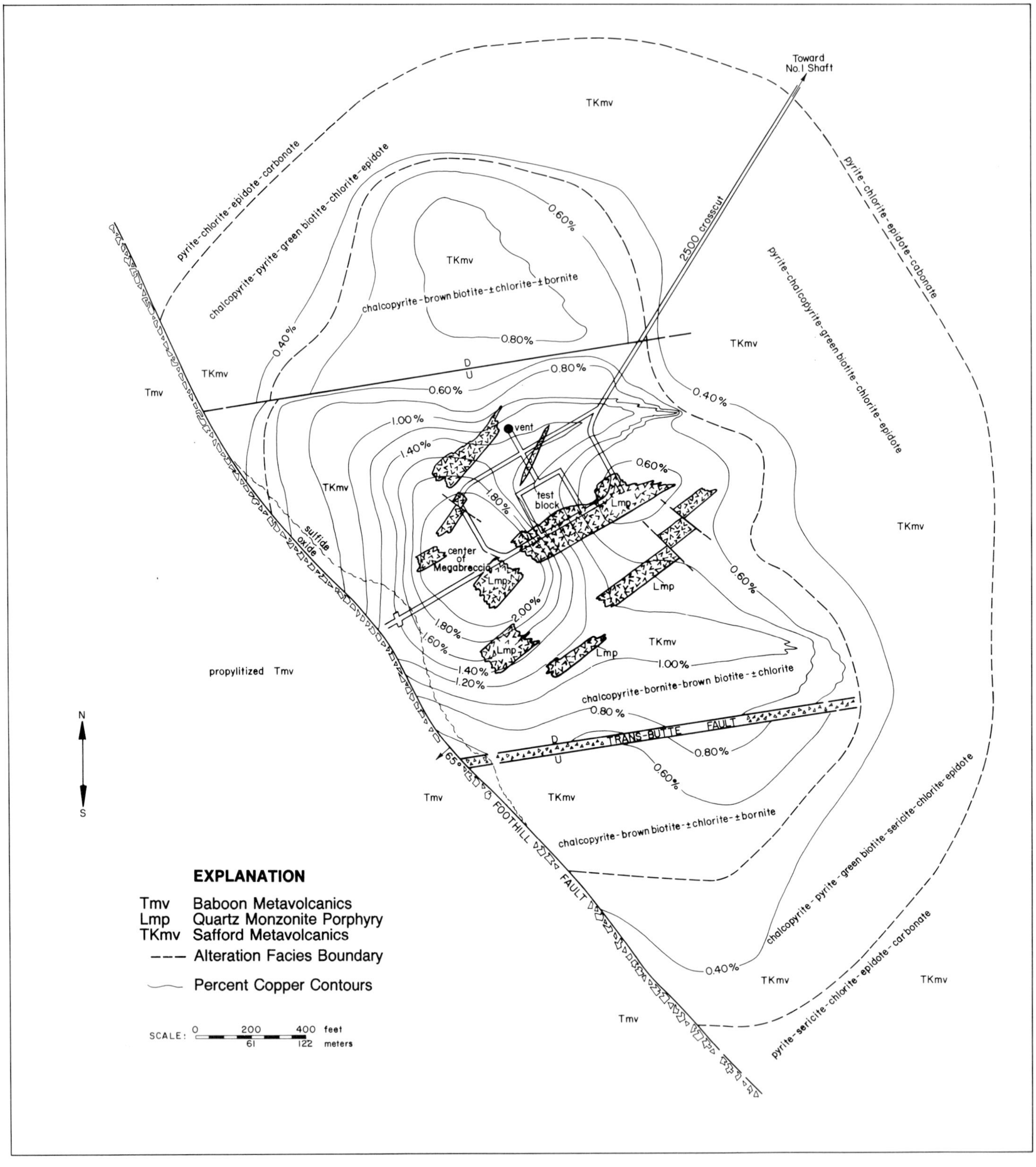

Figure 16.4. Geologic map of 2,500-ft. level. Based on mapping by W. Bowen, R. Boatman, and J. Langton, Phelps Dodge Corp., 1969–1975.

andesites that have been pervasively altered in the vicinity of the orebody. The fragmental nature of the flow breccias is often obscured by metamorphism or hydrothermal alteration, but it may be accentuated by crackling. Contact metamorphism by the parental granodiorite has been clearly dated at 69.8 ± 2.7 m.y.

Productive Porphyries. Some of the higher-grade copper values occur in the dikes or phacoliths in the upper levels of the mine, but with depth the porphyries become progressively lower-grade and relatively barren. It is possible that 2 intrusions invaded the Safford metavolcanics between 47 and 58 m.y. ago, but sufficient information has not been obtained in order to discuss them separately. It will suffice to state that the principal productive porphyry is generally a quartz monzonite, ranging in composition to tonalite or granodiorite. Six drill holes have encountered an apparent stock below the 1,800-ft. elevation in the northwest portion of the orebody (Fig. 16.5), although mapping on the 2,500-ft. level suggests that many of the dikes are detached from this stock (see Fig. 16.4).

Hornblende Andesite Dikes and Sills. Intrusions in the form of hornblende andesite dikes and sills are most obvious in the east-northeast–west-southwest shear zones away from the ore, and most of them are clearly consanguineous with the Baboon volcanics. Large titaniferous hornblende phenocrysts, often more than 1 cm long, suggest that these non-productive intrusions were saturated with water. The dikes, which are evidently late-and post-mineral, acted as dilutents to the ore. Ore grade in their vicinity is invariably lower than in the core of the orebody, where no dikes or sills have been recognized. These intrusions are generally only a few feet thick in the Safford metavolcanics, but they may reach thicknesses of more than 200 ft. in the lower Baboon sequence.

Baboon Metavolcanics. The propylitized andesitic agglomerates, flow breccias, mud flows, and lithic tuffs of the Baboon metavolcanics crop out northeast, north, and northwest of the orebody and thicken to more than 1,500 ft. northwesterly. The sequence has been hydrothermally altered locally, but has not been metamorphosed by either the productive porphyries or the parental pluton(s). Propylitization appears to be autometamorphic away from the east-northeast–west-southwest shear zones, but is clearly hydrothermal toward the orebody. Lower members of these volcanics are intruded by the aforementioned hornblende andesite dikes of late- or post-mineral age, and the upper units contain large xenoliths of the same intrusions, with coronas that indicate the dike fragments were cooling with the flows.

Structure

Two of the most important structures that influence the geometry of the orebody are the Foothill fault and the Dos Pobres anticline (see Fig. 16.3). It was initially thought that folding resulted from older lateral movement along the Foothill fault, but more recent evidence clearly suggests that the drag fold is a secondary feature related to the Valley and Red Dyke faults (see Fig. 16.3). A northwest-southeast cross section parallel to the Foothill fault, demonstrates fold control for the core (see Fig. 16.5).

Low angle faults are present in the orebody, but the significance of these structures has yet to be determined. The strike varies from N40°W to N60°W; dips range between 10° and 40°NE; and the rake is typically N50°E.

Several east-northeast–west-southwest faults have had considerable post-mineral displacement, but these structures were the principal channels for productive porphyries and ore-bearing fluids. Essentially contemporaneous with the major down-throw of the Foothill fault, these veins had recurrent movement and down-faulted the ore in a step-like pattern from southeast to northwest (see Fig. 16.5).

Crackle brecciation constitutes the dominant fracturing in the mine and is most extensive in the metavolcanics, not in the productive porphyries. All of the crackling or fracturing not related to post-mineral faulting appears to be hydrothermal in origin. Simple parting across fragments and large phenocrysts, with virtually no displacement of the respective boundaries, is typical of the character of this fracturing and is seen throughout the orebody.

Contact breccias intimately associated with the porphyries often host the highest-grade ore; these features are more important in the upper portions of the deposit and must have formed early during intrusion. Typically, the upper extremities of dikes grade into the breccias, which are characterized by numerous fragments of metavolcanics embedded in the porphyry.

A later event was the development of a megabreccia, which was apparently related to the de-gassing of the productive rest-magma. This breccia incorporates huge fragments of meta-andesite, productive porphyry, and contact breccia. The overall appearance of the megabreccia suggests "floating" blocks of the porphyry in a crackle breccia (see Figs. 16.4 and 16.5).

Alteration of Porphyry

The productive porphyry at Dos Pobres is generally a quartz monzonite by mode; however, the freshest samples seen tend to be granodioritic, as attested by phenocrysts of embayed β quartz, plagioclase, hornblende, and dark brown biotite. The matrix carries β quartz, plagioclase, hornblende, quartz, and orthoclase. It seems likely that the porphyry was indeed a granodiorite originally, and that it was modified locally and erratically by late magmatic effects.

The productive porphyry is generally seen in the form of dikes or fragments of dikes in the center of the orebody. These dikes have dated at 52.2 ± 2.0 m.y. A more coherent stock of the porphyry, which has been dated at 47.8 ± 1.8 m.y., occurs at depth in the northwest part of the deposit (see Fig. 16.5), and deep drilling here shows a gradual impoverishment in copper values, accompanied by an increase in magnetite and the appearance of pyrrhotite. A downward increase of grain size also has been observed in this drilling.

The earliest change to occur is the replacement of hornblende by biotite flakes, which appear identical in character to the biotite phenocrysts, but which may also crystallize as frilly rings or overgrowths on the larger books themselves. This alteration is surely of late magmatic age. Coarse primary biotite has been deformed by flowage, whereas this new biotite has not. It is probable that, when this biotite alteration was taking place, the wall rocks were undergoing mesozonal metamorphism.

With continued cooling, late magmatic biotite ceased to form and a new assemblage began to crystallize: quartz + orthoclase + magnetite + bornite. Quartz and orthoclase grow in the matrix at the expense of plagioclase and late magmatic biotite. The orthoclase thus formed is clear and generally non-perthitic. At this stage the rock seems quite normal, and one might not suspect any alteration, but the mode is that of quartz monzonite. This metamorphosis probably began as late magmatic but continued into the deuteric stage, for it is often fracture-controlled as well as pervasive. Bornite is seen most often in fractures, with quartz and orthoclase; these veinlets have a distinctly hydrothermal

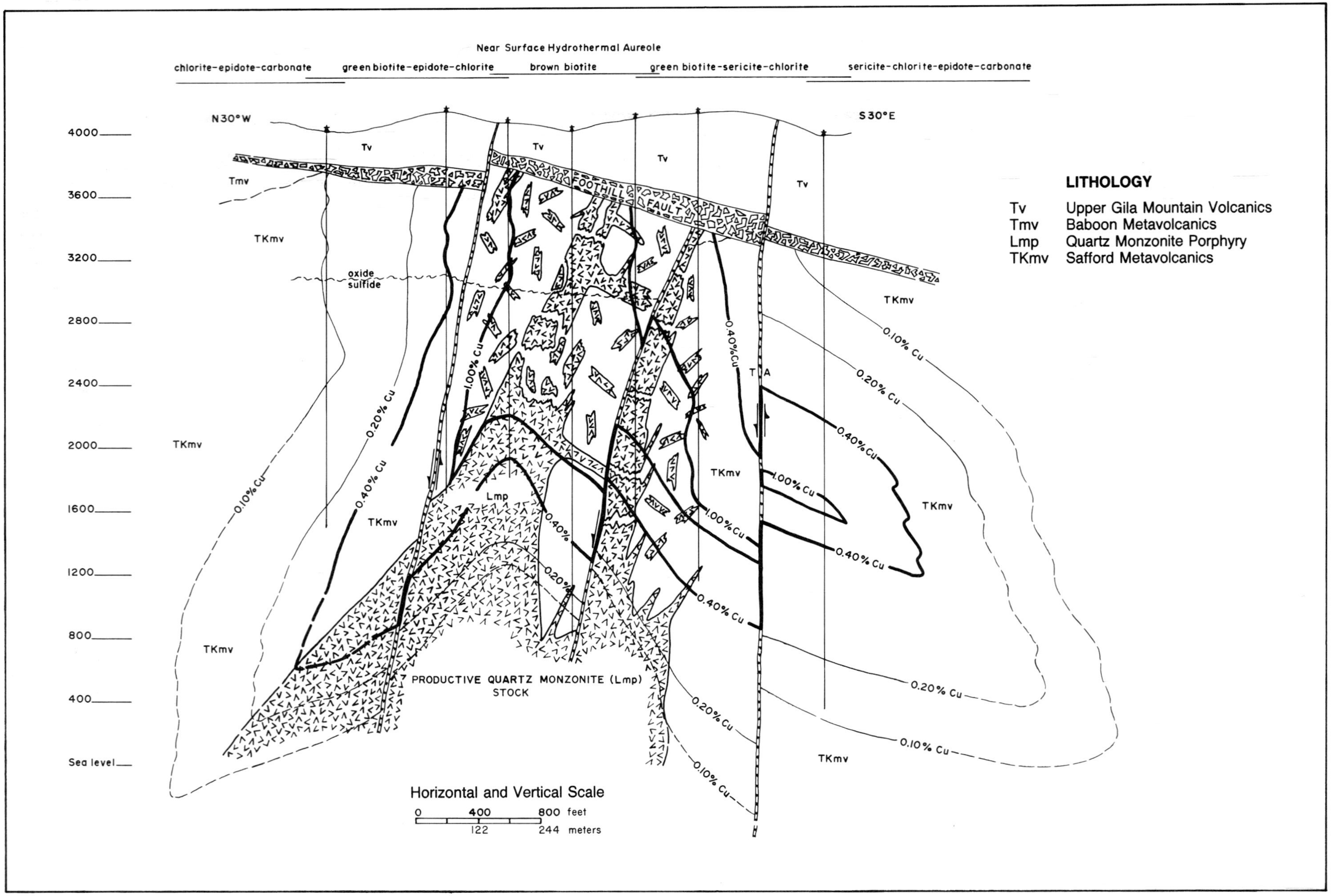

Figure 16.5. Cross section of the Dos Pobres orebody, looking N60°E. Vertical lines descending from the surface mark locations of drill holes.

aspect. This stage of alteration doubtless coincided with the main pulse of mineralization in the wall rocks and with the period of intense K-metasomatism seen in them.

In most places this episode ended, as cooling continued, with simple deuteric alteration. Any biotite surviving, usually the phenocrysts, was partially replaced by coarse clinochlore and blebs of epidote with accessory rutile; the chlorite may be accompanied by minute platelets of hematite. Plagioclase is altered mildly to shreddy sericite and some earthy epidote. Usually only the cores of phenocrysts are so afflicted, and sodic rims remain unchanged. Sulfides remained mobile in veins at this time, with chalcopyrite joining bornite in a gangue of quartz, carbonates, and chlorite. The larger mineralized quartz veins (ca. 1 in.) seen in the mine are closely associated with porphyry dikes and die out away from them. Zeolites may also appear, and some samples have been seen with laumontite attacking plagioclase along the walls of zeolite-sulfide-calcite veins.

In some places, however, the porphyry shows incipient alteration to a quartz-sericite assemblage. This alteration is of deuteric age and occurs in areas where more sulfur was available. While such alteration is seldom complete, the tendency is for groundmass quartz to grow to the point of coalescing, while all remaining feldspars and altered mafites are partially replaced by sericite. Any chlorite that survives is highly magnesian, and even amesite may be present. Pyrite may appear and bornite yields to chalcopyrite. These sulfides occur in quartz veinlets or may be disseminated in sites of former mafites. Alteration of this nature is uncommon and seldom complete, as is typical of low-sulfur porphyry copper systems elsewhere. The best example of such alteration is locally observed on the southeast side of the orebody. It is also in such an alteration assemblage that molybdenum reaches maximum values (0.005–0.015% MoS_2) as shown in Figure 16.6. Molybdenum values are invariably less than 0.005 percent MoS_2 in the core of the orebody.

Chemical analyses for the productive porphyry are presented in Table 16.2. During the series of alteration steps from fresh to deuteric to new biotite, SiO_2 decreases, while Ti, Na, Al, and Fe increase; these changes are due in large measure to the appearance of abundant new biotite. The lack of important changes in K_2O reflects the loss of orthoclase during biotite crystallization and implies no real K-metasomatism within the intrusive. The large amounts of K_2O found introduced in the intrusive walls must have escaped before late magmatic crystallization; otherwise, the intrusive could not have remained so homogenous in this respect. Calcium, on the other hand, is a fugitive of deuteric and late magmatic age and is unique in its strong dependence for mobility on the abundance of species such as CO_3^{-2} and PO_4^{-3}. The low sum of the second column in Table 16.2 reflects the lack of data for CO_2.

Note the relatively similar analyses for the third and fourth columns, with respect to Al, Fe, and K, and the great disparity into Ca values. The elements that show considerable change are those whose mobility is closely tied to the presence of sulfur. Calcium is the best example, for it is quickly removed when sulfur is available; elements such as Si and Al increase only because they are residual, and there is a corresponding decrease in the volume of the original rock. The assemblage quartz-sericite-rutile derives readily from plagioclase-sphene in the presence of sulfur, and the loss of Ca from plagioclase is inevitably the major change.

Alteration of Wall Rocks

The history of events in the andesite pile that hosts the productive porphyries and most of the copper values has been somewhat more complex. The pile exhibits an epizonal metamorphic (alteration) event of almost regional extent that is believed to be the composite effect of two processes. One process was undoubtedly the slow cooling of such a thick, rapidly extruded pile that yielded an autometamorphism or "stewing" in the epizone. We suggest a slowly cooling heat source below as the second cause for the abnormally strong epizonal effects in the volcanic rocks of the district, which are in contrast to those effects in many other thick piles of mafic volcanics. This source of heat must have been the granodiorite or parent pluton of batholithic dimensions (the Lone Star pluton) underlying the district.

As a result of prolonged cooling, the andesites demonstrate an alteration characterized by stability of epidote and pennine. Both minerals may replace mafic minerals completely as coarse-grained epidote prisms embedded in pennine. Epidote singularly replaces plagioclase in part, and the surviving plagioclase is albitic in nature. Excess iron, derived from mafic minerals and accessory magnetite, appears as tiny hematite tablets *in situ.* Although calcite is not abundant, its presence in the volcanics is commonplace, and it may form patchy crystalloblasts in the matrix. In contrast to the dominant andesites in the pile, dacites responded somewhat differently: they were altered to an assemblage of quartz-sericite-calcite-pennine with epidote rare or absent.

The second alteration event, imposed on the volcanics in the aureole around the Dos Pobres deposit, was identical to the first and was due to rising temperatures that resulted from intrusion of the productive magma. Again epidote and pennine formed, often merely as continued development of the same earlier-formed minerals, but with exaggerated growth. Plagioclase may be totally destroyed, and clots or pods of coarse epidote, with interstitial calcite and pennine, spread crystalloblastically and invade the surrounding matrix. It has been observed that any nucleus might have initiated this process, such as a large plagioclase phenocryst or perhaps an especially reactive xenolith or merely a fracture intersection. Some clots do show epidote veinlets leading away in one or two directions. This early zone dies out away from the productive porphyry and merges insensibly into the more regional propylitization of identical mineralogy. Effects cannot be seen with any certainty beyond about 2,000 ft. from the periphery of the orebody.

With continued rising in temperature and final emplacement of the productive magma, mesozonal metamorphism began. The earlier assemblage vanishes and the andesites exhibit abundant secondary actinolitic hornblende and brown biotite, which has been dated at 56.9 ± 2.2 m.y. Both minerals occur as small crystals that vigorously attack both relict plagioclase and hornblende. The new, actinolitic hornblende is not Fe-rich, and disseminated dust-like magnetite

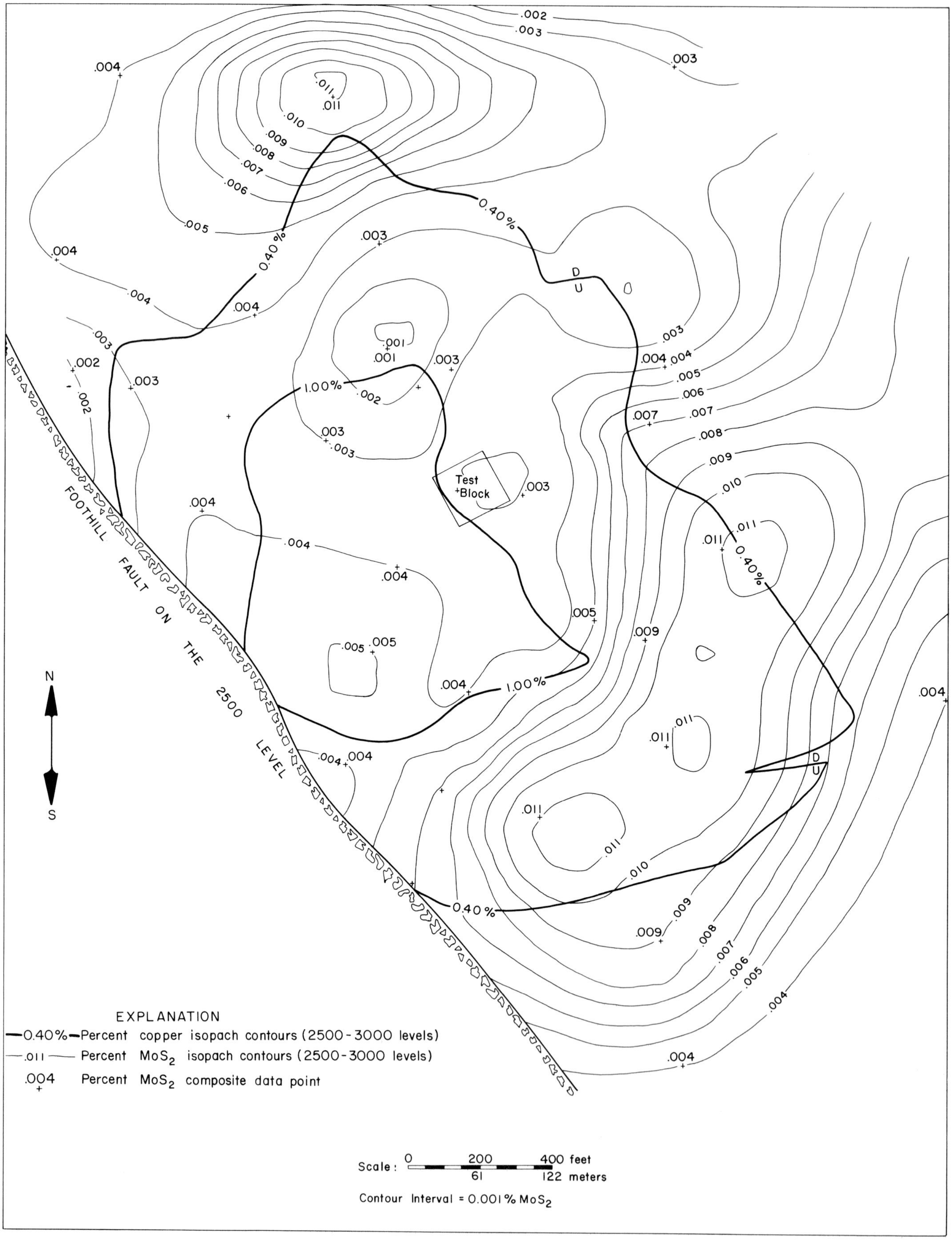

Figure 16.6. Distribution of MoS_2 in the upper lift of the Dos Pobres orebody

TABLE 16.2
Chemical Analysis of Productive Porphyry in the Dos Pobres Orebody

Component	Sample 1 Fresh Porphyry	Sample 2 Deuterically Altered Porphyry	Sample 3 Porphyry With Secondary Biotite	Sample 4 Porphyry Altered to Quartz-Sericite
SiO_2	64.42%	60.95%	56.14%	60.17%
TiO_2	0.50	0.56	0.90	0.66
Al_2O_3	15.69	17.05	18.98	18.94
Fe_2O_3	5.00	5.58	7.79	6.93
CaO	3.54	2.73	4.53	1.46
MgO	0.97	1.05	1.24	1.05
Na_2O	2.56	2.80	3.30	2.44
K_2O	4.04	4.36	3.92	3.82
V_2O_5	0.025	0.020	0.037	0.020
Cl	0.030	0.030	0.041	0.027
Mo	0.016	0.002	0.003	0.008
S	0.41	0.46	0.59	1.94
H_2O^+	2.22	2.23	2.10	2.92
Total	99.421	97.822	99.571	100.38*

NOTE: Analyses performed by A. Dunckhorst of the Phelps Dodge Corporation.

*Values have not been corrected for chlorine identical to oxygen.

is a common accessory in this assemblage. In many samples the disseminated magnetite is concentrated in hazily defined areas suggestive of the outlines of former cognate xenoliths.

Early mesozonal metamorphism was merely a transient stage, for as more K_2O was added during mesozonal conditions, the assemblage yielded to a metasomatic one. The most obvious result of this subtle change was the disappearance of actinolitic hornblende, while ever paler brown biotite continued to crystallize. Ultimately the andesite may consist of some 30 percent by volume of biotite, with tiny crystals scattered evenly in the matrix and more sparingly in phenocrysts. The associated disseminated magnetite is accompanied by bornite, minor chalcopyrite, apatite, rutile, and, occasionally, granular orthoclase. This alteration represents the main pulse of K-metasomatism and mineralization, and, where most intense, it may affect even the productive porphyry dikes. As an end result, these dikes may be so heavily replaced by secondary biotite that they are indistinguishable from the andesites, except for the ghost of biotite phenocrysts. The effect of this strong K-metasomatism is well illustrated by a comparison of Figures 16.7 and 16.8, which suggests enrichment in K_2O and a neutral behavior of SiO_2. Free silica seen in the zone is evidently locally derived from other minerals.

Crackling appears to have been an important mechanism during the mesozonal K-metasomatism, while it was relatively unimportant during the preceding mesozonal metamorphism. The wall rocks were laced with fractures that are now veinlets carrying quartz, orthoclase, apatite, bornite, and chalcopyrite. The bornite: chalcopyrite ratio decreases outward in the mesozonal core; throughout this zone the copper content averages 0.83 percent, while the total content of sulfides is 3 percent by weight. These veinlets probably carry the bulk of the deposit's precious metal content; distribution maps for silver and gold in the Dos Pobres orebody are shown in Figures 16.9 and 16.10, respectively. Both gold and silver show highest values in the central zone of the orebody and both show a relation to bornite distribution. Studies of polished sections reveal minute, smooth, convex blebs of sylvanite and hessite in the bornite. They seem to be centrally located with bornite masses, shunning the bornite that is intimately intergrown with chalcopyrite.

The biotite zone may be seen up to 1,600 ft. from the center of the orebody; then it gradually fades and merges into the surrounding propylitic assemblage. Toward the outer parts of the zone biotite becomes notably paler and assumes a green color. The effect is first shown by biotite formed at the expense of plagioclase, whilst biotite developed in the matrix is still brown; but eventually this, too, assumes a green color.

Chemical analyses of meta-andesites from the core, transition, and outer zones (Table 16.3) reflect a clear loss of CaO in the interior with an enrichment of K_2O. In the zone of 0.2 percent Cu, K_2O averages 2.09 percent; in the range of 0.20 to 0.59 percent Cu, K_2O averages 2.29 percent; and in the 0.6 percent zone, K_2O averages 2.41 percent. These values are for the 1,500-to 1,800–ft. elevations and are relatively higher for K_2O at higher elevations for comparable grades of copper (see Fig. 16.7). As the thermal gradients about the productive stock collapsed, retrograde alteration commenced and another principal stage of metallization evolved. The result of this new mineralization was further enrichment of initial copper values.

In those portions of the wall rocks which show biotitization but which are not fully purged of CaO, epidote reappears in biotite and in remnants of plagioclase. Biotite shows a tendency to alter to clinochlore, in contrast to the more Fe-rich pennines of earlier propylitic assemblages. These effects are only slight to moderate in the biotite zone if the rock mass is devoid of fractures, but the effects are strong in fractures and veins; some of these are clearly reused veins of mesozonal age and others are apparently newly formed at this time.

The veins often carry quartz and important amounts of both chalcopyrite and bornite. Pyrite is rare, but in veins rich in sulfur, it may occur with chalcopyrite. Sericite is apt to form a selvage at the expense of biotite and feldspar remnants. More typically, however, bornite occurs with chalcopyrite, montmorillonite and a myriad of zeolites. Stilbite, laumontite, heulandite, and analcite are most commonly reported. Traces of other minerals have also been observed, and these include barite, fluorite, pumpellyite, and thuringite. It is important to note that these retrograde veins abound in the metasomatic biotite zone but die out, and are rare in or beyond the propylitic zone. As noted previously, however, these veins do extend into the productive porphyry itself, although they are less common there than in its immediate walls.

PETROGENESIS

Considering all available facts from exploratory drill holes and geologic mapping, we propose an orthotectic model for the metavolcanics and an orthomagmatic model for the orebody at Dos Pobres. Although radiometric dates

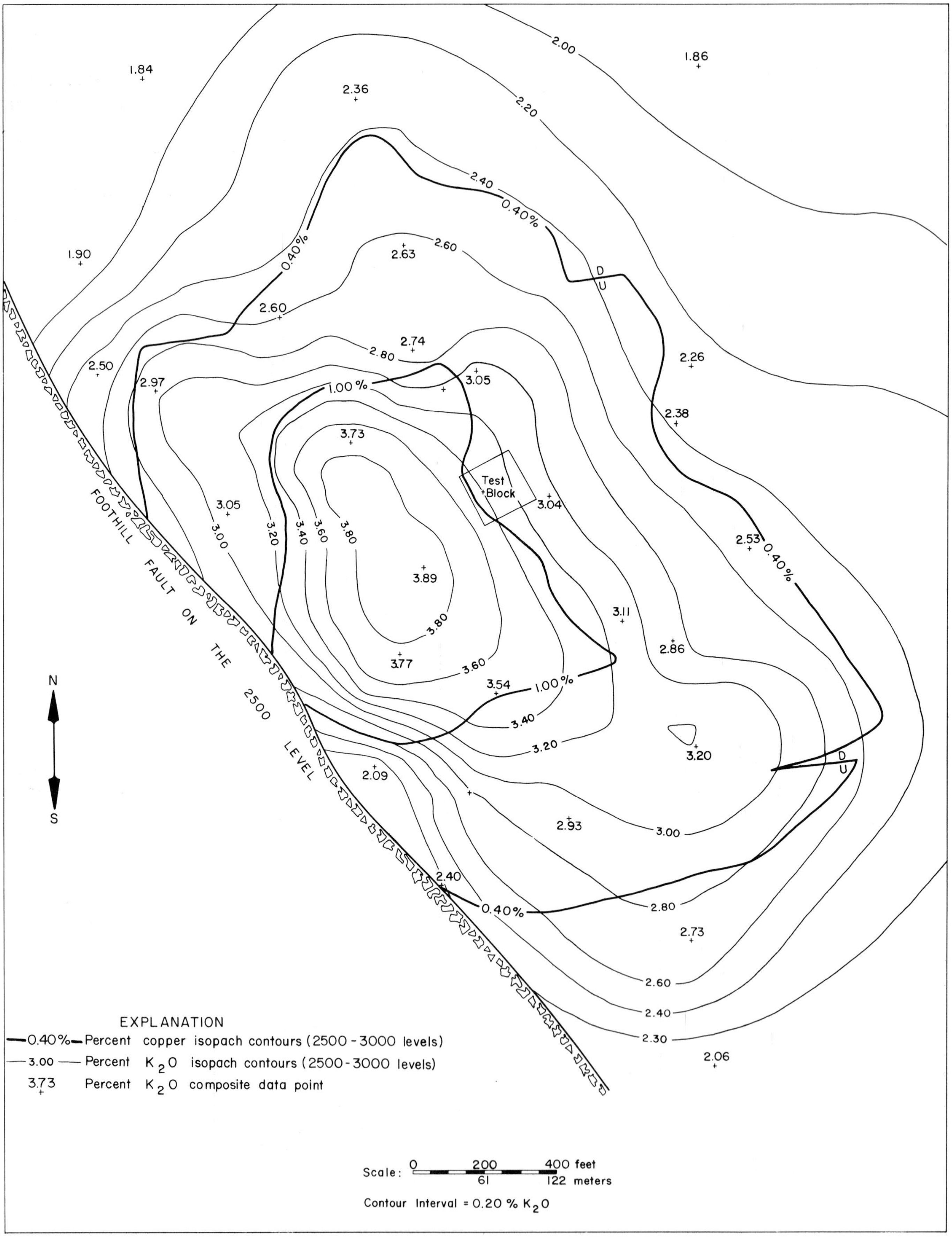

Figure 16.7. Distribution of K_2O in the upper lift of the Dos Pobres orebody

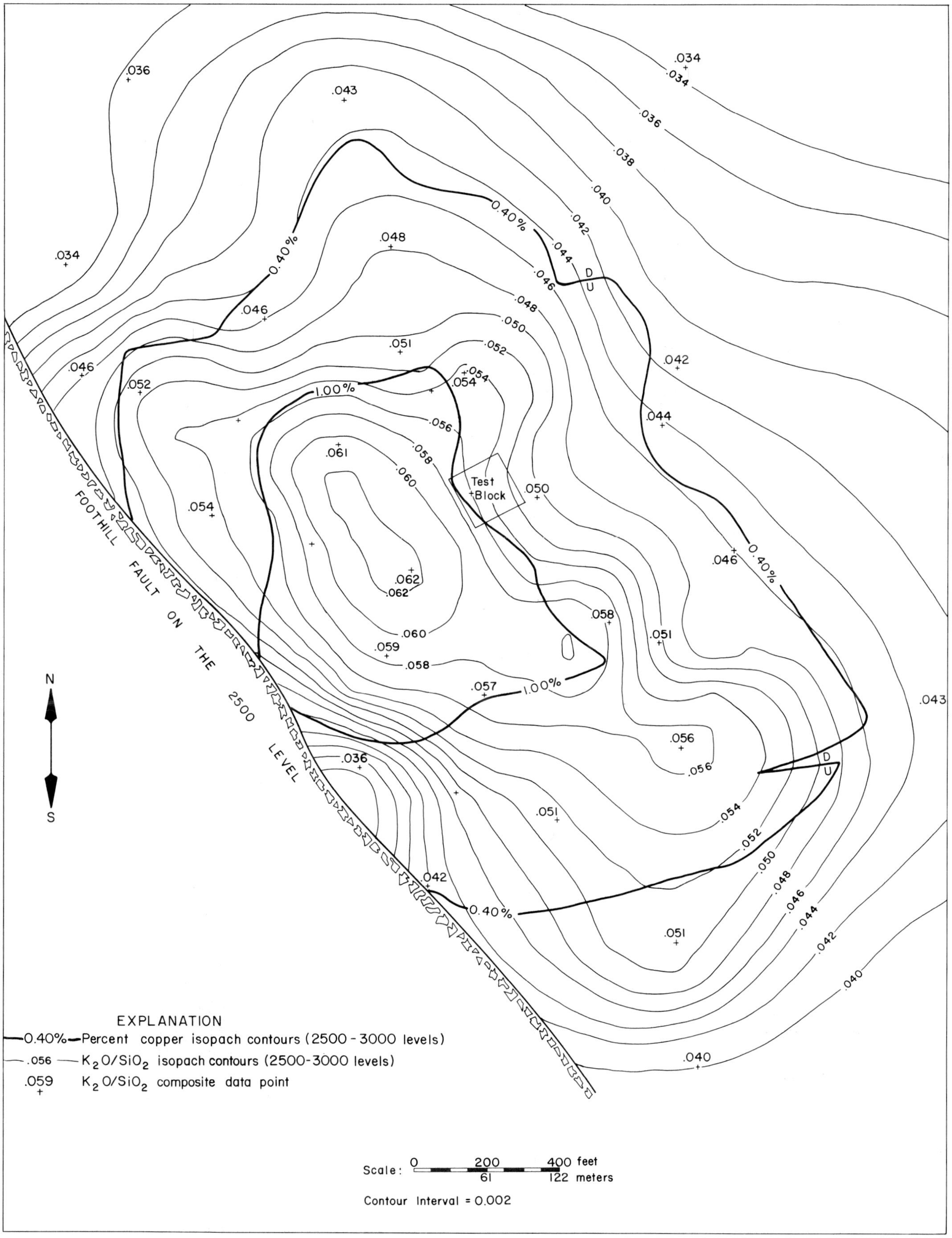

Figure 16.8. Ratios of K_2O to SiO_2 in the upper lift of the Dos Pobres orebody

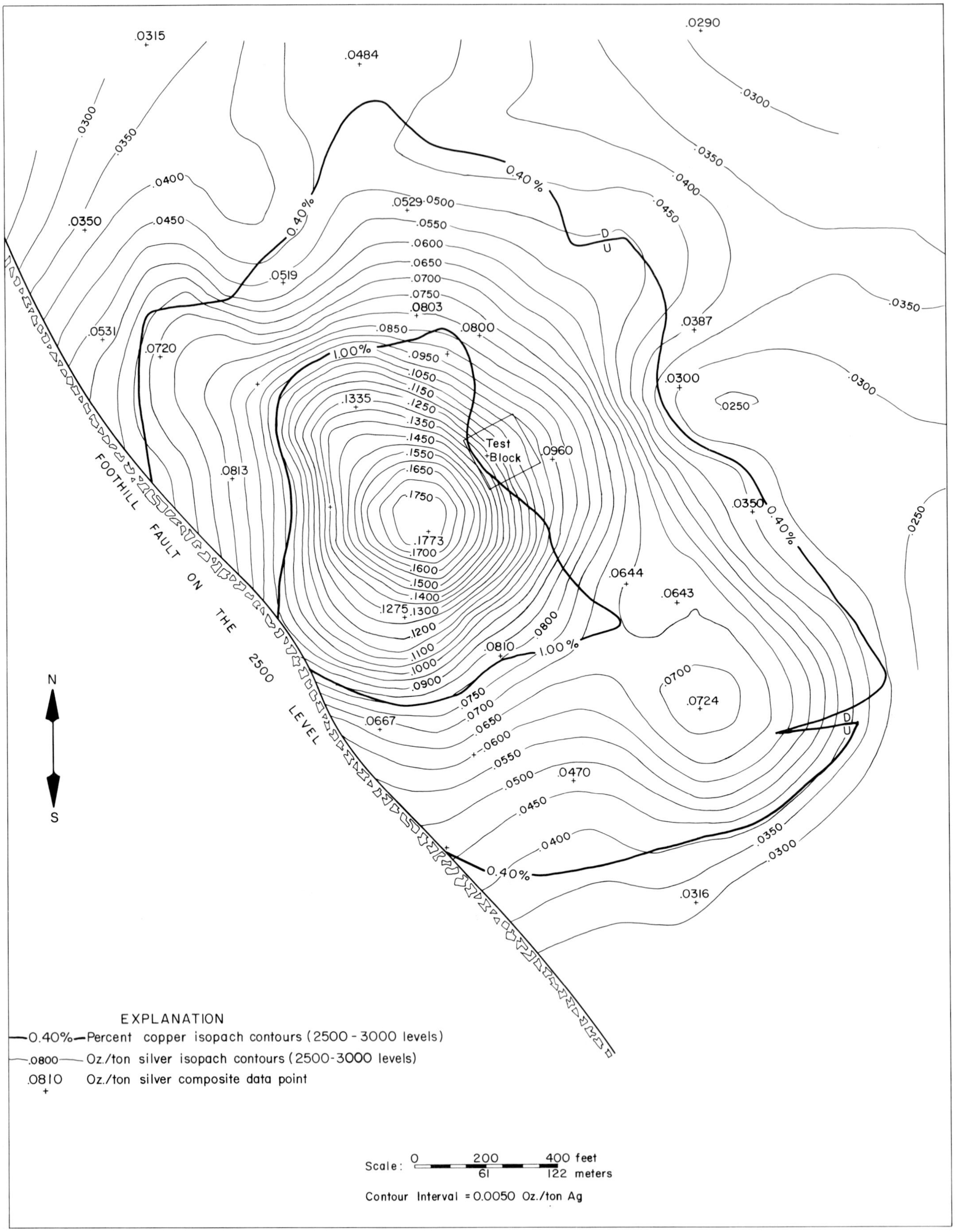

Figure 16.9. Silver distribution in the upper lift of the Dos Pobres orebody

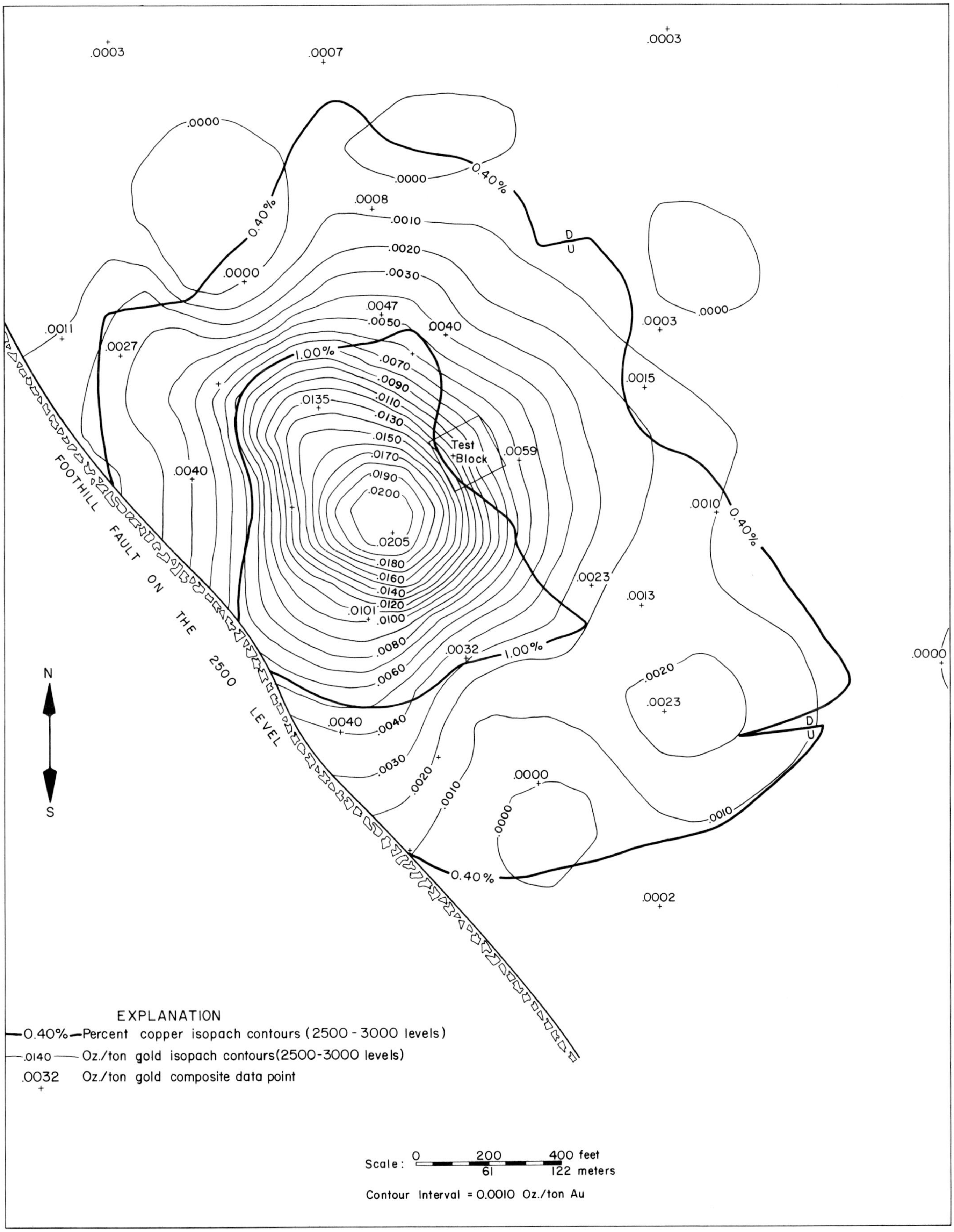

Figure 16.10. Gold distribution in the upper lift of the Dos Pobres orebody

TABLE 16.3
Average Chemical Analysis of Meta-Andesites at the Dos Pobres Orebody

Component	Biotitized Core Zone (+0.60% Cu)	Biotite-Epidote Transition Zone (0.20–0.59% Cu)	Outer Propylitic Aureole Zone (100–2,000 ppm Cu)
SiO_2	55.5%	55.4%	54.0%
Al_2O_3	18.0	20.4	21.3
Fe_2O_3*	4.5	4.9	6.0
CaO	2.66	5.76	7.42
MgO	1.92	3.35	1.45
Na_2O	2.70	3.32	3.46
K_2O	3.07	2.50	2.02

*Total iron reported as Fe_2O_3

are too few to establish firmly the sequence of events, dates that have been obtained and correlated with discernible field relationships provide convincing evidence for establishing a relatively simple geochronology (Table 16.4).

The previously discussed Precambrian xenoliths and the drill-hole intercept of an amphibolite derived from Precambrian(?) sediments furnish the best evidence that Late Cretaceous to Paleocene magma(s) of intermediate composition penetrated the crystalline basement and extruded andesitic lavas on a Precambrian surface. Farther northwest along the Gila Mountain front, however, Middle Tertiary volcanics rest on Paleozoic limestones and occasionally contain rafted blocks of cherty limestone. These phenomena suggest extensive uplift and subsequent erosion which cut through and removed the Paleozoic rocks and exposed the Precambrian basement in the vicinity of the orebody during Mesozoic time.

The parental magma continued rising until it passively intruded its thick andesitic pile and crystallized during Late Cretaceous to Early Paleocene time. The pluton was controlled by north- and northeast-striking shear zones. A broad contact metamorphic aureole that developed around the pluton rendered the Safford volcanic pile into hornfelsic andesites, which vary from an inward amphibolite facies to an outward albite-actinolite-chlorite-epidote facies. Much of the ambiguous, widespread propylitization in the Safford Metavolcanics can be attributed to the quartz diorite–granodiorite pluton or to simple autometamorphism, and it is entirely possible that most of the metavolcanics overlie a single, faulted, tonalitic batholith. An interesting explanation for the

TABLE 16.4
Geochronology of Major Geologic Events in the Lone Star Mining District

Order of Geologic Events	Geologic Age	Dates (m.y.)
1. Uplift, faulting, erosion	Mesozoic	–
2. Intrusion of Lone Star magma(s) into Precambrian metasediments and subsequent contact metamorphism	Upper Cretaceous	69.8* ± 2.7
3. Extrusion of Safford volcanics	Upper Cretaceous–Paleocene	70± – 60±
4. Intrusion of Lone Star magma(s) into Safford volcanics and subsequent contact metamorphism	Upper Cretaceous–Paleocene	69± – 60±
5. Crystallization of Lone Star pluton(s)	Upper Cretaceous–Paleocene	67±* – 60±*
6. Uplift, faulting, northeast-folding, erosion, deposition of volcaniclastic sediments	Paleocene	–
7. Intrusion of productive magma(s)	Paleocene–Eocene	59± – 47±
8. Early pervasive mesozonal contact metamorphism and hydrothermal alteration	Lower Eocene	56.9* ± 2.2
9. Crystallization of productive porphyry dikes	Lower Eocene	52.2* ± 2.0
10. Uplift, faulting, minor folding, continued volcanism	Lower Eocene	–
11. De-gassing and subsequent crystallization of productive rest magma(s) with accompanying hydrothermal phase	Middle Eocene	47.8* ± 1.8
12. Intrusion of hornblende andesite magma(s)	Middle Eocene	47± – 36±
13. Extrusion of Lower Baboon volcanics and pyroclastics	Middle Eocene	47± – 46±
14. Late, prolific retrograde veining	Middle Eocene	46±
15. Extrusion of Upper Baboon agglomerates	Upper Eocene	46± – 36±
16. Hiatus, faulting, minor folding and tilting	Upper Eocene–Lower Oligocene	–
17. Intrusion-extrusion of Gila Mountain Volcanics contemporaneous with development of older pediment	Miocene–Pliocene	–
18. Major Basin and Range gravity faulting, minor tilting, erosion, and oxidation	Miocene–Pliocene	–
19. Basaltic volcanism	Late Pliocene	–
20. Younger pediment, basin fill, and gravel development	Pleistocene–Recent	–

*Specific K-Ar dates, performed by Geochron Labs of Krueger Enterprises, Inc.; all other "dates" are merely inferred from field relations.

proposed stress in the southwest portion of the Morenci-Metcalf district is northeast-southwest dilation resulting from emplacement of this speculated, northwest-trending batholith in the Precambrian basement (Langton, 1973).

Subsequent to crystallization in the upper reaches of the pluton, a drag fold developed in the Safford Metavolcanics along the N60 to 70°W, *en echelon* Red Dyke, Valley, and Foothill faults (see Fig. 16.2). This type of structural pattern, with different orientation, has also been recognized in the vicinity of the North Newman, Bell Copper, South Newman, and Granisle porphyry deposits in British Columbia (Carson and Jambor, 1974). The axial plane of the fold at the Dos Pobres deposit strikes N35 to 40°E, and this secondary structure appears to be the major component for localizing the orebody.

Although the productive tonalite–quartz monzonite–granodiorite porphyry dikes are genetically related to the productive stock and parental pluton, it is doubtful that the productive stocks had an extrusive kindred. Mild folding continued during intrusion and crystallization of the productive dikes and sills, and distribution of the porphyries throughout the Dos Pobres orebody (see Fig. 16.5) provides evidence of this phenomenon. During this time of folding, the first copper protore was formed at Dos Pobres and was evenly disseminated in the porphyries and adjacent meta-andesites. Contemporaneous with, and subsequent to, the final crystallization of the deeper portion of the productive stock, the Baboon volcanics were derived from hornblende andesite magmas that spread over portions of the district and covered the embryonic porphyry copper cell. The consanguinity of the hornblende andesite dikes and sills with the Baboon agglomerates and flow breccias may be easily demonstrated in the field or in drill hole samples. The oldest members of the Baboon flows occasionally contain sub-angular to rounded fragments of the parental pluton, productive porphyries, and biotitized Safford metavolcanics, whereas the upper members contain large xenoliths of the hornblende andesite intrusives.

The first stages of copper mineralization were complete by the time of extrusion of the Baboon volcanics. The additional maturation at the Dos Pobres deposit, culminating in a late period of copper enrichement by virtue of veining, resulted from de-gassing during the middle megabreccia stage. Rejuvenated movement along the east-northeast–west-southwest shear zones apparently facilitated this late mineralization. The Baboon volcanics alone probably sufficed as a relatively impermeable cap that controlled the rate of de-gassing during retrograde alteration and mineralization.

POST-ORE EVENTS

Arguments can be made for tilting and low-angle faulting in the Lone Star mining district, especially at the Dos Pobres deposit. However, any significant tilting that did occur must necessarily have preceded the Miocene extrusive period, as these younger volcanics have an average dip of approximately 12°NE near the orebody. Until further information is obtained, it must be assumed that the Dos Pobres orebody has been tilted between 12 and 25°NE.

Subsequent to tilting, oxidation and erosion were the dominant forces at work during Oligocene and early Miocene times. Also at this time minor supergene enrichment was superimposed on the hypogene ore in the Dos Pobres deposit. The central portion of the Dos Pobres chalcopyrite-bornite ore pipe was partially leached, throughly oxidized, and locally enriched to depths of approximately 1,200 ft. (2,900-ft. level). Sulfides in the periphery of the marginal zone and in the pyritic aureole, however, are often within 300 ft. of the surface on the southeast side of the orebody. Chrysocolla and cuprite are the dominant copper oxides for depths of 1,000 ft. over the center of the sulfide ore, but subordinate amounts of tenorite and brochantite have been recognized. Native copper, chalcocite, and covellite are abundant in the mixed oxide-sulfide zone between the 2,900- and 3,300-ft. elevations. Oxide ore averages 0.62 percent Cu, compared to 0.72 percent for the sulfide ores. Hematite, jarosite, and limonite capping on the southeast side of the orebody also reflects minor chalcocite enrichment in the vicinity of the productive porphyries.

Erosion appears to have been more extensive southeast of the Dos Pobres orebody. The Baboon volcanics are not present 4 miles southeast of the deposit, but they thicken to at least 1,500 ft. northwest of the orebody.

Low-angle faulting has been recognized at the Dos Pobres orebody, but it is most difficult to trace the structures for any distance along strike. This faulting apparently preceded or was contemporaneous with the early stages of Miocene volcanism. As previously mentioned, the significance of these faults is too speculative to pursue in this chapter.

The Oligocene-Pliocene Gila Mountain Volcanics were extruded on an erosional surface that had exposed all of the Laramide intrusives and consanguineous metavolcanics. The source of these volcanics was to the northeast along Bonita Creek, and this arcuate volcanic chain may be mapped in the Peloncillo Mountains as far southeast as Stein's Pass, New Mexico. Contemporaneous with this volcanism, a pediment was forming along the southwest front of the Gila Mountains, and the gravels derived from it thicken rapidly toward the center of the Safford Valley.

Basin and Range block faulting represented the last major tectonic event in the district. The northwest-southeast faults were particularly active, and gravity displacements in excess of 2,000 ft. have been recognized on several of the high-angle structures. Additional adjustments on north-south and northeast-southwest faults also occurred, but apparently they were not of the magnitude of those in the Foothill, Red Dyke, Valley and Butte faults. District tilting of at least 12°NE can be justified during these adjustments. Finally erosion and oxidation of the orebody and development of extensive thicknesses of clay beds, basin fill, terrace gravels, and alluvium during Pliocene and Recent periods established the environment as it now appears.

ACKNOWLEDGMENTS

We are grateful to Phelps Dodge Corporation for permission to publish this research and especially for the opportunity to pursue the study to completion. On a project of such magnitude, numerous people are naturally involved, and we have benefited from prior studies by the following Phelps Dodge geologists: R. W. Ludden, R. E. Geer, and N. J. Theis. Of particular assistance has been the prior work of, and discussion with, R. L. Boatman. During early stages of mapping R. T. Moolick and J. J. Durek were especially helpful, and editorial assistance was obtained from K. C. Bennett and E. M. Schern during preparation of the manuscript.

REFERENCES CITED

Camus, Francisco, 1975, Geology of the El Teniente orebody with emphasis on wall-rock alteration: Econ. Geol., v. 70, p. 1341–1372.

Carson, D. J. T., and Jambor, J. L., 1974, Mineralogy, zonal relationships and economic significance of hydrothermal alteration at porphyry copper deposits, Babine Lake area, British Columbia: Can. Min. and Met. Bulletin, Feb. 1974, 24 p.

Fountain, R. J., 1972, Geological relationships in the Panguna porphyry copper deposit, Bougainville Island, New Guinea: Econ. Geol., v. 67, p. 1049–1064.

Gustafson, L. B., and Hunt, J. P., 1975, The porphyry copper deposit at El Salvador, Chile: Econ. Geol., v. 70, p. 857–912.

Hollister, V. F., 1973, Regional characteristics of porphyry copper deposits of South America: Min. Eng., Aug., p. 51–56.

Langton, J. M., 1973, Ore genesis in the Morenci-Metcalf district: SME Trans., v. 254, p. 247–257.

Robinson, R. F., and Cook, Annan, 1966, The Safford copper district, Lone Star mining district, Graham County, Arizona: in Titley, S. R., and Hicks, C. L., eds., Geology of the Porphyry Copper Deposits, Southwestern North America: Tucson, Univ. Ariz. Press, p. 251–266.

Saegart, W. E., and Lewis, D. E., 1976, Characteristics of Philippine porphyry copper deposits and summary of current production and reserves: SME Preprint, 76-I-79, 47 p.

17

Geology of the Christmas Porphyry Copper Deposit

GILA COUNTY, ARIZONA

Randolph A. Koski and David S. Cook

The Christmas deposit, part of the major porphyry copper province of southeastern Arizona, is located in a steep-sided canyon at the southeast end of the Dripping Spring Mountains in southern Gila County. The closest major porphyry copper deposit is at Ray, approximately 27 km to the northwest. The nearest communities, Winkelman and Hayden, are 8 km to the south, and Globe is 37 km to the north. The mine is accessible by paved secondary road from State Highway 77, which follows the Gila River canyon north of Winkelman. Most of the open-pit mine and support facilities at Christmas are located in the west-central part of the Christmas 7.5-minute quadrangle, but the total area discussed in this study is in the Christmas and Hayden quadrangles (Fig. 17.1).

The colorful, copper-bearing skarns cropping out at the surface in an isolated canyon along the Gila River presented an inviting target for early prospectors. The first mining activity took place in the early 1800s, but territorial land use disputes prevented any substantial development until the enterprising G. B. Chittendon staked the property for the Saddle Mountain Mining Company on Christmas morning, 1902, the day for which the property was named. Underground mining activity by a succession of small and short-lived companies was intermittent during the early 1900s, largely due to unstable economic conditions, low copper prices, lack of sufficient working capital, and geographic isolation. After the depression, production stabilized with the shipment of high-lime fluxing ore to the nearby Asarco smelter at Hayden. Ore mined through 1940 came mainly from replacement beds in the Naco Limestone above the 800-ft. mine level.

During World War II the U.S. Bureau of Mines and the U.S. Geological Survey conducted detailed studies of the skarn orebodies. Deep drilling — below the 800-ft. level — revealed extensive ore horizons in the Escabrosa and Martin limestones. Development of deeper levels, however, did not begin until the property was purchased by the Inspiration Consolidated Copper Company in 1955. Additional exploration by Inspiration confirmed the presence of significant ore reserves at depth, particularly in the rich "O'Carroll bed" at the base of the Martin Limestone. Underground workings were extended to the 1,600-ft. level by 1962. Inspiration began surface mining above the site of the old underground workings in 1965, and shortly afterward underground operations were terminated; by 1981, all production came from an elongate open pit centered on the Naco Limestone-Christmas stock contact.

From the early 1900s through 1966 underground mining of the skarn orebodies at Christmas produced 4.6 million tons of ore yielding 144.5 million pounds of copper. The open pit produced 17.7 million tons of ore and 184.0 million pounds of copper in the period 1966–1979. Small amounts of gold, silver, and selenium were also recovered. In early 1980 production averaged 6,000 tons per day with a stripping ratio of 3.25:1. The open-pit ore, a mixture of 95 percent sedimentary and 5 percent intrusive rock, averaged 0.70 percent Cu. Copper concentrates milled at Christmas were trucked to Inspiration's smelter in Miami, Arizona.

The Inspiration Consolidated Copper Company Annual Report for 1980 listed reserves totalling 701 million pounds of copper, 80 percent of which remained unmined underground. Inspiration also announced (Annual Report, 1974, p. 6) the discovery of a "large low-grade ore body" located "close to the present Christmas open pit mine." The principal host rocks are intrusive and mafic volcanic rocks east of the Christmas-Joker fault system.

The geology, ore deposits, and mining activity of the Ray-Christmas region were first reported by Ransome (1919,

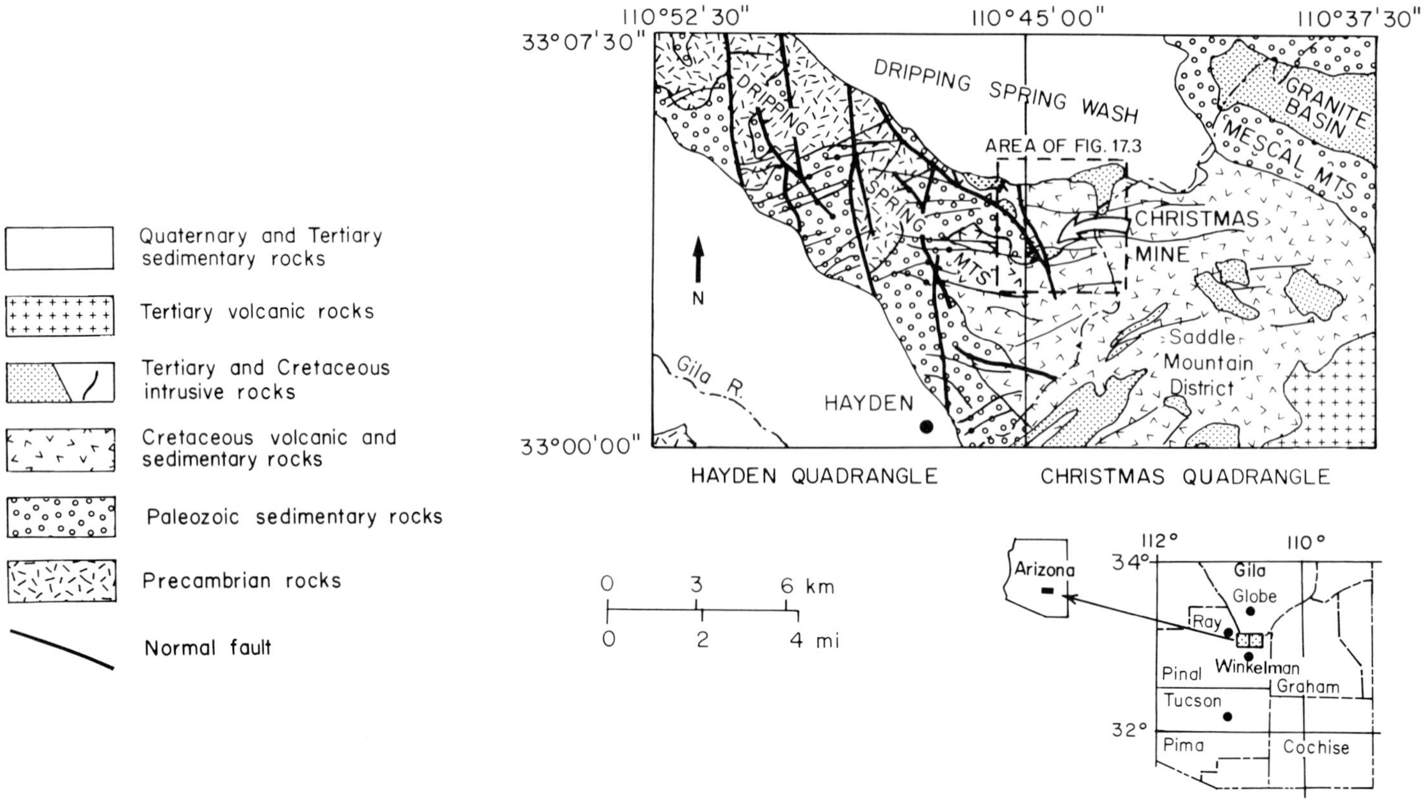

Figure 17.1. Generalized regional geology near Christmas. Geology of the Hayden quadrangle from Banks and Krieger (1977); geology of the Christmas quadrangle from Willden (1964).

1923) and Ross (1925). A mapping program conducted by the U.S. Geological Survey in the Ray-Winkelman-San Manuel area provides a regional geologic framework. Willden (1964) mapped the 15-minute Christmas quadrangle, which includes the Christmas mine and the contiguous Saddle Mountain mining district to the southeast. Near Christmas several 7.5-minute quadrangles have been mapped, including Hayden (Banks and Krieger, 1977), El Capitan (Cornwall and Krieger, 1978), Sonora (Cornwall et al., 1971), Winkelman (Krieger, 1974), and Saddle Mountain (Krieger, 1968). In a detailed field study of the Saddle Mountain mining district, Barrett (1972) established alteration and sulfide mineralization patterns along Laramide dikes intruding Cretaceous volcanic rocks. The Christmas copper deposit has been described in published reports by Peterson and Swanson (1956), Eastlick (1968), and Perry (1969), and in an unpublished thesis by McCurry (1971). These studies have emphasized aspects of mineralization in carbonate wall rocks. Much additional information on the Christmas deposit exists in the form of unpublished maps and reports prepared by the geologic staff of the Inspiration Consolidated Copper Company.

REGIONAL GEOLOGY

The Christmas mine occurs in a zone of topographic transition within the Mountain sub-province of the Basin and Range physiographic province (Ransome, 1923). To the west and north upraised Precambrian and Paleozoic strata form the sharply etched Dripping Spring and Mescal ranges, whereas rolling, subdued topography is characteristic of the terrane developed on overlapping Cretaceous volcanic rocks to the east, south, and southeast. The narrow Gila River canyon is cut perpendicular to the northwest-trending axes of the Dripping Spring and Mescal Mountains and the intervening Dripping Spring Wash. Elevations in the two quadrangles shown in Figure 17.1 range from 1,850 ft. (560 m) at the Gila River to 4,700 ft. (1,430 m) along the crest of the Dripping Spring Mountains.

A composite geologic section for the region is shown diagrammatically in Figure 17.2. Near Christmas only Pennsylvanian and younger rocks are present at the surface; hence, older rocks are treated here briefly. The Precambrian core of the Dripping Spring Mountains and adjacent ranges is composed of the highly deformed Pinal Schist and plutons of batholithic proportions, principally the Ruin Granite. Conglomerate, shale, quartzite, limestone, and basalt flows belonging to the younger Precambrian Apache Group, and the Troy Quartzite unconformably overlie the crystalline basement rocks. Diabase, the youngest rock type of Precambrian age, intrudes all of the previously mentioned rocks, commonly occurring as sills dilating the Apache Group or as tabular masses in the Ruin Granite.

A depositional hiatus of approximately 500 m.y. separates Precambrian rocks from the largely conformable sequence of Paleozoic limestone, dolomite, and sandstone. East of Christmas, Paleozoic rocks are overlain by shallow-water marine sedimentary rocks of the Pinkard Formation. Plant and invertebrate fossils are tentatively assigned an early Late Cretaceous age (Ross, 1925; Hayes, 1970). A diamond drill hole located on the Gila River 1.5 km east of the Christmas

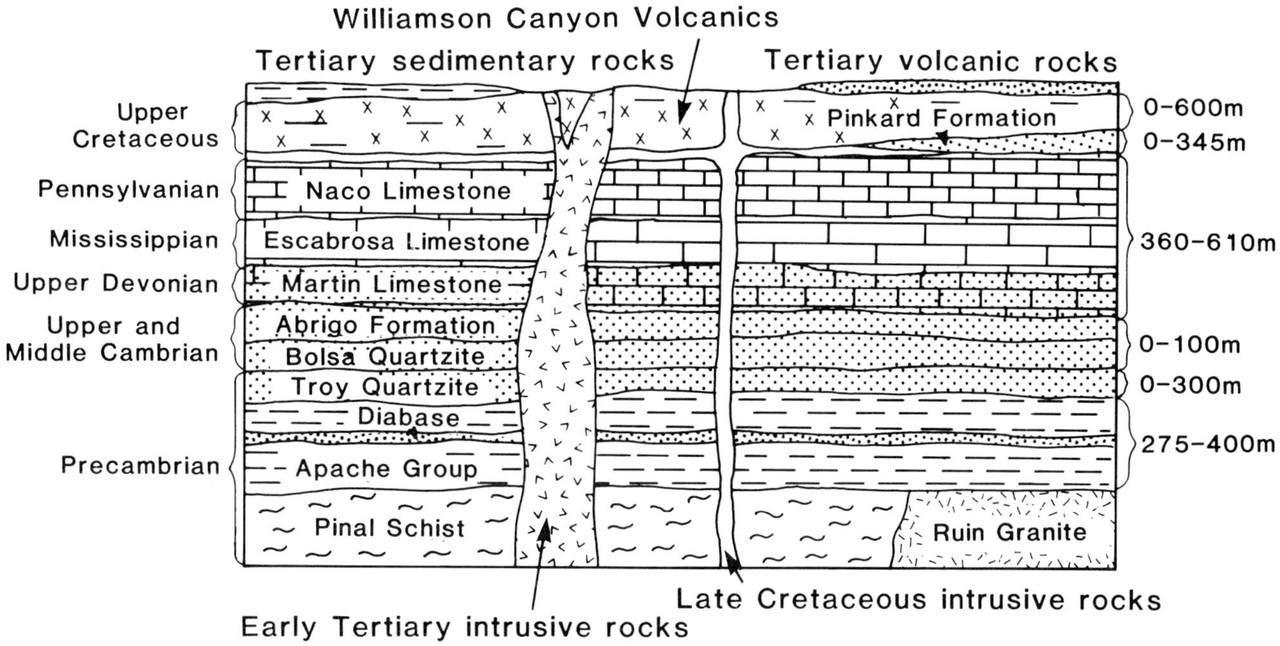

Figure 17.2. Diagrammatic geologic section for the region around Christmas

mine intersected only 12 m of conglomerate above the Naco Limestone, and Pinkard-equivalent sedimentary rocks appear to be absent within, and west of, the Christmas open pit.

The Pinkard Formation or, where the Pinkard is absent, the Naco Limestone is overlain by the Williamson Canyon Volcanics, a thick vent- or cone-complex-facies accumulation of basaltic flows and volcanic breccia with subordinate graywacke and siltstone. Covering approximately 230 km^2, the volcanic sequence ranges in thickness between 750 to 950 m in the Klondyke area (Simons, 1964) and 450 to 600 m where downfaulted at Christmas, but it thins rapidly westward from the Christmas mine. K-Ar ages presented in this report indicate a minimum age for the Williamson Canyon Volcanics of 75 to 80 m.y. before present. This transition from shallow marine sedimentation to subaerial(?) volcanism in Late Cretaceous time is recognized in many areas of southeastern Arizona (Hayes, 1970), and such successions are spatially correlative on a broad regional scale with porphyry copper deposits (Titley, 1972). The post-Laramide rocks shown in Figures 17.1 and 17.2 consist largely of Tertiary basalt-andesite-rhyolite sequences, Miocene and younger basin-filling alluvial and lacustrine deposits, and alluvium deposited along the Gila River drainage.

Precambrian and Paleozoic strata in the Dripping Spring Mountains are folded into a northwest-trending anticline plunging gently to the southeast (Eastlick, 1968; Banks and Krieger, 1977). The Dripping Spring Mountains arch apparently evolved during a period of Laramide compression with maximum stress along an east-west to northeast-southwest axis (Banks and Krieger, 1977; Rehrig and Heidrick, 1972, 1976). Differential uplift and northwest-directed tensional stress resulted in a system of east- to northeast-trending fractures. These extensional structures served as avenues for emplacement of Cretaceous and Paleocene calc-alkaline intrusions, several of which are spatially associated with porphyry-type copper mineralization.

The development of thick Miocene valley-fill deposits indicates a shift from Laramide to basin-and-range tectonics by middle Tertiary time. Although Banks and Krieger (1977) cite evidence for Precambrian, Laramide, and post-Laramide movement along normal range-front faults in the Dripping Spring Mountains, modern basin-and-range physiography in the region reflects, in large part, post–middle Tertiary block faulting.

GEOLOGY OF THE CHRISTMAS MINE AREA

The gently tilted, upper Paleozoic Naco Limestone and the overlying, westward-thinning Williamson Canyon Volcanics of Cretaceous age are intruded by numerous Laramide stocks, sills, and dikes ranging in composition from hornblende andesite porphyry to quartz latite porphyry (Fig. 17.3). The unconformity between limestone and volcanic rocks is occupied in most places by a 5-to-15-m-thick sill of hornblende andesite porphyry. Offsets along high-angle normal faults in the northwest-trending Christmas-Joker fault system combine to downdrop the Williamson Canyon Volcanics nearly 1 km into juxtaposition with the Naco Limestone within the open pit and along the front of the Dripping Spring range, northwest of Christmas (see cross section, Fig. 17.3). Approximately 25 percent of the map area is covered by surficial deposits. Stratified, partly consolidated gravel of Dripping Spring Wash overlies bedrock north of the mine area. On gentle slopes a thin veneer of volcanic rubble thickens toward, and merges with, alluvial deposits in the major drainages. Man-made overburden includes mine dumps, tailings ponds, and road fills.

Naco Limestone

The oldest rock unit exposed at the surface in the mine area, the Naco Limestone, is characterized by thin to medium beds of fossiliferous cherty gray limestone and thin but persistent interbeds of finely laminated calcareous shale and siltstone. Elongate nodules and discontinuous layers of gray, black, and red chert help to define bedding planes where beds are massive. Strata generally strike northeast to east-west and dip 12 to 25° to the southeast or south. Locally, however, minor flexures and drag induced by faulting and small-scale parasitic folding have resulted in steeper dips. Detailed lithologic and paleontologic descriptions of the Naco Limestone in the southern Dripping Spring Mountains can be found in Reid (1966) and Banks and Krieger (1977).

Sections of the Naco Limestone measured by previous workers along the prominent cliffs 1 to 1.5 km northwest of the mine range from 260 to 330 m. Assuming a thickness of 300 m for the highly altered Pennsylvanian limestone in the ore deposit would place the contact between the Naco Limestone and the underlying Escabrosa Limestone at approximately 150 m below the pit bottom in early 1980.

Within the metamorphic aureole adjacent to the Christmas stock, relatively pure limestone beds in the Naco are recrystallized to white marble or converted to andradite exoskarn; shale and siltstone are thermally metamorphosed to diopsidic hornfels. Garnetization of favorable beds extends northwest in the footwall of the Christmas fault for a distance of 750 to 775 m from the Christmas stock.

Individual orebodies in the Naco are typically thin-bedded replacements of limestone, 0.5 to 18 m thick, sandwiched between layers of hornfels and granodioritic sills (Perry, 1969). The principal hypogene sulfide minerals in Naco skarn are chalcopyrite, bornite, pyrite, and sphalerite, with lesser amounts of molybdenite and galena; magnetite is often abundant in garnet-sulfide–rich zones near the intrusive contact. For details of skarn mineralogy and genesis the reader should consult previous publications by Eastlick (1968) and Perry (1969).

Williamson Canyon Volcanics

The Williamson Canyon Volcanics is a monotonous, westward-thinning sequence of dark gray to greenish gray basaltic volcanic breccia and flows and subordinate clastic

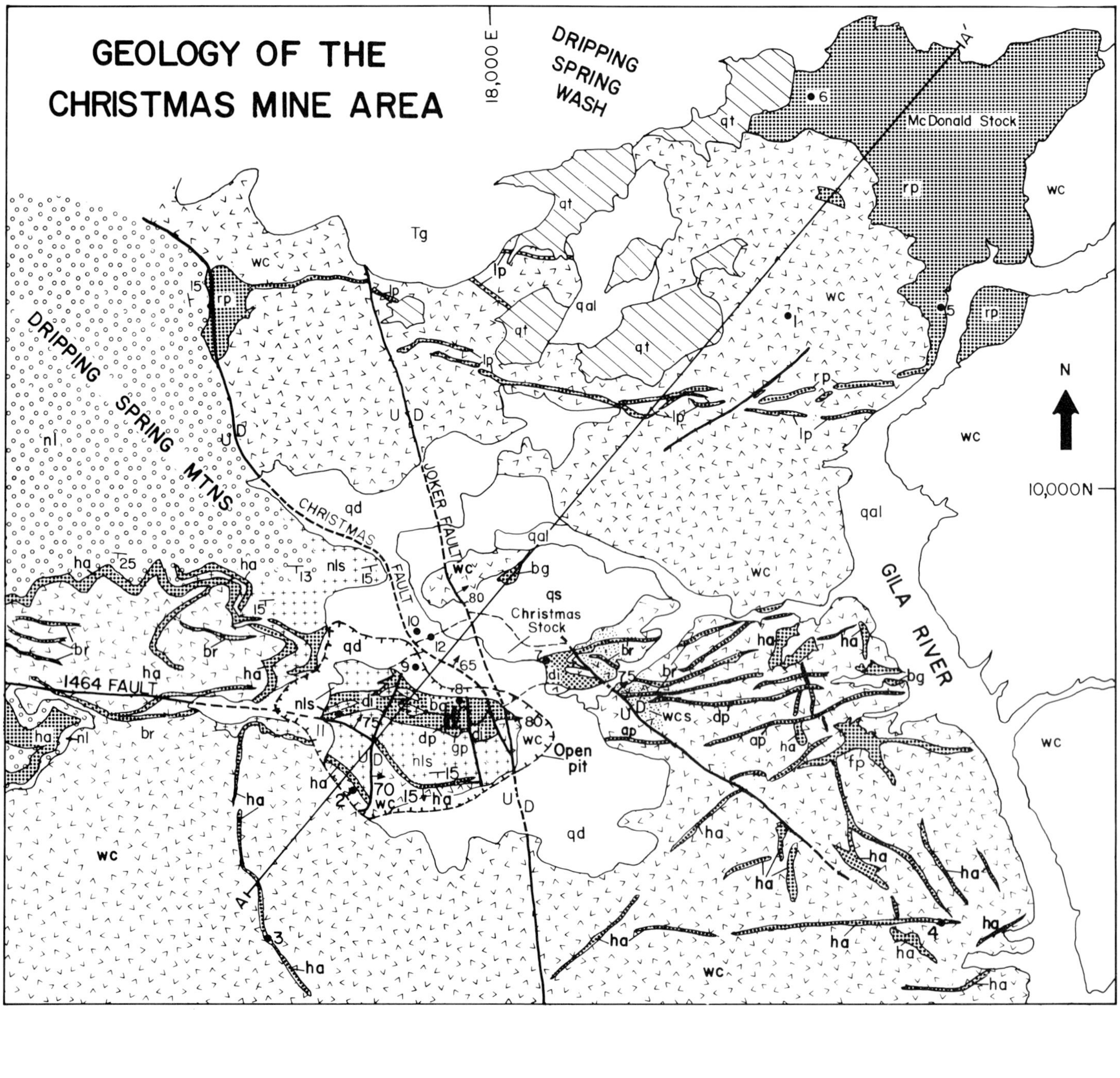

sedimentary rocks. The volcanic pile is 450 to 600 m thick east of the Joker fault and 250 to 350 m thick along the ridge south of the mine, but it wedges out due to erosion 1.5 km west of the Christmas open pit.

Although the details of an internal stratigraphy are obscured by alteration and poor exposure, pyroclastic rocks appear to be more abundant than lava flows in the volcanic section at Christmas. Thoroughly indurated pyroclastic rocks are generally poorly sorted, unstratified lapilli-tuff and tuff-breccia. Sub-angular to sub-rounded blocks and lapilli, mostly of accessory volcanic origin, are enclosed in a crystal-rich tuffaceous matrix. Typically, the fragments have porphyritic or pilotaxitic textures in which 2-mm-long subhedral calcic plagioclase, rounded equant grains and cumulophyric clusters of clinopyroxene (or uralitic amphibole), and granular magnetite are embedded in an intergranular or isotropic brown to black glassy matrix. Fragments with diabasic textures are common. Brown hornblende is a frequent constituent of rock fragments and also occurs as corroded and embayed crystal fragments, occasionally with opacitic rims.

Basalt flows are generally holocrystalline rocks with porphyritic textures. Phenocrysts are well formed and consist largely of rectangular to blocky 1- to 3-mm grains of labradorite and equant grains and glomeroporphyritic aggregates of pale yellow augite set into an intergranular matrix of randomly oriented calcic plagioclase laths (0.1–0.2 mm), interstitial monoclinic pyroxene, and magnetite granules. Plagioclase exhibits normal to oscillatory zoning between core (An_{58-72}) and rim (An_{42-49}). Some samples contain outlines of olivine phenocrysts which have decomposed to aggregates of chlorite-quartz-epidote-sphene or mixtures of epidote, hematite, and smectite. Vesicular horizons suggestive of flow tops or bottoms are not prevalent near Christmas. Locally, however, circular to irregular cavities and gashes are made conspicuous by amygdules of epidote, chlorite, actinolite, calcite, or zeolite (laumontite). Beyond the halo of secondary biotite, the least altered samples of basalt contain weakly saussuritized plagioclase and partially chloritized and epidotized pyroxene.

According to chemical analyses (Table 17.1), the mafic volcanic rocks are quartz-normative, high-alumina ($Al_2O_3 >$ 17 percent), sub-alkaline basalt, with compositions that plot in the calc-alkaline field of an *AFM* diagram (Fig. 17.4*a*) as defined by Irvine and Baragar (1971). The compositions also

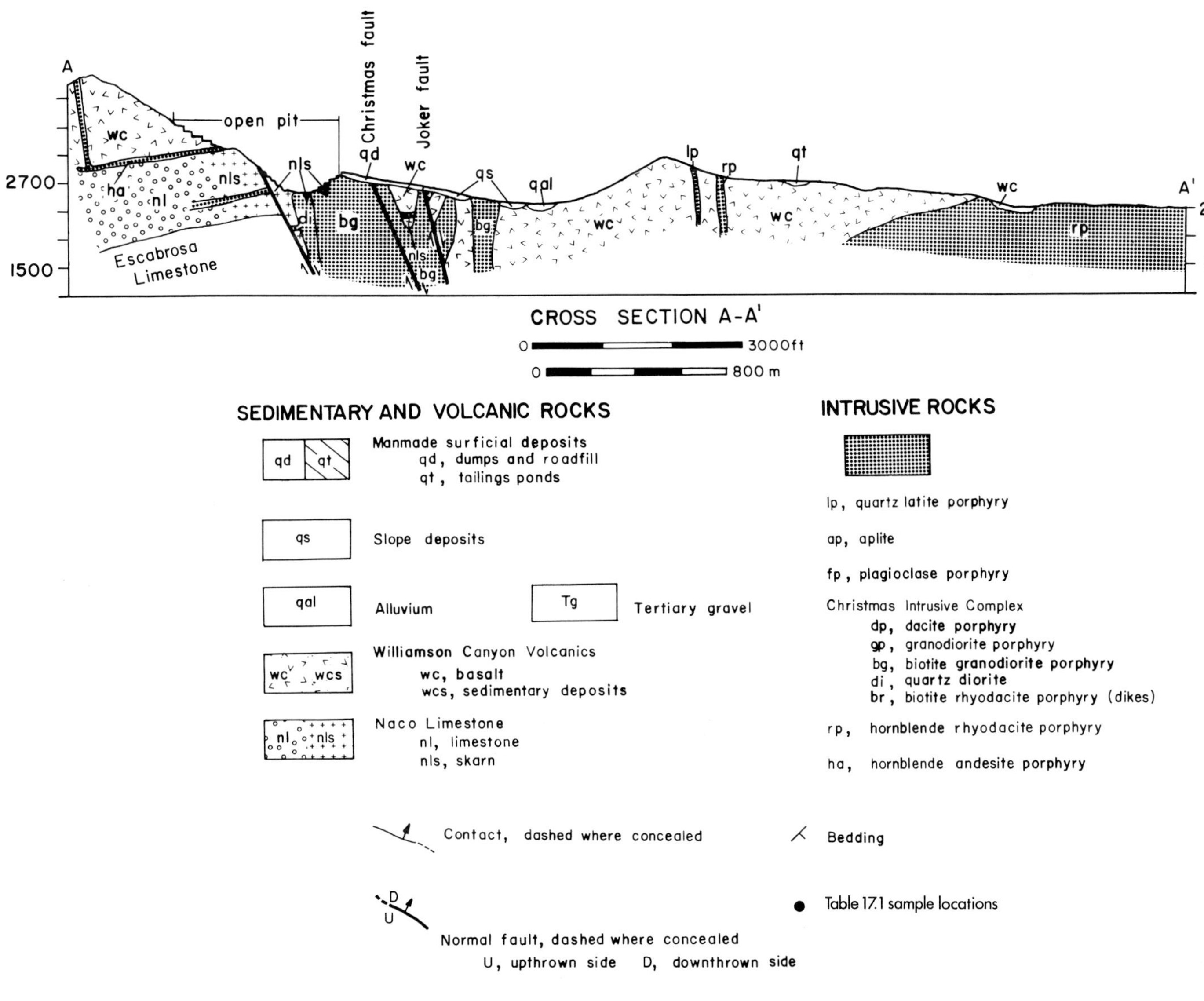

Figure 17.3. Geologic map (*left*) and cross section (*above*) for the Christmas mine area

TABLE 17.1
Chemical Analysis of Selected Rocks at Christmas

	CHEMICAL ANALYSIS (WEIGHT %)											
	Williamson Canyon Volcanics		Hornblende andesite porphyry		Hornblende rhyodacite porphyry		Phases of the Christmas stock			Altered igneous rocks		
*Description number**	1	2	3	4	5	6	7	8	9	10	11	12
Sample number	39AB74	74AB75	54AB75	72AB74	AB64-73A	83AB75	D99-430	AB77-73	D256-148	D237-700	P-30-74	D248-320
Oxides												
SiO_2	49.4	50.8	59.0	56.8	61.9	63.1	63.2	66.5	67.0	64.7	61.9	55.0
Al_2O_3	17.4	16.8	16.7	17.2	15.8	16.0	16.5	15.1	16.3	16.1	16.6	16.8
Fe_2O_3	4.6	4.3	3.7	4.1	2.5	2.5	2.2	2.1	1.3	1.2	4.3	2.4
FeO	5.1	5.4	2.8	2.8	2.0	1.8	2.6	1.9	1.8	2.5	1.6	4.2
MgO	5.8	5.8	2.3	2.4	2.6	2.3	3.6	2.3	2.4	2.1	4.4	6.5
CaO	9.5	10.0	6.5	6.6	4.2	4.0	3.4	3.6	3.5	3.5	.68	4.6
Na_2O	2.2	2.6	4.0	3.8	4.2	4.5	4.1	4.1	4.0	4.0	.26	2.2
K_2O	.90	.89	1.6	2.0	2.4	2.1	2.1	2.1	2.2	2.2	3.3	2.6
H_2O+	2.1	.97	2.0	1.8	2.0	1.6	1.6	.95	1.3	1.4	3.8	3.7
H_2O-	.34	.13	.17	.34	.80	.76	.95	.55	.76	.53	.81	1.7
TiO_2	.95	1.1	.72	.95	.74	.69	.80	.36	.34	.71	.62	.99
P_2O_5	.22	.14	.28	.40	.17	.17	.22	.26	.22	.18	.28	.21
MnO	.10	.12	.11	.10	.06	.06	.04	.00	.00	.05	.00	.07
CO_2	.02	.06	.02	.08	.17	.10	.02	.07	.08	.02	.08	.02
Total	99	99	100	99	100	100	101	101	101	100	99	101
	PARTIAL CIPW NORMS (WEIGHT %)											
Normative minerals												
Q	4.7	3.6	14.2	11.7	16.7	17.9	18.5	23.8	24.2			
OR	5.7	5.5	9.5	12.0	14.4	12.5	12.4	12.4	12.9			
AB	19.8	22.9	33.9	32.5	36.0	38.5	34.6	34.6	33.7			
AN	37.2	32.8	22.9	24.2	17.4	17.4	15.3	15.7	15.4			

NOTE: Chemical analysis made by L. Artis, H. Smith, and F. Brown.

*1 = Flow basalt, 2 = Hornblende-bearing lithic lapilli-tuff, 3 = Fine-grained variety, 4 = Coarse-grained variety, 5 = McDonald stock, 6 = McDonald stock, 7 = Quartz diorite, 8 = Biotite granodiorite porphyry, 9 = Granodiorite, 10 = Biotite granodiorite porphyry, strong secondary biotite, 11 = Quartz diorite, strong quartz-sericite alteration, 12 = Basalt of Williamson Canyon Volcanics, zone of strong biotitization.

plot very near the average value for 141 analyses of circum-Pacific basalts of the calc-alkali series compiled by Hyndman (1972). The basaltic lithology at Christmas contrasts with the section of Williamson Canyon Volcanics described by Simons (1964) in the Klondyke area, which reportedly ranges in composition from hornblende latite to andesite. Neither of these rock types has been recognized at Christmas.

Sedimentary deposits within the Williamson Canyon Volcanics are massive to thinly laminated siltstone, impure feldspathic graywacke, and boulder conglomerate. The restricted vertical and lateral extent and extreme textural variation of these thoroughly indurated epiclastic rocks suggest that they represent shallow basin- and channel-fill deposits interspersed within the volcanic pile. Barrett (1972), however, has described a more widespread continuous sequence of shale, silty sandstone, and conglomerate in the Saddle Mountain district southeast of Christmas. The abundance of quartz, chert, and heterogeneous rock clasts, particularly in coarser sedimentary facies, indicates that much detritus was derived from source areas beyond the limits of the volcanic pile; these sedimentary rocks appear to be only minimally volcaniclastic.

Intrusive Rocks

Sedimentary and volcanic rocks at Christmas are intruded by numerous Laramide-age calc-alkaline dikes, sills, and small stocks. The most prominent of these hypabyssal intrusions, in order of decreasing age, are hornblende andesite porphyry, hornblende rhyodacite porphyry, and the various facies of the granodioritic Christmas intrusive complex. The whole-rock chemical analyses of intrusive rocks listed in Table 17.1 and the triangular variation diagrams shown in Figure 17.4 illustrate a regular and progressive calc-alkaline trend in the southeastern Dripping Spring Mountains. The most differentiated rock phases of the Christmas stock are emplaced along the east-west fracture zone and are spatially related to copper mineralization.

Hornblende Andesite Porphyry. Greenish gray dikes, sills, and irregular pluglike masses of hornblende andesite porphyry are the oldest rocks intruding the Williamson Canyon Volcanics. Hornblende andesite porphyry intrusions become more abundant south and east of the mine, and these bodies are probably equivalent to the swarm of shallow-level andesitic intrusions described in the Saddle Mountain mining district (Willden, 1964; Barrett, 1972). Intrusive rocks of this composition are less common beyond the limits of the volcanic pile west of Christmas.

Several mutually crosscutting textural varieties of hornblende andesite porphyry are recognized. Compositions of the textural variants shown in Table 17.1 suggest a close petrologic affinity. Textures range from strongly porphyritic, with coarse, spindly hornblende phenocrysts up to 2 cm in

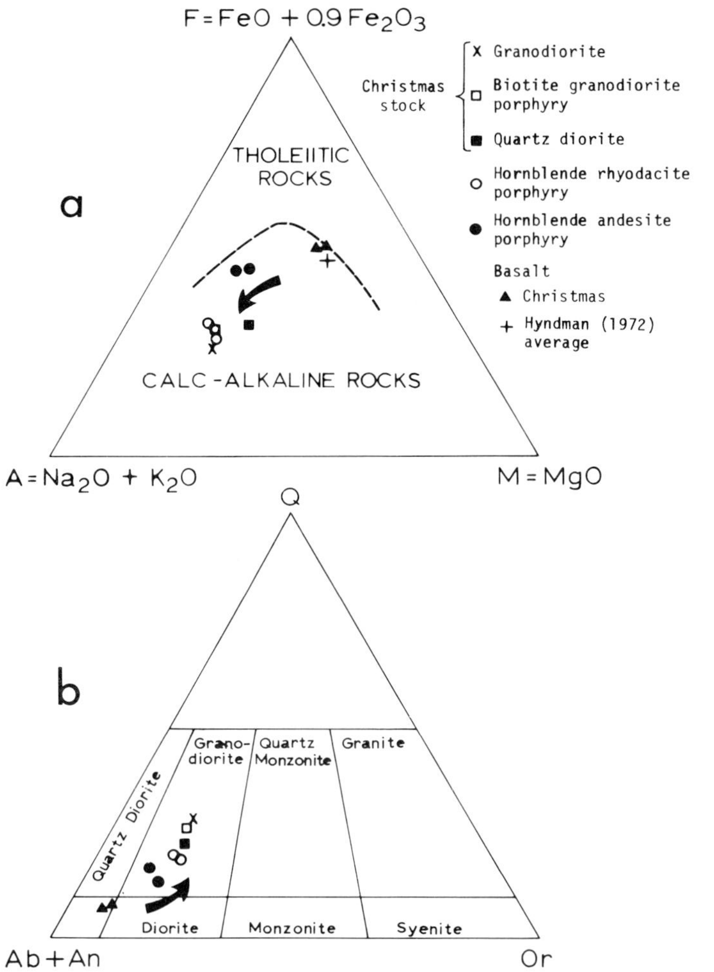

Figure 17.4. Chemical variation diagrams for Christmas igneous rocks: *a*, *AFM* diagram with separation of fields (from Irvine and Baragar, 1971); *b*, normative quartz (*Q*), orthoclase (*Or*), and plagioclase (*Ab* + *An*). Arrows represent trend from older to younger rocks.

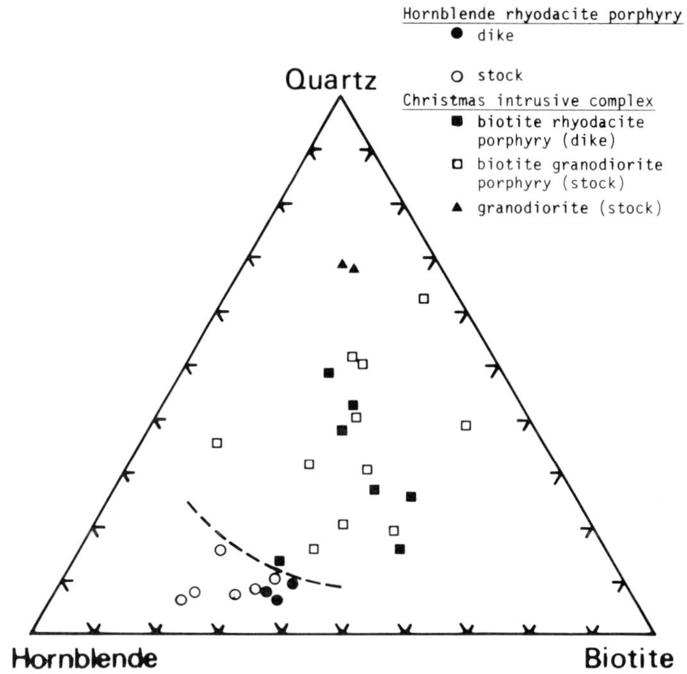

Figure 17.5. Triangular diagram showing relative proportions of quartz, biotite, and hornblende phenocrysts in hornblende rhyodacite porphyry and porphyritic phases of the Christmas intrusive complex. Ratios for the granodiorite phase of the Christmas stock are also included.

length and less conspicuous but more abundant plagioclase (An_{54-62}) in an aphanitic groundmass, to medium-grained, with sub-equant (1–5 mm) plagioclase and hornblende phenocrysts. Magnetite and augite are minor accessory minerals. Groundmasses are felty aggregates of feldspar and interstitial opaque granules.

Andesitic intrusive rocks may represent, at least in part, exhumed feeders for extrusive rocks, perhaps from the upper, more differentiated portion of the Williamson Canyon Volcanics now removed by erosion. The emplacement of hornblende andesite prophyry appears to pre-date copper mineralization at Christmas, and throughout the region.

Hornblende Rhyodacite Porphyry. Hornblende rhyodacite porphyry forms stocks and interconnecting east-west–trending dikes which intrude the Williamson Canyon Volcanics in the northern third of the map area (Fig. 17.3). Diamond-drill and well records indicate that the triangle-shaped stock northeast of Christmas, called the McDonald stock, represents only a portion of a much larger pluton which extends under volcanic and alluvial cover further to the north, east, and southwest. This mass may be directly linked to the petrographically similar laccolith of hornblende rhyodacite porphyry in Granite Basin (see Fig. 17.1) described by Willden (1964).

Whole-rock chemical data (see Table 17.1) reflect the characteristic internal textural and mineralogical homogeneity of hornblende rhyodacite porphyry stocks. Oscillatory-zoned plagioclase (An_{27-44}), prismatic hornblende, and pseudohexagonal books of biotite are the principal phenocrysts; partly resorbed, squarish quartz phenocrysts are sparse and K-feldspar phenocrysts are absent. However, K-feldspar occurs in the aphanitic groundmass with lesser amounts of quartz and plagioclase and small amounts of hornblende and opaque oxides. The phenocryst ratio quartz:hornblende:biotite (Fig. 17.5) shows that hornblende rhyodacite porphyry can be distinguished from megascopically similar porphyritic phases of the Christmas intrusive complex by its greater homogeneity, higher hornblende:biotite ratio, and lower quartz content.

Hornblende rhyodacite porphyry stocks and dikes are massive and appear to be barren of porphyry-type mineralization or alteration. Weak propylitic alteration appears to be the result of pervasive deuteric processes. Rare veins are composed of brown calcite and manganese oxides. Carbonate and volcanic wall rocks along the margins of these intrusions display only minor thermal effects and no evidence of additive metasomatism. According to Willden (1964), the emplacement of the 600-m-thick rhyodacite porphyry laccolith into the Naco Limestone at Granite Basin produced only 16 m of marble.

Christmas Intrusive Complex. The Christmas intrusive complex includes a composite granodioritic stock and peripheral east-west–striking prophyry dikes, all passively emplaced in Paleozoic sedimentary and Cretaceous volcanic rocks. The elongate stock, positioned at the geometric center of the Christmas porphyry copper system, is rather small, measuring 900 m by 450 m at the present level of exposure, and the long horizontal axis trends sub-parallel to the dikes, approximately N80°E. Two northwest-striking normal faults, the Christmas and Joker, bisect the stock, east sides down, with displacements of approximately 400 m and 580 m, respectively. Therefore, rocks in the triangular block between the Christmas and Joker faults and those further east (in the hanging wall) of the Joker fault appear to represent successively higher levels within the stock and within the porphyry copper system.

The stock is best exposed in the open pit and along north-south haulage drifts in the underground workings west (in the footwall) of the Christmas fault. It forms a north-plunging, wedge-shaped mass tapering westward into two dikelike projections separated by a screen of altered country rock. The south contact has an overall steep northward dip of 80°, but it is interrupted by numerous sills and tongues of intrusive rock penetrating the Paleozoic sedimentary section to the south. The north contact between intrusive and sedimentary rocks is more irregular. The northward dip is moderate until it flattens out over a chamber of interconnected sills and dikes approximately 100 m below the present surface. Several large isolated blocks of silicated and mineralized limestone up to 5,400 m^2 in area, and many smaller ones, are engulfed in the western tip of the stock. Relict bedding with xenoliths (even those of relatively small size) is conformable to bedding in the Paleozoic section surrounding the western half of the stock. This feature, along with cleanly truncated, unbrecciated contacts with country rocks, argues strongly for passive emplacement of the Christmas stock by magmatic stoping and, perhaps, partial assimilation.

Although the area northeast of the open pit is covered largely by mine waste and alluvium, drill-hole information indicates that at or near the surface the stock narrows eastward from a maximum width between the Christmas and Joker faults and then flares out into several dikes. A salient of interdigitating intrusive and volcanic rocks extends beneath surficial cover at least 300 m northeast of the central stock. Copper mineralization and the ratio of porphyry:volcanic rock decrease rapidly in drill holes beyond this northeast salient. Occurrences of volcanic rock within the projected surface limits of the stock may represent roof pendants or country-rock partitions between closely spaced dikes.

The Christmas stock can be divided into two groups: (1) early, veined quartz diorite; biotite granodiorite porphyry; and granodiorite; and (2) late, unveined granidiorite porphyry and dacite porphyry. Biotite rhyodacite porphyry dikes extending east and west from the Christmas stock are probably coeval with biotite granodiorite porphyry. Chemical analyses (see Table 17.1) and chemical parameters (see Fig. 17.4) show that phases of the Christmas stock are the most silicic and alkalic members of the suite of calc-alkaline igneous rocks at Christmas.

Seriate-porphyritic quartz diorite forms a discrete phase, 45 to 90 m wide, along the south margin of the stock and is intersected in several drill holes along the projected northern contact with volcanic wall rocks. It apparently forms the bulk of the eastern end of the stock, but the dimensions and distribution of quartz diorite east of the Christmas fault are not well known.

Least-altered samples of quartz diorite consist of blocky plagioclase phenocrysts (up to 1 cm), oscillatory-zoned over the narrow range An_{38-41}; and sparse, corroded biotite books set into an anhedral-granular aggregate of hornblende, plagioclase, quartz, and biotite. Quartz is largely interstitial to the other minerals. The medium to dark gray color of quartz diorite reflects the presence of pervasive, ragged secondary biotite, which is pseudomorphing hornblende and, to a lesser degree, replacing primary book biotite.

Light gray biotite granodiorite porphyry forms the thoroughly veined core facies of the composite stock, and also crops out as several small irregular pluglike masses 1 to 1.5 km east of the mine. This phase is closely related to, but slightly later than, quartz diorite; biotite granodiorite porphyry dikes penetrate quartz diorite with sharp contacts, but without chilled margins. The main contact between quartz diorite and biotite granodiorite porphyry is locally broken and irregular, due to minor offset along numerous north-south faults, interfingering of the two phases, or truncation by still younger intrusive phases. The porphyry core itself is heterogeneous, with many internal contacts between what appear to be individual units or pulses of biotite granodiorite porphyry magma. The internal contacts are difficult to trace for more than a few meters, but they are locally inhabited by quartz-rich veins. Veins are also terminated at these contacts.

Biotite granodiorite porphyry is distinctly porphyritic, with prominent subhedral 0.5- to 10-mm phenocrysts of plagioclase constituting approximately 40 percent of the rock, and coarse, barrel-shaped biotite books, 5 percent. Plagioclase phenocrysts exhibit normal-oscillatory zoning between An_{44-46} at the cores and An_{33-36} near the rims; the average composition is sodic andesine. Less conspicuous are: prismatic hornblende (4%); rounded, occasionally dipyramidal quartz (4%); and disseminated metallic grains—mostly magnetite-ilmenite and chalcopyrite—(1%). In contrast to the nearly complete biotitization of amphibole in quartz diorite, hornblende in biotite granodiorite porphyry is generally partially or totally preserved.

Phenocryst margins are typically scalloped, probably by late reaction with the enclosing melt, which crystallized to form an aplitic groundmass averaging 40 percent quartz, 28 percent plagioclase, 26 percent K-feldspar, and 6 percent biotite. Compositional heterogeneity within the porphyry core is demonstrated by the spread in the phenocryst ratios (see Fig. 17.5).

Granodiorite is distinguished from biotite granodiorite porphyry by its coarser-grained, hypidiomorphic-granular texture; by more abundant quartz and interstitial K-feldspar; and by the paucity of secondary biotite. A representative modal analysis is: plagioclase (53%), K-feldspar (9%), biotite (6%), hornblende (5%), quartz (24%). Accessory minerals are magnetite, apatite, sphene, and occasionally anhydrite. Although not present at the surface, granitoid-textured rock is exposed underground at the 1,600-ft. level near the Number 6 shaft (300 m below minimum pit elevation), and has been intersected in a drill hole in the north-central part of the pit less than 50 m below the surface. No sharp contacts with other intrusive phases have been observed, and coarse-grained, granitoid-textured rocks have not been noted in upper levels of the intrusive complex east of the Christmas fault.

The granodiorite is relatively free of sulfide mineralization, but it is cut by veins of pink K-feldspar and, therefore, appears to have been emplaced before cessation of mainstage, K-silicate, hydrothermal alteration.

Several east- to northeast-trending biotite rhyodacite porphyry dikes extend latitudinally from the Christmas stock. On a regional scale this dike swarm follows the prominent east-west fracture zone across the Dripping Spring Mountains and is related to copper mineralization at the New Year and Chilito mines, 2.5 km and 4 km west of Christmas, respectively (Banks and Krieger, 1977). At Christmas the dikes cannot be traced directly into the central stock, but textural and mineralogical characteristics imply a close genetic relation with biotite granodiorite porphyry. Eastward from the Christmas stock, the dikes show a progressive change from quartz-sericite to propylitic alteration.

The phenocryst content of the dike interiors constitutes 45 to 50 percent of the rock volume and consists of plagioclase, biotite, hornblende, and quartz in roughly the same proportions as biotite granodiorite porphyry in the stock (see Fig. 17.5). Chilling along dike margins diminishes the biotite:hornblende ratio, the quartz content, and the phenocryst:groundmass ratio. In contrast to the simple mosaic groundmass texture of porphyry in the stock, biotite rhyodacite porphyry groundmasses are turbid, fine-grained (0.02–0.05 mm) aggregates of interlocking quartz, feldspar, and chlorite. K-feldspar may constitute up to 50 percent of the total groundmass, producing a strong yellow color in slabs stained with sodium cobaltinitrite.

New exposures in the open pit reveal small unveined bodies of gray to grayish green granodiorite porphyry and dacite porphyry intruding quartz diorite and biotite granodiorite porphyry along the south margin of the stock. K-silicate veins in the latter phases are truncated by the younger porphyries. Where the phases are in contact, granodiorite porphyry shows minor chilling effects and is thought to be the younger rock. East-trending dikes of dacite porphyry also intrude the volcanic pile and crosscut hornblende andesite porphyry dikes east of the Christmas stock.

The younger porphyries are characterized by propylitic alteration and weak, disseminated chalcopyrite-bornite mineralization. Mafic minerals in both phases are typically pseudomorphed by compact, tufted masses of chlorite with lesser amounts of epidote, sphene, and calcite. Plagioclase is partially altered to sericite. The young phases post-date vein-related K-silicate (Stage I) alteration, but their age relative to quartz-sericite (Stage II) alteration and pyritization is unknown.

Minor intrusive rocks. Other Laramide-age intrusive rocks in the mine area include discontinuous dikes of quartz latite porphyry, an irregular plug of plagioclase porphyry, and a prominent 3- to 5-m, east-northeast–trending aplite dike.

Narrow, 0.5- to 1-m dikes of andesite and basalt porphyry represent the youngest igneous activity at Christmas. These dikes strike northwest to northeast and intrude, in part, along steeply dipping fault planes which offset the contact between the Christmas stock and sedimentary rocks.

Breccia

Intrusion Breccia. A steep-walled, pipelike body (30 by 20 m in plan) of poorly sorted, heterogeneous breccia is emplaced between granodiorite porphyry and quartz diorite near the southern edge of the stock in the central pit area. Closely packed, angular fragments up to 10 cm in diameter include quartzite, marble, garnetized limestone, hornfels, and porphyry containing K-feldspar in veinlets. Mineralization is confined to calc-silicate fragments. The matrix material, generally less than 50 percent of the rock, appears to be an igneous porphyry, modified locally by protoclastic deformation.

This fragmental unit appears to be a post-mineral pipe of intrusion breccia consisting largely of the remnants of a shattered block of altered limestone which was engulfed in, and carried upward by, a late surge of magma. This late batch of magma may have been guided by fractures or fault zones, or by intersections of such structures. The body does not appear to represent a mineralized breccia pipe.

Breccia Dikes. Narrow (0.1–2 m), discontinuous, dike-like bodies charged with heterogeneous, rounded to subangular, fragmental debris are termed breccia dikes. Dike segments, 20 to 50 m in length, generally have strikes within a few degrees of east-west and occur most frequently in Cretaceous volcanic rocks between the Christmas intrusive complex and the hornblende rhyodacite porphyry stocks and dikes 1 km to the north. The poorly sorted fragment load commonly includes abrasion-resistant and inert materials, such as quartzite, sandstone, chert, and Precambrian granite, and lesser amounts of diabase, hornblende andesite porphyry, limestone, and calc-silicate hornfels(?). Larger fragments fit tightly within a clastic matrix consisting of abundant angular quartz chips and sparse biotite, feldspar, and sphene grains (0.1 to 0.5 mm across); these fragments are, in turn, enclosed by fine rock dust.

The fine fraction—plagioclase feldspar grains—and some rock fragments are partially to totally replaced by fine-grained epidote or an aggregate of epidote and quartz. A few dikes contain pyrite. Breccia dikes have not been noted in the Christmas stock, and their time of emplacement into volcanic rocks is enigmatic. However, their general occurrence along east-west trends, the fragment load, and the presence of pyrite suggest that their emplacement occurred after emplacement of hornblende andesite porphyry and before cessation of mineralization in the district.

GEOCHRONOLOGY

Eight new K-Ar age determinations for igneous rocks at Christmas and another borrowed from the literature (Creasey and Kistler, 1962) are shown in Table 17.2 and presented graphically in Figure 17.6. Complete sample descriptions and analytical data for Christmas K-Ar ages are

TABLE 17.2
K-Ar Age Dates From the Christmas Mine Area.

Sample Number	Rock Type/Material Dated	Apparent* Age (m.y.)
74AB75	Lithic lapilli tuff from Williamson Canyon Volcanics/hornblende	76.2 ±2.6
54AB75	Hornblende andesite porphyry (fine-grained variety)/hornblende	81.7 ±1.8
72AB74	Hornblende andesite porphyry (coarse-grained variety)/hornblende	76.2 ±1.3
GB–1	Hornblende rhyodacite porphyry (Granite Basin pluton)/hornblende	72.3 ±1.6
83AB75	Hornblende rhyodacite porphyry (McDonald stock)/hornblende	69.8 ±0.9
CS-1-75	K-silicate vein in biotite granodiorite porphyry/biotite (chloritized)	62.8 ±1.1
D148-337	K-silicate vein in biotite granodiorite porphyry/sericite	62.5 ±1.0
AB49-73	Basalt porphyry/whole rock	25.5 ±0.2
KA9†	Biotite granodiorite porphyry/biotite	62

NOTE: Potassium analyses by S. Neil and J. Christie; argon analyses and age calculations by E. H. McKee.

* The ± value is the estimated analytical uncertainty at 1 standard deviation.

† Data from Creasey and Kistler (1962); error estimated at ±4 percent.

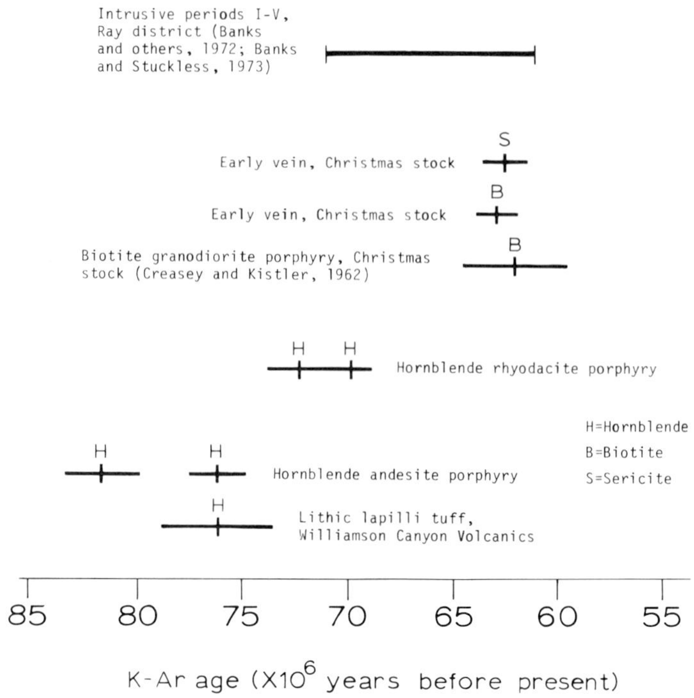

Figure 17.6. K-Ar ages of hornblende, biotite, and sericite from igneous rocks and veins at Christmas. Also included is the period of intrusive activity at Ray. Horizontal bars represent analytical uncertainty.

given in Koski (1978). Also included in Figure 17.6 is the period of intrusive activity in the nearby Ray district taken from K-Ar and fission-track studies by Banks and others (1972) and Banks and Stuckless (1973), respectively. The combined data show that calc-alkaline magmatism in the Dripping Spring Mountains evolved over an extended period from within the Late Cretaceous (~ 75–80 m.y. ago) into the early Tertiary (~ 60 m.y. ago). The sequence of igneous rocks is progressively more silicic, from basalt to diorite-andesite to granodiorite-rhyodacite. Ore deposits were formed at Christmas (~ 63–61 m.y. ago) and at Ray (~ 61–60 m.y. ago) as magmatic activity waned in early Paleocene time.

The single K-Ar age for hornblende from volcanic breccia of the Williamson Canyon Volcanics conflicts with ages for crosscutting hornblende andesite porphyry dikes. Hornblende separated from lapilli tuff occurs as a constituent of accessory rock fragments and as single crystal shards. Crystal margins are rounded and embayed. The rock sample was collected within the hydrothermal aureole of the Christmas stock and thus contains a small amount of fine-grained secondary biotite. Some argon loss may have occurred during a thermal event, possibly the volcanic episode itself or later emplacement of the Christmas stock and circulation of hydrothermal fluids; such a loss would have reset the potassium-argon "clock." Furthermore, S. B. Keith (1976, personal communication) reports that K-Ar age determinations on hornblende from three andesite porphyry-type dikes from nearby Saddle Mountain mining district yielded an average age of 81 m.y. Thus, Keith's results and those of this study show that five hornblende ages from andesite porphyry intruding the Williamson Canyon Volcanics exceed 76 m.y. and four exceed 79 m.y. If the age of hornblende from volcanic breccia is anomalous, the eruption of Williamson Canyon Volcanics and emplacement of some hornblende andesite porphyry dikes occurred prior to 75 to 80 m.y. before present. This period is temporally consistent with early stages of Laramide tectogenesis in southwestern North America, which is thought to have begun approximately 80 m.y. ago (Coney, 1972, 1976).

The K-Ar ages of hornblende from hornblende rhyodacite porphyry plutons near Christmas (69.8, 72.3 m.y.) correlate closely with dates for pre-ore Tortilla Quartz Diorite and Rattler Granodiorite (70 ±1 m.y.) of Intrusive Period I in the Ray district (Banks and Stuckless, 1973). East-west–trending dikes of hornblende rhyodacite porphyry north of the Christmas mine and equivalent dikes with trends N65–70°E in the Hayden quadrangle (Banks and Krieger, 1977) suggest that extension fractures generated by weak, northeast-directed compression may have developed in the Dripping Spring Mountains by approximately 70 m.y. ago (Banks and Krieger, 1977; Rehrig and Heidrick, 1972, 1976).

Two K-Ar ages for vein minerals and a biotite age for their biotite granodiorite porphyry host in the Christmas stock (from Creasey and Kistler, 1962) support the viewpoint derived from field and petrographic observations that emplacement of biotite granodiorite porphyry and early hydrothermal alteration-mineralization are essentially synchronous events. However, the minerals dated—a chloritic biotite and coarse sericite—are not common constituents of early (Stage I) K-silicate vein alteration. No time-limiting brackets can yet be placed on the total episode of intrusion and ore deposition at Christmas. These early Paleocene ages are concordant with the age of the Granite Mountain Porphyry (Intrusive Period III) and the apparent age of the Ray deposit (61–60 m.y.) reported by Banks and others (1972) and Banks and Stuckless (1973).

Laramide age dates for igneous rocks from the Dripping Spring Mountains younger than approximately 60 m.y. were not yet established in 1980. One of several basalt dikes emplaced along a set of northeast- to northwest-trending fractures in the Christmas open pit yielded a whole-rock K-Ar age of ~ 25.5 m.y., which is near the Oligocene-Miocene boundary (see Table 17.2). The pattern of the host structures is diagnostic of late Tertiary Basin and Range tectonism in Arizona (Rehrig and Heidrick, 1976). The 25.5-m.y. date is characteristic of the mid-Tertiary magmatic pulse in Arizona (Damon and Mauger, 1966).

PRE-MINERALIZATION ALTERATION: ACTINOLITE-CHLORITE-EPIDOTE

Dusky green Cretaceous volcanic rocks in the Christmas mine area (see Fig. 17.3) have been subjected to low-grade pervasive alteration, which has resulted in the propylitic assemblage actinolite-chlorite-epidote (-albite-quartz). The distribution of actinolite, epidote, and chlorite is regional, but their occurrence on a local scale is erratic, with no obvious variation in intensity toward the Christmas intrusive complex or other intrusions.

The diagnostic feature of this alteration is the replacement of cumulophyric, phenocrystic, and groundmass clinopyroxene by fibrous, blue-green actinolite. Volcanic breccia appears to be more susceptible to actinolilization than are massive basalt flows. In two-pyroxene basalts clusters of bright green chlorite and grapelike masses of quartz typically occupy the grain sites of original orthopyroxene. The basaltic rocks contain no fresh olivine, but euhedral grain outlines are filled with fine-grained clusters of epidote, chlorite, smectite, and hematite. Plagioclase is partially decomposed to albite, chlorite, epidote, and calcite.

Although ubiquitous in volcanic rocks near Christmas, the most spectacular occurrence of epidote is in distinctive, nearly monominerallic replacement nodules, which range in size from 1 or 2 cm to several meters in diameter. In part the nodules appear to represent replaced breccia fragments, but the mechanism of origin is obscure. This type of epidotization is, however, distinct from vein-related epidote (with attendant sulfide mineralization), which appears to be spatially related to mineralized porphyry of the Christmas intrusive complex. Epidote, chlorite, and actinolite also occur widely as cavity fillings in basalt.

Pervasive propylitization in volcanic rocks appears to pre-date the mainstage of mineralization-alteration. Both actinolite and chlorite were replaced by biotite in the secondary biotite halo around the Christmas stock. Furthermore, actinolite did not develop in any of the early hornblende andesite porphyry bodies that also contain pyroxene. Evidence for burial or regional metamorphism, such as penetrative deformation or metamorphic facies changes, is absent. It is more likely that the alteration resulted from the complex interaction between mafic wall rocks and meteoric and juvenile water circulating within the accumulating volcanic pile. Heat for circulation of fluids and alteration may have been provided by the succession of hypabyssal plutons intruded into the volcanic section, or by a larger body of magma at depth.

PORPHYRY-TYPE MINERALIZATION AND ALTERATION IN IGNEOUS ROCKS

Sulfide Mineralization

The important sulfide minerals in igneous rocks at Christmas are, in decreasing order of abundance, pyrite, chalcopyrite, bornite, and molybdenite. These sulfides have four principal modes of occurrence: (1) ragged disseminations intergrown with secondary minerals, particularly recrystallized biotite phenocrysts; (2) isolated granules and short, disoriented stringers or filaments in veins and wall rock; (3) fracture coatings, less than 1 mm wide, without appreciable carbonate or silicate gangue; and (4) central fracture fillings or seams up to 5 mm wide, typically enclosed by gangue minerals (commonly vuggy) or by alteration envelopes in the host rock. Occurrences (3) and (4) account for the bulk of total sulfide in igneous host rocks.

The generalized distribution of hypogene sulfide minerals is shown in Figure 17.7. In general, mafic volcanic rocks are more strongly mineralized than granodioritic intrusive rocks, and quartz diorite of the Christmas stock has higher copper grades than biotite granodiorite porphyry. Mineralization also increases stratigraphically higher in the porphyry copper system, and, thus, the highest copper values occur in volcanic and intrusive rocks east of the Joker fault zone. Chalcopyrite-bornite-molybdenite is the characteristic sulfide assemblage of the early period of mineralization (Stage I) and is co-extensively distributed with the zone of quartz-rich stockwork veins; both zones are, in turn, centered on the Christmas stock. The low-grade (generally less than 0.1% Cu) core of the stock, exposed in the north wall of the open pit, contains chalcopyrite and bornite as sparse disseminations and minor chalcopyrite deposited along quartz–K-feldspar veins. Molybdenite occurs sporadically throughout the deposit, but it is occasionally concentrated in coarse-grained aggregates with chalcopyrite along the median of quartz veins cutting quartz diorite and biotite granodiorite porphyry. Pyrite is subordinate to copper sulfides in the K-silicate zone. It occurs alone or with chalcopyrite as disseminations or short stringers or filaments along disoriented fractures healed with K-feldspar.

At higher levels in the porphyry copper system east of the Christmas fault, progressively stronger chalcopyrite-bornite mineralization (0.2–0.6% Cu) is present in early (Stage I) veins, fracture fillings, and disseminations in both the Christmas stock and adjacent volcanic rocks. The broad lobe of chalcopyrite-bornite mineralization extending northeast of the stock is related to the distribution of porphyry in the northeast salient. The outer limit of chalcopyrite-bornite mineralization corresponds generally with the outer margin of the strong secondary biotite sub-zone in volcanic rocks. Bornite is typically subordinate to chalcopyrite, and magnetite is a common constituent of Stage I quartz-sulfide veins. Mineralization appears to reach a maximum in strongly shattered zones of mixed volcanic-intrusive country rock, and several rich, pipe-shaped bodies—composed largely of quartz-bornite-chalcopyrite-chalcocite(?) veins—have been described from the hanging wall of the Joker fault (Eastlick, 1968). The pair pyrite-chalcopyrite, occasionally present in

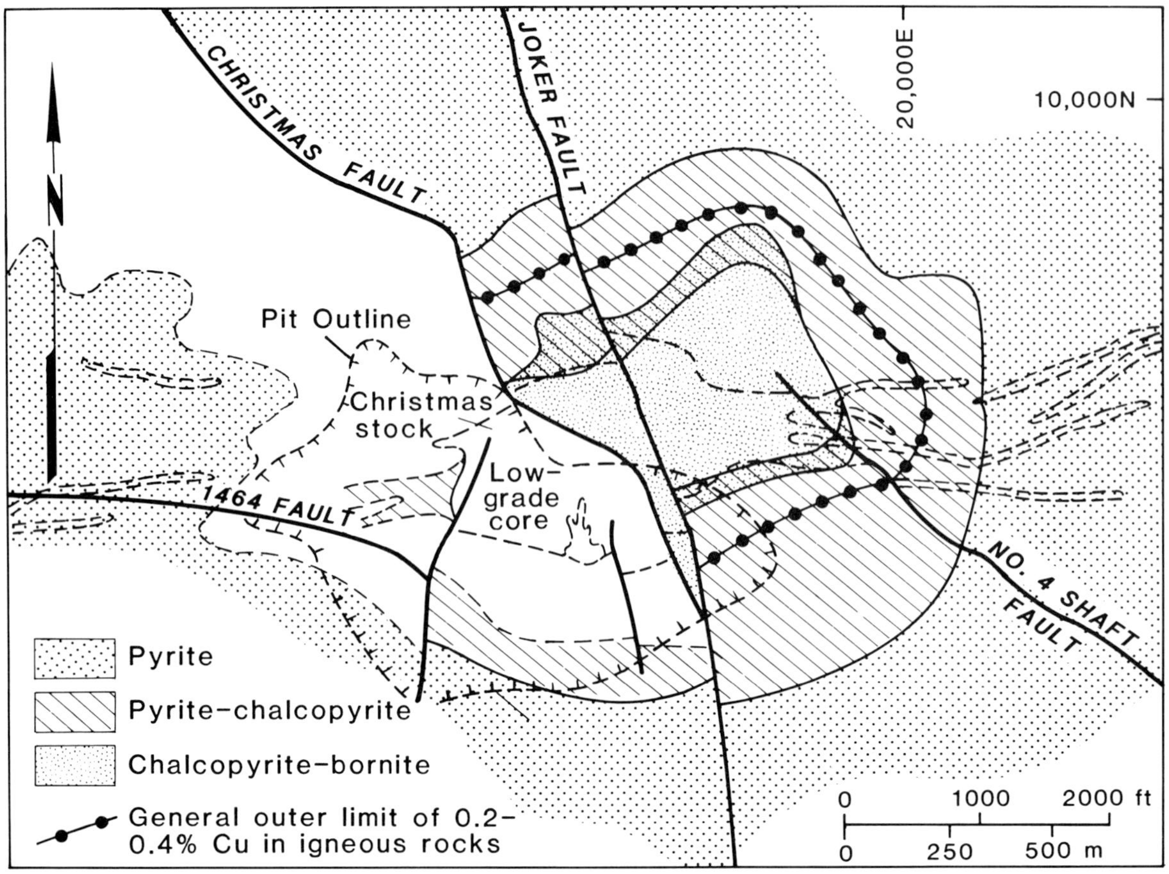

Figure 17.7. Mineral distribution map of sulfide minerals in igneous rocks. Geology generalized from Figure 17.3.

quartz-rich veins in volcanic wall rock, may represent a transitional vein assemblage between Stages I and II.

High total sulfide, pyrite-chalcopyrite mineralization is fracture-controlled, and temporally and spatially associated with younger (Stage II) alteration. The zones of chalcopyrite-bornite and pyrite-chalcopyrite mineralization overlap in a manner analogous to the overlap of central Stage I and peripheral Stage II alteration zones (see Fig. 17.7). In intrusive rocks Stage II sulfides are components of the quartz-sericite alteration zones and consist of 0.5- to 5.0-mm seams of pyrite and subordinate chalcopyrite accompanied by minor quartz and sericite gangue, sandwiched between envelopes of sericitized wall rock. Where pyrite and chalcopyrite are also disseminated between fractures, the total sulfide content may reach 10 percent by volume. Magnetite and bornite are not present in Stage II sulfide veins of the quartz-sericite zone. Molybdenite is occasionally present as finely dispersed grains mixed with quartz and sericite along fractures.

In mafic volcanic rocks the metallic minerals in Stage II veins are, in decreasing order of abundance, pyrite, chalcopyrite, and magnetite; however, sulfide seams, up to 5 mm in width, may exceed 90 percent chalcopyrite. Progressively younger Stage II veins and veins increasingly distant from the stock contain decreasing chalcopyrite:pyrite ratios, resulting in a lower-grade pyritic fringe zone (see Fig. 17.7).

Stage I: K-silicate Alteration

The early period of wall-rock alteration and veining in the stock and adjacent volcanic rocks, referred to as Stage I, was principally an episode of K-metasomatism. This episode was in large part time equivalent with emplacement and consolidation of early intrusive phases, but it preceded intrusion of the granodiorite and dacite porphyries. The principal manifestations of Stage I alteration are: (1) variable pervasive secondary biotite in the stock, (2) biotitization of basaltic volcanic wall rocks, and (3) stockwork veins consisting of relatively early K-feldspar–rich veinlets in the stock and quartz-rich veins in the stock and volcanic rocks.

Mineralization associated with stage I alteration generally has low total sulfide and high copper sulfide:pyrite ratios. The sulfide assemblage chalcopyrite-bornite is characteristic and more abundant than chalcopyrite-molybdenite or chalcopyrite-pyrite. Bornite and pyrite do not coexist in veinlets or as disseminations.

Biotitization of Intrusive Rocks. Early pervasive K-silicate alteration in the Christmas stock is characterized by the partial to total replacement of primary hornblende and biotite phenocrysts by compact, pseudomorphous clusters of fine-grained, leafy biotite and by the presence of small anhedral flakes of biotite in the goundmass. Secondary biotite is optically rather similar to primary biotite and occurs as 0.1- to 0.5-mm anhedral to subhedral plates, either randomly interleaved or gathered into sub-parallel alignment along the prismatic cleavages of the original amphibole crystal. A chemical analysis of strongly altered biotite granodiorite porphyry (see Table 17.1) and a calculation of chemical gains and losses resulting from pervasive biotitization (Table 17.3) suggest that, with the exception of increasing the Fe^{+2}:Fe^{+3} ratio and the hydrogen-ion content, the early pervasive biotitization of porphyry was essentially an isochemical process with respect to the major elements.

TABLE 17.3
Chemical Changes in Biotite Granodiorite Porphyry, Basalt, and Quartz Diorite During Alteration (In Gram Equivalents per 1,000 Cubic Centimeters)

Elements	Biotite Granodiorite Porphyry	Biotite Granodiorite Porphyry (strong secondary biotite)	Change
Si	117.7	114.4	−3.3
Al	25.0	25.0	0.0
Fe^{+3}	2.1	1.2	−0.9
Fe^{+2}	1.4	1.8	+0.4
Mg	3.0	2.7	−0.3
Ca	3.4	3.3	−0.1
Na	3.5	3.5	0.0
K	1.2	1.2	0.0
H	2.8	4.1	+1.3
	Unaltered Basalt	Basalt (strong biotitization)	Change
Si	92.7	97.7	+5.0
Al	28.8	26.4	−2.4
Fe^{+3}	4.8	2.4	−2.4
Fe^{+2}	4.0	3.2	−0.8
Mg	8.0	8.5	+0.5
Ca	9.6	4.4	−5.2
Na	2.0	1.9	−0.1
K	0.5	1.5	+1.0
H	6.6	10.9	+3.3
	Quartz Diorite	Quartz Diorite (quartz-sericite alteration)	Change
Si	110.9	109.9	−1.0
Al	25.5	26.0	+0.5
Fe^{+3}	2.1	4.3	+2.2
Fe^{+2}	3.1	1.1	−2.0
Mg	4.8	5.7	+0.9
Ca	3.2	0.6	−2.6
Na	3.4	0.2	−3.2
K	1.2	1.8	+0.6
H	4.7	11.2	+6.5

NOTE: Calculations made assuming constant total volume during alteration.

Hornblende is more susceptible to replacement than primary biotite, and thus the quartz diorite phase, which initially contained a higher percentage of hornblende, generally contains more abundant secondary biotite than biotite granodiorite porphyry. Furthermore, the completeness of hornblende-destructive biotitization generally increases upward in the composite stock, and in peripheral dikes and sills of biotite granodiorite porphyry. In contrast, samples of quartz diorite recovered from diamond drill holes along the south margin of the stock west of the Christmas fault contain fresh hornblende. Although cut by K-feldspar–bearing veins, the granodiorite phase from the deep core of the intrusion is relatively free of secondary biotite. It appears that the amount of secondary biotite is a function of hornblende content and, to some extent, the time and depth of emplacement in the intrusive complex.

Chlorite is a near-ubiquitous companion of secondary biotite. Where chlorite includes tiny grains of sagenitic rutile and anhedral sphene, it appears to be the encroaching phase. However, where secondary biotite and inclusion-free chlorite are intimately intergrown without bleached grain boundaries, they may have formed simultaneously. The amount of chlorite coexisting with biotite in this fashion is proportionately greater in biotite granodiorite porphyry than in quartz diorite. In general, it appears that main-stage intrusive phases have variable chlorite:secondary biotite ratios; post–main-stage unveined intrusive phases are characterized by chloritic alteration and lack secondary biotite.

The stoichiometric conversion of hornblende to biotite liberates calcium, and small grains of epidote, apatite, and calcite are distributed throughout secondary biotite aggregates. Magnetite and, less commonly, chalcopyrite also form clots and disseminations within clusters of fine-grained biotite. In a few samples opaque grains appear to be aligned along relict cleavage planes of biotite phenocrysts.

Biotitization of the Williamson Canyon Volcanics. Secondary biotite in mineralized mafic volcanic rocks, first noted by Eastlick (1968), occurs within a broad, horseshoe-shaped zone, open to the west, enclosing the Christmas stock. The intensity of biotitization and the grade of copper mineralization vary according to the density of fractures and Stage I veins and reach maximum values adjacent to the Christmas stock east of the Christmas fault. Figure 17.8 shows the sub-division of the biotitization halo—on the basis of rock texture, physical characteristics of the biotite, and associated alteration products—into the outer zone of weak biotitization (fringe zone), the middle zone of moderate biotitization (intermediate zone), and the inner zone of strong biotitization (contact zone). A large part of the area surrounding the mine east of the Christmas fault is buried beneath mine waste and alluvium, and the distribution pattern in that area is partly based on diamond drill core samples. Boundaries between sub-zones are gradational and irregular in detail, and their placement in Figure 17.8 is determined by interpolation between sample locations. The outer limit of biotitization is least clearly defined, but it generally extends between 300 and 750 m north and south of the stock at the present level of exposure. The zone of secondary biotite grades outward into rocks with background actinolite-chlorite-epidote alteration.

Secondary biotite in the fringe zone is pervasive, but its presence is difficult to detect megascopically. In thin section individual biotite grains are minute and exhibit a platy morphology. Grain size ranges between 5 and 20 microns, although a few grains may exceed 75 microns in maximum dimension. The color is generally pale brown to greenish brown, becoming less green and more brown as grain size increases toward the stock.

This incipient biotitization has two principal occurrences. Firstly, anhedral-granular biotite aggregates appear to occupy sites of original olivine and pyroxene phenocrysts and vesicles formerly filled with amygdaloidal minerals. To a lesser extent biotite replaces plagioclase and actinolite. Since no unaltered olivine has been observed in volcanic rocks beyond the biotite zone, it is likely that secondary biotite formed at the expense of minerals originally derived from the decomposition of olivine, such as montmorillonite and chlorite. Likewise, irregular areas with sharp boundaries —probably voids or amygdules in the original rock—are filled with biotite or with mixtures of biotite, chlorite, calcite, and actinolite. The general paucity of chlorite in the fringe

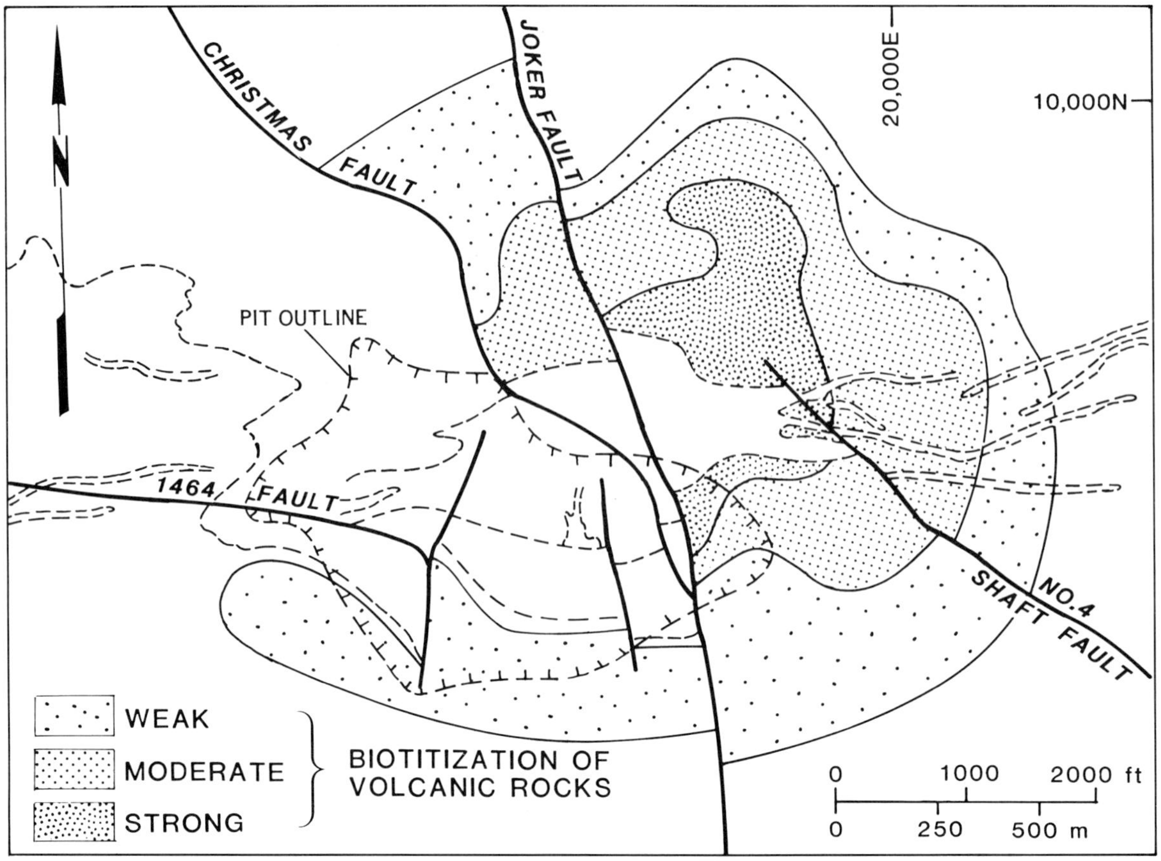

Figure 17.8. Mineral distribution map of hydrothermal biotite in basalt of the Williamson Canyon Volcanics

zone suggests that it has been largely converted to biotite. Secondly, biotite preferentially replaces matrix minerals of accessory volcanic rock fragments in volcanic breccia, often flooding the interstices between intergranular plagioclase laths.

Fracture and vein densities are low in the fringe biotite zone; mineralization consists mainly of pyrite coating fracture surfaces. Consequently, copper grades in the outer zone average less than 0.1 percent Cu.

The outer edge of the zone of moderate biotitization is marked by the appearance of megascopically visible biotite envelopes along mineralized fractures. Typically, the fractures also host Stage II quartz-chlorite-sulfide veins. Areas between fractures have the alteration intensity equivalent to the zone of weak biotitization. As the fracture and vein densities increase approaching the stock-dike complex, the biotite-rich envelopes widen and coalesce, until a continuous network of fine-grained biotite permeates the intervein part of the wall rock.

The increased biotite content (15–55% of the rock) is concentrated in the rock matrix, having formed at the expense of mafic minerals and opaque dust. Only coarser-grained actinolite and plagioclase escape complete destruction. Pale brown to pale greenish brown flakes measure 10 to 60 microns in long dimension, and tight plumose clusters of somewhat coarser tabular crystals are approximately 0.1 mm in length. Hand specimens show little textural modification and the whole-rock color is rendered a dull gray.

The distribution of the inner zone of strong biotitization is spatially related to the location of the Christmas stock and the distribution of Stage I quartz-sulfide veins. For example, the lobe of alteration trending northeast from the stock (see Fig. 17.8) reflects the sub-surface distribution of dikes or tongues of K-silicate–altered biotite granodiorite porphyry in the northeast salient. The wedge block between the Christmas and Joker faults and volcanic rocks along the steeply dipping south contact have very narrow zones of intense biotitization. Thus, the shape of the innermost biotite subzone reflects the sub-surface trend of the Christmas stock.

Basaltic wall rocks in the contact zone adjacent to the Christmas stock are completely recrystallized to an interpenetrating assemblage of biotite–quartz–magnetite–Na-plagioclase ±hornblende(?) ±apatite ±anhydrite ±chalcopyrite ±bornite. All of these minerals except plagioclase also occur in Stage I veins near the stock. In thin section the rock is flooded with anhedral to subhedral flakes of strongly pleochroic brown mica, 0.05 to 0.35 mm across, constituting between 30 and 55 percent of the rock volume. Thus, in volcanic rocks near the stock, increasing grain size, coloration, and content of biotite correlate with increased copper mineralization.

The presence of disseminated quartz suggests addition of silica during biotitization. Pale, nonfibrous amphibole associated with clusters of biotite probably represents altered actinolite. Plagioclase is partially to completely replaced by: (1) numerous tiny crystals of one or more of biotite, quartz, anhydrite, apatite, epidote, and amphibole; and (2) patchy areas of albite, quartz, K-feldspar (rare), and clay minerals. Although fine detail of original-growth zoning and twinning is blurred by these alteration effects, crude measurements of extinction angles on relict albite twin lamellae indicate a composition of sodic to intermediate andesine. Thus, plagioclase may have been enriched in the albite molecule during alteration; such a process is believed to have occurred concomitantly with biotitization of mafic volcanic rocks in some Andean deposits (Gustafson and Hunt, 1975; Camus, 1975). Anhydrite occurs with quartz in Stage I veins and as granular disseminations in the most thoroughly recrystallized rocks adjacent to the Christmas stock east of the Joker fault.

Chemical analyses of strongly biotitized basaltic wall rock (see Tables 17.1 and 17.3) indicate that Si, K, and H were added during formation of quartz and biotite. It is interesting to note that during K-metasomatism significant quantities of H (in terms of gram-equivalents) have also been added. Losses in Fe and Ca are related to the breakdown of pyroxene (or actinolite) and albitization of plagioclase. The alteration of actinolite and, perhaps, chlorite could have released Mg (which shows little variation in Table 17.3), utilized in the formation of secondary biotite. The significant loss of Fe^{+3} may correspond to the destruction of abundant opaque (magnetite-ilmenite?) dust, although ferric and ferrous iron are retained in coarse magnetite, some of which may be secondary. The net loss in total iron suggests that some Fe was actually removed from the wall rock, possibly to be fixed in vein sulfide minerals.

Stockwork Veining. A complex stockwork of Stage I veins, centered on the Christmas stock, consists principally of K-feldspar veinlets and quartz–K-feldspar veins in the intrusive complex and of quartz-sulfide veins in volcanic wall rocks east of the Christmas fault. Other, less common vein types in the core region of the stock are composed of pegmatitic biotite, aplite, and coarse vuggy assemblages of K-feldspar-sericite–chlorite–quartz. The outer limit of Stage I veins (Fig. 17.9) coincides rather closely with the outer limit of strong biotitization (see Fig. 17.8) and chalcopyrite-bornite mineralization (see Fig. 17.7).

Within the stock, Stage I veins penetrate quartz diorite, biotite granodiorite porphyry, and granodiorite but are absent in, and truncated by, dacite and granodiorite porphyry. Early, disoriented 0.5- to 2-mm veinlets of pale pink K-feldspar (generally weakly perthitic orthoclase) are consistently cut by well-defined, often steeply dipping, granular quartz-rich veins up to 5 cm in width. Precipitation of K-feldspar within the veinlets was composite, resulting both from deposition in open channelways and from orthoclazation of phenocrystic and groundmass plagioclase. A typical veinlet has a variable appearance: smooth and continuous when traversing plagioclase grains, diffuse in fine-grained (aplitic) groundmass, and absent or intermittent where the host fracture cuts grains of quartz and biotite. Since K-feldspar veinlets pentrate phenocrysts and locally maintain straight or slightly curvilinear forms, they must have formed, for the most part, after consolidation of the main intrusive phases. A minor amount of K-feldspar, however, particularly in quartz diorite, occurs in irregular swirly masses associated with lenses of granular quartz and apparently crystallized while the magma was still mobile.

The more throughgoing quartz-rich veins typically have sharp contacts against intrusive wall rocks, and contain narrow borders and discontinuous medians of K-feldspar. Many, if not all, zoned quartz-rich veins may have formed along reopened fractures initially healed by K-feldspar. The widest quartz veins have near-vertical attitudes, lack K-feldspar, and cut all other K-feldspar–bearing veins. Therefore, disoriented K-feldspar veinlets and steep quartz veins represent the early and late end members, respectively, of the vein system in the central Christmas stock. Stage I veins offset at junctions with other Stage I veins suggest that structural adjustments continued in the pluton during the period of

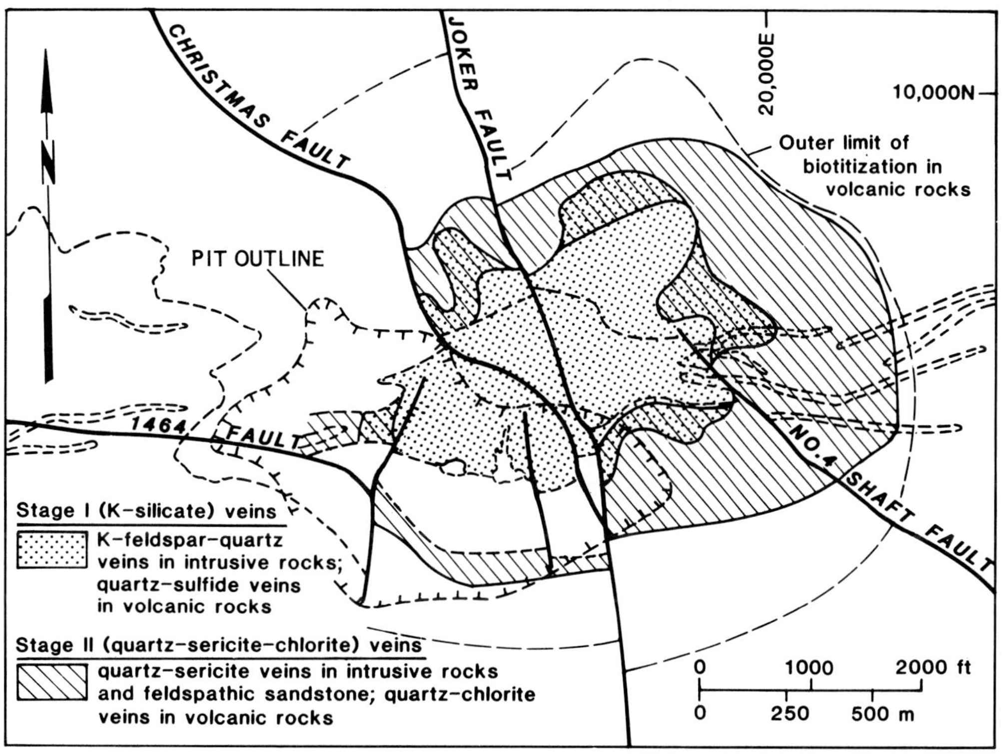

Figure 17.9. Mineral distribution map of vein-related Stage I and Stage II alteration

early veining. In addition to quartz and K-feldspar, Stage I veins in the stock may contain small amounts of calcite, biotite, chlorite, epidote, apatite, stilbite, pyrite, chalcopyrite, bornite, molybdenite, and anhydrite.

Stage I stockwork veins in volcanic rocks are simple aggregates of vitreous quartz and small but significant amounts of chalcopyrite and bornite, which often occur along marginal zones and crosscutting fractures. Anhydrite, an otherwise uncommon mineral in igneous rocks of the Christmas deposit, is abundant in quartz veins near the stock. Other minerals present in sparse amounts are magnetite, molybdenite, chlorite, calcite, biotite, hornblende, and late-forming zeolite. K-feldspar is not a constituent of Stage I veins in volcanic rocks. The contacts between Stage I quartz-sulfide veins and strongly biotitized volcanic wall rock are typically sharp. The vein system consists of steeply dipping, mutually crosscutting veins up to 3 cm in width which anastomose into numerous discontinuous 1-mm veinlets. Typically, veins are offset where intersected by another of the same type. In a few places, the veins are coarse, vuggy aggregates of sugary quartz and sulfide grains, which appear to grade outward into silicified host rock. The vein mineralogy and general style of fracturing and veining suggest that quartz-sulfide veins represent genetically equivalent continuations of Stage I quartz–K-feldspar veins in the stock.

Stage II: Quartz-Sericite-Chlorite Alteration

The second major episode of alteration, Stage II, is characterized by quartz with sericite or chlorite and is accompanied by pyrite and chalcopyrite in composite veins—that is, veins consisting of a central fracture filling and a wider, more diffuse wall rock envelope. Chlorite is the dominant phyllosilicate in Stage II veins in basaltic volcanic rocks, while sericite is dominant in intrusive and clastic sedimentary rocks. Stage II alteration assemblages represent an episode of retrograde hydrogen metasomatism during the evolution of the Christmas porphyry copper deposit.

Quartz-Sericite Alteration in Intrusive Rocks. K-silicate–altered rocks in the main body of the stock are flanked east and west by zones of structure-controlled quartz-sericite alteration (see Fig. 17.9). Within the western apex of the stock, quartz, sericite, pyrite, and chalcopyrite are concentrated in closely spaced, steeply dipping sheet fractures; chlorite is less common, and apatite is a rare constituent. Any K-feldspar originally present along these fractures has now been entirely replaced. Total sulfide is high (up to 10% by volume) with a high ($>$ 10:1) pyrite:chalcopyrite ratio.

In bleached vein envelopes enclosing the fractures, plagioclase phenocrysts and groundmass feldspar are replaced by fine-grained sericite, and mafic minerals (both primary phenocrystic and secondary biotite) are replaced by pale chlorite and sericite. Where fracture density is high, alteration envelopes overlap, and sericitization becomes pervasive. Relict outlines of biotite and plagioclase phenocrysts remain, but only quartz, apatite, and zircon of the original rock are visibly unaltered. Plagioclase between encroaching sericitized vein envelopes is altered to montmorillonite.

A chemical analysis of pervasively sericitized quartz diorite has been presented in this study (see Table 17.1, no. 11). The gain-loss calculation for quartz diorite (see Table 17.3) shows that the principal chemical changes during quartz-sericite alteration involve leaching of Na and Ca, conversion of Fe^{+2} to Fe^{+3}, and strong hydrogen metasomatism.

Mineralized fractures in the western apex of the stock are oriented parallel to the margins of the intrusion—that is, nearly east-west, with near-vertical dips. The intensity of alteration decreases eastward toward the interior of the intrusion, and the quartz-sericite zone merges gradationally with the central K-silicate zone over a distance of 50 to 100 m. Thus, the transition from K-silicate alteration in the stock to sericitic alteration is also a structural transition from stockwork fractures to closely spaced vertical sheet fractures conformable with the intrusive-metasedimentary rock contact.

The eastern sericitic zone centers on rhyodacite porphyry dikes but extends laterally into porous beds of feldspathic sandstone and siltstone in the Williamson Canyon Volcanics. The transition from K-silicate alteration to sericitic alteration, like that in the western zone, corresponds with the change from stockwork to vertically parallel fracturing in the intrusive complex. The development of vertical sheeting and related alteration reaches a maximum intensity approximately 125 to 175 m east of the stock. With increasing distance away from the stock, fracturing in the dikes diminishes and sericitic alteration yields to alteration of the propylitic type.

The strong vertical deformation is internal to the dikes. Strong parallel fractures are typically 1 to 5 cm apart, and the intervein parts of rhyodacite are converted to thoroughly bleached, light gray to buff quartz porphyries. Large blebby quartz eyes and compact felted masses of sericite (after plagioclase) and sericite intergrown with colorless to pale green chlorite (after mafic minerals) are set in a field of fine-grained sericite and quartz. Sites of original book biotite are marked by rods, needles, and anhedral grains of rutile all of which are often aligned along relict basal cleavages. At the surface, sulfides are converted to yellow to reddish brown oxidation products, principally colloform jarosite and goethite; the resulting gossan is characteristic of dikes in the eastern sericitic zone.

Quartz - Chlorite - Sulfide Veins in Volcanic Rocks. Stage II quartz-chlorite-pyrite-chalcopyrite veins in volcanic rocks contribute to ore-grade mineralization east of the Christmas fault in a zone overlapping with, but largely peripheral to, the zone of Stage I veining (see Fig. 17.9). Where overlap occurs, Stage II quartz-chlorite-sulfide veins crosscut Stage I quartz-sulfide veins.

Unlike sheeted Stage II veins in intrusive rocks, Stage II veins in volcanic rocks form an intricate stockwork. Quartz-chlorite-sulfide veins are superimposed on earlier biotitization. Where earlier biotic alteration is not pervasive (that is, where biotite occurs only along fractures), the Stage II veins are separated from fresh volcanic wall rock by a relict fringe of biotitization. Bleached, light gray to grayish green envelopes enclosing the central fracture mark the outwardly encroaching zone of biotite-destructive chloritization. Chlorite within the vein envelope does not generally extend beyond the limit of biotitization, although patchy chloritization between veins may be a contemporaneous product of Stage II alteration. Disseminated quartz, sericite, calcite, and sulfides also occur with chlorite in the vein envelope, and plagioclase is converted to albite. The bulk of Stage II sulfides appears to be confined largely to veins.

The central fracture filling varies in width between 1 mm and 3 cm, and is commonly zoned with chlorite (occasionally with sericite) at the margins; it is zoned with sulfides, magnetite, quartz, calcite, and calcium zeolites at the center. The infilling material often occurs in separate bands of sulfides, magnetite, chlorite, and quartz and implies successive periods of fracturing, deposition, and refracturing. Pyrite and chalcopyrite are present in all proportions, but the pyrite: chalcopyrite ratio is generally high and increases outward, where veins become less abundant and narrower.

Propylitic Alteration

Beyond the pyritic east and west quartz-sericite zones, grayish green biotite rhyodacite porphyry dikes host the propylitic assemblage epidote-chlorite-albite-sphene. The transition outward from quartz-sericite to propylitic alteration is gradational and coincides with the diminution of steep, parallel sheet fractures. Propylitic alteration is pervasive and mafic-destructive, as barrel-shaped book biotite is pseudomorphed by leafy chlorite enclosing lenses of granular epidote, anhedral sphene, and minute rod-shaped clusters of rutile. Where epidote is less abundant or absent, chloritized biotite may contain small amounts of interleaved prehnite. Hornblende and plagioclase are converted to aggregates of epidote plus chlorite and epidote plus albite, respectively. Coarse, bladed epidote originates in plagioclase as a small kernel near the grain perimeter and expands (as alteration proceeds) to consume the entire phenocryst and adjacent parts of the groundmass.

Pyrite may occur as scattered blebs or coatings on microfractures and is more abundant than chalcopyrite. However, the amount of total sulfide is low, generally less than 1 percent of the rock volume. Cu values approach trace levels.

In volcanic rocks near the deposit, but largely peripheral to the zone of Stage II quartz-chlorite-sulfide veins, epidote-quartz veins are narrow (< 1 cm), with diffuse epidotized reaction selvages in adjacent wall rock. Pyrite and traces of chalcopyrite occur within the veins and along fractures in nearby host rocks. At greater distances from the deposit, weakly banded, vuggy veins of coarse epidote and milky quartz occupy fractures, shear zones, and faults. Calcite and zeolite (laumontite) are commonly present as cavity linings and interstitial fillings between prismatic epidote crystals. Single veins are discontinuous and generally less than 10 cm wide; in aggregate they may constitute zones 1 m across. Scattered blebs and veins of oxidized sulfide, probably pyrite originally, are common, and copper oxide staining is present at a few localities. Semi-quantitative spectrographic analyses of samples from two epidote-quartz veins indicate the presence of small amounts of Mn, Cu, Pb, and Zn.

Summary of Zonation

The alteration-mineralization pattern at Christmas is a composite of two distinct levels and environments—the higher, intrusive-mafic volcanic zone, and the deeper, intrusive-sedimentary zone. The zones are juxtaposed by approximately 1 km of near-vertical displacement along the Christmas-Joker fault system.

When zonation is considered along an east-west to northeast-southwest axis through the Christmas stock-dike complex west of the Christmas fault (the eastward extension is at depth), it conforms to the concentric zonation pattern expressed in the Lowell-Guilbert (1970) model. Relatively low-grade (0.05–0.1% Cu), low-total sulfide (less than 1% by volume) chalcopyrite-bornite-molybdenite mineralization in the K-silicate–altered core yields outward to high-total sulfide (1–10%) pyrite-chalcopyrite mineralization in the zone of quartz-sericite alteration. Total sulfide content and the chalcopyrite:pyrite ratio diminish rapidly toward background values in propylitically altered dike rocks. This zonation corresponds closely to the structural transition from stockwork to vertical sheet fracturing which, in turn, yields to unfractured dike rock. The absence of steeply dipping sheet fractures along the north and south margins of the stock may have been a major factor inhibiting the development of quartz-sericite alteration in those areas.

West of the Christmas fault, K-silicate and sericitic alteration zones terminate abruptly at contacts with carbonate wall rocks. The formation of calc-silicate mineral assemblages in limestone and dolomite—what Titley (1973) refers to as the pyrometasomatic type of alteration—may be temporally equivalent to higher-temperature alteration types (early K-silicate) in igneous rocks. Retrograde actinolite veinlets cutting diopsidic hornfels in the Naco Limestone may, however, be contemporaneous with K-metasomatism in intrusive rocks (M. T. Einaudi, 1977, personal communication).

The higher-level zonation pattern in the Christmas porphyry copper deposit east of the Christmas fault is developed across silicate wall rocks of contrasting compositions. The broad K-silicate zone encompasses pervasive biotitization and K-feldspar–bearing stockwork veins in the stock, and quartz-sulfide veins and widely dispersed biotitization in the mafic volcanic environment. The widespread distribution of biotite in basalt is an expression of the fundamental control of wall rock composition. The Fe-Mg–rich basaltic rocks were a sensitive environment for crystallization of biotite during Stage I potassium metasomatism. Both fracture density and the intensity of biotitization decrease outward from the stock. The occurrence of secondary biotite beyond the zone of high fracture density might indicate that additional structural controls, such as vesicular zones or high-porosity horizons in poorly sorted volcanic breccia, may have been effective in transmitting hydrothermal fluids.

The zone of quartz-chlorite veins overlaps the zone of strong biotitization (and Stage I quartz-sulfide veins) but does not appear to extend to the outer limit of the fringe biotitization zone. Unlike the relations predicted by the Lowell-Guilbert model, K-silicate alteration (although weak) extends beyond the outer limit of the quartz-chlorite, or phyllic, zone. Furthermore, an argillic zone has not been identified in volcanic rocks, and the inner limit of vein-related epidotization may coincide generally with the outer limit of the quartz-chlorite zone. Thus, some overlap of propylitic and biotitic alteration (not allowed in the typical zonation model) is necessary, although the relative ages of these types of alteration are still uncertain. No discrete outer limit of the propylitic zone can be established because of the widespread regional epidotization of the Williamson Canyon Volcanics.

The level of exposure east of the Joker fault intersects a high level—possibly the roof zone of the stock—and the domed top of the ore zone which spans the somewhat irregular contact between intrusive and volcanic rocks. Early, low total sulfide (Stage I) chalcopyrite-bornite, and later, high total sulfide (Stage II) pyrite-chalcopyrite mineralization are telescoped in the chemically reactive basaltic wall rocks. The sulfide zonation derived from these superimposed mineralization episodes (moving away from the Christmas stock) is: chalcopyrite-bornite, chalcopyrite-bornite plus chalcopyrite-pyrite, pyrite-chalcopyrite, and pyrite. The presence of Pb, Zn, and Cu in outlying epidote-quartz veins may signify a larger-scale, base-metal zonation.

Vertical zonation of sulfide mineralization is also evident in the stock. In contrast to the nearly sulfide-barren deep core of the intrusion west of the Christmas fault, the upper level east of the Joker fault contains ore-grade copper mineralization. Adjacent country rocks at both levels are heavily mineralized, but the limit of ore is well within the outer limit of hydrothermal alteration. The reconstructed, pre-fault form of the orebody (ignoring, for purposes of this discussion, irregularities relating to dikes and apophyses of the stock) might then approximate a dome or an inverted cup, similar to the geometric model for mineralization zonation in certain porphyry copper deposits as suggested by James (1971). These observations underline the importance of considering depth of erosion when evaluating zonation in porphyry-type deposits.

SUPERGENE ALTERATION

The principal consequence of supergene alteration in igneous rocks at Christmas is the near-surface oxidation and total leaching of sulfides in the highly fractured, pyritic quartz-sericite alteration zones. Steeply dipping sheet fractures originally occupied by pyrite and chalcopyrite now contain crusty, yellowish brown (jarositic) to reddish brown (geothitic) seams of limonite, quartz, and gypsum. Sericite between fractures is variably altered to kaolinite or, less commonly, montmorillonite; the ultimate product of intense leaching is a compact, massive aggregate of kaolinite and quartz.

The development of gossan in intrusive rocks is a very shallow phenomenon, and limonite-rich fractures exposed near the western rim of the Christmas pit are transitional downward to pyritized fractures over a vertical interval of 20 to 50 m. Pyrite and chalcopyrite immediately below that level are commonly coated with a thin film of chalcocite, but copper enrichment is minimal.

In basaltic volcanic rocks east of the Christmas fault, supergene alteration has an erratic distribution. Fresh pyrite and chalcopyrite are abundant in veins and fractures in many samples of drill core within a few meters of the surface, but assays of other samples show significant copper oxide values to depths of 330 m. Sulfide minerals are altered to iron oxides and small amounts of cuprite, malachite, and native copper. Chrysocolla commonly forms as a fracture coating in intrusive rocks. Concentration of copper by supergene processes in volcanic rocks also appears to be insignificant.

FLUID-INCLUSION PETROGRAPHY

A reconnaissance study utilizing petrographic techniques and a classification scheme outlined by Nash (1976) has established the presence of three types of fluid inclusions in quartz from the Christmas porphyry vein system. Type I, or moderate-salinity inclusions, contain a liquid water phase and a relatively small vapor bubble occupying between 5 and 30 percent of the inclusion volume. Halite is absent, but one or more tiny daughter minerals may be present, including orange-red hematite. Type II, or gas-rich inclusions, contain low- or moderate-salinity liquid and greater than 50 percent vapor phase; this variety is generally believed to represent entrapment of dense steam (Roedder, 1971; Nash, 1976). Opaque daughter minerals (hematite?) are observed when the bubble is significantly smaller than the inclusion volume. All gradations appear to exist between Type I and Type II fluid inclusions, and they commonly occur together within the same host crystal.

Type III, or high-salinity inclusions, are the least abundant and contain a liquid phase, a 5 to 20 percent gas phase, and a cube of halite. Other daughter minerals are invariably present, but only hematite can be identified with confidence. The number of solid phases usually ranges between three and five, but as many as nine have been observed crowded into one inclusion.

Early Stage I stockwork veins are characterized by low to moderate populations of moderate-salinity and gas-rich fluid inclusions, and minor but ubiquitous halite-bearing inclusions. The ratio of gas-rich to moderate-salinity inclusions in both major veined phases of the stock is generally < 1, but the gas-rich variety is dominant in quartz–K-feldspar and quartz-sulfide veins east of the Christmas fault. Type I and Type II inclusions are less abundant in Stage II veins, and Type III inclusions are not present.

The greater abundance of Type II fluid inclusions and the higher Type II:Type I ratios in Stage I veins in the hanging wall of the Christmas fault may reflect increasing boiling in response to a decreasing pressure gradient at progressively higher elevations in and above the epizonal Christmas stock.

SEQUENCE OF EVENTS

Stage I: Intrusion and Early Alteration-Mineralization

Following deposition and actinolite-chlorite-epidote alteration of the Late Cretaceous Williamson Canyon Volcanics, the basaltic volcanic pile was intruded by a succession of Laramide calc-alkaline stocks, dikes, and small pluglike bodies. In early Paleocene time ($\sim$ 62 m.y ago) the Christmas intrusive complex was passively emplaced at shallow depth along east-northeast– to east-west–trending fractures which had formed in response to northeast-directed regional compression and differential uplift in southeastern Arizona (Rehrig and Heidrick, 1972, 1976; Banks and Krieger, 1977).

The spatial configuration of the reconstructed Christmas intrusive complex, viewed along a north-south cross section at approximately 18,000E, is shown schematically in Figure 17.10*a*. Seriate-porphyritic quartz diorite was intruded first, either as a thick tabular mass or a series of narrower, closely spaced dikes. Following at least partial consolidation, the quartz diorite was intruded and breached by numerous surges of biotite granodiorite porphyry, which in aggregate form the core of the complex. One or more pulses of magma ultimately migrate outward along the fracture zone to form rhyodacite porphyry dikes, and also pushed outward into volcanic rocks to form the northeast salient.

Intrusion of quartz diorite and biotite granodiorite porphyry, K-silicate alteration, and associated chalcopyrite-bornite mineralization are believed to be broadly contemporaneous events. K-Ar ages for Stage I vein minerals (see Table 17.2) are within error limits of the determined age of primary biotite from biotite granodiorite porphyry. Early alteration-mineralization, however, did not evolve in a static system, but rather during a period of repeated surges of magma, particularly within the core of the stock.

Pervasive, and nearly isochemical, hornblende-destructive biotitization, accompanied by precipitation of small amounts of sulfide and magnetite, occurred, at least in part, under late magmatic or deuteric conditions. Pervasive propylitic alteration in peripheral rhyodacite porphyry dikes may have been a contemporaneous process. K-feldspar did not form with secondary biotite during deuteric alteration, but began to replace plagioclase along newly generated disoriented fractures. Thus, plagioclase-destructive alteration appears to have been triggered by a change in confining pressure. The random, fine-scale brecciation within each intrusive phase and in superjacent volcanic rocks may have been generated by an internal process, such as the explosive escape of volatiles during periods of retrograde boiling (Burnham, 1967; Phillips, 1973) or differential thermal expansion of pore fluids (Knapp and Knight, 1977).

Subsequently developed fractures were progressively more throughgoing and steeply dipping. This change in fracture style, whether caused by external tectonic stress, the pressure of upwelling magma on consolidated rock, hydraulic action of hydrothermal fluids, or some other mechanism, coincided with the formation of increasingly quartz-rich, K-feldspar–poor veins. Although veins were becoming wider, K-feldspar envelopes remained narrow. Minor amounts of chalcopyrite and, locally, molybdenite were deposited in the core of the complex, but increasing quantities of chalcopyrite with bornite were precipitating in upper levels of the Stage I vein system, perhaps in response to a steeper temperature gradient. The presence of both primary and secondary gas-rich fluid inclusions in Stage I quartz veins indicates that boiling was a recurring event.

The proposed direction of movement of Stage I fluids and the geometry of early alteration-mineralization is shown in Figure 17.10*b*. As potassic fluids emanating from or passing through the stock encountered basaltic volcanic rocks, K, Si, H, Cu, and S were added during a nearly complete recon-

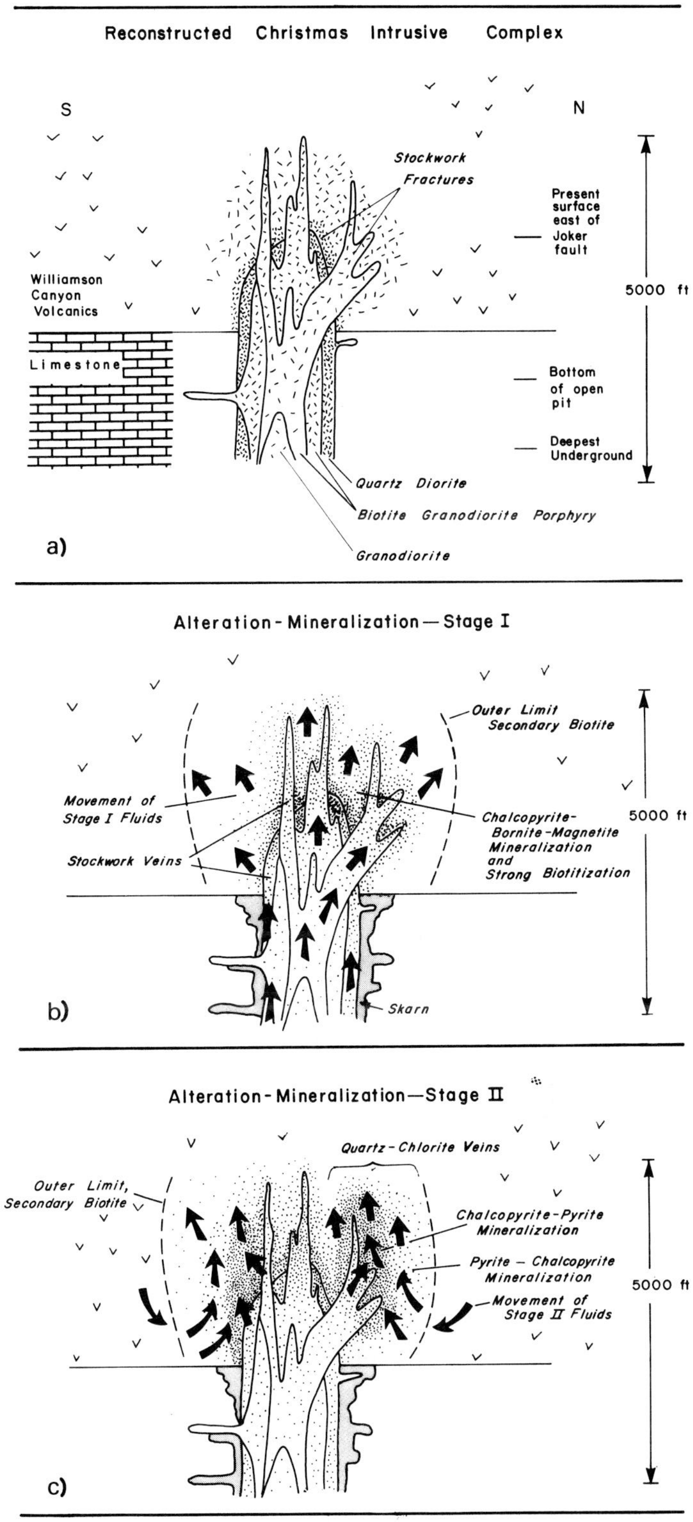

Figure 17.10. Diagrammatic configuration of the Christmas intrusive complex, viewed along a north-south section at approximately 18,000E, showing: *a*, the general sequence of emplacement of main stage intrusive phases and the fracture distribution pattern; *b*, Stage I alteration and mineralization; and *c*, a convection model for Stage II alteration and mineralization. Arrows indicate movement of magmatic-hydrothermal and meteoric-hydrothermal fluids.

stitution of the assemblage biotite-quartz-sodic plagioclase-hornblende(?)-chalcopyrite-bornite-magnetite. The biotitic alteration and mineralization centered on the network of quartz-rich stockwork veins that were developing upward in the volcanic pile. The distribution of strong biotitization was further controlled by the configuration of genetically related intrusive rocks. Whereas a narrow zone developed along the steep south contact, a broad lobe of intense biotitization formed over shallow apophyses of porphyry in the northeast salient.

Stage II: Late Alteration and Mineralization

After the formation of quartz-rich Stage I veins, a fundamental change occurred in the nature of fluid–wall-rock interaction, as K-metasomatism diminished relative to processes that were predominantly hydrolitic in character. The mineral assemblages, distribution patterns of fracture-controlled chloritic alteration in mafic volcanic rocks and sericitic alteration in felsic intrusive and clastic sedimentary rocks, and fluid-inclusion populations in all types of Stage II veins suggest that these types of alteration resulted from the same hydrothermal process acting contemporaneously in host rocks of contrasting composition.

The transition to Stage II quartz-sericite-chlorite alteration, largely a function of decreasing K:H ratio and/or cooling of the hydrothermal fluids (Hemley and Jones, 1964; Meyer and Hemley, 1967), probably commenced with the first significant incursion of meteoric water into the porphyry system. The general model shown in Figure 17.10*c* may reasonably account for the overlapping zonal distribution of vein-related alteration in Stages I and II. This hypothetical meteoric-hydrothermal model is similar to that proposed for porphyry copper deposits in general by Taylor (1974).

The flow of meteoric water was guided by an extensive system of fractures which were particularly abundant near the stock. A circulatory system may have evolved after the last major surge of magmatic-hydrothermal fluid from the cooling intrusive center. As cool meteoric water and fluids from the magma began to intermix, sulfide solubilities decreased and pyrite and chalcopyrite were dumped along irregular fractures. The Mg^{+2}:H^{+} ratio in the fluids was high enough and K^{+}:H^{+} ratios low enough to produce chlorite from earlier-formed secondary biotite. Fluids near the stock were depositing more chalcopyrite relative to pyrite than fluids in distal parts of the convection cell.

As the intrusive center continued to cool, the convection cell was drawn inward toward the stock, and the result was an overlap of Stage I and Stage II alteration-mineralization. Meteoric-hydrothermal fluids were able to penetrate the intrusive complex only along closely spaced vertical sheet fractures, leaching Ca, Na, and Fe from the wall rock, in exchange for H. The sheet fractures effectively channeled a volume of fluid large enough to permit expansion and, ultimately, coalescence of vein envelopes. Since the outer limit of quartz-sericite alteration in intrusive rocks was also fracture controlled, the zone of Stage II alteration developed in an intermediate position between zones of K-silicate and propylitic alteration.

After emplacement of quartz diorite and biotite granodiorite porphyry, granodiorite and dacite porphyry intruded the south margin of the stock with sharp contacts. These phases appear to post-date K-silicate alteration in the stock, but their temporal relation with quartz-sericite-chlorite alteration and pyritization is unknown. The chlorite-epidote alteration in these late phases is most reminiscent of the low-grade alteration prevalent in the McDonald stock northeast of the Christmas mine. However, the presence of disseminated bornite and chalcopyrite indicates that substantial concentrations of metals and sulfur were present in the late-forming magmas or where introduced during late propylitic alteration in the Christmas stock.

IMPLICATIONS AND SUGGESTIONS FOR EXPLORATION IN THE REGION

The nature of hydrothermal alteration and mineralization in the Williamson Canyon Volcanics at Christmas is an important consideration for regional exploration. Two observations should be emphasized. Firstly, the volcanic rocks are basaltic in composition and a major host for copper ore. The chemical reactivity of thoroughly fractured basalt has induced telescoped Stage I and Stage II alteration and sulfide assemblages and has, thereby, upgraded copper values. Laramide-age mafic and intermediate volcanic sequences should be given high priority as favorable host rocks for ore.

Secondly, the increased stability of biotite in a mafic rock environment undergoing K-metasomatism considerably expanded the dimensions of the K-silicate zone. The zone of secondary biotite in basalt extends beyond the zone of quartz-sericite-chlorite alteration, and well beyond the limits of ore-grade mineralization. Where propylitic alteration related to mineralization may be obscured by low-grade propylitic alteration of regional extent, biotitization may be the more reliable porphyry-related fringe alteration in mafic volcanic terranes. In addition, biotite halos may effectively increase the dimensions of reliable prospecting targets.

Biotitization of basalts and andesites has been recognized as porphyry-type alteration at Safford, Arizona (Robinson and Cook, 1966); El Salvador (Gustafson and Hunt, 1975) and El Teniente (Camus, 1975), Chile; and at the La Florida prospect in Sonora, Mexico (Theodore and DeWit, 1976). Although the occurrency of secondary biotite in volcanic rocks is not in itself *prima facie* evidence that ore-grade mineralization exists nearby, its presence is a positive indication of porphyry-type hydrothermal alteration. It is equally important to note that no biotitization has been observed in basaltic country rocks adjacent to barren granodioritic stocks near Christmas.

Although the presence of fine-grained, disseminated biotite in basalts may escape detection, particularly during reconnaissance mapping programs, chip samples can be checked quickly in the field office with a binocular microscope. If identification is still uncertain, X-ray diffraction provides a rapid, accurate, and inexpensive method of analysis. The presence of biotite in altered basalts may also be indicated by anomalous potassium values in chemical analyses. Considering the number of Laramide volcanic fields in southeastern Arizona with co-magmatic or younger intrusive rocks, the recognition and interpretation of secondary biotite should be an important contribution to future exploration for porphyry copper deposits.

ACKNOWLEDGMENTS

We are indebted to the following for their helpful guidance and stimulating suggestions during various stages of this investigation: Marco T. Einaudi, Konrad B. Krauskopf, and Juhn G. Liou of Stanford University; Henry R. Cornwall, Cyrus Creasey, and Norman G. Banks of the U.S. Geological Survey; and John T. Eastlick of the Inspiration Consolidated Copper Company. Careful reviews by Marco T. Einaudi, Norman G. Banks, and William J. Moore greatly improved the manuscript.

REFERENCES CITED

Banks, N. G.; Cornwall, H. R.; Silberman, M. L.; Creasey, S. C.; and Marvin, R. F., 1972, Chronology of intrusion and ore deposition at Ray, Arizona: Part I, K-Ar ages: Geol. v. 67, p. 864–878.

Banks, N. G., and Krieger, M. H., 1977, Geologic map of the Hayden quadrangle, Gila and Pinal Counties, Arizona: U.S. Geol. Survey Map GQ-1391, 1:24,000.

Banks, N. G., and Stuckless, J. S., 1973, Chronology of intrusion and ore deposition at Ray, Arizona: Part II, Fission-track ages: Econ. Geol., v. 68, p. 657–664.

Barrett, L. F., 1972, Igneous intrusions and associated mineralization in the Saddle Mountain mining district, Pinal County, Arizona: Utah Univ., Unpub. M.S. Thesis, 90p.

Burnham, C. W., 1967, Hydrothermal fluids at the magmatic stage, *In* Barnes, H. L., ed., Geochemistry of Hydrothermal Ore Deposits: New York, Holt, Rinehart and Winston, p. 34–76.

Camus, Francisco, 1975, Geology of the El Teniente ore body with emphasis on wall-rock alteration: Econ. Geol., v. 70, p. 1341–1372.

Coney, P. J., 1972, Cordilleran tectonics and plato motion: Am. Jour. Sci., v. 272, p. 603–628.

———, 1976, Plate tectonics and the Laramide Orogeny, *in* Woodward, L. A., and Northrop, S. A., eds., Tectonics and mineral resources of southwestern North America: New Mex. Geol. Soc. Spec. Pub. 6, p. 5–10.

Cornwall, H. R.; Banks, N. G.; and Phillips, C. H., 1971, Geologic map of the Sonora quadrangle, Pinal and Gila Counties, Arizona: U.S. Geol. Survey Map GQ-1021, 1:24,000.

Cornwall, H. R., and Krieger, M. H., 1978, Geologic map of the El Capitan quadrangle, Gila County, Arizona: U.S. Geol. Survey Map GQ-1442, 1:24,000.

Creasey, S. C., and Kistler, R. W., 1962, Age of some copper-bearing porphyries and other igneous rocks in southeastern Arizona, *in* Geological Survey research 1962: U.S. Geol. Survey Prof. Paper 450-D, p. D1–D5.

Damon, P. E., and Mauger, R. L., 1966, Epeirogeny-orogeny viewed from the Basin and Range province: AIME-SME Trans., v. 235, p. 99–112.

Eastlick, J. T., 1968, Geology of the Christmas mine and vicinity, Banner mining district, Arizona, *in* Ridge, J. D., ed., Ore deposits of the United States, 1933–1967: AIME, v. 2, p. 1191–1210.

Gustafson, L. B., and Hunt, J. P., 1975, The porphyry copper deposit at El Salvador, Chile: Econ. Geol., v. 70, p. 857–912.

Hayes, P. T., 1970, Cretaceous paleogeography of southeastern Arizona and adjacent areas: U.S. Geol. Survey Prof. Paper 658-B, 42p.

Hemley, J. J., and Jones, W. R. 1964, Chemical aspects of hydrothermal alteration with emphasis on hydrogen metasomatism: Econ. Geol., v. 59, p. 538–569.

Hyndman, D. W., 1972, Petrology of igneous and metamorphic rocks: New York, McGraw-Hill, 533p.

Irvine, T. N., and Baragar, W. R. A., 1971, A guide to chemical classification of common volcanic rocks: Canadian Jour. Earth Sci., v. 8, p. 523–548.

James, A. H., 1971, Hypothetical diagrams of several porphyry copper deposits: Econ. Geol. v. 66, p. 43–47.

Knapp, R. B., and Knight, J. E., 1977, Differential thermal expansion of pore fluids: Fracture propagation and microearthquake production in hot pluton environments: Jour. Geophys. Res. v. 82, p. 2515–2522.

Koski, R. A., 1978, Geology and porphyry copper-type alteration-mineralization of igneous rocks at the Christmas mine, Gila County, Arizona: Stanford Univ., Unpub. Ph.D. Diss. 196p.

Krieger, M. H., 1968, Geologic map of the Saddle Mountain quadrangle, Pinal County, Arizona: U.S. Geol. Survey Map GQ-671, 1:24,000.

———, 1974, Geologic map of the Winkelman quadrangle, Pinal and Gila Counties, Arizona: U.S. Geol. Survey Map GQ-1106, 1:24,000.

Lowell, J. D., and Guilbert, J. M., 1970, Lateral and vertical alteration-mineralization zoning in porphyry ore deposits: Econ. Geol., v. 65, p. 373–408.

McCurry, W. G., 1971, Mineralogy and paragenesis of the ores, Christmas mine, Gila County Arizona: Arizona State Univ., Unpub. M.S. Thesis.

Meyer, Charles, and Hemley, J. J., 1967, Wall rock alteration, *in* Barnes, H. L., ed., Geochemistry of Hydrothermal Ore Deposits: New York, Holt, Rinehart and Winston, p. 166–235.

Nash, J. T., 1976, Fluid-inclusion petrology—data from porphyry copper deposits and applications to exploration: U.S. Geol. Survey Prof. Paper 907-D, p. D1–D16.

Perry, D. V., 1969, Skarn genesis at the Christmas mine, Gila County, Arizona: Econ. Geol., v. 64, p. 255–270.

Peterson, N. P., and Swanson, R. W., 1956, Geology of the Christmas copper mine, Gila County, Arizona: U.S. Geol. Survey Bull. 1027-H, p. 351–373.

Phillips, W. J., 1973, Mechanical effects of retrograde boiling and its probable importance in the formation of some porphyry ore deposits: Inst. Min. Metall. Trans., v. 82, p. B90–B98.

Ransome, F. L., 1919, The copper deposits of Ray and Miami, Arizona: U.S. Geol. Survey Prof. Paper 115, 192p.

———, 1923, Description of the Ray quadrangle: U.S. Geol. Survey Geol. Atlas Folio 217, 24p.

Rehrig, W. A., and Heidrick, T. L., 1972, Regional fracturing in Laramide stocks in Arizona and its relationship to porphyry copper mineralization: Econ. Geol., v. 67, p. 184.

———, 1976, Regional tectonic stress during the Laramide and Late Tertiary intrusive periods, Basin and Range province, Arizona: Arizona Geol. Soc. Digest X, p. 205–228.

Reid, A. M., 1966, Stratigraphy and paleontology of the Naco Formation in the southern Dripping Spring Mountains near Winkelman, Gila County, Arizona: Univ. Ariz., Unpub. M.S. Thesis.

Robinson, R. F., and Cook, Annan, 1966, The Safford copper deposit, Lone Star mining district, Graham County, Arizona, *in* Titley, S. R., and Hicks, C. L., eds., Geology of the Porphyry Copper Deposits, Southwestern North America: Tucson, Univ. Ariz. Press, p. 250–266.

Roedder, Edwin, 1971, Fluid inclusion studies on the porphyry-type ore deposits at Bingham, Utah; Butte, Montana; and Climax, Colorado: Econ. Geol., v. 66, p. 98–120.

Ross, C. P., 1925, Ore deposits of the Saddle Mountain and Banner mining districts, Arizona: U.S. Geol. Survey Bull. 771, 72p.

Simons, F. S., 1964, Geology of the Klondike quadrangle, Graham and Pinal Counties, Arizona: U.S. Geol. Survey Prof. Paper 461, 173p.

Taylor, H. P., Jr., 1974, The application of oxygen and hydrogen isotope studies to problems of hydrothermal alteration and ore deposition: Econ. Geol., v. 69, p. 843–883.

Theodore, T. G., and de Wit, M. P., 1976, Porphyry-type metallization and alteration at La Florida de Nacozari, Sonora, Mexico: U.S. Geol. Survey Open-file Rept. 76–760, 28p.

Titley, S. R., 1972, Some geological criteria applicable to the search for southwestern North American porphyry copper deposits: AIME, MMIJ Preprint GI2, p. 1–16.

———, 1973, "Pyrometasomatic"—an alteration type: Econ. Geol. v. 68, p. 1326–1329.

Willden, Ronald, 1964, Geology of the Christmas quadrangle, Gila and Pinal Counties, Arizona: U. S. Geol. Survey Bull. 1161–E, 64p.

18

Geology of the Poston Butte Porphyry Copper Deposit

PINAL COUNTY, ARIZONA

Philip W. Nason, Allen V. Shaw, and Kent D. Aveson

In 1969 Conoco geologists recognized the mineral potential of the Florence area, based on a systematic examination of regional geology. A small outcrop of leached capping at the foot of Poston Butte (2.5 miles northwest of Florence, Arizona) indicated that a porphyry copper orebody could lie somewhere beneath the overburden adjacent to the surface exposure. Upon the recommendation of Conoco geologist B. F. Kern, land acquisition began in late 1969, and a drilling program was started in the spring of 1970. In the summer of that year the interception of the first ore proved the above hypothesis based on the tiny outcrop.

Early exploration consisted of rotary drilling through the overburden and examination of bedrock spot cores. Results were favorable enough to continue exploratory drilling on a triangular drill grid; rotary drilling was used to bedrock, followed by diamond drilling. Initial drilling (with 1,000-ft. drill-hole spacing) before 1972 outlined the discovery; further drilling through 1973 reduced the spacing to 500 ft. and defined more details of the geology. Drilling the pattern with 250-ft. spacing in 1974 and 1975 corroborated earlier interpretations and improved confidence in geologic mapping and projections. The core was photographed, logged, and prepared for assay on the property. Early in the exploration program a geological logging system was adopted which put the raw geologic data, including assays, into standardized, easily codable form for computer use.

The exploration drilling program that was begun in 1970 completed 659 rotary drill holes and 396 diamond drill holes, with a total footage of 299,838 ft. and 306,019 ft., respectively. In 1974 Conoco developed a single-level, underground, pilot mine through two 700-ft. bored shafts to examine the ore for metallurgical, mining, and geological studies. The establishment of more than a mile of drifts and cross cuts allowed access to both oxide and sulfide ore zones for firsthand examination of rock in place. Over 50,000 tons of ore were mined for pilot-plant feed. The exploration and development drilling programs and pilot-mine studies have supplied geologic and analytical information to prove the existence of a major porphyry copper ore deposit.

REGIONAL GEOLOGY

The generalized geology of the area is shown in Figure 18.1. Precambrian metamorphic and igneous rocks, intruded by diabase dikes and Laramide intrusive rocks, crop out extensively east and west of the deposit. The Precambrian and Laramide rocks are cut by Tertiary hypabyssal intrusives that range in composition from basalt to quartz latite. Unconformably overlying Precambrian and Laramide rocks are Tertiary and Quaternary gravels and volcanic rocks. The region has been broken into a series of horsts and grabens by Basin and Range orogenesis.

Precambrian Rocks

The oldest local Precambrian unit is the Pinal Schist, which crops out 3.5 miles north of the deposit and is not mineralized. Intruding the Pinal Schist is the Precambrian Oracle Granite batholith, locally a quartz monzonite porphyry to quartz monzonite, which is the major host for copper mineralization at Florence. Outcrops of the Oracle are sparse in the immediate area but do exist at the base of Poston Butte and at sites ¾ of a mile east and 2 miles north of the deposit. Precambrian diabase dikes intrude both the Oracle Granite and Pinal Schist. Outcrops of diabase are found north of the deposit, and numerous diabase dikes have been intersected by drilling in the orebody.

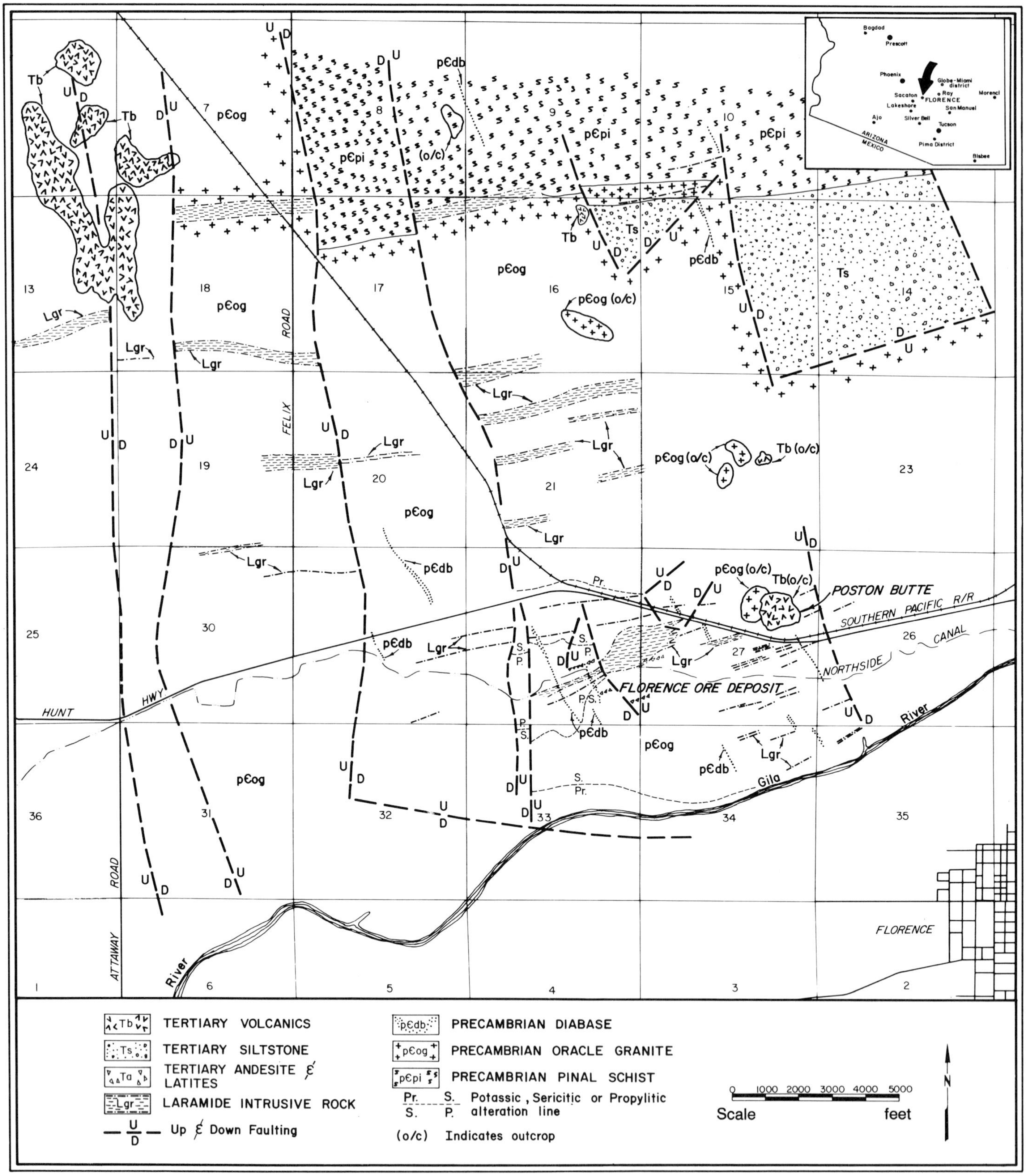

Figure 18.1. Generalized, sub-surface geology map of Poston Butte area (showing outcrops)

Laramide Rocks

A large Laramide granodiorite intrusion, the Sacaton Peak stock, is exposed 4 miles west of the deposit (Balla, 1972) and may be genetically related to the Laramide intrusions at Florence. At least three textural phases of Laramide intrusive granodiorite porphyries are known from drill core data and pilot-mine intersections, but there are no known outcrops of these rocks in the immediate area. An age-date (K-Ar) of 62.0 ± 1.0 m.y. has been obtained on the mineralized granodiorite porphyry. (Data from Conoco. All age-dates in this chapter are from Conoco, unless otherwise noted.) The interrelationship among the various phases of granodiorite is uncertain, but they appear to be co-magnetic.

Tertiary-Quaternary Rocks

Post-mineral dikes of several compositions intruded the granodiorites and the quartz monzonite porphyry during the Tertiary Period. The unmineralized dikes are latite-dacite (60.3 ± 1.3 m.y.), andesite (55.8 ± 1.1 m.y.), and basalts (5.86 ± 0.14 m.y.). Determining the orientations of these dikes is difficult, even with closely spaced drilling. The andesite and latite dikes appear to be quite narrow, striking east-northeast and dipping steeply to the northwest.

During Tertiary-Quaternary times siltstones, sandstones, and locally derived gravels were deposited unconformably on the Oracle Granite. A poorly to moderately indurated, poorly sorted conglomerate composed of angular and sub-angular, igneous pebbles in a brown, arkosic matrix covers bedrock in the grabens west of the orebody. It contains very few fragments of volcanic material.

One mile northwest of the deposit, in a graben, a thick sequence of interbedded sandstone and gypsum has been intersected by drill holes. Steeply dipping bedding in this unit is thought to be the result of local slumping. Based on pollen analysis, the sandstone has an age range of late Cretaceous to mid-Tertiary. The conglomerate and playa deposit are interpreted to be part of the Whitetail (?) Conglomerate (Ransome, 1903). Unconformably overlying the sandstone and gypsum units is an 89-ft.-thick basalt flow which compares with the "Blue Basalt" described by Blucher (Sell, 1968). A thin, red, "baked" zone occurs at the base of the basalt.

Overlying the porphyry deposit and the Whitetail (?) Conglomerate is a poorly indurated and poorly sorted alluvial deposit, consisting of pebbles and cobbles of a variety of rock types—including volcanic material. Flat-lying basalt flows are interbedded with these sediments. This formation correlates with the Big Dome Formation (Krieger et al., 1974). An ash-flow tuff within the Big Dome Formation north of the porphyry deposit has been K-Ar dated at 17.6 ± 0.4 m.y. This age correlates with that of a tuff unit within the Big Dome Formation at its type locality near Kearny (Krieger et al., 1974). A palynological age of Pliocene, however, has been obtained from a near-horizontal, areally extensive, clay layer in the formation at Poston Butte 60 ft. above granite bedrock.

Throughout the region, numerous basalt outliers rest directly on Precambrian and Laramide rocks. Potassium-argon dates of the Poston Butte basalt and a basalt dike intersected by drilling are 7.9 ± 0.3 m.y. and 5.86 ± 0.14 m.y., respectively. These basalts may correlate with the volcanic sills within the Big Dome Formation, but the exact relationship is not known.

REGIONAL STRUCTURE

Because few outcrops are present in the Florence area, the regional structure is interpreted from extensive drill-hole data in the orebody, assessment drilling beyond the orebody, underground geology, and projection of known structures. The Poston Butte deposit is associated with Laramide intrusions that possibly were emplaced at the junction of conjugate faults. The most evident structures in the Florence area are related to the Basin and Range orogenesis. One of these features is the Party Line fault, which strikes N35°W and dips 45 to 55°SW. This major fault on the east side of the deposit has a vertical displacement of over 1,000 ft. West of the Party Line fault is a series of *en echelon* normal faults striking north to northwest and dipping west. The Florence deposit is within a complex, north-trending horst block.

SUMMARY OF GEOLOGIC HISTORY

The geologic events recognized or inferred at Florence from late Jurassic to the present are summarized below:

1. Nevadan and Laramide movement on the Florence uplift (Turner, 1962), with erosion of Mesozoic, Paleozoic, and possibly Precambrian sediments and exposure of part of the Precambrian Oracle batholith
2. Intrusion of the Sacaton Peak stock (Balla, 1972) and granodiorite porphyries of the Florence deposit during Laramide time
3. Alteration and mineralization of the Oracle Granite (locally quartz monzonite porphyry), granodiorite porphyries, and diabases, probably penecontemporaneous with the intrusion of the granodiorite at about 62 ± 1.0 m.y. ago
4. Intrusion of unmineralized Tertiary andesite and quartz latite dikes
5. Uplift, erosion, and development of the oxide and enriched zones, creating a sub-horizontal oxide-sulfide interface
6. Burial of the deposit by Whitetail (?) Conglomerate
7. Basin and Range faulting in middle Miocene, which displaced Whitetail (?) Conglomerate, bedrock, and the oxide-sulfide interface
8. Erosion of the Whitetail (?) Conglomerate except in grabens
9. Further oxidation of deposit
10. Deposition of the Big Dome Formation with interbedded basalt flows, filling basins and covering the deposit during late Miocene
11. Continued oxidation at least into upper Pliocene as evidenced by chrysocolla in a basalt dike that is 5.86 ± 0.14 m.y. old
12. Regional uplift upon which the present topography was formed

OREBODY GEOLOGY

Rock Units

Plutonic and hypabyssal rocks compose the mineralized rock suite of the Florence copper deposit. Approximately 90 percent of the mineralization is contained in quartz monzonite porphyry and granodiorite porphyry. Other igneous rocks associated with the deposit are diabase, aplites, diorite, latite, dacite, andesite, and basalt.

Precambrian rocks include quartz monzonite porphyry (Oracle Granite), which forms the host rock for the deposit, and Precambrian diabase dikes. Aplite dikes, schlieren of biotite, and metasomatized inclusions are common within the quartz monzonite porphyry, and the nature of their contacts suggests a close genetic relationship. A gradational change occurs in the quartz monzonite porphyry toward the western end of the deposit, as the porphyritic texture gradually changes to an equigranular texture and the sphene content increases. This equigranular quartz monzonite is believed to be a phase of the quartz monzonite porphyry (or vice versa), rather than a separate intrusion.

Quartz monzonite porphyry in the deposit consists of coarse-grained, subhedral, locally perthitic, twinned K-feldspar phenocrysts (25–35%) embedded in a medium-grained, hypidiomorphic to xenomorphic matrix of quartz (15–30%), plagioclase (20–35%), and biotite (5–8%). Graphic and myrmekitic textures are locally developed. Textures indicative of strain deformation are common as strained quartz, deformed biotite books, and bent plagioclase twin lamellae. Some of the deformation may be protoclastic, although the major strain features are probably cataclastic. Deuteric effects are also noticeable as redistribution of K-feldspar and quartz. Microcline twinning is observed in quartz monzonite porphyry samples along the unaltered periphery of the deposit. Lack of microcline twinning in the K-feldspar phenocrysts of the main portion of the deposit may indicate a zone of re-equilibration, with a transition from microcline to orthoclase. Plagioclase grains are commonly compositionally zoned and range from andesine (An_{38}) to oligoclase (An_{26}). Accessory minerals include apatite, rutile, sphene, zircon, and magnetite. Pleochroic halos associated with zircon inclusions in biotites are common.

Quartz monzonite porphyry is the major host for mineralization. Fracturing, brecciation, and the creation of permeable zones, all related to the intrusion of Laramide granodiorite porphyry, controlled the distribution of mineralization. Chalcopyrite, the principal copper mineral, occurs in veins, veinlets, and disseminations within biotite. Mineralization is generally more intense near the contacts with granodiorite porphyry.

Diabase dikes are probably Precambrian in age. Inclusions of these mafic rocks in the quartz monzonite porphyry have been observed, but generally they were intruded along north-northwest planes of weakness. The diabase dikes are fine-grained, dark, and dense, with drill hole intercepts ranging from a few inches to tens of feet. Petrographically these rocks consist of plagioclase laths embedded in a mafic matrix. These mafic rocks are mineralized, and the locally altered varieties contain 10 to 15 percent chalcopyrite.

Laramide igneous activity is represented by granodiorite porphyry as dikes and irregular hypabyssal bodies. The granodiorites associated with the deposit are subdivided into three petrographic varieties: Granodiorite porphyry Type I is a light grey, medium- to fine-grained rock with quartz, plagioclase, and biotite phenocrysts set in a xenomorphic matrix of quartz and K-feldspar. Modal ranges are quartz (15–20%), plagioclase (40–50%), K-feldspar (15–20%), and biotite (5%). Graphic and myrmekitic textures are locally developed. Plagioclase phenocrysts tend to be compositionally zoned and range from An_{30} to An_{40}. Accessory amounts of rutile, apatite, zircon, and magnetite are also present. Granodiorite Type I is the main intrusive mass and composes some 20 percent of the deposit.

Granodiorite porphyry Type II is a grey, more mafic, and finer-grained rock than granodiorite porphyry Type I and is generally found as narrow dikes. Quartz, biotite, and plagioclase phenocrysts are set in a very fine-grained xenomorphic matrix of quartz, K-feldspar, biotite, and plagioclase. Modal composition is quartz (20%), plagioclase (50%), K-feldspar (15–20%), and biotite (5–10%). Plagioclase phenocrysts are zoned with an average composition in the andesine range. Accessory minerals include zircon, apatite, and magnetite.

Granodiorite porphyry Type III is a greenish grey, very fine-grained rock which contains only quartz and plagioclase phenocrysts. This variety forms a dike about 100 ft. thick in the northern portion of the deposit; it strikes east-northeast and dips south. A modal composition for this variety is quartz (15–20%), K-feldspar (15–20%), biotite (5–10%), and plagioclase (49–55%). The characteristics of the granodiorite types and the geometry of their placement indicate that the Type II dikes predate—or overlap with—the massive Type I intrusion, which was followed by intrusion of the Type III dike.

Mineralization in the granodiorite porphyries is less well developed than in the quartz monzonite porphyry. This weaker mineralization may be a function of both composition and fracture intensity. Due to the nature of contact mineralization and the geometry of the granodiorite in relation to ore, the intrusion must have played a fundamental structural role in the development of mineralization.

Dikes and sills of Tertiary hypabyssal rocks have been intersected in drill cores. These younger units were devoid of primary copper mineralization, but, during subsequent oxidation, quartz latite, andesite, and basalt acted as local precipitating hosts to copper-bearing solutions. During Tertiary-Quaternary time faulting and burial occurred. The major portion of the deposit, between the Sidewinder fault and the Party Line fault, was buried under 500 to 550 ft. of flat-lying conglomerate and 50 to 70 ft. of recent fluvial deposits and caliche. The conglomerate is a poorly sorted terrestrial deposit consisting of sub-angular fragments of many different rock types. Volcanic clasts are numerous. This formation, correlative with the Big Dome Conglomerate near Kearny, is continuous over the orebody. Basalt flows are locally interbedded with the conglomerate.

Structure

Since the deposit is entirely covered by conglomerate and alluvium, all structural interpretation has been made using vertical drill hole data and mapping in the underground pilot mine. Structures have been determined by offsets and irregularities in bedrock, the oxide-sulfide interface, dikes, and orezone boundaries. Depth to bedrock is uniform over most of the deposit, with downward displacement in the west and southwest, forming a graben. The oxidation surface in most cases reflects the contour of bedrock depth. Depressions in the interface are caused by weathering along fractures and breccias. These depressions, along with displacements in the oxide-sulfide interface, are used as indicators of structure.

The continuity of dikes between drill holes has been

difficult to establish. The granodiorite porphyry Type III dike, striking east-northeast and dipping steeply south, is the most consistent and reliable marker unit in the deposit. Other granodiorite porphyry dikes and intrusions, along with a few diabase and andesite dikes, have been delineated, but their lateral extent is somewhat localized. Offsets of ore-grade material in areas where uniformity was expected have yielded evidence for the location of structure. Faulting and fracturing observed underground in the pilot mine (Fig. 18.2) show a preferred east-northeast orientation, but no major offsets are apparent. The most evident period of faulting in the deposit is associated with Basin and Range orogenesis. This stage of faulting was responsible for north and northwest-trending faults, downthrown to the west.

The east boundary of the orebody is defined by the Party Line fault, which strikes N35°W and dips 45 to 55° SW. Drilling through the Party Line fault has intersected gouge material up to 100 ft. thick, and major changes in rock type, alteration, and/or mineralization have been encountered. High permeability along the fault plane resulted in a depression of the oxide-sulfide interface, with isolated pockets of oxide and sulfide materials in the hanging wall (Fig. 18.3). The Party Line fault has a strike length of 3,600 ft. (extending outside drilled areas) and a vertical displacement exceeding 1,000 ft. Minor offsets of andesite dikes indicate several stages of movement. Late Tertiary basalts were intruded along the fault zone.

Two thousand feet west of the Party Line fault, a zone of *en echelon,* normal, north-striking faults dips 45°W and vertically displaces the deposit downward as much as 1,200 ft. This zone can be projected three miles north of the deposit; displacement of 800 to 1,500 ft. has been found in the zone. The footwall boundary of this zone is known as the Sidewinder fault and is defined by differential displacements of bedrock, lithologic units, and mineralization. At the north edge of the deposit bedrock appears to be displaced 250 ft., whereas some dikes have been vertically dropped 1,200 ft. Displacements diminish toward the south edge, indicating possible hinge movement. Seven hundred feet west of the Sidewinder fault bedrock has been offset as much as 1,400 ft., west side down.

Offsets of dikes between drill holes indicate possible additional faulting in the deposit, but the existence of displacing structures has not been determined with any reliability. Analysis of underground mapping of joints and faults and computer search through drill-hole geologic logs for planar surfaces have revealed that there is a close correlation between joint and fault attitudes. The broad, large-scale structures, like the Party Line and Sidewinder faults, strike north to N50°W and dip 45 to 55° west to southeast. Older structures striking N70°E and dipping steeply have been offset by these features and are generally less persistent. The permeability created by this fault pattern seems to be responsible for the irregular oxide-sulfide contact that is encountered in pilot mining.

Rotation or tilting of the orebody is a possibility, but present information is inconclusive. If rotation of the orebody did take place, it must have been before oxidation occurred and prior to, or contemporaneous with, deposition of the Whitetail (?) Conglomerate, because the oxide-sulfide interface is nearly horizontal.

The Party Line and Sidewinder faults divide the orebody into three parts. On the east in the footwall of the Party Line fault, it is 400 to 600 ft. thick toward the north, and its subtle layers of varying grade are horizontal. Most of the orebody is contained in a central block between the Party Line and Sidewinder faults, where the thickness of the ore zone exceeds 2,000 ft. In it, the layers of varying grade are conformable with the granodiorite. On the far west, in the hanging wall of the Sidewinder fault, the grade layers dip westerly with the fault and are terminated by a bedrock-conglomerate (fault scarp) contact. Here the alluvium-conglomerate overburden thickens to 1,250 ft.

Alteration Zones

Intense hydrothermal alteration accompanied metalization and apparently had a genetic relationship with the complex granodiorite porphyry intrusions. The alteration zone boundaries were evidently not strongly affected by contacts between the quartz monzonite host and the granodiorite porphyry complex. Alteration in the granodiorite porphyries seems to be more strongly veinlet-controlled than that in the quartz monzonite porphyry. The alteration zoning pattern is roughly concentric and symmetrical around the deposit in plan, as well as in cross section (see Fig. 18.2). The pattern is interrupted by erosion and bedrock displacement due to faulting.

The types of alteration in the rocks composing the ore deposit are classified on the basis of the dominant species in assemblages of secondary minerals, as follows: potassic zone (quartz-orthoclase-biotite-sericite), sericitic zone (quartz-sericite-pyrite), propylitic zone (calcite-chlorite-epidote), and argillic zone (kaolinite-montmorillonite-sericite). Volumetrically, the potassic zone predominates.

Potassic Zone. Dimensions of the potassic zone in plan view exceed 3,600 ft. in an east-northeast direction and 3,000 ft. north-northwest at the widest point. The maximum vertical dimension reaches 2,500 ft. Longitudinally, the zone is shaped like a prolate ellipsoid, being thin or non-existent in the north-northeast, thicker in the center, and thinning again to an undetermined thickness in the west as a result of post-ore faulting. The zone dips gently to the southwest as a cylinder enveloped by sericitic alteration. Alteration is distinguished by pervasive and/or veinlet-controlled replacement of the primary minerals by secondary orthoclase, biotite, sericite, rutile, magnetite, and chlorite. There is a high chalcopyrite:pyrite ratio, and molybdenite is commonly present. Alteration is characterized by a large-scale addition of potassium occurring with microveinlet quartz as orthoclase fillings in primary rocks. Primary orthoclase is flesh-colored; secondary orthoclase is slightly orange with a cloudy texture. Plagioclases are commonly replaced along corroded edges by irregularly shaped orthoclase lenses.

Secondary biotite in the potassic zone occurs as brown or green, shreddy anhedral clusters, and replaces plagioclase phenocrysts and groundmass feldspars. It is also associated with sulfides in thin, discontinuous zones along microveinlets. Biotite-chlorite microveinlets with magnetite, sulfides,

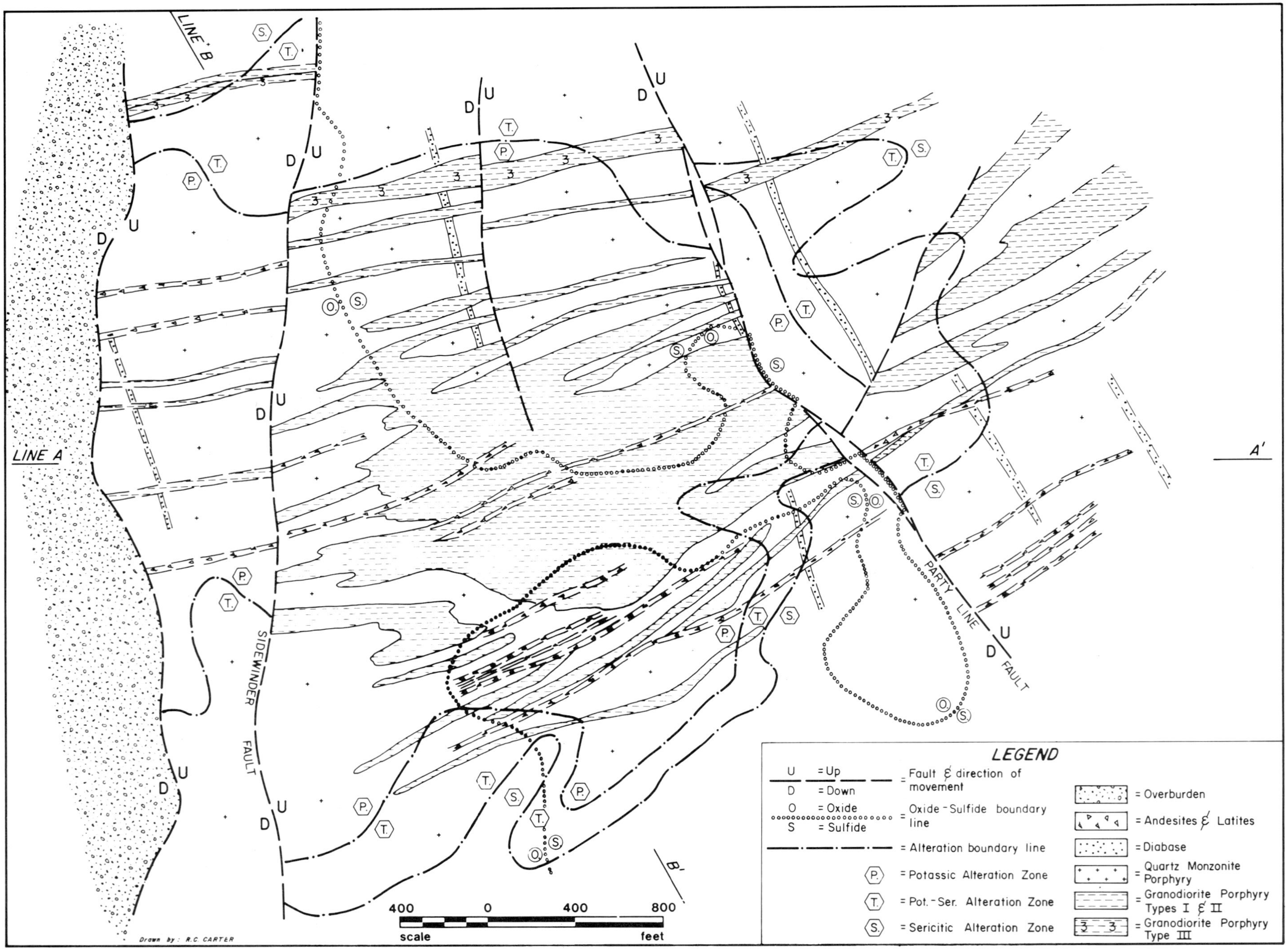

Figure 18.2. Generalized geology of 600-ft. elevation, Poston Butte porphyry copper deposit

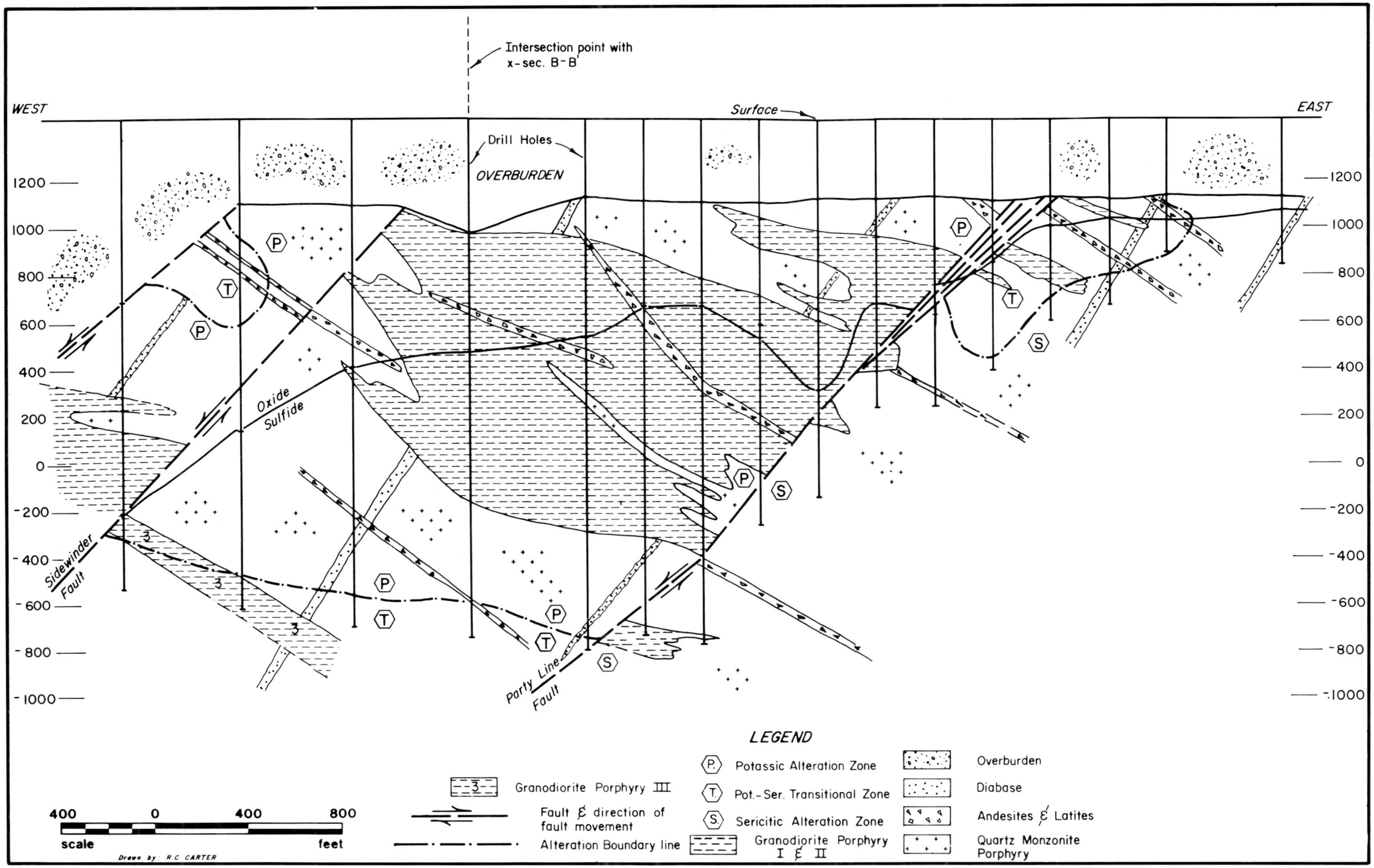

Figure 18.3. Generalized geologic cross section along line A-A', Poston Butte porphyry copper deposit

and rutile are sparingly encountered. Black, euhedral grains have been megascopically observed rimming secondary orthoclase, which, in turn, rims primary orthoclase. Chlorite intergrowth with biotite is common. Plagioclases are partially altered to fine sericite and carbonate, and replacement by secondary orthoclase along crystal edges is also common. Carbonate is a vein component associated with opaques; it is also an alteration product of plagioclase. Minor anhydrite is associated with carbonate in quartz veins.

Sericitic Zone. A sericitic alteration zone envelops the potassic zone, except where it has been planed off by erosion. It is represented by a mineralogic assemblage of quartz, sericite, pyrite, and minor rutile and apatite. Horizontal widths of the envelope vary from 500 ft. at the southern edge to 2,500 ft. at the eastern and northwestern edges. The vertical extent is unknown, due to its erosion from above the potassic zone, but at depth it has been encountered for 2,300 ft. below the potassic zone in the footwall of the Party Line fault. It is co-extensive with abundant pyrite, which generally occurs as vein material or as replacement aggregates in biotite sites. Chalcopyrite and molybdenite contents are low and variable, occurring in limited amounts in pyrite-quartz-sericite veinlets. Fine-grained sericite completely replaces plagioclase, orthoclase, and biotite and also forms alteration halos about quartz-pyrite veins. The degree of sericitization is gradational between potassic/sericitic and sericitic/propylitic "transition" zones. Total sulfide content increases with higher pyrite:chalcopyrite ratios.

Propylitic Zone. The propylitic zone represents the fringe alteration of the orebody. Its limits, although not delineated, appear extensive. This alteration is weaker in degree than the potassic and sericitic alterations and is lowest in total sulfides, averaging 1 percent pyrite. The mineralogic assemblage consists of epidote, sericite, carbonate, chlorite, and quartz. Accessories are rutile, magnetite, pyrite, adularia, and zeolites. Plagioclases are 10 to 70 percent altered to sericite and quartz, with minor amounts of carbonate and epidote along cleavage boundaries. Fine-grained pyrite is found as an alteration product and as vein material. Pyrite is disseminated in the wall rock, replacing magnetite and, locally, biotite. Traces of chalcopyrite are found in association with pyrite along thin veinlets.

Argillic Zone. Late-stage argillic alteration is present as a superposition of clays and sericite upon pre-existing alteration types. It is extensive throughout the oxidized zone as a response to oxidation of sulfides and the conversion of sericite to clay under acidic supergene conditions. It is characterized by the conversion of plagioclases to montmorillonite and kaolinite. Orthoclase is stable, except in cases where argillization is superimposed upon sericitic alteration and orthoclase has previously been destroyed. Other supergene clay minerals rarely present are halloysite, allophane, and illite. Argillization is found to be most prevalent along fractures in all alteration zones.

Mineralization

The deposit is divided into two major mineralogical zones, oxide and sulfide, with a thin irregular zone of secondary enrichment at the oxide-sulfide contact. The oxidized copper-bearing material makes up roughly one-third of the total thickness of the deposit and about one-half the total volume. The average thickness of the oxide zone is 400 ft., with a range of 100 to 1,000 ft. Many faults have been postulated from the linearity of the contact, but only two (Sidewinder and Party Line) have been confirmed through drilling. Permeable fault zones allowed meteoric waters to percolate into the mineralized ground locally, creating mixed, supergene oxide, and sulfide ores.

The most common type of copper oxide mineralization occurs as fine-grained chrysocolla adsorbed on the surface of residual clays after plagioclase. This material is easily leached and does not appear to be a replacement phenomenon. Massive chrysocolla occurs on fractures or as vein fillings. In some instances it forms botryoidal coatings in vugs along fractures. Minor oxide minerals are cuprite, native copper, azurite, brochantite, and shattuckite. "Copper wad" occurs as dendritic, occasionally reniform, sooty coatings on fracture surfaces. It is composed of an amorphous-appearing mixture of hydrous manganese oxide and copper. Rarely are there coatings more than ⅛-in. thick.

Deposition of oxide mineralization is dependent on the porosity and permeability of the host rock. Minute fractures in the quartz monzonite and granodiorite allowed leach solutions access to the primary sulfide minerals and the feldspar sites. Fractures and some late, hypabyssal intrusions commonly have high copper values in the oxide zone but are barren in the sulfide zone. Where fracturing is weak, there is a gradational infusion of copper oxides into a barren core.

The grade of the oxidized ore at Florence is nearly the same as that of the primary ore. The reason for this is the low total sulfide content and low pyrite:chalcopyrite ratio. Only minor addition or subtraction of copper took place, except in the sericitic zones, where the pyrite:chalcopyrite ratio was higher. Chalcocite mineralization as much as 300 ft. thick has been encountered.

The thin, secondarily enriched zone, which does not exceed 40 ft. except along faults, is testimony that little mobility has taken place in the oxidation process. Hypogene alteration of the rock exposed in the pilot mine is potassic, and the pyrite content is low.

It was observed in underground development that the oxide-sulfide interface was more irregular than had been projected from drill-hole core samples. The east-west drift at the 800-ft. level was in and out of sulfide-oxide material for a length of 500 ft. Small, structural features in this zone had strong, localized effects on the distribution of oxidation. Oxide mineralization at the interface is characterized by chrysocolla, native copper, "copper wad", limonite, and abundant cuprite and chalcotrichite. The cuprite is usually smeared on fracture surfaces. Secondary sulfides—in the form of black, sooty, chalcocite coatings replacing pyrite and chalcopyrite in fracture fillings—frequently admix with oxides and silicates.

The main mass of granodiorite porphyry intrusions is almost completely within the potassic zone (Fig. 18.4). Although chalcopyrite:pyrite ratios are essentially the same in the granodiorite porphyry as in the quartz monzonite porphyry, total sulfide distribution is significantly different.

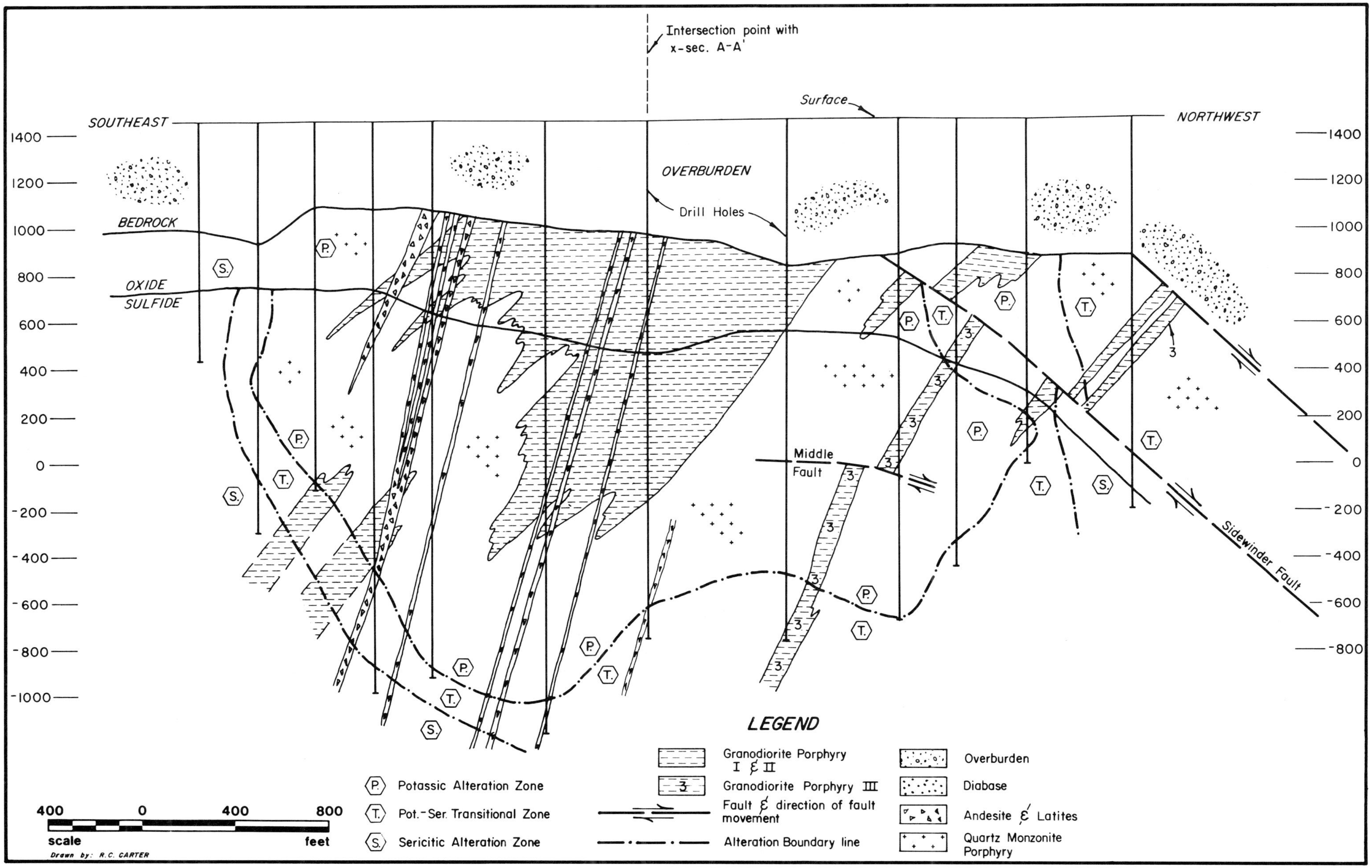

Figure 18.4. Generalized geologic cross section along line B-B', Poston Butte porphyry copper deposit

Grades of ore in quartz monzonite porphyry adjacent to the granodiorite porphyry are usually better than grades in the granodiorite, by a factor of two. The higher copper grades found in the mixed zones at the contact between granodiorite porphyry and quartz monzonite porphyry indicate that the granodiorite porphyry emplacement controlled the distribution of primary-grade copper to a high degree.

Sulfide mineralization is very simple, consisting of chalcopyrite, pyrite, and molybdenite, with minor quantities of chalcocite and covellite. Bornite, galena, and sphalerite have been recorded but are very rare. Pyrite and chalcopyrite occur as veins and veinlets along fracture surfaces and as disseminated grains, often intimately associated with biotite. Mapping in the pilot mine has indicated that most mineralized fractures trend to the northeast. Specularite and vuggy quartz are common in these fractures. Microveinlets of chalcopyrite frequently cut orthoclase phenocrysts in the quartz monzonite porphyry. Veins containing chalcopyrite, pyrite, and molybdenite are commonly high in quartz and rimmed with secondary potassic feldspar and sericite.

Ore-Localizing Factors

Regional structures and their intersections suggest possible zones of weakness which could have influenced emplacement of the granodiorite porphyry complex and succeeding mineralizing fluids. The ore at Florence is in siliceous rock, but physical structures seem to have controlled the copper mineralization. The fractured contacts between the granodiorite porphyry and the quartz monzonite porphyry appear to have been the main *loci* for better mineralization. It is suggested that the ore solutions were channeled through highly fractured contact zones and dissipated through a narrowing stockwork away from the contacts.

Underground mapping indicates that northeasterly oriented fractures seem to be preferentially, but not exclusively, mineralized. Dissemination of the ore leads to the conclusion that hydrothermal ore solutions were also introduced along grain boundaries and cleavages after complete crystallization of the granodiorite porphyry. The Florence orebody is also a result of supergene factors. Pre-oxide faulting and fracturing were of paramount importance to the distribution of oxidation.

Orogenesis

Radiometric dating has placed the intrusion of the granodiorite complex in the Laramide Revolution (62 m.y. ago); this date is similar to other porphyry deposits related to the Sonoran Copper subprovince (Titley, 1972). Emplacement of the granodiorite probably took place under pressure along pre-Laramide linear structures. The porphyritic nature of the granodiorite indicates two stages of crystallization: a deep phase yielding medium-grained plagioclase crystals, followed by rapid injection to shallow depths with a sharp drop in pressure and temperature creating a fine groundmass.

Fracturing, related to the intrusion of the granodiorite and possibly superimposed on earlier regional structures, created stockwork channels that opened the way for hydrothermal solutions. It is possible that upon emplacement of the granodiorite, solidification commenced rapidly at the contacts followed by slower crystallization in the center. Textural differences within the granodiorite porphyry complex could be attributed to fluctuations in magma pressure. Local narrow breccia pipes have been noted, especially along contacts, which could be the result of pressure fluctuations and local slumping or collapse. Upon cooling there was probably differential contraction between the granodiorite porphyry and the quartz monzonite porphyry, which created innumerable thin cracks throughout both rock types, but especially at their contacts.

During the final stages of crystallization of the molten granodiorite, copper, iron, and sulfur were concentrated into a residual aqueous solution. Distribution of the ore and hydrothermal alteration zones followed the zones of weakness described above. The fluids migrated through the more permeable zones and precipitated primarily in the quartz monzonite porphyry.

SUMMARY

A small outcrop of leached capping focused the attention of Conoco geologists on the Florence deposit in 1969. Since that time 273,000 feet of vertical drill core and a mile of underground drifting have exposed an orebody which is structurally complex but remarkably uniform and consistent in mineralogy and grade.

The deposit is totally covered by post-mineral conglomerates and recent alluvium. Primary ore controls are predominantly structural and are numerous and complex. The oldest unit is a Precambrian quartz monzonite porphyry, which is part of the Oracle Granite batholith. This unit was intruded by diabase dikes of late Precambrian age. Subsequent emplacement of the Laramide granodiorite porphyries (about 62 m.y. ago) and the associated hydrothermal alteration and mineralization were followed by the introduction of a variety of hypabyssal rocks, including basalt, andesite, and felsic units of Tertiary age. The hypabyssal rocks are devoid of primary copper mineralization.

Porphyry copper mineralization is associated with both supergene and hypogene alteration zones. Hydrothermal alteration patterns are elliptical in plan and show distinct patterns similar to those in other porphyry copper deposits (Lowell and Guilbert, 1970). Hypogene alteration above the ore-bearing core is complicated by faulting, tilting (?), and oxidation.

Supergene alteration in the deposit is shown in a well-developed argillic zone, where weathering produced clays, iron oxides, and acid-soluble copper silicates and oxides. The oxide ore is composed mainly of chrysocolla and copper-bearing clays, with minor amounts of cuprite and "wad"; mineralization is distributed along veinlets in fracture fillings and in replaced plagioclase sites.

The oxide and sulfide portions of the orebody are discrete, but there is a narrow zone of mixing and chalcocite enrichment at the interface. Primary sulfide minerals include chalcopyrite, pyrite, molybdenite, and some minor amounts of bornite. They are distributed in stockwork veinlets and disseminations in quartz monzonite porphyry, granodiorite porphyry, and diabase.

ACKNOWLEDGMENTS

Appreciation is expressed to Bill F. Kern, Conoco Senior Geologist, and the late Robert E. Anderson, exploration Project Manager, whose team of geologists laid the interpretive groundwork of the Florence porphyry copper deposit geology. Acknowledgment is made to Adolph V. Mitterer, Manager of Mining and Milling; W. A. Petersen, Manager of Metallics Exploration; and Alex F. Bissett, Project Manager, Florence, for generously giving their time for review of this study. Credit is also given to Rikard C. Carter, who drafted the illustrations. The writers wish to thank the Continental Oil Company for permission to publish.

REFERENCES CITED

Balla, J. C., 1972, The Relationship of Laramide stocks to regional structure in central Arizona: Unpub. Ph.D. Diss., Univ. of Ariz., 138p.

Krieger, M. H.; Cornwall, H. R.; and Banks, N. G., 1974, The Big Dome Formation and revised Tertiary stratigraphy in the Ray-San Manuel area, Arizona: U.S. Geol. Survey Bull. 1394-A, p.A54–A62.

Lowell, J. D., and Guilbert, J. M., 1970, Lateral and vertical alteration-mineralization in porphyry ore deposits: Econ. Geol., v. 65, p.373–408.

Ransome, F. L., 1903, Geology of the Globe copper district, Arizona: U.S. Geol. Survey Prof. Paper 12, 168p.

Sell, J. D., 1968, Correlation of some post-Laramide Tertiary units, Globe (Gila County) to Gila Bend (Maricopa County), Arizona, *in* Titley, S. R., ed., Southern Arizona Guidebook III: Arizona Geol. Soc., p.69–74.

Titley, S. R., 1972, Some geological criteria applicable to the search for southwestern North American porphyry copper deposits: AIME-MMIJ Joint Meeting, Tokyo, Japan, May 24–27, Preprint GI2, New York, N.Y., AIME, 12p.

Turner, G. L., 1962, The Deming Axis—southeastern Arizona, New Mexico and Trans-Pecos, Texas: *in* Weber, R. G., and Pierce, H. W., eds., Guidebook of the Mogollon Rim Region, East-Central Arizona: New Mex. Geol. Soc., 13th Field Conference, p.59–71.

19

Some Features of Tectonic History and Ore Genesis in the Pima Mining District

PIMA COUNTY, ARIZONA

Spencer R. Titley

The Pima mining district, located near the Sierrita Mountains some 20 miles southwest of Tucson, Arizona, is one of the premier porphyry copper districts in the world. The deposits of the district are an important source not only of copper and molybdenum, but also of silver and—of potential importance in the 1980s—tungsten. A measure of the size and potential of the orebodies is provided by Greeley's (1978) estimate of designed copper capacity for 6 operations in the district: 371,000 tons of copper per year. In 1976 the mines of the district produced 303,000 short tons of copper (Greeley, 1978). This production was greater than that of any other district in North America. Totals of 67 years of production are shown on Table 19.1.

HISTORY

Extraction of the porphyry-related ores, in great part the result of discoveries since 1950, represents only the most recent activity in this old district. Situated on the west side of the valley of the Santa Cruz River (Fig. 19.1), the Pima district lies within a region, the Pimería Alta, that was extensively explored by the first Europeans who came north from Mexico in the seventeenth century. It may be among the oldest known mineral-bearing regions of North America. Documentation of mining activity in this region that may be of even earlier vintage is a difficult task. Minerals of value to native Americans, such as hematite and secondary copper minerals used as pigment, were and remain widely scattered in outcrop; some turquoise was present in the leached capping above the Esperanza Orebody. Notwithstanding Hinton's (1878, p. 116) statement that "Traces are not wanting of their [the ores] having been worked even anterior to the Spanish conquest of Mexico," made in his account of early Arizona, it seems unlikely that there was mining of any consequence prior to the arrival of the Spanish because most of the oxidized ores of the district required metallurgical beneficiation.

Table 19.1
Metal Production of the Pima Mining District
Pima County, Arizona
(1908–1975)

Cu (Tons)	Pb (Tons)	Zn (Tons)	Mo (Tons)	Ag (Tr. Oz.)	Au (Tr. Oz.)
2,842,498	43,587	116,564	91,592	40,361,000	58,668

Source: Data from Keith, et al., (1978).

The "Jesuit Fathers were the pioneer miners of Arizona" (Hamilton, 1884, p. 144), and discoveries made during their tenure in the valley during the eighteenth century apparently resulted in widespread prospecting and mining. It may be inferred that parties working out of the missions at Guevavi, Tumacacori, and San Xavier del Bac in the late 1600s and early 1700s ranged widely and explored the Santa Rita, Cerro Colorado, and Sierrita Mountains (see Fig. 19.1). However, only a few discoveries may be specifically related to this early activity, and it is not certain that the exposures of ores in the Sierrita Mountains were among them. Hamilton (1884, p. 144) has stated that there is reason to believe that the early mining was prosecuted on an "extensive scale," as evidenced from the presence of old tunnels and shafts located in the mountains surrounding these missions. It "is known that Jesuits opened mines in the latter part of the eighteenth century" (Hamilton, 1884, p. 226), and the presence of arastres at the Guevavi Mission, which was abandoned before 1784, indicates that ores were beneficiated in those early times—perhaps as early as 1748, when the first records of mining indicate the San Pedro mine to have been worked by the Spanish (Hinton, 1878).

Mining and exploration activity in the Santa Cruz valley and adjacent regions flourished and waned through many cycles that marked political, economic and social change. These events included the effects of orders and regulations promulgated when the region was part of New Spain. During this period, the Jesuits were expelled by royal order and replaced by Franciscian friars; Kessel (1976) has noted, however, that there is no evidence that the Franciscans were less zealous than the Jesuits in any of their endeavors. Other changes included the revolt of 1810, which resulted in the separation of Mexico from Spain; the treaty of Guadalupe Hidalgo in 1848, which ceded lands north of the Gila River to the United States; the American Civil War; and intermittent periods when Apache Indian attacks forced halts in mining and prospecting. Following the time of the Gadsden Purchase, when the region became part of the United States,

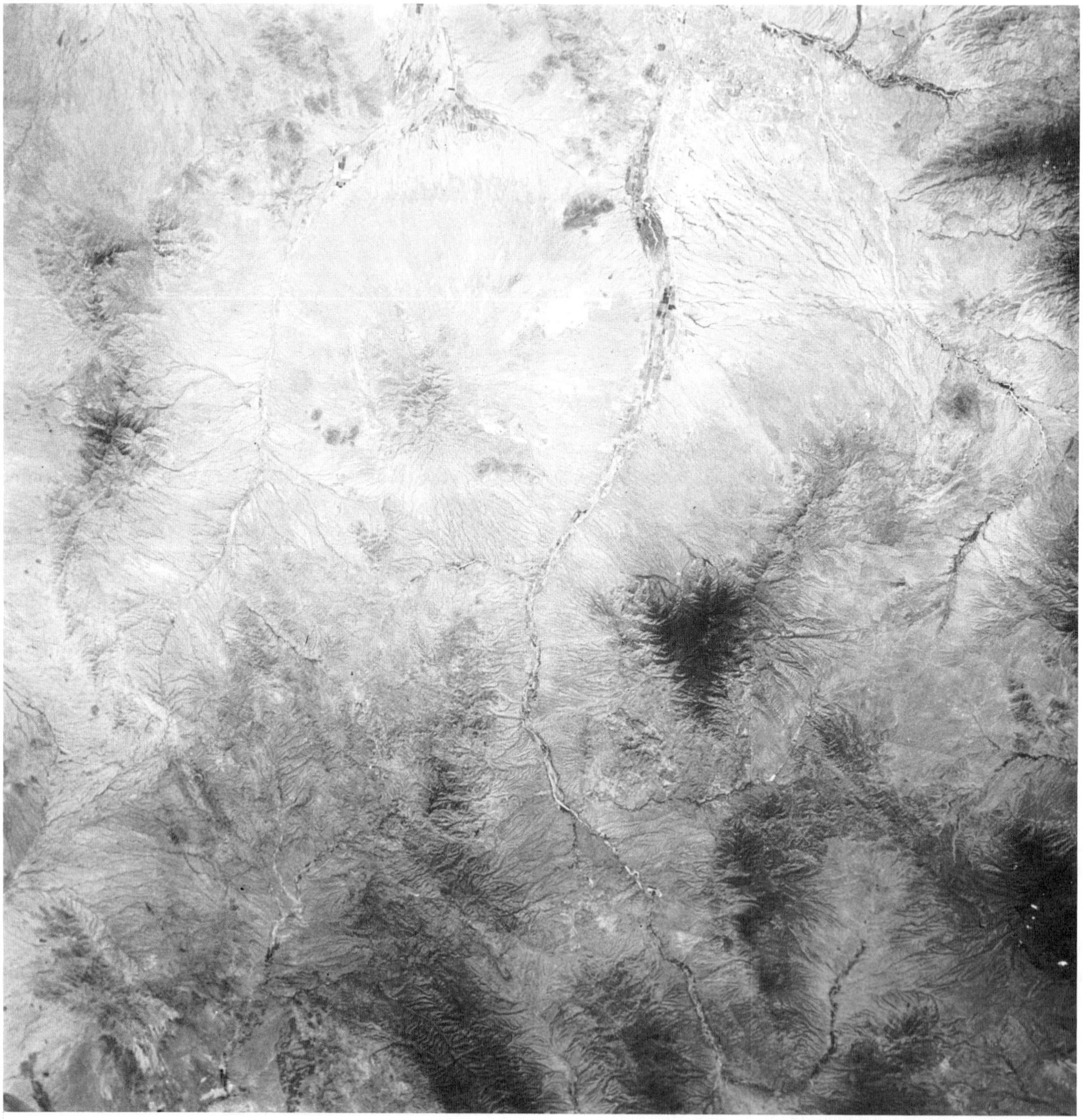

Figure 19.1. The Pima mining district and surrounding area: *above,* aerial photograph taken on the Gemini IV Mission (1964); *right,* planimetric map of the area shown in photograph (same general orientation). The photograph predates stripping for the Twin Buttes and Sierrita mines. White patches on the eastern flank of the Sierrita Mountains are dumps from the Pima-Mission complex (north) and the Esperanza mine (south). Locations of the missions shown on the map are from the data of Kessell (1970).

and extending to about the time of the beginning of the American Civil War when protection of troops was withdrawn, mining in the Sierrita Mountains and nearby ranges recommenced. The Cerro Colorado mine, south of the Sierritas, once again became active. First discoveries in the San Xavier lode are not recorded, but this old mine, said by Hinton (1878, p. 119) to have been "long known and partially worked by Mexicans," may have been a site of renewed mining activity. By 1859 the company operating the San Xavier mine was doing satisfactorily (Wagoner, 1975). The "modern" period of mining did not begin until pacification of the Apache Indians and their movement onto reservations in 1874. The Pima mining district was formally established in 1877 (Mayuga, 1942).

For the next 35 years, mines of the district were operated at modest to intense scales. Claims were staked in the north

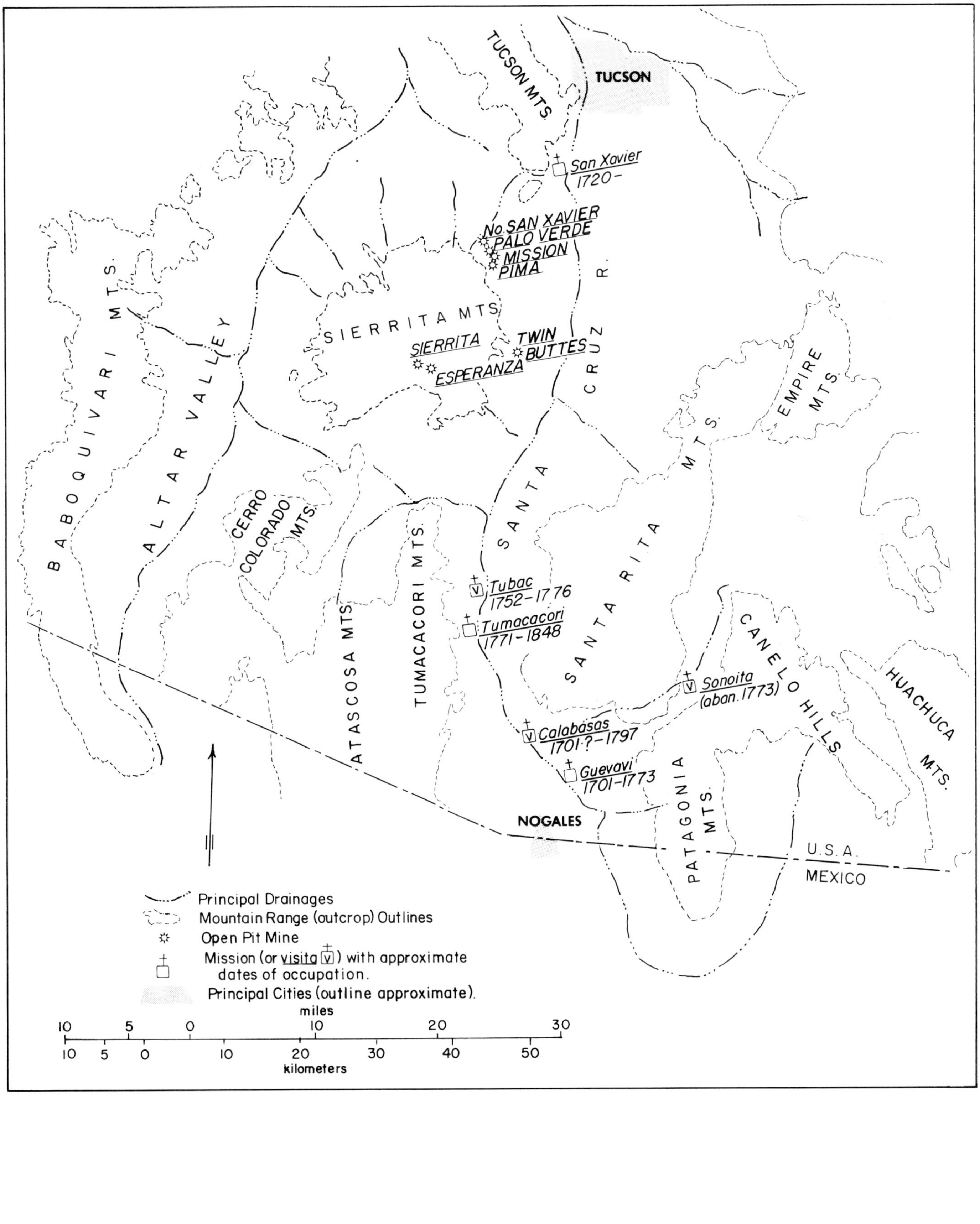

part of the district at Mineral Hill by 1882, and the San Xavier mine continued in operation. Orebodies in the south part of the district, at Twin Buttes, were discovered and under active exploitation by 1907. At the same time as the discovery and working of the carbonate-hosted replacement ores at Mineral Hill, San Xavier, and Twin Buttes, copper-lead-silver veins in volcanic rocks were being worked at these three deposits; the Olivette and Annette Groups were located in 1886. Mayuga (1942) has noted that the activity in the district of the early 1880s seems to have coincided with waning activity at Tombstone, when prospectors turned their efforts elsewhere.

By the time of Ransome's (1922) visit to the district in 1920 much activity had ceased and, although the San Xavier mine continued to operate intermittently during the next 35 years, it was not until 1950, when the Banner Mining Company purchased and took up extensive claim holdings in both north and south ends of the district that activity was renewed on a large scale. The Mineral Hill mine was put back into production and exploration recommenced in the Twin Buttes mines. In 1950, the Pima Orebody was discovered beneath alluvium by geophysical methods (Thurmond et al., 1954) and was stripped for open-pit mining by 1955. This discovery heralded a decade of widespread exploration in the district. By 1960, the Banner Mining Company had drifted 1,500 ft. eastward on the 500-ft. level of the Copper Glance mine (Kalt, 1968) and had drilled through alluvium into the disseminated copper mineralization of the Twin Buttes Orebody. The Duval Corporation had begun mining the Esperanza Orebody and the Mission mine was under development. Several other discoveries were made and developments were undertaken in the period of the mid-1950s to 1960s, including the Palo Verde Orebody and San Xavier Extensions of the Mission Orebody in the northern part of the district and the Sierrita mine in the southern part of the district. Thus, the period since 1950 marks the latest chapter of many in the history of this old district. The history reveals the building of one discovery upon another, and this process, combined with advances in technology and changing economic conditions, has brought the district through a typical sequence of exploration and exploitation. This sequence ranges from the early stages of mining shallow precious metal ores, through underground mining of complex base and precious metal ores, to the mining of disseminated copper ores based on advanced technology for handling bulk materials.

GEOLOGIC SETTING

The Pima mining district occurs in a faulted complex of sedimentary, volcanic, and plutonic rocks that lies along the eastern pediment surface of the Sierrita Mountains. The mountain range is distinguished from adjacent and nearby ranges not only by the wealth of copper that was deposited, but also by the presence of many regionally anomalous geologic characteristics. The topographically elevated mass of the central part of the range consists chiefly of Mesozoic volcanic and sedimentary rocks, with smaller exposures of Laramide plutonic rocks and remnants of older Mesozoic plutons. The major porphyry copper deposits of the district occur in close association with Laramide plutons in the rock complex. This succession of rocks is topographically depressed and is exposed along the edge of the pediment bedrock surface as groups of ridges and isolated hills. With the exception of rocks at the Sierrita-Esperanza deposit, which are exposed high on the pediment, all other porphyry copper deposits and their faulted parts were buried beneath 60 to 125 m of poorly indurated, poorly sorted slope debris and alluvium of Holocene and Pleistocene(?) age that overlie thin, indurated beds of possible Miocene-Pliocene age.

The mountain range is anomalous if compared with the prevailing geomorphology of the region. The range, as expressed by topography and outcrop, is roughly circular and does not reveal the pronounced NNE-N-NNW elongation of Basin and Range land forms that lie east, north, and west of it (see Fig. 19.1). Further, the low, relatively subdued topography of the mountains and their low relief (ca. 1 km) contrasts with the prominent ridges and higher relief (ca. 2 km) of adjacent ranges. Although the response to weathering of the granodiorite core of the Sierrita Mountains may have been different from that of the igneous rocks of the cores of nearby mountains, the morphology of the range is not readily explainable in the context of prevailing ideas of Basin and Range tectonism, a tectonic framework that resulted in development of generally narrow, north-trending, fault-block mountains.

Contrasted further, the Sierrita Mountains are the site of an unusually complete succession of the thick volcanic and clastic rock sequences representing all systems of the Mesozoic. This complete sequence occurs in very few ranges of southeastern Arizona. The Mesozoic rocks present reveal a history of episodic volcanic activity, and the southeastern part of the mountain range has been the site of repeated emplacement of plutons and batholiths representing at least four periods of intrusive activity since the Late Triassic. Field and radiometric age data also reveal evidence for repeated tectonic activity that resulted in numerous angular unconformities within the section during the Mesozoic, in Laramide time, and in the Cenozoic. Although some of the tectonic activity may be ascribed to movement along some less well exposed faults, the mountain range is bisected by the projection of a major regional fault whose trace is exposed– both as a fault zone and as a series of inherited structures— southeast of the district. (see Fig. 19.1). This structure, the Sawmill Canyon fault, was active at various times during the Mesozoic.

Precambrian basement is exposed in a few places in the district, and where present it consists of granitoid rocks. However, the district lies in a part of southern Arizona where Pinal schist (ca. 1,620 m.y. old [Silver, 1978]) is believed to have been widely present (Titley, 1982). Remnants of the schist may now be present as inclusions of roof pendants in younger (ca. 850 ±100 m.y. old [Marvin et al., 1973]) Precambrian intrusions. In the Santa Rita Mountains, adjacent to the east, a similar-appearing granitic rock, the Continental Granodiorite, occurs which has been dated radiometrically at 1,360 to 1,450 m.y. (Marvin et al., 1973). The younger date for the intrusion in the Sierrita Mountains may be a result of resetting.

During the Paleozoic, the region of the Sierrita Mountains lay on the periphery of a basin to the east. The strata of the deeper parts of this basin attained a thickness of up to 2,000 m of carbonate-dominated sedimentary rocks. Isopachs of the Paleozoic suggest that a thickness of 1,500 to 1,700 m of Paleozoic rocks occured over the present location of the Sierrita Mountains. Even though the Paleozoic is thinner in the Pima district, most formations of this era present elsewhere in southeastern Arizona are present, including those of youngest recognized Permian age. An additional noteworthy feature of the Paleozoic is the presence of a section of interlayered dolomite and anhydrite in the Permian section. These rocks are part of the mineralized Paleozoic section in the Twin Buttes and Mission deposits. The deposits of the Pima District are interpreted as lying along the edge of a northwest-trending Permian basin in which the evaporites were accumulated (Butler, 1971; Titley, 1982).

Regional distribution of Mesozoic rocks is shown in Figure 19.2. The pattern of their distribution hints strongly at structural control—in the case of Triassic and Jurassic sections, by a regional fault, and, for the Lower Cretaceous strata, by a deep basin possibly controlled by basement tectonics. In the Sierrita Mountains, the thickness of the Mesozoic section is unknown but may exceed 6,000 m (Cooper, 1971). The Sawmill Canyon fault appears to have influenced the distribution of thick Triassic-Jurassic volcanic and clastic sequences. The fault extends, by projection, into the Sierrita Mountains, where the continuation of that control is expressed in the influence on Mesozoic outcrop distribution. Rare and thinned exposures of these early Mesozoic rocks occur north of the Sawmill Canyon fault, but the thick sections and the most extensive exposures all lie south of the fault.

Lower Cretaceous strata correlative with the Bisbee Group (Hayes, 1970) occupy a deep basin whose western terminus lies some 25 km east of the Pima district (see Fig. 19.2). Possible lower Cretaceous strata are present in the Sierrita Mountains and are probably correlative with rocks of Bisbee Group age (Cooper, 1971), but, because of their marked difference from Bisbee Group lithologies—principally in their volcanic component—these rocks have been interpreted as foreland facies (Titley, 1972*a,* 1976). It is this foreland upon which many porphyry copper deposits of the region have evolved (Anderson, 1966; Titley, 1972*a*).

The Pima district is, thus, similar to other porphyry copper districts of southeastern Arizona in its setting on the edge of the basin of thick, lower Cretaceous strata. It is atypical, however, because of the presence of an unusually thick and complete section of Mesozoic strata, together with numerous volcanic sequences and plutons of pre-Laramide age. Further, it is one of the few districts in the Southwest where major linear structures may be shown to project into the location of a complex of igneous intrusions. Although these features may be shown on a regional scale and the

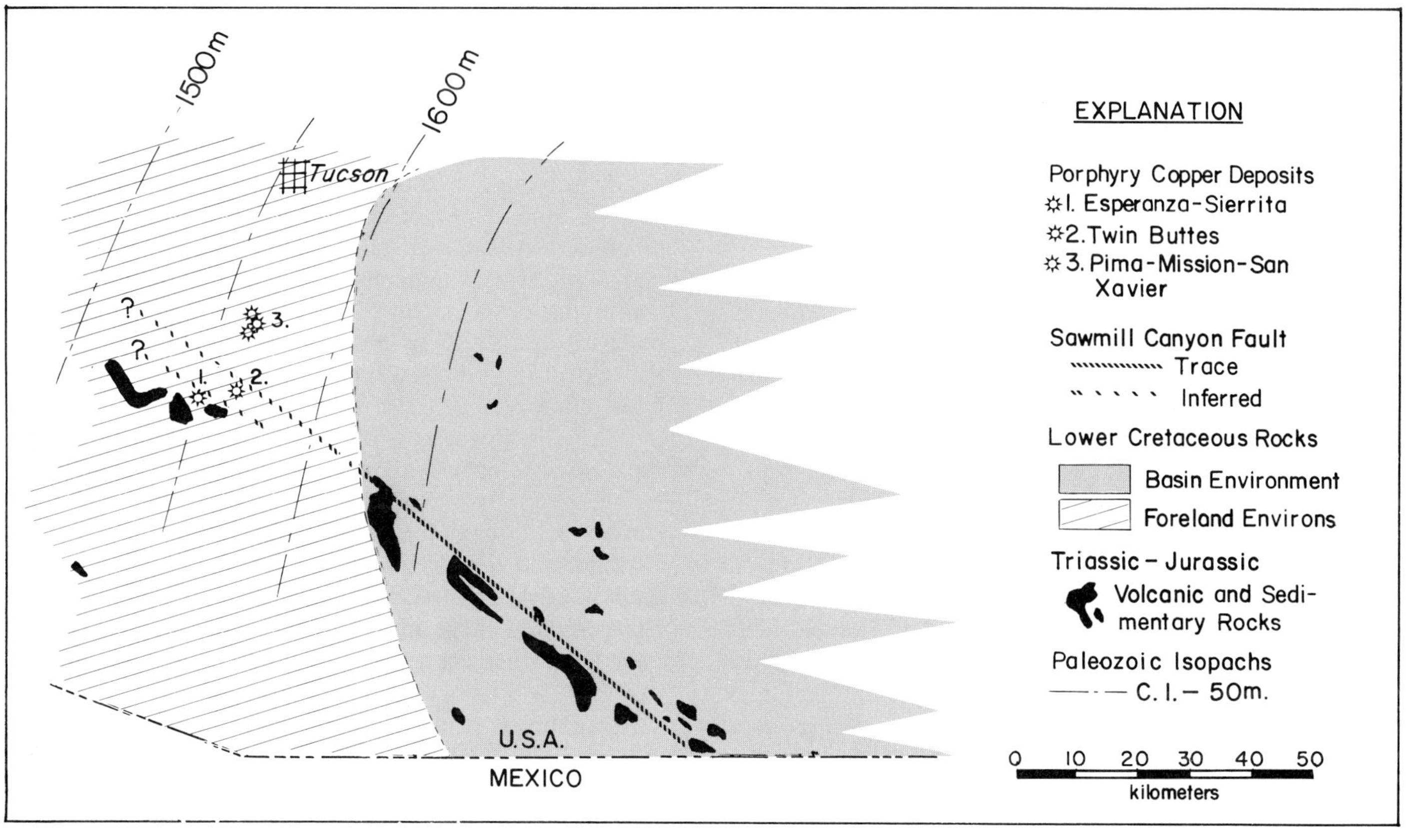

Figure 19.2. Principal characteristics of the pre-ore Phanerozoic geology of the Sierrita Mountains and adjacent environments. Paleozoic isopachs are modified from Titley (1982); distribution of Triassic and Jurassic strata includes some data from Hayes and Drewes (1978); and the distribution of Cretaceous strata is adapted in part from Hayes (1970) and Titley (1972*a*). Location and projection of the Sawmill Canyon fault based upon studies by the author.

relationship of the Pima district to them outlined, details of the geology of the district are complex and reflect the results of several episodes of igneous activity and tectonism.

PIMA DISTRICT GEOLOGY

A substantial body of geologic formation has been developed for the Pima mining district. Many papers have discussed ore deposit geology, as well as the stratigraphy of various parts of the Phanerozoic section. Because of the economic importance of post-ore deformation, numerous studies have dealt with the nature of Tertiary magmatism and faulting. Extensive radiometric age dating has been carried out on intrusions in the district and the results reported in many publications. The eastern part of the Sierrita Mountains, the Pima district, and parts of the district have been mapped at different scales and in varying detail. A geological map covering most of the district and adapted from many sources, but chiefly those of Cooper (1960, 1973), is shown in Figure 19.3.

Because of the existence in the district of plutons of older Mesozoic age and because of the presence of mid-Tertiary igneous rocks, mineralization episodes that may be both older and younger than the Laramide are suspect but have not been substantiated, even though some equivocal geologic relationships exist. The evidence developed through the 1970s indicates only one major metallization episode, that one in the Laramide: host rocks to mineralization are all of Laramide age or older. The Laramide event resulted in the evolution not only of the porphyry copper ores of the district, but also of other genetic types. These include both massive replacement and vein-controlled base and precious metal deposits in pyrometasomatically altered carbonate host rocks, replacement ores in clastic rocks, and vein-or vein-breccia–controlled deposits of silver-rich base metal ores in volcanic and volcaniclastic strata. Evolution of these genetic types appears to be in part related to some regional zoning, as well as to be controlled by host-rock type.

Following formation of the porphyry ores in the Laramide, the orebodies were faulted and displaced, probably since about 25 m.y. ago. Movement took place on a low-angle fault surface, the San Xavier "thrust" fault, and is interpreted to have transported the upper part of the Twin Buttes Orebody to the north some 10 km (Cooper, 1960). The upper part of this orebody is now interpreted to comprise the Pima–Mission–Palo Verde orebody complex. The base of this complex lies in low-angle to flat fault contact with granitic rock (cf. Jansen, 1982). These northern orebodies lie within an allochthonous plate whose southern edge lies just north of the Twin Buttes (see Fig. 19.3). The Twin Buttes and Sierrita-Esperanza orebodies are interpreted as authochthonous. Thus, consideration of Laramide and pre-Laramide tectonics and stratigraphy requires that the rocks of the allochthonous plate be restored to a position approximately 10 km south of their present location.

The geology of the Paleozoic for southeastern Arizona has been reported in many studies that consider a wide scale of detail and interpretation. This section occurs in the Pima district. Similarly, general features of the Precambrian for this same region have been reported. For these reasons, the following sections omit detailed consideration of these rocks and focus primarily upon Mesozoic and Tertiary rocks and their structural geology.

Mesozoic Stratigraphy and Geochronology

The Mesozoic column comprises volcanic, volcaniclastic, and immature clastic rock successions, as well as three recognized periods of intrusive igneous activity. The stratigraphic succession present in the eastern and southern Sierrita Mountains has been studied and mapped by various workers (the most encompassing synthesis is by Cooper [1971]). A summary that is more regional in scope and that includes rocks of the Sierrita Mountains has been prepared by Hayes and Drewes (1978). A summary of the named formations and intrusions, together with suggested stratigraphic correlations, and of Pima district intrusions and temporal intrusive correlatives is shown in Figure 19.4. Radiometric age assignments of Pima district strata are based mostly upon a correlation between lithologies of rocks in the Sierrita Mountains and dated rocks and strata of nearby ranges. Somewhat surprisingly, no radiometric ages had been reported for the variety of Mesozoic volcanic rocks of the Pima district by the end of the 1970s. However, the lithologic similarities, the stratigraphic succession of those rocks, and the limiting ages of the strata—based upon relationships to dated intrusions—bear strong similarities, if not identities, with dated rock sequences elsewhere; the age assignments and correlations appear to be generally consistent and are tentatively interpreted as valid.

Cooper (1971) suggested a dichotomy of Mesozoic strata based upon differences in units exposed in the northern and southern parts of the district. The separation, based upon differences in rocks present on the upper and lower plates of the San Xavier fault, was interpreted as resulting from different depositional environments on the southwest and northeast sides of a zone of active tectonism. Although such a separation may still be valid on the basis of distribution of one or two stratigraphic units, it is less distinctly so, because continuing development of exposures in open pits in both northern and southern parts of the district has revealed a wider distribution of strata than that originally interpreted from outcrop.

Triassic Rocks. In much of southeastern Arizona the Paleozoic-Mesozoic contact is marked by only a slight angular unconformity or a disconformity. In the Pima district the contact is a pronounced angular unconformity between the Permian and the Triassic and Triassic(?). The base of the section consists of a sequence of volcanic flows and pyroclastic rocks that range in composition from rhyolite through dacite and that are assigned to the Ox Frame Formation (Thoms, 1966; Cooper, 1971). This formation, known only in the southern part of the district, is correlated with the Mt. Wrightson Formation (Cooper, 1971), which has an imprecise age of 220 m.y. (Marvin et al., 1973). In the Twin Buttes mine, rocks possibly correlative with the Ox Frame Formation lie southeast of the main mass of mineralized rock (Barter and Kelly, 1982). West of the mine, however, and exposed in several areas of the southern Sierrita Mountains, the Ox Frame Formation is present, and it comprises an important

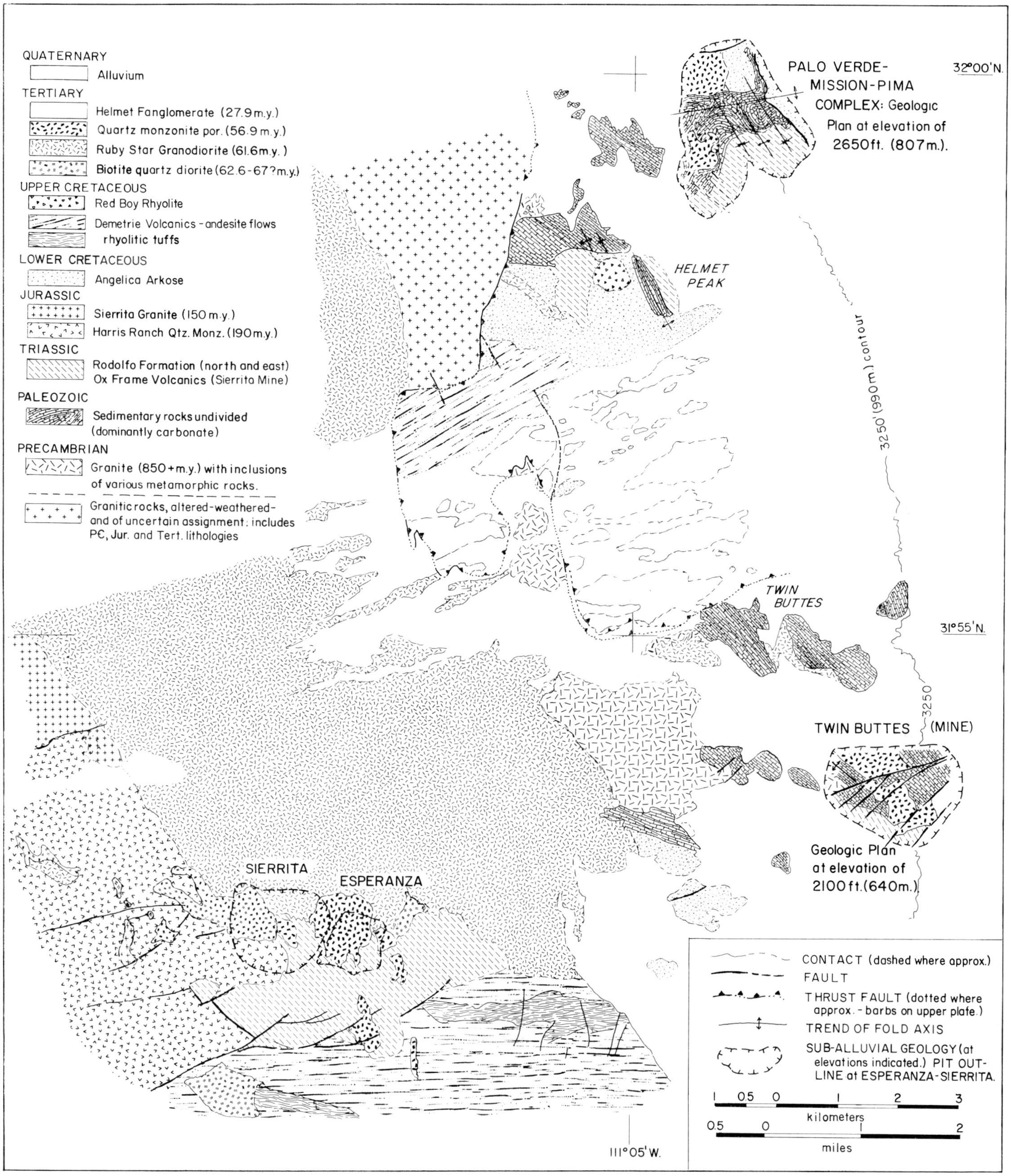

Figure 19.3. Geologic map of part of the Pima mining district. The map does not show the North San Xavier Orebody, which lies several km north of the area shown. The map base is that of Cooper (1973), with geologic modifications by the author from Barter and Kelly (1982), Cooper (1960, 1973), Jansen (1982), Lacy (1959), Lacy and Titley (1959, 1962), Langlois (1978), and Mayuga (1942).

INTRUSIONS: Temporal Correlatives — Radiometric Age	INTRUSIONS: Temporal Correlatives — Name	INTRUSIONS: Pima Mining District — Radiometric Age	INTRUSIONS: Pima Mining District — Name	STRATA: Pima Mining District — Name	STRATA: Stratigraphic Correlatives — Name	STRATA: Stratigraphic Correlatives — Radiometric Age	Geologic Age
	Many	53-58 58-61 63-67	Quartz monzonite porphyry Ruby Star Granodiorite Biotite quartz diorite				PALEOCENE
				Red Boy Rhyolite	Cat Mountain Rhyolite Roskruge Rhyolite Salero Formation (upper part)	66-70 69-74 72.5	UPPER CRETACEOUS
				Demetrie Volcanics	Salero Formation (lower part) Silver Bell Formation	— —	
				Angelica Arkose Whitcomb Quartzite	Amole Arkose		LOWER CRETACEOUS
145-160 150	Squaw Gulch Granite Dikes, Tucson Mtns.	140-150	Sierrita Granite				
				Stevens Mountain Rhyolite[(a)]	Canelo Hills Volcanics (in part)	ca. 173	JURASSIC
				Tascuela Red Beds[(b)]	do.	do.	
178 186-188	Gleeson Quartz Monzonite Juniper Flat Granite (Bisbee)	190	Harris Ranch Quartz Monzonite				
				Rodolfo Formation[(c)]	Gardner Canyon Formation Recreation Red Beds	192	TRIASSIC
				Ox Frame Volcanics[(d)]	Mt. Wrightson Formation	220	
				Rain Valley Formation	Rain Valley Formation		PERMIAN

NOTES: (a,b) Units of southwestern Sierrita Mtns.; assigned to Pima district by inferrence from presence of regional correlatives but eroded before deposition of Whitcomb Quartzite.
(c) Presence known only on upper plate of San Xavier fault in north part of district and in Twin Buttes deposit.
(d) Presence known only in south part of district.

Stratigraphic correlations suggested from associations reported by Cooper (1971, 1973). Additional data from Anderson (1968), Barter and Kelly (1982), Creasey and Kistler (1962), Damon (1968), Drewes (1971), Hayes and Drewes (1978), Lacy (1959), Marvin et al. (1973, 1978), Shafiqullah and Langlois (1978), and Thoms (1966).

Figure 19.4. Suggested correlation diagram of igneous and sedimentary rocks of the Pima district, together with some radiometric age data

host to mineralization in the Esperanza Mine (see Fig. 19.3). Its base is not exposed.

Weathering of the Ox Frame Volcanics produced distinctive fragments that make up the basal unit of the overlying Rodolfo Formation. This unit, of Triassic(?) age, was named from exposures in the vicinity of Helmet Peak (see Fig. 19.3), where the clasts are often of chert, and where it lies in angular unconformity on the Rain Valley Formation (Permian). Originally observed by Cooper (1971) on the upper plate of the San Xavier fault, the unit is now recognized to occur, probably in angular unconformity, on Paleozoic rocks in the Twin Buttes Orebody (Barter and Kelly, 1982); it is, thus, on the lower plate as well. Strongly metamorphosed or hydrothermally altered siltstone and arkose overlie parts of the Paleozoic section exposed in the Pima and Mission mines and are interpreted as possibly correlative with the Rodolfo Formation (Himes, 1973; Jansen, 1982).

In the area of the Pima-Mission mine, these altered rocks, interpreted as Rodolfo Formation, lie in depositional contact with *overturned* Paleozoic strata, while at Twin Buttes, Rodolfo correlatives overly vertically dipping Paleozoic strata. The Rodolfo-Paleozoic contact at Twin Buttes is apparently depositional, and restoration of a reasonable pre-Rodolfo configuration of this contact indicates that these Triassic sediments were deposited on overturned Permian strata (C. F. Barter, 1981, personal communication). In the Mission Orebody, evidence for depositional contact seems straightforward; to the southwest, in the contiguous Pima Orebody, the contact is interpreted as faulted (Langlois, 1978). These relationships are important for two reasons: first, although Cooper (1973) has mapped the contact as a thrust fault, the evidence accumulated from study of exposures widened in the process of mining shows an absence of any deformational fabric at most contacts; and second, the deposition of Triassic(?) strata on overturned Paleozoic successions, which reveals the existence of a major orogen at that time in this part of southeastern Arizona, appears to corroborate the interpretation of Permo-Triassic tectonic activity in the Santa Rita Mountains made by Drewes (1972).

Southeastern Arizona was the site of Late Triassic–Early Jurassic intrusive activity. One intrusion of this epoch is the Harris Ranch Quartz Monzonite, an important host to ore in the Sierrita Orebody. The Harris Ranch rocks have yielded a K-Ar age of about 190 m.y. (Cooper, 1973), which corresponds closely to the age of the Juniper Flat Granite at Bisbee and to the age of the Gleeson Quartz Monzonite at Courtland-Gleeson, Arizona (Anderson, 1968). There is no certain evidence that intrusions of this age were progenitors to porphyry copper deposits in the regions cited, but mineralization at Bisbee unequivocally pre-dates lowermost Lower Cretaceous rocks (i.e., older than ca. 140 m.y.). Copper mineralization at Sierrita is of Laramide age, and there is no evidence that the Harris Ranch Quartz Monzonite is more than a host rock to porphyries and mineralization of Laramide age. The evidence at Courtland-Gleeson is equivocal, since the district is also the site of a major Laramide volcanic and intrusive episode.

Jurassic Rocks. A sequence of volcanic rocks and red beds is exposed in the southwestern and western Sierrita Mountains. These units, the Tascuela Red Beds and Stevens

Mountain Rhyolite, have lithologic and stratigraphic correlatives in the Canelo Hills to the east that have been dated at about 173 m.y. (Cooper, 1971). The Tascuela and Stevens Mountain units may have overlain the Sierrita mine area, but deep erosion of these strata, which extended into the subjacent Ox Frame Volcanics, took place there before deposition of Lower Cretaceous strata (Thoms, 1966). The contact of the Tascuela Red Beds and the Ox Frame Volcanics is disconformable (Thoms, 1966), and the deep, pre–Upper Cretaceous erosion resulted in the removal of much of the superjacent Stevens Mountain Rhyolite prior to deposition of Upper Cretaceous arkose and volcanic rocks. These relationships are analogous to those interpreted for correlative units in the Huachuca Mountains and Canelo Hills (Hayes and Drewes, 1978). The Jurassic strata of the Sierrita Mountains and of the Canelo Hills and Huachuca Mountains may be remnants of an episode of volcanic activity localized along or near the Sawmill Canyon fault.

Remnants of a Jurassic intrusion, the Sierrita Granite, are exposed in several areas of the district, but none are known in close proximity to the orebodies. The granite, dated at about 150 m.y. (Cooper, 1971), is conspicuously different from other intrusions of the district because of the presence of large (up to 1 cm), isolated, and equant quartz crystals or masses of quartz. The unit is exposed in faulted contact with the Harris Ranch Quartz Monzonite west of the Sierrita mine, and it probably makes up much of a mass of weathered granite west of the San Xavier mine. Although slightly altered, both by hypogene and supergene effects, the granite is not known to have either hosted or given rise to any mineralization of the district; it is known only on the autochthonous plate.

Cretaceous Rocks. Rocks of Lower Cretaceous age (the Bisbee Group) are widely exposed in southeasternmost Arizona, where they were deposited in a restricted northwest-trending basin. In the Pima district, strata probably correlative with Bisbee units are exposed on both upper and lower fault plates and in close proximity to the Twin Buttes and Pima-Mission complexes. These rocks, the Angelica Arkose, are host to mineralization in the Twin Buttes and Pima-Mission mines, where they overlie Triassic strata in angular unconformity, and may be, in part, deposited directly upon Paleozoic strata. The unit is not reported in the Sierrita-Esperanza area.

The Angelica Arkose is conformably overlain by a thick (ca. 2,500 m) succession of Upper Cretaceous volcanic rocks, the Demetrie Volcanics. This unit, of inferred Late Cretaceous age (Hayes and Drewes, 1978) consists of andesite and dacite flows, lahars, and pyroclastic rocks; in the southern part of the district, it contains interlayered rhyolite flows and tuffs. The unit has numerous compositional and stratigraphic counterparts in and around many porphyry copper districts of the Southwest. The nature and significance of these rocks were first noted by Courtright (1958) and Richard and Courtright (1960) from studies initiated at Silver Bell. Detailed studies of these volcanic and volcaniclastic strata have been reported from two mineralized areas—one in the Santa Rita Mountains, where a thick (1,500 m) section of the Salero Formation is present (Drewes, 1971), and the other near Christmas, in the Williamson Canyon volcanics (Koski and Cook, 1982). The Demetrie Volcanics bear strong similarities in lithology to these and other volcanic units in similar stratigraphic positions. The scattered outcrops of these volcanic rocks in southeastern Arizona and contiguous regions are, in many locations, closely associated with dated Laramide intrusions. Richard and Courtright (1960) have noted some of these associations and have commented that such volcanic rocks marked a "pronounced shift" in the style of geologic evolution, which had been dominated by sedimentation during the Lower Cretaceous. The Demetrie and correlative rocks may likely be the volcanic precursors of more extensive igneous activity, which gave rise to the porphyry copper plutons. Demetrie rocks in the Sierrita Mountains lie in part on the Ox Frame Volcanics and are overlain by a still younger Laramide rhyolite unit. Because the Demetrie thins to the north beneath the rhyolite, Cooper (1971) has suggested that the unit was deposited on a basement that was being uplifted and was near the present core of the Sierrita Mountains. Thus, the southern Sierrita Mountains are a region unique in their manifestation of probable Laramide mountain building.

In the Pima district and in many nearby ranges—especially in the Silver Bell, Tucson, Santa Rita, and Roskruge Mountains—the Cretaceous section is capped by rhyolite flows and pyroclastic rocks. A thick (ca. 300 m) section of such rocks, the Red Boy rhyolite, is present a few kilometers west of the Sierrita Orebody. Within the exposures are outcrops of vertically structured rhyolite bodies that Cooper (1971) has interpreted as necks. Since these uppermost pre-ore volcanic units have been subjected to a long period of erosion, the original thicknesses are solely a matter of speculation; upper units of the Salero Formation, of the Santa Rita Mountains, which are considered to be correlative (Cooper, 1971), attain thicknesses of up to 700 m (Drewes, 1971). It is presumed that erosion has thinned the Red Boy volcanic rocks and that the unit was originally more widely distributed. Although rhyolitic rocks are not commonly present as the youngest pre-ore volcanic rocks in many porphyry copper districts of the American Southwest, their absence may be a result of erosion from their vulnerable position at the top of volcanic sections. Rhyolitic rocks of close pre-ore age are present in many districts and are conspicuously present in the southern part of the Sierrita Mountains. The geotectonic implication of the presence of andesites and their relationships to different kinds of ore deposits, including porphyry copper deposits, have been discussed by Sillitoe (1980).

Cretaceous–Early Tertiary Intrusions

A group of Laramide-aged intrusions occurs in the Pima district. Their radiometric ages have been reported and summarized by Shafiqullah and Langlois (1978). A spread of K-Ar dates from about 67 m.y. ago to about 57 m.y. ago brackets the principal episode of intrusive activity, during which at least three distinct kinds of plutons were emplaced. In the Sierrita mine area, the relationships among intrusive rock types and their relationships to times of mineralization seem straightforward, with the youngest of three Laramide intrusive types apparently genetically related to copper mineralization. At Twin Buttes, however, an intrusive complex exists within which field evidence indicates a history of protracted intrusion of pre-, inter-, and possibly post-ore plutons (Barter and Kelly, 1982). Except for some of the intrusions at Twin Buttes, general descriptions of the plutons in the district are outlined below.

The oldest of the intrusive types is a fine-grained, in some phases nearly microcrystalline, equigranular plagioclase-hornblende-biotite rock that Cooper (1973) has termed a biotite diorite. Locally it contains over 10 percent quartz; where it lies within the aureole of potassic alteration at Sierrita, its biotite content is augmented by alteration of hornblende (Preece, 1979). The rock occurs in several small (less than 1 km diameter), irregularly shaped, but commonly northwest-aligned bodies. It is intrusive into the Harris Ranch Quartz Monzonite and the Ox Frame Volcanics. The rock bears strong textural and mineralogical resemblance to fine-grained andesite (dacite) and it is suggested here that the small intrusive bodies, many of which occur along a northwest belt (see Fig. 19.3) west of the Sierrita Orebody, may be remnants of andesitic volcanic columns. The age of about 69 m.y. places these intrusions in about the same range of age interpreted for the Demetrie Volcanics, which lie to the southeast of the intrusions on the authochthonous plate. The diorite is an important host to copper mineralization in the Sierrita Orebody.

Emplacement of the Ruby Star Granodiorite followed at about 60 to 63 m.y. ago. This body of this rock, of near batholithic dimensions, extends from the vicinity of the Sierrita mine northwestward through the mountain range for a distance of over 20 km. The rock consists of two phases, the most widespread of which is an equigranular, holocrystalline, biotite granodiorite. Less common, and apparently restricted to small and irregular areas near the southern edge of the body, is a porphyritic granodiorite phase, characterized by large (1–2 cm) conspicuous phenocrysts of orthoclase. Although exposures are inadequate to assess the relationships accurately, the porphyritic phase of the Ruby Star Granodiorite may be transitional into a still younger granodiorite porphyry that appears genetically related to mineralization at Sierrita, Esperanza, and Twin Buttes. The Ruby Star Granodiorite and its associated porphyries have been revealed, through continued development and drilling at Sierrita, to underlie at least some of the Harris Ranch Quartz Monzonite. At least some of the intrusions—and perhaps some of the sedimentary and volcanic rocks of the southern Sierrita Mountains—may, thus, be interpreted as rafted on the younger intrusive mass.

The porphyry plutons of the district are exposed or known near or within the principal orebodies. Except at Sierrita, where a relatively large mass of only weakly altered quartz monzonite porphyry is present, most other exposures are of strongly mineralized or hydrothermally altered porphyritic rocks. The age of the porphyry bodies—possibly as young as about 55 m.y., but more likely near 58 m.y.—places them within the youngest major intrusions of the Laramide rock suite. Radiometric age dates are mostly from weakly altered rocks, but the correspondence between porphyry ages and mineralization ages (ca. 58–60 m.y.) as determined from alteration products (Shafiqullah and Langlois, 1978) suggests that the porphyry intrusions within the ore deposits are genetically related to mineralization and alteration. As noted, the porphyry bodies occur both on the allochthonous and autochthonous plates. On the lower plate, the bodies are exposed around the southern lobe of the Ruby Star pluton. Restoration at the Mission-Pima complex of the upper plate to a position near the Twin Buttes Orebody places the porphyry masses of those bodies in a similar location with respect to the southern lobe of the Ruby Star pluton.

Mesozoic and Early-Tertiary Structural Geology

The pre–mid-Tertiary structural complexity of the Pima district is revealed in the stratigraphic succession, where cycles of volcanism and intrusion are represented as variations in characteristics of contacts that range from marked, deep disconformities to profound angular unconformities within the Mesozoic column. The arguments and interpretations that follow are premised upon four bases of evidence: first, the reasonably well-established and well-documented idea that the Paleozoic and Mesozoic strata of the allochthonous plate were originally parts of exposures now present in the Twin Buttes area; second, that so restored, the Mesozoic strata became parts of the belt of thick Mesozoic rocks that extends to the southest (see Fig. 19.2); third, that folding of Paleozoic strata may be unequivocally demonstrated to have occurred during at least two times during the Mesozoic, and that such folding may be interpretable in the context of transport; and fourth, that the history of movement on the Sawmill Canyon fault, as deduced from evidence in the Santa Rita Mountains, is permissively consistent with interpretations that may be drawn for the Mesozoic tectonic history of the Pima district.

The structural history of the Pima district is revealed by the characteristics of Paleozoic and Mesozoic rock relationships. In the Twin Buttes Orebody, Rodolfo strata (Triassic[?]) were deposited across overturned and eroded upper Paleozoic strata (Barter and Kelly, 1982). Similarly, the Rodolfo is deposited on an erosion surface cut across the same overturned upper Paleozoic strata in the Mission mine (Jansen, 1982). No evidence is yet known to assess the relationship of lowermost Triassic strata (Ox Frame Volcanics) with the Paleozoic of the district. It is apparent, nonetheless, that folding and erosion of the Paleozoic took place at a very early time in the Mesozoic or during latest Paleozoic. A lack of stratigraphic symmetry in the folds at Twin Buttes, noted by Barter and Kelly (1982), suggests faulting associated with folding there and the further probability of recumbent folds developing at this early time. These researchers have also noted that some asymmetry may be the result of plastic deformation of some Permian strata. The interpretation advanced here, however, is that at least some of the folding represents translation and that some of the Paleozoic of the Twin Buttes Orebody, particularly that south of the Twin Buttes fault, is allochthonous.

Drewes (1972) has showed that the northeast side of the Sawmill Canyon fault in the Santa Rita Mountains was uplifted at least 1.5 km, and possibly as much as 3 km, in order to permit stripping of the Paleozoic to expose Precambrian rocks in the Early Triassic. If extended to the Pima district, a relief of this order along the projection of the

Sawmill Canyon fault would certainly promote movement of the Paleozoic to the south from an uplifted area to the northeast. Because of still younger folding and implied transport of the Paleozoic and Mesozoic rocks of Twin Buttes, the early transport direction has not been determined. No autochthonous Paleozoic in the district is recognized north of the exposure of the mid-Tertiary San Xavier fault.

Accumulation of thick columns of Triassic, Jurassic, and mid- to late-Cretaceous strata took place south of the Sawmill Canyon fault in the Santa Rita Mountains (Drewes, 1972). The same distribution of Mesozoic volcanic and sedimentary rocks (on the basis of restoration of the San Xavier nappe) is present south of the projection of the Sawmill Canyon fault through the district.

In the Mission mine, the overturned Paleozoic, together with its Mesozoic cover, was deformed by a group of parallel, northwest-striking folds that controlled distribution and grade of ore (Jansen, 1982). These folds, which involve uppermost Lower Cretaceous strata (Angelica Arkose), formed some time during the Upper Cretaceous. A similar geometry of folding involves the Angelica Arkose in the San Xavier North Orebody (King, 1982). At Twin Buttes northwest-striking folds, grossly concordant with the strike of the Paleozoic section, but also folding the Angelica strata, have been reported by Barter and Kelly (1982). Comparison of trends of fold axes in the Pima-Mission block with those of the Twin Buttes Orebody shows a difference of about 10°. The significance of this variation, beyond that of a rotation of the allochthonous block, is not known. Nevertheless, the Paleozoic section at Twin Buttes, overturned in the Triassic(?) and covered with Mesozoic and volcanic and clastic sediments, was further folded during the Late Cretaceous. Stress directions during this later time were compressive and oriented northeast-southwest.

Northeast-southwest–directed compression that crossed southern Arizona and adjacent regions during the Laramide has been recognized by many workers and its effects have been interpreted in different ways. Thrust faulting has been interpreted in many field studies from the widespread presence of northwest-oriented folds. The magnitude of interpreted transport varies from great distances (tens of kilometers), premised upon regional overthrust models (Drewes, 1978), to shorter distances (kilometers), based upon uplift and gravity-induced fault models (Jones, 1966). Davis (1979) has proposed basement-cored uplifts with overthrust faults that resulted in northwest-trending folds along edges of the uplift. The southwestern edge of one such uplift shown by Davis is the Sawmill Canyon fault; geologic interpretations by Davis have extended no further west than the Santa Rita Mountains, but extension of the fault into the Pima district is proposed (see Fig. 19.2). If, as Davis (1979) has suggested, in the Santa Rita Mountains the north side of the fault was up during the Laramide, the edge of the uplifted block would lie just north of, but near, the Twin Buttes exposures, and the transport direction would be to the southwest.

It bears repeating at this point that Cooper (1971) has interpreted uplift of the southern Sierrita Mountains during or before the time of Red Boy Rhyolite (Laramide). Such an interpretation requires faults southwest of the Sierrita mine that are not now obvious but that may be represented by the belt of northwest-striking exposures of mid-Tertiary volcanic rocks. A solution to the tectonic problem remained evasive in the late 1970s. The regional nature of the Sawmill Canyon fault and its wide exposure in the Santa Rita Mountains, where its complexity is manifest, suggests that a zone of faulting—kilometers wide—rather than a single break may pass through the southern end of the Pima district. Although there are probably many features of structural geology in this part of the district that may be inherited from regional faulting, their recognition is profoundly complicated by the presence of features related to both pre- and post-Laramide tectonism.

Numerous faults are exposed on the autochthonous block and in the transported rocks of the Mission-Pima complex. A dominance of northwest and east-northeast strikes on these structures is apparent. The northwest trend may be inherited from effects of pre-Laramide tectonics (Titley, 1976), and the east-northeast faults are probably a distinct phenomenon of Laramide stresses (Rehrig and Heidrick, 1972; Heidrick and Titley, 1982). Sense of movement on the two sets of faults is not always obvious; however, Lacy (1959) noted that left slip was the probable sense on the northwest-striking set. In Sawmill Canyon, Drewes (1972) observed drag folding that was also suggestive of left slip on that fault; he proposed the folding to be of Paleocene to Oligocene age. At Twin Buttes, the northeast-and east-northeast–striking faults are characterized by normal movement, with the southeast side down (Barter, 1981, personal communication). Although it is possible that some Laramide folding may be related to left slip along the northwest-striking projection of the Sawmill Canyon fault, documenting such a relationship remains a formidable task.

The control of ore grades by Laramide folds reported at Mission (Jansen, 1982), suggests that ore-formation followed folding and that folding may possibly pre-date intrusion. The temporal relationships of Laramide folding and intrusion are not understood elsewhere in the district, however. Many Laramide intrusions are grossly oriented, with their long axes northwest; the distribution of biotite-diorite bodies in the Sierrita mine area appears to follow such a trend. The orientation is generally concordant with the orientation of Laramide folds, and they are probably related.

In summary, the Pima district manifests complex structural geology involving, at various times, each successive rock system that was deposited. A major tectonic event resulted in recumbent(?) folds in earliest Mesozoic time, followed by a period of erosion. Disconformities and angular unconformities within the Mesozoic section indicate episodic tectonic activity, culminated by a major episode of block movement during latest Cretaceous that was associated with widespread emplacement of porphyry plutons. It is noteworthy that this small part of Arizona was a site of continuous tectonic instability and a site of intrusion of stocks of several ages. In this sense, the district reveals a history similar to that of the Courtland-Gleeson district of the Dragoon Mountains to the northeast. That district lies along the northeastern edge of Davis' basement uplift and also reveals episodic

Mesozoic intrusive activity, as well as faulting, interpretable in the context of uplift and gravity tectonics (Gilluly, 1956; Keith and Barrett, 1976; Davis, 1979).

CENOZOIC GEOLOGIC HISTORY

Following emplacement of porphyries and the evolution of hydrothermal ores (i.e., since about 58 m.y. ago), the Sierrita Mountains were the site of at least two further episodes of igneous activity. The district also experienced renewed tectonic activity, which resulted in faulting of the Laramide orebodies at Twin Buttes. This history has been summarized by Shafiqullah and others (1976) and Shafiqullah and Langlois (1978).

Radiometric ages determined for many granitic rocks and porphyries in the Pima district range from about 57 to 36 m.y. old (Shafiqullah and Langlois, 1978). These ages pre-date a conspicuous igneous event that resulted in emplacement of andesite dikes, one of which, dated at 24 m.y. old, has been mapped by Cooper (1973) in the autochthonous block. Elsewhere, the andesite dikes are known in the San Xavier nappe, from the Twin Buttes area, and from drill hole intersections. The older Tertiary ages are primarily from rocks than cannot be distinguished lithologically from the suite of Laramide intrusions, and the younger ages may represent resetting of K-Ar ages by the mid-Tertiary event. However, there are ages of about 52 m.y. from pegmatoid bodies in the Ruby Star Granodiorite and an age of about 36 m.y. from a muscovite granite beneath the San Xavier North Orebody. There, thus, remain geologic features and a thermal history requiring further study and understanding.

The early Tertiary geologic history of the Twin Buttes and Sierrita areas is obscure, but it is logical to assume that it was a time of weathering of the sulfide orebodies, with both erosion and initiation of secondary enrichment above some parts of the porphry copper bodies. Between about 27.9 and 30.7 m.y. ago (Cooper, 1973), a thick sequence of clastic and volcanic rocks accumulated—according to most interpretations, in the southern part of the district. These rocks described by Cooper (1960), make up the helmet Fanglomerate, a unit in excess of 3,200 m thick. The fanglomerate is characterized by conglomerate, landslide blocks, volcanic flows, tuffs, breccias, arkose and arkosic sandstone, and locally, thin beds of well-sorted, layered, fine-grained sediment. Evidence from the vicinity of the CWT mine, where arkosic rocks of Cretaceous(?) age are overlain in angular unconformity by the fanglomerate, suggests that the debris of the fans covered at least part of the Mesozoic section exposed in the southern part of the district (see Figs. 19.5 and 19.6). The clastic rocks and landslide blocks are interpreted by Cooper (1960) as having been derived from a highland to the west, on the basis of distribution of large (up to 10 m) blocks within the fanglomerate. The fanglomerate is known to be exposed only in the 3- to 5-km interval between the deposits of the north and south parts of the district, where it makes up the great preponderance of rocks in the allochthonous plate.

The Helmet Fanglomerate is floored by a nearly flat fault surface that has been termed the San Xavier thrust fault (Lacy, 1959). Evidence for existence of a faulted contact between the fanglomerate and subjacent units is unequivocal for exposures east of the Ruby Star fault, but it is less certain for those exposures to the west. Preceding sections of this chapter have based interpretations upon the concept of a transport direction on the fault that was to the north, with a translation of about 10 km. This premise is based upon Cooper's (1960) work, and, although it was generally widely accepted in 1981, there still remained unsolved problems, controversies, and alternative hypotheses.

The arguments of Cooper (1960) are based primarily upon the similarity between the two ends of the district in outcrop geometry, in distribution of Paleozoic and Mesozoic rocks within those outcrops, and in structural features. Restoration of the volcanic, clastic, and carbonate rocks of the Pima-Mission-San Xavier block fits the relative positions of exposures of the same rocks, with respect to a center on the Twin Buttes Orebody, in a remarkable way (see Fig. 19.3). The interpreted transport direction, based upon fracture orientations measured in large blocks in the fanglomerate (Cooper, 1960), likewise suggests movement of the upper plate in the proper direction to accomplish a "fit," provided the fractures measured are not of a different age (see Fig. 19.5*A*).

Alternatively, Weaver (1965, 1971) has proposed that coherent blocks of pre-ore strata from a high area to the west moved eastward, where they came to rest upon granitic basement. Based upon extensive drill hole information, Weaver has concluded that they were then covered by the fanglomerate that was deposited into the present location of the unit; in this interpretation no movement of a fault plate is required in the sense suggested by Cooper (see Fig. 19.5*B*). Lacy and Titley (1962) have proposed similar eastward movement during the Laramide, and, although the timing suggested for that interpretation has been invalidated by radiometric age dates, the mechanism described is similar to that of Weaver (1965, 1971). Further definition of the nature of the fanglomerate and faulting style has been proposed by Lukanuski and others (1976). Their interpretations have suggested that at least some of the exposed length of the San Xavier fault, as defined by Cooper (1960), west of the Ruby (Star) fault, is characterized by undeformed sedimentary strata—in the base of the fanglomerate—that lie in contact with Precambrian(?) or Laramide(?) granitic rocks (see Fig. 19.5*C*). They have further interpreted that the San Xavier fault in its southern expression dies out against the north-striking, normal Ruby Star fault. Exposures of the fanglomerate are controlled by the normal fault, whose extension may be projected into the thrust at the north end of the district, as mapped by Cooper (1960)—compare parts *A* and *C* in Figure 19.5.

These studies, carried out in great part since Cooper's original (1960) work continue to develop further details and ideas on this complex and economically important problem. Notwithstanding other ideas of the provenance of the San Xavier nappe and its nature, the original comparison of geometry and structure outlined by Cooper remains a strongly compelling argument for his interpretation of the origin of the fanglomerate to the south and southwest and of its northward transport, in whole or in part, to its present location. Timing of the movement has been interpreted by

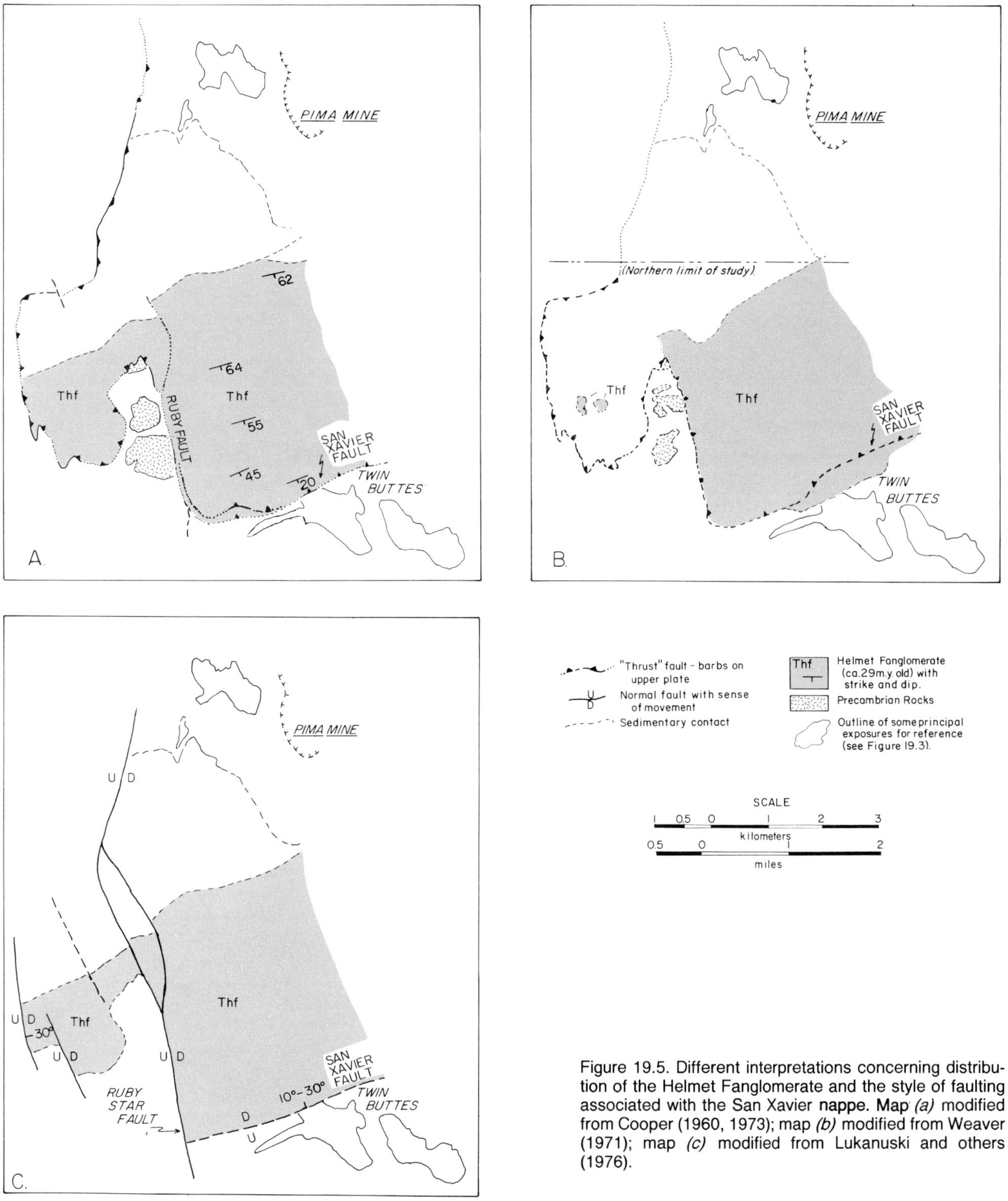

Figure 19.5. Different interpretations concerning distribution of the Helmet Fanglomerate and the style of faulting associated with the San Xavier **nappe. Map** *(a)* modified from Cooper (1960, 1973); map *(b)* modified from Weaver (1971); map *(c)* modified from Lukanuski and others (1976).

Shafiqullah and Langlois (1978) as late Oligocene or early Miocene, on the basis of radiometric ages of dikes cut by the fault, and by Barter and Kelly (1982) as between 28 and 24 m.y. ago.

Following transport, the orebody at Mission and Pima was exposed and eroded to a nearly flat surface. It was then covered by a thin (1–3 m) layer of conglomerate, which is now well-indurated, and then by over 65 m of poorly consolidated slope wash and alluvium. In this connection it should be noted that, with the exception of the San Xavier North Orebody (King, 1982), there is no significant secondary sulfide enrichment of orebodies in the district. In other

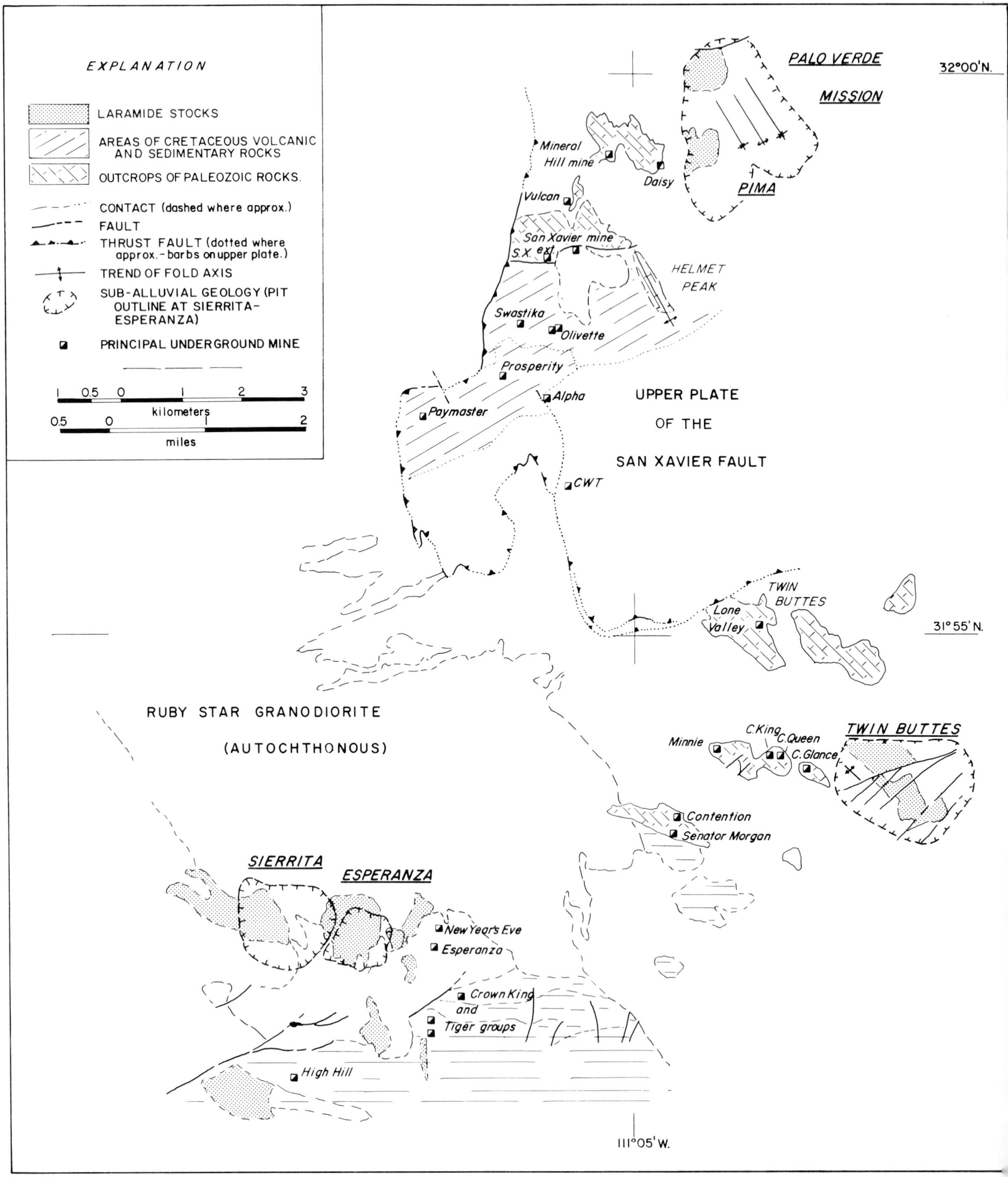

Figure 19.6. Location map of certain outcrops, plutons, and open pits, as well as older underground mining operations, in the Pima district. Base map is the same as in Figure 19.3, and details are keyed to features shown on that map.

districts of the Southwest, enrichment is interpreted to have taken place in the Early Tertiary (Livingston et al., 1968).

One final tectonic episode resulted in development of north-striking normal faults (possibly the Ruby Star fault and similar structures). These normal faults (extensional, east side down) are of possible mid-Miocene to Pliocene age—i.e., concurrent with the time of Basin and Range tectonism. As earlier noted, however, the Sierrita Mountains do not reflect the characteristic form of other mountain ranges believed to have formed at that time; it seems likely that north-striking faults of basin and range nature resulted in depression of the flanks of the Sierrita Mountains that were already in existence as a topographic high.

ORES AND ORE GENESIS

The Pima district is the location of several different genetic types of orebodies, each of which is characterized by its own host rocks, ore control, and metal content or metal ratios. The wealth of information that exists concerning many aspects of ore deposits in this district allows a generalized picture to be drawn of the features of a large, metallized district with disseminated copper deposits at its core and with other genetic types of ores and contrasting metals and metal ratios at its fringe.

Production and reserves of the disseminated ores in the district may be contrasted with those of vein and replacement orebodies. Viewed from this perspective, the contrast is also historical, because the vein and replacement ores were mined before the porphyry ores were discovered. Further, the perspective allows consideration of the nature of ores as related to host rocks and structural control. Because of the closely similar distribution of porphyry ores and fringe mineralization in deposits of both the upper and lower plates of the San Xavier fault, it is further possible to compare vein and replacement ores in the two plates as they relate to different host rocks. Production figures for 29 mines of the district (excluding the open pits) are compared in Table 19.2. These data are separated on the basis of volcanic and clastic host rocks (Mesozoic) and carbonate host rocks (Paleozoic); and on the basis of occurrence in the northern and southern blocks. The table includes figures since about 1878, when production records began. Little production from the ores in clastic and volcanic rocks, except for the Paymaster mine near the San Xavier Group (see Fig. 19.6), has been recorded since about 1920. Ores in carbonate rocks at Twin Buttes and in the north end of the district have been mined since the 1890s and were mined at the Mineral Hill and San Xavier mines during the early history of extraction of the disseminated ores—i.e., in the period 1955 to 1965.

Some contrasts in metal associations may be seen from the grade averages in Table 19.2. The ores in volcanic and clastic host rocks are relatively richer in lead and silver than the replacement ores in carbonate rocks and, although most of the lead-silver ores are presumed to have been enriched, the values are probably representative of primary sulfide compositions. The relatively high lead and zinc averages from carbonate-hosted ores in the north block reflect the production of only the San Xavier mine. Other carbonate-hosted ores in both north and south blocks tend toward values high in copper and silver, and may be approximated by the copper and silver values shown for carbonate-hosted ores of the south block. Most of the carbonate-hosted ores to which data refer were hypogene.

These data for vein and replacement ores may be contrasted with the production from disseminated ores in the district, as summarized in Table 19.3. The disseminated ores of the district are unusual in some respects. For example, silver values (up to 0.1 oz. Ag per ton at Mission, where calc-silicate altered limestones host mineralization; 0.3 oz.

TABLE 19.2
Production and Grade of Vein and Replacement Ores, Pima Mining District, Pima County, Arizona (ca. 1878 through 1972)

TYPE OF ORE	PRODUCTION						GRADE			
	Number of Mines	Ore (s.t. × 10^3)	Cu (t. × 10^3)	Ag (Tr. oz. × 10^3)	Pb (t. × 10^3)	Zn (t. × 10^3)	Cu (%)	Ag (Tr. oz./ton)	Pb (%)	Zn (%)
Vein Ores in Volcanic and Clastic Host Rocks										
Allochthon (northern part of district)	8	101	4.71	480	1.141	0.15	4.7	4.75	1.1	0.15
Autochthon (southern part of district)	6	8.21	0.256	34.27	0.083	trace	3.1	4.17	1.0	—
Replacement Ores in Carbonate Host Rocks										
Allochthon (northern part of district)	8	2,444	58.89	3,514.1	48.14	85.65	2.4	1.44	2.0	3.5
Autochthon (southern part of district)	7	479.3	26.42	1,381.5	trace	1.53	5.5	2.75	—	0.3
Totals		3,032.5	90.28	5,409.87	49.36	87.33				

Source: Data, which exclude open-pit mines, are calculated from values in Keith (1974).

Ag per ton in 1 percent copper ore in the altered Epitaph limestone at Twin Buttes (Barter and Kelly, 1982); and within the range of 0.03 to 0.04 oz Ag per ton for ores in non-carbonate host rocks at Twin Buttes) are high compared to reported grades of the metal in other deposits of this type. The large tonnage of porphyry ores mined, and the modest silver values in the vein deposits have combined to make the district a major silver producer. Further, the district contains orebodies richer by nearly a factor of 2 in their molybdenum content than most other mines in this region, as described by Lowell and Guilbert (1970).

Contrasting the metal contents of the disseminated ores with the other genetic types in the district—even though the volumetric bases for grade comparison is greatly different—shows that some metal zoning may correspond to changes in depositional environments away from the porphyry centers. Vertical zoning of the system is likewise indicated by changes in copper and silver compositions; if the ores of the San Xavier nappe were restored to a position above those of the southern block, a measured vertical span of mineralization in excess of a kilometer would exist. The silver values in ores of the Pima and Mission bodies, at reported recovered grades of 0.06 to 0.07 oz. Ag per ton, are somewhat lower than the ores of Twin Buttes (see Table 19.3).

Veins in Volcanic and Clastic Rocks

Mesozoic andesite, dacite, and arkose host groups of veins that lie southwest of the San Xavier mine in the northern part of the district and southwest of the Twin Buttes mine to the south (see Fig. 19.6). The exotic blocks of outcrop that host the veins in the northern part of the district are floored by granitic rocks at the fault contact. It is presumed that these ores are of Laramide age, or at least that they pre-date the age of the San Xavier fault; this presumption is based upon the absence of evidence that the veins cross the flat fault into subjacent granites. However, no radiometric age dating of the vein ores had been reported by 1980, and verification of their age awaits further study.

In a general way, the geometry and mineralization of the orebodies and the character of ores are similar for vein-related ores at both ends of the district, although the preponderance of production has been from the north end. A summary of production reported from the vein ores in Mesozoic rocks is shown in Table 19.2, and tonnage and grades of vein ores reported for three of the larger mines in the north end are shown in Table 19.4. No rigorously determined thermometry has been reported for the veins, but in other characteristics the ores and environment are typically epithermal. The ores are mineralogically complex and consist of quartz-pyrite gangue, with accessory base and precious metal sulfides and sulfosalts. In addition to galena, sphalerite, and chalcopyrite, which are commonly present, these ores also contain argentite and argentiferous galena. Widescale propylitization of volcanic and arkosic host rocks is present, as is weak quartz-sericite alteration of arkosic hosts. Veins in the northern block extend to a depth of about 150 ft. (ca. 45 m)

TABLE 19.3
Production (1955–1976) and Reserves (1977) of Porphyry Copper and Related Ores
Pima Mining District, Pima County, Arizona

DEPOSIT	PRODUCTION				RESERVES		
	Ore (t. × 10^6)	Cu (lbs. × 10^6)	Mo (lbs. × 10^6)	Ag (Tr. oz. × 10^6)	Ore (t. × 10^6)	Cu (%)	Mo (%)
Southern Half of District							
Twin Buttes	69.3	102.4	11.62	6.93[a]	329 (S at 0.2% cutoff) 57 (O at 0.6% cutoff)	0.67 1.10	0.03
Sierrita	224.75	1,208.1	98.98	6.74[b]	459.8	0.32	0.033
Esperanza	86.34	693.6	35.61	3.45[c]	21.85	0.42	0.022
Northern Half of District							
Mission	108.9	1,364.7	20.36	7.3	104.46	0.73	0.019
Pima	199.8	1,907.6	16.56	12.08	146	0.48	ND
Palo Verde	.47	19.5	ND	ND	125(AN) 31.5(AS)	0.61 0.70	ND
San Xavier	2.7	42.15[d]	ND	ND	166.9(S) 1.05(O)	0.52 1.48	ND
Totals	692.26	5,338	183.13	36.5	1,384.5 (915.1)	0.51[e]	(0.030[f])

Source: Data from Keith and others (1978) unless otherwise noted.

KEY: AN = ANAMAX; AS = ASARCO; ND = no data available; O = oxide; S = sulfide

[a] Production estimate based upon grade of 0.1 oz./ton (from Keith, 1974).
[b] Production estimate based upon grade of 0.03 oz./ton (from Keith, 1974).
[c] Production estimate based upon grade of 0.04 oz./ton (from Keith, 1974).
[d] Production figures from Greeley (1978).
[e] Tonnage and grade totals calculated on basis of sulfide ores.
[f] Tonnage and grade for copper-molybdenum ores as tabulated.

TABLE 19.4
Production and Grade of Major Non-Porphyry Mines in the Pima Mining District, Pima County, Arizona (ca. 1880–1974)

MINES	PRODUCTION	GRADE			
	Ore (s.t.)	Ag (oz./t.)	Cu (%)	Pb (%)	Zn (%)
Twin Buttes Area (Southern Part of District)					
Replacement Ores in Carbonate Host Rocks					
Copper Glance Mine	186,000	1	7	ND	ND
Copper Queen Mine	122,000	1	4.2	ND	ND
Senator Morgan Mine	100,000	9	4	ND	ND
Minnie Mine	63,000	1.5	6.5	ND	ND
Contention Mine	8,000	2	2	1	11
Mineral Hill–San Xavier Area (Northern Part of District)					
Replacement Ores in Carbonate Host Rocks					
San Xavier Mine	800,000	3	0.7	6	10
Mineral Hill Mine	605,000	0.5	2.0	ND	ND
Daisy Mine	522,000	0.5	3.0	ND	ND
CWT Mine	69,000	0.5	—	trace	4
Vein Ores in Clastic and Volcanic Host Rocks					
Alpha Mine	70,000	1	6.0	ND	ND
Paymaster Mine	13,000	20	2	3	ND
Olivette-Annette Group	10,000	10	ND	5	1

Source: Data from Keith, 1974.
NOTE: ND = no data available.

in the Paymaster Group at the edge of the plate (Waller, 1960) and to a depth of at least 350 ft. (ca. 106 m) in the Prosperity Group, where exploration to depths of 600 ft. (ca. 180 m) has been reported (Wilson, 1950). Only shallow workings are reported for the few mines on veins in Mesozoic rocks of the southern part of the district. If mineralization pre-dates movement on the San Xavier fault as is seemingly the case, mineralization exposed in the southern part of the district may represent roots of the epithermal veins present to the north.

Structural control of vein mineralization is complex, as reported by Mayuga (1942), Wilson (1950), Waller (1960), and Nye (1961). Predominant vein strikes are east-northeast or north-northwest, with dips tending to flatten with depth in some veins. Control is exerted by changes in dip and by structural intersections. Of the kinds of structural intersections present, those of steep faults are reported to be most important, but a secondary control exerted by low angle (<30°) faults has been observed locally (Waller, 1960; Nye, 1961). Within andesite and dacite hosts, widescale brecciation, as in the Paymaster Group, may locally act in conjunction with faulting to control distribution of lower-grade mineralization in fault walls.

Replacement Ores in Carbonate Rocks

The predominant non-porphyry ore production of the district has come from the relatively higher-grade ores deposited in the Paleozoic sections near the disseminated ore centers at both ends of the district. These replacement ores, dominated by pyrometasomatic-altered carbonate rocks and sulfide volumes on the order of 10 to 20 percent, consist of two mineralogical types. One of these is characterized by copper-silver mineralization, e.g., the Copper Glance, Senator Morgan, Mineral Hill, and Daisy orebodies; the other consists of the zinc-rich ores exemplified by the San Xavier, CWT, and Contention mines (see Table 19.4). Grades shown for the replacement ores in carbonate host rocks in Table 19.4 indicate similar copper : silver ratios for ores at both ends of the district, but the grades of copper and silver differ for most of the production by a factor of 2 between the two ends of the district.

Replacement ores at Twin Buttes were mostly localized in silicated Paleozoic rocks along pre-minerization faults. These ores formed at least a hundred meters from the contact of the Ruby Star Granodiorite (C. F. Barter, 1981, personal communication). In these sites they comprised numerous rich, but relatively small, bodies of copper and silver in skarns (Ransome, 1922). Skarn-related ores were also developed in the orebodies of the Daisy and Mineral Hill mines and, similarly, were formed in favorable Paleozoic strata, where faulting served to localize mineralization at sites up to 75 m away from igneous contacts. Access to most of these older mines was not possible in the late 1970s and thus, inspection of the nature of rocks and alteration was not possible; evidence from outcrop, however, reveals that igneous rocks present are mostly of Precambrian age. Laramide porphyries nearby are only weakly mineralized, but they contain abundant fractures and are altered (cf. Heidrick and Titley, 1982); circulation of mineralizing fluids through plutons is, thus, inferred to have taken place. An additional noteworthy feature of these ores in the carbonate section is the widespread presence of scheelite, some of which was produced from the Senator Morgan mine (Keith, 1974). Its presence seems to be due not only to the existence of tungsten in the

systems but also to the abundance of calcium-rich host rocks.

Carbonate-hosted ores of the San Xavier and CWT mines differ from the copper-silver ores of Mineral Hill and Twin Buttes in an important way—they contain relatively much richer zinc and, locally, lead (see Table 19.4). Only sparse information concerning habits of the ore in the CWT mine was available by the late 1970s, but Keith (1974) has reported that the occurrence was characterized by irregular replacement lenses and fractures in Paleozoic host rocks at the base of the San Xavier nappe. The genetic type is, thus, uncertain. However, the ores of the San Xavier mine have been studied and described (Mayuga, 1942; Wilson, 1960). Sulfide ores there occurred in pyrometasomatically altered carbonate rocks at a contact with Mesozoic clastic rocks that are of probable Triassic or Cretaceous age (see Fig 19.6). The succession has been warped into a steeply plunging syncline, with the locus of metallization and alteration forming an open, canoe-shaped zone of mineralization draped beneath the folded contact. No evidence has been developed to indicate that mineralization of either the San Xavier or the CWT mines lies in close proximity to an intrusion. Rather, the mineralization appears to be the product of solutions of more obscure parentage and history than those forming copper-silver ores in close proximity to intrusions. These solutions produced pyrometasomatic alteration phenomena in carbonate rocks associated with zinc-rich ores similar to those in the same host rocks associated with copper-silver ores. The reasons for the different ore types are uncertain, but the differences may be tentatively interpreted as a manifestation of district-wide metal zoning. Most of the zinc-dominated metal assemblages are located farther from intrusion contacts than are the ores dominated by copper.

Disseminated (Porphyry-Related) Ores

Some features of the disseminated ores (discussed in detail in following chapters) merit brief mention in the context of district-wide considerations of ore genesis. Two major kinds of orebodies occur in the district and are separable on the basis of host rock compositions, alteration types, and metal content. In the southern part of the district the contrast between the features of the Twin Buttes and the Esperanza-Sierrita ore systems is striking. Pyrometasomatically altered carbonate rocks are hosts to copper-molybdenum-silver-(tungsten) mineralization, centered on porphyries of several textural varieties at Twin Buttes (Barter and Kelly, 1982; Einaudi, 1982). At Esperanza-Sierrita, porphyry plutons that are texturally similar to, and of about the same ages as, those at Twin Buttes have focussed copper-molybdenum-(silver) mineralization in a variety of non-carbonate host rocks. These include felsic igneous intrusions and the volcanic and clastic rock sequences of the Ox Frame Volcanics. Alteration zoning is only weakly developed, but it is manifested in potassic, propylitic, and phyllic mineral assemblages (West and Aiken, 1982) typically of those commonly present in host rocks of such compositions.

Comparison of production and reserve figures for these two deposits in the southern part of the district (see Table 19.3) reveals that mined copper grade at Sierrita is about half of that at Twin Buttes but that molybdenum assays, which are relatively high (0.03%) are about the same. Silver content of ores at Twin Buttes is higher than that at Sierrita by a factor of about 3 as reported by Keith (1974) and as shown on Table 19.3 (see footnotes *a* and *b*). The metal content of ores at Twin Buttes contrasts further with the content of metal in the ores at Mission and Pima, which are orebodies that were, presumably, detached from the higher parts of the original Twin Buttes system. Silver and molybdenum values are somewhat lower in these orebodies of the northern half of the district.

The only orebody in the area in which secondary enrichment is significant and economically important in this district is the North San Xavier Orebody, described by King (1982). This orebody, interpreted as detached from the upper portion of the Mission system and moved even further north, would, if restored as interpreted, occupy the highest and most exposed part of the original Twin Buttes system. Ores at North San Xavier occur in the arkose of Cretaceous age and reflect secondary sulfide and oxide enrichment. Although some sulfide enrichment is reported at Twin Buttes (Barter and Kelly, 1982), it is neither extensive nor economically important. Silver content of these secondary ores has not been sufficient to warrant reporting its value (Greeley, 1978).

District-Wide Zoning

Certain interpretations of district metal zoning may be suggested on the presumption that the ores present are part of one metallizing event. It is re-emphasized, however, that the only radiometric ages determined in the district are those of rocks and minerals closely associated with the porphyry-related ores. Simultaneity of mineralization during the Laramide of all ores described here may only be inferred, although the basis for that inference seems substantial. If the inference is correct, then zoning may be viewed as related both to the position of porphyry intrusions and to the geologic coincidence of location of host rocks with different mineralogical compositions and physical properties. Viewed from this perspective, metal composition of the Pima district ores may be seen to grade from large centers of (mesothermal) disseminated copper-molybdenum-silver ores, outward to replacement copper-silver ores in carbonate hosts (mesothermal), to replacement zinc or zinc-lead orebodies with minor copper, to "fringe" mineralization (epithermal) characterized by copper-bearing silver-lead veins and breccia fillings. Although such a pattern may be proposed for those orebodies presumably related to the Twin Buttes system, the placement of the Sierrita Orebody in such a framework remains enigmatic. The ore system, located some 9 km west of Twin Buttes, is regionally anomalous in its relatively high (0.033%) molybdenum content and relatively low (0.32%) copper content. Data available and interpretations based on that data pointed in the late 1970s to the existence of two separate centers of ore formation along a profound regional structure, and, although there may be a deeper or more fundamental relationship between the orebodies of the autochthonous block, it has not been recognized.

ACKNOWLEDGEMENTS

The continuing study of orebodies and of the geology of the Pima District has been facilitated over many years by the cooperation and courtesy of management and the geologic staffs of the Anaconda Company, ANAMAX, ASARCO, Banner Mining Company, Cyprus Pima Company, Duval Corporation, and McFarland & Hullinger. Our understanding of the geology of this extremely complex and important copper district continues to evolve, but it would not do so without the continuing production of high-quality data and the interpretations of operating staffs. Similarly, the work of researchers at the U.S. Geological Survey, particularly that of J. R. Cooper, established a district-wide geologic framework from which much subsequent study has proceeded.

Discussions of mine geology over a period of many years with operating geologists have provided continuing stimulus for new ideas and interpretations. Among those geologists are: L. J. Jansen of ASARCO; D. M. Aiken, C. D. Iles, R. A. Metz, and R. J. West of Duval; J. D. Langlois and J. A. Journeay of Pima; F. D. MacKenzie of Banner; and C. F. Barter and J. L. Kelly of ANAMAX. While all contributed in some way to ideas presented here, it should be emphasized that some geologic interpretations in the district remain equivocal and that there may not be concurrence concerning some important subjects, particularly structural geology. Considerations of some features of ore genesis have benefited through study and discussion with R. W. Beane. Finally, I acknowledge with thanks a review and discussion of this chapter by C. F. Barter.

REFERENCES CITED

Anderson, C. A., 1966, Areal geology of the Southwest, *in* Titley, S. R., and Hicks, C. L., eds., Geology of the Porphyry Copper Deposits, Southwestern North America: Tucson, Univ. Ariz. Press, p. 3–16.

———, 1968, Arizona and adjacent New Mexico, *in,* Ridge, J. D., ed., Ore Deposits of the United States, 1933–1967: New York, AIME, p. 1163–1190.

Barter, C. F., and Kelly, J. L., 1982, Geology of the Twin Buttes mineral deposit, Pima County, Arizona, *in* Titley, S. R., ed., Advances in Geology of the Porphyry Copper Deposits, Southwestern North America: Tucson, Univ. Ariz. Press, Chap. 20.

Butler, W. C., 1971, Permian sedimentary environments in southeastern Arizona: Ariz. Geol. Soc. Digest IX, p. 71–93.

Cooper, J. R., 1960, Some geologic features of the Pima mining district, Pima County, Arizona: U.S. Geol. Survey Bull. 1112–C, p. 63–103.

———, 1971, Mesozoic stratigraphy of the Sierrita Mountains, Pima County, Arizona: U.S. Geol. Survey Prof. Paper 658-D, 42 p.

———, 1973, Geologic map of the Twin Buttes Quadrangle, southwest of Tucson, Pima County, Arizona: U.S. Geol. Survey Map I-745.

Courtright, J. H., 1958, Progress report on investigation of some Cretaceous-Tertiary formations in southeastern Arizona: Ariz. Geol. Soc. Digest I, p. 7–9.

Creasey, S. C., and Kistler, R. W., 1962, Age of some copper-bearing porphyries and other igneous rocks in southeastern Arizona: U.S. Geol. Survey Prof. Paper 450-D, p. D1–D5.

Damon, P. E., 1968, Application of the potassium-argon method to the dating of igneous and metamorphic rock within the basin ranges of the Southwest: Ariz. Geol. Soc. Guidebook II, p. 7–20.

Davis, G. H., 1979, Laramide folding and faulting in southeastern Arizona: Am. Jour. Sci., v. 279, p. 543–569.

Drewes, Harald, 1971, Mesozoic stratigraphy of the Santa Rita Mountains, southeast of Tucson, Arizona: U.S. Geol. Survey Prof. Paper 658-C, 81 p.

———, 1972, Structural geology of the Santa Rita Mountains, southeast of Tucson, Arizona: U.S. Geol. Survey Prof. Paper 748, 35 p.

———, 1978, The Cordilleran orogenic belt between Nevada and Chihuahua: Geol. Soc. America Bull., v. 89, p. 641–657.

Einaudi, M. T., 1982, Descriptions of skarns associated with porphyry copper plutons, southwestern North America, *in* Titley, S. R., ed., Advances in Geology of the Porphyry Copper Deposits, Southwestern North America: Tucson, Univ. Ariz. Press, Chapter 7.

Gilluly, James, 1956, General geology of central Cochise County, Arizona: U.S. Geol. Survey Prof. Paper 281, 169 p.

Greeley, M. N., 1978, The primary copper industry of Arizona in 1975–1976: Ariz. Dept. Mineral Res., Spec. Rept. No. 2, 87 p.

Hamilton, Patrick, 1884, The Resources of Arizona, 3rd Edition: San Francisco, A. L. Bancroft and Co.

Hayes, P. T., 1970, Cretaceous paleogeography of southeastern Arizona and adjacent areas: U.S. Geol. Survey Prof. Paper 658-B, 42 p.

Hayes, P. T., and Drewes, Harald, 1978, Mesozoic depositional history of southeastern Arizona, *in* Land of Cochise, Southeastern Arizona: New Mex. Geol. Soc., Ariz. Geol. Soc. Guidebook, 29th Field Conf., p. 201–207.

Heidrick, T. L., and Titley, S. R., 1982, Fracture and dike patterns in Laramide plutons and their structural and tectonic implications, American Southwest, *in* Titley, S. R., ed., Advances in Geology of the Porphyry Copper Deposits, Southwestern North America: Tucson, Univ. Ariz. Press, Chapter 4.

Himes, M. D., 1973, Mineralization and alteration at Pima mine, a complex porphyry copper deposit: AIME, SME Trans., v. 254, p. 166–174.

Hilton, R. J., 1878, The Handbook to Arizona: San Francisco, Payot, Upham and Co.

Jansen, L. J., 1982, Stratigraphy and structure of the Mission copper deposit, Pima County, Arizona, *in* Titley, S. R., ed., Advances in Geology of the Porphyry Copper Deposits, Southwestern North America: Tucson, Univ. Ariz. Press, Chapter 22.

Jones, R. W., 1966, Differential vertical uplift—a major factor in the structural evolution of southeastern Arizona: Ariz. Geol. Soc. Digest VIII, p. 97–124.

Kalt, W. D. Jr., 1968, Awake the Copper Ghosts! The History of Banner Mining Company: Banner Mining Co. Publication, 100 p.

Keith, Stanton B., 1974, Index of mining properties in Pima County, Arizona: Ariz. Bur. Mines Bull., 189, 156 p.

Keith, Stanley B., and Barrett, L. F., 1976, Tectonics of the central Dragoon Mountains: a new look: Ariz. Geol. Soc. Digest X, p. 169–204.

Keith, Stanley B.; Lehman, N. E.; Sell, J. D.; and Wilt, J. C., 1978, Supplemental road log no. 1: Tucson to Benson via Nogales, Patagonia, Sonoita and Whetstone Junction, *in* Land of Cochise, Southeastern Arizona: New Mex. Geol. Soc., Ariz. Geol. Soc. Guidebook, 29th Field Conf., p. 88–104.

Kessell, J. L., 1970, Mission of Sorrows, Jesuit Guevavi and the Pimas, 1691–1767: Tucson, Univ. Ariz. Press, 224 p.

———, 1976, Friars, Soldiers, and Reformers: Hispanic Arizona and the Sonora Mission Frontier: Tucson, Univ. Ariz. Press, 347 p.

King, J. R., 1982, Geology of the San Xavier North porphyry copper deposit, Pima mining district, Pima County, Arizona, *in* Titley, S. R., ed., Advances in Geology of the Porphyry

Copper Deposits, Southwestern North America: Tucson, Univ. Ariz. Press, Chapter 23.

Koski, R. A., and Cook, D. S., 1982, Geology of the Christmas porphyry copper deposit, Gila County, Arizona, *in* Titley, S. R., ed., Advances in Geology of the Porphyry Copper Deposits, Southwestern North America: Tucson, Univ. Ariz. Press, Chapter 17.

Lacy, W. C., 1959, Structure and ore deposits of the east Sierrita area: Ariz. Geol. Soc. Guidebook II, p. 184–192.

Lacy, W. C., and Titley, S. R., 1959, Structure and ore deposits of the east side of the Sierrita Mountains, Trip I, Road Log: Ariz. Geol. Soc. Guidebook II, p. 207–217.

———, 1962, Geological developments in the Twin Buttes district: Min. Congr. Jour., April, p. 62–65.

Langlois, J. D., 1978, Geology of the Cyprus Pima mine, Pima County, Arizona: Ariz. Geol. Soc. Digest XI, p. 103–113.

Livingston, D. L.; Mauger, R. L.; and Damon, P. E., 1968, Geochronology of the emplacement, enrichment, and preservation of Arizona porphyry copper deposits: Econ. Geol., v. 63, p. 30–36.

Lowell, J. D., and Guilbert, J. M., 1970, Lateral and vertical alteration mineralization zoning in porphyry ore deposits: Econ. Geol., v. 65, p. 373–408.

Lukanuski, J. N.; Nevin, A. E.; and Williams, S. A., 1976, Locomotive-type post-ore fanglomerates as exploration guides for porphyry copper deposits: AIME-SME Trans., v. 260, p. 326–331.

Marvin, R. F.; Stern, T. W.; Creasey, S. C.; and Mehnert, H. H., 1973, Radiometric ages of igneous rocks from Pima, Santa Cruz, and Cochise counties, southeastern Arizona: U.S. Geol. Survey Bull. 1379, 27 p.

Marvin, R. F.; Naeser, C. W.; and Mehnert, H. H., 1978, Tabulation of radiometric ages—including unpublished K-Ar and fission-track ages—for rocks in southeastern Arizona and southwestern New Mexico, *in* Land of Cochise, Southeastern Arizona: New Mex. Geol. Soc., Ariz. Geol. Soc. Guidebook, 29th Field Conf., p. 243–252.

Mayuga, M. N., 1942, The geology and ore deposits of the Helmet Peak area, Pima County, Arizona: Unpub. Ph.D. Diss., Univ. Ariz., 124 p.

Nye, T. S., 1961, Geology of the Paymaster mine, Pima County, Arizona: Ariz. Geol. Soc. Digest IV, p. 161–168.

Preece, R. K. Jr., 1979, Paragenesis, geochemistry, and temperatures of formation of alteration assemblages at the Sierrita deposit, Pima County, Arizona: Tucson, Unpub. M.S. Thesis, Univ. Ariz. 106 p.

Ransome, F. L., 1922, Ore deposits of the Sierrita Mountains, Pima County, Arizona: U.S. Geol. Survey Bull., p. 407–428.

Rehrig, W. A., and Heidrick, T. L., 1972, Regional fracturing in Laramide stocks of Arizona and its relationship to porphyry copper mineralization: Econ. Geol., v. 67, p. 198–213.

Richard, Kenyon; and Courtright, J. H., 1960, Some Cretaceous-Tertiary relationships in southeastern Arizona: Ariz. Geol. Soc. Digest III, p. 1–17.

Shafiqullah, M.; Langlois, J. D.; and Damon, P. E., 1976, Chronology of tectonic events in the Pima mining district, southern Arizona: Geol. Soc. America, Ann. Mtg., Abs. with Programs, v. 8, no. 6, p. 1100 (abs.).

Shafiqullah, M., and Langlois, J. D., 1978, The Pima mining district, Arizona—a geochronologic update, *in* Land of Cochise, southeastern Arizona: New Mex. Geol. Soc., Ariz. Geol. Soc. Guidebook, 29th Field Conf., p. 321–327.

Sillitoe, R. H., 1980, Are porphyry copper and Kuroko-type massive sulfide deposits incompatible?: Geology, v. 8, p. 11–14.

Silver, L. T., 1978, Precambrian formations and Precambrian history in Cochise County, southeastern Arizona, *in* Land of Cochise, southeastern Arizona: New Mex. Geol. Soc., Ariz. Geol. Soc. Guidebook, 29th Field Conf., p. 157–163.

Thoms, J. A., 1966, The geology and ore deposits of the Tascuela area, Sierrita Mountains, Pima County, Arizona: Unpub. Ph.D. Diss., Univ. Michigan, 371 p.

Thurmond, R. E.; Heinrichs, W. E. Jr.; and Spaulding, E. D., 1954, Geophysical discovery and development of the Pima mine, Pima County, Arizona—a successful exploration project: AIME Trans., 199 p.

Titley, S. R., 1972*a*, Pre-ore environment of southwestern North American porphyry copper deposits: Int. Geol. Congr., 24th, Montreal, Proc. Sect. 4, p. 252–260.

———, 1972*b*, Some geological criteria applicable to the search for southwestern North American porphyry copper deposits: MMIJ-AIME Joint Mtg., Tokyo, May 24–27, Preprint G-I-2.

———, 1976, Evidence for a Mesozoic linear tectonic pattern in southeastern Arizona: Ariz. Geol. Soc. Digest X, p. 71–101.

———, 1982, Geologic setting of porphyry copper deposits, southeastern Arizona, *in* Titley, S. R., ed., Advances in Geology of the Porphyry Copper Deposits, Southwestern North America: Tucson, Univ. Ariz. Press, Chapter 2.

Wagoner, J. J., 1975, Early Arizona: Prehistory to Civil War: Tucson, Univ. Ariz. Press, 547 p.

Waller, H. E., 1960, The geology of the Paymaster and Olivette mining areas, Pima County, Arizona: Unpub. M.S. Thesis, Univ. Ariz., 48 p.

Weaver, R. R., 1965, Geologic interpretation of the Ruby Star ranch area, Twin Buttes mining district, Pima County, Arizona: Unpub. M.S. Thesis, Univ. Ariz., 74 p.

———, 1971, Uplift and gravitation adjustment, Ruby Star ranch area, Pima mining district, Arizona: Ariz. Geol. Soc. Digest IX, p. 197–211.

West, R. J., and Aiken, D. M., 1982, Geology of the Sierrita-Esperanza deposit, Pima County, Arizona, *in* Titley, S. R., ed., Advances in Geology of the Porphyry Copper Deposits, Southwestern North America: Tucson, Univ. Ariz. Press, Chapter 21.

Wilson, C. A., 1960, Ore controls of the San Xavier mine, Pima County, Arizona: Unpub. M.S. Thesis, Univ. Ariz., 58 p.

Wilson, E. D., 1950, Pima district, Arizona Zinc and Lead Deposits, Pt. I: Ariz. Bur Mines Geol. Ser., no. 18, Bull. 156, p. 39–50.

20

Geology of the Twin Buttes Mineral Deposit

PIMA MINING DISTRICT, PIMA COUNTY, ARIZONA

Charles F. Barter and James L. Kelly

The Twin Buttes mine is one of the more recently developed large copper mines in the United States. It is located some 25 miles (40 km) south of Tucson in the Pima mining district, Pima County, Arizona. The mine is on the west side of the Santa Cruz River and is situated on the eastern pediment of the Sierrita Mountains at an elevation of approximately 3,300 ft. (1,007 m). In 1982 the property was owned and operated as an open-pit mine by the Anamax Mining Company. A sulfide ore concentrator and an oxide ore leaching plant were also part of the Twin Buttes operations.

Other copper-producing mines in the district are the Esperanza-Sierrita mining operation, five miles (8 km) to the southwest, and the Pima and Mission mines, seven miles (11.3 km) to the north. The district's copper production during the late 1970s was about 30 percent of that produced in Arizona and nearly 17 percent of the production from the United States. The Pima district, with a substantial contribution from the Twin Buttes mine, thus ranks as one of the major copper-producing areas in the country.

HISTORY AND DEVELOPMENT OF THE TWIN BUTTES AREA

The recorded mining history of the Twin Buttes area dates from about 1870, and for the first 30 years or so there was only limited production of copper ore from shallow mine workings. Soon after the turn of the century, concerted mining efforts got under way and continued intermittently until 1928. A 24-mile (38.6 km.) railroad, completed from Tucson to the mines in 1906, provided part-time service until it was finally dismantled in 1935 (Murphy, 1964).

A smaller smelter, built several miles northeast of the mines near the Santa Cruz River, treated Twin Buttes copper ore during much of the year 1911. Most of the ore mined at Twin Buttes in the early years, however, was shipped to smelters at Hayden and Douglas, Arizona, and El Paso, Texas. The bulk of the production came from the old Copper Glance, Copper Queen, and Copper King mines, located about 1 mile (1.6 km) west of the Twin Buttes pit. Peak production probably was attained during World War I.

The district was essentially dormant between 1930 and 1950, when the Banner Mining Company first acquired mining claims in the area and soon thereafter started an investigation that continued intermittently for about twelve years (Kalt, 1968). During this time Banner reopened the Copper Glance mine and did considerable drilling in the alluvium-covered area from Glance Hill to the Twin Buttes and extending about one mile (1.6 km) easterly, toward the Santa Cruz Valley (Fig. 20.1).

The Anaconda Company, following execution of a long-term lease agreement with Banner Mining Company, started an intensive surface drilling campaign in 1963. From 1963 to 1967 this investigation was augmented by underground development and drilling from cross-cuts and drifts driven from the Twin Buttes No. 1 Shaft (Kelly, 1971). This exploratory, development, and test work culminated in the initiation of an open-pit mining operation (Knaebel, 1970). Under the management of The Anaconda Company, overburden stripping, which signaled the start-up of the Twin Buttes open pit, got under way in mid-1965, and bedrock was first exposed in December, 1967. The sulfide concentrator began operation in September, 1969.

Following the acquisition of the Banner Mining Company by AMAX, ownership and operation of the Twin Buttes mine was vested in the Anamax Mining Company, a partnership formed in 1973 by AMAX, Inc., and The Anaconda Company. Construction of a leaching plant to treat copper oxide ore was started soon thereafter, and the first

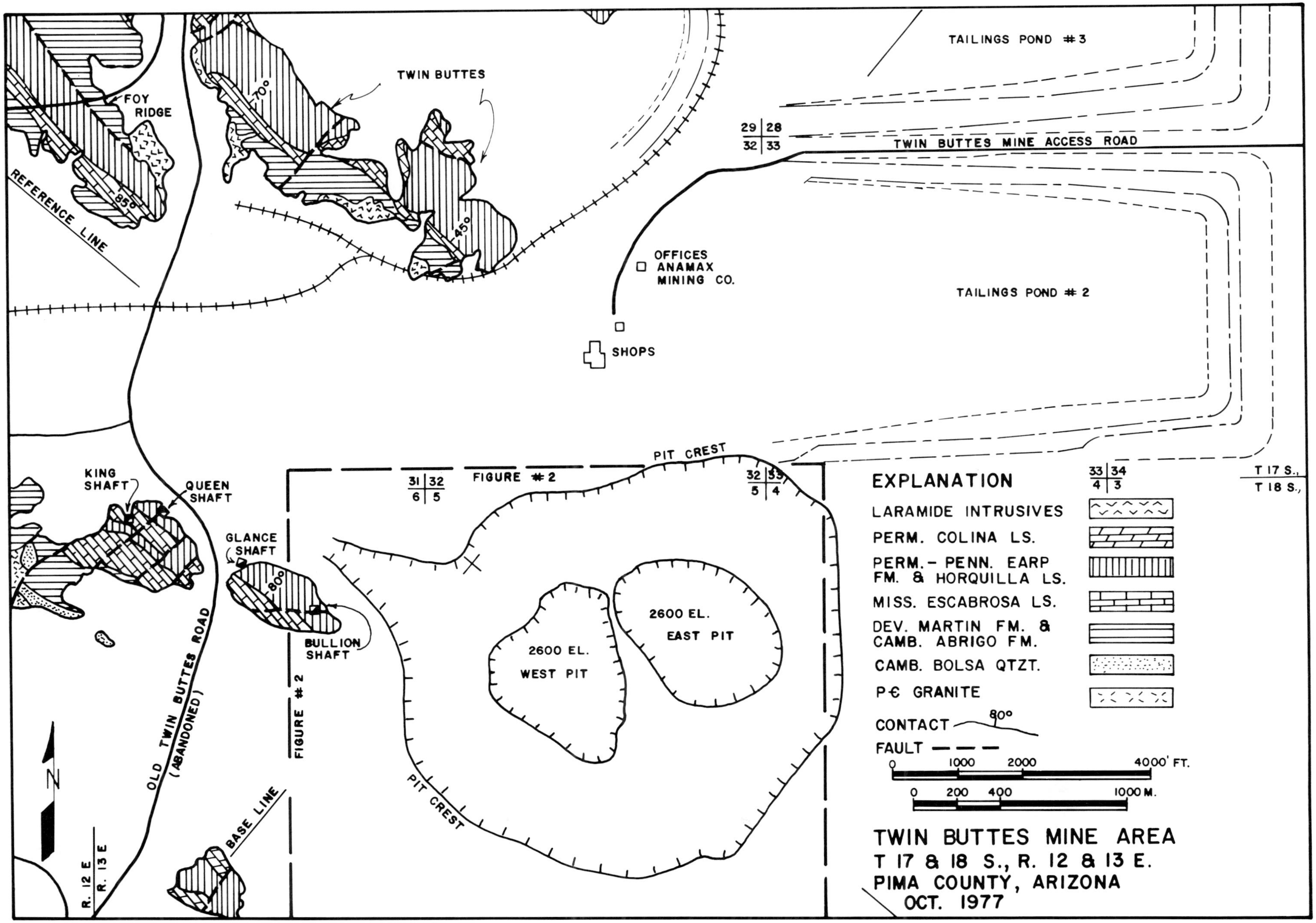

Figure 20.1. Outcrop geology and surface features in the Twin Buttes mine area

production of electrolytic copper from this plant was in August, 1975.

Total material removed from the open pit from inception to January 1, 1981, including alluvial overburden, rock waste, and ore, was approximately 1.26 billion short tons (1.14 billion metric tons). The sulfide concentrator has treated nearly 98 million short tons (88.9 million metric tons), and the oxide leaching plant has processed about 19 million short tons (17.2 million metric tons).

F. L. Ransome (1922) of the U.S. Geological Survey made an early geologic study of the Twin Buttes area as part of a broader investigation of the Sierrita Mountains. Later work by the U.S. Geological Survey which included the Twin Buttes area was done by J. R. Cooper (1960, 1971, 1973). The U.S. Geological Survey geology map of the Twin Buttes quadrangle, field mapping by Cooper and others, was prepared for publication by Drewes and published in 1973. The U.S. Geological Survey has contributed to the knowledge of the area geology also through its water supply paper on the Tucson basin by E. S. Davidson (1973). Publications and theses by faculty members and students of the University of Arizona Geology Department have made significant contributions to the recorded observations of the Twin Buttes area geology. Among those touching directly on the area, are R. L. Brown (1926), E. R Gordon (1922), W. C. Lacy (1959), D. J. Lootens (1965), and R. R. Weaver (1965). Others listed in the bibliography have been drawn upon for information pertinent to the district geology.

Since the start of the development at Twin Buttes, there has been a great amount of geologic work accomplished by members of The Anaconda Company and Anamax Mining Company Geological Departments. The results of some of this work have been recorded in unpublished company reports cited throughout this chapter. There is also a wealth of geologic information in the Anamax company files, prepared principally by Anaconda and Anamax geologists, consisting of geologic maps, sections, drill hole logs, petrographic descriptions, memoranda, notes, etc. This information is, in fact, the most important data base for this paper.

REGIONAL AND DISTRICT GEOLOGY

The Twin Buttes mineralization center is one of two known porphyry copper centers located in an area of moderate to sparse outcrop in the foothills and on the mostly buried, eastern pediment of the Sierrita Mountains. Duval's Sierrita-Esperanza mine complex is located at the other center (Pima-Mission, North San Xavier, and West San Xavier are herein considered allochthonous). Some 12 miles (19.3 km) east of the relatively low-lying Sierrita Mountains is a major, north-flowing drainage, the Santa Cruz River, which generally parallels a fault of early to mid-Tertiary age (Davidson, 1973). Between the Sierritas and the Santa Cruz, are a number of northeast- to north-northeast—trending faults with apparent southeast-side-down movement. The latest significant activity along these structures is post-Laramide and pre-Pliocene in age. The cumulative structure relief attributable to this set of faults is probably greater than 12,000 ft. (3,358 m).

The Helmet Fanglomerate and the Tinaja Formation, which are Oligocene and Miocene alluvial fan deposits with intercalated volcanic rocks, occur in scattered parts of the Pima mining district (Cooper, 1973). These deposits are local accumulations of detritus derived directly from the older rocks that comprise the Sierritas: presumably, they were formed in response to an early to middle Tertiary positive structural anomaly in the general Sierrita Mountains area. In response to this unstable relief, a large fault block of Precambrian through Oligocene rocks moved several miles northward. A low-angle fault, called the San Xavier thrust by Lacy (1959), is at the base of this block. The fault was active between 24 and 28 m.y. ago, as limited by a 28 m.y. rhyolite tuff (Mauger, 1966) intercalated in the allochthonous Helmet Fanglomerate and by the reasonably inferred cross-cutting relationship of a 24-m.y.-old andesite dike (Creasey and Kistler, 1962) which occurs west of Twin Buttes and which probably penetrates the fault.

Cooper (1960) has hypothesized that the movement on the San Xavier thrust is about 6½ miles (10.5 km) to the north-northwest, based on matching rock units, structural features, and mineral occurrences in the allochthonous and autochthonous blocks. Therefore, it can be postulated that the Twin Buttes deposit was segmented and that the upper part moved north to the Pima-Mission mine area along this fault in Middle Tertiary time.

The central mass and the eastern side of the Sierrita Mountains are mainly composed of volcanic, fluvial clastic, and acidic to intermediate intrusive rocks of Triassic through Laramide age. Much of the extensive eastern pediment of the range is carved on the Ruby Star Granodiorite, dated at 54 to 62 m.y. (Cooper, 1973). Lesser amounts of Precambrian and faulted and folded Mesozoic and Paleozoic rocks also occur in small hills and low-lying outcrops which protrude through the alluvial cover. This alluvium becomes thicker and more extensive eastward, toward the Santa Cruz Valley.

The outcrop of the Ruby Star Granodiorite has a north to north-northwest trend. Beneath the alluvium, portions of this batholith extend southeasterly into the Twin Buttes mineralization center. At Twin Buttes the complex set of Laramide intrusions, bedding in the Paleozoic and Mesozoic rocks, multiple fold axes, and mineralized structures have N35° to 70°W trends. This trend is coincident with the strike and projection of the Sawmill Canyon fault zone from the Santa Rita Mountains, some 20 miles (32 km) to the southeast. Titley (1976), Lutton (1958), and Drewes (1972) have discussed the nature of this fundamental crustal break and they have postulated a long history of activity. At Twin Buttes there is considerable evidence that this major structural element plays an important role in controlling Mesozoic sedimentation, the emplacement of Laramide intrusions, and mineralization. Northeast fracturing, parallel to the major post-mineralization faults, is a significant mineralization control in the Pima district and apparently influences at least the later stages of mineralization at Twin Buttes.

GEOLOGY OF THE MINE AREA

A set of southeasterly-trending intrusions, which are genetically related to the Ruby Star Granodiorite batholith, occupies the central portion of the Twin Buttes mineralized

zone. On the northeast and southwest sides and locally over these intrusions, are altered Paleozoic sedimentary rocks, altered Mesozoic sedimentary and volcanic rocks, early Laramide intrusions, and pre-Laramide intrusions. The Paleozoic metasedimentary rocks strike northwesterly and have vertical to moderate northeast dips. On the southwest side of the mine area, the altered Paleozoic strata are overlain across an angular unconformity by a sequence of Mesozoic metasedimentary and metavolcanic rocks, which strike northwesterly and are folded into an open syncline. These groups of rocks have been segmented by nearly vertical, northeasterly trending faults. The mineralized zone has been eroded, oxidized, and enriched, and all but the northwestern fringes were buried beneath 300 to 800 ft. (92 to 244 m) of post-mineralization alluvial materials.

The higher-grade, hypogene mineralization (i.e. >0.4% Cu) is generally confined to occurrences in the Precambrian granite, the rhyodacite, the Angelica Arkose, and the metasedimentary rocks with some original carbonate content. The areas of higher-grade mineralization are segmented by faulting and are partly separated by the lower-grade central intrusive mass. This separation of grade zones has led to a mine designation of orebodies as follows (Fig. 20.2):

1. The Northwest Orebody is located northwest of the Twin Buttes fault and southwest of the porphyritic quartz monzonite. Better grade areas occur in metacarbonate

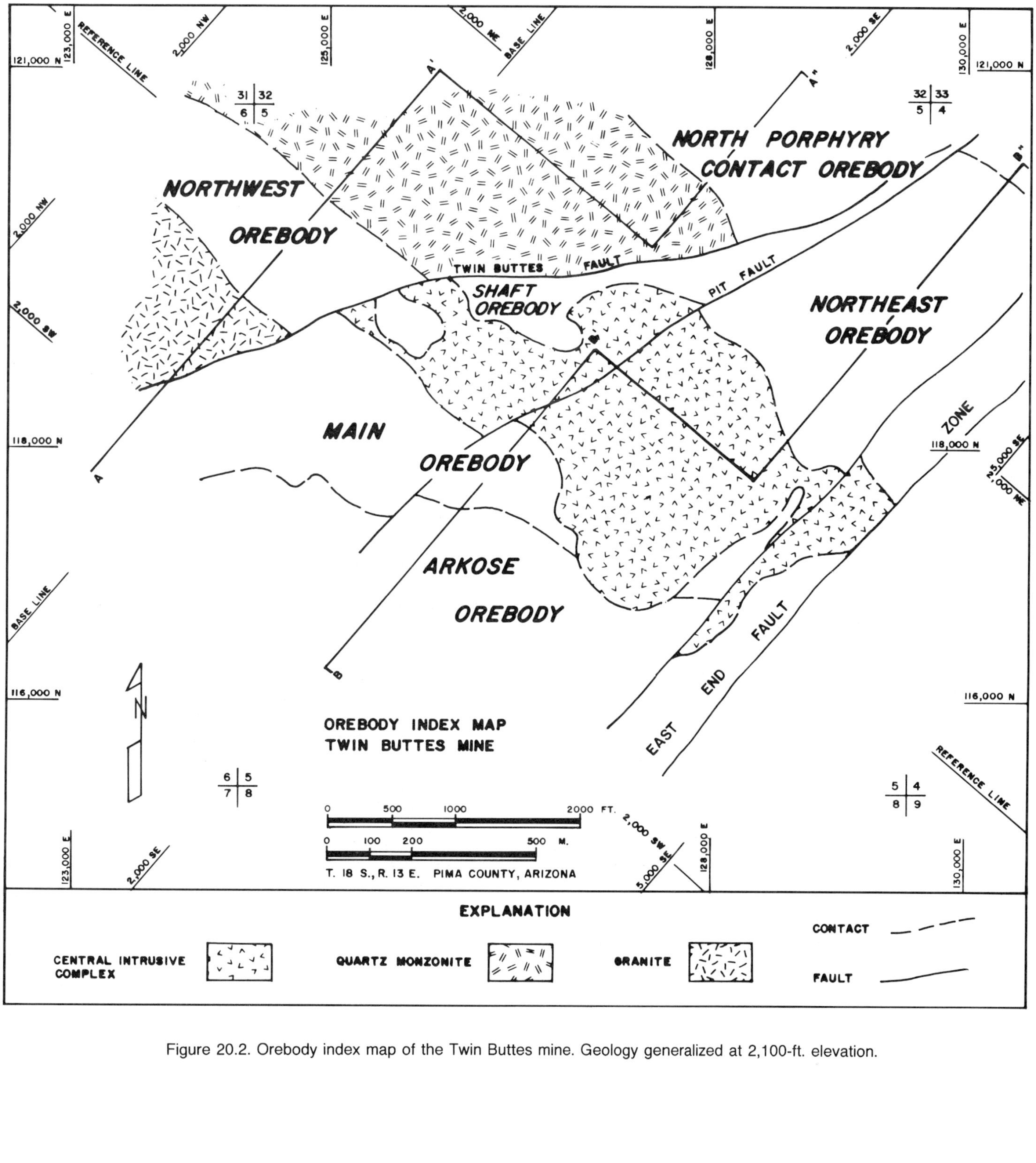

Figure 20.2. Orebody index map of the Twin Buttes mine. Geology generalized at 2,100-ft. elevation.

rocks of the Abrigo Formation, Martin Formation, and Escabrosa Limestone.

2. The North Porphyry Contact Orebody is also northwest of the Twin Buttes fault but is on the northeast side of the porphyritic quartz monzonite, in Pennsylvanian and Permian metasedimentary rocks.
3. The Main Orebody is southeast of the Twin Buttes fault, northwest of the East End Fault, southwest of the central intrusive complex, and is in Permian and Triassic metasedimentary rocks.
4. The Arkose Orebody extends about 1,900 ft. (579 m) northwest of the East End fault on the southwest side of the central intrusive complex. It is principally confined to the Late Cretaceous Angelica Arkose.
5. The Shaft Orebody is between the Twin Buttes and Pit faults and north of the central intrusive complex. Permian and Pennsylvanian rocks are well mineralized in this area.
6. The Northeast Orebody is principally in Permian metasedimentary rocks. It is bounded by the Pit fault and the East End fault zone and extends northeastward from the central intrusive complex.

Metasedimentary and Metavolcanic Rocks

Fundamental to the understanding of the distribution of metal values at Twin Buttes is a detailed knowledge of the pre-Laramide stratigraphy. This knowledge must be used within the context of the patterns of hypogene and supergene alteration. The eastern pediment and foothills of the Sierrita Mountains have a rather complete stratigraphic column of partly metamorphosed sedimentary and volcanic rocks, ranging from Cambrian through Late Cretaceous in age. All periods of the Mesozoic are represented, and, with the exception of the Ordovician and Silurian, formations of all the Paleozoic periods are found.

Most of the pre-Laramide rocks in the vicinity of the Twin Buttes mineralization center are at least weakly recrystallized and often are silicated or otherwise altered. Therefore, in many cases it has been necessary to consider stratigraphic sections many miles distant in order to establish a data base adequate for comparison and identification of the mappable lithologic units. The prime sources considered for establishing such a data base, in addition to the Twin Buttes Geology Department's detailed Pima mining district mapping, are: Britt (1973), Bryant (1955), Butler (1969, 1971), Luepke (1971), and Wilt (1969) for the Permian system; Britt (1955), Bryant (1968), Lodewick (1970), McClymonds (1959), Nations (1961), and Wright (1964) for data on the Cambrian through Pennsylvanian systems; and Cooper (1971) and Drewes (1971) for rocks of the Mesozoic.

Certain formation breaks used at Twin Buttes vary somewhat from type sections. These differences occur either because the alteration in the mine area precludes recognition of the original lithology distinctive of a particular formation, or because the lithologic facies locally present are not definitive of those present in the type section.

Table 20.1 summarizes the stratigraphy in the Twin Buttes area. A thorough stratigraphic description of the Paleozoic and Mesozoic at Twin Buttes is beyond the scope of this chapter, so the following discussion is confined to a general description of the strata shown in Table 20.1 and to notation of particularly interesting or anomalous features of the pre-Laramide stratigraphy.

Paleozoic. The content of the Cambrian Bolsa Quartzite with Precambrian granite in the Pima district is locally marked by a thin conglomerate with abundant quartz pebbles and occasional clasts of granite. At other locations, the granite appears to intrude the Bolsa. These apparently contradictory observations are best explained by partial assimilation of the quartzite during the Jurassic or Laramide, which were periods of extensive igneous activity and metamorphism.

In the Twin Buttes mine area, the lithologies and thicknesses of the Cambrian Bolsa Quartzite and Abrigo Formation, the Devonian Martin Formation, and the Mississippian Escabrosa Limestone are generally quite predictable from less altered occurrences near and within the Pima district.

Another conglomerate, the Black Prince, is locally found between the Mississippian Escabrosa Limestone and Pennsylvanian Horquilla Limestone. This chert and limestone pebble to cobble conglomerate is quite irregular in thickness, i.e., 2 to 20 ft. (0.6–6.1 m), and detailed mapping indicates that it was deposited on karst topography developed on the upper Escabrosa Limestone. A ferruginous shale included in the Black Prince occurs less frequently in the Pima district than does the conglomerate.

A considerable range in the thickness of the Horquilla Limestone is shown on Table 20.1. This variation is partially due to difficulty in identifying the upper and lower contacts. If the Black Prince is missing or not identifiable, as is often the case, the lower contact cannot be located with certainty because of the similarity of the rocks in the lower Horquilla and upper Escabrosa. The contact of the Horquilla to the Earp Formation is also difficult to identify, particularly where extensively silicated.

The thicknesses and interpreted original lithologies of the Colina Limestone, Epitaph Formation, and Scherrer Formation are quite compatible with those predicted from other sections. The considerable variation in some of the member thicknesses may be due to significant stratigraphic thickening within the Twin Buttes mineralized zone or to erroneous inclusion of structurally thickened sections.

The upper portion of the Colina Limestone as defined at Twin Buttes is somewhat more thin-bedded and locally contains more anhydrite and quartzose clastic rocks than the lower part. A traditional location of the top of the Colina would probably place this more thinly-bedded section in the basal portion of the Epitaph, but at Twin Buttes the altered lithologies are much more akin to altered lithologies correlated with the Colina.

The position selected for the top of the Epitaph Formation may also vary somewhat from typical sections. In the mine area the upper member of the Epitaph, Pe_4, is usually an altered siltstone with altered carbonate beds, but locally the siltstone portion varies to mixed siltstone and very fine-grained quartzite. This portion of the Epitaph may be comparable to the lower portion of the Scherrer Formation as described by Luepke (1971).

The Scherrer Formation in the Main Orebody varies little in its mean thickness of 460 ft. (140 m). The thickness of the Scherrer Formation in the Northeast Orebody is considered to be about 280 ft. (85 m). In addition, the lower member of the Scherrer, Ps_{1-2}, in the Northeast Orebody contains significant altered carbonate rocks, whereas in the

TABLE 20.1
Stratigraphic Summary of the Twin Buttes Area

Era	Age	Formation	Members	Description	Thickness Feet	Thickness Meters	Age Dates (m.y.)
Cenozoic	Holocene through Pliocene	"Alluvium"		Sands, gravels, caliche conglomerate at base	0–1000**	(0–305)	
Cenozoic	Miocene	Formation of Tinaja Peak		Volcanics, gravel, and sands	?		
Cenozoic	Miocene			Andesite dike			23.6 (K-Ar, B)
Cenozoic	Oligocene	Helmet Fanglomerate		Fanglomerate, andesite flow, tuffs, and monolithic breccias	10,500	(3200)	27.9 (K-Ar, B) tuff 20.7 (K-Ar) andesite
Cenozoic	Paleocene	Quartz monzonite porphyry		Variable texture, Twin Buttes mine intrusives			56.9 (K-Ar, B) 58.6 (K-Ar, B)
Cenozoic	Paleocene	Biotite rhyolite		Quartz latite tuff with lithic fragments	?		57 and 58 (K-Ar, B)
Cenozoic	Paleocene	Ruby Star Granodiorite		Granodiorite, quartz monzonite and aplite			57.1, 58.7, 59, 61.4 (K-Ar, B)
Mesozoic	Late Cretaceous	Red Boy Rhyolite		Rhyolite flows and tuffs	700–1000	(214–305)	
Mesozoic	Late Cretaceous	Demetrie Volcanics		Basal conglomerate, andesite flows and breccia, local rhyolitic tuff	8000	(2440)	
Mesozoic	Early Cretaceous	Angelica Arkose	Ma_3*	Arkose and siltstone with beds conglomerate	to 1300**	(to 397)	
Mesozoic	Early Cretaceous	Angelica Arkose	Mac*	Conglomerate, volcanic clasts	50–300**	(15–92)	
Mesozoic	Jurassic (?)	Whitcomb Quartzite	Ma_2*	Quartzite and arkose	10–270**	(3–82)	
Mesozoic	Jurassic (?)	Whitcomb Quartzite	Mav*	Quartzite and acidic volcanics	0–190**	(0–58)	
Mesozoic	Jurassic (?)	Whitcomb Quartzite	Mv*	Rhyodacite tuff, partly welded	0–280**	(0–67)	
Mesozoic	Jurassic (?)	Whitcomb Quartzite	Ma_1*	Quartzite and acidic volcanics	0–220**	(0–67)	
Mesozoic	Jurassic	Sierrita Granite		Granite, aplite, and gneiss			140 (Rb-Sr, WR) 150 (Pb-a, Z)
Mesozoic	Triassic	Harris Ranch Monzonite		Monzonite, granite, and quartz monzonite			190 and 210 (Pb-a, Z)
Mesozoic	Triassic	Rodolfo Formation	M_{sv}*	Siltstone and volcanics	0–1000**	(0–305)	
Mesozoic	Triassic	Rodolfo Formation	M_L*	Conglomerate, carbonate-rich	0–250**	(0–76)	
Mesozoic	Triassic	Ox Frame Volcanics		Rhyolitic to dacitic volcanics and quartzite	4000+	(1200+)	

Era	Period	Formation	Member	Lithology	Thickness (ft)	Thickness (m)	Age
Paleozoic	Permian	Rain Valley Formation		Limestone, minor sandstone beds	+400**	(122)	
		Concha Limestone		Cherty limestone	+480**	(146)	
		Scherrer Formation	Ps_4*	Quartzite, local carbonate beds	50–120**	(15–37)	
			Ps_3*	Dolomite, local beds sandstone	80–140**	(15–37)	
			Ps_1*	Quartzite, partly bimodal; minor carbonate beds	150–320**	(46–98)	
		Epitaph Formation	Pe_4*	Interbedded siltstone and limestone, local anhydrite and quartzite	90–150**	(27–46)	
			Pe_3*	Limestone, minor siltstone and anhydrite	100–270**	(31–82)	
			Pe_2*	Interbedded siltstone, dolomite, limestone, and anhydrite	100–350**	(31–107)	
			Pe_1*	Siltstone, minor anhydrite	150–380**	(46–116)	
		Colina Limestone		Limestone, thin beds siltstone, anhydrite, and local quartzite	230–370**	(70–113)	
	Permian / Pennsylvanian	Earp Formation		Siltstone and sandstone, partly limy and dolomitic; beds limestone and shale	300(?)–500**	(92(?)–153)	
	Pennsylvanian	Horquilla Limestone		Limestone, beds siltstone, quartzite near base	550(?)–980	(168(?)–299)	
		Black Prince Limestone		Chert and limestone pebble to cobble conglomerate, local ferruginous shale	0–32	(0–10)	
	Mississippian	Escabrosa Limestone		Limestone, partly cherty	200–450	(61–137)	
	Devonian	Martin Formation		Dolomite, limestone and local siltstone	±240**	(±73)	
	Cambrian	Abrigo Formation	€al*	Interbedded limestone and siltstone	290–350**	(+85)	
			€aq*	Interbedded quartzite, shale, and siltstone	+280**	(+85)	
		Bolsa Quartzite		Quartzite, local basal conglomerate	170–290**	(52–88)	
Precambrian		Granite		Granite, locally gneissic; local Pinal Schist inclusions			850 (Pb-a, Z)

*Member nomenclature, as on Twin Buttes maps.

**Thickness in Twin Buttes mine.

Main Orebody no carbonate beds have been found. This change in thickness and lithology of sections of the same formation in such close proximity suggests that at the time of deposition they may have been much further apart. Faulting of pre-Laramide or Laramide age combined with folding is a feasible means of moving these sections to their present positions.

Northeast of, and stratigraphically above, the Scherrer Formation of the Northeast Orebody are some 880 ft. (268 m) of altered carbonate rock with local, thin beds of silty sandstone. This structurally isolated and poorly known block is divided into 480 ft. (146 m) of Concha Limestone and some 400 ft. (122 m) of the Rain Valley Formation. In the Main Orebody only 250 ft. (76 m) of skarn, assigned to the Concha, has been definitely identified above the Scherrer Formation.

Mesozoic. Above the nearly vertical, Paleozoic, metasedimentary rocks in the Main Orebody and below the distinctly Mesozoic, siliceous, clastic rocks, there is a discontinuous unit composed of altered carbonate rock, siltstone, and quartzite (Barter, 1974). Where the rocks are less altered, coarse clastic textures have been identified in this unit. These textures suggest that the basal member of the Mesozoic is often a conglomerate, composed mainly of carbonate rock with blocks of siltstone and shattered and brecciated quartzite. The character of these altered rocks indicates a local derivation from an erosion surface developed on the Paleozoic strata during the earliest Triassic or late Paleozoic. This conglomerate unit, designated M_L at Twin Buttes (see Table 20.1), varies from 0 to 250 ft. (0–76 m) in thickness, is conformable with the lowermost siliceous, clastic rocks of the Mesozoic, and forms an angular unconformity of 30 to 80° with the underlying Paleozoic metasedimentary rocks. M_L has been correlated with the basal conglomerate of the Rodolfo Formation because the rocks above the conglomerate are predominately silty, siliceous, clastic rocks that are best correlated with the siltstone member of the Rodolfo (Cooper, 1971).

In the Sierrita Mountains the Ox Frame Volcanics occur below the Rodolfo Formation, but in the immediate Twin Buttes mine area, rocks possibly correlative with the Ox Frame are known only within, and southeast of, the East End fault zone. In this sparsely drilled and structurally complex area, several hundred feet (?) of biotitized, pyritic, quartz, and feldspar porphyry occur stratigraphically below(?) arkose, conglomerate, and quartzite correlated with the Angelica Arkose and the uppermost Whitcomb Quartzite.

In the area of the Main Orebody, M_L, where present, or Paleozoic metasedimentary rocks are overlain by siliceous, very fine-grained, often strongly biotitized, clastic rocks with included volcanic detritus (Barter, 1972). These rocks are correlated with the siltstone member of the Rodolfo Formation. Within 20 to 50 ft. (6 to 15 m) of the base of this unit is a local, lenticular, altered carbonate unit up to 40 ft. (12 m) thick. Southeast of the Main Orebody, the silty clastic rocks of the Rodolfo, M_{sv}, reach a recognized maximum thickness of 450 ft. (137 m). This unit decreases rapidly in thickness to the northwest, along strike, to a point near the Pit fault where M_{sv} does not occur, and younger Mesozoic strata are found directly over M_L.

A sequence of altered quartzite, partly welded pyroclastic rocks, volcanic flows, arkosic conglomerate, and arkose is stratigraphically above M_{sv}, across an apparent angular unconformity (Barter, 1972). This series of clastic and volcanic rocks has been divided into six mapping units at Twin Buttes. All six are conformable, and on the south side of the Main Orebody they are folded into an open syncline. The lower four units are interbedded volcanic rocks and quartzite and are correlated with the Jurassic or Early Cretaceous (Cooper, 1971) Whitcomb Quartzite. Over the Whitcomb Quartzite is a tuff, pebble-rich, arkosic conglomerate which varies in thickness from 50 to 300 ft. (15 to 91 m). This conglomerate and the overlying arkose are correlated with the Early Cretaceous Angelica Arkose, a Bisbee Group equivalent.

In the central portion and eastern foothills of the Sierrita Mountains, andesitic and rhyolitic volcanic rocks overlie the Angelica Arkose. These rocks, named the Demetrie Volcanics and the Red Boy Rhyolite (Cooper, 1971), do not occur in the pit, but drilling southwest of the Main Orebody has penetrated lithologies similar to those described by Cooper (1971) for these Late Cretaceous rocks. Since structural complications have not been resolved in the area where these rocks occur, their relationship to the Angelica Arkose is uncertain and a positive identity is not possible.

Intrusive Rocks

The Pima mining district contains intrusive rocks of Triassic through Miocene, as well as Precambrian, age (Cooper, 1973). At Twin Buttes the Laramide intrusive rocks associated with the Ruby Star Granodiorite are by far the most common, but both younger and older intrusions occur in or near the mineralized zone.

Figure 20.3 shows six types of Laramide intrusive rock in the Twin Buttes mine area. These six have been recognized as having significant volume and as being separate intrusions, rather than internal variations or alteration zones in a single contemporaneous mass. Other compositional and textural variants similar to quartz monzonite porphyry exist in the mineral zone, and more basic intrusive rocks are known to occur. However, these are not of sufficient size to be shown in Figure 20.3; some of the smaller intrusions will be noted in the ensuing descriptions.

Precambrian Granite. The oldest igneous rock in the Pima mining district and in the immediate area of the Twin Buttes mine is Precambrian granite. This rock is coarse-grained and locally ranges to a quartz monzonite in composition. Quartz and feldspar constitute 90 to 95 percent of this rock. Very fine-grained, felty biotite occupies most of the intergranular space, along with minor amounts of magnetite, sphene, apatite, and zircon. The feldspar and quartz are strained and often appear crackled. The quartz occasionally has the distinctive bluish-gray color frequently found in coarse detrital grains of the Bolsa Quartzite. Inclusions of biotite-rich Pinal Schist are common throughout the district. The granite near the Northwest Orebody averages 0.2 to 0.3 percent copper over large areas, and there are scattered, small zones of about 0.4 percent copper.

The contact relationships of the Bolsa Quartzite and other lower Paleozoic formations with rocks similar to this

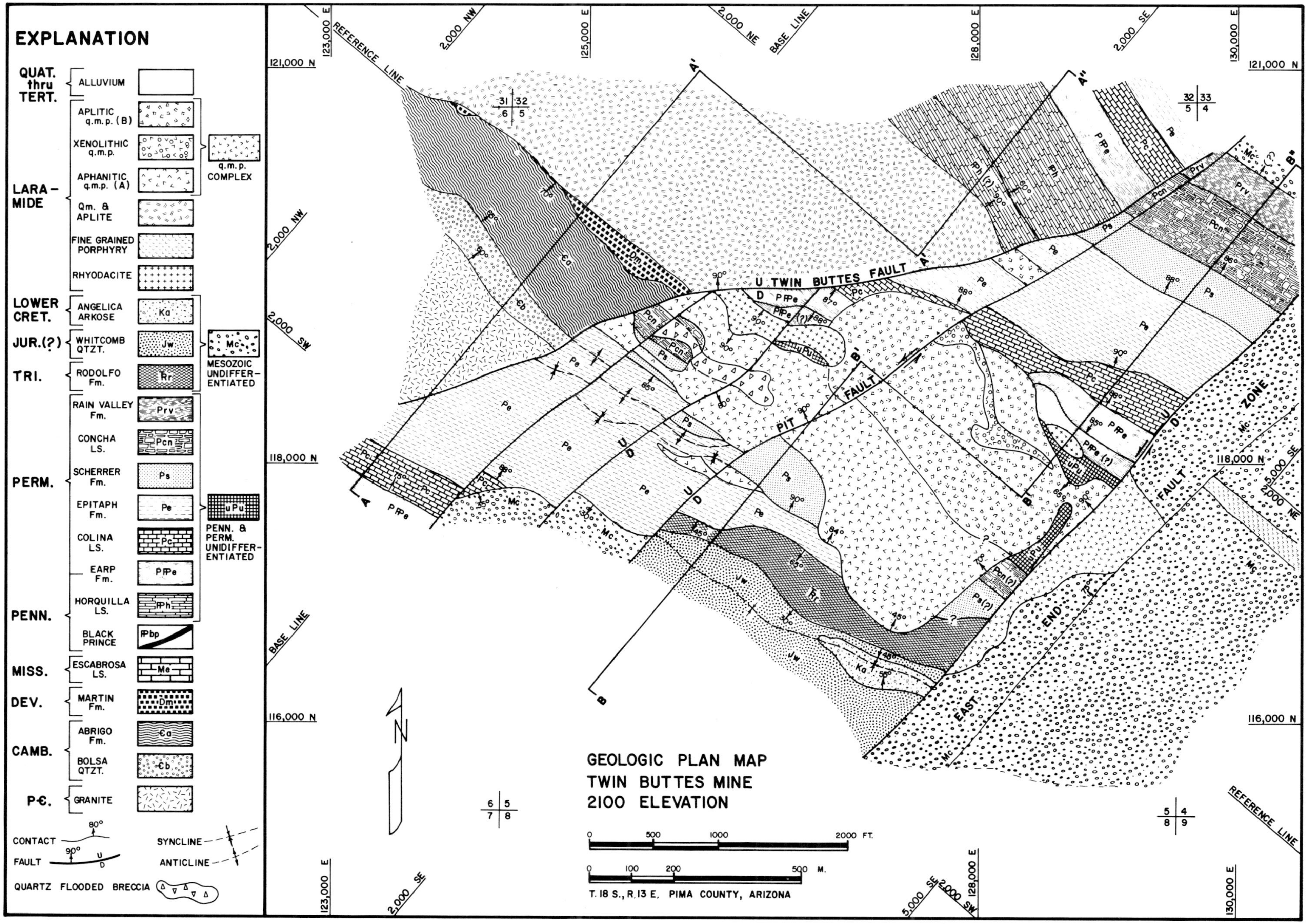

Figure 20.3. Geologic plan map of the Twin Buttes mine, 2,100-ft. elevation

granite have been a traditional problem near Twin Buttes and in nearby mountain ranges. One such contact, exposed in a low hill near the mine, is marked by a 1- to 3-ft. (0.3 to 0.9 m) conglomerate with abundant quartz pebbles and a rare pebble of probable granite. Geologists of the U.S. Geological Survey (Cooper, 1973) and Anaconda have mapped this contact as sedimentary. Exposures of the contact along the southeast side of Foy Ridge, northwest of the mine, and on a hill half a mile west of the mine were interpreted first as sedimentary (Cooper, 1960) and later as faults (Cooper, 1973) by the U.S. Geological Survey. These contacts have been considered to be sedimentary and sedimentary with local intrusive features, respectively, by the Twin Buttes Geology Department. In drill penetrations near the Northwest Orebody, the contact has generally been described as intrusive or gradational.

The Pima district granite and regional equivalents have been deeply buried and have been subjected to as many as three periods of reheating and partial recrystallization. Such metamorphism is indicated by the strained quartz, foliation, felty biotite, and the multiple age dates recorded for the regional equivalents (Marvin et al., 1973). It seems quite reasonable that under the described conditions partial assimilation of the Bolsa Quartzite may have occurred. Limited assimilation should explain many, but not all, such granite-to-Paleozoic contacts in the Pima district and regionally.

Laramide Rhyodacite. One of the earliest porphyries in the mine area is the rhyodacite, sometimes referred to as diorite porphyry (Kelly, 1977). This rock is very strongly altered in its principal occurrence, a northwest-trending dike which is intruded parallel with, or at a low angle to, bedding. The dike has a well-defined, undulating top within the mineralized zone. Much of the rock within this approximately 300-ft. (91-m)-wide dike is completely recrystallized, strongly biotitized, and shows evidence of extensive orthoclasization (McAleer and Barter, 1973). Other, less altered, narrow, northwest-trending dikes, which are presumed correlative to the rhyodacite, occur throughout the altered sedimentary rocks of the mineralized zone. Significant volumes of the main dike assay 0.4 to 0.6 percent copper. The sulfides occur principally in quartz veins in which chalcopyrite is more abundant than pyrite.

Laramide Fine-Grained Porphyry. Fine-grained porphyry is a name assigned to a little-studied type of porphyry which has been found only within, and southeast of, the East End fault zone. This rock contains fine-grained quartz and feldspar phenocrysts and is very strongly sericitized. The sulfide mineralization is dominantly pyrite, and copper grades are generally less than 0.1 percent.

Laramide Porphyritic Quartz Monzonite. Beneath the alluvial cover northwest of the Twin Buttes fault, is a large mass of porphyritic quartz monzonite which is flanked on the southwest by the Northwest Orebody. Drilling has established a physical connection between this intrusion and outcrops of Ruby Star Granodiorite a mile northwest of the mine (Cooper, 1960). Fresh biotite from exposures of quartz monzonite in the mine has been dated at 57.1 ±2.1 m.y. (Kelly, 1977), and an age of 54 m.y. has been determined from drill core samples of the quartz monzonite 2,000 ft. (610 m) northwest of the mine (Damon and Mauger, 1966). This rock has a few large K-feldspar phenocrysts (up to 4 cm long) in a medium-grained groundmass of quartz, plagioclase, microcline, and orthoclase. The feldspars are in part weakly altered to sericite and clay. Biotite books up to 2 mm are often partly altered to chlorite, and euhedral sphene crystals to 1 mm in length are common. Adjacent to the Northwest Orebody, where areas of aplite and quartz monzonite porphyry are known to occur, the enriched sulfide grade of this rock is frequently between 0.1 and 0.2 percent copper; other areas contain less than 0.1 percent copper. Much of the sulfide is along quartz veinlets with sericite. Quartz-sulfide veinlets with K-feldspar halos are less common. Pyrite is considerably more abundant than chalcopyrite.

Laramide Quartz Monzonite Porphyry Complex. The central intrusive mass, or quartz monzonite porphyry complex, contains three principal classifications of porphyry. The aphanitic style is considered the oldest of the three, followed by the xenolithic quartz monzonite porphyry, and then by the aplitic quartz monzonite porphyry. The major occurrence of the aphanitic style is on the southwestern side of the central intrusive mass, while the aplitic style occurs on the northeastern side. The contact between these two types is occasionally marked by a one- to ten-ft.-wide zone of coarse crystalline quartz and K-feldspar. The xenolithic style is adjacent to and included within the larger mass of aplitic quartz monzonite porphyry. Contacts of xenolithic porphyry to aphanitic porphyry have not been observed.

The aphanitic variety of porphyry has been dated at 58.6 ±2.5 m.y. (Kelly, 1977). This rock consists of fine- to coarse-grained phenocrysts of plagioclase, quartz, and orthoclase, with 1- to 2-mm biotite books in a groundmass of quartz and K-feldspar. The groundmass appears nearly aphanitic in hand specimen and frequently contains enough extremely fine-grained magnetite, ilmenite, and chlorite to impart an overall medium to dark gray color. The rock is, in general, only weakly altered, with partial chloritization of the biotite and weak sericite and clay alteration of the feldspar. Pyrite and chalcopyrite, in approximately equal portions occur as disseminations and in quartz veinlets. These veinlets may have K-feldspar halos or bleached, sericite-rich halos. The average hypogene copper grade for this rock is approximately 0.2 percent.

The xenolithic quartz monzonite porphyry occurs primarily on the north side of the complex and is intruded by the aplitic quartz monzonite porphyry. This intrusion contains few to abundant, often angular fragments of altered Paleozoic and Mesozoic rocks and other intrusions. The xenoliths are of a wide variety of sizes and frequently have reaction rims that separate them from the variable-textured quartz and feldspar groundmass. Pyrite and chalcopyrite occur as disseminations in the xenoliths and groundmass and as veinlets, some of which are terminated in the xenoliths.

The aplitic quartz monzonite porphyry has medium- to coarse-grained phenocrysts of quartz, plagioclase, and orthoclase in a very fine-grained to fine-grained aplitic groundmass of quartz and K-feldspar. Biotite books, partly altered to chlorite, are common. The plagioclase and K-feldspar are weakly altered to clay and sericite. Pyrite is more abundant than chalcopyrite, and both occur as disseminations and along quartz veinlets, partly with sericite halos. The average grade of this rock is near 0.1 percent copper.

Laramide Breccia. A pipe-like, quartz-flooded breccia is partially exposed in the West pit (Kelly, 1977) and has been further defined by drilling. Fragments of quartz monzonite porphyry, the Epitaph Formation, Scherrer Formation, and Concha Limestone are present in the brecciated mass. The fragments are angular, up to several ft. long, and have been slightly rotated. Minor mixing of adjacent rock types has occurred. Stratigraphic units in the breccia walls can be traced through the breccia. The fragments are cemented by coarse-crystalline, vuggy quartz, with sparse occurrences of pyrite, chalcopyrite, and molybdenite. The total sulfide content of the breccia is low. Small, irregular, quartz-flooded breccia zones, containing minor sulfide materials, have also been observed in the quartz monzonite porphyry in the East pit at Twin Buttes.

Other Intrusive Rocks. A northwest-trending dike of hornblende diorite, up to 90 ft. (27 m) wide, intrudes the Mesozoic rocks of the Arkose Orebody. Where it appears in drill holes below the zone of oxidation and enrichment, this rock may assay 0.2 to 0.3 percent copper. Pyrite is much more abundant than chalcopyrite, and epidote, K-feldspar, and chlorite are common alteration products.

Coarse-grained, mafic-poor intrusions of quartz monzonite to quartz diorite composition are frequently encountered as short intercepts in drill core samples at deep levels in the Main Orebody. These intrusions are erratically mineralized and, near their contacts with the altered sedimentary rocks, often have textures suggesting both endoskarn and envelopment of a pre-existing skarn.

Other types of intrusive rocks noted in the mineralized zone at Twin Buttes include dacite, hornblende quartz monzonite porphyry, and andesite. A post-sulfide andesite dike has been exposed in the pit, where it intrudes the porphyritic quartz monzonite near the Twin Buttes fault. This andesite may be correlative with Miocene dikes found in the Pima and Mission mines and other places in the district.

Folding

A number of the outcrops near Twin Buttes are of folded Paleozoic sedimentary rocks (Cooper, 1973). The axes of these folds trend northwesterly, and the dips on fold limbs vary from shallow to overturned. Folding of this style is not immediately obvious in the Paleozoic rocks of the mine area, but it seems reasonably certain that the style persists and that the mine strata are parts of limbs of large folds.

The style of fold mapped in the Paleozoic rocks in the mine is shown by the Scherrer Formation to Epitaph Formation contact in Figure 20.4. Near the 1,500-ft. (457-m) elevation, the Scherrer Formation, predominantly a competent quartzite, is vertical with a flat "step" fold, and the less competent Epitaph Formation has been deformed to fill the area beneath the "step." On nearby sections, the Scherrer Formation is again vertical on the northeast side of this fold; whereas in Figure 20.4, the intrusion is shown cutting out this portion of the "step." This particular fold has amplitudes of as much as 400 ft. (122 m) and occurs along strike for a distance of 3,000 ft. (914 m) in the Main Orebody. Other smaller folds of this style, with amplitudes of 20 ft. (6 m), have been observed in pit exposures.

The same Permian formations occur in the Northeast and Main orebodies (see Fig. 20.4), and in both areas southwest is stratigraphically down. The strike of the Paleozoic rocks in these two areas is N50 to 70°W, and their dip is nearly vertical. Intrusions generally occupy the zone between the two orebodies, but along and northwest of the East End fault (see Fig. 20.3) the two orebodies are nearly connected by altered sedimentary rocks that are, as yet, of uncertain identity. Faulting alone could account for such a relationship; however, a combination of folds with steep to overturned limbs and northwest-trending faults is more likely. Similar structural patterns are known to occur elsewhere in the district.

The Earp Formation in the Northeast Orebody has a top near the 2,400 ft. (732 m) elevation. This top persists with a similar configuration to that portrayed on Figure 20.4 for several hundred feet along strike. Internal stratigraphy of the Earp does not permit making it the center of an isoclinal fold, and such an abrupt lithologic facies change, i.e., from predominantly quartzose clastic to carbonate, seems unlikely. Other explanations are possible. Foremost among these are: faulting now obscured by alteration, destruction of characteristic Earp lithologies by metamorphism, or the Earp Formation top represents the end of a boudin. This last explanation is preferred.

Folding of the Mesozoic strata is considerably simpler than that of the Paleozoic. In Figure 20.4 an open set of folds is shown in the Mesozoic section, and a gentle plunge to the southeast is indicated in Figure 20.3. This plunge may be real, or the occurrence of the Mesozoic strata at progressively deeper levels to the southeast may be due to a series of small faults with southeast-side-down movement.

Faulting and Fracturing

In the southern Pima mining district there are three prominent directions of faulting (Cooper, 1973). These directions are N40 to 60°W, N40 to 75°E, and N5 to 20°E. Of these, N40 to 75°E is by far the most commonly measured direction along post-sulfide fault clays and slickensided surfaces in the Twin Buttes mine.

Northeast Faulting. A number of northeast-trending, near-vertical faults (shown in Fig. 20.3) cut the intrusive complex and segment the mineralized zone. The most northwesterly of these is the Twin Buttes fault. At the 2,100-ft. (640-m) elevation (see Fig. 20.3) this structure has placed the upper portion of the Epitaph Formation against the Bolsa Quartzite, which is some 3,500 ft. (1,067 m) of apparent stratigraphic displacement (Fig 20.5). This displacement of 3,500 ft. is the minimum offset on the Twin Buttes fault, as the overall attitude of beds southeast of the fault is vertical and, northwest of the fault, dips are about 60°. Relationships outside of the mine area suggest that post–Late Cretaceous movement on this structure was essentially vertical. In the mine the Twin Buttes fault is a structure of one or more strands with heavy clays and much adjacent brecciation. At least the last major movement was post-mineralization.

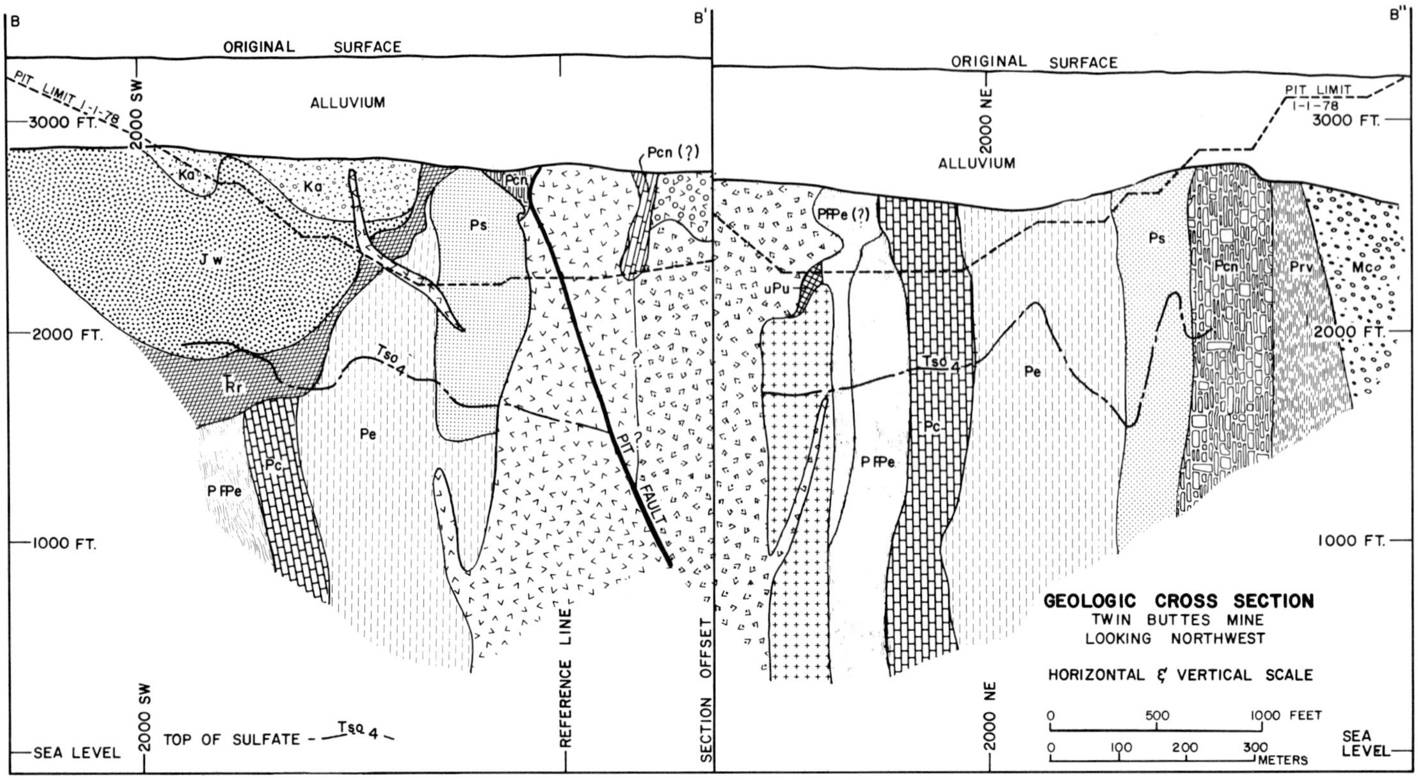

Abbreviations:

Jw = Jurassic (?) Whitcomb Quartzite
Ka = Lower Cretaceous Angelica Arkose
Mc = Mesozoic undifferentiated
Pc = Permian Colina Limestone
Pcn = Permian Concha Limestone
Pe = Permian Epitaph Formation
Prv = Permian Rain Valley Formation
Ps = Permian Scherrer Formation
PPe = Permian and Pennsylvanian Earp Formation
Tr = Triassic Rodolfo Formation
Tso_4 = top of sulfate zone
uPu = Permian and Pennsylvanian undifferentiated

Figure 20.4. Geologic cross section through the Main Orebody *(B-B')* along 2,000 SE and the Northeast Orebody *(B'-B")* along 3,600 SE. Line of section is shown in Figures 20.2 and 20.3.

There is some suggestion in sulfide and skarn zoning patterns that breaking along the Twin Buttes fault zone may have influenced the movement of hydrothermal fluids (Smith, 1977), but the evidence is not compelling.

Southeast of the Twin Buttes fault and northwest of the Pit fault is a series of near vertical, northeast-trending faults with southeast-side-down movement. Only two of the more significant of these structures have been shown in Figure 20.3. The cumulative offset attributed to the fault system is 450 to 550 ft. (137 to 168 m).

The Pit fault is the next significant structure encountered to the southeast. The movement on this nearly vertical fault is 500 ft. (152 m) southeast-side-down and approximately 100 ft. (30 m.) left lateral.

Between the Pit fault and East End fault zone, are several northeast- to east-trending faults of small displacement. These structures are insignificant from the standpoint of a geologic reconstruction or grade projection, but some are quite significant in determining the angle to which the pit walls can be safely and economically mined.

The most southeasterly of the northeast-trending faults shown in Figure 20.3 is the East End fault zone. On the northwest side of the zone is a set of thick, vertical to northwest-dipping fault clays which strike N40 to 50°E. Southeast of these clays are a number of 1-inch (2.54-cm)- to 1-foot (30.5-cm)-wide, clay-rich fault breccias that dip 60 to 75° to the northwest and that strike parallel to the vertical clays. Within the zone, brittle rocks are intensely shattered over large areas, and clay alteration is extensive. The movement across the zone is thought to be several hundred feet of left lateral slip and a few thousand feet of southeast-side-down displacement.

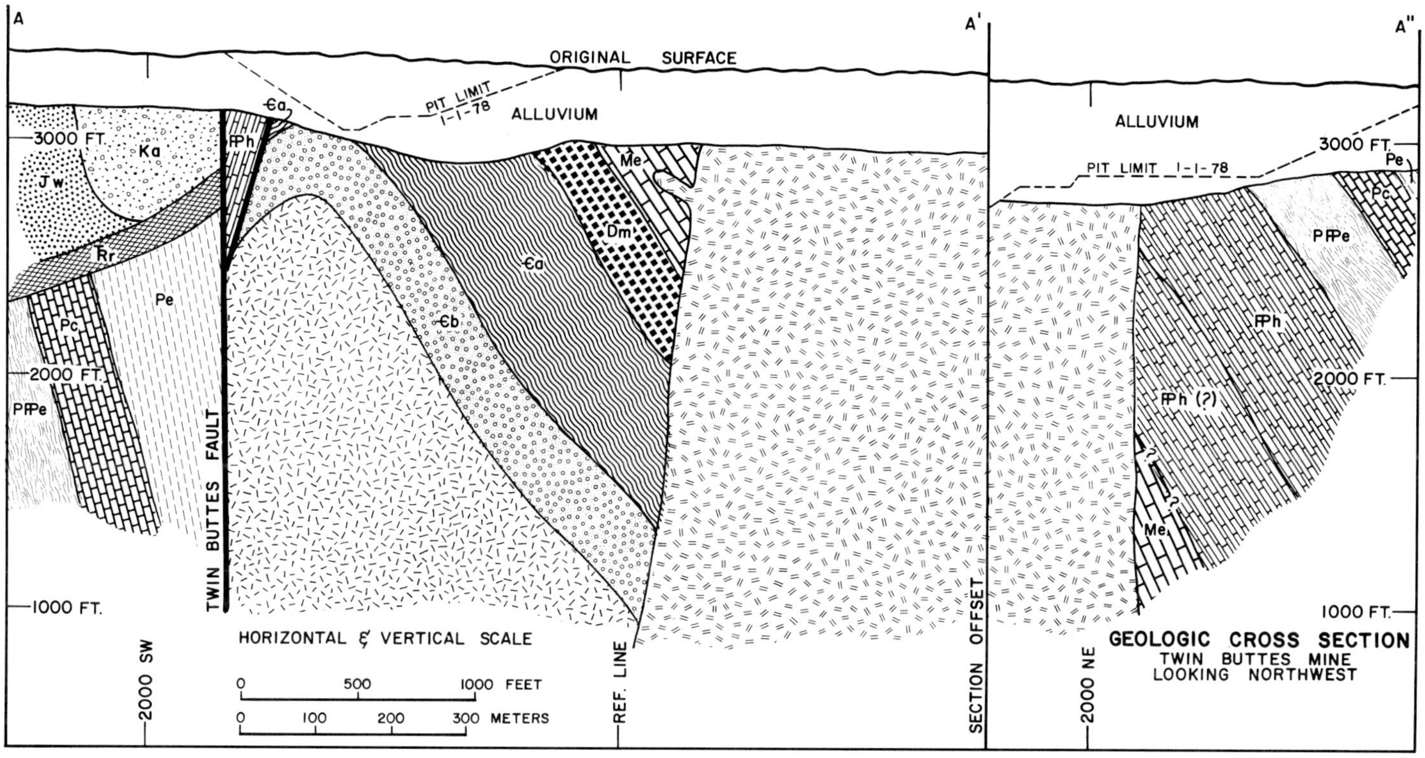

Abbreviations:

€a = Cambrian Abrigo Formation
€b = Cambrian Bolsa Quartzite
Dm = Devonian Martin Formation
Jw = Jurassic (?) Whitcomb Quartzite
Ka = Lower Cretaceous Angelica Arkose
Me = Mississippian Escabrosa Limestone
Pc = Permian Colina Limestone
Pe = Permian Epitaph Formation
PPe = Permian and Pennsylvanian Earp Formation
Ph = Pennsylvanian Horquilla Limestone
Tr = Triassic Rodolfo Formation

Figure 20.5. Geologic cross section through the Northwest Orebody *(A-A')* and the North Porphyry Contact Orebody *(A'-A")*. Line of section is shown in Figures 20.2 and 20.3.

Northwest Faulting. Northwesterly faults are much less common in the mine area than northeasterly faults. The pre-mineralization age of many of the northwest structures in the Pima district probably explains this fact. Northwest structures would have been obscured or obliterated by intrusion, alteration, and mineralization. The northwesterly trend of the Laramide intrusions and the numerous veins of this attitude suggest significant structural control, particularly in the area now occupied by the central intrusive complex. Mineralized, northwest-striking, near vertical faults occur in the Glance Hill area and on Foy Ridge west of the pit.

Fracturing. Two dominant orientations of fractures—strike N55°E, dip 75°NW; and strike N77°E, dip 45°NW—have been recorded in the area of the Main and Arkose orebodies (Seegmiller, 1971). The next most frequent orientations are strike N60°W, dip 39°NE; and strike N60°W, dip 77°NE. These less common fracture orientations approximate bedding trends in the Mesozoic and Paleozoic rocks, respectively.

Tilting

Some evidence can be cited for 10 to 25°, southeast-side-down, post-mineralization tilting of the Twin Buttes mineralized zone. The northeast fault system is a set of southeast-side-down faults with near vertical dips. It seems reasonable that these originally were typical normal faults with dips no more than 70° to the southeast. The southeastern portion of the central intrusive complex between the Pit fault and the East End fault zone spread horizontally from a more vertical mass below. Because this flattened shape is not observed nearer the Pit fault, a southeastward tilt is suggested. The axis of the fold in the Angelica Arkose, southwest of the central intrusive complex, apparently plunges 10° to 15° to the southeast. None of these data is particularly compelling, but tilting is a parameter that should be considered in reconstructions of the geology of the mine area.

Post-Mineralization Sediments

The bedrock surface, i.e., the top of Laramide or older rocks, at Twin Buttes is an erosion surface of moderate to severe relief with an overall easterly slope. From a high at the crest of the Twin Buttes, elevation 3,740 ft. (1,140 m), the top of bedrock drops to near the 2,400-ft. (732-m) elevation on the eastern side of the mine area. A number of paleostream channels are cut into the bedrock surface, and abrupt changes in the elevation of this interface locally occur. Fault offsets of the bedrock surface have been observed in the pit, and steep-sided depressions exist over what was once an anhydrite-rich unit of the Epitaph Formation, Pe_2.

Some 300 to 800 ft. (91–244 m) of post-mineralization sediments occur above the bedrock surface in the Twin Buttes pit. Three units are recognized, the oldest of which occurs infrequently in the bottom of the deeper channels in the bedrock surface. This unit consists of poorly consolidated, dark reddish brown sand and conglomerate. The conglomerate has a silt, sand, and clay matrix, and numerous angular pebbles, frequently of silicated rocks. The dips in this older unit are steeper than the nearly flat attitudes of the intermediate sequence and have been measured as high as 35°. These older, post-mineralization sediments are probably correlative with the Helmet Fanglomerate or the Tinaja Formation, and so are either Oligocene or Miocene in age.

The intermediate unit of post-mineralization sediments is usually found in direct contact with bedrock but, in isolated areas, is separated from bedrock by a few feet of older sediments. The unit is up to 700 ft. (214 m) thick in the immediate mine area and consists of tan to brown, poorly consolidated, partly cemented sand, silt, and gravel. Pebbles and cobbles are of all older rock types in the district, but clasts of granite are probably the most abundant. Individual beds are a few inches to a few feet thick, and the dips are very gentle to the east. Paleochannels are present throughout the sequence. Varying amounts of calcium carbonate cement occur in much of the sediments. The zone directly over bedrock or over the older red sediments is frequently very well cemented and is locally called the caliche conglomerate. This well-cemented zone varies up to 100 ft. (30 m) in thickness. Occasional faults of small magnitude have been observed in the intermediate sequence. The lowermost portion of this unit may be correlative with the Tinaja beds (Harshbarger and Associates, 1972); but most is equivalent to the Fort Lowell Formation of Pleistocene age.

The uppermost unit of the post-mineralization sediments consists of very poorly compacted red and brown, silty, coarse sand with beds of silt and gravel. The unit varies in thickness from a few feet to as much as 100 ft. (30 m) on the eastern side of the pit.

MINERALIZATION AND ALTERATION

The Twin Buttes mineralization center was formed during the Laramide along a major, northwest-trending fault zone which had affected Precambrian through Cretaceous rocks. Adjacent to the Twin Buttes center, the Ruby Star Granodiorite batholith was emplaced. A southeasterly trending limb of this batholith extends into the immediate area of the mineralized center. The center is presently occupied by the limb of the granodiorite and a series of genetically related, porphyritic intrusive rocks.

A zone of thermally metamorphosed rocks several thousand feet wide occurs adjacent to the granodiorite and porphyries. Internal to this zone a metasomatic aureole developed around the Twin Buttes mineralization center. The aureole has an elliptical horizontal outline, elongate parallel to the northwesterly bedding and fault trends. A number of elements—Si, Al, Fe, S, K, Mg, Cu, Zn, and Mo in particular—were added to the rocks within the aureole. As the hypogene fluids invading the wall rock evolved with the changing physical and chemical conditions, the original alteration minerals locally became unstable and were replaced by a second or even a third generation of alteration mineralogy. The fluids providing the transport medium were channeled by a changing system of conduits consisting of faults, fractures, and permeable strata. As the alteration process took place, the intrusions of the central intrusive complex were emplaced, and significant masses of the early metasomatic aureole were probably engulfed.

Erosion and oxidation of the upper part of the metasomatic aureole began during or after the end of the hypogene alteration process. Subsequently, the upper part of the Twin Buttes mineralized zone, including a large block of sulfide, was removed along the San Xavier thrust. This décollement was followed by continued erosion and a second stage of oxidation. The irregular upper surface of the sulfide zone at Twin Buttes is the product of this second stage of oxidation and enrichment.

Thermal Metamorphism

The effects attributed to thermal metamorphism—namely, recrystallization and regrouping of the chemical constituents of the wall rock—occur within, and external to, the zone of metasomatic calc-silicate formation and the frequently congruous edge of metallization.

Widespread metamorphic assemblages are known beyond the presumed limits of metasomatic effects. Marmorization of calcitic limestones, such as the Escabrosa and Concha Limestones and parts of the Epitaph and Colina Formation, is extensive but is not a pervasive occurrence in the Pima district. Wollastonite frequently forms around chert nodules in these marbles. Of similar district extent to the marmorization is the formation of diopside, tremolite, and serpentine in silty and dolomitic carbonate, as often occurs in the Martin Formation. Complex, flinty or sandy, calc-silicate hornfelses result from the metamorphism of the ferruginous, calcareous shales and siltstones of the Earp, Abrigo, and Horquilla formations. These and other formations contain bands of biotitized, siliceous rocks, located at considerable distances from known metasomatic centers, as alteration equivalents of quartzose clastic beds. In many instances this biotitization is thought to be a product of thermal metamorphism; in others, where the original chemistry is not compatible, it is necessary to invoke metasomatic processes to explain the secondary micas.

Recrystallized minerals are the residual products within the metasomatic aureole that are often attributable to thermal metamorphism. Calcite, quartz, and feldspar are the notable minerals which can be found occurring within the zone of metasomatism as recrystallized equivalents of the same pre-alteration minerals.

Marble is frequently found in the mineralized zone at Twin Buttes completely or partly surrounded by metasomatic silicate and sulfide minerals. This phenomenon usually occurs where the Paleozoic sequence contains a thick carbonate unit bounded on both sides by a quartzose clastic rock, which presumably acted as an effective channelway for the hypogene fluids. The marble, therefore, appears to be a residual alteration product that was not completely destroyed by encroaching calc-silicate alteration.

Much of the pre-alteration quartz in rocks of the metasomatic aureole has, to some degree, been recrystallized. Comparison of altered quartzose sedimentary rocks to their less-altered or unaltered equivalents indicates that the amount of quartz in the altered rock, exclusive of quartz in veins and intercrystalline spaces, is much the same as the amount of quartz, exclusive of chert, in the unaltered rock. Quartz coarser than fine to medium silt in the metasedimentary rock often accurately reflects the size of quartz in the unaltered rock (McAleer and Barter, 1973). These observations indicate that through the alteration process little happened to sedimentary quartz except for *in-situ* recrystallization. Furthermore, detrital quartz that is as coarse as, or coarser than, fine sand frequently retains its pre-alteration shape.

Hypogene Alteration and Mineralization

Most of the available detailed information concerning hypogene alteration and mineralization at Twin Buttes has come from studies conducted in the Arkose, Main, and Northeast orebodies. Additional observations in other parts of the Twin Buttes mineralized zone indicates that the same alteration and mineralization patterns exist throughout, but, in some instances, these observations are limited.

Within the tested portions of the Twin Buttes mineralized zone, considerable horizontal and local vertical variation in alteration products is known to occur. Within the context of these variations, analysis and definition of the metasomatic effects are made considerably more difficult by the complex stratigraphy of the rocks within the aureole and by the fact that their bedding attitudes are frequently parallel to the postulated alteration patterns. In addition, Laramide intrusions occupy a large volume within the mineralized zone. These intrusions have contacts which are often sub-parallel to the alteration patterns, and the largest mass of intrusive rock has obliterated the early center of mineralization that has been postulated for the area.

The basic categories of hypogene alteration types at Twin Buttes are as follows: (1) alteration in the Mesozoic siliceous volcanic and clastic rocks; (2) alteration in the quartzose Paleozoic clastic rocks; (3) early, anhydrous alteration of the carbonate rocks; (4) later, hydrous alteration of the carbonate rocks: (5) alteration in miscellaneous sedimentary rocks; (6) alteration in intrusive rocks. In general, metallization, a specific classification of hypogene alteration, also fits conveniently into these categories.

Figure 20.6 is a portrayal of the postulated original lithology and the products of hypogene alteration and metallization of a particularly well mineralized and economically very significant part of the Twin Buttes mineralized zone. Much of the data in this figure are composited from a number of drill penetrations in the altered Paleozoic sedimentary rocks. The drill penetrations used are limited to those above the 1,000-ft. (305-m) elevation along and near the 2,000 SE Section in the Main Orebody and the 3,600 SE Section in the Northeast Orebody. A geologic section of the rocks portrayed in Figure 20.6 is shown in Figure 20.4.

The composited data presented in Figure 20.6 are derived in a number of ways. The reconstruction of original lithology was based on mapping by Twin Buttes geologists in the Pima district and from projection of published and unpublished data originating with many workers. The rock mineralogy was established by hand specimen identification of the minerals in drill core samples in conjunction with the study of numerous thin sections and considerable X-ray analysis. The weight percentage copper and molybdenum was determined by averaging assay data from a number of nearby drill holes. Pyrite : chalcopyrite ratios were determined by visual estimates of the amounts of these minerals in the drill cores. The volume percentage of pyrite and chalcopyrite is a calculated value. Only data from areas below any supergene effects were used in Figure 20.6 if such data were available. Anhydrite beds are shown, but hypogene anhydrite, which occurs in variable amounts in nearly all of the rock, is not.

Feldspar, mostly K-feldspar, occurs in many of the altered quartzose clastic rocks and some skarns shown in Figure 20.6. The origin of the feldspars is frequently ambiguous, and they usually can be identified only in thin section. Feldspar, therefore, is not indicated in this portrayal.

Neither color nor composition of garnet is indicated on Figure 20.6. These are important in the understanding of the alteration process, and, where known, they are noted in the descriptions that follow. The few unit cell measurements of garnet at Twin Buttes, made by The Anaconda Company's geological laboratory, suggest that medium to dark brown and reddish brown garnets have a larger mole percentage andradite than grossularite and that pale brown, green, and cream-colored garnets have a larger mole percentage grossularite.

Mesozoic Siliceous Volcanic and Clastic Rocks. Three distinct sedimentary rock types, in addition to the layers of siliceous volcanic rocks, occur in the Mesozoic sequence at Twin Buttes above the basal conglomerate of the Rodolfo

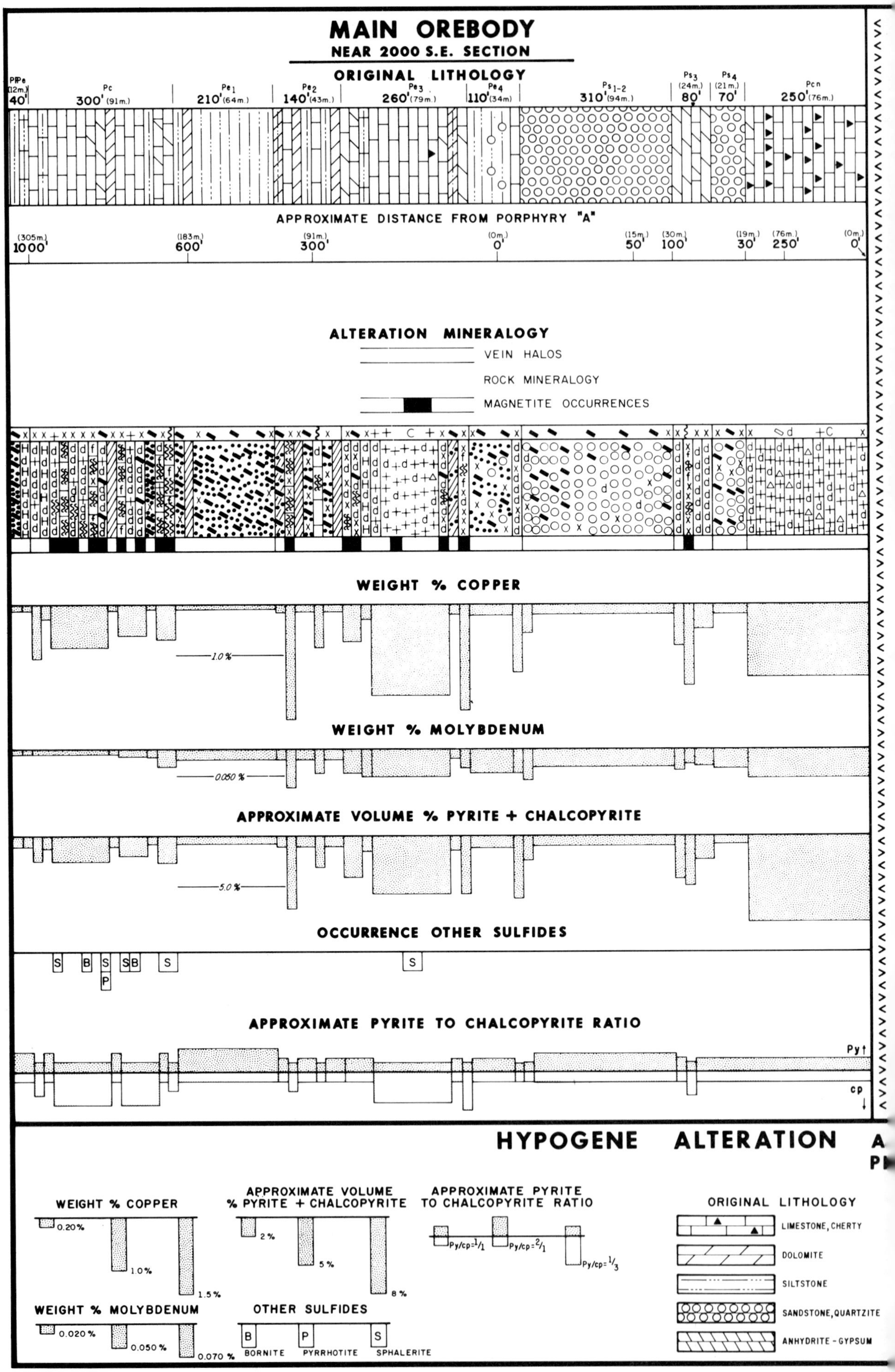

Figure 20.6. Hypogene alteration and mineralization in the Main and Northeast orebodies of the Twin Buttes mine

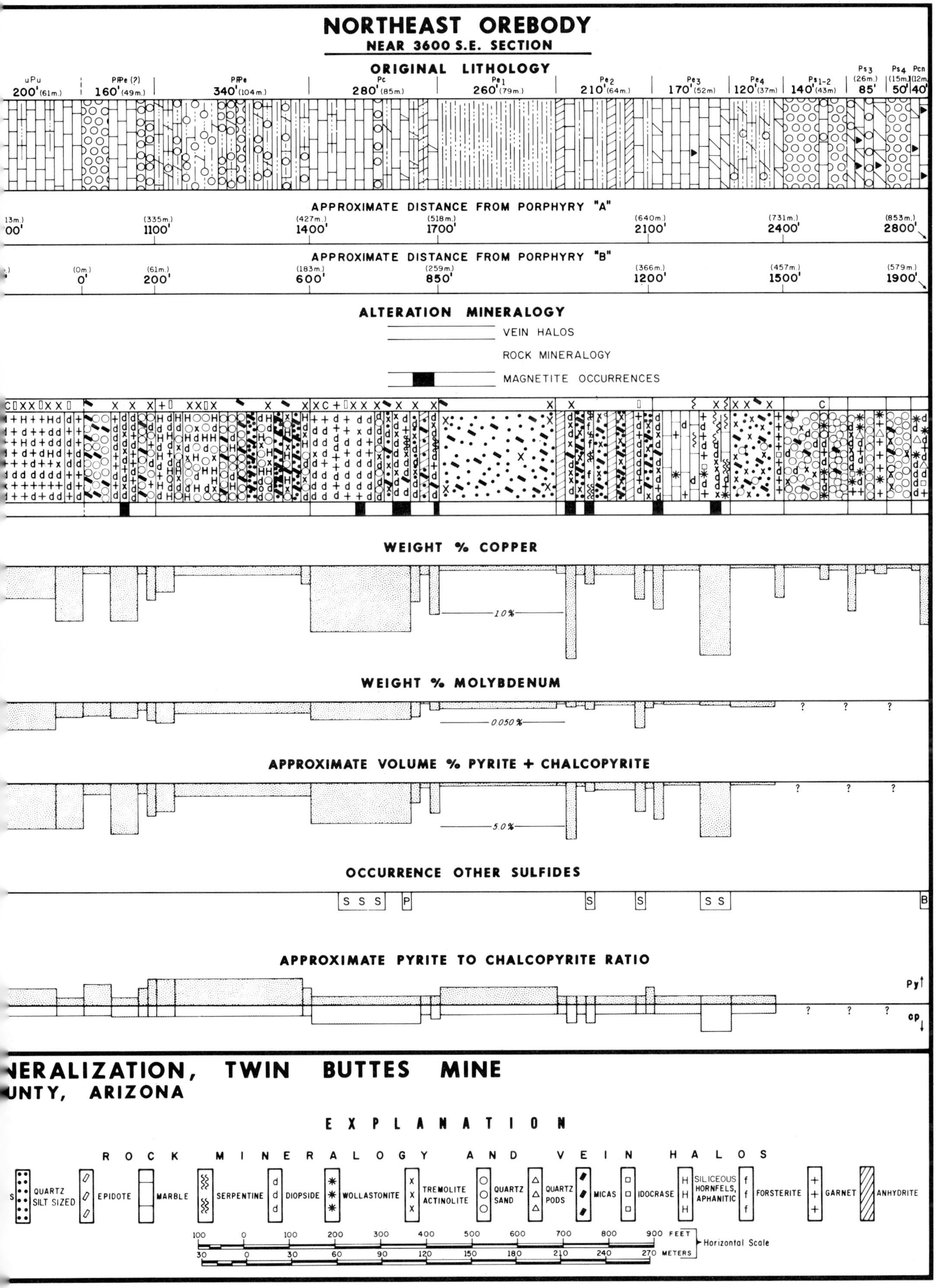
NORTHEAST OREBODY
NEAR 3600 S.E. SECTION
ORIGINAL LITHOLOGY
uPu 200' (61m.)
PPe (?) 160' (49m.)
PPe 340' (104m.)
Pc 280' (85m.)
Pe1 260' (79m.)
Pe2 210' (64m.)
Pe3 170' (52m)
Pe4 120' (37m)
Ps1-2 140' (43m)
Ps3 (26m.) 85'
Ps4 (15m.) 50'
Pcn (12m.) 40'
APPROXIMATE DISTANCE FROM PORPHYRY "A"
(335m.) 1100'
(427m.) 1400'
(518m.) 1700'
(640m.) 2100'
(731m.) 2400'
(853m.) 2800'
APPROXIMATE DISTANCE FROM PORPHYRY "B"
(0m.) 0'
(61m.) 200'
(183m.) 600'
(259m.) 850'
(366m.) 1200'
(457m.) 1500'
(579m.) 1900'
ALTERATION MINERALOGY
VEIN HALOS
ROCK MINERALOGY
MAGNETITE OCCURRENCES
WEIGHT % COPPER
1.0%
WEIGHT % MOLYBDENUM
0.050%
APPROXIMATE VOLUME % PYRITE + CHALCOPYRITE
5.0%
OCCURRENCE OTHER SULFIDES
S S S
P
S
S
S S
B
APPROXIMATE PYRITE TO CHALCOPYRITE RATIO
Py
cp
NERALIZATION, TWIN BUTTES MINE
UNTY, ARIZONA
EXPLANATION
ROCK MINERALOGY AND VEIN HALOS
QUARTZ SILT SIZED
EPIDOTE
MARBLE
SERPENTINE
DIOPSIDE
WOLLASTONITE
TREMOLITE ACTINOLITE
QUARTZ SAND
QUARTZ PODS
MICAS
IDOCRASE
SILICEOUS HORNFELS, APHANITIC
FORSTERITE
GARNET
ANHYDRITE
100 0 100 200 300 400 500 600 700 800 900 FEET
30 0 30 60 90 120 150 180 210 240 270 METERS
Horizontal Scale

Formation. These three types of altered rock are quartzite, meta-arkose, and metasiltstone.

Partly sandy, black, biotitized metasiltstone comprises most of the upper part of the Rodolfo Formation, M_{sv}, in the mineralized zone and occurs as thin beds in both the Whitcomb Quartzite and Angelica Arkose. The unaltered equivalents of these rocks are partly sandy, argillaceous, red siltstones, locally containing much volcanic debris.

The metasiltstones of the Rodolfo Formation consist of fine-grained quartz and occasional plagioclase and K-feldspar grains set in a microcrystalline matrix of quartz, K-feldspar, brown to green biotite, and occasionally significant amounts of chlorite, sericite, magnetite, and actinolite. Textures vary from granoblastic to clastic and probable modified pyroclastic. These metasiltstones have been strongly biotitized, and considerable K-feldspar has been added along sulfide veins and throughout the unit. Sericite halos, often formed at the expense of the earlier secondary biotite, are also common along quartz-sulfide veins. This style of alteration is much the same as that of other Mesozoic metasiltstones within the metasomatic aureole. The copper content of these metasiltstones is generally less than 0.10 percent. Molybdenum grades in M_{sv} are often anomalously high, greater than 0.030 percent, when compared to the amount of copper and the low total sulfide content.

The altered Whitcomb quartzites typically consist of fine- to medium-grained, detrital quartz set in a microcrystalline, granoblastic matrix of sericite and K-feldspar. The intergranular material often includes considerable epidote and small amounts of actinolite. Copper grades in the quartzite are usually near 0.2 percent, and the pyrite:chalcopyrite ratio is relatively high.

The siliceous volcanic flows and pyroclastic rocks interlayed with the Whitcomb quartzites are strongly recrystallized and have been variably biotitized and sericitized. The groundmass of these rocks contains much feldspar, but the amount of this mineral that is of metasomatic origin is not known. Copper grades are infrequently greater than 0.1 percent.

Much of the greater than 0.4 percent hypogene copper in the siliceous Mesozoic rocks occurs in the Angelica Arkose, which essentially constitutes the Arkose Orebody. These arkoses and conglomerates on the southwest side of the mine area consist of detrital grains of quartz and K-feldspar with sparse to numerous plagioclase grains and rock fragments in a microcrystalline, granoblastic matrix of quartz and K-feldspar. The distinctly detrital K-feldspar is often weakly altered to clay and sericite. Early, pervasive biotitization, with later biotite destructive vein halos, is a commonly observed alteration pattern in the Angelica Arkose. Biotite, sericite, epidote, actinolite, and chlorite occur along and adjacent to quartz-sulfide veinlets and in the matrix. Some quartz-sulfide veins contain K-feldspar and have K-feldspar halos. Hypogene metallization in the Angelica Arkose consists of pyrite, chalcopyrite, and molybdenite occurring along quartz veinlets or as disseminations. Pyrite is usually more abundant than chalcopyrite.

Quartzose Paleozoic Sedimentary Rocks. The quartzites and siltstones of the Scherrer and Epitaph Formations are the Paleozoic quartzose sedimentary rocks that are most abundant and that have been most thoroughly investigated. The lower Epitaph siltstone in both the Northeast and Main orebodies is altered to a dark brown, strongly biotitized, very fine-grained quartz and K-feldspar rock. The quartz is partly recrystallized, and at least some of the K-feldspar is presumed to be an alteration product. Biotite destructive, sericite-rich halos are common along quartz-sulfide veins.

In the Main and Northeast orebodies, the Scherrer quartzites occur at significantly different distances from the central intrusive complex. In both areas, much of the finer-grained component of these rocks is recrystallized and the fine to medium, rounded quartz grains are little changed from their original detrital shapes. Biotite and sericite are pervasive alteration products and simply diminish in amount at greater distances from the intrusive complex. Sericite is the most common mineral in vein halos in the biotitized portion of the quartzites.

On both sides of the central intrusive complex, the siltstones of the middle and upper part of the Epitaph Formation, Pe_2 and Pe_4, are rather uniformly altered to a tan or brown, micaceous, tremolite siltstone. The micas are biotite, sericite, and phlogopite. Some K-feldspar has been noted in thin sections of these rocks. Halos along quartz-sulfide veins are commonly of sericite in biotite-rich portions of the rock and of biotite in tremolite-rich portions.

The Earp Formation, Abrigo Formation, and Bolsa Quartzite also contain or are composed of quartzose sedimentary rocks. Biotite is the most apparent alteration product in the silty, quartzose, clastic rocks in the Earp and Abrigo Formations. The Bolsa is, in part, recrystallized and sericitized where it occurs adjacent to the Northwest Orebody.

Sulfides in these altered clastics are more commonly found along veins with quartz and anhydrite than disseminated. Copper values are rarely more than 0.3 percent except where the rocks contain significant amounts of calc-silicate. Molybdenum values are also usually low, but a ratio of molybdenum:copper is frequently higher in these quartzose rocks than in adjacent skarns. Pyrite:chalcopyrite ratios are uniformly higher in the low calc-silicate rocks than in nearby skarns.

Carbonate Rocks (Anhydrous Phase). Most of the unaltered carbonate rocks in the Twin Buttes area have high calcium:magnesium ratios and small amounts of quartz. Those carbonate rocks known to contain considerable amounts of magnesium are the Martin Formation, the upper part of the Colina Limestone, the uppermost beds of the upper Epitaph limestone (Pe_3), the middle Scherrer carbonate, and beds in the Rain Valley Formation. Comparison of the original composition of the carbonate rocks to the anhydrous skarns, formed as early alteration products, indicates the addition of Mg, Al, and Si, followed by addition of Fe.

The oldest suite of skarn minerals in the Main and Northeast orebodies includes diopside, wollastonite, green and pale brown garnet, and forsterite. Of these, diopside is by far the dominant mineral, and it occurs throughout the metasomatic aureole with essentially all other calc-silicate minerals. The few determinations of diopside composition at Twin Buttes indicate that all of this pyroxene is low in mole percentage hedenbergite. These determinations have been done by Husian Salek of The Anaconda Geological Laboratories.

The amount of forsterite formed during this early stage of metasomatism is obscured, because it readily changes to serpentine during later alteration. Forsterite is a notable occurrence in various altered carbonate rocks, but it usually constitutes only a small percentage of the high-magnetite, magnesium-rich mineral assemblages (see Fig. 20.6).

Pale brown and green garnets are common at many places in the metasomatic aureole. They occur in association with diopside and with wollastonite as an alteration of carbonate rocks.

Wollastonite is an alteration product of the calcitic limestones at Twin Buttes and usually occurs with pale garnet, idocrase, diopside, chert, and calcite. It is presently found at the outer edge of the metasomatic aureole in calcitic limestone and near or at marble to skarn contacts which occur within some of the thicker carbonate units. This early silicate is not particularly common, and the pattern of its occurrence suggests that it was once much more abundant.

Darker brown garnet veins and replaces diopside and paler garnet, and forms the outer growth rings on pale brown and green garnet throughout the mineralized zone. Reddish brown, presumably more Fe-rich garnet is particularly abundant throughout the inner alteration zones, in Pe_3 of the Epitaph Formation and the Concha Limestone, where they occur in the Main Orebody, and in the undifferentiated Permian and Pennsylvanian rocks and Earp Formation in the Northeast Orebody. The alteration of carbonate rocks to andraditic garnet marks the start of significant Fe metasomatism, which continues through the hydrous stage of calc-silicate alteration.

Considerable chalcopyrite and less pyrite and sphalerite were deposited nearly coeval with, but possibly somewhat later than, the formation of the Fe-rich garnets. These early sulfides occur as disseminations and, less frequently, in veins with quartz and anhydrite.

Scheelite occurs with some frequency in the altered mine rocks. This mineral has been noted as disseminations in skarn, along veins with quartz and sulfide, and in vein halos. There is a fair correlation between garnet (presumably darker garnet) and higher WO_3 assays (Wright, 1971). Values of 0.02 to 0.04 percent WO_3 are rather common, and the darker garnetite often has values in the range of 0.05 to 0.07 percent WO_3.

Carbonate Rocks (Hydrous Phase). With the exception of garnet, the anhydrous phase minerals were, to varying degrees, altered to hydrous, usually more iron-rich assemblages. This alteration took place along fractures, shear zones, and permeable strata—principally the quartzose Paleozoic and Mesozoic clastic rocks. The hydrous assemblages are now seen both as vein halos and as pervasive alteration affecting large areas of the metacarbonate rocks. Hydrous alteration locally extends to and beyond the front of anhydrous alteration. Consequently, both groups of minerals can be found at silicate to marble contacts. The pattern of hydrous alteration is shown for a part of the mineralized zone in Figure 20.6. Notable in these relationships is the essential absence of anhydrous calc-silicates in altered quartzite and siltstone.

The earlier skarn minerals alter to specific, and frequently diagnostic, hydrous assemblages at Twin Buttes. Sulfide veins in diopside often have vein halos of actinolite and nontronite and, less frequently, of epidote. Also, diopside is, to varying degrees, pervasively altered to nontronite, phlogopite-magnetite, and tremolite-magnetite. (Very little diagnostic chemistry has been done on tremolite-actinolite at Twin Buttes, and the distinctions in this chapter are based on color—i.e., actinolite is medium to dark green and tremolite is white or very light greenish gray). Forsterite is usually found as remnant microscopic grains scattered in a serpentine-magnetite rock. Wollastonite alters to montmorillonite clays. Garnet locally contains veins with epidote halos.

Pyrite and chalcopyrite are the dominant sulfide minerals associated with the hydrous alteration stage. These sulfides occur in quartz-anhydrite and anhydrite veins, in vein halos, and as disseminations. The pyrite : chalcopyrite ratio for veins with hydrous alteration halos is often much greater than this ratio for the earlier, disseminated sulfides in the rock through which the vein passes. Also, the pyrite : chalcopyrite ratio of disseminated sulfides associated with hydrous calc-silicates is frequently higher than this ratio in earlier deposited sulfides.

Miscellaneous Sedimentary Rocks. Beds of anhydrite up to 40 ft. thick occur in the Epitaph Formation and in the upper portion of the Colina Limestone. In the Northeast and Main Orebodies, below the lower limit of supergene effects, these beds consist of medium- to coarse-crystalline, light gray to translucent or pale purple anhydrite. The small amount of sulfides in these sulfate beds occurs as disseminations or as sparse veins, partly with associated calc-silicates. Copper and molybdenum grades are very low in pure anhydrite.

The altered Earp Formation in the Northeast Orebody and the North Porphyry Contact Orebody contains numerous beds of flinty to very fine-grained, siliceous, calc-silicate hornfels. Similar rocks are also found in the Abrigo Formation of the Northwest Orebody. These hornfelses contain considerable quartz, K-feldspar, plagioclase, and a variety of calc-silicate minerals, the most common of which are diopside and tremolite-actinolite. Calcareous shales and siltstones are found in the unaltered Earp Formation in nearby mountain ranges, and the hornfelses are presumably alteration products of one or both of these rock types.

Intrusive Rocks. The character of alteration in the intrusive rocks at Twin Buttes depends on the pre-alteration rock mineralogy, proximity to the mineralization center, and the time of emplacement of a particular intrusive mass in relation to the age of the alteration. The granite is clearly older than any events in the metasomatic process, and the pervasive potassic alteration in the main dike of the rhyodacite indicates that it also pre-dates much of the Laramide alteration. A third type of early intrusive rock is the coarser, well-mineralized, and partly calc-silicated intrusions occurring in deeper portions of the Main Orebody.

The next younger age group of intrusions includes much

of the central intrusive complex and the porphyritic quartz monzonite. Hypogene alteration in these rocks generally consists of partial chloritization of the biotite books and development of sericite and K-feldspar as halos along quartz-sulfide veins.

Some 700 ft. (213 m) southwest of the central intrusive complex is a hornblende diorite dike. This rock is moderately to strongly altered to an epidote-pyrite-chlorite assemblage, and it contains only minor chalcopyrite. Potassium feldspar–epidote vein halos are common. The time of emplacement of this rock is uncertain, and the degree to which the alteration of the dike is a function of its age is not known.

Small masses of a dacite porphyry occurring in the central intrusive complex and an exposure of andesite along the Twin Buttes fault zone comprise the known post-mineralization intrusive rocks at Twin Buttes. The dacite is extremely fine grained, and the only obvious alteration in this rock is weak clay development on fractures and in the feldspars. The andesite has been significantly altered to clay as a result of exposure to the supergene fluids.

The early intrusions often have higher hypogene copper grades, higher total sulfides, and lower pyrite:chalcopyrite ratios. The central intrusive complex, emplaced after much of the anhydrous alteration, is characterized by K-feldspar and sericite halos along veins, low hypogene copper grades, and relatively high pyrite:chalcopyrite ratios.

Silicate Alteration Patterns. The dominant, overall pattern of change in the alteration-metallization process is one of decreasing intensity of metasomatism outward from the mineralization center, the early location of which has been occupied by genetically related intrusive bodies. This dominant pattern is significantly modified by the availability of conduits to provide access to reactive lithologies at any given time during the alteration process. The most rapid and radical changes in the products of alteration occur within the original carbonate lithologies, but changes, primarily in degree, also occur in the quartzose sedimentary rocks.

The occurrence of marble in the mineralized zone constitutes one of the more dramatic and informative variations in the alteration products of the carbonate units. In the northwest portion of the Main Orebody, a large block of black to gray and white, fine- to coarse-crystalline marble occurs in a structurally thickened portion of Pe_3. This marble zone is about 1,200 ft. (366 m) long and terminates against the Twin Buttes Fault. It expands in width to the northwest and is bordered on both sides by diminishing widths of skarn. A variety of calc-silicate materials vein, interfinger with, and border this marble. A garnet-wollastonite-idocrase assemblage with bornite, chalcopyrite, and sphalerite is common adjacent to the marble contact, as is garnet-diopside-chalcopyrite-pyrite. High copper grades locally occur in the garnet-diopside rocks directly adjacent to the marble contact.

The upper Epitaph limestone, Pe_3, in the Northeast Orebody contains a zone of black to white marble. This marble zone is canoe-shaped in plan, cut off on the southeast by the East End fault. The marble is surrounded, except on the southeast, by skarns developed in Pe_3. The zone is widest on the southeast and narrows gradually northwestward to a point, located some 600 ft. (183 m) northwest of the East End fault, where the entire 170-ft. (52 m) width of Pe_3 is silicated. Both garnet and diopside occur at the marble contact. Near the western limit of the marble, zones of high copper grade occur in a garnet-diopside-chalcopyrite-pyrite assemblage. Further westward, toward the Pit fault, and beyond the marble, the silicated Pe_3 contains a wollastonite-garnet-idocrase assemblage with bornite, chalcopyrite, sphalerite, and molybdenite.

The altered Colina Limestone and narrow altered carbonate beds near the southwest contact of Pe_2 in the Main Orebody have similar northwest to southeast and vertically oriented changes in silicate and sulfide patterns. Near the 2,000 SE Section of the Main Orebody (see Figure 20.4, Section B-B') and for at least a few hundred feet along strike, these carbonate rocks are rather pervasively altered to tremolite-serpentine-magnetite and diopside. In addition, they contain local areas of partly silicated, fine-crystalline, gray marble. Further along strike, away from the 2,000 SE section, there is an increased amount of marble and less pervasive silication, mostly serpentine-magnetite, which occurs predominantly as veins and vein halos with sulfides. Paralleling this decrease in silication is a general decrease in copper grade and an increase in the pyrite:chalcopyrite ratio.

In one of the altered carbonate beds near the southwestern contact of Pe_2 in the Main Orebody, a significant and rapid change in the intensity of silicate and sulfide alteration products occurs in a vertical direction (Smith, 1977). Near the upper contact of this bed with the Mesozoic rocks, the bed is more pervasively silicated and has a higher copper grade, a lower pyrite:chalcopyrite ratio, and higher total sulfide content than occur at greater distances from the contact. This pattern of decreasing abundance of alteration products away from the Mesozoic to Paleozoic contact also has been noted at other places in the Main Orebody.

The pattern of occurrence of dark brown or reddish brown, presumably more iron-rich garnet in the skarns of the Main and Northeast orebodies is particularly significant because of the frequently parallel pattern of increased chalcopyrite. This dark garnet and other, later, generally hydrous alteration products occur in rocks presumed to have been previously altered to marble, diopside, forsterite, wollastonite, and grossular garnet. The darker garnet is the dominant skarn material or is a significant part of the dominant assemblage in altered carbonate rocks which are now near the central intrusive complex. Beyond these occurrences to near the outer edge of silication, darker garnet is found as veins, vein halos, and irregular masses.

The dominant hydrous alteration minerals in the altered carbonate rocks are tremolite-actinolite and serpentine. These minerals often exist in close proximity, but serpentine, usually with magnetite, is locally found beyond any other obvious silication products as veins and vein halos in dolomite or marble.

Drilling during the late 1970s, mainly in the oxide zone of the Northeast Orebody, extended the data base some 250 ft. (76 m) beyond the edge of information portrayed on Figure 20.6. This drilling has indicated that pervasive silication, with diopside, partly clay-altered wollastonite, idocrase, and pale garnet, extends 50 to 80 ft. (15–24 m) northeast of the upper Scherrer quartzite. Beyond the pervasive silication is a zone of white marble containing patchy wollastonite-clay and minor diopside, idocrase, and pale garnet. This zone extends about 250 ft. (76 m) northeast from Ps_4 where dark to medium gray marble, with trace amounts of silication, is encountered.

It is not known whether significant changes in kind, as well as degree, of alteration occur in the quartzose clastic rocks of the Main and Northeast orebodies. The little change documented is primarily in the abundance of biotite and sericite in the Scherrer quartzites. These rocks in the Northeast Orebody have discernably fewer secondary mica minerals than the Scherrer quartzites of the Main Orebody, which are close to the central intrusive complex.

The patterns of silicate alteration in the metasedimentary rocks at Twin Buttes are complicated, and the relationship of these patterns to the central intrusive complex is a continuing problem. Significant variation in alteration products often takes place over short distances along northeast-southwest–oriented traverses, essentially at right angles to the skarn-to-intrusion contact. Equally significant changes in alteration products also occur along lines that are subparallel to the intrusive-to-metasedimentary rock interface, but these changes usually occur over longer distances. In the Northeast and Main orebodies, changes of a few hundred feet in the position of the intrusions with respect to a particular stratigraphic unit may not be accompanied by significant changes in the alteration assemblages. Conversely, variations in the alteration assemblage within a particular stratigraphic unit frequently occur at constant distances from the intrusive contact. The conclusion inferred from these patterns, when considered with other data, is that the central intrusive complex was intruded after formation of many of the observed alteration patterns. It is believed that much of the parallelism between the alteration patterns and the edges of the central intrusive mass occurs because both were generally controlled by the same structural entities.

Patterns of Hypogene Sulfide Occurrences. Pyrite and chalcopyrite are by far the dominant hypogene sulfide minerals in the Twin Buttes mineralized zone. Other, at least locally important, sulfides include sphalerite, molybdenite, bornite, pyrrhotite, chalcocite, and galena. These sulfides occur as disseminations, in discontinuous hairline fractures, and in a wide variety of veins.

The patterns of sulfide occurrences at Twin Buttes are dependent on various factors, among which rock mineralogy is considered to be dominant. This factor is determined by original mineralogy and access and reactivity to the mineralizing fluids. Another, and in part redundant parameter, is proximity to the mineralization center and access to the principal channelways for movement of the mineralizing fluids. A third significant factor is the relative age of formation of the particular set of sulfides.

The patterns include variation in total sulfide percentage, variation in mineral or metal ratios, the local presence of a particular sulfide which may be exclusive of some other mineral, and the mode of occurrence of a single sulfide or a group of sulfides. Particular sulfide assemblages are often associated with specific and predictable groups of alteration minerals. Knowledge of these associations is useful in both identification of sulfide or silicate minerals and in projection of metal values. Figure 20.6 deals with many of these parameters, but shows essentially one dimension in space and portrays only the final product of a lengthy evolutionary process.

In the altered wall rock at Twin Buttes, the amount of sulfide decreases away from the central portion of the mineralized zone. In general, the amounts of molybdenum and copper also decrease away from the central intrusive mass. The pyrite : chalcopyrite ratio increases away from the intrusive center, but less obviously so. These conclusions are based on comparison of rocks with the same or similar original character at varying distances from the central intrusive complex.

In considering each of these sulfide patterns, the general variations outward from the center of the mineralized zone are frequently much less significant than the variation between adjacent altered quartzose and carbonate rocks. The amount of sulfide and copper is much greater in the skarns than in adjacent altered quartzose rocks, and pyrite : chalcopyrite ratios are usually higher in the quartzose rocks when compared to the skarns.

In the rocks of the Main Orebody occurring within approximately 250 ft. (76 m) of the central intrusive complex (Fig. 20.4), the products of silication and metallization remain similar to those shown in Figure 20.6 for many hundreds of feet along the strike of a particular lithologic unit. But a few hundred feet away from the 2,000 SE Section (see Fig. 20.4 and 20.6, Main Orebody) in the Colina Limestone, there is a rather rapid decrease in copper grade caused by an increase in pyrite : chalcopyrite ratio and a decrease in total sulfide. Similar patterns can be seen in altered carbonate beds near the southwestern contact of Pe_2 in the Main Orebody, but to a large degree, such variations are obscured by the vertical variations in both skarn and sulfide alteration products (Smith, 1977). Downward, away from the Mesozoic contact in the altered carbonates of Pe_2, the pyrite : chalcopyrite ratio increases from approximately 1 : 8 to 2 : 1, and there is a parallel decrease in total sulfide and copper grade.

One of the more economically significant variations in the patterns of sulfide occurrence is the abrupt increase in both sulfide and copper percentage often found in skarn adjacent to marble contacts. This alteration feature is well portrayed in Figure 20.6 only in Pe_3 of the Northeast Orebody. Marble to skarn contacts occur with some frequency at Twin Buttes and usually, but not always, have accompanying high copper grade. It has been our experience that copper grade and amount of sulfide may vary radically within short distances along these contacts.

Quartz veining in altered carbonate rocks decreases significantly within a few hundred feet of the central intrusive mass. In the quartzose metasedimentary rocks such a decrease may also occur; if so, it is much more gradual. A significant percentage of the molybdenum in the Twin Buttes mine area occurs along veins, mostly with quartz. The amount of molybdenum is frequently higher in a skarn if compared to an adjacent quartzose rock. But, if a molybdenum : copper ratio of the adjacent rock types is compared, the ratio in the quartzose rock is nearly always higher. These patterns in molybdenum mineralization are, at least in part, dependent on the amount of quartz veining.

The occurrence of bornite, sphalerite, pyrrhotite, hypogene chalcocite, and galena in the Twin Buttes mine area is not of particular economic significance at this time. However, these minerals provide some insight into the mineralization process. Sphalerite, the most widespread of these sulfides, occurs in at least small amounts throughout the skarns in the metallized zone and, infrequently, in veins in the quartzose rocks. Only persistent occurrences of relatively large amounts of sphalerite are shown in Figure 20.6. Sphalerite is common in the high chalcopyrite zones in Pe_3 of the Main Orebody and in this location frequently contains exsolution blebs of the copper sulfide. Small amounts of sphalerite occur with bornite and chalcopyrite in the Colina Limestone of the Main Orebody and in the Concha Limestone of the Northeast Orebody. Large amounts of sphalerite also occur with pyrrhotite and magnetite in the two known occurrences of this assemblage in the Colina Limestone of the Northeast and Main orebodies. Microscopic exsolution blebs of sphalerite have been observed in chalcopyrite (McCurry, 1971).

The occurrence of bornite in the Twin Buttes mineralized zone is quite restricted. It is found associated with wollastonite, montmorillonite, idocrase, green and minor brown garnet, diopside, chalcopyrite, sphalerite, molybdenite, and pyrite in the Concha Limestone and Pe_3 of the Northeast Orebody. In the Main Orebody minor bornite occurs in diopside-altered rocks adjacent to marble in the Colina Limestone, and also in a structurally thickened portion of Pe_3, as disseminations and in veins, with garnet-idocrase-wollastonite-montmorillonite, that penetrate the marble. In the latter case, bornite is associated with chalcopyrite, primary chalcocite and sphalerite. Bornite is also known in the Northwest Orebody, where it occurs adjacent to marble in the Escabrosa Limestone.

Economically significant amounts of silver occur in the Twin Buttes mineralized zone, but only small amounts of two silver minerals, tetrahedrite and matildite (Salek, 1976), have been identified. The principal known occurrences of tetrahedrite are along the outer periphery of sulfides and in northeast-trending, late veins with calcite, quartz, pyrite, chalcopyrite, galena, sphalerite, and fluorite. Microprobe work by The Anaconda Company's geological laboratory has proven that most of the silver, at least in the higher-grade portions of the Main Orebody, occurs in chalcopyrite, with lesser amounts in sphalerite (Salek, 1976). In the Epitaph Formation skarns of the Main Orebody, there is a correlation between silver and copper content. The silver grade at 1.0 percent copper averages 0.32 ounces per ton of ore, and for each decrease or increase of 0.5 percent copper there is a parallel change in silver of approximately 0.1 ounce per ton.

Summary. The following are some of the salient features of the products of the alteration-mineralization process at Twin Buttes.

1. The products of alteration at Twin Buttes necessitate the addition of significant amounts of Si, Mg, Fe, S, Al, K, Cu, Zn, and Mo to the original lithology.
2. Carbonate beds form skarns or marble within the metasomatic aureole.
3. The amount of quartz in an altered sedimentary rock, excluding that quartz occurring as veins or within intercrystalline spaces, accurately reflects the amount of quartz in the unaltered rock. Chert is wholly or partly destroyed in the more intense alteration zones.
4. Quartz coarser than medium-grained silt in the altered sedimentary rock, even if recrystallized, often reflects the size of quartz grains in the unaltered rock.
5. The amount of sulfides, the copper and molybdenum grade, the intensity of silication, and the amount of vein quartz generally decrease outward from the mineralization center, and the pyrite:chalcopyrite ratio shows a parallel increase. A high total sulfide, pyritic halo has not been recognized at Twin Buttes (Baker, 1968).
6. A comparison of closely adjacent quartzose metasedimentary rocks and skarns shows that skarns invariably have the higher copper grade, higher total sulfide percentage, and lower pyrite:chalcopyrite ratio.
7. Quartzose medisedimentary rocks with minimal calc-silicates never contain large tonnages which average more than 0.3 percent primary copper. The single known exception is the Angelica Arkose.
8. The later silicate and sulfide assemblages contain significantly more iron than those formed earlier in the metasomatic process. The earlier formed silicates were calcium-, magnesium-, and aluminum-rich, while the early sulfides were copper-rich.

Supergene Alteration and Mineralization

The depth of penetration and the products of the supergene processes at Twin Buttes are quite variable. The depth below the bedrock to which supergene processes affect the rocks is dependent primarily on hypogene alteration mineralogy and on permeability. Supergene effects penetrate much deeper into siliceous rocks than into adjacent skarns because of the greater degree of fracture permeability in the siliceous rocks and the smaller amount of minerals which react to the supergene fluids.

Supergene effects at Twin Buttes can be divided into three zones. The deepest of these has undergone removal of sulfate and has some clay alteration of the silicates, but the sulfides have remained essentially unaffected. Above the zone of sulfate removal is a middle zone of increased clay alteration and formation of supergene sulfides, mostly chalcocite, which to varying degrees replace the hypogene sulfides. The uppermost zone is the zone of oxidation and leaching.

Lowermost Supergene Zone. The deepest penetration of the supergene process is marked by the uppermost occurrences of anhydrite (Gustafson and Hunt, 1975). Above the top of hydrothermal anhydrite and anhydrite occurring as beds in the Permian strata, there is a zone a few inches to tens of feet thick in which the anhydrite is hydrated and converted to selenite or satin spar. The upper limit of occurrences of satin spar, selenite, and anhydrite is shown as Tso_4 in Figure 20.4, which is the top of the sulfate zone. Below the top of the sulfate zone, permeability is extremely low, as essentially all voids are filled with these sulfates. Above the top of the sulfate zone, there is an immediate and significant increase in porosity and permeability and often a marked decrease in the competence of the rock.

Essentially all the mineralized zone rocks occurring below the top of the sulfate zone have some anhydrite or gypsum, and in the Permian section there may be beds as much as 40 ft. (12 m) thick of nearly pure anhydrite. The removal of a small percentage of anhydrite from a garnetite usually does little more than produce a vuggy rock with lower *in-situ* density, but removal of beds of anhydrite in a section of interbedded siltstone and variably altered carbonate rocks produces a collapse breccia (Barter, 1976). Such breccias are common at Twin Buttes and can be tracked vertically above beds of anhydrite through all of the supergene zones to the bedrock surface, where its subcrop may be marked by a paleostream channel or a bedrock depression.

A further effect sometimes noted immediately above the top of the sulfate zone is one of copper grade enhancement; this effect is not because of supergene enrichment, but because of selective removal of the sulfate, which increases the sulfide : gangue ratio. This effect is most significant in a section of the Epitaph Formation, which, below the top of the sulfate zone, may contain as much as 50 percent anhydrite. Here, grade enhancement approaches 100 percent.

In the zone above the top of sulfate and below the occurrence of supergene sulfides, the removal of sulfate is the most significant supergene effect, but selective clay alteration of the silicate minerals is also common. Magnesium-rich montmorillonite may form after diopside and other calcium-magnesium silicates; feldspars may be partly clay-altered, particularly if they have undergone some hypogene alteration; and wollastonite apparently alters to a distinctively colored montmorillonite.

Middle Supergene Zone. The middle zone in the supergene alteration pattern is the zone of supergene sulfide deposition. Nearly all of the supergene copper sulfide at Twin Buttes is chalcocite. Small amounts of covellite have been reported (McCurry, 1971), and bornite tarnish on primary chalcopyrite is known. The thickness and elevation of the middle supergene zone is widely variable, and the amount of secondary copper sulfides in the zone generally increases upward until the lower fringes of oxidation are encountered. The percentage increase of copper grade in the chalcocite zone is often considerably more in quartzose rocks than in skarns and is probably more in garnetites than in diopside rocks.

Upper Supergene Zone. The elevation above which significant amounts of supergene oxide minerals formed varies nearly 1,000 ft. (305 m) in the immediate mine area. The base of significant oxides is as high as the 2,775-ft. (846-m) elevation, 25 ft. (7.6 m) below the bedrock surface, in garnetite in the Main Orebody; and as deep as the 1,800-ft. (549-m) elevation, 800 ft. (244 m) below bedrock surface, in siltstone in the Northeast Orebody.

Copper, iron, and manganese oxides are found in abundance and wide variety in the uppermost supergene zone. Chrysocolla is widespread, as is a black copper-iron-manganese wad. Brochantite, tenorite, cuprite, and native copper are locally common, and there are lesser amounts of azurite, malachite, and medmontite. The iron and manganese oxides have not been studied at Twin Buttes, but they are known to encompass the more common types, including limonite, hematite, geothite, and pyrolusite. Occurrences of the molybdenum oxides, wulfenite, powellite, and ferrimolybdite are known.

A crude zoning based on the abundance of various copper minerals in the oxide zone is present at Twin Buttes. Such zoning has been most frequently observed in calc-silicate rocks, but it also occurs, at least locally, in siliceous rocks. Directly above the supergene chalcocite zone, native copper and cuprite are common, and native copper occurs essentially nowhere else in the oxide zone. Above this near-sulfide band, is a zone with abundant chrysocolla and black copper-manganese-iron wad or tenorite. Progressing upward, the amount of black, copper-bearing oxide often decreases and the amount of chrysocolla increases.

Clay alteration attributed to supergene processes is essentially pervasive in susceptible rocks in the oxide zone. Diopside is particularly affected, as are some feldspars, but garnet seems relatively unaffected.

GEOLOGIC HISTORY OF THE TWIN BUTTES AREA

Only isolated remnants of Pinal Schist, quartzite, and mafic-rich intrusions remain, as inclusions in the granite (see Table 20.1), to indicate the character of the earlier portion of the Precambrian in the Twin Buttes area. Most of the rock assigned to the Precambrian is a coarse granite, which has been dated at 850±100 m.y. (Pb-α, zircons [Cooper, 1973]) and which is indicative of a deep-seated intrusive event. This is an anomalous cooling date in the Precambrian of Southeastern Arizona (Damon, 1968; Marvin et al., 1973), and the granite was presumably emplaced considerably earlier, ca. 1,400 m.y. After emplacement, it was metamorphosed, producing the steep, northwesterly foliation common to this rock in the Pima district.

During the Middle Cambrian the Bolsa Quartzite was deposited on an erosion surface developed on the Precambrian complex (Bryant, 1968). The Bolsa is the earliest record of the beginning of the tectonically quiescent Paleozoic Era. The Paleozoic is characterized in the Twin Buttes area and over much of southeastern Arizona by shallow shelf, marine deposition, with interspersed shorter periods of sub-aerial exposure, erosion, and continental sedimentation. A notable hiatus in the quite continuous Paleozoic sedimentary record occurs in the Ordovician and Silurian, but in the Pima district only a discontinuity marks the contact of the Devonian Martin Formation and the underlying Cambrian Abrigo Formation. A period of sub-aerial exposure and erosion occurred early in Pennsylvanian time when the chert pebble conglomerate and red shales of the Black Prince were deposited on a low-relief, karst surface developed on the Escabrosa Limestone. Submergence and periods of continental sedimentation are indicated for the remainder of Pennsylvanian by the marine limestones and deltaic deposits (Lodewick, 1970) of the Horquilla and Earp Formations respectively.

At least by the time of deposition of the Permian Colina Limestone, the northwest-trending Pedregosa Basin was well established in southeastern Arizona (Butler, 1971). This elongate feature influenced the sedimentation style for the remainder of the Paleozoic. Twin Buttes is located in what usually was a shallow shelf area, northwest of the deeper portions of the basin. The character of the sediments deposited in this Permian basin had a major influence on the occurrence of metal values in the Twin Buttes mine.

Near the end of the Permian, the area was uplifted and the onset of Triassic volcanism marked the start of the tectonically active Mesozoic Era. The oldest Triassic rocks in the Pima district are the Ox Frame Volcanics. These rocks may occur on the eastern side of the mine area, but where the Paleozoic to Mesozoic contact is best known, on the southwest side of the pit, the Permian strata are overlain across an angular unconformity by a strongly altered unit. This unit is interpreted to be a conglomerate of local derivation, containing clasts of many Paleozoic formations. The conglomerate is correlated with the basal conglomerate of the Rodolfo Formation. If this correlation is correct, as much as 5,000 ft. (1,524 m) of the Ox Frame Volcanics were eroded from the immediate Twin Buttes mine area before the Middle (?) Triassic.

The contact of Paleozoic strata to the conglomerate, M_L, is an unconformity of high angularity. The large blocks of Scherrer quartzite in M_L, along with this high angularity (an apparently anomalous condition in southeastern Arizona), suggest that an erosion surface of high relief was locally developed on deformed Paleozoic sedimentary rocks. To achieve the angularity, 30 to 80°, the Paleozoic strata must have been folded or at least significantly tilted in the interval between Permian Rain Valley deposition and accumulation of Triassic Rodolfo Formation sediments. The sequence of events preferred to explain local geological conditions across this important Permian-Triassic boundary began with gentle uplift near the end of the Permian, resulting in sub-aerial exposure and erosion of the upper Permian strata; then came volcanism and accelerated deformation with shearing along northwest faults and production of northwest-trending folds; the final event was extensive erosion of the early Triassic sedimentary and volcanic rocks. Erosion locally continued into the Paleozoic rocks, and then the basal conglomerate of the Rodolfo Formation (M_L) was deposited on the deformed Paleozoic strata during a tectonically active period.

The Mesozoic rocks overlying M_L at Twin Buttes consist of a clastic and volcanic sequence, with an angular unconformity at the base of the Jurassic(?) Whitcomb Quartzite and a disconformity at the base of the Early Cretaceous Angelica Arkose. The mine section is only a portion of the Mesozoic record in the southern Pima district (Cooper, 1971). This record indicates repeated volcanism and intrusion, significant deformation, periodic uplift and erosion, and accumulation of considerable thicknesses of sediments and volcanic rocks through the Late Cretaceous when the Demetrie Volcanics and Red Boy Rhyolite were extruded. This Late Cretaceous volcanic event has not been isotopically dated in the Pima district, but lithologic and age equivalents in surrounding mountain ranges have dates between 66 and 74 m.y. (Cooper, 1971; Marvin et al., 1973).

Folding took place possibly as early as the end of the Lower Cretaceous, but more likely after formation of the Red Boy Rhyolite. The obvious result of this folding is the open syncline occurring in the Angelica Arkose southwest of the intrusive complex. There is no evidence at Twin Buttes that the Laramide porphyries were emplaced before this folding, but such folding could have been contemporaneous with intrusion.

Alteration and metallization of rocks near the Twin Buttes mineralization center began after extrusion of the Late Cretaceous volcanic rocks and apparently before intrusion of the porphyries of the central intrusive complex. The rhyodacite is the first of the Laramide intrusions emplaced along northwest-trending faults in the mineralized zone, and it is thought to have been intruded before the onset, or early in the process, of alteration. Alteration and metallization patterns in the porphyries of the central intrusive complex and adjacent wall rocks indicate that this set of Laramide intrusions was emplaced well after the onset of metasomatic processes. The only age date of a metasomatic mineral at Twin Buttes is 66.8 ±2.5 m.y. (dated in 1973 by Geochron Laboratories for The Anaconda Company) on coarse, green phlogopite occurring in a skarn. Reasonable isotopic ages for cooling of the Ruby Star Granodiorite and related porphyries vary from 54 m.y. to 62 m.y. (Damon and Mauger, 1966; Cooper, 1973; Marvin et al., 1973); many fall near 58 m.y. The biotite rhyolite, which has been found only in the allochthonous block of the San Xavier fault, has also been isotopically dated at 57 (dated in 1973 by Geochron Laboratories for The Anaconda Company) and 58 m.y. (Cooper, 1973). This rock is presumed to be, in part at least, an extrusive equivalent of one of the porphyries occurring at or near the copper centers of the Pima district.

After the end of the Laramide extrusive, intrusive, and metasomatic events, there is an apparent gap in the Pima district stratigraphic record, as the next rock encountered directly above the biotite rhyolite is the Oligocene (Cooper, 1973) Helmet Fanglomerate, a Pantano Formation equivalent. This fanglomerate is of local derivation and is the product of very rapid sediment accumulation in alluvial fans. Since the age of the lower portion of the Helmet Fanglomerate is uncertain, it is quite possible that the hiatus in the stratigraphic record is short and that these alluvial fan deposits record the uplift, onset of erosion, and oxidation of the mineralization centers which presumably occurred during the Early Tertiary. This uplift was accomplished by faulting, much of which must have been of a northeasterly trend in the Pima district.

During the Oligocene and Miocene, there was continued rapid accumulation of fanglomerates and repeated volcanism, as evidenced by the andesitic to rhyolitic volcanics occurring within the Helmet Fanglomerate and the Formation of Tinaja Peak (Cooper, 1973). Mineralized landslide blocks and lenses with abundant mineralized fragments in the Helmet Fanglomerate offer further evidence that the mineralization centers, Twin Buttes in particular, were periodically uplifted. Approximately 26 m.y. ago, the San Xavier thrust, here considered to be a gravity glide fault, was active. Along this décollement surface, the upper portion of the Twin Buttes mineralization center was apparently moved, within a large allochthonous block, some 6½ miles (10.5 km) northward to the present position of the Pima-Mission-Palo Verde deposit. After décollement, there was continued erosion and oxidation of the Twin Buttes deposit, and sediments resembling the mid-Tertiary fanglomerates were deposited over at least part of the area.

Over the bedrock surface at Twin Buttes or over the

sparse occurrences of the older, reddish, post-mineralization sediments are a few hundred feet of flat-lying Pliocene and Pleistocene sands and gravels, the lower portion of which may be as old as Miocene. These alluvial sediments, the product of erosion of block-faulted mountain ranges, were deposited on a pediment surface. The bedrock surface, cemented conglomerate, and the lower portion of the nearly flat alluvial sediments are minimally offset by faults. At the top of the flat-lying alluvium, are reddish and dark brown sediments which blend with the recent fluvial channel sands.

ACKNOWLEDGMENTS

The writers wish to thank Anamax Mining Company for permission to publish this chapter. They also are indebted to the many co-workers who have made significant contributions to the better understanding of the geology of the Twin Buttes copper deposit and who participated in the preparation of this chapter.

REFERENCES CITED

The Anaconda Company, Geologic maps of the Helvetia and Pima mining districts, Pima County, Arizona: unpublished company maps, repository at Twin Buttes.

Baker, R. C., 1968, Preliminary geologic report on the Twin Buttes mine, Pima County, Arizona: unpublished report, The Anaconda Company, 26 p.

Barter, C. F., 1972, Mesozoic stratigraphy of the Twin Buttes ore zone, Pima County, Arizona: unpublished report, The Anaconda Company, 18 p.

———, 1974, Second progress report, Twin Buttes mine, Pima County, Arizona: unpublished report, The Anaconda Company, 40 p.

———, 1976, Occurrences of anhydrite and gypsum in the Twin Buttes mineralized zone, Pima County, Arizona: unpublished report, The Anaconda Company, 8 p.

Britt, T. L., 1955, Geology of the Twin Peaks area, Pima County, Arizona: unpublished M.S. thesis, Univ. Ariz., 58 p.

———, 1973, Preliminary composite section Empire Mountains, Pima County, Arizona: unpublished measured section, The Anaconda Company.

Brown, R. L., 1926, Geology and ore deposits of the Twin Buttes district: unpub. M.S. thesis, Univ. Ariz., 40 p.

Bryant, D. L., 1955, Stratigraphy of the Permian System in southern Arizona: unpubl. M.S. thesis, Univ. Ariz., 209 p.

———, 1968, Diagnostic characteristics of the Paleozoic formations of southeastern Arizona: Ariz. Geol. Soc., Southern Ariz. Guidebook III, p. 33–47.

Butler, W. C., 1969, The upper Paleozoic stratigraphy of Total Wreck Ridge, Pima County, Arizona: unpublished M.S. thesis, Univ. Ariz., 138 p.

———, 1971, Permian sedimentary environments in southeastern Arizona: Ariz. Geol. Soc. Digest, v. IX, p. 71–94.

Cooper, J. R., 1960, Some geological features of the Pima mining district, Pima County, Arizona: U.S. Geol. Survey Bull. 1112-C, p. 63–103.

———, 1971, Mesozoic stratigraphy of the Sierrita Mountains, Pima County, Arizona: U.S. Geol. Survey Prof. Paper 658-D, 42 p.

———, 1973, Geologic map of the Twin Buttes quandrangle southwest of Tucson, Pima County, Arizona: U.S. Geol. Survey, Misc. Geol. Inv., Map I-745.

Creasy, S. C., and Kistler, R. W., 1962, Age of some copper-bearing porphyries and other igneous rocks in southeastern Arizona: U.S. Geol. Survey Prof. Paper 450-D, p. D1–D5.

Damon, P. E., 1968, Application of the potassium-argon method to the dating of igneous and metamorphic rock within the basin ranges of the Southwest: Ariz. Geol. Soc., Southern Arizona Guidebook III, p. 7–20.

Damon, P. E., and Mauger, R. L., 1966, Epeirogeny-orogeny viewed from the Basin and Range Province: SME Trans., v. 235, no. 1, p. 99–112.

Davidson, E. S., 1973, Geohydrology and water resources of the Tucson Basin, Arizona: U.S. Geol. Survey Water Supply Paper 1939-E., 81 p., 7 pls.

Drewes, Harald, 1971, Mesozoic stratigraphy of the Santa Rita Mountains, southeast of Tucson, Arizona: U.S. Geol Survey Prof. Paper 658-C, 81 p.

———, 1972, Structural geology of the Santa Rita Mountains, southeast of Tucson, Arizona: U.S. Geol. Survey Prof. Paper 748, 35 p.

Gordon, E. R., 1922, The geology of the Twin Buttes mining district: unpub. M.S. thesis, Univ. Ariz., 12 p.

Gustafson, L. B., and Hunt, J. P., 1975, The porphyry copper deposit at El Salvador, Chile: Econ. Geol., v. 70, p. 857–912.

Harshbarger, J. W., and Associates, 1972, Sahuarita-Continental critical groundwater area: report prepared for the Anaconda Company, 113 p.

Kalt, W. D., Jr., 1968, Awake the Copper Ghosts! The History of the Banner Mining Company and the Treasure of Twin Buttes: copyright, Banner Mining Company.

Kelly, J. L., 1971, Geological development and general geology of the Twin Buttes orebody: unpublished paper, presented to Ariz. Sec., AIME, Mining Geology Div., 16 p.

———, 1977, Geology of the Twin Buttes copper deposit, Pima County, Arizona: SME-AIME Trans., v. 262, p. 110–116.

Knaebel, J. B., 1970, Development of the Twin Buttes mine for production: AIME Preprint No. 70-A0-58, 63 p.

Lacy, W. C., 1959, Structure and ore deposits of the east Sierrita area: Ariz. Geol. Soc., Southern Arizona Guidebook II, p. 185–192.

Lodewick, R. B., 1970, The petrology and stratigraphy of the Earp Formation, Pima and Cochise Counties, Arizona: unpub. Ph.D. diss., Univ. Ariz., 194 p.

Lootens, D. J., 1965, Structure and petrography of the east side of the Sierrita Mountains, Pima County, Arizona: unpub. Ph.D. diss., Univ. Ariz., 227 p.

Luepke, G., 1971, A re-examination of the type section of the Scherrer Formation (Permian) in Cochise County, Arizona: Ariz. Geol. Soc. Digest, v. IX, p. 245–257.

Lutton, R. J., 1958, Some structural features in southern Arizona: unpub. M.S. thesis, Univ. Ariz., 138 p.

McAleer, J. F., and Barter, C. F., 1973, 1st progress report, Twin Buttes area, Pima County, Arizona: unpublished report, The Anaconda Company, 37 p.

McClymonds, N. E., 1959, Paleozoic stratigraphy of the Waterman Mountains, Pima County, Arizona: Ariz. Geol. Soc., Southern Arizona Guidebook II, p. 67–76.

McCurry, W. G., 1971, Some mineralogy and alteration features at the Twin Buttes mine: unpublished paper, presented to Ariz. Sec., AIME, Mining Geology Div., 9 p.

Marvin, R. F.; Stern, T. W.; Creasey, S. C.; and Mehnert, H. H., 1973, Radiometric ages of igneous rocks from Pima, Santa Cruz, and Cochise Counties, southeastern Arizona: U.S. Geol. Survey Bull. 1379, 27 p.

Mauger, R. L., 1966, A petrographic and geochemical study of Silver Bell and Pima Mining Districts, Pima County, Arizona: unpubl. Ph.D. diss., Univ. Ariz., 140 p.

Murphy, J. M., 1964, The Twin Buttes railroad: Arizonian, v. 5, n. 1, p. 20–34, and n. 2, p. 12–25.

Nations, J. D., 1961, The Black Prince Limestone of southern Arizona: unpubl. M.S. thesis, Univ. Ariz., 52 p.

Ransome, F. L., 1922, Ore deposits of the Sierrita Mountains, Pima County, Arizona: U.S. Geol. Survey Bull. 725, p. 407–428.

Salek, H., 1976, The silver occurrence study of a sample from the Twin Buttes project, Pima County, Arizona: unpublished report, The Anaconda Company, 2 p.

Seegmiller, B. L., 1971, Rock slope stability of the south and northwest slopes, Twin Buttes pit, Sahuarita, Arizona: unpublished report, The Anaconda Company, 75 p.

Smith, G. E., 1977, Skarn and sulfide mineral zonation patterns in band 3 of the Main ore zone, Twin Buttes: unpublished report, The Anaconda Company, 21 p.

State of Arizona, Department of Mineral Resources, 1975, 1974 tabulation of ore, copper, and molybdenum production from Arizona mining operations, 2 p.

Titley, S. R., 1976, Evidence for a Mesozoic linear tectonic pattern in southeastern Arizona: Ariz. Geol. Soc. Digest, v. X, p. 71–102.

Weaver, R. R., 1965, Structural interpretation of the Ruby Star Ranch area, Pima mining district, Pima County, Arizona: unpub. M.S. thesis, Univ. Ariz., 74 p.

Wilt, J. C., 1969, Petrology and stratigraphy of the Colina Limestone (Permian) in Cochise County, Arizona: unpub. M.S. thesis, Univ. Ariz., 117 p.

Wright, J. J., 1964, Petrology of the Devonian rocks in eastern Pima and Cochise Counties, Arizona: unpub. Ph.D. Diss., Univ. Ariz., 153 p.

Wright, W. A., 1971, Geology of the Twin Buttes orebody: unpublished report, The Anaconda Company, 14 p.

21

Geology of the Sierrita-Esperanza Deposit

PIMA MINING DISTRICT, PIMA COUNTY, ARIZONA

Richard J. West and Daniel M. Aiken

The Sierrita-Esperanza complex is located 40 km south-southwest of Tucson, Arizona, on the southeast flank of the Sierrita Mountain Range. Eight km to the east lies the Twin Buttes deposit and about 19 km to the northeast, the Pima-Mission orebodies. The Sierrita and Esperanza deposits were brought into production as separate open pits within parts of a single, large, mineralized system and have been integrated into one of the world's largest copper-molybdenum operations. Worked sporadically since 1895, the Esperanza property was acquired by Duval Corporation in 1955 on the recommendation of Dr. Harrison A. Schmitt, consulting geologist. Duval was initially attracted to the Esperanza deposit by features of the prominent leached capping and, under Dr. Schmitt's direction, an exploratory drilling program delineated a well-developed chalcocite blanket below the capping. Pre-mine stripping began in 1957 and, following completion of the 12,000 ton-per-day milling facilities, production started in 1959.

With the beginning of stripping in early 1968 and the start of mill operations in March, 1970, the Sierrita mine became one of the lowest-grade porphyry copper–molybdenum mines in the world. The success of this operation was due to a combination of factors, including thorough preliminary geologic work and engineering design, favorable financing conditions, and technological advances. Development of the $190-million Sierrita project was made possible through a program initiated by the General Services Administration to encourage additional domestic copper production in the interest of developing strategic mineral reserves. The property was recommended for this program and a contract with the U.S. government was signed on November 28, 1967. The GSA program called for an $83-million advance against future copper deliveries priced at 38¢ per pound. The GSA also agreed to guarantee a privately advanced loan. The remaining costs of the project were covered by Duval Corporation.

HISTORY AND DEVELOPMENT

Esperanza

Claims in the Esperanza area were first located and recorded in 1895 by P. H. Chambers (Anderson and Kupfer, 1944). Sporadic underground mining of high-grade base and precious metal veins was undertaken. Exploration was also conducted to locate near-surface copper carbonates. The New Year's Eve mine (known then as the Red Carbonate mine and located in what became the Esperanza pit) was extensively developed by the Calumet and Arizona Mining Company in 1907–1908. According to Lynch (1967, p. 6), ". . . about 2,000 tons of carbonate ore, averaging four percent copper, were shipped between 1912 and 1916. In 1912, 30 tons of sulfide ore, averaging ten percent copper, were also shipped."

During the 1930s and 1940s, several companies examined the New Year's Eve mine as a potential source of molybdenum. Interest in the deposit was particularly stimulated in the early 1940s by W. J. Vanderwilt, consulting engineer, at a time when molybdenite was found in quantities of commercial value in few locations. Based substantially on Vanderwilt's recommendations, the U.S. government showed interest in the property as an additional source of molybdenum against possible war shortages. The U.S. Bureau of Mines and the U.S. Geological Survey were requested by the War Production Board to examine the underground workings of the New Year's Eve deposit and to explore the Esperanza claims. Both properties then belonged to the Amargosa Molybdenum and Copper Corporation. The

USGS conducted geologic studies and prepared topographic maps of the area in 1943 and logged core samples from 3 holes drilled by the Bureau of Mines in 1944 in conjunction with the Bureau's preliminary engineering examination.

In the early 1950s, the Duval Sulphur and Potash Company (later Duval Corporation) began searching for major copper deposits. Dr. Harrison A. Schmitt, consulting geologist, was retained to locate possible targets. Following an examination of the Esperanza deposit by Dr. Schmitt, Duval acquired the claims in February, 1955, from C. D. Wilson, who had leased them from the Sierrita Mining and Ranching Company. After completion of preliminary geologic mapping and a geochemical survey, 28 diamond and churn drill holes were drilled to delineate mineralization. The chalcocite orebody was determined to contain 52 million tons of ore at 0.62 percent copper. By mid-1981, about 350 exploration and development holes, totaling approximately 225,000 ft. (68, 580 m), had been drilled at Esperanza.

Pre-mine stripping began in 1957, production in 1959. Additional exploratory drilling immediately northwest of Esperanza developed the West Esperanza extension, and pre-mine stripping started there in 1963, with production in 1965.

The ore grade of Esperanza averaged 0.5 percent copper and 0.028 percent molybdenum from the start of operations to the end of 1977. Ore reserves for Esperanza in 1981 were about 55 million tons, with grades of 0.27 percent copper and 0.033 percent molybdenum. Daily mill capacity in 1981 was 18,000 tons of ore, with a stripping ratio of 1:1.

Sierrita

The first serious exploration work west of Esperanza started in early 1959 when a major mining company initiated an exploration program in the Sierrita–Lofton Peak area. Extensive geochemical sampling, ground geophysics, and surface geologic mapping were done during the next two years. The project entailed the drilling of 64 diamond drill holes, totaling 32,146 ft. (9,800 m). The average depth of these holes was 502 ft. (153 m); the deepest was 2,322 ft. (708 m). It was decided that the values encountered were not of sufficient economic interest to warrant additional expenditures at that time.

In 1963, Duval Corporation acquired an option to purchase the property. Approximately 58 percent of the orebody was obtained by the purchase of 143 unpatented mining claims (the remaining 42 percent of the property was controlled by mining claims already owned by Duval). An additional 87 diamond drill holes, totaling 86,965 ft. (26,507 m), were drilled to further delineate the mineralization, to confirm the accuracy of the previous holes, and to test proposed dump areas. As of mid-1981, some 680 holes, totaling about 950,000 ft. (137,160 m), had been completed. The Sierrita property encompasses approximately 13,000 acres (5,261 ha.), including land for tailings disposal, water fields, pipeline rights-of-way, a railroad spur, mill sites, dump, and maintenance facilities.

Pre-mine stripping began in 1968, with initial production in mid-1970. Ore mined at Sierrita averaged 0.39 percent copper and 0.028 percent molybdenum from 1970 to 1977. Daily production in 1979 was 92,000 tons (84,000 metric tons) ore and 120,000 tons (109,000 metric tons) waste. Exploration and development drilling through 1980 established total ore reserves of 399 million tons (363 million metric tons), with a grade of 0.30 percent copper and 0.035 percent molybdenum. Silver content was approximately 3 ounces per ton of copper concentrate.

GEOLOGIC SETTING

The Sierrita-Esperanza copper-molybdenum deposit is associated with a Laramide-aged, porphyritic facies of a large north-northwest–trending granodiorite batholith, which comprises the eastern flank of the Sierrita Mountains. The range, also trending north-northwest, is approximately 14 miles (22.5 km) in length and varies in width from 2 to 5 miles (3 to 8 km). It consists of a central core of calc-alkaline series intrusive rocks ranging from Precambrian to Oligocene in age and is bordered on the east and west by Mesozoic felsic to mafic volcanic and Paleozoic sedimentary rocks.

Extensive, high-angle faulting and folding occurred throughout the range. Late Cretaceous and early- to mid-Tertiary thrust faulting occurred locally in response to weak, northeast-directed, regional compressive forces. Pre-Laramide deformation is not obvious, as most was destroyed or concealed by Laramide tectonism (Drewes, 1973). Tertiary volcanism and Basin and Range activity also obliterated much of the pre-Laramide and Laramide structural record.

Lootens (1966) has reported that regional structural trends include: (1) "discrete" high-angle faults trending N70°W; (2) "diffuse" high-angle fault zones trending N60 to 80°E; and (3) poorly developed north-south–trending faults.

ROCK TYPES

The Sierrita-Esperanza deposit is composed principally of Mesozoic and Tertiary igneous rocks. The Triassic, Ox Frame Volcanics are the oldest unit in the mine area. This unit was intruded by the Harris Ranch Quartz Monzonite and overlaid later by the Late Cretaceous Demetrie Volcanics. Late Cretaceous to Early Tertiary intrusive rocks—including biotite quartz diorite, Ruby Star Granodiorite, and Ruby Star Quartz Monzonite Porphyry—invaded the preexisting volcanic and intrusive rocks to complete the premineral profile. The locations and relationships of the rock types present in the area are shown in Figure 21.1 and in the cross sections of the mines in Figures 21.2 and 21.3. A description of these rocks is presented in Table 21.1.

Ox Frame Volcanics

The Ox Frame Volcanics are composed of mainly tuffaceous rhyolite flows. The unit covers much of the terrain west of Sierrita pit and forms the upper levels of the south and east Esperanza pit. It is believed to be 2,000 ft. thick in the mine area (Cooper, 1960), and appears to dip eastward. The lower member of the Ox Frame Volcanics does not crop out in the vicinity of the mine. Subdivisions of the formation present at the property are reviewed below. For a complete discussion

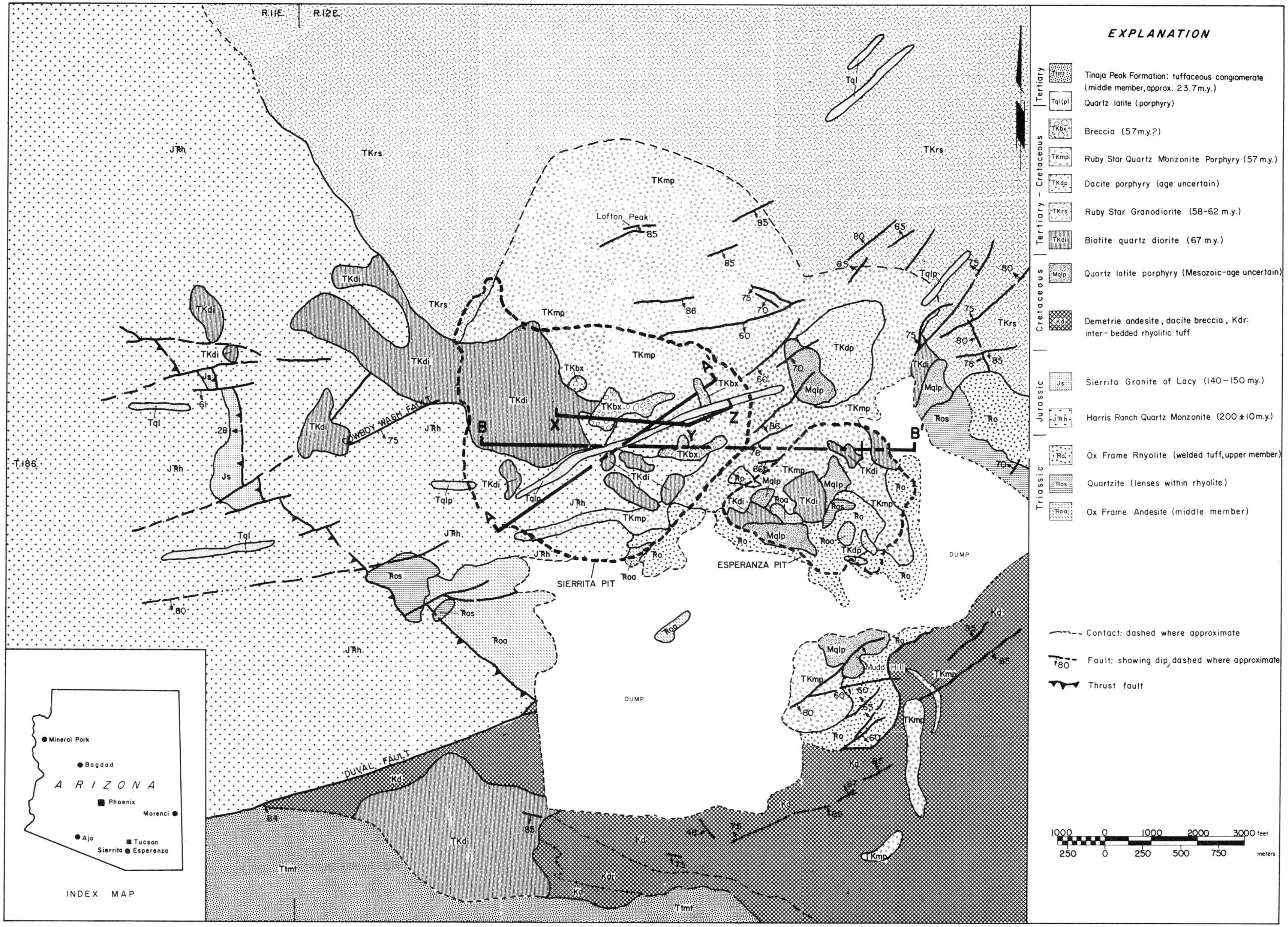

Figure 21.1. Generalized geologic map of the Sierrita-Esperanza area. Modified after Cooper (1973).

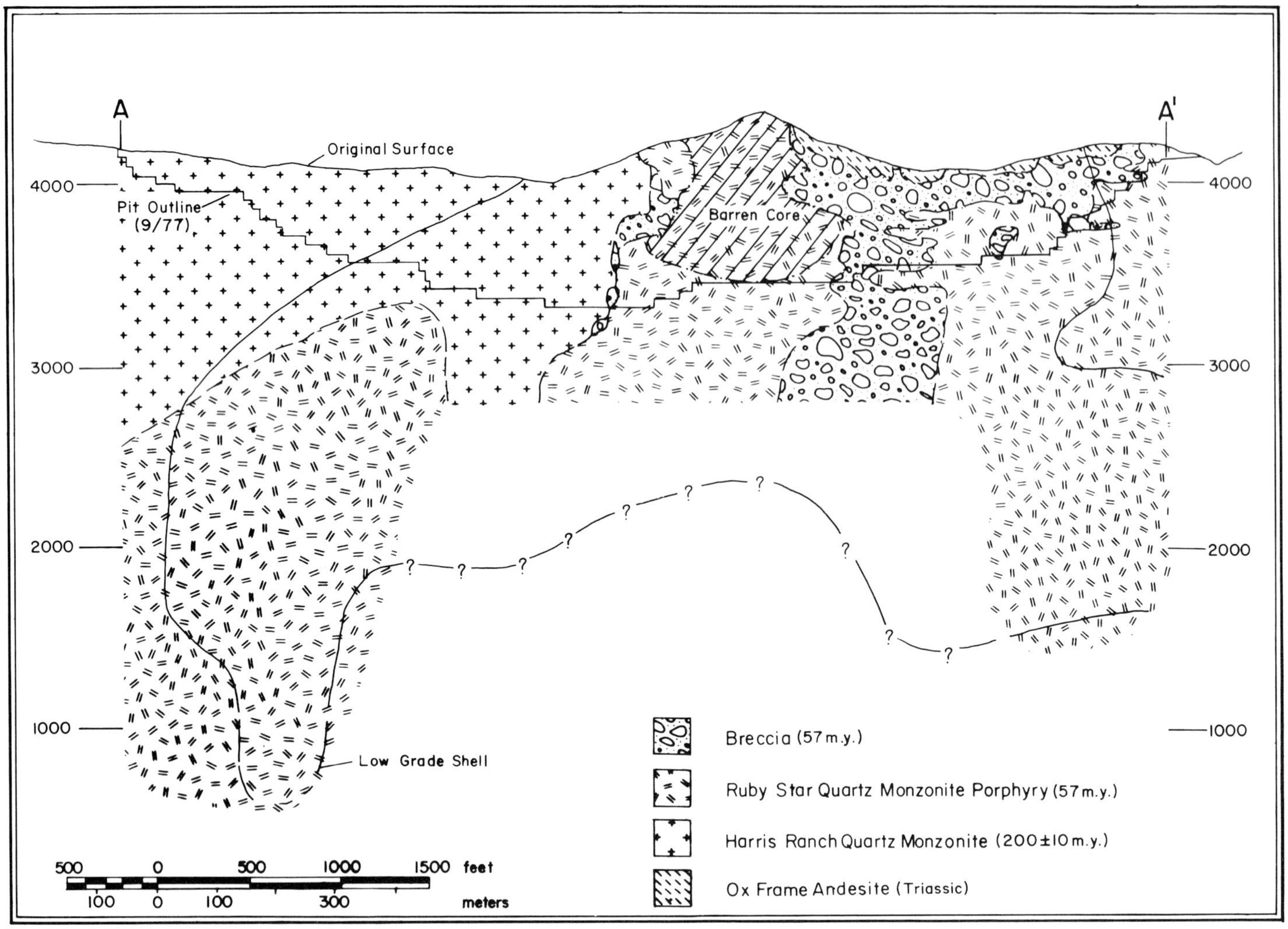

Figure 21.2. Geologic section *A-A'*, trending N55°E through Sierrita

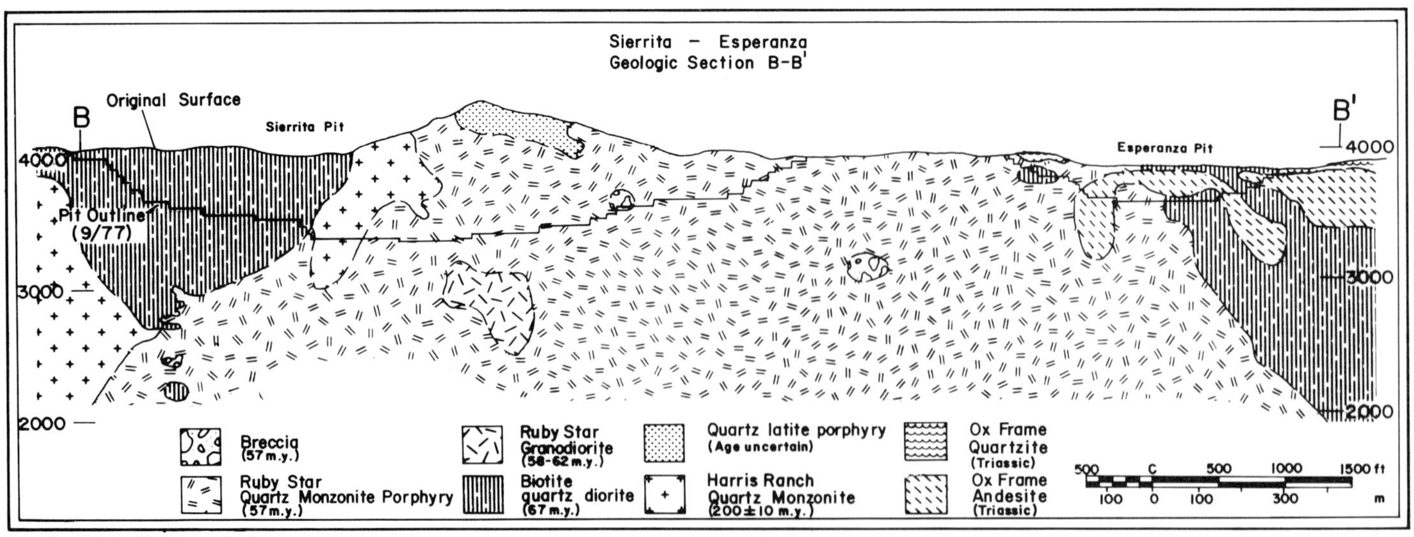

Figure 21.3. Geologic section *B-B'*, trending east-west through Sierrita and Esperanza

TABLE 21.1
Description of Mesozoic and Tertiary Rocks in the Sierrita-Esperanza Area

	Name	Age	Description and Occurrence
Tertiary	Tinaja Peak Volcanics	23.7 m.y. (lower member)	Breccia tuffs and flows of intermediate composition; part of the Basin and Range epoch
	Quartz latite (porphyry)	Eocene (?)	Pods and high angle dikes (weakly mineralized)
	Breccia	Eocene 57.0 m.y.	Irregular, pipe-like bodies; large discontinuous masses; dikes
	Ruby Star Quartz Monzonite Porphyry	Eocene 53.5 m.y. (Damon, 1966) 56.0 m.y. (Creasey and Kistler, 1962) 56.9 m.y. (Cooper, 1973)	Stocks and plugs (probable source of metal-bearing hydrothermal solutions)
	Dacite porphyry	Eocene-Paleocene	Dikes and irregularly shaped bodies, probably genetically related to quartz monzonite porphyry
	Ruby Star Granodiorite	Paleocene 58.7 m.y. (Damon, 1966) 59.0 m.y. (Damon, 1965) 61.6 m.y. (Cooper, 1973)	North-northwest–trending batholith considered to be source magma for quartz monzonite porphyry and mineralization
	Biotite quartz diorite	Paleocene(?) to Late Cretaceous 67.0 m.y.* (Cooper, 1973)	North-northwest–trending, rectangular stock and smaller bodies (excellent host for mineralization)
?	Quartz latite porphyry	Uncertain	Principally plugs at Esperanza with associated hybridized zones and thin flows(?) or sills, extending from the vicinity of Esperanza to central Sierrita; occurrence in the central Sierrita pit may represent a chilled fringe or strongly supergene-altered phase of quartz monzonite porphyry.
Mesozoic	Demetrie Volcanics	upper Upper Cretaceous Older than 75 m.y.; (Drewes, 1973)	Sequence of andesitic and dacitic breccias and flows located south and east of Esperanza mine
	Sierrita Granite	Jurassic 140 m.y. (Damon, 1966) 150 m.y. (Cooper, 1973)	Located west and north of Sierrita-Esperanza
	Harris Ranch Quartz Monzonite	Jurassic to Triassic 190 m.y. 210 m.y. (Cooper, 1973)	Northwest–trending stock (excellent host for mineralization); found in Sierrita pit and west of mine area
	Ox Frame Volcanics	Triassic	Rhyolite flows, tuffs, and tuff breccias with intercalated lenticular beds of sandstone/quartzite, and andesite/dacite flows, with a few flow breccias

* Additional radiometric dates of 47.0 m.y., 56.0 m.y., and 60.0 m.y. (Cooper, 1973) have been obtained from minerals in quartz veinlets in diorite; vein emplacement may be related to Ruby Star Granodiorite intrusion.

of the Ox Frame Volcanics, the reader is referred to Lynch (1967), Cooper (1971) and Smith (1975).

Andesite. Ox Frame Andesite is the middle member of the extrusive sequence. It occurs as a mass bordering the Sierrita pit on the south and as pods within rhyolite welded tuff at Esperanza. It is also prominent as xenoliths of variable size in the younger intrusive rocks at Sierrita.

The andesite is dark gray to greenish black, with 15 to 36 percent albite microphenocrysts, 1 to 5 mm long. Albite, an alteration product, occurs locally with epidote, sericite, and clay minerals. Sparse actinolite and epidote are pseudomorphic after augite(?). The groundmass is composed of albite, actinolite, and magnetite microphenocrysts, with interstitial cryptocrystalline "felsite." Epidote, sericite, chlorite, calcite, and minor tourmaline are scattered throughout the andesite.

Andesite was a good host for hypogene and supergene copper metallization. Groundmass biotite and hornblende grains were often a good site for sulfide deposition.

Rhyolite Welded Tuff. Rhyolite welded tuff is the upper member of the Ox Frame Volcanics. The unit is exposed across many benches in the southern part of the Esperanza mine, and originally it extended into the Sierrita mine, where xenoliths are present at depth in younger intrusions.

The welded tuff commonly has a flinty groundmass, with little trace of bedding, and is variable in color, ranging from pink or white to dark gray. Several workers have subdivided the unit based on textural contrasts, degree of welding, and compositional differences. Some important sub-facies include Lynch's (1967) vitric tuff, fragmental tuff, siliceous-aphanitic tuff and Smith's (1975) rhyolite tuff breccia, rhyolite crystal tuff and quartz latite crystal tuff. Zebra quartz (Lynch, 1967), a related textural variation, was formed when rhyolite welded tuff was shattered in place (possibly by emplacement of quartz monzonite porphyry) and then injected with late magmatic(?) quartz along sub-parallel fractures.

A eutaxitic texture is prominent in welded facies of the rhyolite welded tuff and is characterized by alternating bands of quartz-albite and quartz-orthoclase of variable grain size, averaging 0.02 mm.

Because the rhyolite welded tuff was relatively unreactive and poorly fractured, it was not an important host for hypogene mineralization.

Quartzite. Quartzite occurs as isolated pods and irregular masses interbedded with the rhyolite welded tuff at Esperanza and west of Sierrita. In most cases, definite contacts with welded tuffs are hard to identify, due to the effects of alteration which commonly sweep through contact zones. The quartzite may have been derived from pre–Ox Frame rocks. It was perhaps rafted into place as blocks within younger lava flows or deposited by streams during intervals of volcanic inactivity (Cooper, 1971). The unit sometimes shows relict sandstone texture and is locally cross-bedded (Metz, 1977, personal communication).

The quartzite is hard, white to medium gray, and generally very fine-grained. Smith (1975) describes it as a feldspathic sandstone composed of 60 to 70 percent rounded, elongated quartz grains, with 24 to 30 percent interstitial albite and orthoclase of 0.1 mm size. The rock is about 5 percent Mg-chlorite, with less than 1 percent pyrite, rutile, calcite, and a trace of zircon. Recrystallization of quartz grains, which sealed off many micro-fracture systems, made the rock impervious to ore solutions; veins and disseminations of metallic sulfides, therefore, are rare.

Harris Ranch Quartz Monzonite

The Harris Ranch Quartz Monzonite crops out extensively near its type locality ½ to 1 mile west of the Sierrita mine. An extension of the southeast end of the stock crops out in the southwestern part of the Sierrita pit (see Fig. 21.1) but does not reach the Esperanza pit. The rock is characterized by medium-grained, purple-gray, subhedral perthitic orthoclase, which comprises about ⅓ of the rock (Tables 21.2 and 21.3). Aggregates of subhedral to anhedral biotite flakes are also widespread but may be absent in the more granular aplitic facies occurring locally in west Sierrita. In the pit, biotite content is more variable, due to local absorption of andesite xenoliths and to introduction of groundmass biotite derived from the later intrusion of quartz diorite and attendant fluids.

Tourmaline is common in the Harris Ranch Quartz Monzonite above the 3,900-ft. level and west of the mine. Thin section studies of a sample from the 4,050-ft. bench have identified as much as 4 percent tourmaline (Laine, 1973). Field observation has identified some tourmaline veining. However, tourmaline content diminishes toward the contact with the Laramide intrusions. The tourmaline alters to biotite, chlorite, or sericite near Laramide contacts.

Table 21.2 presents an average composition based on thin section data for 6 specimens sampled from the 4,000 to 4,150-ft. levels (Laine, 1973). These samples were taken from the propylitic zone and are consistent in most respects with analyses of Harris Ranch Quartz Monzonite samples from depth. However, sericite and albite percentages increase with depth, reflecting increased alteration. The average sericite content for ten samples collected on the 3,350 to 3,650-ft. benches is 6 percent. Albite averages 1 to 2 percent, but ranges up to 5 percent. Contrasts in values shown in Tables 21.2 and 21.3 illustrate the variability of the Harris Ranch Quartz Monzonite; Figure 21.4 also shows the wide compositional range of the unit. Thin section study of one sample taken from the 3,400-ft. level of Sierrita inside the potassic zone shows 45 percent orthoclase and only 13 percent plagioclase; these figures reflect up to 80 percent replacement of plagioclase by secondary orthoclase (Dewhurst, 1977). Phenocryst content in the rock is also quite variable. Pheno-

TABLE 21.2
Ranges of Mineralogical Composition of Representative Samples of Harris Ranch Quartz Monzonite (In Percent)

Composition	Average Range of Samples Shown	Sample Numbers					
		S-2	S-3	S-1	S-6	S-40	S-41
Minerals							
Quartz	23	10	42	25	30	20	10
Oligoclase-Andesine	24	35	3	22	15	30	40
K-spar	35	35	35	31	34	40	35
Biotite	3	—	10	—	10	—	—
Actinolite	1	4	—	—	—	—	—
Tourmaline	1	4	—	—	Trace	Trace	—
Sericite	3	—	Trace	15	1	—	—
Epidote Group	4	6	4	<1	4	3	8
Chlorite	2	2.3	3	2	4	3	—
Montmorillonite	1	—	—	—	3	—	4
Pyrite	1	1	1.5	3	<1	2	—
Chalcopyrite	0.7	0.5	1	1	<1	1	—
Calcite	Trace	<1	<1	<1	—	—	—
Anhydrite	Trace	—	—	—	—	—	—
Sphene	Trace	—	—	—	—	Trace	—
Leucoxene	Trace	—	—	1	—	—	—
Limonites	—	—	—	—	—	—	3
Phenocrysts	—	39	65	0	0	0	0
Alteration Minerals	—	11	20	28	37	14	15

Source: After Laine (1973).

crysts are absent in some specimens but range up to about 70 percent in other samples. This irregularity of composition and texture affected the rock's receptivity to alteration and mineralization.

The Harris Ranch Quartz Monzonite was not originally recognized as an important host for mineralization, but exploration by deep drilling in the west-central area of the Sierrita pit delineated an extensive ore zone several hundred feet below the original surface. The Harris Ranch Quartz Monzonite in this vicinity is well broken and formed an extensive, strongly altered crackle zone which was very receptive to ore deposition.

Quartz Latite Porphyry

Quartz latite porphyry intrudes the Ox Frame Volcanics on the southwest side and central part of the Esperanza deposit; a similar unit is recongized north of Esperanza (see Fig. 21.1 and Table 21.1). This porphyry is light colored, with phenocrysts which are 25 to 30 percent anhedral to subhedral perthite, 0.5 to 3 mm in size. Albite clots (An_{6-10}), 0.5 to 2 mm in diameter, are present locally, with uncommon quartz eyes of 2 to 3 mm. The aphanitic groundmass (0.02 to 0.25 mm) varies from light brown to brownish red; it is composed of anhedral quartz, albite, variable amounts of orthoclase, and variable (but generally minor) amounts of chlorite. Epidote, calcite, rutile, pyrite, and apatite occur as accessories.

The quartz latite porphyry was a favorable host for primary copper and molybdenum and secondary enrichment in the mine. However, because of its limited areal extent, it is not an important source of ore. Field relationships indicate that this rock type is younger than the Triassic volcanic rocks but suggest that it may pre-date quartz monzonite porphyry. It has tentatively been designated Mesozoic.

TABLE 21.3
Modal, Normative, and Chemical Compositions of Representative Samples of Harris Ranch Quartz Monzonite (In Percent)

	Sample Numbers		
	4429	4426	4427
Minerals	**Modal Composition**		
Quartz	15.8	23.1	22.8
K-spar	20.6	61.0	32.3
Plagioclase	61.0	12.8	40.1
Biotite	0.8	1.7	3.8
Chlorite	1.8	0.7	0.4
K-mica	—	0.3	—
Epidote	—	—	—
Pyrite	0.6	0.1	0.6
Chalcopyrite	0.3	0.3	—
Molybdenite	—	—	—
Minerals	**Normative Composition**		
Quartz	33.40	29.66	26.92
Orthoclase	25.06	34.28	25.14
Albite	25.81	22.09	32.49
Anorthite	10.17	6.16	8.04
Hypersthene	1.72	1.63	2.64
Corundum	1.77	—	1.41
Hematite	2.08	3.74	3.09
Wollastonite	—	1.20	—
Enstatite	—	1.03	—
Components	**Chemical Composition**		
SiO_2	69.60	68.00	69.50
Al_2O_3	14.44	12.10	15.05
Total Fe	1.99	3.58	3.03
MgO	0.66	1.01	1.04
CaO	1.96	1.72	1.57
Na_2O	2.92	2.46	3.77
K_2O	4.05	5.47	4.22
Cu	—	—	—

Source: From Hillman (1972).

Biotite Quartz Diorite

A northwest-trending, irregular-shaped remnant of a late Cretaceous biotite quartz diorite pluton occurs northwest of the Sierrita Mine. It extends into north Sierrita pit and is wedge-shaped, with numerous marginal dikes that trend N60°E (see Figs. 21.1 and 21.3). The unit is also present in the western half and the north-central part of the Esperanza Mine, where it forms an extensive hybrid zone with the quartz monzonite porphyry. Rock in the hybrid zone is characterized by engulfed plagioclase and orthoclase phenocrysts and by intermixed lithic fragments and irregular replacement features. Smith (1975) has distinguished a "leuco-quartz diorite porphyry" in the northwest corner of Esperanza. His analysis of the unit suggests that it is not a distinct lithology but rather hybridized quartz diorite–quartz monzonite porphyry–dacite porphyry(?).

The unit is variably black to dark green; this color range reflects the presence of groundmass secondary biotite, amphiboles, and chlorite. It shows a salt and pepper texture in most weathered or strongly altered exposures. The groundmass texture of the diorite is generally fine grained (0.5 mm) except in related dikes (see Fig. 21.1), where it is often aphanitic. It is typically equigranular but has a low percentage of phenocrysts (1 to 4 mm), which are variably biotitized clusters of hornblende or hornblende after pyroxene(?). Plagioclase grains are sub-parallel, and other grains are randomly oriented. A poikiloblastic habit is observed in certain ferromagnesian minerals which bear inclusions of magnetite, sphene, and epidote.

Tables 21.4 and 21.5 present average and representative quartz diorite modal compositions with normative and chemical determinations. Figure 21.4 shows the petrologic compositional range of the rock, and indicates its regularity within the quartz–plagioclase–K-feldspar system.

The quartz diorite was an excellent host for hypogene copper-molybdenum mineralization. Moderate shattering, probably associated with quartz monzonite porphyry intrusive activity, prepared the chemically receptive rock for the invasion of hydrothermal solutions which accompanied the young Laramide intrusions.

Ruby Star Granodiorite

The Paleocene Ruby Star Granodiorite composite intrusion (see Table 21.1) is a northwest-trending batholith that makes up much of the eastern flank of the Sierrita Mountain Range. The two major facies which comprise the Ruby Star Granodiorite include a central porphyritic phase and an equigranular border phase. These have been described by several

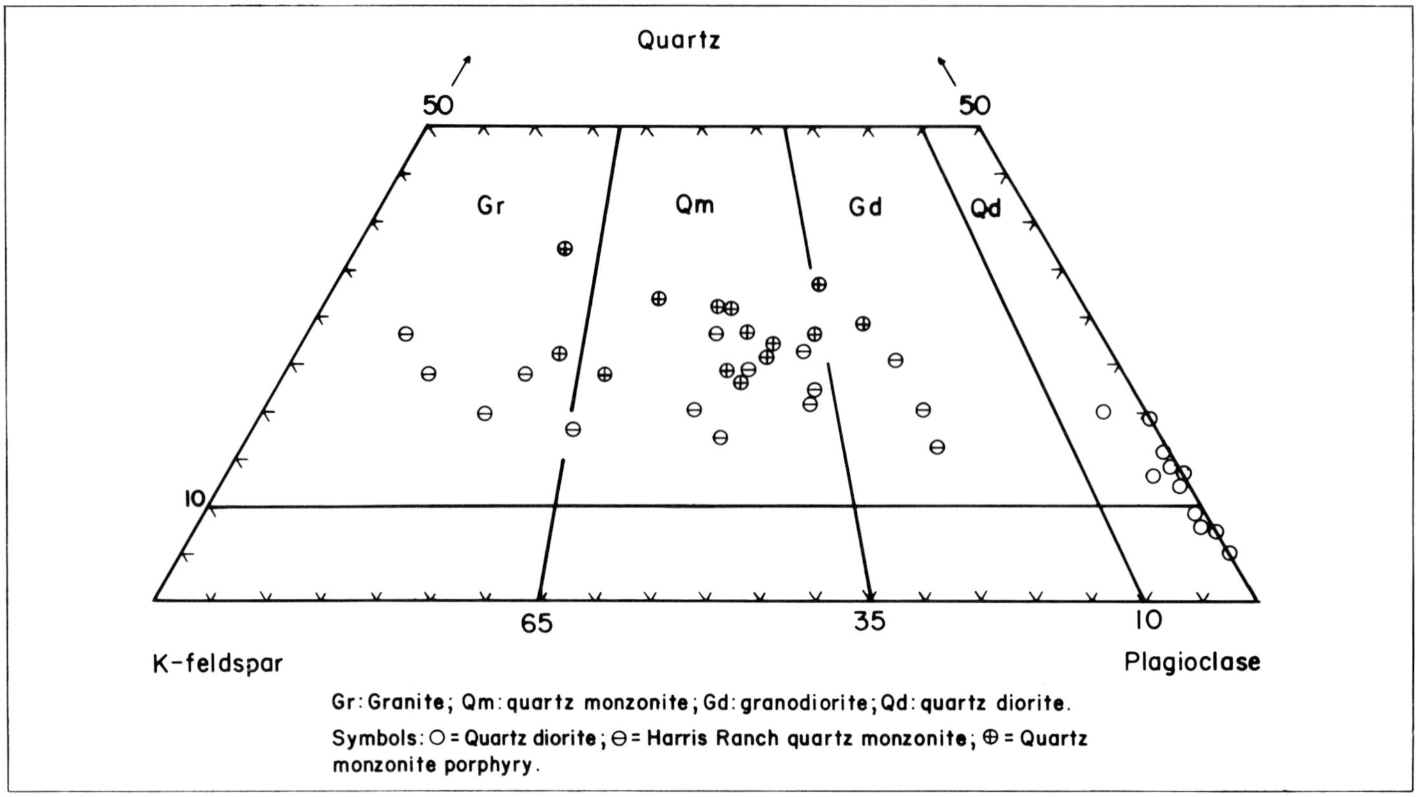

Figure 21.4. Quartz-Orthoclase-Plagioclase diagram of rock compositions, showing modal plots of quartz diorite, Harris Ranch Quartz Monzonite, and Ruby Star Quartz Monzonite Porphyry from Sierrita. After Hillman (1972).

TABLE 21.4.
Ranges of Mineralogical Compositions of Representative Samples of Quartz Diorite (In Percent)

Composition	Average Range of 14 Samples	Selected Representative Samples — Sample Numbers		
		S-4	S-16	S-8
Minerals				
Quartz	7	1–2	5	10
Andesine	32	45	24	30
K-spar	8	<1	15	4.5
Biotite	24	25	23	15
Actinolite	6	13	—	—
Hornblende	13	—	28	5
Magnetite	1	—	—	—
Epidote Group	2	5	2	6
Chlorite	2	2	3–4	6
Montmorillonite	2	2	2–3	12
Pyrite	2	2.5	Trace	6
Chalcopyrite	1	2.5	Trace	4
Molybdenite	Trace	—	Trace	—
Calcite	Trace	—	—	—
Sphene	Trace	1	—	1
Apatite	Trace	—	—	—
Bassanite	Trace	—	—	—
Labradorite	Trace	—	—	—
Phenocrysts	—	0	1	0
Alteration Minerals	—	14	8	42

Source: After Laine (1973).

workers (Lutton, 1958; Cooper, 1960, Lootens, 1965; and Lovering, et al. 1970). Lootens has classified the two varieties as a single unit, stating that the textural differences may represent different phases of a magmatic surge. In addition, no radiometric dates have been reported to indicate any age differences between the two varieties. Contacts between the two facies are generally gradational.

The equigranular border phase is a light gray, medium-grained rock, characterized by visible quartz, plagioclase, potash feldspar, brown biotite, hornblende, and small, honey-colored crystals of sphene (Table 21.6, Analysis *A*). Pink to white potash feldspar megacrysts, comprising up to 25 percent of the rock, are the most distinctive feature of the porphyritic variety. Lovering and others (1970) have shown that the porphyritic core phase trends roughly parallel to the long dimension of the Ruby Star batholith. Porphyritic rocks continue southward into the Ruby Star Quartz Monzonite Porphyry and crop out at Sierrita-Esperanza. This distinctive trend to the southeast, which cuts the two Ruby Star lithologies, may represent a principal axis of Laramide intrusive activity.

Ruby Star Quartz Monzonite Porphyry

The Ruby Star Quartz Monzonite Porphyry is a porphyritic, monzonitic differentiate of the batholithic Ruby Star Granodiorite, bordering the southwest fringe of the batholith as a stock with several associated plugs (see Fig. 21.1). These plugs are irregularly shaped and trend northwestward, reflecting a major regional structural trend. Both the lateral and vertical extent of the porphyry are much greater than

TABLE 21.5
Modal, Normative, and Chemical Compositions of Representative Samples of Quartz Diorite (In Percent)

	Sample Numbers	
	4448	4449
Minerals	**Modal Composition**	
Quartz	10.0	2.7
K-spar	0.7	—
Plagioclase	62.5	57.7
Biotite	0.7	24.2
Chlorite	22.8	12.2
K-mica	1.2	—
Epidote	1.0	—
Pyrite	1.2	3.3
Chalcopyrite	—	—
Molybdenite	—	—
Minerals	**Normative Composition**	
Quartz	18.67	14.34
K-spar	11.73	13.42
Albite	18.95	31.05
Anorthite	32.94	18.30
Hyperstene	7.47	5.71
Corundum	0.94	—
Hematite	9.73	8.31
Wollastonite	—	4.75
Enstatite	—	4.10
Components	**Chemical Composition**	
SiO_2	51.30	58.40
Al_2O_3	16.72	14.65
Total Fe	8.65	8.01
MgO	2.67	3.80
CaO	5.90	5.76
Na_2O	1.99	3.54
K_2O	1.69	2.19
Cu	—	—

Source: From Hillman (1972).

might be inferred from surface exposures, because the stock has generally not penetrated through the older volcanic and intrusive rocks in the southern part of the mine area. The contact on the north between quartz monzonite porphyry and parent granodiorite is gradational in most cases. There, the two units are most definitively identified by modal analyses, but they may usually be distinguished in the field by the presence or absence of sphene, a characteristic mineral of the granodiorite. The quartz monzonite porphyry is intimately associated with mineralization and alteration in the Sierrita-Esperanza system, and is considered to be the source of metal-bearing hydrothermal solutions.

Features common to most quartz monzonite porphyry varieties include: (1) subrounded to hexagonal quartz "eyes," which are preserved even in intensely weathered and altered rock; (2) euhedral orthoclase phenocrysts ranging up to 5 cm in length; and (3) honeycomb texture resulting from the weathering out of plagioclase phenocrysts. The existence of several textural and compositional varieties of quartz monzonite porphyry at Sierrita-Esperanza suggests that several geologic processes may have occurred. Among these processes are successive periods of igneous activity, fractional crystallization of both granodiorite and quartz monzonite porphyry, and development of zonal variations within a single cooling magma. Contacts between quartz monzonite porphyry textural varieties have been observed in drill core samples and are usually sharp. The criteria used to distinguish facies include:

1. *Phenocryst composition, abundance and size.* Orthoclase, plagioclase, quartz, and biotite phenocrysts are common, but may be locally scarce. Plagioclase grains are uniform in size overall, while orthoclase may attain megacryst dimensions.
2. *Groundmass grain size.* The porphyry groundmass ranges from aphanitic to phaneritic, and occasionally approaches pegmatitic dimensions.
3. *Overall rock composition.* The abundance of major minerals in representative samples of each facies is presented in Table 21.6; chemical analysis is shown in Table 21.7.

Based on the features noted above, at least five principal "facies" of quartz monzonite porphyry are recognized: aphanitic porphyry, phaneritic porphyry, aplite, dacite porphyry, and quartz latite porphyry.

Aphanitic Porphyry. This particular unit (see Table 21.6, Analyses *C* through *F*) is rarely observed at the mines. According to Lynch (1966), the surface and near-surface exposures of quartz monzonite porphyry had a dense, aphanitic groundmass, with small phenocrysts. The variety could be a peripheral chilled facies or the result of rapid nucleation induced by a drop in pressure caused by a breach of the magma chamber (Mauger, 1966).

The unit is light to pinkish gray on fresh exposures. Visible phenocrysts compose up to 50 percent of the rock. Most of these phenocrysts consist of 0.5 to 6 mm andesine (An_{36-42}), along with some quartz and microperthitic orthoclase megacrysts. Many of the orthoclase megacrysts exhibit a rapakivi texture, wherein orthoclase cores are rimmed by an andesine myrmekitic rind (Smith 1975). Orthoclase phenocrysts can be homogeneous or perthitic and show an internal layered structure in samples from Esperanza (Mauger 1966). Various minerals, including albite, biotite, and quartz, are localized as fine-grained inclusions along contacts between these internal layers. The groundmass is a holocrystalline aggregate of grains composed principally of orthoclase and quartz, with accessory untwinned plagioclase (Cooper, 1960). Groundmass grain size varies from 0.02 to 0.5 mm.

Phaneritic Porphyry. More typical of the quartz monzonite porphyry observed in the mine areas is the medium-grained porphyry facies (see Table 21.6, Analyses *H* through *K*). The phenocryst population is composed of 2- to 7-mm grains of oligoclase (An_{26-28}), sub-rounded quartz "eyes," biotite books, and 1- to 3-cm orthoclase megacrysts. The myrmekitic rind—present in the aphanitic porphyritic facies, as well as in the dacite porphyry—is visible in some of the orthoclase megacrysts. One- to 5-mm subhedral plagioclase, 0.5 to 3 mm anhedral orthoclase, and quartz with minor sericite, calcite, and rutile comprise the bulk of the groundmass.

Textural variations in the phaneritic porphyry facies are considerable, due mainly to differences in the type, size, and percentage of feldspar phenocrysts present in a given hand specimen. For example, in central and west Sierrita, the

TABLE 21.6
Modal Analysis of Ruby Star Granodiorite (GD) and Quartz Monzonite Porphyry (QMP) Facies

Analysis Letter	A	B	C	D	E	F	G	H	I	J	K	L	M
Type of Facies	Equigranular GD (Lovering et al., 1970)	Porphyritic GD (Lovering et al., 1970)	Aphanitic QMP (Lovering et al., 1970)	Aphanitic QMP (Cooper, 1960)	Aphanitic QMP (Smith, 1975)	Aphanitic QMP (Mauger, 1966)	Aplitic QM (Lovering et al., 1970)	Phaneritic QMP (Smith, 1975)	Phaneritic QMP (Dewhurst, 1977)	Phaneritic QMP (Hillman, 1972)	Phaneritic QMP (Laine, 1974)	Rhyodacite Porphyry (Smith, 1975)	Dacite Porphyry (Smith, 1975)
No. of Samples	3	2	3	1	11	?	1	4	1	19	23	8	1
Quartz	25.10	33.20	27.40	27.70	25.70	22.68	26.40	28.20	30.00	26.20	26.00	22.60	33.70
Orthoclase	20.60	19.20	35.40	32.50	27.00	34.83	30.10	31.60	21.00	32.70	29.00	13.20	5.00
Plagioclase	45.00	42.80	33.50	34.00	41.60	34.66	38.30	33.40	31.00	35.50	31.00	55.80	52.50
Biotite	5.90	3.40	2.80	4.20	4.80	1.03	3.70	4.20	2.00	4.20	3.90	5–10	8.14
Chlorite	5.90	3.40	2.80	4.20	—	2.40	3.70	—	3.00	0.37	1.60	—	—
Muscovite	—	—	—	—	—	1.66	—	—	5.00	0–26.70	0–25.00	—	—
Hornblende	2.00	—	—	—	—	—	—	—	—	—	—	—	—
Apatite	0.20	0.10	—	Trace	Trace	0.17	Trace	Trace	0.50	—	0.20	0.15	Trace
Zircon	0.20	0.10	—	0.40	Trace	—	Trace	Trace	—	—	—	Trace	Trace
Hematite	—	—	—	0.40	Trace–3.90	—	—	—	—	—	0–4.00	—	—
Epidote	—	—	0.20	0.40	—	0.39	0.40	—	3.00	—	0–5.00	—	—
Leucoxene	—	—	0.20	—	—	—	0.40	—	0.50	—	0–1.00	—	—
Magnetite	0.80*	0.80*	0.80*	—	—	—	1.00*	Trace	0.50	—	0–0.75	0–1.80	—
Calcite	—	—	—	—	—	0.40	—	—	0.50	—	0–3.00	—	—
Chalcopyrite	—	—	—	—	—	0.58	—	0.07	—	0.55	0.10	—	0.80
Pyrite	—	—	—	—	—	1.16	—	—	3.00	0.28	0–3.50	0–3.00	0.80
Clay	—	—	—	—	—	—	—	—	—	—	0–6.00	—	—
Sphene	0.40	0.20	—	—	—	—	0.10	—	—	—	—	—	—

NOTE: Samples with asterisk were analyzed as "opaques." Dash indicates that the mineral is not present.

TABLE 21.7
Chemical Analysis Of Ruby Star Quartz Monzonite Porphyry (QMP) Facies (In Weight %)

Analysis Letter*	F	J	K	E, H	L	M
Type of Facies	Aphanitic QMP (Mauger, 1966)	Phaneritic QMP (Hillman, 1972)	Phaneritic QMP (Laine, 1974)	Aphanitic, Phaneritic QMP (Smith, 1975)	Rhyodacite Porphyry (Smith, 1975)	Dacite Porphyry (Smith, 1975)
No. of Samples	?	18	23	6	3	1
SiO_2	62.00	72.08	70.60	66.59	62.73	70.89
Al_2O_3	16.00	14.85	15.44	15.58	16.09	13.63
K_2O	4.70	4.11	5.79	5.08	4.65	2.30
Na_2O	3.80	3.34	3.18	3.09	3.43	4.70
CaO	2.60	2.18	1.47	1.74	2.02	2.00
MgO	1.10	0.82	0.72	1.24	2.32	1.85
FeO (as silicates)	0.10	No Analysis	2.31	1.93	3.46	1.52
TiO_2	Trace	No Analysis	0.47	0.34	0.583	0.362
MnO	No Analysis	No Analysis	0.02	0.042	0.084	0.034
Fe_2O_3 (as silicates)	Trace	2.63	No Analysis	No Analysis	No Analysis	No Analysis
P_2O_5	0.10	No Analysis	No Analysis	No Analysis	No Analysis	No Analysis
H_2O	0.40	No Analysis	No Analysis	No Analysis	No Analysis	No Analysis
CO_2	0.20	No Analysis	No Analysis	No Analysis	No Analysis	No Analysis
S	1.40	No Analysis	No Analysis	No Analysis	No Analysis	No Analysis
ZnO_2	Trace	No Analysis	No Analysis	No Analysis	No Analysis	No Analysis
F	Trace	No Analysis	No Analysis	No Analysis	No Analysis	No Analysis
Fe (as sulfide)	1.30	No Analysis	No Analysis	No Analysis	No Analysis	No Analysis
Cu	0.30	No Analysis	No Analysis	No Analysis	No Analysis	No Analysis

*Refer to Table 21.6.

phenocryst population is composed primarily of white euhedral plagioclase, which is typically 20 percent of the rock mass. In eastern Sierrita, Esperanza, and the area to the north and east of the mine complex, orthoclase phenocrysts and megacrysts predominate, often comprising 50 percent of the rock. This high-orthoclase phase corresponds to the porphyritic zone (approximately 1 to 2 miles wide), which extends from the mine area northward through the core of the granodiorite (Fig. 21.5).

Aplite. Irregular bodies of aplite (see Table 21.6, Analysis *G*) have been reported by various workers (Anderson and Kupfer, 1944; Metz, 1969; Lovering et al., 1970). The report by Anderson and Kupfer noted considerable variation in the quartz monzonite porphyry (then called granodiorite). The intrusion was observed to grade from a normal, granular granodiorite to porphyritic granodiorite to local masses with rare biotite and aplitic texture. Based on their field work, Anderson and Kupfer believed that the various facies grade from one to the other and "do not represent separate intrusions."

In any case, most of the aplite occurrences appear to be localized near the top of the Sierrita-Esperanza system, as observed in drill holes and pit mapping. This suggests that the facies is a chilled border of the quartz monzonite porphyry complex. No modal analyses for the aplite are available.

Dacite Porphyry. Dacite porphyry (see Table 21.6, Analyses *L* and *M*) is considered by Lynch (1966) to be younger than the quartz monzonite porphyry. However, the frequent occurrence of dacite xenoliths in quartz monzonite porphyry at Sierrita, the close spatial relationship of dacite pods with the quartz monzonite porphyry masses, plus the presence of rock which is texturally transitional between the two lithologies strongly suggest that the dacite porphyry is a facies of the Ruby Star composite intrusion.

As is the case with other quartz monzonite porphyry facies, phenocryst composition in the dacite porphyry (Smith's "rhyodacite porphyry") is variable, but it includes zoned plagioclase and myrmekitic orthoclase megacrysts (Smith, 1975). Phenocrysts comprise about 20 percent of the rockmass. It is interesting to note that orthoclase megacrysts in the dacite porphyry are confined to those plugs and dikes located within and near Esperanza.

Lynch (1966) describes a typical dacite porphyry specimen as "dark gray to dark gray-green in color, [exhibiting] a very hard, aphanitic groundmass." The groundmass consists of grains of quartz, orthoclase, oligoclase, and biotite averaging less than 1 mm in diameter.

Quartz Latite Porphyry (Laramide). At Sierrita, Tertiary quartz latite porphyry dikes cut all rock types, including the Ruby Star intrusions. These dikes, 1 to 12 feet (0.3 to 2 m) in width, represent the second period of quartz latite

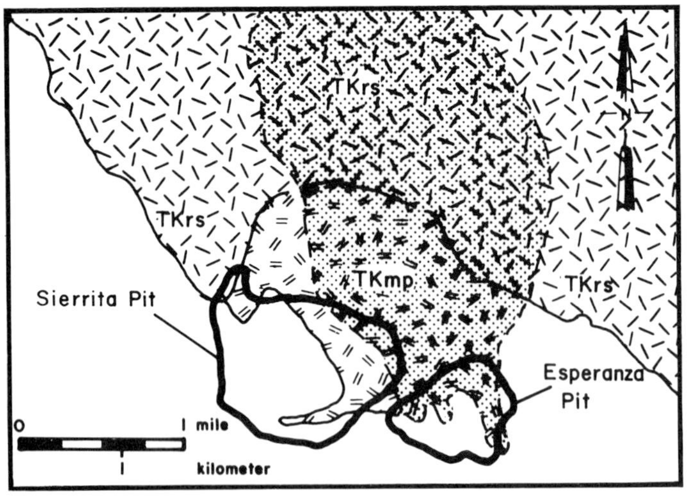

Figure 21.5. Ruby Star Granodiorite *(TKrs)* and Quartz Monzonite Porphyry *(TKmp)*, with porphyritic facies represented by shaded area. Adapted from Lovering and others (1970).

porphyry magmatism in the Sierrita-Esperanza mine area and are believed to be a late-stage surge of Ruby Star Quartz Monzonite Porphyry.

The dikes are mineralized with weak pyrite-chalcopyrite fracture coatings and fine-grained disseminated pyrite. They are cut by occasional quartz-pyrite-chalcopyrite ±orthoclase veinlets of approximately 1-mm thickness, but the general absence of alteration envelopes and groundmass replacement features suggest that the unit intruded following the major episodes of alteration.

Quartz latite porphyry exhibits both light and dark phases. Its mineralogy is characterized by widespread plagioclase phenocrysts, 2 to 4 mm, and locally common orthoclase phenocrysts, 2 to 7 mm, set in a light to dark gray aphanitic quartz-feldspar groundmass. Biotite phenocrysts, 1 mm in size, are spotty in occurrence.

Sierrita Intrusive Breccia

Several irregular breccia masses occur in the eastern portion of the Sierrita pit. These are remnants of a much larger, roughly east-west–trending body (Fig. 21.6). In the upper levels of Sierrita, clasts derived from Ox Frame volcanic rocks, Harris Ranch Quartz Monzonite, Ruby Star Quartz Monzonite Porphyry, and biotite quartz diorite are commonly observed in the breccia. The lower part of the breccia, as exposed on the 3,600-ft. level is composed of sub-angular fragments, typically of Ruby Star Quartz Monzonite Porphyry. The clasts generally become more angular toward the edges of the breccia zone; locally they resemble a crackle breccia, with little or no movement of fragments. However, well-rounded fragments up to 10 in. (25 cm) in diameter are commonly observed near its western edge in upper levels of the mine.

The zone of brecciation expands laterally along rock contacts near the 3,900-ft. elevation (see Fig. 21.2) and fingers out in Ox Frame Andesite, biotite quartz diorite, and other units which cropped out on the pre-mine surface. This intertingering may explain the relative abundance of intermediate to mafic fragments in upper breccia occurrences noted earlier. The breccia extended up to 2,500 ft. (760 m) across and from 600 to 1,000 ft. (180 to 300 m) in width in the upper body, but it narrows below the 3,750-ft. bench into discontinuous bodies of variable size.

The breccia is generally characterized by moderate sericite alteration of plagioclase in fragments, by biotite flow features around clast edges, and by relatively large fragments with little microbrecciation. The matrix, which is dark and dense, is composed mainly of fine-grained biotite, silica, rock flour, and minor local magnetite. Open channels and vugs are rare. Copper and molybdenum mineralization in the breccia, good in upper levels of Sierrita, diminishes with depth. Both Cu and Mo isograds closely follow the breccia–quartz monzonite porphyry contact in upper Sierrita, with overall grade increasing 3- to 4-fold in and near the breccia. The increased grade in the upper part of the breccia appears related to the abundance of receptive fragments of Ox Frame Andesite, biotite quartz diorite, and Harris Ranch Quartz Monzonite.

Breccia Pipe Formation. The Sierrita breccia pipe formed during the Ruby Star Quartz Monzonite Porphyry intrusive cycle, early in the history of hydrothermal activity. Two hypothetical modes of formation have been proposed. The first model involves development of the pipe as a vent in a narrow consolidated crust or hood of quartz monzonite porphyry that occurred high in the magma chamber. In this hood, fracture systems developed, and the relatively shallow depth at which the breccia pipe dies out may correspond to the width of the hood. According to this model (Fig. 21.7), volatiles from the magma chamber vented into several irregular conduits. Solutions migrated upward and outward into quartz diorite, Ox Frame Andesite, and Harris Ranch Quartz Monzonite above the Ruby Star Quartz Monzonite Porphyry.

Pore spaces and joints within pre-pipe quartz monzonite porphyry contained scattered ore fluids. Some of these fluids may have been drawn from the rock to the breccia by the lower pressure in the pipe environment; such fluids were probably joined by ore material derived from depth. This process may have been responsible for developing the "barren core" central to the breccia (see Figs. 21.2 and 21.6). Another major influx of ore solutions occurred following consolidation of the breccia. This episode, the main mineralization event, accompanied renewed quartz monzonite porphyry magmatism. Mineralized porphyry dikes cut upper portions of the pipe.

The breccia presented highly favorable depositional conditions, since it was reactive and permeable, with a predominantly biotitic matrix. During the breccia formation, large volumes of mafic units were stoped back into the pipe, where hornblende and biotite recrystallized as secondary biotite. The secondary biotite, with silica, mobilized around fragments and formed flow bands within the breccia matrix.

The quartz monzonite porphyry generally underwent post-pipe pervasive sericitization, overprinting earlier groundmass alteration. Fragments of this rock were in apparent equilibrium with the pipe-forming fluids, for they exhibit almost no alteration effects distinctive from unbrecciated quartz monzonite porphyry. Barren quartz-orthoclase vein-

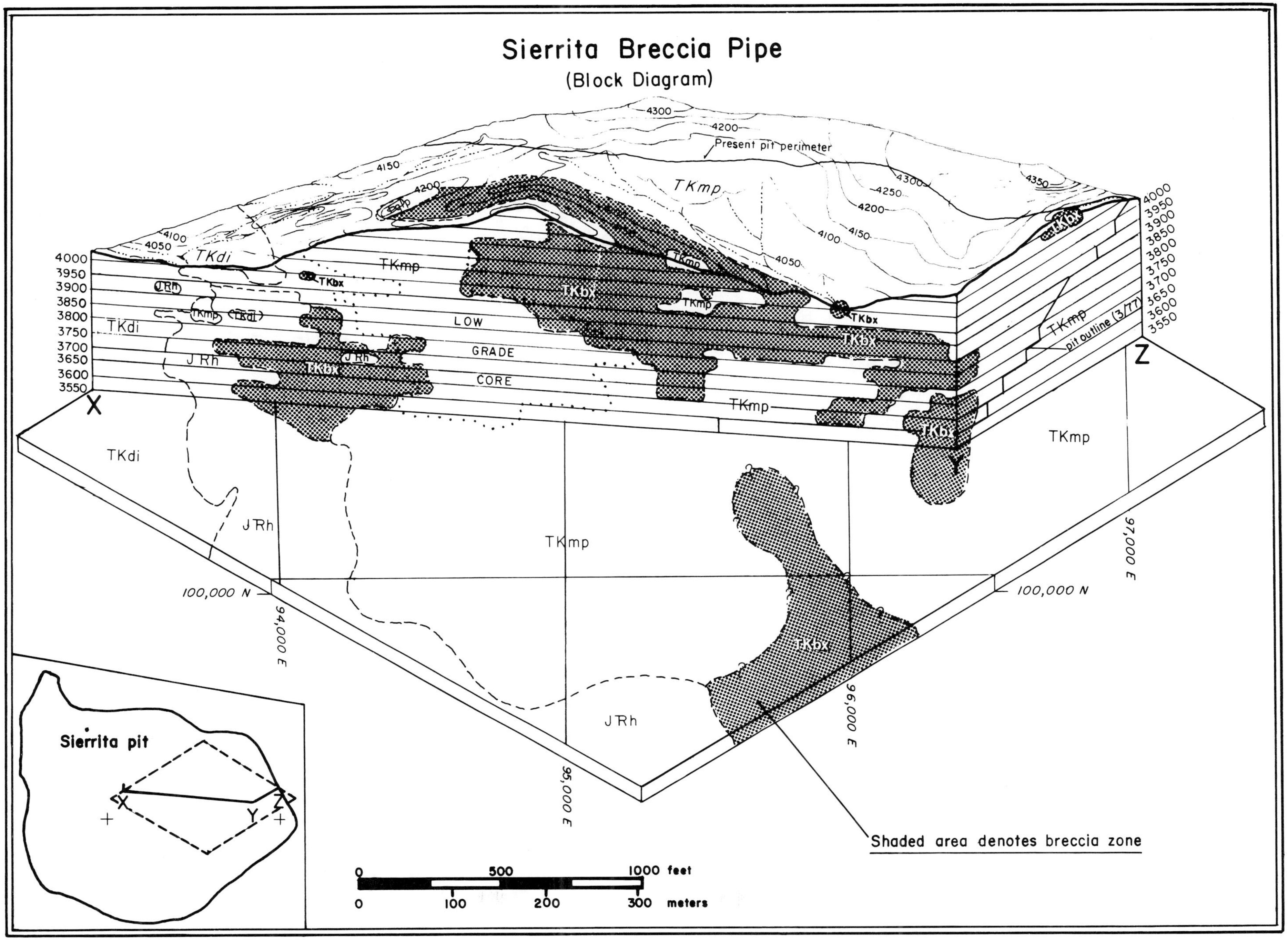

Figure 21.6. Block diagram of Sierrita breccia pipe, looking north-northwest. Key: *JRh* = Jurassic-Triassic Harris Ranch Quartz Monzonite Porphyry, *Tkbx* = Tertiary-Cretacious breccia, *TKdi* = Tertiary-Cretaceous diorite, *TKmp* = Tertiary-Cretaceous Quartz Monzonite Porphyry, *Tqlp* = Tertiary quartz latite porphyry.

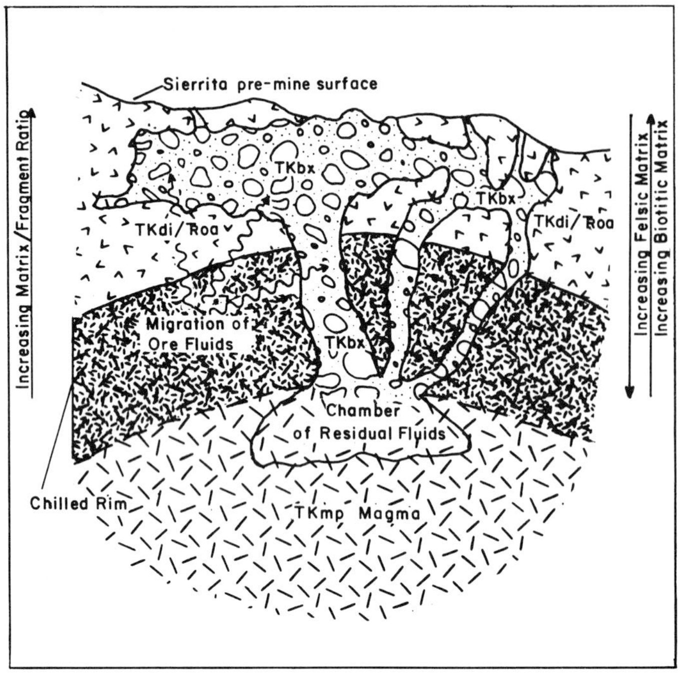

Figure 21.7. Evolution of Sierrita breccia pipe. Key: *TKbx* = Tertiary-Cretaceous breccia, *TKdi* = Tertiary-Cretaceous diorite, *TKmp* = Tertiary-Cretaceous Quartz Monzonite Porphyry, *TRoa* = Triassic Ox Frame Andesite.

lets, which represent a period of very early hydrothermal alteration, have been observed in pre-pipe breccia fragments. Metallization is pervasive in the matrix and along post-breccia crosscutting fractures.

An alternate model of breccia pipe development involves the discontinuous nature of breccia at depth and origins of the barren core. A barren facies of post-breccia quartz monzonite porphyry is conjectured to have invaded the breccia, perhaps following a weak zone established by the breccia. (This later intrusion occurred when the pipe was more fully developed than the model discussed above.) The intrusion assimilated the lower extremities and interior of the pipe and masked its original extent. This concept would account for the peripheral arrangement of breccia north and east of the Sierrita barren core or barren facies (see Figs 21.2 and 21.6). It would also explain the origin of the barren core (simply a barren intrusive phase) and the source of dikes cutting the breccia locally. However, certain observations may discount this idea. Thin section studies, core logging, and pit mapping show no difference in mineralogy or texture to distinguish a barren facies quartz monzonite porphyry from other Sierrita-type phaneritic porphyry. Further, breccia inclusions or biotite zones suggestive of breccia assimilation have generally not been encountered in diamond drill cores or pit mapping the barren core area, except locally in upper contact zones. In addition, the barren core becomes economic at about the same level at which breccia volume drops off (with an accompanying drop in the ratio of matrix to fragments). These facts suggest the following conclusions:

1. Loss of matrix caused a loss of permeability at depth and made the breccia a poor host for ore solutions circulating in surrounding rock. This forced ore fluids to deposit in the quartz monzonite porphyry at depth rather than in breccia, and suggests that a barren facies did not exist, but was only stripped of its mineralization in proximity to matrix-rich breccia.
2. General absence of included breccia blocks or remnants within quartz monzonite porphyry at depth indicates that the breccia, rather than being assimilated, simply grades into unbrecciated porphyry.

REGIONAL STRUCTURE

Diverse primary and secondary structural features occur in the intrusive rocks of the Sierrita-Esperanza mine area. These include flow layering, foliation, dikes, veins, joints, and faults. Various workers have interpreted these features in order to identify principal structural trends and their chronology. Fracturing associated with the development of the Sierrita-Esperanza Orebody has been found by Haynes (1980) to have extended about 4.5 km north of the hydrothermal system into the Ruby Star Granodiorite. Haynes's study of integrated fracture densities has shown that values of 0.2 to 0.3 cm^{-1} occur near the center of the system and decrease to 0.03 cm^{-1} or less outside the area of hydrothermal activity.

A study conducted by Rehrig and Heidrick (1972) on the structural control of porphyry copper deposits in Arizona has indicated the presence of an orthogonal regional fracture pattern that trends roughly ENE and NNW (±20°). The study has pointed out that this structural fabric is imprinted on Laramide stocks throughout the Basin and Range province of Arizona. Their findings have shown the east-northeast–trending set to be dominant, especially in terms of larger structural features, such as dikes and major veins.

Lutton (1958) has mapped trends of fractures, foliation, and layered rocks in the vicinity of Esperanza which agree substantially with those of Rehrig and Heidrick. The presence of these attitudes at Sierrita-Esperanza is further supported by the structural studies undertaken by the Duval geology staff.

Titley (1976) has suggested that the Sierrita Range is transected by one of the six major linear tectonic discontinuities which he has identified in southeastern Arizona. This major, N55°W break is the Sawmill Canyon discontinuity (Lutton, 1958). Titley (1976) has classified it as a "fundamental crustal lineament." Evidence for its existence includes broad zones of strong, northwest-oriented faulting and fracturing. In the Sierrita Mountains, the trend is more specifically reflected by conspicuous northwest-trending contacts bounding the Upper Cretaceous and Jurassic stocks which appear to have intruded along it. According to Titley (1976) the Sawmill Canyon fault forms the southwest boundary of a graben that may have been active from early Mesozoic through Tertiary time. Lutton (1958) has suggested that the fault was active during the Precambrian. A north-south–trending joint set was formed after the principal trends noted above as the result of late doming in the Sierrita Mountains (Lootens, 1965) combined with Basin and Range faulting in the Santa Cruz Valley.

LOCAL STRUCTURE

Faults, joints, and mineralized fractures are prominent structural features within the Sierrita-Esperanza system. Results of deposit-wide structure studies are illustrated in Figure 21.8. Principal trends for both pits reflect the observed regional patterns noted by Rehrig and Heidrick (1972, 1976) and discussed in the preceding section. Other important sets of structures were superimposed over the regional grain as diversely oriented (stockwork) fractures. Their formation appears to be caused by stresses developed during the period of intrusion, consolidation, and cooling of the quartz monzonite porphyry. Generally, stockwork fracture density increases with proximity to the center of the deposit and is influenced by the character of host rocks.

Pre-Mineral Structure

In detail, pre-mineral structures at Sierrita and Esperanza exhibit certain strong differences in orientation, and these are shown in Table 21.8. Most notable of these is the flatter attitude of dips measured for Esperanza faults, joints, and veins. Average dips of fractures are 45 to 50° at Esperanza, whereas they average 70 to 80° at Sierrita. Also, the orientation of strikes at Esperanza is much more random than at Sierrita. The distinctive difference between the structural setting of the two pits suggests that Esperanza had a more complex tectonic history. It has also been speculated that the whole Sierrita-Esperanza deposit could be slightly tilted to the southeast, with Esperanza representing the upper portion of the entire deposit.

A study of fractures in Sierrita drill core samples has yielded additional information in the third dimension. Dips for four structure types (faults, veins, joints, and contacts) compiled from 163 drill holes at Sierrita are illustrated in Figure 21.9; they represent 6,000 structures. Faults, veins, and joints show similar orientations. This similarity is the apparent result of two processes. First, tensional joints formed within intruding and host rocks in response to the stresses set up by early phases of quartz monzonite porphyry magmatic activity. Second, a portion of these same joints subsequently became mineralized or faulted (or both).

The average Sierrita dip angle (greater than 70°) reported in Figure 21.8 differs from that reported in Figure 21.9 (roughly 45°); the nature of development drilling is responsible for this variation. Drill holes at Sierrita are all vertical, approximately 250 ft. apart. Therefore, high-angle joints or faults are rarely encountered in drill core. In addition, many of the faults analyzed in this study are actually faulted veins of typically low angle, showing only minor, post-mineral movement. This fact tends to further distort the importance of lower-angle faulting as reported in Figure 21.9 with respect to high-angle faults of greater movement.

Post-Mineral Structure

Two structural trends developed after the main mineralizing event at Sierrita-Esperanza. These are post-mineral phases of well-expressed, regional trends. The two varieties are as follows:

1. The northeast trend is represented by aplite and (quartz) latite dikes. These dikes are weakly mineralized and represent a late surge of magmatic activity; their formation followed the main stage of hydrothermal alteration and mineralization.
2. Prominent, flat-lying joints located in the uppermost Sierrita pit were possibly formed by load removal during erosion of overlying rocks. The flat-lying set is obscured at Esperanza because of the well-developed leach cap.

HYPOGENE MINERALIZATION AND ALTERATION

Hypogene sulfide mineralization in the Sierrita-Esperanza deposit consists of pyrite, chalcopyrite, molybdenite, and lesser pyrrhotite, with comparatively minor amounts of galena, spalerite, magnetite, tennantite-tetrahedrite, and rare marcasite, cubanite, and bornite(?). Within the ore zone, the pyrite:chalcopyrite ratio is roughly 1:2; total sulfide content is normally 2 to 3 percent or less and seldom exceeds 4 percent by volume. This ratio increases to greater than 20:1 in the propylitic zone, with total sulfide content estimated at 2 to 4 percent.

The Sierrita-Esperanza mineralized system occurs within a zone of three major regional trends, oriented east-northeast, west-northwest, and north-northwest. The east-northeast grain is the most prevalent in the mine area. The dominant "ore trends" (Fig. 21.10*a*) are sub-parallel to, if not coincident with, a regional structural fabric of northwest trend. However, on a more local scale, mineralized trends are often transverse to the northwest trend. This orientation is consistent with Lootens's observation (1965) that the Duval and Cowboy tank faults, two major N60–80°E breaks intersecting the deposit (see Fig. 21.1), represent a "major regional control for copper-molybdenum mineralization." The north-northwest regional system acted as a principal conduit for several episodes of magmatism. However, the northeast "plumbing system" was important in localizing the hydrothermal solutions which formed the Sierrita-Esperanza deposit.

The overall northwest trend of the orebody (see Fig. 21.10*a*) is, in large part, related to chemically and mechanically receptive rocks, such as quartz diorite (Fig. 21.10*b*). Linear mineralized zones parallel or girdle fault trends and intrusive contacts between quartz monzonite porphyry and older, typically northwest-trending tabular intrusions. Pre-Laramide rocks, with the exception of the Ox Frame Formation, were moderately shattered by the intruding quartz monzonite porphyry; this shattering facilitated the influx of sulfide-bearing fluids. The Ox Frame Rhyolite may have been shattered as well, but was then sealed by subsequent silicification.

Iles (1973) defined 4 mineralized zones in the Sierrita-Esperanza orebody; these zones are illustrated in Figure 21.10*a* and in the cross sections in Figures 21.11 and 21.12. Two principal zones at the Sierrita pit, the Amargosa and Sierrita, are sub-parallel, trending N40–60°W. These zones are positioned on the northeast and southwest sides of the pit, but they do connect in northwestern Sierrita via a third major

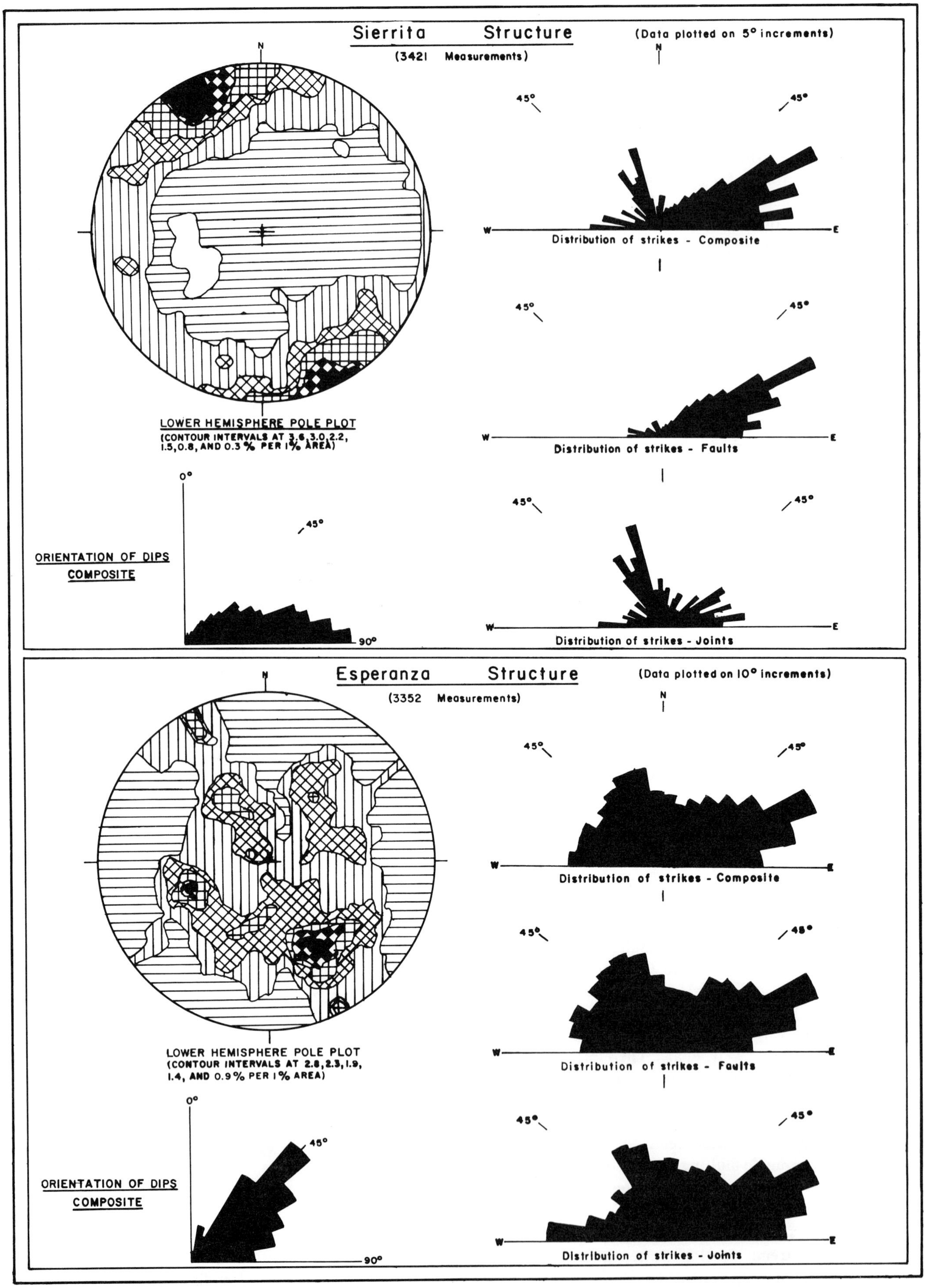

Figure 21.8. Diagrams showing fault and joint orientations in the structure of Sierrita *(top)* and Esperanza (*bottom*)

TABLE 21.8
Strikes of Dominant Pre-Mineral Structures at Sierrita-Esperanza
(In Decreasing Order of Abundance)

	Faults	Joints	Veins (undifferentiated)
	Strike and Dip	Strike and Dip	Strike and Dip
Sierrita	N65°E; 70–83°SE	N23°W; 82°NE	N55°E; 80°NE–SW
	N59°E; 70–80°NW	N72°E; 83°SE	N15°E; 25°SE
	N82°W; 74°NE	N70°E; 75°NW	N55°E; 55°SE
	N18°W; 83°NE	N82°W; 64°NE	N5°W; 60°NE
	N57°W; 63°W	N2°W; 85°SW	
	N5°E; 46°NW	N43°E; 12°NW (variable)	
Esperanza	N66°E; 44°NW	N65°E; 49°NW	N52°W; 43°NE
	N25°W; 50°SW	N62°E; 46°SE	N60°E; 45°NW
	N30°W; 47°NE	N14°W; 70°SW	N30°W; 37°SW
	N60°E; 53°SE	N50°W; 42°NE	N2°W; 32°SW
	N55°W; 50°SW	N50°E; 65°SE	N62°E; 40°SE
	N65°W; 49°NE	N20°E; 72°NW	
	N32°E; 64°NW		
	N86°W; 26°NE		
	N9°E; 38°NW		
	N60°E; 75°NW		

ore trend, the northeast-bearing Cross zone. The Amargosa zone extends southeastward into the Esperanza pit and intersects the N40°E-trending Esperanza zone, which is the fourth principal ore zone at Sierrita-Esperanza. The southeastern limit of the Sierrita zone has not been established.

Deep drilling indicates that the Sierrita Zone plunges steeply westward 60 to 80°. The Amargosa Zone has a configuration similar to the Sierrita Zone but dips eastward. The orebody at Sierrita, therefore, has a semi-oval cross section (see Fig. 21.11), with gradational boundaries. The trend of the Esperanza Zone is less well defined, because the presence of diverse lithologies within the zone has caused widely variable receptivity to mineralization.

The interconnected Sierrita-Esperanza ore trends form an irregular mineralized shell (see Fig. 21.10*a*) peripheral to a central, low-grade core (ridge) which trends southeastward. The low-grade core has a copper equivalent of less than 0.20 percent and is roughly 900 ft. (275 m) long and 600 ft. (180 m) wide (see Figs. 21.2 and 21.6). It is characterized by low fracture density and fresh- to weakly sericitized groundmass alteration, with light quartz-orthoclase veining. Below the 3,500-ft. level, mineralization in the core increases to economic grade.

Hypogene alteration assemblages in the Sierrita-Esperanza system were developed by late magmatic and hydrothermal fluids evolved during emplacement of the Ruby Star Quartz Monzonite Porphyry. Pervasive and vein-type alteration in the quartz monzonite porphyry are primarily the end products of its magmatism and partitioning of the aqueous phase with mineralizers, metals, volatiles, and felsic components into fracture systems. Host rocks were penetrated by fluids of composition initially the same as those fluids altering the porphyry. However, the more mafic hosts —specifically quartz diorite, Ox Frame Andesite, and also Harris Ranch Quartz Monzonite—reacted with the fluids to modify alteration mineral assemblages that were formed during rock alteration. The nature and distribution of hypogene alteration is described in Table 21.9 and in Figures 21.13 and 21.14.

Figures 21.13 and 21.14 show the distribution of principal vein-type and pervasive alteration. As indicated in Table 21.9, particular varieties of pervasive alteration are strongly associated with certain rock types. Vein systems, however, tend to be widespread, although they vary in the abundances of characteristic minerals from one rock type to the next. For example, orthoclase is generally spotty in quartz-orthoclase veins occurring in biotite quartz diorite, but it is plentiful in veins in the Harris Ranch Quartz Monzonite and quartz monzonite porphyry. Conversely, accessory epidote in quartz-orthoclase veining achieves its greatest abundance in quartz diorite, but it is much less common in quartz monzonite porphyry (see Fig 21.13*b*).

Potassic and phyllic alteration zones are locally telescoped around the breccia pods at Sierrita. Generally, however, alteration effects tend to emanate broadly from the quartz monzonite porphyry into the older rocks. Alteration

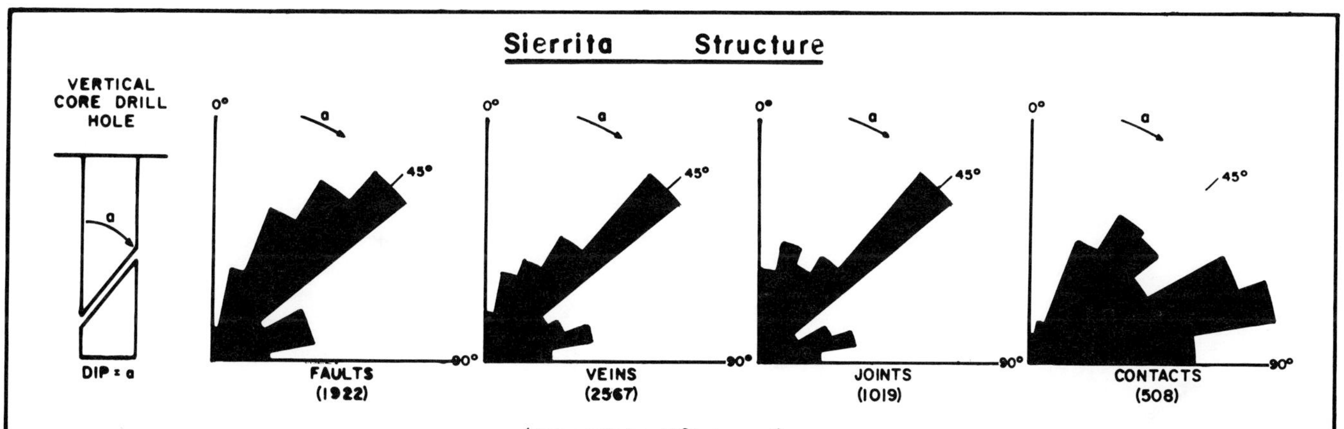

Figure 21.9. Structure to core-axis angles of faults, veins, joints, and contacts measured in drill cores at Sierrita

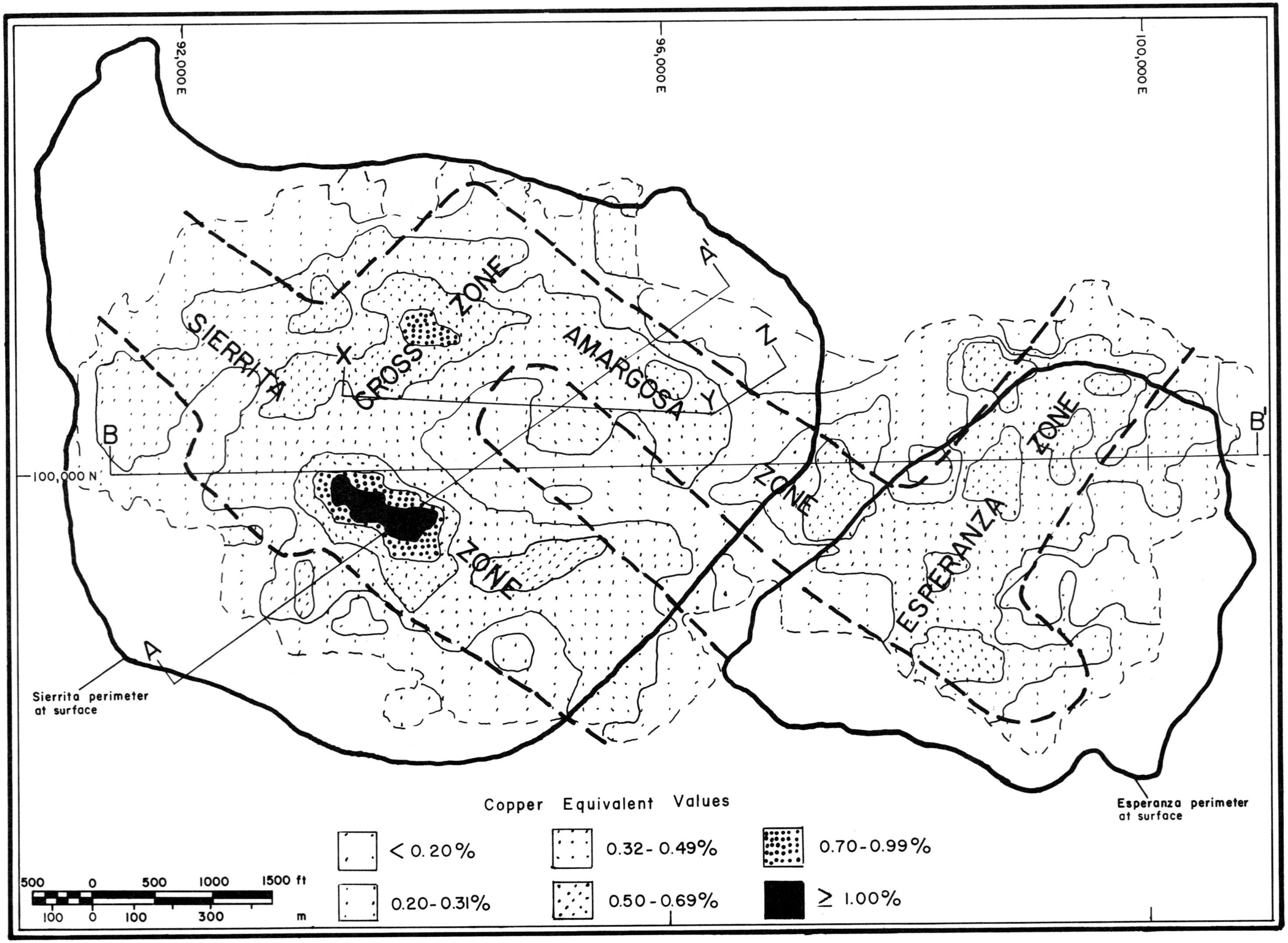

a

Figure 21.10. Mineralized zones *(a)* and geology *(b)* of the Sierrita-Esperanza system at the 3,200-ft. bench

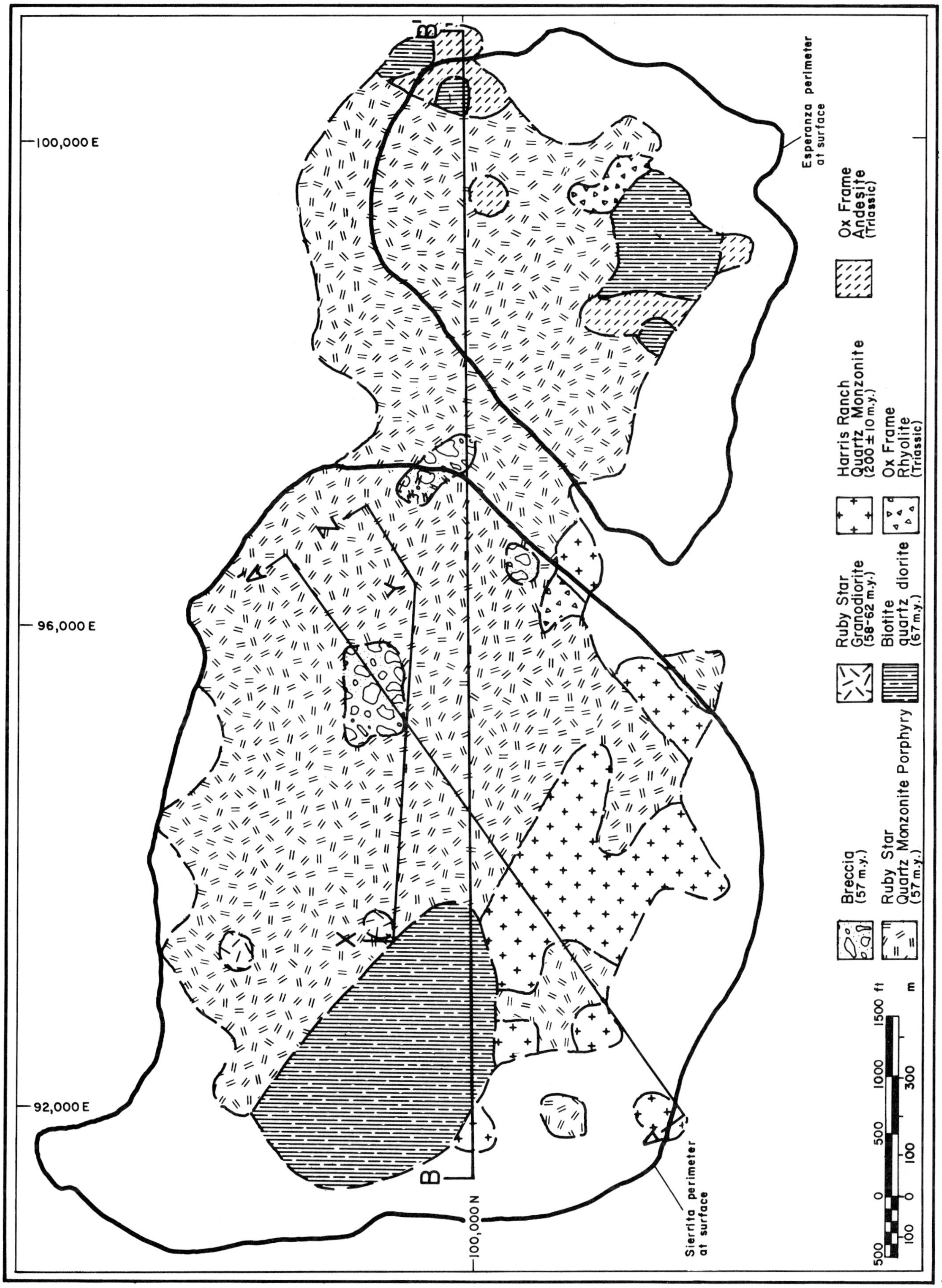

100,000 E
96,000 E
92,000 E
100,000 N
B
B'
Esperanza perimeter at surface
Sierrita perimeter at surface
Breccia (57 m.y.)
Ruby Star Quartz Monzonite Porphyry (57 m.y.)
Ruby Star Granodiorite (58-62 m.y.)
Biotite quartz diorite (67 m.y.)
Harris Ranch Quartz Monzonite (200 ± 10 m.y.)
Ox Frame Rhyolite (Triassic)
Ox Frame Andesite (Triassic)
500 0 500 1000 1500 ft
100 0 100 300 m

b

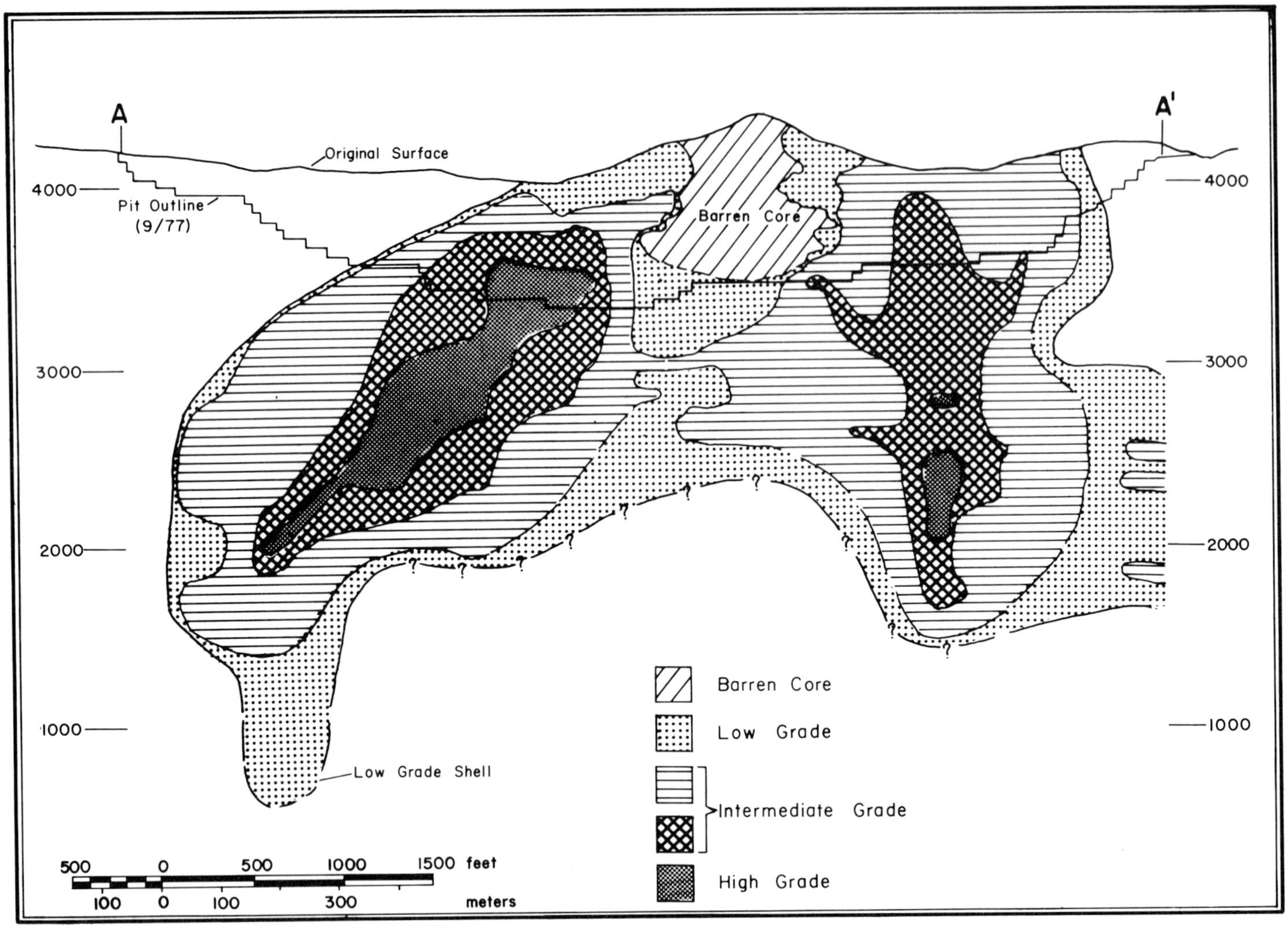

Figure 21.11. Copper-molybdenite grade at cross section *A-A′*, trending N55°E through the Sierrita pit

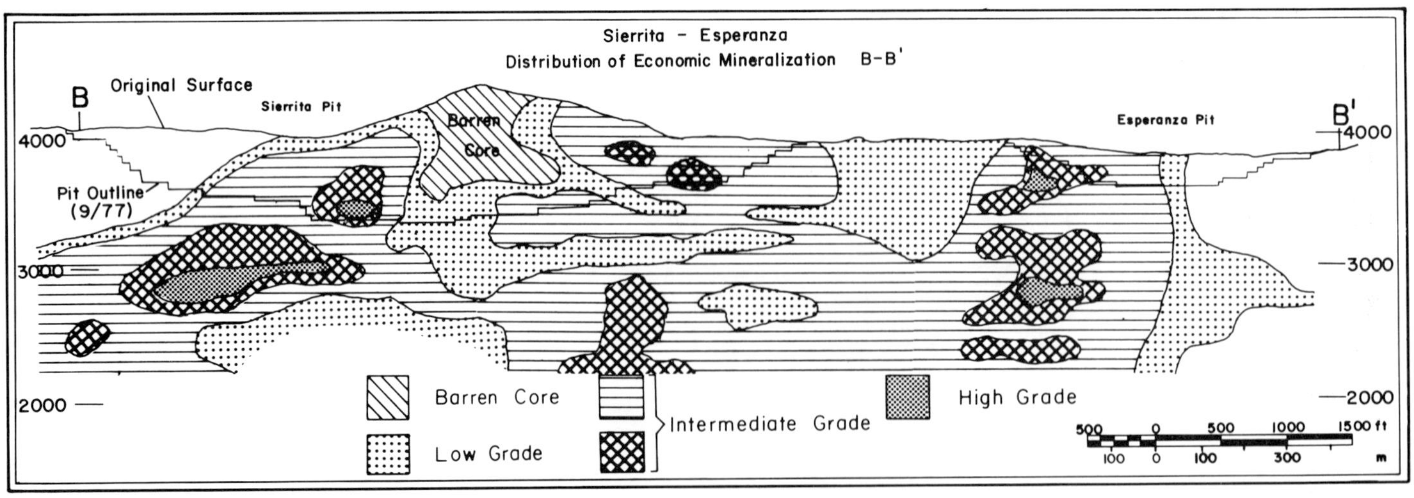

Figure 21.12. Copper-molybdenite grade at cross section *B-B′*, trending east-west through the Sierrita and Esperanza pits

intensity within pre-Laramide units can be correlated with proximity to quartz monzonite porphyry contacts, which underlie and cut the older rocks.

Hydrothermal Alteration

Hydrothermal alteration consists of several distinctive alteration types and is widespread as a fracture-related phenomenon in the orebodies at Sierrita.

Potassic—Early Stage. The first stage of hydrothermal alteration in the area was initiated by migration of pore and residual fluids into fracture systems within the consolidated quartz monzonite porphyry and host rocks. This episode, the main mineralizing event, developed widespread potassic alteration, principally in the form of quartz-orthoclase-chalcopyrite-pyrite-molybdenite-(pyrrhotite) vein-selvage assemblages, with groundmass and veinlet biotitization (see Fig. 21.13*a, b;* see Geochemistry section for further discussion of secondary biotite.) Potassic veining also persisted into otherwise fresh-appearing rock to the north and east of the mines and at depth. Chlorite, epidote, sericite, albite, calcite, and purple anhydrite are prominent accessory minerals that occur with quartz-orthoclase, and magnetite occurs with biotite. The presence of epidote with quartz-orthoclase-chlorite sulfides is atypical of conventional potassic assemblages. Titley (1975) has commented that the occurrence of orthoclase veining with attendant epidote in diorite rocks is known at Sierrita but not common in North America. This observation indicates the important role of host rock mineralogy in influencing constituents of the potassic alteration suite at Sierrita-Esperanza. The occurrence of chlorite and epidote is generally consistent with high a_{K^+}/a_{H^+} and high Ca^{++} activity locally, with availability of ferric iron, and with temperatures below 475°C (Smith 1975). Studies of fluid inclusions (Denis, 1974), Sierrita geochemistry (Hillman, 1972; Laine, 1974), and Esperanza host-rock composition (Smith 1975) indicate that these conditions existed during the first stage (potassic) hydrothermal event, particularly in quartz diorite and Harris Ranch Quartz Monzonite.

Preece and Beane (in press) have reported that ore-bearing potassic fluids first entered the biotite quartz diorite at about 420°C and deposited quartz and orthoclase. As the vein temperature cooled to about 380°C, epidote, chlorite, and sulfides (chalcopyrite, molybdenite, pyrite) were formed from the Ca^{++}, Mg^{++}, Fe^{+++}, and other ions released by the biotite quartz diorite wall rock. As new fracture episodes occurred, new fluids entered the biotite quartz diorite and formed the same assemblages noted above, but these formed at progressively cooler temperatures. Preece and Beane (in press) have observed that the 400°C fluids that had produced quartz and orthoclase then cooled to 350°C and deposited epidote, chlorite, and sulfides, with chlorite and epidote. In hand specimen, epidote may replace orthoclase partially or wholly, or may be intergrown with it.

Albite alteration is an additional, but less significant manifestation of first-stage alteration. Albite may occur as fracture fillings enclosed within earlier-formed, quartz-orthoclase veining or as chessboard albite selvages along quartz-albite veinlets. Two workers (Mauger 1966; Smith 1975) have reported albite at Esperanza, but its occurrence at Sierrita, mainly in Harris Ranch Quartz Monzonite and quartz diorite, is not abundant (Dewhurst, 1977). Variable alteration (see Fig. 21.14) resulted from widely irregular penetration by alteration fluids into strongly fractured rocks of mixed composition. Thus, plagioclase grains that were weakly replaced by sericite and calcite accompany other plagioclase grains which have been wholly replaced by orthoclase. Epidote and chlorite occur abruptly within biotite masses. These effects, particularly common in Esperanza, are probably controlled by networks of microfracturing that are superimposed on rocks of mixed mafic and felsic compositional elements.

Phyllic—Middle Stage. Intermediate-stage alteration is characterized by variously constituted quartz veins—with accompanying sulfides (chalcopyrite, pyrite ±molybdenite)—typically sheathed in a quartz-sericite envelope (see Fig. 21.13*c*). These veinlets as a group are widespread but not so abundant as early-stage veining. The veins reflect what Preece and Beane (in press) have called the quartz-muscovite-sulfide assemblage, which developed below 300°C. A last stage of quartz-sericite-sulfide assemblages, including chalcopyrite, were deposited at 190°C. Smith (1975) believes the quartz-pyrite-sericite vein-selvage assemblage was developed by intermixture of convective meteoric waters with magmatically derived waters. A chronology and summary of the several intermediate stage hydrothermal veins are shown in Table 21.9.

Pervasive "Green" Phyllic Alteration. A late-stage, widespread type of phyllic alteration developed in the quartz monzonite porphyry and to a lesser extent in the Harris Ranch Quartz Monzonite (see Fig. 21.13*d*). This alteration is referred to in the mine as "greenite" (alluding to its green to blue color). On fresh breaks it is often more blue-green. This alteration occurs in the heart of the deposit and extends outward to its margins and to depth.

The alteration type appears to have formed from relatively low-temperature waters migrating through a weak but very widespread system of microfractures. Fluid inclusion studies (Beane and Abramson, 1979, personal communication) have placed the fluid temperature at about 200°C during evolution of this alteration; this temperature indicates that it was nearly contemporaneous with a late-stage chalcopyrite-pyrite mineralizing event and roughly contemporaneous with the phyllic alteration discussed above.

The mineral assemblage is principally sericite, which occupies both the calcic zones (or cores) of plagioclase and small discontinuous fractures in the mineral grains or rock. In addition, calcite is a prominent constituent, as is chlorite-muscovite alteration of biotite. Clay also occurs in small but varying amounts.

Propylitic Stage. Epidote veining—commonly associated with granular pyrite, calcite, quartz, and chlorite—is widespread in the upper benches and fringes of the Sierrita deposit, particularly in Harris Ranch Quartz Monzonite and quartz diorite (see Fig. 21.13*e*) A regional epidote-pyrite aureole extends eastward from Esperanza toward the Twin Buttes deposit and the Santa Cruz Valley, where drill cuttings show epidote-pyrite alteration in rocks beneath the alluvial cover.

Epidote ±pyrite, calcite, chlorite, and quartz penetrated

TABLE 21.9
Nature and Distribution of Hypogene Alteration of Sierrita-Esperanza

	Alteration Type	Ruby Star Quartz Monzonite Porphyry	Harris Ranch Quartz Monzonite	Biotite Quartz Diorite	Quartz Latite Porphyry (Mesozoic)	Ox Frame Rhyolit Welded Tuff
Pre-Laramide	Tourmaline Vein-Groundmass		Tourmaline			
	Biotitization I		Biotite			
Magmatic	Biotitization II Pervasive-Vein	Phlogopite (Esperanza)	Biotite	Biotite, magnetite ± sulfides		
Potassic-Early Hydrothermal	Quartz-Orthoclase Vein Type	Quartz, orthoclase, chalcopyrite, pyrite ± molybdenite, chlorite, sericite, albite, calcite, anhydrite	Quartz, chlorite, orthoclase, pyrite, chalcopyrite, epidote ± calcite, anhydrite, albite, sericite	Quartz, orthoclase, chalcopyrite, pyrite, epidote, chlorite ± molybdenite, anhydrite, calcite	Orthoclase, quartz, chalcopyrite, pyrite ± molybdenite, anhydrite, apatite, calcite	Quartz, orthoclase, chalcopyrite, pyrite ± calcite
	Orthoclase Flood Type	Orthoclase, quartz, sericite, chalcopyrite, pyrite ± molybdenite, chalcopyrite, epidote, anhydrite, calcite	Orthoclase, quartz, sericite, chalcopyrite, pyrite ± molybdenite, chlorite, epidote, anhydrite, calcite			
	Albite Vein Type	Quartz, albite, orthoclase ± pyrite, chalcopyrite, molybdenite, epidote, chlorite		Albite, quartz, orthoclase, chlorite ± pyrite, calcite, epidote		
Variable	Variable Pervasive				± Sericite, chlorite, orthoclase, calcite, pyrite, albite, rutile	± Sericite, chlorite, o clase, calcite, pyrite, bite, rutile
Phyllic-Middle Hydrothermal	Quartz-Chalcopyrite-Sericite Vein Type	Quartz, chalcopyrite, sericite ± pyrite	Quartz, chalcopyrite, sericite ± pyrite			
	Quartz-Molybdenite Vein Type	Molybdenite ± quartz, orthoclase, sericite	Molybdenite ± quartz, orthoclase, sericite	Molybdenite ± quartz, orthoclase, sericite (less common)	Molybdenite ± quartz, orthoclase, sericite	Molybdenite ± quart thoclase, sericite
	Quartz-Pyrite-Sericite Vein Type	Quartz, pyrite, sericite ± rutile	Quartz, pyrite, sericite ± rutile	Quartz, pyrite, sericite, (less common)	Quartz, pyrite, sericite, (less common)	Quartz, pyrite, serici (less common)
	Sericitization Pervasive-(Fractured) "Greenite"	Sericite ± calcite, chalcopyrite, chlorite muscovite, clay	Sericite ± calcite, chalcopyrite, clay		Sericite ± calcite, montmorillonite	Sericite ± calcite, mo morillonite
Propylitic	Epidote Vein Type	Epidote ± pyrite, calcite, quartz (less common)	Epidote ± pyrite, calcite, quartz	Epidote ± pyrite, calcite, quartz (albite?)		Epidote ± pyrite, cal quartz (less commor
Late Hydrothermal	Quartz-Sphalerite-Calcite Vein Type	Quartz, sphalerite, galena ± chalcopyrite, pyrite, chlorite	Quartz, sphalerite, galena ± chalcopyrite, pyrite, chlorite	Quartz, sphalerite, galena ± chalcopyrite, pyrite, chlorite		Quartz, sphalerite, g ± chalcopyrite, pyri chlorite
	Gypsum	Gypsum ± stilbite, calcite, clay, fluorite	Gypsum ± stilbite, calcite, clay, fluorite	Gypsum ± stilbite, calcite, clay, fluorite	Gypsum ± stilbite, calcite, clay, fluorite	Gypsum ± stilbite, ca clay, fluorite
Miscellaneous	Crackle Zone	Chlorite, sericite, hematite clay, calcite ± fluorite	Chlorite, sericite, hematite, clay, calcite ± fluorite	Chlorite, sericite, hematite, clay ± fluorite (not common)		

Hybrid Zones	Time/Space	Replacement Sequence	Vein Size	Halo Size	Characteristics
	Pre-Laramide		$\frac{1}{8}$–$\frac{1}{4}$ in.		Occurs as sprays within groundmass and as narrow veins.
te	In Harris Ranch Quartz Monzonite–Ox Frame Andesite and Harris Ranch Quartz Monzonite–Biotite quartz diorite contact zones				Associated with syntexis related to assimilation of Ox Frame Andesite during Harris Ranch Quartz Monzonite emplacement; local biotitization in Harris Ranch Quartz Monzonite–Biotite quartz diorite hybrid zones in vicinity of contacts.
	Near contemporary with orthoclase alteration	Biotite, hornblende, actinolite, tourmaline → hydrothermal biotite + magnetite	$\frac{1}{32}$–12 in.		Developed in transitional magmatic to hydrothermal environments; formation of phlogopite in high pH, high K^{+}, locally high Mg^{++} fluids at Esperanza (Sierrita?).
		Plagioclase, magnetite, biotite → orthoclase, sulfides, chlorite	$\frac{1}{16}$–4 in.	$\frac{1}{16}$–>12 in. orthoclase	The first major hydrothermal vein system, developed in temperatures ranging from 350 to 400°C (Denis, 1974); up to 420°C (Preece and Beane, in press).
		Plagioclase, magnetite, biotite → orthoclase, sulfides, chlorite		1–50 ft.	Occurs in restricted zones—marginal to pods of Sierrita breccia pipe, Esperanza quartz blowout, Ruby Star Quartz Monzonite Porphyry megacryst zones; called "orthoclase metasomatite" by Smith (1975).
	Weak to moderate at Esperanza	Plagioclase → albite	$\frac{1}{32}$–$\frac{1}{4}$ in.	$\frac{1}{16}$–$\frac{1}{4}$ in. quartz-orthoclase	Albite veinlets form numerous assemblages of limited distribution.
icite, chlorite, or- ase, calcite, pyrite, , rutile	Hybrid zones occur in contact zones of all rocks	Ferro-magnesian → pyrite, chlorite, rutile, epidote, calcite, plagioclase → sericite + calcite → orthoclase + albite			Variable fragment size and composition plus irregular fracturing in Ox Frame Rhyolite Welded Tuff and hybrid zones caused wide variation in intensive, extensive, pervasive alteration parameters.
	Irregular distribution, cut previous veins	Orthoclase, plagioclase, biotite → quartz, sericite, chalcopyrite	$\frac{1}{16}$–3 in.	$\frac{1}{4}$–4 in. quartz-sericite	Scattered system of veins, which make significant local additions to ore grade.
	Throughout deposit, in all major rock types		$\frac{1}{32}$ in.	$<\frac{1}{32}$ in. orthoclase	Veins consistent in size from one rock to another; moly may be injected along narrow fractures, often in well-sericitized, calcite-chlorite–bearing zones.
	Post–economic mineralization	Orthoclase, plagioclase, biotite, magnetite, chalcopyrite → quartz, sericite, pyrite	$\frac{1}{16}$–3 in.	$\frac{1}{4}$–4 in.	Developed by circulation of heated convective water; mineral deposition occurred near 210°C.
	Late stage/very wide spread	Plagioclase, pyroxene, biotite → sericite, calcite, chlorite			Developed by hydrothermal fluids, 200°C, circulating through weak, widespread microfractures during late stage chalcopyrite-pyrite mineralization.
te ± pyrite, calcite, z	In fringes of ore shell into margins of deposit		$\frac{1}{64}$–$\frac{1}{2}$ in.		Epidote veins are typically marginal to ore shell but penetrate into potassic zone, establishing cross-cutting relationships with quartz-orthoclase veins.
	In fringes of ore shell		3 in.–10 ft.		Late-stage hydrothermal veins, which develop locally high lead and zinc values in ore.
ım ± stilbite, cal- lay, fluorite	Joint-cavity fillings, widespread		$\frac{1}{32}$–2 in.		Selenite, alabaster, satinspar occur as hydrothermal veins, products of anhydrite alteration, supergene alteration of metalliferous rock and calcium-bearing mineral species.
	Developed in well-fractured Harris Ranch Quartz Monzonite–Ruby Star Quartz Monzonite Porphyry contact zones			1–75 ft.	Variable width; well-developed in monzonites more than diorite; hydrothermal fluids reacted more pervasively with calcic plagioclase than with sodic plagioclase and orthoclase.

into the potassic zone at depth, in possible response to: (1) collapsing physical conditions in a dying hydrothermal system, (2) the presence of a weak or deep-seated hydrothermal pulse (R. A. Metz, 1976, personal communication), or (3) resurgent heating of pore fluids. In any case, these veins established crosscutting relationships with earlier formed assemblages, most notably the quartz-orthoclase ±sulfide-chlorite-epidote-calcite-anhydrite. In such associations, two independent stages of epidote may be observed, and apparent "retrograde propylitic" effects (R. A. Metz, 1975, personal communication) have been noted, such as epidote locally replacing orthoclase.

The propylitic veining is generally most abundant in rocks with plagioclase of relatively high anorthite content. Thus, at depth, quartz monzonite porphyry may be devoid of epidote, but crosscutting mafic dikes and inclusions will commonly exhibit epidote veining.

Late Stage. Late-stage hydrothermal alteration features diverse vein selvage varieties which are probably typified best by their crosscutting, fracture-filling habit and their general

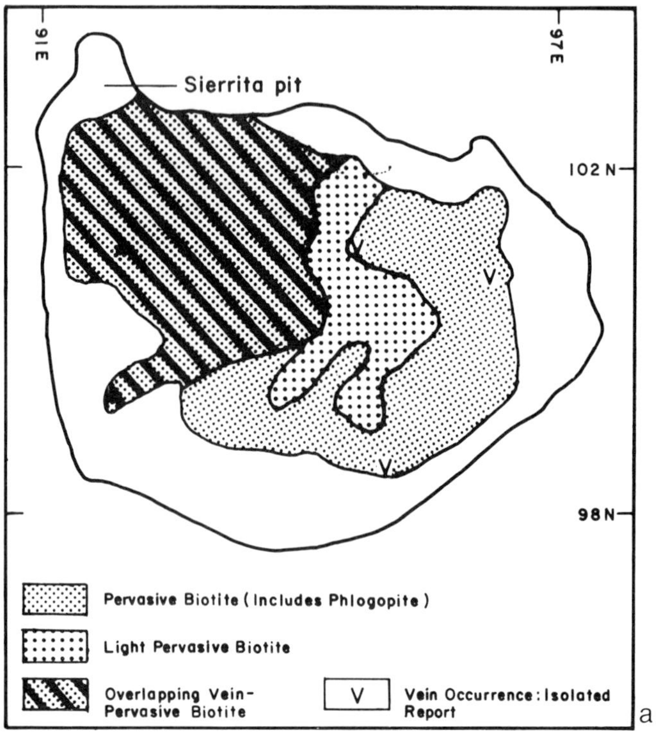

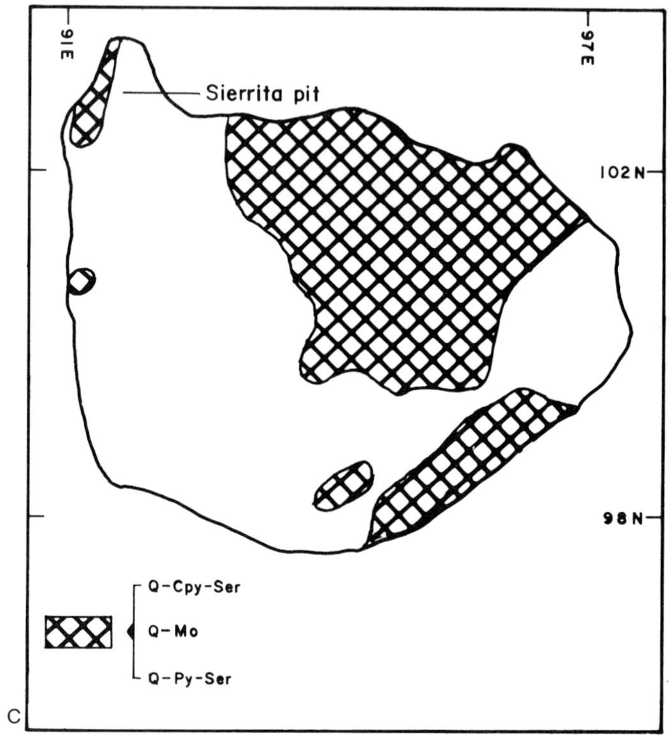

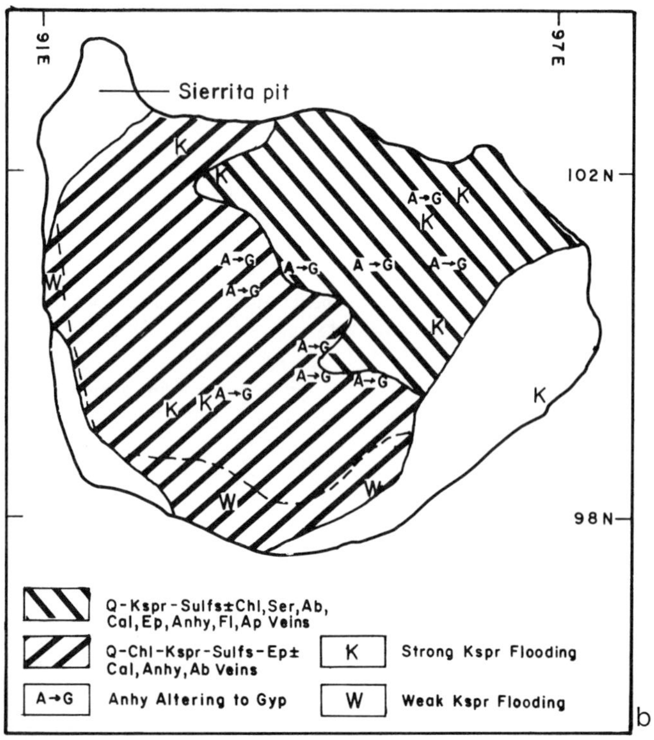

Key to Minerals
Ab = albite
Anhy = anhydrite
Ap = apatite
Cal = calcite
Chl = chlorite
Cpy = chalcopyrite
Ep = epidote
Fl = fluorite
Gyp = gypsum
Kspr = orthoclase
Mo = molybdenite
Musc = muscovite
Py = pyrite
Q = quartz
Ser = sericite
Sulfs = sulfides

Figure 21.13. Major vein and pervasive alteration types at Sierrita: *a*, biotite alteration; *b*, orthoclase stage alteration; *c*, quartz-sulfide vein distribution; *d*, pervasive sericite alteration; *e*, epidote-calcite-quartz veins.

association with partially decomposed rock groundmass. These fillings commonly have not healed the fractures in which they occur. Quartz-sphalerite-galena vein materials tended to inject along fractures that were mobilized or remobilized during subsequent faulting. Molybdenite paint of uncertain age filled narrow joints in hydrous mineral zones. Gypsum, in addition to replacing anhydrite and occurring near and along strongly altered contact zones, filled joints and commonly crystallized as satin spar veinlets in complex fault zones, often with stilbite.

Crackle-Zone Alteration. Crackle-zone alteration, a miscellaneous category which includes crackle-zone and fault-related alteration, developed initially in the Harris Ranch Quartz Monzonite and Ruby Star Quartz Monzonite Porphyry in areas of mutual contact. The Harris Ranch Quartz Monzonite, being older and well-fractured by the emplacement of both quartz diorite and quartz monzonite porphyry, developed crackle-zone alteration most broadly. The alteration is centered around near-vertical Laramide faults connected by smaller, more lateral or radial-trending structures. These conduits provided high penetrability for early hydrothermal solutions concentrated on the fringes of the quartz monzonite porphyry stock. The solutions reacted extensively with the plagioclase-biotite groundmass of both Harris Ranch Quartz Monzonite and quartz monzonite porphyry. Chlorite and sericite are both widespread, and abundant calcite and lesser amounts of montmorillonite and hematite occur with residual rock orthoclase and quartz.

SUPERGENE ENRICHMENT

As mentioned above, interest in the Esperanza area was the result of leached-capping interpretation (Fig. 21.15). The distribution and relative abundance of certain limonites offered good evidence for the existence of an underlying supergene copper blanket. By 1957 development drilling had proved a supergene enriched zone of chalcocite consisting of 52,416,000 tons (47,551,000 metric tons) with a grade of 0.62 percent copper and 0.025 percent molybdenum; this zone was mined out by about 1965, although zones of chalcocite continued to be encountered during stripping of upper benches. The principal supergene mineral at Esperanza is digenite, Cu_9S_5 (R. L. Flagg, 1976–1977, personal communications); however, the term "chalcocite" is used in the text to be consistent with previous usage.

Enriched Blanket

The supergene enriched zone in the Esperanza area varied in thickness from 30 to 150 ft. (9 to 45 m) but averaged about 100 ft. (30 m). The blanket was roughly conformable to pre-mine topography (see Fig. 21.15), yet varied locally; it was found at greater depth under extreme local relief (300 ft. (91 m) or more) and closer to the surface where topography was deeply incised by stream erosion. The configuration of the supergene blanket was influenced by structure and rock chemistry. According to Lynch (1967) a well-developed set of east-west–trending joints, dipping 45 to 50° north, was important in supergene ore localization, serving as channels for the downward-percolating solutions.

As with many supergene deposits, rocks at Esperanza are not homogeneous, and fracturing and alteration effects are not consistent from one rock type to another. These factors contributed to the irregular fashion in which solutions penetrated rock masses. Nevertheless, a saturation level (water table) was recognized (Lewis 1959) at the 3,935-ft. level of Esperanza. Little variation was evident in mid-1981 in this water table, which appeared to be perched in rock with low

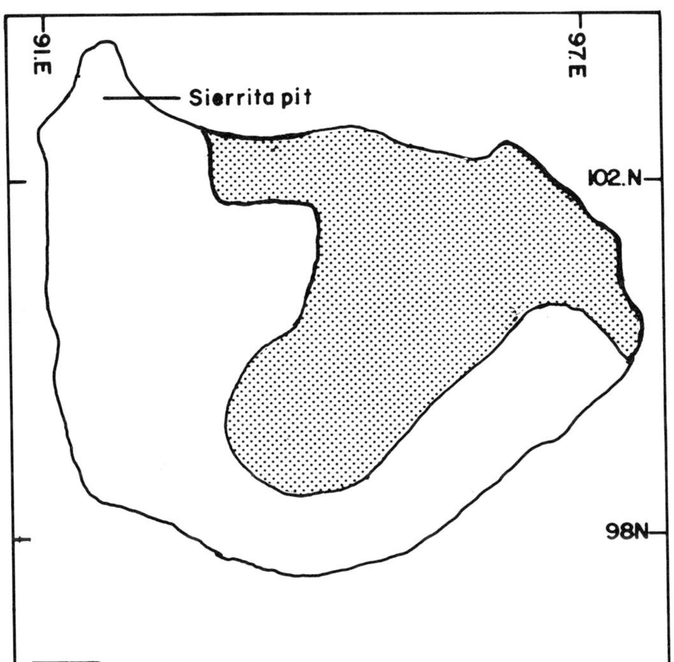

d

e

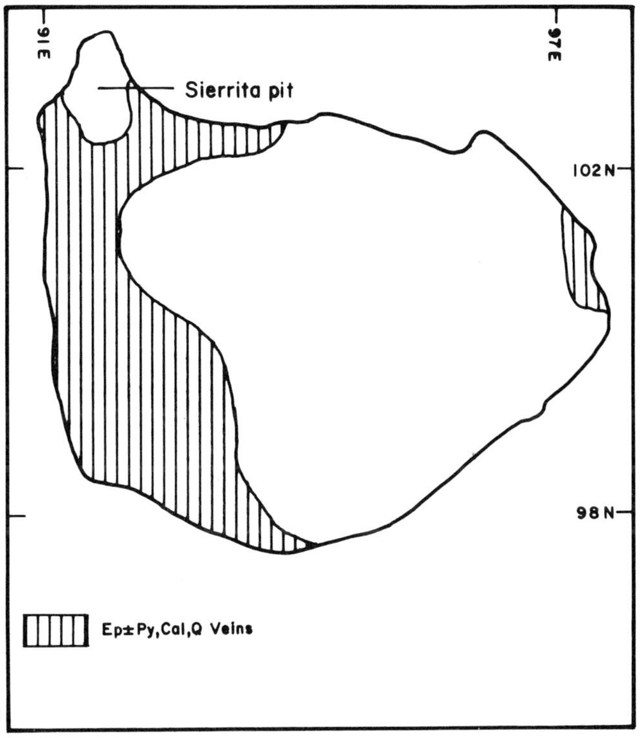

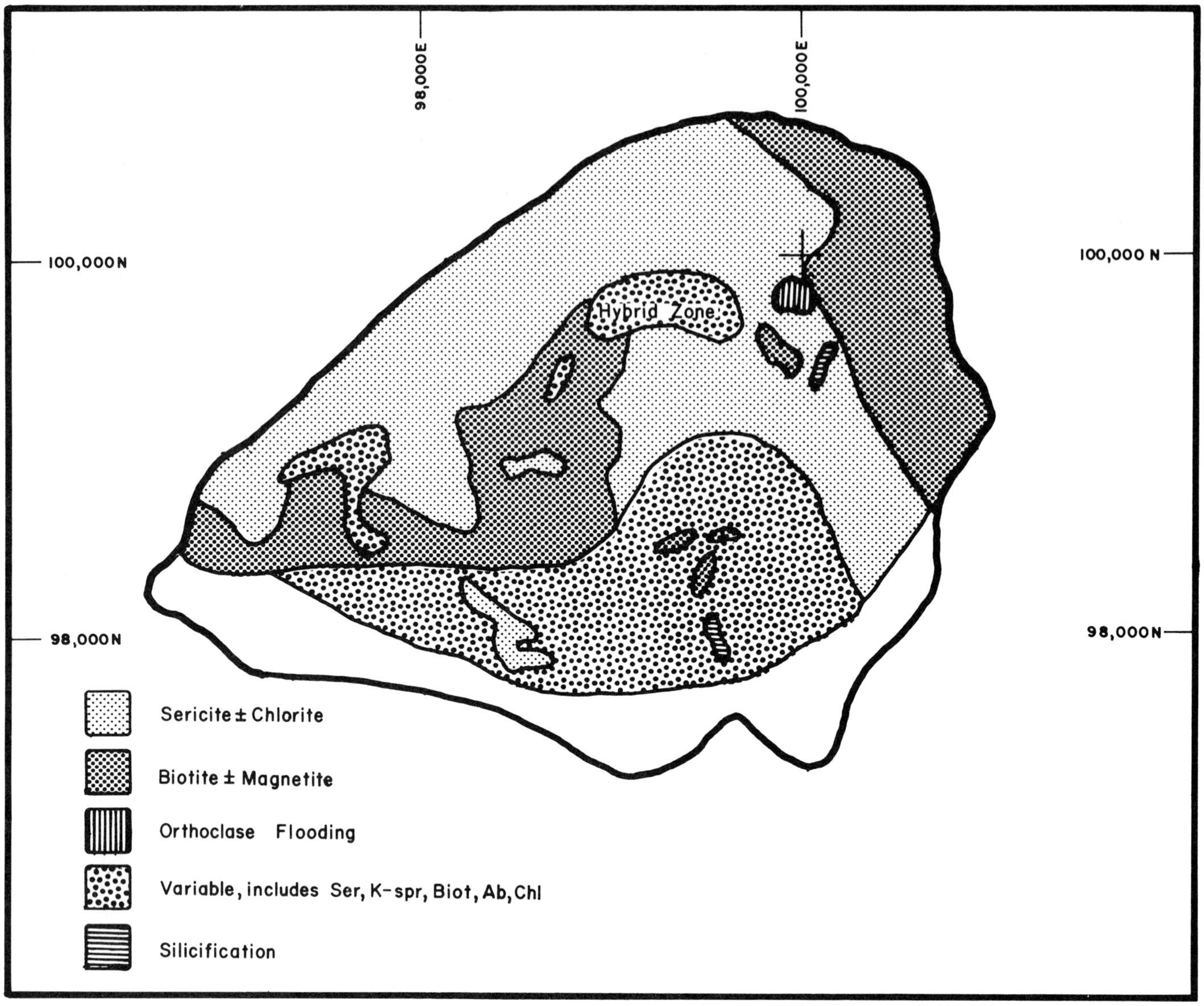

Figure 21.14. Generalized distribution of pervasive alteration at Esperanza

permeability in which fractures had been cemented with gypsum and other minerals.

In the capping the extent of sulfide decomposition locally ranged from light oxidation to total disintegration. Replacement of pyrite and chalcopyrite by chalcocite in the enriched zone was usually incomplete. The majority of chalcocite ore shows remnant pyrite centers (Lynch, 1967). From the 4,005-ft. bench to the 3,970-ft. bench, chalcocite and chalcopyrite are roughly equal in volume; below 3,970 ft. chalcopyrite predominates (Lynch 1967). Covellite is a common mineral in both the oxide and supergene zones, where it coats pyrite, chalcopyrite, and chalcocite.

Mafic units, particularly the andesite (porphyry), were highly receptive to deposition of chalcocite (Lynch 1966). This receptivity was due to several characteristics of the andesite: (1) highly shattered, it offered easy access to the copper-bearing solutions; (2) moderately reactive locally, due to the presence in certain areas of abundant calcite in the groundmass and along fractures, it provided an environment for neutralizing supergene solutions; and (3) because it generally contained above-average concentrations of chalcopyrite and pyrite on fractures, it provided sites for chalcocite deposition under proper conditions.

Certain other rock types were conducive to formation of oxide mineralization. Tenorite, azurite, and malachite are encountered to a depth of 350 ft. (110 m) within quartz monzonite porphyry of northern Esperanza (Lynch 1967), probably as fault-related occurrences. Fracturing also played an important roll in mineralizing the generally impervious quartzite; the quartzite hosts large concentrations of azurite, moderate amounts of malachite, and minor cuprite and chalcotrichite. Additional oxidation products occurring in minor quantities included native copper, turquoise, ferrimolybdite, akaganeite[β-FeO(OH,Cl)], ilsemannite, torbernite, marcasite, chrysocolla, lampadite, libethenite, antlerite, and brochantite. Many of the oxidation products occurred sporadically within the enriched zone and deeper in the system in association with faults.

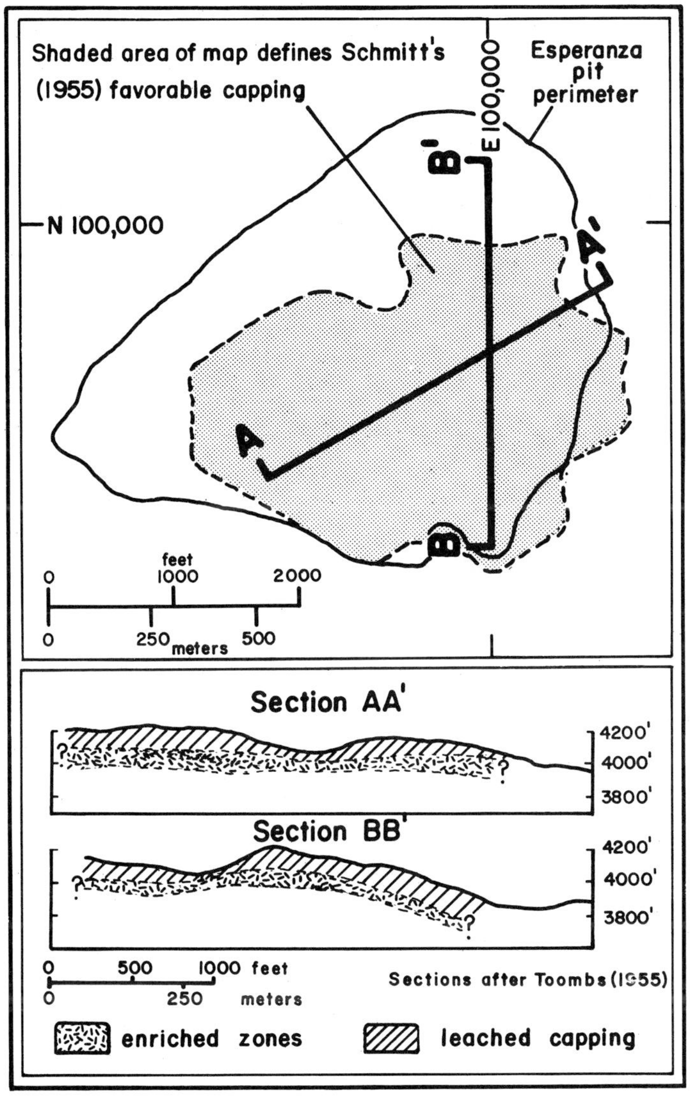

Figure 21.15. Plan map and sections (after Toombs, 1955) of favorable leached capping and enriched zones at Esperanza

Leached Capping

The thickness of the oxidized capping at Esperanza was variable, ranging from 10 to 180 ft. (3 to 55 m) (see Fig. 21.15). Lewis describes the colors of iron oxides over the chalcocite orebody as reddish orange–brown in volcanics and orange-brown in quartz monzonite porphyry; such colors are due to the presence of hematite, the dominant limonite in outcrop, which is followed in abundance by goethite and then jarosite. Some occurrences of indigenous relief limonite after chalcocite and covellite(?) were reported (Lewis, 1959) with admixed goethite, and similar occurrences have been observed in the vicinity of Mudd Hill, ½ mile to the south. However, Lewis points out that much of the limonite on joint surfaces is transported. In the less reactive rocks, Ox Frame Rhyolite in particular, limonitic solutions apparently traveled for considerable distance. Limonite stains after pyrite are widely present in rhyolite outcrops above the orebody at Esperanza.

In reference to hematitic limonite replacing chalcocite and covellite(?) Lewis (1959) has noted that the process seems to have gradually lowered the upper boundary of secondary enrichment. In the late 1970s a prominent leached hematitic horizon was present in the uppermost levels of Esperanza in Ox Frame Rhyolite and offered evidence of a limited, two-cycle supergene blanket, as discussed by Mitcham (1977). This two-cycle blanket probably developed most extensively in rocks susceptible to primary mineralization, enrichment, and subsequent erosion—particularly in the quartz monzonite porphyry, quartz diorite, and Ox Frame Andesite. The limited, two-cycle enrichment process generally augmented the grade of primary copper (chalcopyrite) by a factor of 1.5 to 2, but locally it achieved a 5-fold increase.

Despite evidence of a two-cycle blanket, leaching at Esperanza must have generally been a slow process. Overall primary sulfide content in the Esperanza system averages only 3 to 4 percent, with a pyrite:chalcopyrite ratio of 1:1 to 2:1 (which may range as high as 50:1 in the Ox Frame Rhyolite). This generally low ratio inhibited the formation of acid, which would have transported limonite constituents away from the point of oxidation; the effectiveness of acid was further retarded in moderately reactive gangues—specifically the quartz monzonite porphyry, which is rich in reactive alkali feldspars and clays. Under such conditions the enriched blanket and leached cap were probably less well developed than would have been achieved with higher initial copper grade and greater pyrite:chalcopyrite ratio.

Supergene alteration in the leached capping is variably argillic to sericitic and overlaps moderate to heavy hypogene phyllic alteration. However, supergene sericite is typically coarser than hypogene sericite, and it commonly occurs as solitary fracture coatings without quartz or other vein fillings. Supergene argillic alteration usually affected plagioclase in all rock types and concentrated in fault zones, intermixing with limonite staining.

West Esperanza. During reconnaissance in the early 1950s, Schmitt outlined a zone of favorable capping northwest of the Esperanza pit. The results of a drilling program in 1961 delineated an economic copper-enriched zone (known as West Esperanza) of several million tons of ore with a grade similar to that of Esperanza.

The thicknesses of both the leached cap and the enriched zone at West Esperanza were highly irregular. This condition may have been due to the fact that much of the chalcocite (digenite) occurred in strongly fractured quartz monzonite porphyry and breccia. The permeability of the breccia itself was variable and resulted in variable total sulfide content. A high-angle, northeast-trending fault system provided plumbing for percolating supergene solutions and extended enrichment to greater depth locally. The West Esperanza Orebody was incorporated into the Sierrita pit by 1971.

Sierrita. A minor oxidized cap was developed over the Sierrita deposit, ranging in thickness from 0 to 75 ft. (0 to 23 m), but averaging 50 ft. (15 m). Typical oxide minerals found at Sierrita, such as azurite, malachite, tenorite, and melaconite, are localized in highly shattered rock or fault zones. Goethite as well as akaganeite and jarosite compose the dominant limonite stains coating fracture surfaces; boxworks are rare. Ferrimolybdite and primary sulfides, inculding pyrite and chalcopyrite, were exposed at the pre-mine surface relatively untouched by oxidation processes. Where limonites are observed in quartz-sulfide veinlets, they typically occur as very thin layers on individual sulfide grains. The moderately reactive feldspathic quartz monzonite porphyry and Harris Ranch Quartz Monozonite generally neutralized acid solutions fairly close to the source sulfides, and often created yellowish aureoles several inches wide around sulfide veins. The relationship was enhanced by the low pyrite : chalcopyrite ratio.

GEOCHEMISTRY

Several studies have indicated a correlation between concentrations of Na_2O and K_2O in the Sierrita and Esperanza pits (Hillman, 1972; Laine, 1974; Smith, 1975; Anderson, 1975). According to Hillman (1972), there is a correspondence of areas of high K_2O concentration and enrichment with areas of low Na_2O and low CaO concentration and Na_2O and CaO depletion (Fig. 21.16). He has concluded that the hydrothermal fluids enriching portions of Sierrita were leaching Na_2O and CaO simultaneously. Laine (1974) has found that SiO_2 was also removed from areas of potassic alteration. Figure 21.17 represents the composition of altered Sierrita rocks in terms of potassic minerals versus sodic-calcic feldspar; this distribution further illustrates the inverse relationship between K and Na-Ca occurrences.

Two major K_2O enrichment zones in the upper benches of the central and north Sierrita pit (see Fig. 21.16*a*) correspond to rocks of relatively high Cu grade. As delineated in Cu contour plan maps, K_2O enriched rocks correlate with 0.30 to 0.39 percent Cu isograds, which represent well-mineralized rock at this level in the hypogene system. These enriched zones are reflected in the pit by strong potassic metasomatism in the form of widespread orthoclase and biotite flooding and veining.

Smith's (1975) study of "leuco" quartz diorite samples shows chemical trends that may be correlated with abundance of orthoclase veins, as well as with abundance of sericite. One sample (3655–6) is characterized as "least altered," with 3.53 percent K_2O, 2.69 percent CaO, and 3.20 percent Na_2O. "Most altered" varieties are represented by sample 3655–9, which has 6.65 percent K_2O, 1.55 percent CaO, and 2.48 percent Na_2O. These results in Esperanza parallel Hillman's (1972) findings in Sierrita.

Leaching of CaO and Na_2O during potassic metasomatism promotes formation of epidote, calcite, anhydrite, albite, and fluorite in fracture-filling assemblages. Zeolites and montmorillonite are other products of CaO and Na_2O leaching, although they develop later.

Chemical data indicate that, as potassic alteration intensity increases in the quartz monzonite porphyry, there occur substantial decreases in Fe, Mg, Mn, Ca, Sr, and Na, with slight decreases in Si and Ti. Predictably, K content is increased markedly, as is Al (Hillman 1972; Smith; 1975). Rb shows an enrichment pattern which parallels K (constant K:Rb ratio). Rb content in the Esperanza quartz monzonite

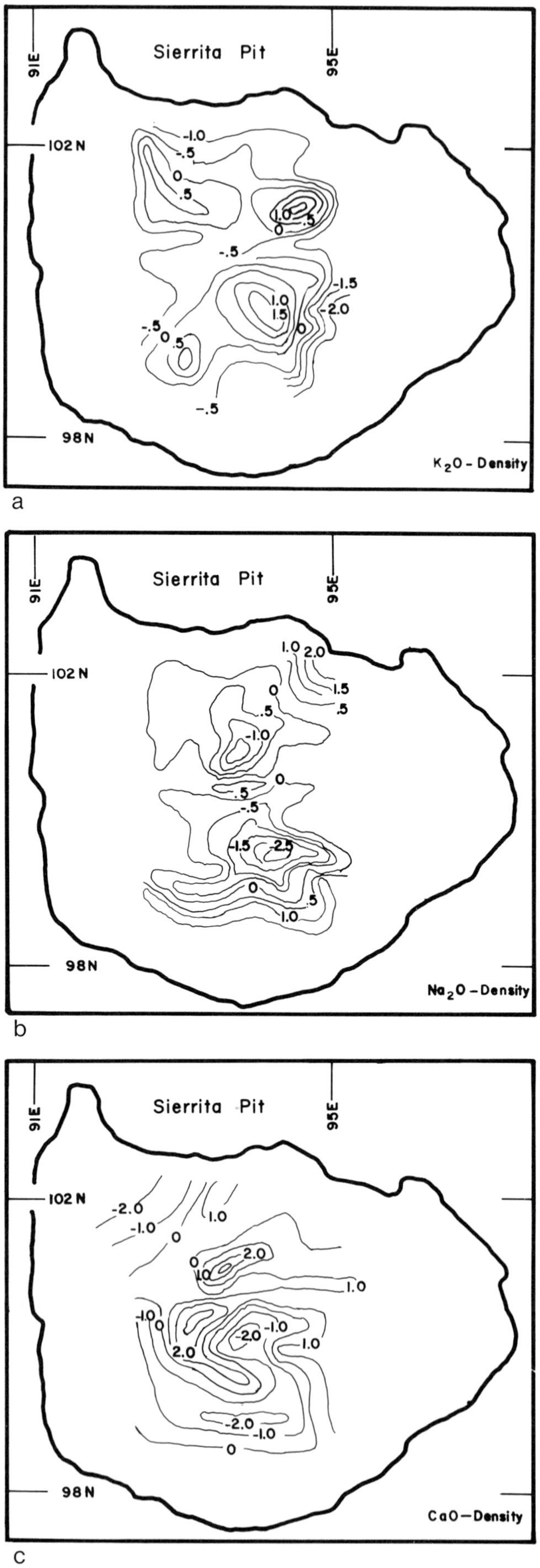

Figure 21.16. Density plots of the Sierrita pit: *a,* density of K_20; *b,* density of Na_20; *c,* density of Ca0. Modified after Hillman (1972).

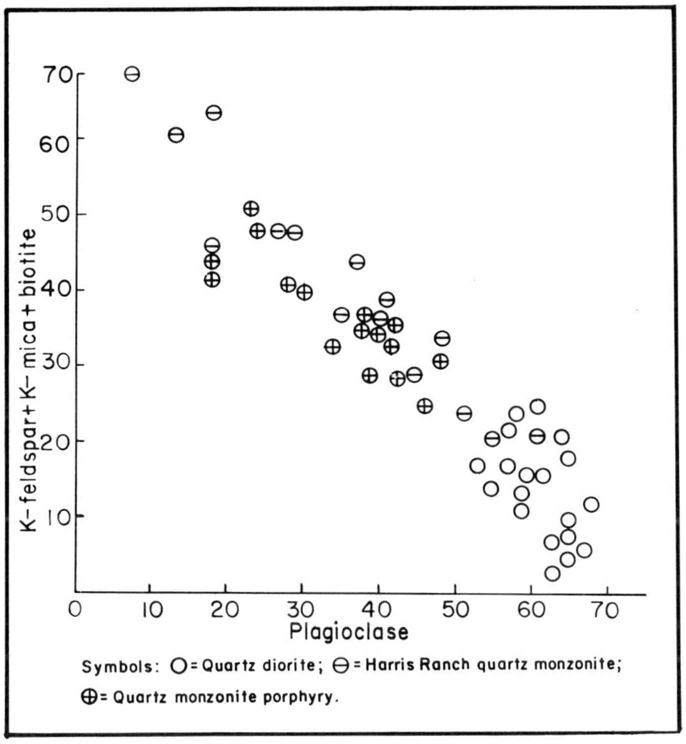

Figure 21.17. Plot of altered Sierrita rocks in terms of K-feldspar + K-mica + biotite vs. plagioclase. After Hillman (1972).

porphyry ranges from 183 ppm in low K rock (4.40%) to 262 ppm in higher K rock (5.24%). Ca is depleted most rapidly from light-colored rocks overall, whereas Sr is removed preferentially from quartz diorite (Smith; 1975). Ba and Pb correlate positively with potassic alteration in quartz diorite. For a group of Esperanza quartz diorite samples collected progressively closer to the quartz diorite–quartz monzonite porphyry contact, Smith notes a general increase in overall alteration intensity and a correlative decrease in Fe, Mg, and Mn. According to Hillman (1972), MgO distribution in Sierrita quartz diorite is a result of redistribution of the component within the diorite rather than of its introduction from an outside source.

Phyllic alteration enriches quartz monzonite porphyry in H_2O and Si and removes Mn, Ti, and Mg. Al is decreased slightly. Phyllic alteration in quartz diorite is characterized by Be, Pb, Cu, S, and H_2O deposition and Cl, Sr, Fe^{+3} and Ca depletion (Laine, 1974).

Beane (1974) has noted that alteration of biotite to chlorite in quartz diorite tends to liberate Mg and fix Fe. This appears to occur for biotite altering to chlorite also in quartz monzonite porphyry (Table 21.10, Analyses 2 and 3). Alteration biotite is widespread, as indicated by thin section studies (Dewhurst, 1977; Smith, 1975) and field work which have identified similarities in color and texture shared by both groundmass and vein biotite. Beane (1974) has reported that environments producing igneous biotite and alteration biotite are geochemically distinct: the molecular ratios of Mg : Fe in igneous biotites is usually <1.0, while in alteration biotites the ratios are >1.5.

It is believed the igneous biotite at the Sierrita-Esperanza deposit widely altered to phlogopitic biotite under temperatures thought to be transitional between magmatic and hydrothermal conditions. A review of biotite chemical analyses (Table 7, Analyses 1 and 2) from the western part of Esperanza pit shows that both biotite samples are actually phlogopites in which the Mg:Fe ratio is greater than 2:1. Such an alteration environment is thought to be characterized by high fS_2 and low fO_2 with Fe^{+3}:Fe^{+2} less than 1:3 (Beane, 1974).

TABLE 21.10
Biotite and Chlorite Analyses of Esperanza Quartz Monzonite Porphyry (In Percent)

Components	Analysis #1 Biotite With Rutile Clots and Needles	Analysis #2 "Fresh" Biotite	Analysis #3 Chlorite Pseudomorphs After Biotite
SiO_2	38.91	40.40	28.80
Al_2O_3	16.64	16.92	20.09
TiO_2	1.85	2.11	—
MgO	20.25	19.51	23.94
FeO	5.70	6.19	14.34
Na_2O	0.24	0.27	—
K_2O	9.86	10.19	—

Source: From Smith's (1975) analyses of Sample 3760–6.

REVIEW OF FLUID INCLUSION STUDIES

The following discussion is based on findings of other workers in this field (Wheeler, 1971; Denis, 1974; Smith, 1975). From study of such fluid inclusion research, some generalizations about the Sierrita system can be suggested. Early Sierrita fluids contained little copper. Denis (1974) found that chalcopyrite in the inclusions rarely exceeded 250 ppm, quite a low number in comparison with two other deposits, Butte and Sar Chesmeh (Iran), which he also discussed. He analyzed fluid inclusions of several types for dissolved Na^+, K^+, Ca^{++}, Mg^{++} Cl^-, and $SO_4^=$ in the aqueous phase. It was found that the solutions were essentially sodium and chloride rich, with potassium always present, but in amounts much weaker than sodium. The other ions tested (Ca^+, Mg^{++}, $SO_4^=$ showed little prominence.

Preece (1979) has studied fluid inclusions in the two older intrusions at Sierrita—the biotite quartz diorite and the Harris Ranch Quartz Monzonite. He has found that early alteration in these rocks was developed from two chemically distinct fluids that ranged in temperature from 300°C to 430°C and differed in salinities. "The earliest veining observed was associated with hypersaline brines (approximately 12 molal NaCl equivalent), which was followed by an initially hotter, locally boiling 2 molal NaCl equivalent solution" (Preece, 1979, p. ix). The 2 molal NaCl equivalent solution boiled in the range 410–440°C suggesting a pressure of about 330 bars. Preece (1979) concluded that most mineralization in the biotite quartz diorite and Harris Ranch Quartz Monzonite was deposited by the low salinity fluid, at 320°C to 370°C.

According to Smith (1975) and Wheeler (1974) several generalizations can be made regarding the fluid inclusions observed at Sierrita. Most inclusions have been observed in quartz, and inclusions in quartz-orthoclase veins are abundunt. Quartz within albite-quartz veinlets contains inclusions which may possess slightly larger vapor phases than observed in other veinlets. Quartz from quartz-sericite-pyrite veinlets contains very small, 1- to 2-phase inclusions; most samples do not reveal a fluid phase within quartz-sericite-pyrite vein material. Inclusions are normally 1 to 10 microns, but can be up to 30 microns wide in unusual specimens; fluid inclusions in Harris Ranch Quartz Monzonite and biotite quartz diorite are commonly 10 to 25 microns.

Aqueous inclusions with two fluid phases, according to Denis (1974), are characterized at Sierrita by an unsaturated liquid phase and a vapor phase that occupies generally only 5 to 10 percent of the total volume of the inclusion. This type comprises about 90 percent of those studied. Studies of these inclusions indicate that temperatures of fluids range from 120°C to 420°C.

Aqueous inclusions with several fluid and solid phases (multiphased) comprise about 5 percent of the group observed by Denis (1974). These are characterized by a vapor phase representing 5 to 10 percent of the total volume. Smith (1975) has reported that this vapor phase comprises 15 to 25 percent of this multiphased group. Also noted by Denis (1974) was a supersaturated liquid phase and one or several solid phases (daughter minerals)—chiefly halite and hematite, with occasional chalcopyrite; according to Smith (1975), these minerals can also include (rarely) anhydrite and sylvite. Preece and Beane (in press) have noted that the vapor bubble observed in this type occupied 10 to 40 percent of the inclusion volume.

Rarely observed were CO_2 inclusions, characterized by three fluid phases, composed of CO_2 gas, CO_2 liquid, and an aqueous phase unsaturated in salts.

ENGINEERING GEOLOGY

In addition to addressing problems related to ore genesis and deposition, geologic studies at Sierrita-Esperanza have been directed at a number of problems related to engineering and mine operations. Among the more important of these are slope stability and rock comminution.

Slope Stability

The excavation at the Sierrita pit was down to the 2,900-ft. elevation (a depth of approximately 1,400 ft. below the pre-mine surface) in mid-1981; Esperanza pit was down to the 3,400-ft. elevation (a depth of approximately 900 ft. below the pre-mine surface). The projected ultimate depth of the combined Sierrita-Esperanza complex as of June, 1981, was approximately 2,300 ft. below the pre-mine surface, to the 2,000-ft. elevation. Consequently, pit slope angles had to be designed to minimize the stripping ratio while at the same time promoting safe mining conditions.

The Sierrita-Esperanza mines had 9 major areas of pit slope instability in 1981 (Fig. 21.18). These slope failures were caused by a combination of factors, predominantly by the removal of lateral confinement (daylighting) at the toe of

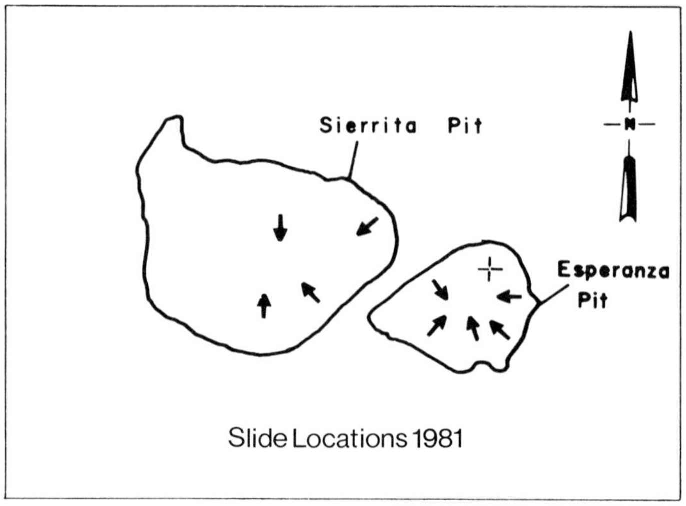

Figure 21.18. Locations of major slides at the Sierrita and Esperanza pits in 1981.

slopes in structurally adverse and lithologically incompetent areas. Renewed slope movement is often triggered by heavy rainfall.

Rock failure at Sierrita-Esperanza occurs in step failure, in translational, wedge, and pseudo-rotational modes, and as ravelling. The vectors of pitwall movement have been established (as generalized on Fig. 21.18). Rates of failure have been recorded by extensometers and pit monitors, as well as by other methods. Features of certain failures have been mapped in detail. These include tension cracks, toe heave, zones of mass movement, fracture densities, types of fracture fillings, and extent of alteration. Diamond drill logs have been utilized to determine the nature of the subsurface in critical areas. In particular, rock quality and structural data have been examined to help identify incompetent zones. Special attention has been given to identifying the extent of gypsum, chlorite, molybdenite, sericite, and clay fracture coatings because of their low shear resistance in water-impregnated fracture systems.

Rock Comminution at Sierrita

The various rock and alteration types at the mines have produced some special problems in comminution. The crushing index (W_i) for ore at Sierrita is high compared to average test values for similar materials. For example, an average W_i value for diorite is 19.4; for granite, 14.4 (F. C. Bond, 1960, personal communication to Duval Corporation). Undifferentiated Sierrita ore from January 16, 1976, has a W_i of 22.8 (R. N. Woody, 1976–1977, personal communications). Equipment parts that come into contact with abrasive rock material have, since the beginning of mine operations, been observed to wear out exceptionally fast (R. N. Woody, 1975–1977, personal communications).

As noted in a paper by Dirks (1975, ms.), "ore type affects total crusher production in the amount of fines removed before secondary crushing. Uneven feed distribution to the tertiary crushers results in power draft fluctuations, cyclic mechanical stresses and uneven concave wear." Sierrita ore is composed of two general types: quartz diorite and quartz monzonite (including Harris Ranch and Ruby Star).

Rocks representative of these two types are contrasted in the following outlines to highlight the major lithologic variations which control comminution, particularly in the ore shell–crackle zone.

Compared to quartz monzonite, quartz diorite in the ore shell–crackle zone has: (1) less degenerative alteration of groundmass, fewer broken zones, and less jointing; (2) greater compositional regularity; (3) greater evenness in groundmass grain size; and (4) intergranular bonds of more uniform strength.

In contrast to the quartz diorite, Harris Ranch Quartz Monzonite in the ore shell is characterized by: (1) more breakdown of rock, due to groundmass sericite, chlorite, clay, etc.; numerous intensely altered fault zones; and a habit of liberating abundant quartz, and orthoclase grains when crushed; (2) considerable compositional variation possible from one area to another; (3) wide variation in relative grain sizes and dimensions; and (4) less regular lines of weakness as influenced by the above factors.

Conditions in quartz diorite lead to: (1) coarser, blockier muck; (2) relative uniformity of feed size to crusher; (3) regularity of the various crushed quartz diorite product sizes; and (4) greater crushing and milling work requirements for rock particles after easy flaw structures have been exploited.

On the other hand, physical properties of the Harris Ranch Quartz Monzonite result in: (1) finer, more abrasive muck, a source of unusual wear on shovels; (2) irregular feed textures and fragment sizes, abundant fines commonly mixed with less altered, competent blocky muck; (3) wide variation in the various product sizes, due to wide variation in feed size and hardness; and (4) diverse milling problems caused by abundance of platy minerals.

CONTRASTING AND PERIPHERAL FEATURES OF THE SIERRITA-ESPERANZA DEPOSIT

Despite many similarities and the closeness of the two operations, Sierrita and Esperanza present numerous contrasts, which show notable differences in magmatic history and in the development of ore zones, alteration, and other features. At Sierrita, the major host rocks are intrusions; at Esperanza the major hosts are both intrusions and extrusive volcanic rocks. At Sierrita the intrusive rock associated with mineralization is a porphyry; at Esperanza the texture of this intrusive phase ranges from porphyry-textured to porphyritic. Hybridized rocks are restricted to limited contact zones of intrusive brecciation and mixed lithologies at Sierrita, whereas at Esperanza, hybrid zones are more extensive and characterized by major zones of replacement and flooding.

A late stage of volatile fluids is strongly evident at Esperanza, as shown by pegmatitic textures, zones of orthoclase megacrysts, quartz pods, silicified shatter zones, and K^+- and H_2O-enriched rock. These types of features are generally absent from Sierrita. Both Cu and Mo are important at Sierrita and Esperanza. A well-developed chalcocite blanket was associated with Esperanza and with areas marginal to that pit, while most of the Sierrita pit did not have a well-developed supergene horizon. Finally, as shown in Table 21.8, at Esperanza there is a greater prevalence of relatively low-angle dips on structures and, generally, a much higher fracture density than at Sierrita.

Knowledge of the nature and distribution of alteration and mineralization is chiefly confined to the economic portions of the system. However, information gained from scattered diamond drill holes encompassing the lateral and vertical pit limits gives a more complete indication as to the nature of the deposit. Certain deep holes have probed mineralization at least 1,500 ft. (450 m) below the ore shell to determine possible irregularities in the distribution of economic mineralization. These drill holes have identified certain features and changes beyond the ore shell laterally and vertically. For example, copper grade typically decreases by 75 percent across a distance of 100 to 150 ft. (30–45 m) from the lower limit of the ore shell (economic cutoff = 0.32 copper equivalent). Molybdenite grade typically decreases 50 to 90 percent across this same distance, but values may be erratic. Disseminated molybdenite is rare at depth and in the ore shell. Both Cu and Mo are present in quartz monzonite porphyry at the maximum depths drilled (i.e., elevations of 345 ft. [105 m] below sea level). Grades there average 0.05 Cu and 0.005 Mo. Pyrite content is typically 5 to 6 percent or less but ranges up to 10 percent south, west, and east of Esperanza.

Sulfide mineralization in the ore shell is predominantly associated with quartz as fracture fillings and coatings. However, below the ore shell, dissemination is locally the dominant mode of deposition. The predominant vein type alteration in the orebody is potassic, whereas groundmass alteration is fresh to weakly sericitic. These alteration types accompany mineralization to the maximum depths drilled. Rock texture within individual quartz monzonite porphyry facies remains uniform with increasing depth, but it may change abruptly to associated textural varieties. However, the trend does not consistently change to coarser- or finer-grained phases. Rock competency increases with depth as the result of decreased fracture density and lack of soft, hydrous alteration minerals in the groundmass.

The Sierrita deposit exhibits both hood and root zone characteristics. Hood zone characteristics include the presence of a porphyritic mineralizing intrusion (Ruby Star Quartz Monzonite Porphyry), which extends to depth at least 4,000 ft. below the pre-mine topography. A breccia is present and well developed near the pre-mine surface. The size of the ore zone increases with depth and expands laterally (see Fig. 21.11). Propylitic alteration on the surface partially overlies potassic alteration at depth. In addition, large galena-sphalerite veins are most strongly developed marginal to the higher-grade ore shell. Very fine grained background Pb (roughly 0.01%) is found in ore and waste zones at depth.

EPIZONAL AND MESOZONAL FEATURES OF THE SIERRITA-ESPERANZA DEPOSIT

The Sierrita-Esperanza deposit manifests both epizonal (0–4 miles [0–6.4 km]) and mesozonal (4–8 miles [6.4–12.9 km]) characteristics. The system is developed substantially in a composite intrusion, the Ruby Star Granodiorite and Quartz Monzonite Porphyry with associated facies. The contact zones of the Ruby Star Quartz Monzonite Porphyry show both chilled and phaneritic textures. Contacts are not always sharp but range from sharp welded borders separating distinct bodies to diffuse contacts of variable widths. Genetically related volcanic rocks may have been eroded off or may include the Demetrie Volcanics, but no clear-cut correlation has been perceived between the Ruby Star units and volcanic rocks. Weak contact effects are exhibited by contact-related alteration, with a low-grade alteration aureole widespread but no evidence of regional metamorphism in the mine area; however, Drewes (1973, p. 2–3) uses the terms "possibly tectonically metamorphosed" and "thermal metamorphism" to describe the effects associated with structural and intrusive activity in the area. Late-stage dikes are present, composed of quartz latite porphyry and aplite. Small patches of pegmatitic material are locally present in upper levels of the Sierrita-Esperanza system. Planar foliation is generally most common on the dike margins and in breccia matrix.

At the Sierrita and Esperanza deposit, contacts are variable; assimilation is widespread, reflecting disintegration of stoped blocks and xenoliths, intrusion brecciation, and biotite enrichment. The affected contacts include Harris Ranch Quartz Monzonite–Ox Frame Andesite, Ruby Star Quartz Monzonite Porphyry–quartz diorite, and Ruby Star Quartz Monzonite Porphyry–quartz latite porphyry. The Ruby Star units comprise a composite intrusion in which foliation is generally not well developed; regional green-schist metamorphism is not present. No genetically related volcanic rocks have been observed, but a well-developed hydrothermal aureole does occur around the Ruby Star Quartz Monzonite Porphyry. Some dikes occur adjacent to plutons, notably biotite quartz diorite and quartz latite porphyry dikes. Aplites and lesser pegmatites commonly occur in border zones, particularly those marginal to the Ruby Star Quartz Monzonite Porphyry. Miarolitic cavities are absent.

ACKNOWLEDGMENTS

The authors would like to thank Verl Smith, James Savely, Roger Laine, Barry Hillman, Michel Denis, John Cooper, Spencer Titley, Richard Mauger, Joanna Dewhurst, and Richard Beane, Richard Preece, and Beth Abrams for their valuable research and assistance, which enlarged the scope of this chapter.

Special thanks go to Robert A. Metz for his ideas regarding various aspects of the deposit and for his critical review of the manuscript. Thanks are also given to the previous members of the Sierrita and Esperanza geology staff for their accumulated data and ideas, which have formed the basis for much of the material presented in this report; in particular, we wish to thank D. W. Lynch, R. A. Metz, C. D. Iles, C. A. Oakley, A. H. James, F. W. Mack, E. H. Lewis, H. A. Schmitt, and B. L. Wilhelm. Other staff members including J. C. Morgan, S. C. Hintze, and J. J. Regan have also aided this effort. R. K. Riebel is acknowledged for her contribution to the final typing of the manuscript.

The authors express their appreciation to Harry L. Shively, General Manager, Duval Corporation; Dr. John I. Sharpe, Manager, Duval Exploration; Ken L. Lamb, Manager of Mining, Duval Corporation; and to Duval Corporation for permission to prepare and publish this study.

REFERENCES CITED

Anderson, C. A., and Kupfer, D. H., 1944, Report of the properties of the Amargosa Molybdenum and Copper Corporation, Pima County, Arizona: U.S. Geol. Survey Strategic Minerals Inventory.

Beane, R. E., 1974, Biotite stability in the porphyry copper environment: Econ. Geol., v. 69, p. 241–256.

Cooper, J. R., 1960, Some geologic features of the Pima mining district, Pima County, Arizona: U.S. Geol. Survey Bull. 1112-C, 103 p.

———, 1971, Mesozoic stratigraphy of the Sierrita Mountains, Pima County, Arizona: U.S. Geol. Survey Prof. Paper 658-D, 42 p.

———, 1973, Geologic map of the Twin Buttes Quadrangle, southwest of Tucson, Arizona: U.S. Geol. Survey Misc. Geol. Inv. Map I-745.

Creasey, S. C., and Kistler, R. W., 1962, Age of some copper-bearing porphyries and igneous rocks in southeastern Arizona: U.S. Geol. Survey Prof. Paper 450-D, p. D1–D5.

Damon, P. E., Compiler, 1965, Correlation and chronology of ore deposits and volcanic rocks: Univ. Ariz. Geochronology Lab., Ann. Prog. Rept., COO-689-50.

———, 1966, Correlation and chronology of ore deposits and volcanic rocks: Univ. Ariz. Geochronology Lab., Ann. Prog. Rept., COO-689-50.

Denis, Michel, 1974, Alterations et Fluides Associés dans le Porphyre Cuprifère de Sierrita (Arizona, Etats-Unis): Unpub. Ph.D. Diss., Univ. Nancy (France), 146 p.

Dewhurst, Joanna, 1977, Supplemental petrographic report on Sierrita-Esperanza samples: Unpub. report to Duval Corp.

Dirks, M. S., 1975, Sierrita crushing plant: Ariz. Sec. AIME, Spring Meeting.

Drewes, Harald, 1973, Structural geology of the Sierrita Mountains: Abstract of talk presented at AIME symposium on Sierrita Mountains, Apr. 13.

Haynes, F. M., 1980, The evolution of fracture-related permeability within the Ruby Star Granodiorite, Sierrita porphyry copper deposit, Pima County, Arizona: Unpub. M.S. Thesis, 48 p.

Hillman, B. A., 1972, Research in hydrothermal activity as related to ore deposition at the Sierrita porphyry copper deposits, Arizona: Unpub. M.S. Thesis, Univ. Cincinnati, 69 p.

Laine, R. P., 1973, Sierrita open-pit petrography progress report: Unpub. report to Duval Sierrita Corp.

———, 1974, Geological-geochemical relationships between porphyry copper and porphyry molybdenum ore deposits: Unpub. Ph.D. Diss., Univ. Ariz., 326 p.

Lewis, E. H., 1959, Résumé of the geology of the Esperanza mine: Unpub. report to Duval Corp.

Lootens, D. J., 1965, Structure and petrography of the east side of the Sierrita Mountains, Pima County, Arizona: Unpub. Ph.D. Diss., Univ. Ariz., 199 p.

———, 1966, Geological and structural environment of the Sierrita Mountains, Pima County, Arizona: Ariz. Geol. Soc. Digest VIII, p. 33–56.

Lovering, T. G.; Cooper, J. R.; Drewes. Harald; and Cone, G. C., 1970, Copper in biotite from igneous rocks in southern Arizona as an ore indicator: U.S. Geol. Survey Prof. Paper 700-B, p. B1–B8.

Lutton, R. J., 1958, Some structural features in southern Arizona: Unpub. M.S. Thesis, Univ. Ariz., 138 p.

———, 1961. A lensoidal rhyolite near Twin Buttes, Arizona: Ariz. Geol. Soc. Digest IV, p. 43–49.

Lynch, D. W., 1966, The economic geology of the Esperanza mine and vicinity, *in* Titley, S. R., and Hicks, C. L., eds., Geology of the Porphyry Copper Deposits, Southwestern North America: Tucson, Univ. Ariz. Press, p. 267–280.

———, 1967, The geology of the Esperanza mine and vicinity, Pima County, Arizona: Unpub. M.S. Thesis, Univ. Ariz., 61 p.

Mauger, R. L., 1966, A petrographic and geochemical study of Silver Bell and Pima mining districts, Pima County, Arizona: Unpub. Ph.D. Diss., Univ. Ariz. 140 p.

Metz, R. A., 1969, General geology of the Sierrita orebody: Unpub. report to Duval Sierrita Corp.

Preece, R. K. III, 1979, Paragenesis, geochemistry, and temperatures of formation of alteration assemblages at the Sierrita Deposit, Pima County, Arizona: Unpub. M.S. Thesis, Univ. Ariz., 106 p.

Preece, R. K. III, and Beane, R. E., in press, Contrasting evolutions of hydrothermal alteration in quartz monzonite and quartz diorite at the Sierrita porphyry copper deposit, Arizona: Econ. Geol., v. 76.

Rehrig, W. A., and Heidrick T. L., 1972, Regional fracturing in Laramide stocks of Arizona and its relationship to porphyry copper mineralization: Econ. Geol., v. 67, p. 198–213.

———, 1976, Regional tectonic stress during the Laramide and late Tertiary intrusive periods, Basin and Range province, Arizona: Ariz. Geol. Soc. Digest X, p. 205–228.

Smith, V. L., 1975, Hypogene alteration at the Esperanza mine, Pima County, Arizona: Unpub. M.S. Thesis., Univ. Ariz. 161 p.

Titley, S. R., 1976, Evidence for a Mesozoic linear tectonic pattern in southeastern Arizona: Ariz. Geol. Soc. Digest X, p. 71–101.

Toombs, H. B., 1955, Cross sections of Esperanza leached cap: Unpub. Maps, Duval Corp.

Wheeler, D. P., 1971, Brief review of fluid inclusions in some Sierrita rocks: Umont Mining Company Report.

22

Stratigraphy and Structure of the Mission Copper Deposit

PIMA MINING DISTRICT, PIMA COUNTY, ARIZONA

Louis J. Jansen

The Mission copper deposit is one of five orebodies located in the northeastern part of the Pima district that were originally recognized as distinctly separate orebodies. Results of mining, continued exploration since its discovery in 1954, and information developed from nearby orebodies since that time have revealed that Mission is an ore system contiguous with those of Pima, Palo Verde, and San Xavier South. The San Xavier North orebody to the northwest of Mission remains separate, but it is interpreted as an original part of the whole that was displaced by low-angle faulting.

Data published by Keith and others (1978) indicate that the Mission mine produced 108.9 $\times$ 10^6 tons of ore with calculated grades of 0.62 percent Cu, 0.019 percent Mo, and 0.11 oz./s.t. Ag. Reserves in 1977 were about 135 $\times$ 10^6 tons of 0.73% Cu. Ore tonnages of the contiguous orebodies, Pima and Palo Verde, have been given at about 470 $\times$ 10^6 tons, mined and in reserve (Keith et al., 1978); thus, Mission constitutes a third of the total tonnage of this complex. As a major producer in one of the largest porphyry copper districts in the United States, Mission is an important deposit. Even more importantly in the context of the subject of this volume, Mission is a copper orebody at one end of a depositional spectrum, as its ores were deposited almost entirely in sedimentary rocks, dominated by a carbonate section. Further, Mission and contiguous orebodies are suggested to be klippe, shed from a site to the south following mineralization; thus, geologic studies of this orebody assume major importance in clarifying not only the mineralization history, but also the tectonic history, of this region during the mid-Tertiary.

Since the discovery of the Pima and Mission orebodies in the early 1950s, many geological studies have been carried out in the Pima mining district. Those of particular relevance to Mission orebody geology include regional studies by Cooper (1960, 1973), a description of the orebody as it was known shortly after initiation of mining (Kinnison, 1966), a study of the geology and skarn alteration (Gale, 1965), a study of the geology of the Pima mine (Himes, 1973) and a summary of radiometric age dates reported by Shafiqullah and Langlois (1978). As many aspects of area geology and general mine geology have been reported, they will be only briefly mentioned here. The principal focus of this chapter is a summary of the nature and geometry of stratigraphy in the Mission mine as it was worked out during the 1970s and an assessment of the resulting stratigraphy in the overall context of mineralization and structural history of the Mission orebody.

GENERAL GEOLOGY

The Mission orebody occurs in an overturned sequence of Upper Paleozoic strata which lie in fault contact with subjacent granitic rocks of unknown age. The inverted Paleozoic strata are, in turn, overlain by Mesozoic clastic rocks on an angular unconformity which progressively cuts across the section to the east. The sedimentary sequence has been deformed into broad, gentle, northwest-trending folds. In the mine area, one mass of quartz monzonite porphyry occurs as a sill-like intrusion into the sedimentary rocks near the western limits of the orebody. Radiometric age dates of about 58 m.y. (Shafiqullah and Langlois, 1978) indicate a Laramide age for the quartz monzonite from samples at the San Xavier North mine (King, 1981)—the quartz monzonite interpreted as correlative with that in the Mission Mine.

Mineralization in the Mission orebody occurs as disseminated and veinlet controlled sulfides in a wide variety of calc-silicate altered sedimentary rock types. Development of the skarn alteration assemblages was controlled by original rock lithologies (Gale, 1965); both hydrous and anhydrous mineral assemblages are present, with the hydrous assemblages commonly occurring as veinlet alteration selvages along fractures cutting older anhydrous skarn. A secondary control of alteration and of copper grade may have been exerted by primary sedimentary structures; this point will be more fully developed in sections of the chapter that follow.

Viewed from the perspective of district geology (Fig. 22.1), the Mission, Pima, Palo Verde Extension (of Mission), and San Xavier North orebodies lie some 6 miles (10 km) north of the Twin Buttes porphyry copper deposit. The orebodies were discovered beneath some 200 ft. (60 m) of alluvium that covered them and remains as cover above much Mesozoic and Paleozoic strata of this part of the district. They are further separated from the Twin Buttes orebody by exposures of the mid-to-late-Tertiary Helmet Fanglomerate (Cooper, 1960), which are about 28.5 m.y. old (Shafiqullah and Langlois, 1978).

The Paleozoic, Mesozoic, and Cenozoic strata of this interval, together with the orebodies within them, are interpreted as lying within a large (ca. 60 mi^2) (155 km^2) allochthonous plate which had its origin to the south; the Twin Buttes orebody is interpreted as the "root" of the Mission and contiguous ore systems (Cooper, 1960, 1971, 1973). Interpreted geology of this interval is shown on the cross sections of Figure 22.1. The allochthonous block, the upper

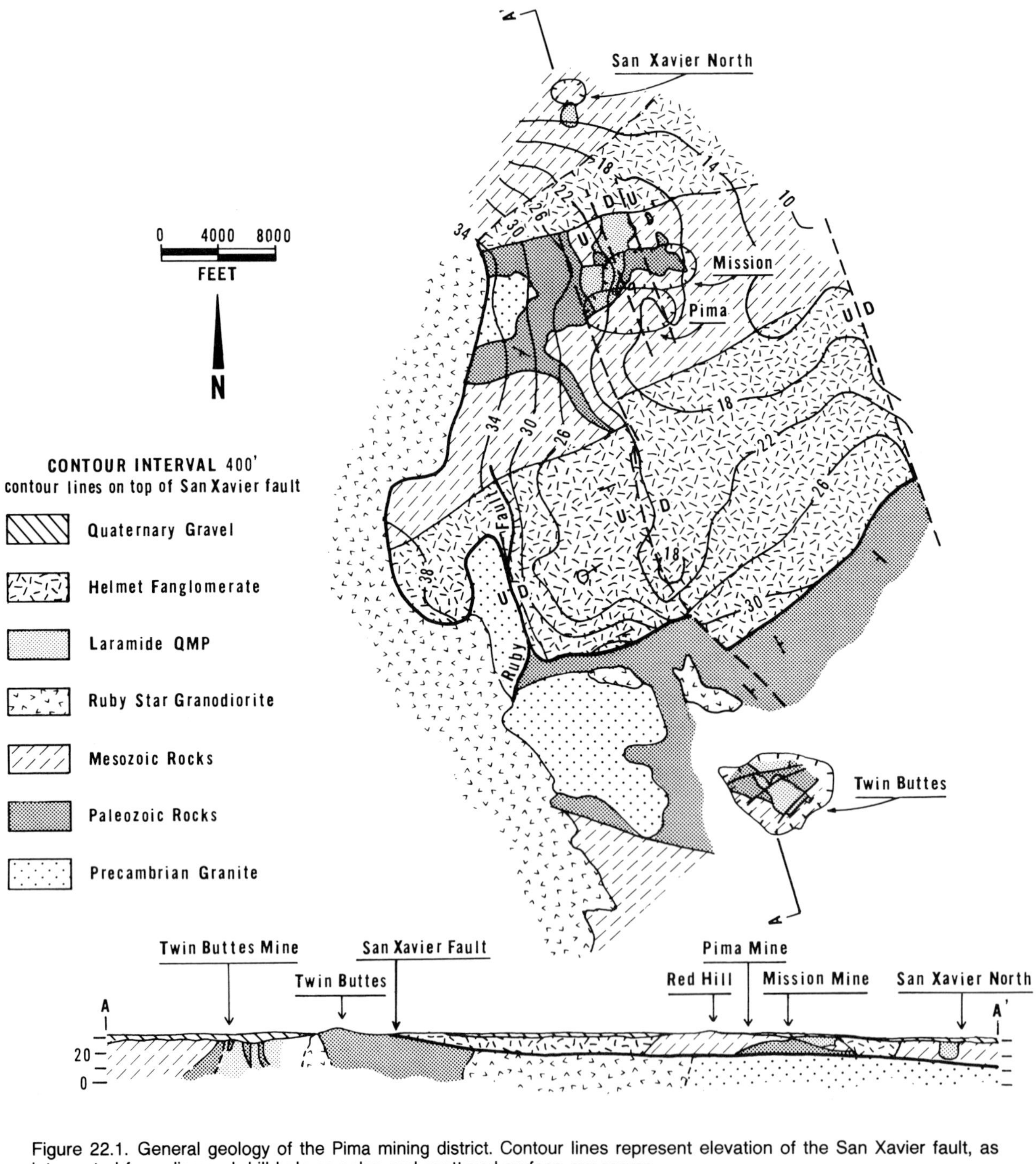

Figure 22.1. General geology of the Pima mining district. Contour lines represent elevation of the San Xavier fault, as interpreted from diamond drill hole samples and scattered surface exposures.

plate of the San Xavier gravity fault, is interpreted from many drill hole samples; interpreted contours of its lower surface are shown in Figure 22.1. This surface is a major, low angle, undulating feature on the northeastern pediment of the Sierrita Mountains. It separates mineralized rock of the upper plate from unmineralized rock in the subjacent rocks. As presently exposed and interpreted, the upper plate of the fault ranges in thickness from a few tens of feet up to 2,000 ft. (ca. 600 m) and is composed of rocks ranging in age from Precambrian to the late Tertiary. Interpretations drawn from certain features of the stratigraphy and structural geology in this upper plate (further considered below) lend credence to the interpretation of the northward direction of movement and the displacement of 6.2 miles (10 km) suggested by Cooper (1960).

MISSION MINE STRATIGRAPHY

The Mission deposit occurs in a sequence of Permian sedimentary rocks overlain by Mesozoic clastic rocks (Fig. 22.2). In the central and western parts of the deposit, 3 Permian formations are present but the Paleozoic-Mesozoic unconformity has cut away all but 1 in the eastern part of the orebody. Mesozoic clastic rocks are present as sub-horizontal strata in depositional contact with the overturned Paleozoic sequence and compose the upper stratigraphic unit in the mine sequence. All of the units show the effects of hydrothermal activity and mineralization. The central part of the Mission orebody occupies a structural trough which is characterized by the presence of the 3 Permian formations (from oldest to youngest: the Epitaph Dolomite, the Scherrer Formation, and the Concha Limestone).

Epitaph Dolomite

Gilluly and others (1954) described and defined the Epitaph Dolomite from exposures in central Cochise County, Arizona. The 750 ft.-section (ca. 250 m) present in the type locality is thinned to about 250 ft. (ca. 80 m) in the mine sequence. Five mappable units are recognizable in the Mission deposit, but they bear only scant resemblance to the units in the type section, owing to pronounced lateral variations in the composition of the formation in this part of Arizona (Butler, 1971). The principal basis of correlation is the presence, within the unit at Mission, of beds of anhydrite, which are unique in this part of the section to the Epitaph Dolomite.

At Mission the oldest (topographically highest) unit is limestone, varying from 35 to 70 ft. (ca. 10–22 m) thick, which is commonly altered to brown garnet tactite. The basal unit is overlain by about 70 ft. (22 m) of light to dark green siltstone and marl. Limestone beds within this unit are locally altered to a distinctive light brown garnet tactite. The middle unit consists of 15 to 35 ft. (5–12 m) of limestone, altered to light brown garnet tactite. The next higher unit, probably originally a mixed clastic and carbonate unit, consists of 20 to 30 ft. (6–10 m) of a green-brown colored, epidote-garnet tactite, and the uppermost unit consists of 40 to 60 ft. (13–20 m) of anhydrite. These characteristics, of both the altered

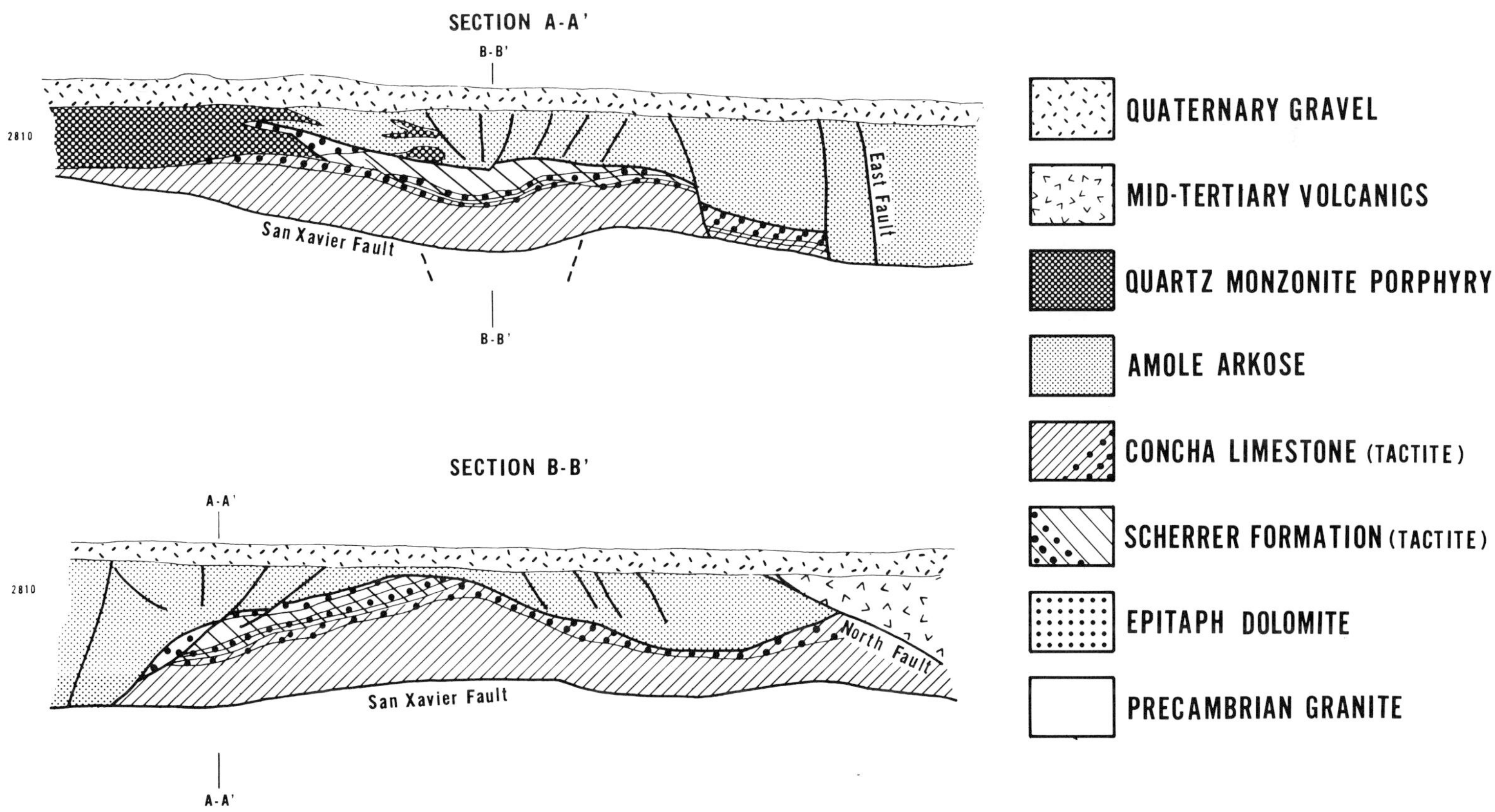

Figure 22.2. Geologic cross sections through the Mission mine and vicinity

facies and the unaltered facies of the unit, are diagnostic of the Epitaph Dolomite in the mine area. Drill hole intercepts, as well as bench face exposures, reveal either the entire sequence or recognizable parts of it which allow the interpretations made here.

Scherrer Formation

The Scherrer Formation has been described and defined in the Gunnison Hills by Gilluly and others (1954). In most exposures, the Formation is characterized by 4 alternating units of sandstone and carbonates, but the thickness of the type section is considerably thinned in the Mission mine and in other exposures west of the type locality. The 680 ft. (210 m) of strata at the type locality consist of an upper sandstone overlying gray limestone. These overlie a 270-ft. (90 m) sequence of monotonous sandstone and a basal unit of bright red sandstone. Nearer to the Pima district, Jansen (1973) recognized only a threefold division of the section in the Tucson Mountains. The members consisted of a lower, light-colored orthoquartzite, 100 ft. (30 m) thick; a middle unit of gray limestone, 10 to 35 ft. (3–12 m) thick; and an upper, gray to brown orthoquartzite, also 10 to 35 ft. (3–12 m) thick.

Three members of the Scherrer Formation are present in the central part of the Mission deposit where they are overturned. The lower quartzite member (topographically highest) is a clean, light-colored quartzite, ranging up to 160 ft. (ca. 50 m) thick. Its contact with the Epitaph Dolomite is commonly faulted. However, numerous mapped exposures in the east-central part of the mine show the stratigraphic contact. The intermediate unit, which was probably a dolomite correlative with the silty dolomite of McClymonds (1957) in the Waterman Mountains and the intermediate limestone of the Tucson Mountain Section (Jansen, 1973), is a fine-grained, compact, light to dark green diopside tactite. It ranges from 30? to 50 ft. (10?–16 m) thick. The upper unit (topographically lowest) lies in conformable contact with the middle dolomite member and consists of 30 to 50 ft. (10–16 m) of gray to brown quartzite. The Scherrer Formation ranges from 240 to 260 ft. (ca. 80 m) thick in the Mission deposit and correlates with high certainty with nearby sections. The consistent stratigraphy of the three members and the presence of the Epitaph Dolomite provide a strong basis for the interpretation of stratigraphic inverson.

Concha Limestone

The youngest Permian unit present in the Mission mine, the Concha Limestone, was named from type localities in Cochise County (Gilluly et al., 1954). In measured sections of southeastern Arizona, the formation is dominated by various cherty, dark-gray, finely crystalline limestone units and its thickness—500 to 550 ft. (ca. 165 m)—is relatively constant. This figure is about that measured for sections in the Mission mine. Although both the Epitaph and Scherrer units were affected by Mesozoic erosion and thinned in the mine, the Concha Limestone was relatively unaffected because of its topographically lower position and maintained a uniform thickness. The lower part of the section (topographically highest and in contact with the Scherrer Formation) is a garnet tactite ranging from 80 to 160 ft. (26–50 m) thick, which is characterized by variations in garnet compositions and which contains local zones of hematite that Gale (1956) considers hypogene. The upper part of the formation is thick-bedded marble with zones of wollastonite, which is probably correlative with chert-bearing strata in the original limestone.

Mesozoic Rocks

Triassic and Cretaceous clastic rocks (Cooper, 1971) lie on the overturned Permian section above an angular unconformity. In the Pima mine, contiguous to the Southwest, Himes (1973) described rocks belonging to the Rodolfo Formation described by Cooper (1971) and proposed that rocks there correlated with Cooper's middle siltstone member of that Formation. The siltstones extend to the northeast into the Mission deposit, where they attain a thickness of up to 1,000 ft. (320 m). The rocks of this unit present in the Mission mine comprise fine-grained, compact, siliceous argillites, arkose, and local basal pebble conglomerates. At the northern end of the Mission deposit, interbedded sandstones, siltstones, and massive arkose units occur which are tentatively correlated here with the Cretaceous Angelica Arkose of Cooper (1971). In both the Pima and Mission mines, the Rodolfo Formation is an important host to sulfide ores, and in the North San Xavier deposit, the Angelica Arkose was a host to sulfide ores, which were later oxidized (King, 1981).

STRUCTURAL GEOLOGY OF THE MISSION OREBODY

Geologic cross sections (see Fig. 22.2) illustrate the tabular nature of Mission orebody geology and the overall boundaries. These include the post-mineral North fault and the San Xavier fault, as well as the pre-mineral East fault. Figure 22.3 shows the position of the Mission pit with respect

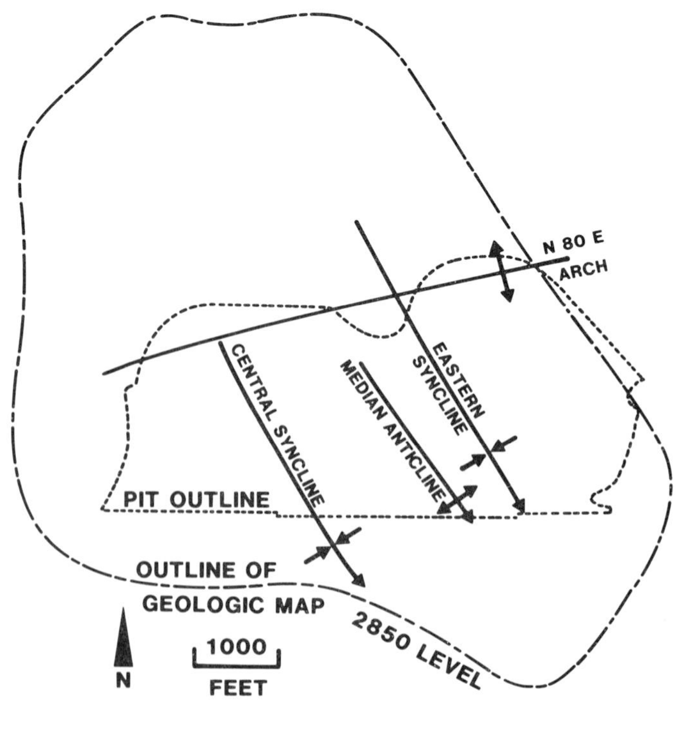

Figure 22.3. Correlation diagram between pit outline at the Mission mine and distribution of geologic data shown in Figures 22.4, 22.5, and 22.6

to the outline of the entire deposit, while the shape and internal structure of separate stratigraphic units in the deposit are detailed in the structural contour maps and ispoach (thickness) maps of Figure 22.4. These maps and cross sections reveal broad northwest- and northeast-striking folds present in the Mesozoic and Paleozoic rocks.

The earliest deformation recorded in the rocks at Mission is the overturning of the Paleozoic section. Precise dating of this event is not possible but the fact that Rodolfo strata lie above an unconformity places the time of deformation early in the Mesozoic or in the very latest Paleozoic. Large errors in the Pb-alpha dates cited, and recognized, by Cooper (1971) as evidence for the age of the Rodolfo Formation allow only a broad bracket of time to assign a youngest age for the event during the Triassic. However, the stratigraphic relationships of the unit with the subjacent Paleozoic are consistent with similar relationships reported elsewhere in the Pima district by Cooper (1971). The overturned Paleozoic strata of the Mission orebody persist in the inverted sequence to the west, where the lower part of the section is exposed on Mineral Hill (Cooper, 1973).

In the Pima mine, the Rodolfo Formation may, at least in part, lie in fault contact with the Paleozoic section along the unconformity (Langlois, 1978). In the Mission mine, the basal unit of the Rodolfo is a mineralized pebble conglomerate, exposed in many places, and in the western part of the mine, there is local strong shearing at that contact. Elsewhere, however, the contact appears to be sedimentary and the evidence for early Mesozoic deformation and erosion is substantial.

Structural events that may have taken place through the middle Mesozoic are not recorded in the rocks at Mission, and the Rodolfo is overlain along a diffuse contact by the Angelica Arkose. There appears to have been erosion of the upper units of the Rodolfo and possibly of substantial amounts of Triassic and Jurassic strata whose presence can only be inferred from the occurrence of these strata elsewhere in the Pima district.

Northwest-trending folds and faults form the dominant pre-mineral structural elements in the Mission mine rocks. The age of much of this deformation is unknown but, because of the influence of these structures on ore grades, there is good evidence for their pre-ore age. Structural contour maps (see Fig. 22.4) show the folding to be continuous through the entire section; therefore, the folds are at least as young as the Angelica Arkose (Lower Cretaceous). The northwest-striking folds have been modified by still younger arching along a N80°E axis, causing the older folds to plunge gently away from the arch. This young arch is of post-ore age and may be either the result of the movement of the upper plate of the San Xavier Fault over a ridge in the basement or the result of still younger block faulting in the basement rocks. The effects of both the pre-ore, northwest-trending folds and the post-ore, northeast-trending fold on stratigraphic thicknesses are shown in Figures 22.2 and 22.4. Three geologic bench maps are shown in Figure 22.5. The 2850-ft. (above sea level) bench map shows the influence of the northwest pre-mineral structures and the east-northeast arch on rock distribution. The two synclines and the median anticlines of northwest trend are clearly revealed, as are the effects of young arching. On the 2650 bench, the northeast arch assumes increasing prominence, with the effects of the northwest folds subdued. On the 2450 bench map the western and eastern synclines and the northeastern arch are prominent.

The occurrence of the Epitaph Dolomite and the Scherrer Formation are restricted to, and thicken toward, the trough of the western syncline, while Mesozoic strata and the Concha Limestone thicken in several locations along the axis of the eastern syncline. It is noteworthy that copper grades show trends parallel to the northwest structural grain. Isograde maps of the individual units recognized in mine mapping are shown on Figure 22.4. The grades may correspond to the strike of the Paleozoic-Mesozoic unconformity, but there is also strong correspondence to the strike of the pre-mineral folds, which strongly suggests ore controls related to both sedimentary structure and lithology.

Post-mineral tectonics included the evolution of the San Xavier fault and related imbricate structures, together with Basin and Range normal faults. Shafiqullah and Langlois (1978) have determined an age of younger than 26 m.y. for the most recent movement along the San Xavier fault, based on the offset of a dated andesite dike in the Pima mine. A similar andesite dike is truncated by the North fault at the northern end of the Mission deposit. The structural contour map of the San Xavier fault shown on Figure 22.1 indicates a low angle structure beneath the northeastern pediment of the Sierrita Mountains. Most of the data used to compile the map were from diamond drill hole records from ASARCO, Inc., and Cyprus Pima Mining Company. Extensive drilling of the upper plate of the fault in the late 1970s yielded a number of intercepts of the top of the lower plate that were used to further detail the surface of the fault.

Two main structural directions are present in this fault system. One is a N45°E-trending trough which plunges gently northeastward; the other is a system of N10°W-striking normal faults. The trough contains the thick continental deposits of Tertiary Helmet Fanglomerate (Cooper, 1960; Weaver, 1965; Jansen, 1978). Surface mapping has revealed several N10°W-striking normal faults which, when overlaid on the San Xavier fault structural contour map, project vertically to steep gradients on the contoured surface of the San Xavier fault; the assumption is made here that these normal faults offset the San Xavier fault at depth. Two such normal faults border a graben which passes beneath the Mission and Pima mines (Section A-A', Fig. 22.2).

Two additional N10°W-striking faults—the Ruby fault and a central, unnamed fault—appear to die out to the north (Fig. 22.1) but show increased displacements along their southern extensions. The removal of the scissor displacement along the southern extension of these faults would change the present northeast dip of the San Xavier fault surface to a gently northward-dipping surface, thereby approximating the interpreted original paleosurface of the San Xavier fault.

It follows implicitly from these interpretations and the data that the Mission mine and contiguous orebodies have been moved northward from an original site of ore formation in the proximity of the Twin Buttes orebody. The presence of a "basement fault" was noted in the first reports of Mission geology (Richard and Courtright, 1959). The interpretation

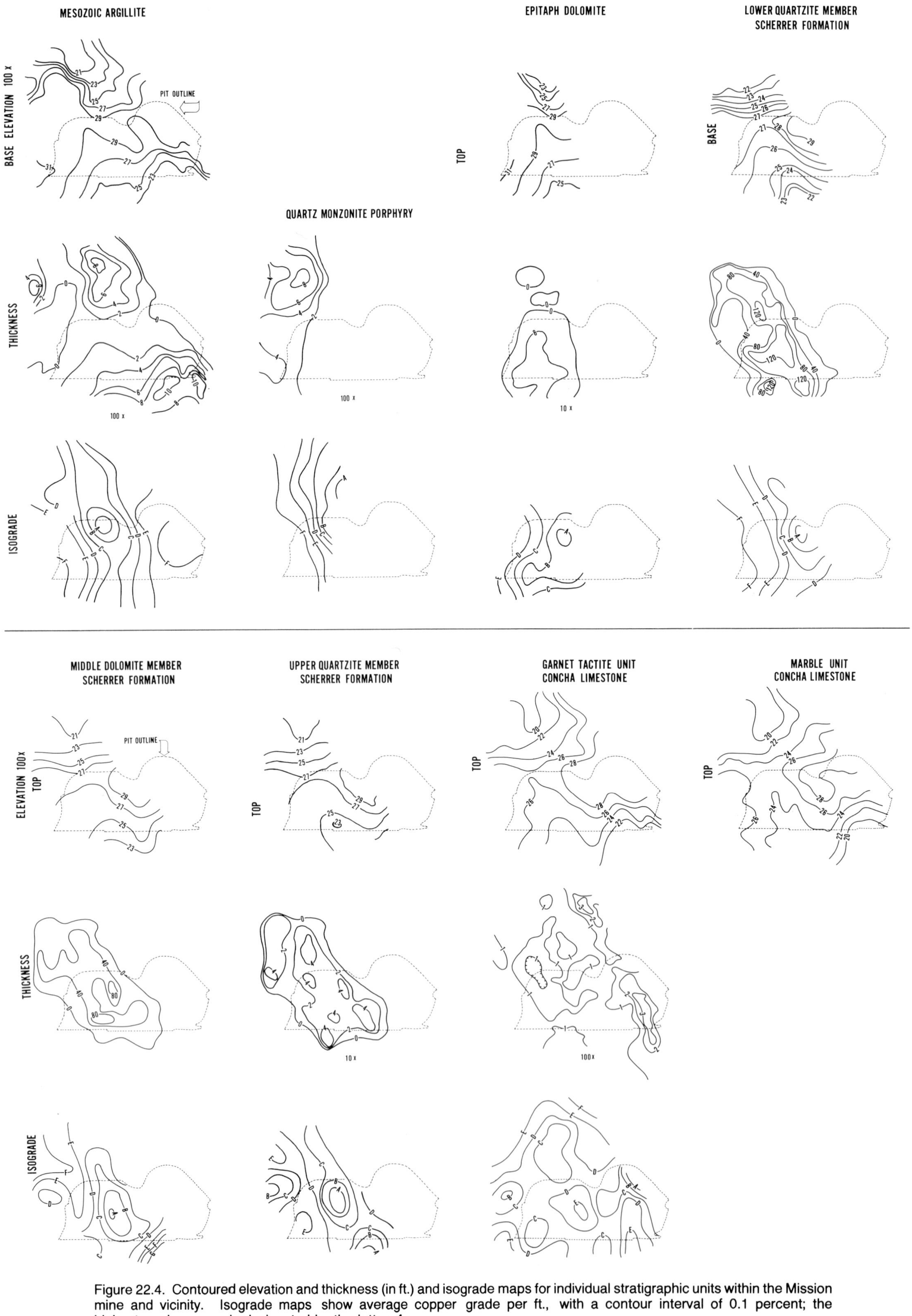

Figure 22.4. Contoured elevation and thickness (in ft.) and isograde maps for individual stratigraphic units within the Mission mine and vicinity. Isograde maps show average copper grade per ft., with a contour interval of 0.1 percent; the highest-grade copper is designated by the letter *A*.

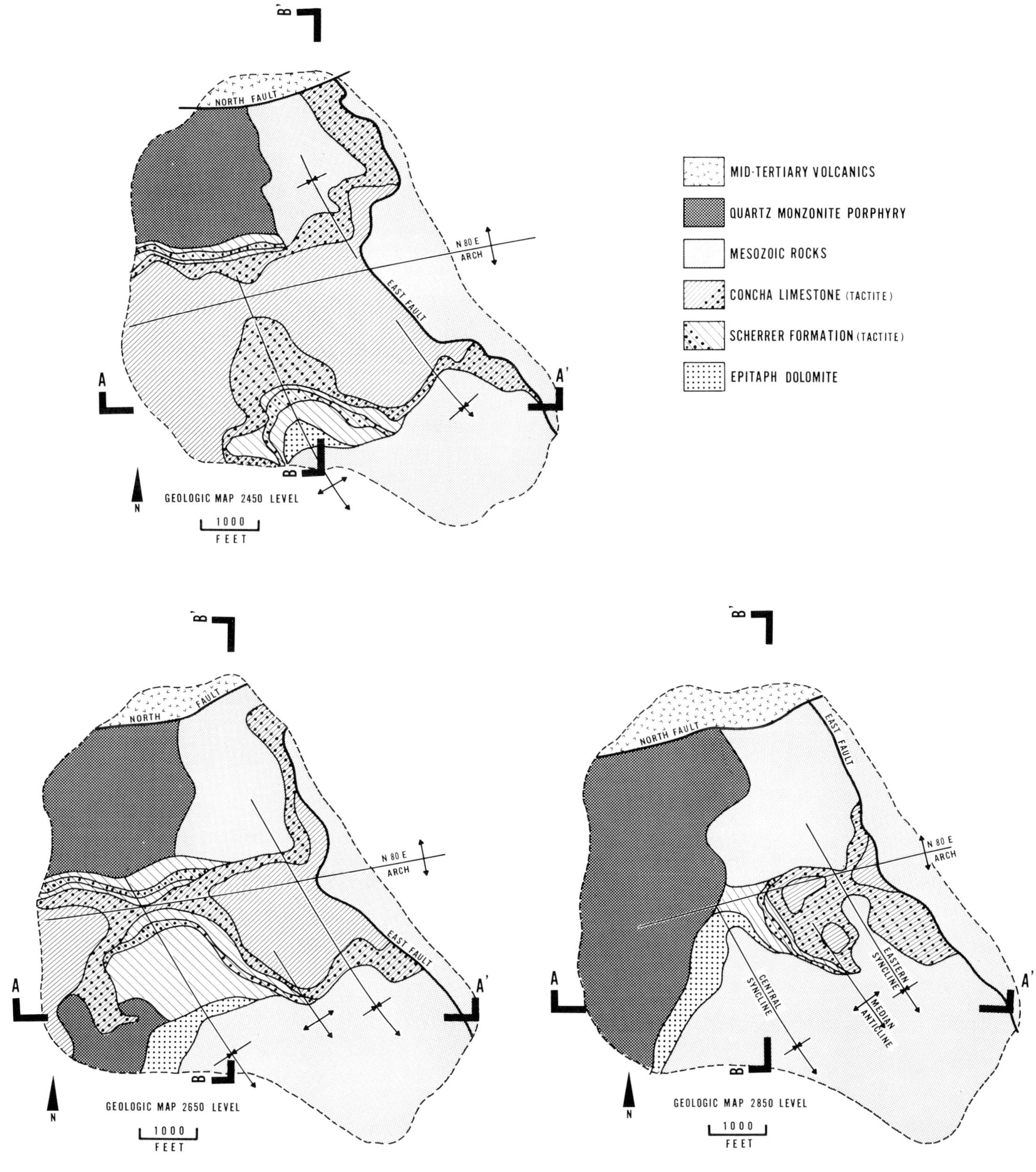

Figure 22.5. Geologic bench maps of selected levels in the Mission mine and vicinity. Refer to Figure 22.2 for cross sections and stratigraphic section. Refer to correlation diagram in Figure 22.3 for relationship to contour maps in Figures 22.4 and 22.5.

of the nature of the San Xavier thrust was advanced in considerable detail, including the suggestion of an undulating surface, by Cooper (1960). Among the points in evidence cited by Cooper was the apparent correspondence of Paleozoic strata in the north end of the district (the Mission mine, Mineral Hill and Banner mine area) with strata exposed in the region of Twin Buttes to the south. There was correspondence not only in formation types, but also in structures and in types and styles of mineralization. Projection of the sole of the thrust, which is exposed north of the Twin Buttes orebody, places it an unknown height above the present surface. The presence of northwest-striking fold axes in the Twin Buttes orebody (Barter and Kelly, 1981) corresponds to the pre-ore folding recognized in the Mission mine. The existence of an identical style of alteration and mineralization in the same parts of the Permian section at both ends of the district, in the Mission and Twin Buttes orebodies, lends further support to permissive interpretation of a common genesis.

SUMMARY

The structural history of the Mission orebody is outlined as follows:

1. Late Paleozoic or early Mesozoic orogenic events resulted in some folding and overturning of the Upper Paleozoic section. At this time, or at least prior to deposition of the middle units of the Rodolfo Formation (Triassic), the Paleozoic section of the Mission mine was inverted. The interpretation of post-ore movement of the block suggests that this folding took place in the vicinity of the Twin Buttes orebody and was involved in structures which developed there.
2. Following folding and weathering, deposition of the Rodolfo Formation took place on an angular unconformity.
3. Another period of weathering ensued during the middle Mesozoic and was followed by deposition of the Lower Cretaceous strata of the Angelica Arkose.
4. Emplaced into the strongly deformed Upper Paleozoic section and the overlying Mesozoic rocks were plutons of Laramide age. The closely similar radiometric age dates of quartz monzonite porphyry at San Xavier North (58.0 ± 1.2 m.y [Shafiqullah and Langlois, 1978] and at Twin Buttes (58.6 ± 2.5 m.y [Barter and Kelly, 1981]; 58.4 ± 2.1 m.y [Kelly, 1976]) are noteworthy. The interpretation of common sites of emplacement is permitted. Mineralization of the sedimentary section and, to a considerably less degree, of the porphyries took place.
5. Deposition of the Helmet Fanglomerate took place about 28.5 m.y. ago (Damon and Bikerman, 1964) following a period of uplift and weathering.
6. Movement of the San Xavier thrust commenced shortly after deposition of the Helmet Fanglomerate and presumably following further local uplift of the system to allow gravity gliding to take place. The Mission orebody reached its present position above the sole of the thrust about 26 m.y. ago (Barter and Kelly, 1981) but minor adjustments by movement ensued since then (Langlois, 1978).
7. Further weathering followed, accompanied (?) by faults striking north-northwest, a direction which corresponds to that suggested for the mid-Tertiary by Rehrig and Heidrick (1976). Since the Late Tertiary, evolution of the Sierrita pediment took place, with burial of the Mission and Pima deposits by about 200 ft. (65 m) of alluvium.

ACKNOWLEDGMENTS

The author wishes to thank Asarco geologists Dr. F. T. Graybeal and Mr. S. A. Anzalone for their critical review of this manuscript, and Asarco management for permission to publish. Responsibility for gathering and interpreting the data remains with the author.

REFERENCES CITED

Barter, C. F., and Kelly, J. L., 1982, Geology of the Twin Buttes mineral deposit, Pima mining district, Pima County, Arizona: *in* Titley, S. R., ed., Advances in Geology of the Porphyry Copper Deposits, Southwestern North America: Tucson, Univ. Ariz. Press, Chapter 20.

Butler, W. C., 1971, Permian sedimentary environments in southeastern Arizona: Ariz. Geol. Soc. Digest, v. IX, p. 71–93.

Bryant, W. H., 1959, Marker zones in the Permian Formations in southern Arizona: Ariz. Geol. Soc., Southeastern Ariz. Guidebook II, p. 38–42.

Cooper, J. R., 1960, Some geologic features of the Pima mining district, Pima County, Arizona: U.S. Geol. Survey Bull. 1112-C, p. 63–101.

———, 1971, Mesozoic stratigraphy of the Sierrita Mountains, Pima County, Arizona: U.S. Geol. Survey Prof. Paper 658-D, 42 p.

———, 1973, Geologic map of the Twin Buttes Quadrangle southwest of Tucson, Pima County, Arizona: U.S. Geol. Survey Map I-745.

Damon, P. E., and Bikerman, M., 1964, Potassium-argon dating of post-Laramide plutonic and volcanic rocks within the Basin and Range province of southeastern Arizona and adjacent areas: Ariz. Geol. Soc. Digest, v. VII, p. 63–78.

Gale, R. E., 1956, Geology of Mission copper Mine, Pima mining district, Arizona: Unpub. Ph.D. Diss., Stanford Univ., 140 p.

Gilluly, J.; Cooper, J. R.; and Williams, J. W., 1954, Late Paleozoic stratigraphy of Central Cochise County, Arizona: U.S. Geol. Survey Prof. Paper 266, 49 p.

Himes, M. D., 1973, Mineralization and alteration at Pima mine—a complex porphyry copper deposit: AIME Trans., v. 254, p. 166–174.

Jansen, L. J., 1973, Geology of the Sus Hills, Pima County, Arizona: Unpub. M.S. Thesis, Univ. Ariz., 33 p.

———, 1978, The San Xavier fault, Pima mining district, Arizona: Ariz. Geol. Soc. Digest, XI, (abs.), p. 99–100.

Keith, S. B.; Lehman, N. E.; Sell, J. D.; and Wilt, J. C., 1978, Supplemental road log no. 1; Tucson to Benson via Nogales, Patagonia, Sonoita and Whetstone Junction: Land of Cochise, N. Mex. Geol. Soc., Ariz. Geol. Soc., 29th Field Conf. Guidebook, p. 88–104.

Kelly, J. N., 1976, Geology of the Twin Buttes copper deposit, Pima County, Arizona: AIME Preprint 76-I-3, 23 p.

King, J. R., 1982, Geology of the San Xavier North porphyry copper deposit, Pima mining district, Pima County, Arizona, *in* Titley, S. R., ed., Advances in Geology of the Porphyry Copper Deposits, Southwestern North America: Tucson, Univ. Ariz. Press, Chapter 23.

Kinnison, J. E., 1966, The Mission copper deposit, Arizona; *in* Titley, S. R., and Hicks, C. L., eds., Geology of the Porphyry Copper Deposits, Southwestern North America: Tucson, Univ. Ariz. Press, p. 281–287.

Langlois, J. D., 1978, Geology of the Cyprus Pima mine, Pima County, Arizona: Ariz. Geol. Soc. Digest, v. XI, p. 103–113.

McClymonds, N. E., 1957, The stratigraphy and structure of the southern portion of the Waterman Mountains, Pima County, Arizona: Unpub. M.S. Thesis, Univ. Ariz., 157 p.

Rehrig, W. A., and Heidrick, T. L., 1976, Regional tectonic stress during the Laramide and Late Tertiary intrusive periods, Basin and Range Province, Arizona: Ariz. Geol. Soc. Digest, v. X, p. 205–228.

Richard, K. E., and Courtright, J. H., 1959, Some geologic features of the Mission copper deposit: Ariz. Geol. Soc., Southeastern Arizona Guidebook II, p. 200–204.

Shafiqullah, M., and Langlois, J. D., 1978, The Pima mining district, Arizona—A geochronologic update: Land of Cochise, N. Mex. Geol. Soc., Ariz. Geol. Soc., 29th Field Conf. Guidebook, p. 321–327.

Weaver, R. R., 1965, Geologic interpretation of the Ruby Star Ranch area, Twin Buttes mining district, Pima County, Arizona: Unpub. M.S. Thesis, Univ. Ariz., 74 p.

23

Geology of the San Xavier North Porphyry Copper Deposit

PIMA MINING DISTRICT, PIMA COUNTY, ARIZONA

John R. King

The San Xavier North porphyry copper deposit is located on the Papago Indian Reservation, 15 miles south of the city of Tucson, in the Pima mining district. It is shown on the Index Map (Fig. 23.1), along with the other major copper producers of the district (the Sierrita-Esperanza, Twin Buttes, and Mission-Pima mines). The San Xavier North porphyry copper deposit was discovered in 1955, when Asarco geologists found two small, altered and mineralized outcrops surrounded by alluvium. These outcrops, although leached of sulfides, were correctly interpreted as porphyry copper mineralization. Exploration diamond drilling began in mid-1957 after successful competitive bidding with the Papago Indians and was discontinued in 1958 because the deposit, as outlined on a 600-ft. triangular grid, was marginal at the then-existing copper price. In 1965, after a sharp rise in the price of copper, interspaced drilling on a 300-ft. equilateral triangular grid was initiated to define the size and economic viability of the deposit. In all, over 60 holes, averaging in depth between 600 and 700 ft., have been drilled in the San Xavier North copper deposit.

Open-pit mining began in 1968 with the production of copper-bearing silica flux, which was refined at Asarco's Hayden and El Paso smelters. In 1973 copper oxide ore production began at a rate of approximately 4,000 tons per day. Oxide ore is transported 2 miles south to the Mission Mine, where the ore is crushed, placed in vats for leaching, and finally recovered as cement copper.

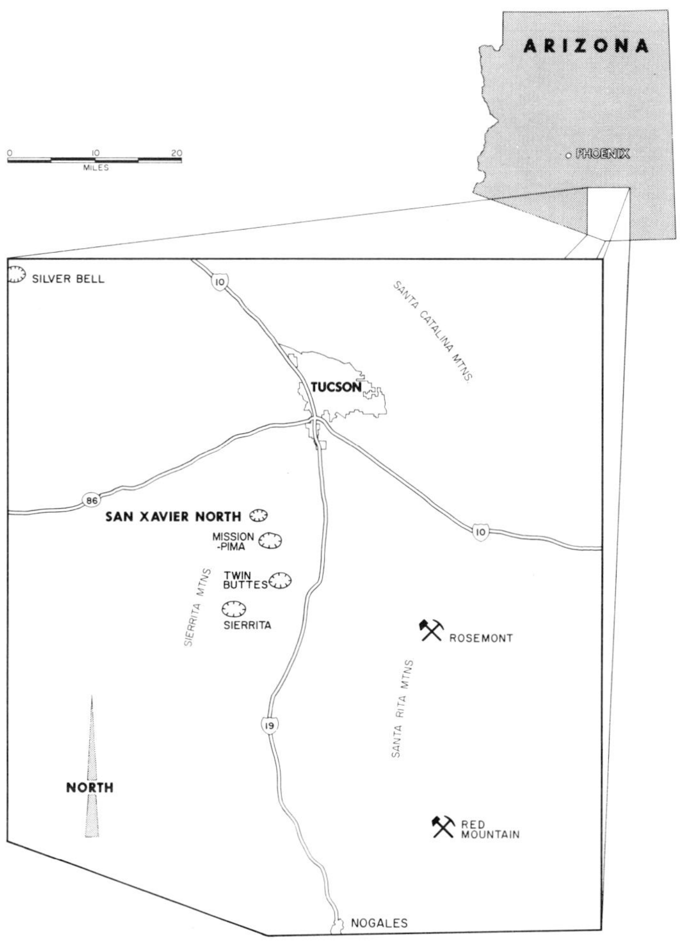

Figure 23.1. Index map, San Xavier North

REGIONAL SETTING

The San Xavier North deposit is situated at the northern boundary of the Pima mining district, which has been described and discussed by several authors, including J. R.

Cooper (1960, 1973), J. E. Kinnison (1961, 1966), and L. J. Jansen (1978). The generalized regional geology of the Pima mining district is shown on Figure 23.2. The alluvial cover has been removed and the "bedrock" geology simplified, showing only the following units: Precambrian granite; Paleozoic rocks, undifferentiated; Mesozoic clastic and volcanic rocks; Laramide granodiorite and quartz monzonite porphyry; and the post-mineral, mid-Tertiary Helmet Fanglomerate. The San Xavier fault is the major structural feature of the district, and all rocks shown on Figure 23.2, including the Helmet Fanglomerate, which lie to the east and north of the surface trace are bottomed by this low-angle structure. At the end of the 1970s only barren autochthonous Precambrian granite and Laramide quartz monzonite, K-Ar dated at 49.9 m.y. (Langlois, 1978), had been found below the fault.

As the San Xavier fault also bounds the Helmet Fanglomerate (28 m.y.), the age of movement along the structure is established as syn- or post-formation of the fanglomerates. My interpretation is that San Xavier Fault movement coincided with the deposition of the Helmet Fanglomerate and that, as movement occurred, a rotational basin was created in which deposition of the fanglomerates was restricted to the forming basin. With continued fault displacement the dip of the fanglomerates will always be in the opposite direction of the dip of the fault surface. If this is the correct interpretation, the strike of east-northeast and average dip of +30° to the south of the fanglomerates demand that the direction of movement along this antithetic fault be in a north-northwest direction. This direction of movement is the same as that proposed by both Cooper (1960) and Kinnison (1961), who have also proposed that the Pima-Mission ore zone is a simple slide block, representing the upper part of the Twin Buttes deposit. My speculation, however, is that the Mission-Pima allochthon originated as a complex (multiple-plated) gravity slide, possibly tearing off from the eastern flank of the Twin Buttes deposit. The San Xavier North allochthon is believed to have been faulted away from either the top

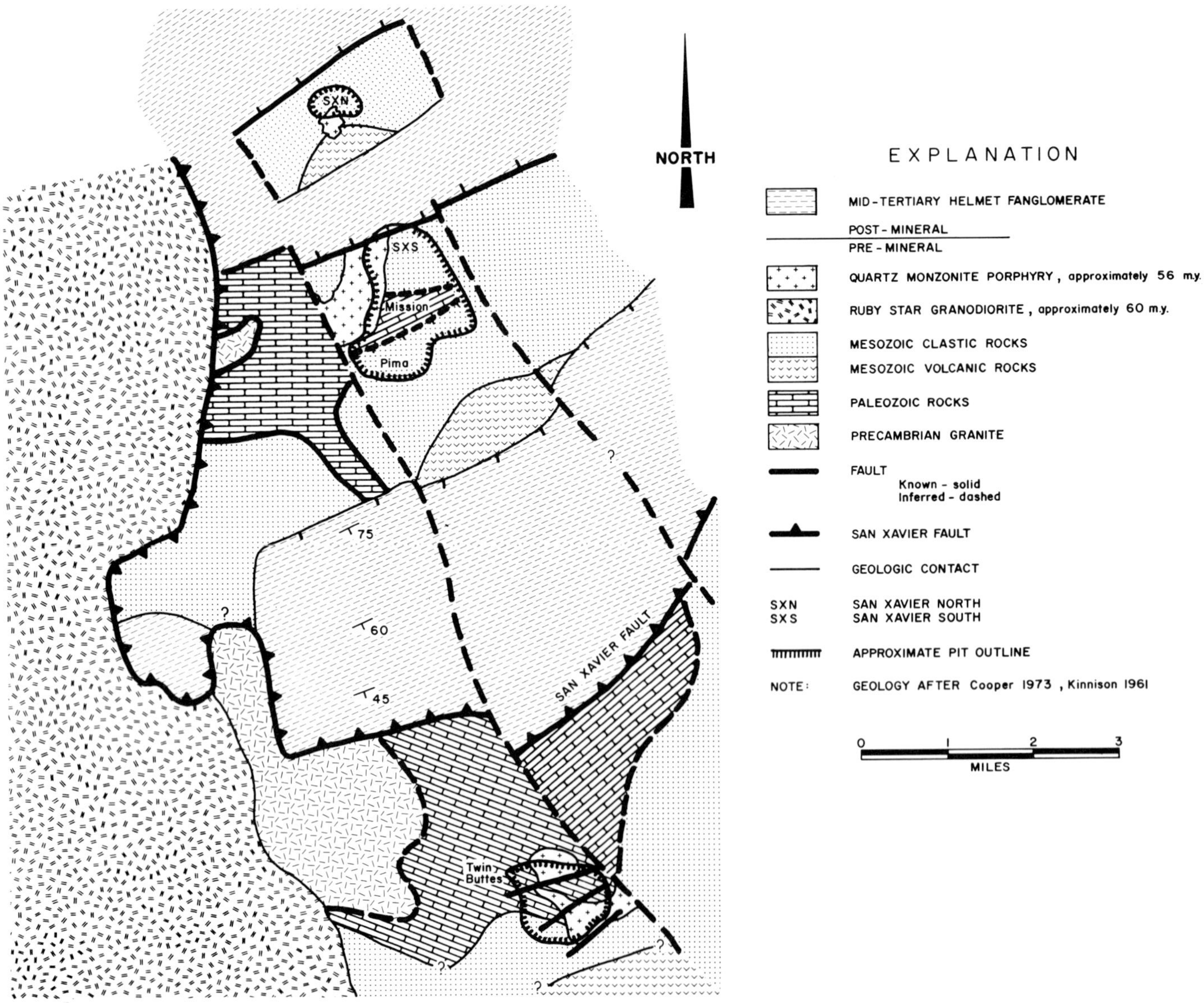

Figure 23.2. General regional geologic map of the Pima mining district

or the northern side of the Mission-Pima ore zone by gravity movement along an imbricate fault split of the San Xavier fault, the North fault of Jansen (1978).

Regardless of finer details of where the Mission-Pima roots are, the preponderance of geologic evidence indicates that the Twin Buttes, Mission-Pima, and San Xavier North ore zones were once part of a single, very large porphyry copper system in which over 90 percent of the economic-grade copper mineralization was contained within Paleozoic and Mesozoic sedimentary rocks.

GEOLOGY

The San Xavier North porphyry copper deposit consists of three mineralogic entities (oxide copper zones, supergene chalcocite, and hypogene sulfides), all contained in Cretaceous clastic rocks and intrusive quartz monzonite porphyry. Figure 23.3 is a plan map of the general geology at the San Xavier North mine. The clastic units depicted are defined by the preponderance of a particular sediment grain size and, therefore, represent only the gross-bedding character of that sedimentary unit.

Throughout the deposit the clastic rocks are an intimately interbedded sequence of mudstones, siltstones, fine- to coarse-grained sandstones, and an occasional pebble conglomerate; most of these beds are arkosic in modal composition. The sandstones are generally less than 20 ft. thick, with an occasional bed showing either graded bedding or sediment laminations. The sandstones consist of clastic quartz grains (40–65%), feldspar grains (20–40%), and an argillaceous matrix (5–15%). According to Travis's (1955) classification, these clastic rocks are mostly arkoses and argillaceous arkoses, which grade locally to feldspathic sandstones. The occasional pebble conglomerate is interbedded within the sandstones and consists of poorly-sorted, sub-rounded to rounded pebbles set in a matrix of sand and minor argillaceous cement. The pebbles consist of quartzite, feldspathic sandstones and siltstones, occasional microcline granite fragments, and even rarer silic volcanic clasts. The siltstones and mudstones are argillaceous and locally contain thin laminae of fine sand having the same appearance as adjacent sandstone beds. Individual mudstone beds are always less than 20 ft. thick and are frequently found as interbeds less than 1 ft. thick. The thicker mudstone beds occasionally display calcareous nodules up to 1/2 in. in diameter. Sedimentary features have yet to be found which can be used to identify the tops and bottoms of individual beds.

The sedimentary rocks at San Xavier North are probably correlative with the Early Cretaceous Amole Arkose of the Tucson Mountains and the Early Cretaceous Angelica Arkose of the Sierrita Mountains (Cooper, 1971) and, thus, are part of the Cretaceous Bisbee Group. Similar stratigraphic sections are described at the Pima mine (Himes, 1972; 1974; Langlois, 1978) and at the Twin Buttes mine (Kelley, 1976; Barter, 1978).

Intruding the clastic section are a number of quartz monzonite porphyry dikes and a single, larger mass of quartz monzonite porphyry. The larger mass of porphyry lies to the south of the present pit (see Fig. 23.3) and has been only partially delineated by drilling. Only a couple of small porphyry dikes are exposed within the present pit. The porphyry intrusives are composed of subhedral phenocrysts of plagioclase, orthoclase, and quartz ±biotite set in a fine-grained groundmass consisting essentially of quartz and orthoclase. Closely associated with the quartz monzonite porphyry both in time and space are intrusive and intrusion breccias, in which abundant clastic rock fragments and occasional porphyry xenoliths are sealed in an igneous matrix. Most of the breccias mapped and logged are contact intrusion breccias with a quartz monzonite matrix. The quartz monzonite porphyry intrusions at San Xavier North are identical to the quartz monzonite porphyry at the Mission and Pima mines and are quite similar to the quartz monzonite porphyry described at Twin Buttes (Kelley, 1976). The porphyries at San Xavier North are thus assumed to have a similar age (56 m.y., Pima district [Creasey and Kistler, 1962]; 58 m.y., Twin Buttes [Kelley, 1976]).

As interpreted from detailed pit mapping, and displayed simply on Figures 23.2 and 23.3, the sedimentary rocks are asymmetrically folded, with fold axes that plunge to the northwest and with axial planes that trace approximately N15°W and dip approximately 70° to the southwest. Within the pit three relatively large folds have been defined; two anticlinal folds (with one having a slightly overturned limb) and an intervening syncline. A multitude of smaller, discontinuous folds have been mapped; however, these structures are related to drag along minor faults and, because of their discontinuity, they are not depicted on Figure 23.3. The three larger folds displayed on the map are interpreted to be a result of regional tectonism prior to quartz monzonite porphyry intrusion. Evidence for this interpretation is shown on the cross section, where a porphyry dike clearly cuts the anticlinal and synclinal structures. Geologic work at Mission (Jansen, 1976) and at Twin Buttes (Kelley, 1976) also points to a structural event that is post-Bisbee Group and pre-Laramide intrusion in age.

The only major fault encountered at San Xavier North is the low-angle San Xavier fault. The depth to this structure is 2,010 ft., as determined from drill hole 2SC-18, the only hole drilled to depth. Sympathetic, low-angle shearing occurs for over 100 ft. above the fault and for about 30 ft. below the structure. Typical, fresh Precambrian granite exists below the fault. A structurally important feature encountered in this drill core is the presence of a fault slice, or wedge, of Paleozoic marble existing at depth from 2,000 ft. (the structural bottom of Cretaceous rocks) to 2,010 ft. (the top of the San Xavier fault). This marble wedge is identical to the marble exposed at the Mission mine and in the footwall of the North fault (Jansen, 1978).

Many other faults have been mapped in the pit and logged in the core; however, only those faults with interpretable and significant displacement ($\geq$50 ft.) are shown on the geologic map (Fig. 23.3). All faults mapped are not only post-mineralization but also post-supergene enrichment in age. The most significant fault delineated within the pit is a west-northwest–trending fault that is exposed in the southern part of the pit. This fault dips steeply to the south and the movement is clearly reverse.

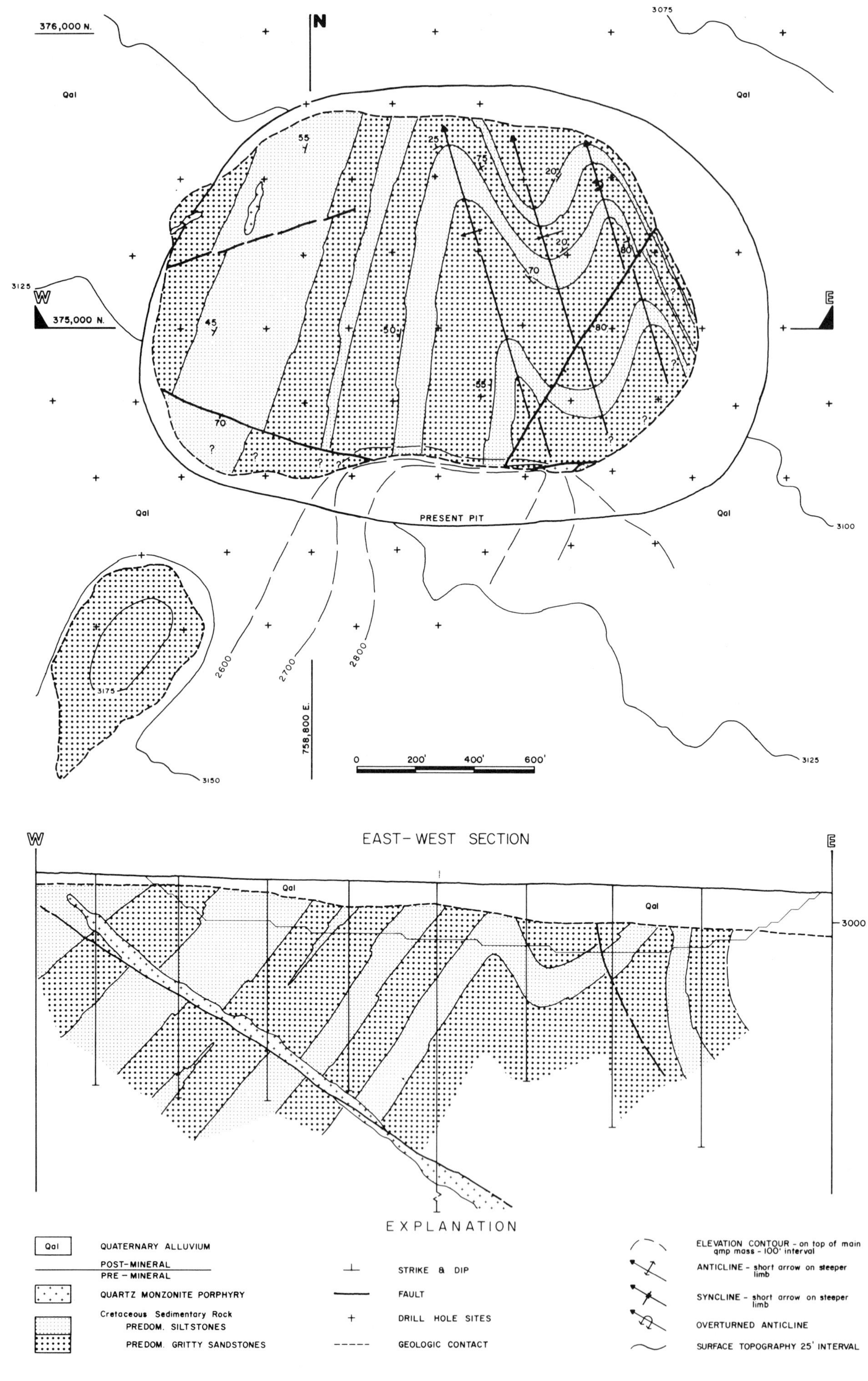

Figure 23.3. General geologic map and section of San Xavier North orebody

Post-mineral rocks exposed in San Xavier North pit consist of Pliocene to Pleistocene alluvial gravels. The Helmet Fanglomerate is not exposed in the pit, although it has been encountered in scout hole drilling both to the north and to the south of the pit. Andesite dikes, probably related to the adensite volcanism of the Helmet Formation, have been encountered in several of the drill holes east of the present pit.

HYPOGENE MINERALIZATION

Hydrothermal mineralization and alteration at San Xavier North were contemporaneous, spatially interrelated, and formed as part of a continuing chemical process that resulted in a zonal distribution of both sulfide and alteration minerals. Figure 23.4 is the plan map at an elevation of 2,800 ft., showing zonal distribution of the primary sulfide system. Hypogene, ore-grade (approximately 0.5% copper) mineralization is developed entirely within the central ore zone area. This ore zone is characterized by a low total sulfide content (1–3% by volume) and a low pyrite to chalcopyrite ratio that varies between 1 : 1 and 1 : 3. Sulfide minerals include, in order of abundance, chalcopyrite, pyrite, molybdenite, bornite, sphalerite, and galena. Mineralization occurs as disseminations, as fracture fillings without significant gangue quartz, and as discrete grains within quartz veins. A direct relationship exists between disseminated and veinlet sulfide grain size and grain size of the sedimentary host. In other words, the finer-grained the sedimentary host, the finer-grained is the sulfide.

Anomalous silver (+1 ppm) and molybdenite (+100 ppm) mineralization is associated with the ore zone. Molybdenite commonly occurs either as aggregates of crystals within late-forming quartz veins or as films along fractures; it appears to be slightly younger than the main pyrite-chalcopyrite event. The higher MoS_2 assays are consistently displayed in the quartz monzonite porphyry intrusives.

The total character of mineralization of the ore zone as described above is displayed by both sedimentary and igneous rocks; however, the main quartz monzonite porphyry mass rarely makes an economic copper grade. Within the ore zone better-grade copper mineralization is primarily controlled by proximity to the main quartz monzonite porphyry mass. Figure 23.5 displays this relationship by showing the outline of quartz monzonite porphyry and the distribution of +0.3 percent copper value, averaged from the 2,800 elevation (below the lower limit of chalcocite) to the final depth of all drill holes.

Copper mineralization is secondarily influenced by stratigraphy. A statistical study comparing assays to individual stratigraphic beds demonstrates that the finer-grained sediments display a greater chalcopyrite content than coarser-grained sediments. The mudstones and siltstones were found to average over 0.4 percent copper, whereas medium- to coarse-grained sandstones average less than 0.3 percent copper. The reason for this secondary distribution is probably the combined result of rock chemistry and rock preparation. The finer-grained sediments display not only a slightly higher $CaCO_3$ content but also a higher concentration of parting, both along bedding and as cross-fracturing, than the sandstones.

Surrounding the ore zone is an area of higher volume, pyrite mineralization (henceforth referred to as the pyrite shell) that is typified by a total sulfide content of 2 to 4 percent (by volume) and a pyrite to chalcopyrite ratio varying from 10 : 1 to 3 : 1. Sulfide mineralization in this zone is primarily pyrite, with minor occurrences of chalcopyrite, sphalerite, galena, and molybdenite. Pyrite occurs as disseminations, as thin fracture fillings, as discrete grains in the occasional quartz veins, and as prominent veins (up to 1 in. thick) without significant addition of gangue quartz. Molybdenum and silver mineralization average 10 ppm and 0.2 ppm, respectively. In the pyrite shell the control of stratigraphy on disseminated, sulfide grain size remains the same as described for the ore zone, although this distribution is partially masked by an increase in sulfide vein thickness. The differential distribution of copper content with respect to stratigraphy is such that copper values vary from 0.2 percent Cu for siltstones to less than 0.1 percent Cu for sandstones.

The area of change from the pyrite shell to the ore zone is transitional over a distance of approximately 100 ft., and is labeled "transition zone" on the map and cross section in Figure 23.4. As shown in the east-west section, the transition zone is relatively symmetrical about a vertical axis. However, in a north-south section the zone is not symmetrical about a vertical axis but dips steeply to the north and gently to the south. This asymmetry may indicate post-mineral rotation of the San Xavier North deposit.

Within the transition and ore zones a multiple sequence of vein relationships and paragenesis is markedly displayed and by its nature illustrates the continuing, complex, chemical evolution typical of porphyry copper systems. At San Xavier North disseminated mineralization appears to be closely associated with the earliest of the numerous cross-cutting, sulfide veins. As the hydrothermal system evolved, the younger veins became noticeably thicker, richer in gangue quartz, with wider alteration selvages. The final phases of hydrothermal mineralization are characterized by multiple, cross-cutting, quartz-rich veins, most of which carry not only pyrite and chalcopyrite but also molybdenite.

HYDROTHERMAL ALTERATION

Associated with both of the above-described mineral zones is classic hydrothermal phyllic alteration, which in itself is internally zoned in a manner sympathetic with the mineral zoning. Propylitic and potassic alteration zones are present but have yet to be delineated, due to the lack of both deep and peripheral drilling. Figure 23.6 depicts the alteration zoning at the 2,800-ft. elevation and in cross section, as determined both from core logging and pit mapping. The distribution patterns are determined by the abundance and pervasiveness of hydrothermal sericite and the relative abundance of quartz veining.

In the general area of the pyrite shell the alteration is classified as weak to moderate phyllic, displaying 5 to 20 percent hydrothermal sericite, minor epidote, kaolinite, and virtually no quartz veining. Hydrothermal sericite is pervasive throughout the groundmass of all rock types and is present as partial replacement (less than 50%) of the clastic feldspar grains of the sandstones. In the groundmass of the

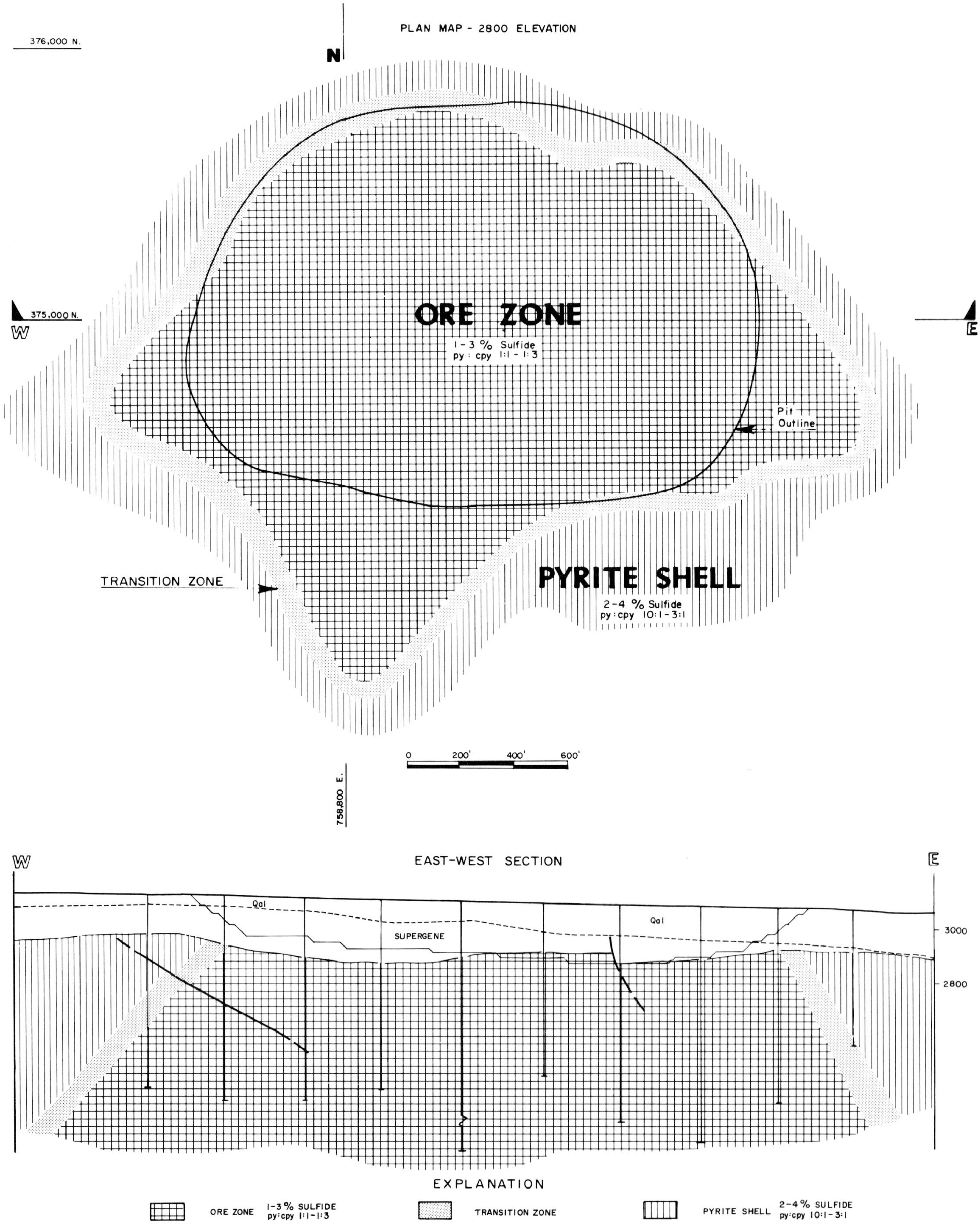

Figure 23.4. Hypogene mineral zoning, San Xavier North orebody

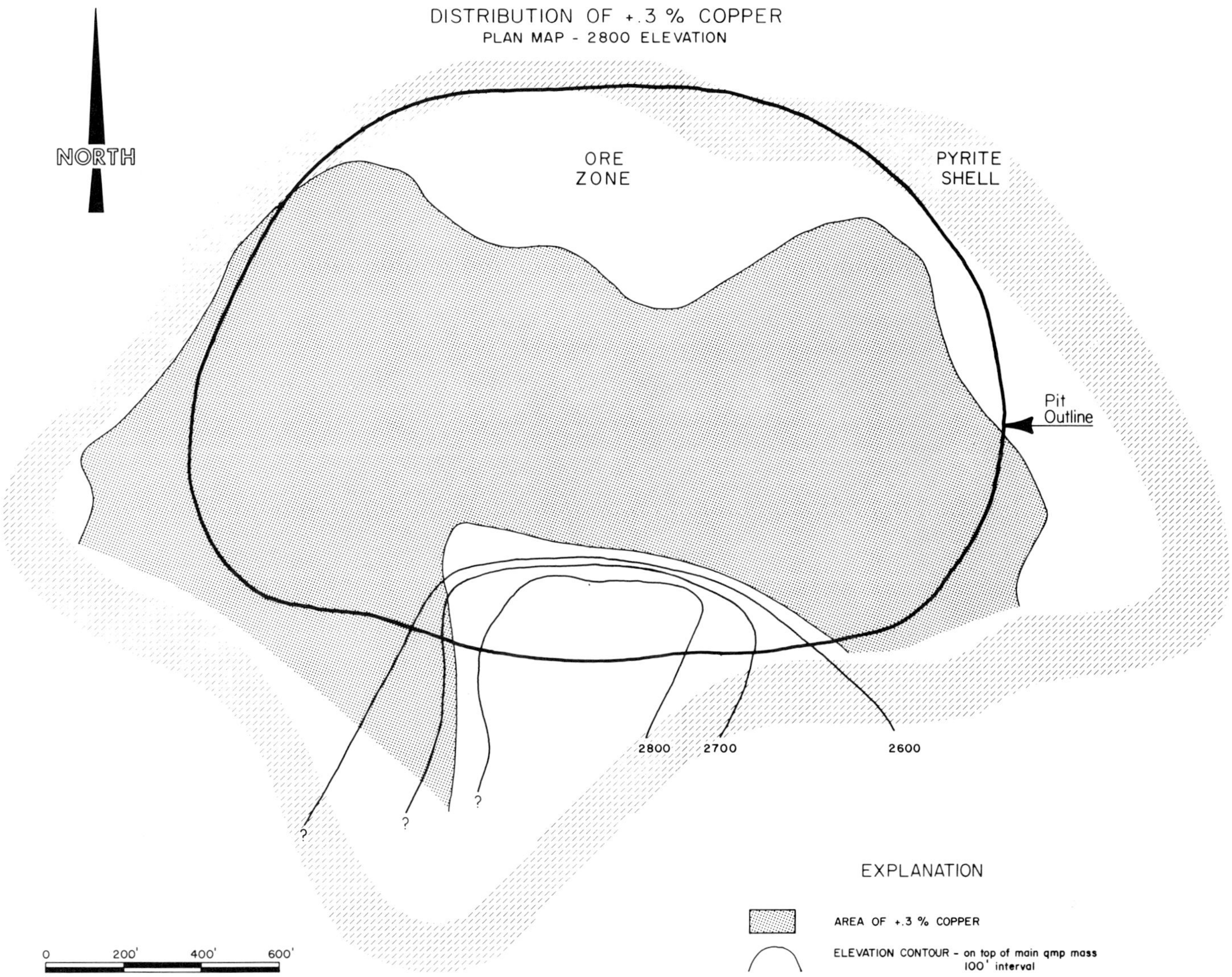

Figure 23.5. Grade distribution map, San Xavier North orebody

mudstones and finer-grained siltstones, sericite is closely associated with fine-grained hydrothermal chlorite, actinolite, and minor epidote. Detrital quartz in the sandstones displays minor silica overgrowths and suturing between adjacent grains. The silica overgrowths display a rind of opaque dust and fluid inclusions at the original quartz-grain boundary, and the secondary silica is in optic continuity with the original clastic quartz. Late hydrothermal calcite (up to 2% by volume) occurs throughout this alteration zone as both vein and disseminated calcite pervasive to all rocks. Trace amounts of pyrite occur with the carbonate veins. In this zone of weak to moderate phyllic alteration and pyritic mineralization, fluid inclusions within detrital quartz are abundant, predominantly gas rich, and, for the most part, are secondary or pseudosecondary in character.

In an area that encompasses the mineral transition zone, phyllic alteration is totally pervasive and classified as moderate to intense. Hydrothermal sericite comprises from 15 to 40 percent of the rock. The plagioclase and—to a lesser extent—the orthoclase feldspars are from 60 to 99 percent converted to an exclusive assemblage of sericite and minor quartz. In the mudstones and fine-grained siltstones the groundmass still exhibits a mix of hydrothermal sericite and chlorite; however, now epidote and actinolite are absent. Adjacent detrital quartz grains show strong sutured boundaries and no direct evidence of silica overgrowth, as the opaque dust and fluid inclusions are more or less evenly distributed through the quartz. Hydrothermal quartz is present both in numerous veins and as weak silicification of the groundmass. The quartz veins show several different paragenetic relationships, with the thicker, molybdenite-bearing veins being the youngest. Disseminated and vein calcite and minor dolomite are overprinted on this phyllic alteration and in thin section they comprise up to 3 percent of the rock. Minor pyrite and chalcopyrite are associated with the carbonate veins.

Central to the above alteration zones and, thus, characteristic of the ore zone is a hydrothermal alteration suite characterized by 15 to 30 percent sericite, minor groundmass silicification, and a moderate abundance of quartz veins.

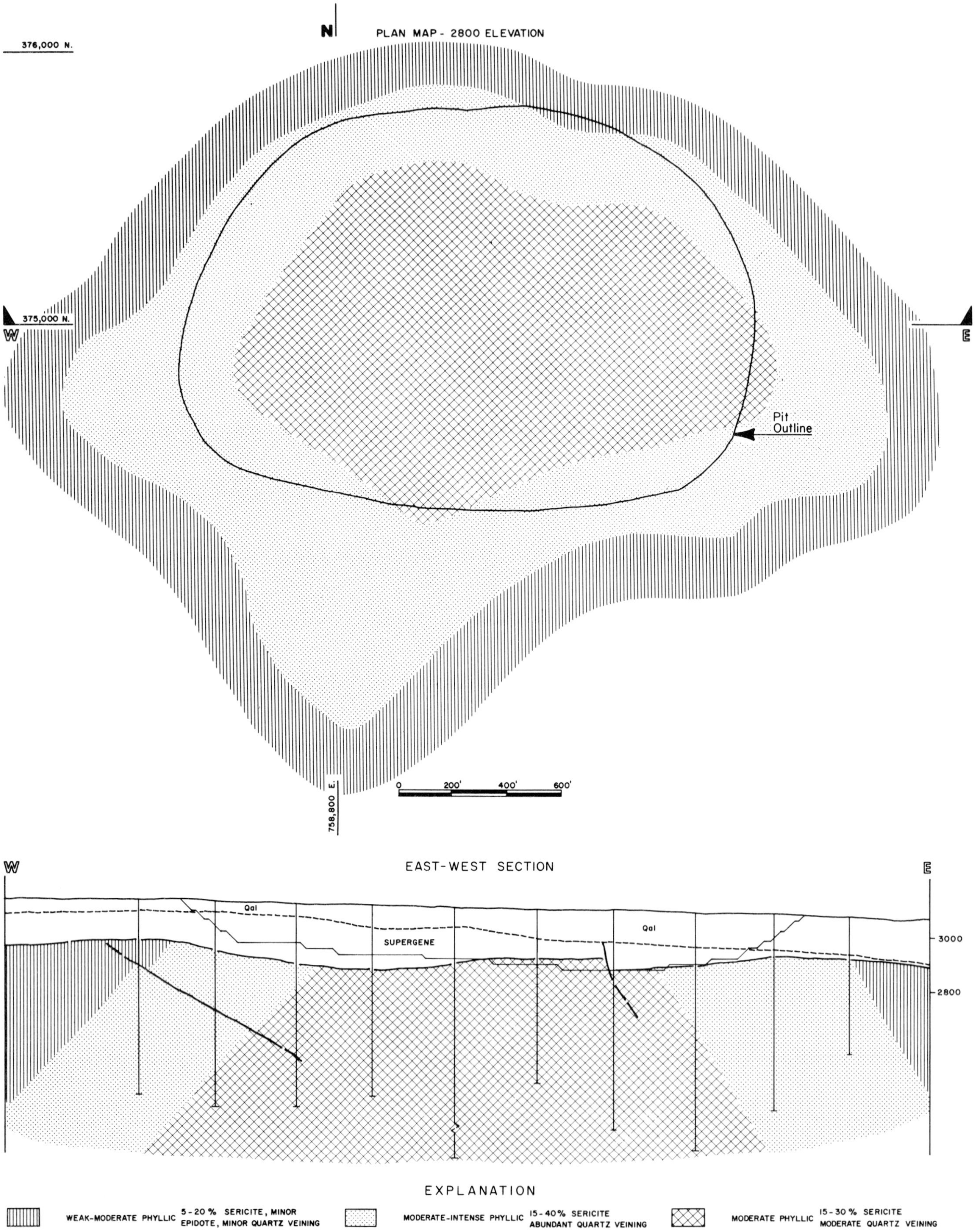

Figure 23.6. Map and section of hypogene alteration zoning, San Xavier North orebody

Plagioclase feldspars are pervasively altered and are from 40 to 95 percent converted to sericite and minor quartz. Potassium feldspars are relatively stable, being only from 5 to 30 percent sericitized. In the groundmass of the mudstones and fine-grained siltstones, up to 50 percent of the chlorite is converted to very fine-grained biotite. Detrital quartz grains exhibit recrystallization and strong suturing of grain boundaries, not only with adjacent clastic grains but also with the secondary silica in the groundmass. Late hydrothermal calcite and dolomite comprise up to 4 percent of the rock. Within this central phyllic zone fluid inclusions in the detrital quartz are still predominantly gas-rich and abundant; however, over 50 percent of the inclusions appear to be primary in character. Gas-poor and saline fluid inclusions are occasionally present. The daughter minerals in the saline-inclusion type are halite, unidentified opaques, and minor hematite.

Although a zone of potassic alteration has yet to be defined, it is worth noting that one of the deeper drill holes bottomed in mixed potassic and phyllic alteration. This alteration is characterized by less than 20 percent sericite; 1 to 2 percent biotite and chlorite as thin veins and disseminations in all clastic rocks; up to 4 percent potassium feldspar as an occasional vein, vein selvage, or overgrowth on stable grains of detrital potassium feldspar; and 1 percent anhydrite occurring as thin veins and as disseminated grains in all rock types. The fluid inclusions in the potassic-altered rocks show an increase in abundance of saline inclusions and a decrease in size and abundance of gas-rich inclusions.

SUPERGENE MINERALIZATION-ALTERATION

The supergene character of the San Xavier North deposit is depicted in E-W cross section (Fig. 23.7). The supergene system consists of leached capping, two different oxide copper zones, an economically significant chalcocite blanket, and a lower limit of supergene chalcocite. The upper zone of oxide copper is contained within the capping and represents a totally oxidized chalcocite zone that was stranded during the main period of leaching and enrichment. Chrysocolla is the dominant oxide mineral, with varying lesser amounts of malachite, azurite, neotocite, and melaconite. The occurrence of these copper minerals is predominantly as fracture coatings, which vary in thickness from less than 1/64 in. to a maximum of 1 in., the average being less than 1/16 in. In general the black oxides (neotocite and melaconite) occur along the outer edge of the fracture, and the green and blue oxides (malacite, azurite, and chrysocolla) occur as central fillings of the fracture. Pit mapping and blast-hole assaying demonstrate that stratigraphy influences the distribution of the oxide copper. The siltstones display a high copper grade, with most of the values being distributed along fractures. The sandstones generally contain a lower total copper grade. A somewhat higher percentage of the copper value is contained within the rock as disseminations and as absorbed copper oxide in altered feldspars.

As shown on the cross-section (Fig. 23.7), the upper zone of oxide copper exists at the bedrock-alluvial interface and, thus, appears to have been subjected to partial erosion. At this erosion surface chrysocolla is by far the prevalent copper oxide; however, with increasing depth from this surface, copper carbonates become more noticeable. It is the opinion of the author that the chrysocolla is replacing pre-existing copper carbonate. This association suggests that, in the upper zone at least, the chalcocite oxidized to form a copper carbonate ore zone which, in turn, was almost wholly replaced by copper silicates.

In the lower zone oxide copper is intermixed with chalcocite and occurs at the base of the leached capping. This zone of mixed oxide-sulfide mineralization is the product of erosion and partial oxidation of the main chalcocite blanket. With the exception of minor occurrences of native copper and cuprite, the oxide copper minerals of the lower zone are the same as those described for the upper zone, although in the lower zone the copper carbonates (malachite and azurite) are equally as abundant as the copper silicate (chrysocolla). Again, chrysocolla appears to be replacing the copper carbonate minerals.

As can be seen in cross section (Fig. 23.7), significant chalcocite ($\geq$25% of sulfide present as Cu_2S) is developed only where the hypogene ore zone was exposed by pre-fault erosion to oxidation and leaching. Typically the chalcocite selectively replaces chalcopyrite in preference to pyrite. Enrichment is at most two-fold and is the result of an apparent single cycle of enrichment, as the remaining capping displays a gradual increase of hematitic limonites with depth. Figure 23.8 shows the distribution of the remaining chalcocite blanket, the area of partial erosion of this blanket, the bedrock topography, and the position of the two discovery outcrops.

Stratigraphy appears to influence the thickness of chalcocite formation. The siltstones and mudstones exhibit a high degree of chalcocite replacement, because of the combined effect of their finer-grained hypogene sulfides, higher chalcopyrite content, and prevalence of fracture-controlled sulfides. Because of this high degree of total sulfide replacement by chalcocite, the blanket in siltstone horizons is relatively restricted in thickness. The sandstones, on the other hand, show a lower percentage of chalcocite replacement but develop a chalcocite enrichment zone over a greater thickness. This development is the result of the greater porosity of the sandstones, the larger sulfide grains, and the possible presence of more pyrite relative to chalcopyrite.

The leached capping, as exposed by mining over the last several years, has proven to be difficult to rationalize, in that the limonite mineralogy does not always predict the underlying sulfide compositions. Above the chalcocite blanket, mudstone and siltstone beds exhibit a false leached cap that shows essentially no evidence of disseminated mineralization, virtually no goethitic limonites or boxworks after chalcopyrite, and only minor hematite. Thus, of the limonites present, most are on fractures and most show an inordinately high frequency of jarosite. The adjacent sandstones, however, display a true capping, in which the limonites and boxworks are indicative of the known supergene and hypogene mineralization below.

Typical supergene alteration products seen in the leached capping are alunite, kaolinite, halloysite, and dickite(?). The alunite is extensively abundant in the siltstone

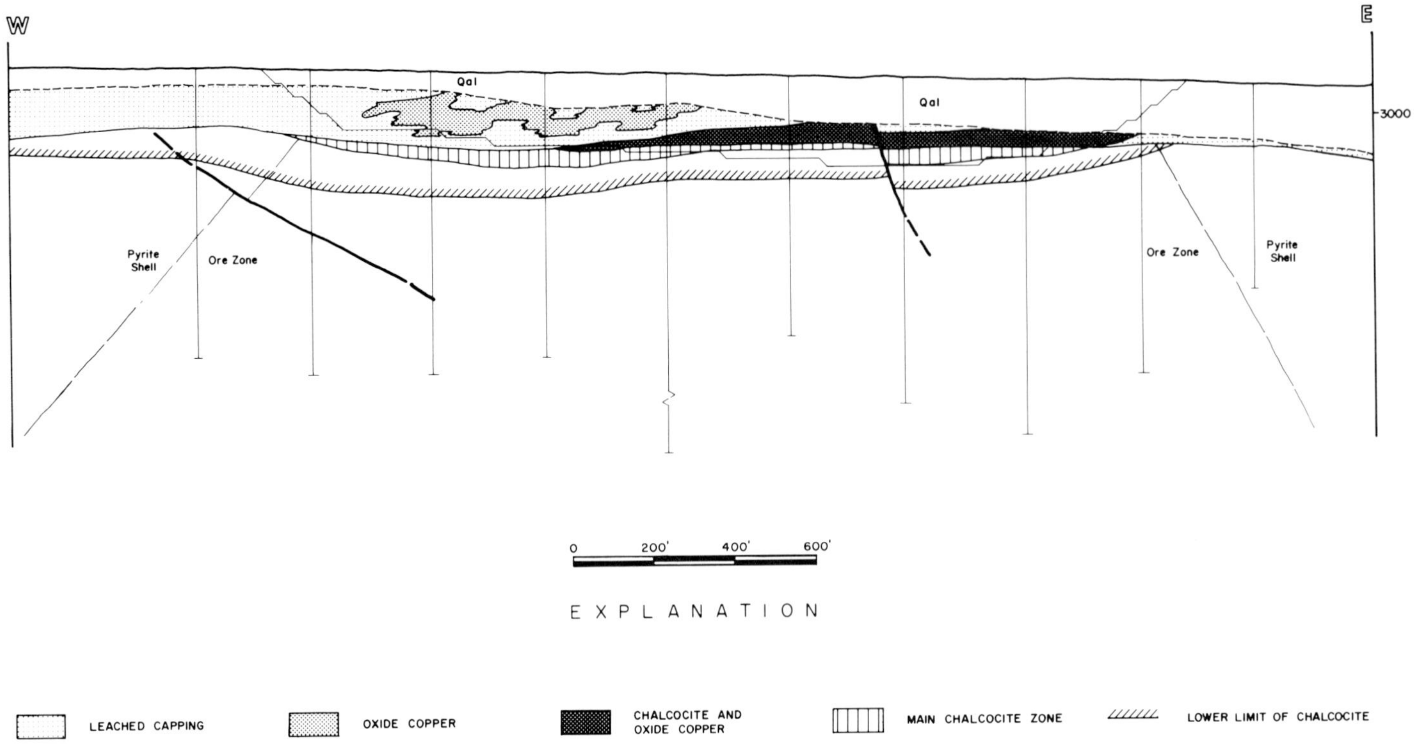

Figure 23.7. East-west cross section of supergene mineral zoning, San Xavier North orebody

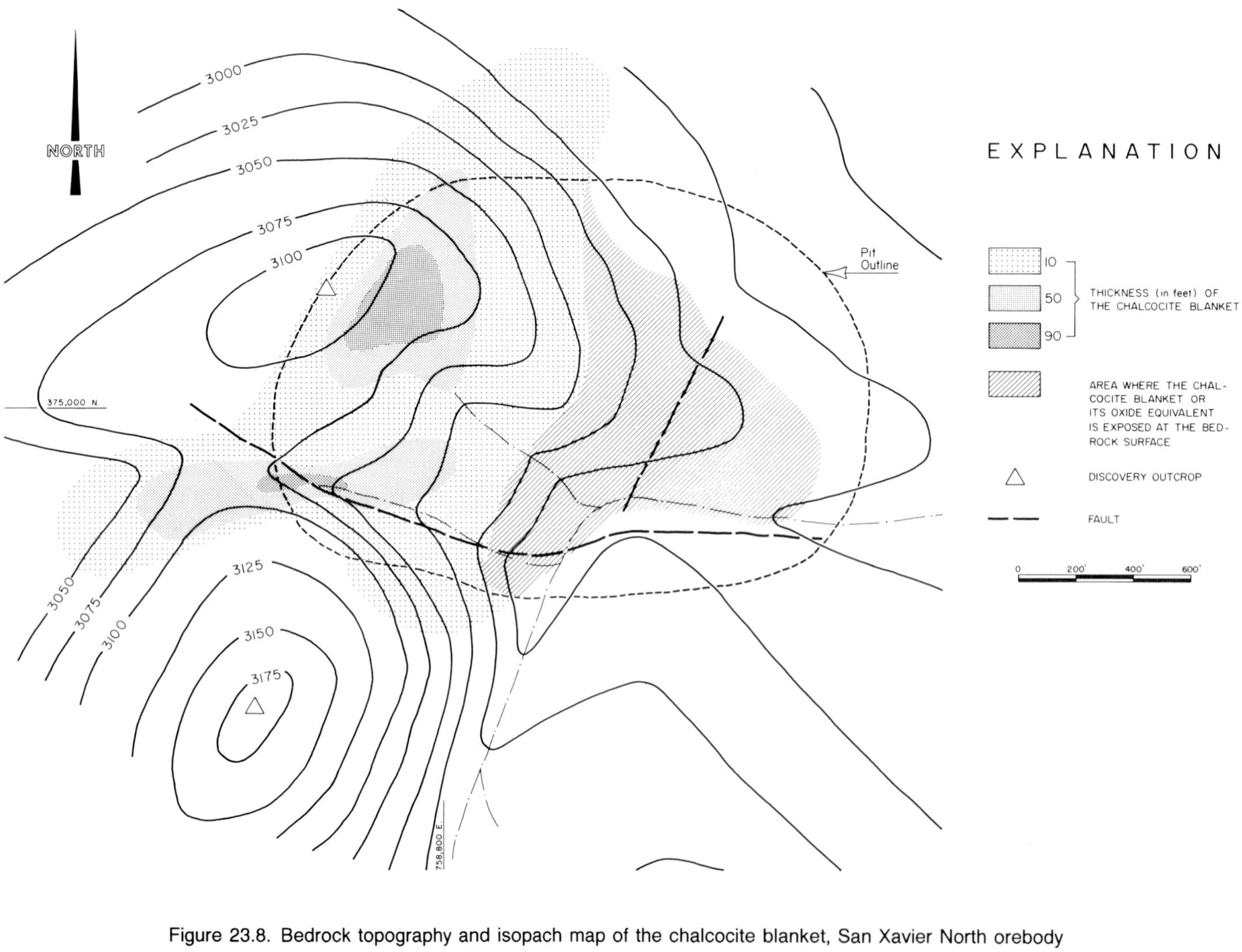

Figure 23.8. Bedrock topography and isopach map of the chalcocite blanket, San Xavier North orebody

and mudstone horizons, and its abundance may be the result of sulfide oxidation and iron leaching in a high aluminum environment.

ACKNOWLEDGMENTS

The author began his work at San Xavier North in 1973, and this report is the compilation of pit mapping, at a scale of 1 : 600, and relogging of much drill core. Previous workers at the San Xavier North deposit include K. Richard, J. H. Courtwright, J. E. Kinnison, S. A. Anzalone, D. Hall, and L. J. Jansen. Review and encouragement by Asarco management and geologists are gratefully acknowledged. However, this report is solely the responsibility of the author.

REFERENCES CITED

Barter, C. F., 1978, Stratigraphy, alteration and ore controls in the Main Ore Zone, Twin Buttes Mine, Pima County, Arizona: Ariz. Geol. Soc. Digest XI, p. 115–116.

Cooper, J. R., 1960, Some geologic features of the Pima mining district, Pima County, Arizona: U.S. Geol. Survey Bull. 1112-C, 103 p.

———, 1971, Mesozoic stratigraphy of the Sierrita Mountains, Pima County, Arizona: U.S. Geol. Survey Prof. Paper 658-D, 42 p.

———, 1973, Geologic map of the Twin Buttes Quandrangle southwest of Tucson, Pima County, Arizona: U.S. Geol. Survey Misc. Geol. Inves. Map I-745.

Creasey, S. C., and Kistler, R. W., 1962, Age of some copper-bearing porphyries and other igneous rocks in southeastern Arizona: U.S. Geol. Survey Prof. Paper 450-D, p. D1–D5.

Himes, M. D., 1974, Mineralization and alteration at Pima Mine—a complex porphyry copper deposit: Soc. Min. Engrs. AIME Trans., v. 254, p. 166–174.

———, 1972, Geology of the Pima Mine, Pima County, Arizona: Unpub. M. S. Thesis, Univ. Ariz.

Jansen, L. J., 1978, The San Xavier Fault, Pima mining district: Ariz. Geol. Soc. Digest XI, p. 99–100.

Kelley, J. L., 1976, Geology of the Twin Buttes copper deposit, Pima County, Arizona: AIME, SME Preprint 76-I-3, 23 p.

Kinnison, J. E., 1961, Cholla Flat-Twin Buttes area, Pima County, Arizona: Private Report, ASARCO, Inc., April.

———, 1966, Cholla Flat-Twin Buttes area, Pima County, Arizona, Exploration Review, San Xavier Indian Reservation: Private Report, ASARCO Inc., November.

Langlois, J. D., 1978, Geology of the Cyprus-Pima mine; Ariz. Geol. Soc. Digest XI, p. 103–114.

Travis, R. B., 1955, Classification of Rocks: Quarterly, Colo. Sch. of Mines, v. 50, no. 1.

24

Geology of the El Tiro Area

SILVER BELL MINING DISTRICT, PIMA COUNTY, ARIZONA

Frederick T. Graybeal

The Silver Bell mining district is located 35 miles northwest of Tucson on the south side of the Silver Bell Mountains at elevations varying from 2,500 to 3,000 ft. Recorded mining activity began in 1865 with the discovery of an altered limestone outcrop near El Tiro pit which contained up to 17 oz. Ag and mixed copper oxides. Further exploration located massive chalcopyrite pods in skarn which were mined until 1930. Production for the period 1865–1930 is estimated at 1,400,000 tons averaging 3.5 percent Cu.

An extensive churn drill program was started in 1909 to investigate the possibility of disseminated copper mineralization in the igneous rocks and resulted in the discovery of the Oxide and El Tiro deposits, which were then submarginal. ASARCO acquired control of the district in 1917 and did some mining until 1930. The district was inactive until 1948, when check drilling confirmed the existence of two separate deposits of disseminated chalcocite ore. Production began in 1954 at an annual rate of 18,000 tons of copper and for the time period 1954–1977 yielded 75,655,000 tons averaging 0.80 percent Cu, 0.07 oz. Ag, and 0.022 percent MoS_2. In the late 1970s some production was derived from disseminated chalcopyrite in skarn in the eastern portion of El Tiro pit.

The first geologic study of the Silver Bell district was by Stewart (1912). This was followed by Kingsbury and others (1941), who mapped the El Tiro-Oxide area in detail; Richard and Courtright (1966), who published the only general study of the geology and mineralization in the Silver Bell district; Kerr (1951), who studied hydrothermal alteration; Watson (1964), who studied the Mesozoic stratigraphy and structure in the area east of the pits; Cummings (1973), who made the first attempt to define hypogene zoning patterns; and Davis (1977), who mapped the North Silver Bell area.

About 1970 mining reached the base of the chalcocite blanket and it became possible to study hypogene mineral assemblages previously masked by strong supergene alteration. It is the purpose of this chapter to report and interpret data on these assemblages with respect to modern concepts of porphyry copper zoning and genesis. The study is restricted to the El Tiro area (Fig. 24.1), which forms a center of mineralization separate from the Oxide area. Emphasis is on the entire hydrothermal system rather than geology within the pit walls. The El Tiro area was selected because of the abundance of exposures below the chalcocite blanket where hypogene patterns are best preserved. The data are primarily the result of detailed field mapping at scales larger than 1 in. = 1,000 ft. supplemented by chemical analyses and petrographic studies.

GENERAL GEOLOGY

Rocks which vary in age from Precambrian to Recent are exposed in the Silver Bell Mountains. These rocks are cut by an elongate zone of pyritic mineralization more than 8 miles long, which varies from 200 ft. to 2 miles wide. East of Oxide pit the pyrite zone is linear, with a strike of N80°W. In the El Tiro area the pyrite zone strikes N5°W. Although sulfide mineralization is continuous, the pyrite zone is very narrow between the two pits, and it is clear that two separate centers of mineralization are present. Control of the mineralization is attributed by Richard and Courtright (1966) to a well-developed fault zone. Northeast of the fault zone Paleozoic sedimentary rocks and Mesozoic volcanic and minor clastic rocks form a gently northeast-dipping homocline. Southwest of the fault zone Mesozoic clastic rocks are intruded by a large pluton of alaskite, and volcanic rocks are mostly absent. Dikes, sills, and small stocks of quartz

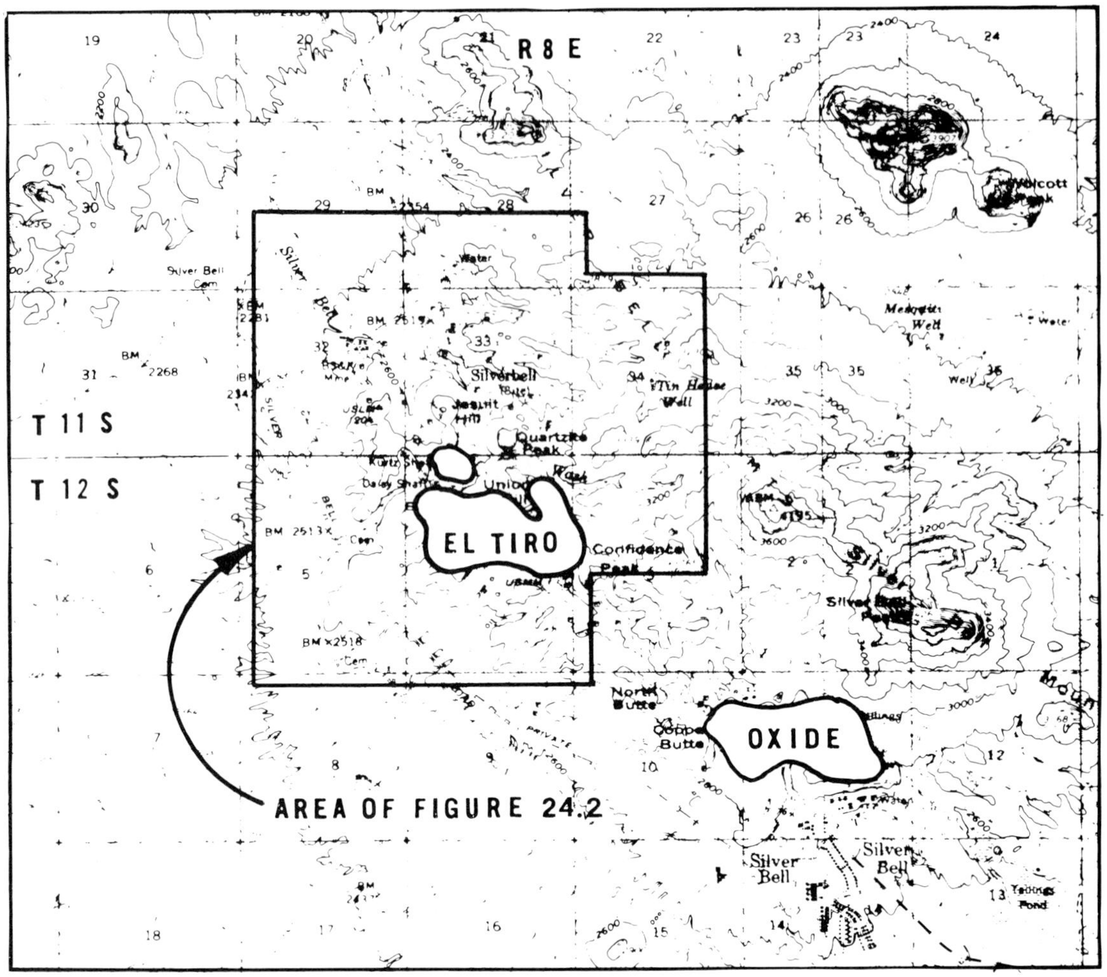

Figure 24.1. Location map of the El Tiro area in the Silver Bell mining district (from portions of the Vaca Hills and Silver Bell Peak 15' Quadrangles)

monozonite porphyry and related intrusive rocks are most abundant near the contact of the alaskite and adjacent volcanic rocks.

ROCK TYPES

The distribution of rocks in the El Tiro area is shown on Figure 24.2. The rock types discussed are those in and immediately adjacent to the El Tiro alteration halo and represent only a small portion of the rocks exposed in the Silver Bell Mountains.

Paleozoic

Identification of Paleozoic rocks in the El Tiro area is complicated by pervasive thermal metamorphism and hydrothermal alteration. Quartzite is present on several hills north of El Tiro pit. Although it is generally thought to be Cambrian Bolsa Quartzite, it bears some resemblance to quartzites in the Dripping Spring Formation and in the Scherrer Formation.

The Cambrian Abrigo Formation was tentatively identified in the eastern portion of El Tiro pit by Merz (1967) where thin, greenish, siltstone lenses are interbedded with altered limestone and thicker, gray, siltstone beds. Similar lithologies were reported by McClymonds (1959) for the middle and upper members of the Abrigo Formation in the Waterman Mountains, roughly 5 miles to the southeast. There the Abrigo is roughly 700 ft. thick. In El Tiro pit the existence of additional carbonate rocks at depths below the 1,250-ft. dacite porphyry sill shown on Figure 24.3 may require unreasonable thicknesses for the Abrigo and suggests the identification may be in error.

Other Paleozoic formations have been identified on the basis of lithologic similarity to rocks in the Waterman Mountains, interpreted through the alteration, and their spatial relationship to what was thought to be the Abrigo Formation. As these interpretations may be partly in error, the individual formations have not been shown separately on Figures 24.2 and 24.3. Although the Paleozoic carbonate rocks are good hosts for hypogene ore, the degree to which they are mineralized appears to be a function of both proximity to the Imperial quartz monozite porphyry stock and intrinsic factors.

The thickness of the Paleozoic rocks cannot be accurately determined due to extensive silication, faulting, and dilation by irregular sills of intrusive rocks. Their distribution is quite linear and closely coincides with the contact of the alaskite and dacite. In addition, although strikes are variable, dips are mostly gentle and folding is absent. These rocks appear to have been engulfed by the dacite, and some offsets

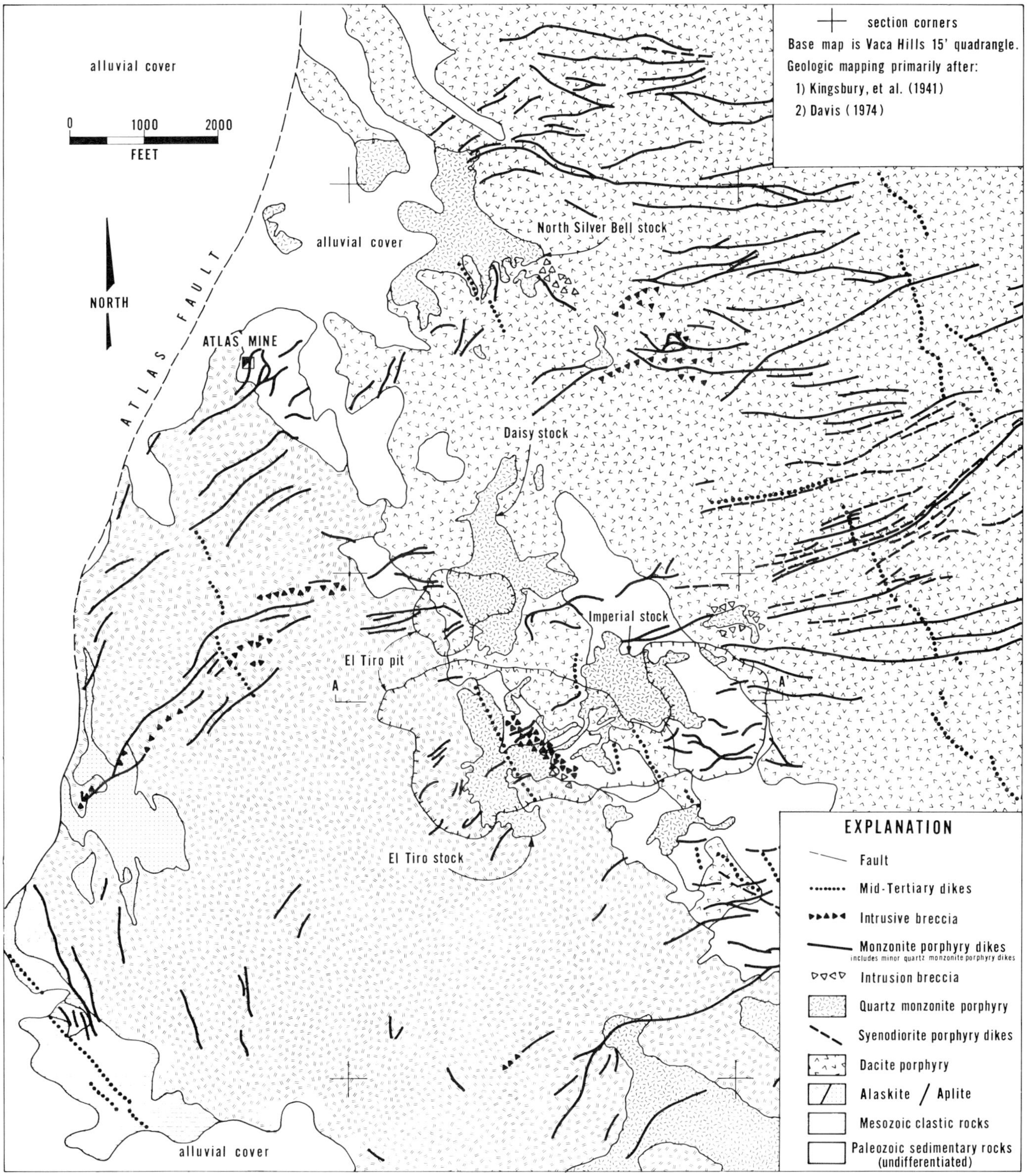

Figure 24.2. Geologic map of the El Tiro area (geology projected through dump areas)

which have been interpreted as faults may instead be fractures along which large blocks have been pulled apart during emplacement of the dacite.

Mesozoic

Clastic rocks are exposed in the southwestern corner of the area mapped in Figure 24.2. They consist of well-sorted and bedded arkoses with minor siltstone and pebble conglomerate units, all varying in color from buff to maroon. They generally dip 20 to 40° SW and are locally contorted where cut by later igneous rocks.

Alaskite underlies the western half of the El Tiro alteration zone. It is a buff-colored, medium- to coarse-grained, generally equigranular intrusive rock which contains 25 percent quartz, 54 percent weakly perthitic orthoclase, 18 percent oligoclase, 2 percent biotite, and traces of zircon, apatite,

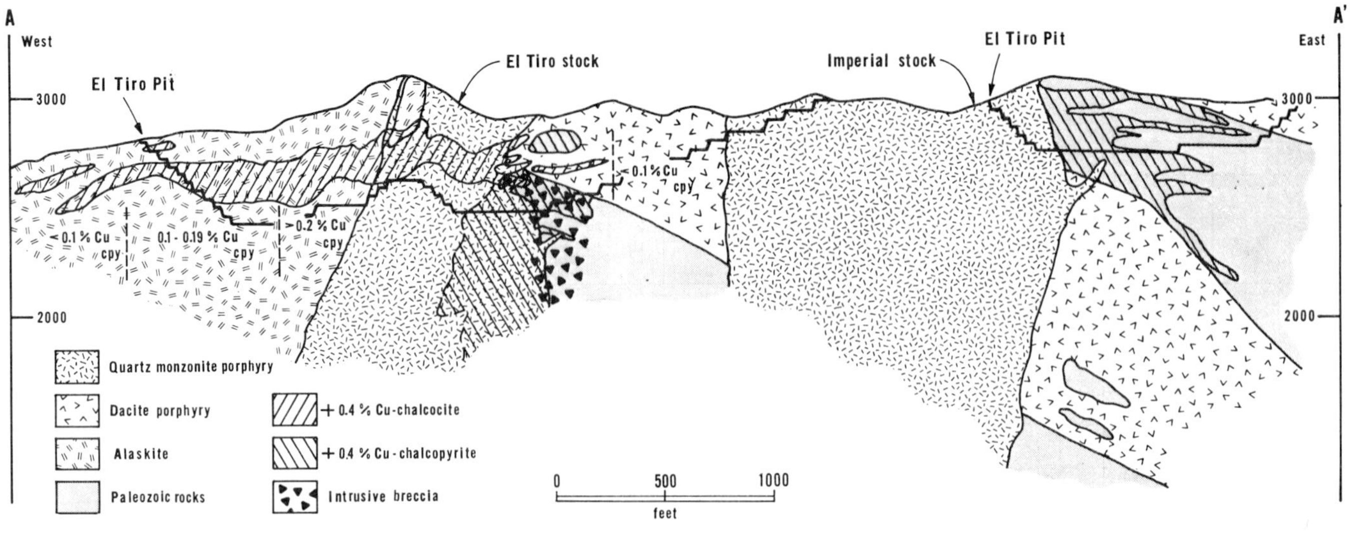

Figure 24.3. East-west cross section through the central portion of the El Tiro area, looking north (see Fig. 24.2 for location)

and opaques. The biotite and feldspar contents are locally variable, but within the mapped area the alaskite does not generally attain a quartz monzonite composition as described by Banks and Dockter (1976). Thin aplite dikes are found throughout the alaskite in small amounts and a large aplitic mass has been mapped 1 mile west of El Tiro pit. The Mesozoic age of the alaskite is well established where alaskite dikes and contact-related hornfels cut Mesozoic clastic rocks. Attempts to refine the age by isotopic dating have not been successful. The alaskite is an important host for chalcocite ore, although the underlying hypogene grades are generally less than 0.2 percent Cu. The alaskite was intruded earlier than and is genetically unrelated to the mineralization in El Tiro pit.

The dacite porphyry underlies the eastern half of the El Tiro alteration zone. It has been mapped by Watson (1964), who believes it has the form of a sill-like intrusion, possibly 3,400 ft. thick near El Tiro pit, which thins to the northeast. It is a dark-colored, porphyritic rock with a phenocryst:matrix ratio of 50:50. Phenocrysts are quartz (15%), andesine (30%), and biotite (5%)—all occasionally reduced by variable amounts of sanidine, orthoclase, opaques, and xenoliths, and all set in a cryptocrystalline matrix of either devitrified glass or ash. The quartz phenocrysts are usually rounded, resorbed, and often strongly broken; flow structure is commonly observed in thin section. The proportion of broken to intact phenocrysts and the abundance of lithic clasts both increase to the east. Using a cobaltinitrite stain, Watson found significant amounts of K-feldspar in the matrix indicating the composition of the rock may be quartz latitic. However, the term "dacite porphyry" was correctly retained by Watson to eliminate confusion in the literature. Dacite porphyry dikes cut Mesozoic clastic rocks and are cut by quartz monzonite porphyry. Attempts to date the dacite porphyry isotopically have been unsuccessful. Although hypogene grades are low, the dacite porphyry is a host for some low-grade supergene ore.

Syenodiorite porphyry dikes, which are probably the earliest members of the Laramide intrusive porphyry suite, cut dacite porphyry and Paleozoic carbonate rocks in the eastern portion of the El Tiro alteration zone. The syenodiorite porphyry is a dark-colored, strongly porphyritic rock which contains 2 percent quartz, 15 percent orthoclase, 70 percent andesine, and 12 percent biotite and hornblende. Phenocrysts form roughly 35 percent of the rock, and all minerals occur both as phenocrysts and in the matrix. The distribution and orientation of the syenodiorite porphyry dikes and the monzonite porphyry dikes are similar, and, in areas where the two dikes occur in mutual contact, the monzonite porphyry dikes are chilled against the earlier syenodiorite porphyry dikes.

Rocks of quartz monzonitic composition, which comprise over 95 percent of the Laramide intrusive porphyry suite, are confined to irregular stocks close to the contact between the alaskite and dacite porphyry and to rare dikes of roughly similar composition which extend outward from these stocks. The most abundant rock in this suite is a quartz monzonite porphyry, which occurs in large and small stocks throughout the alteration zone. Although referred to as monzonite by Richard and Courtright (1966), these rocks are always quartz-rich and porphyritic. The quartz monzonite porphyry contains roughly 20 percent quartz, 28 percent orthoclase, 44 percent andesine, 5 percent biotite, and 1 percent hornblende with accessory magnetite, zircon, sphene, and apatite. The phenocryst : matrix ratio is 55 : 45, with rounded quartz (4%), anhedral orthoclase (2%) euhedral plagioclase (43%), biotite (5%), and hornblende (1%) phenocrysts in a medium- to fine-grained matrix of equant quartz and orthoclase. Within El Tiro pit several less well mineralized zones in the quartz monzonite porphyry grade into either a seriate porphyritic texture, with less quartz and more orthoclase than is typical, or a granodioritc phase which varies from equigranular to porphyritic with up to 75 percent phenocrysts.

Orthoclase quartz monzonite porphyry is locally abundant as dikes and small stocks and is easily distinguished by the presence of 1 to 5 percent euhedral orthoclase phenocrysts up to 1 in. long and 2 to 10 percent rounded quartz phenocrysts up to 3/8 in. in diameter. In thin section this rock is hard to distinguish from the quartz monzonite porphyry unless the large phenocrysts are present. In El Tiro pit the two rock types appear to be gradational phases of a single intrusive event and are important hosts for hypogene and supergene ore.

A single small exposure of a hydrothermal biotite-rich quartz monzonite porphyry with minor associated fine-grained dikes exists on a deep bench at the south end of El Tiro pit, and it may be a separate intrusive phase younger than the orthoclase quartz monzonite porphyry. It contains 20 to 25 percent fine- to medium-grained biotite, which occurs as disseminated grains and in massive aggregates (probably as an alteration product of pre-existing hornblende—which is rarely present in the aggregates—and biotite). The quartz content averages about 10 percent, all in the matrix. This rock exhibits the strongest biotitic alteration and the highest hypogene grades of any of the porphyries. Although the strong biotite alteration, abundant chalcopyrite, and location in the center of the El Tiro hydrothermal zones suggest the rock is an alteration phase of the quartz monzonite porphyry, sharp contacts with adjacent porphyries argue that it is a separate intrusive phase. The abundance of alteration biotite indicates the rock may have contained 10 to 20 percent mafic minerals before alteration, which would suggest a separate, more mafic rock type than the other porphyries.

The existence of several quartz monzonite porphyry phases has not previously been described at Silver Bell, largely due to extensive supergene alteration and chalcocite enrichment, which masked hypogene alteration and sulfide mineral zoning. These rocks are believed to be the source of the alteration and copper mineralization. At the end of the 1970s mining had not progressed deeply enough below the chalcocite blanket to permit detailed mapping of the distribution and relative abundance of the various phases, and it is possible that as-yet-unrecognized intrusive phases remain to be described. Mauger (1966) has reported a K-Ar age of 65.5 ± 2 m.y. on biotite from quartz monzonite porphyry in El Tiro pit.

Small, dark-colored porphyritic dikes of granodioritic composition with up to 10 percent matrix hornblende cut unmineralized alaskite southwest of the pit. These dikes are probably related to the large porphyry stock south of El Tiro pit and are not separated on Figure 24.2

Monzonite porphyry occurs as abundant dikes which extend outward from the central portion of the El Tiro area. It contains an average of 4 percent quartz, 53 percent orthoclase, 38 percent andesine, and 4 percent biotite, with accessory hornblende and opaques. The phenocryst : matrix ratio is 30:70, with rounded quartz (2%) and euhedral plagioclase (28%) phenocrysts in a fine-grained matrix of somewhat variolitic orthoclase. The relatively uniform composition and texture of the monzonite porphyry suggest it is not gradational with the quartz monzonite porphyry. Its age relative to the other porphyries is unclear, but it may be younger, and it is not an important host for ore.

Cenozoic

Several post-mineral dike rocks of presumed mid-Tertiary age occur in the El Tiro area. Near-vertical, dark gray-green, continuous dikes up to 10 ft. wide of andesitic composition strike N20°W across the central portion of El Tiro pit. Biotite phenocrysts are occasionally present and Watson (1964) found pyroxene and hornblende phenocrysts in similar dikes east of the pit. Several resistant quartz latite porphyry dikes up to 200 ft. thick, with a N20°W strike, were also mapped by Watson east of El Tiro pit. Numerous light to dark gray northwest-striking dikes of latitic(?) composition with 10 to 20 percent white feldspar phenocrysts have been mapped in the Mesozoic clastic rocks southwest of the alaskite. The area west of the Atlas fault is underlain by a coarse, often unsorted, variably caliche-cemented conglomerate presumably equivalent in age to the Gila Conglomerate.

STRUCTURE

Faults are not well exposed or preserved in the El Tiro area. The northeast contact of the alaskite is virtually a straight line which strikes N40°W and dips at a high angle to the southwest. This line is inferred by Richard and Courtright (1966) to have been a fault between the Paleozoic rocks and Mesozoic clastic rocks which was largely destroyed by later intrusive activity. This fault appears to have controlled the emplacement of the alaskite, the dacite porphyry, some of the quartz monzonite stocks, and ensuing alteration and mineralization. The fault, referred to here as the El Tiro fault, is poorly preserved in El Tiro pit due to later intrusions of porphyry and intrusive breccia. Well-developed fault-gouge zones up to 15 ft. wide with steep westerly dips are probably remnants of the original structure. Maps of some of the underground workings indicate that quartz monzonite porphyry dikes locally parallel the fault, attesting to its pre-mineral age.

A probable second structure in this area is defined by a line striking N5°W which passes through the Daisy and El Tiro stocks. This line is parallel to the direction in which these stocks are elongated and is roughly parallel to the direction in which these two stocks and the North Silver Bell stock are aligned. The alteration and sulfide mineral zones are also elongate in this same direction. The intersection of the N5°W and N40°W structures occurs roughly in the center of El Tiro pit and coincides with the area of highest hypogene grades in silicate host rocks in the El Tiro area. The nature of this second structure is unclear; its relatively low deviation from the strike of the northeast contact of the alaskite suggests it may be a split off the El Tiro fault.

The largest post-mineral structure is the Atlas fault which brings Gila Conglomerate into fault contact with earlier rocks west and north of El Tiro pit. The strike of this fault varies within 20° of NS, and dips vary from 45°W to nearly vertical. A large number of post-mineral faults have been mapped in the pit, where they offset dikes and sulfide veins. Most of these faults are thin and discontinuous, with offsets less than 10 ft., and are not shown on Figure 24.2.

Pebble dikes occur in limited amounts throughout the Silver Bell district and are most common in the alaskite and dacite along the monzonite porphyry dike swarm northwest and northeast of El Tiro pit, where they typically occur as the outward and/or upward (from mineralized centers) manifestation of monzonite porphyry dikes. In this area porphyry and pebble dikes often occupy the same fissure, and occasionally fragments of porphyry occur as clasts in the pebble dikes, indicating that the gas which formed the pebble dikes was probably derived from the porphyry dikes. The pebble dikes tend to bulge irregularly and contain a relatively limited assortment of angular to subrounded clasts up to 6 in. across set in a gritty matrix. In many places the angularity is such that the term "breccia dike" would be equally accurate. They are collectively shown on Figure 24.2 as intrusive breccia.

A particularly large breccia mass is exposed in the southeast wall of El Tiro pit, along the approximate trace of the El Tiro fault. The size of the breccia is unclear, but it appears to be at least 500 ft. long, 500 ft. high, and from 0 to 250 ft. wide. As seen in the pit wall, it appears to terminate upward in a series of dike-like extensions into the roof rocks. Diamond drilling suggests a somewhat dome-shaped upper limit in places. The near absence of any outcrops at the present surface suggests the breccia never vented to the original surface. A second, apparently similar, mass of breccia was described in underground workings 1,500 ft. north of the present exposures by Kingsbury and others (1941). Fragments are mostly angular, vary from 1/4 to 6 in. in size, and are contained in a medium-fine-grained, gritty matrix which forms 5 to 80 percent of the breccia. Rare larger clasts are also present. Although some vertical banding suggestive of flow structure is present, rounding is absent. Fragments of quartz monzonite porphyry with quartz veins which terminate at the edge of the fragment establish a late-mineral age for the breccia. The dome-shaped geometry interpreted in places from diamond drilling suggests that collapse may have been involved in the origin of this feature. However, the lack of vugs; the mixing of alaskite, quartz monzonite porphyry, and skarn; the flow banding; and the dike-like penetrations of intrusive breccia into the walls above the main breccia mass suggest that the latest stage in its evolution resulted from the entrainment and transport of rock material in a rapidly moving fluid—a process generally termed "fluidization." One pebble dike exposed in El Tiro pit contains altered limestone clasts derived from a block of skarn approximately 200 ft. east of the exposure, which gives some indication of the intrusive mobility of these features.

Several siliceous, occasionally vuggy breccias are exposed in El Tiro pit and in the dacite northeast of the pits. These breccia masses vary in size from 50 to 300 ft. across and are always near the contact of a quartz monzonite porphyry stock. The relationships suggest these are intrusion breccias related to emplacement of the stocks. The intrusion breccias are texturally characterized by occasional vugs, often pervasive silicification, a low abundance of grit or rock flour between the clasts, and an absence of mixing of different rock types. Although they appear to be pre- or early mineral, they are not notably more mineralized than the adjacent unbrecciated rocks.

The El Tiro area occurs roughly at the intersection of the N50°W-striking El Tiro fault and the northeast-striking porphyry dike swarm. Watson (1968) refers to this as a structural intersection, and the possibility exists that the porphyry dikes follow a pre-mineral structure which may have been an ore control. East of El Tiro pit in the dacite porphyry the dike swarm maintains an extremely linear pattern, roughly one mile wide, striking N65 to 80°E over a distance of more than 2 miles. West of El Tiro pit the dike swarm is weakly developed in the alaskite and the few dikes present define an arcuate pattern convex to the west, which subtends an arc of roughly 90°. Outcrops throughout the area are sufficiently well exposed to preserve some evidence of pre-mineral structures into which the dikes were emplaced, but none has been observed.

An alternative to the concept of a pre-mineral structural intersection is suggested by Heidrick (1974). He proposes a model for the development of fractures and emplacement of dikes and veins which involves hydraulic fracturing by water-saturated magmas. The hydraulic fracturing model is attractive in that it does not require the presence of a pre-existing permeable structure along which a dike may be emplaced. Although this model does not explain the arcuate dike pattern west of El Tiro pit, a detailed analysis of joint and vein patterns in El Tiro pit reveals that northeast-striking fractures acquire a more northerly orientation, averaging about 5°, when they extend westerly from the quartz monzonite porphyry into the alaskite. This change in strike of the fractures is in the same direction as the dikes. These arcuate patterns may be in part related to a difference in the index of refraction of the alaskite as compared to the porphyries. The dikes do not appear to define an inward-dipping cone sheet.

METAMORPHISM

Textural and mineralogical changes which occurred with relatively minor chemical changes and which contain no sulfide minerals are present in several rock types and are believed to be a result of thermal metamorphism. Southeast of El Tiro pit thin beds in the Paleozoic limestones have been recrystallized to a largely anhydrous assemblage of lime-silicate minerals. The mineralogy has not been carefully studied, but various minerals carefully preserve the bedding down to a scale of a few inches. This metamorphism has clearly resulted in the movement of some silica, although shaly partings are present in the section, so bulk movement over significant distances was not required. The metamorphism appears to weaken to the northeast, notwithstanding local effects related to the emplacement of the dacite porphyry. The heat for this metamorphism may have been supplied during emplacement of the alaskite.

A second type of metamorphism consists of a white to dark gray, siliceous, flinty hornfels up to 500 ft. wide, which has formed in the Mesozoic clastic rocks along the southwest contact of the alaskite. The hornfels has been intruded and brecciated by fresh quartz monzonite porphyry dikes which establish a minimum age limit for the metamorphism. It consists primarily of quartz, sericite, chlorite, orthoclase, and epidote, with minor garnet and diopside in limy units and hornblende and diaspore in argillaceous units. Mineralogical banding preserves former bedding down to the scale of a thin section.

HYDROTHERMAL ALTERATION-MINERALIZATION

Alteration and sulfide minerals occur in consistent, well-defined assemblages at Silver Bell and are discussed together. The names used will be those summarized by Lowell and Guilbert (1970) for alteration zones in porphyry copper deposits. Although their paper treated alteration and mineralization zones separately, the sulfide minerals were discussed according to the alteration zone in which they occurred—an implicit recognition that silicate and sulfide minerals should be treated together as specific assemblages. The assemblages present in silicate rocks are biotite-potassic, in which chalcopyrite is the dominant sulfide; K-feldspar-potassic, in which chalcopyrite, molybdenite, and pyrite are all important phases; phyllic, in which pyrite is the dominant sulfide; and propylitic, in which pyrite is the only sulfide.

Alteration Assemblages

Rock type has a strong influence on both the type of alteration assemblage developed and the form in which the minerals occur. The potassic and propylitic alteration minerals occur largely as selective replacements of mafic minerals and plagioclase; thus, their distribution is very uniform in the dacite porphyry and in the quartz monzonite porphyry suite, but extremely erratic in the alaskite. Phyllic alteration occurs in all these rocks, but is best developed in the alaskite. Skarn assemblages are restricted to the Paleozoic carbonate rocks, and the alteration in the quartzites is limited to minor recrystallization. The occurrence of alteration minerals may also depend on rock type. Regardless of the alteration zone, the ratio of disseminated:vein-controlled alteration and sulfide minerals appears highest in the dacite porphyry, intermediate in the quartz monzonite porphyry, and lowest in the alaskite.

Potassic Assemblage. The potassic assemblage most closely associated with hypogene copper is centered on the elongate El Tiro quartz monzonite porphyry stock and consists of biotite-chalcopyrite ± quartz ± pyrite. Exposures of this assemblage are best preserved in the bottom of El Tiro pit. Biotite and sulfides occur both as disseminations and as thin veins or joint coatings; quartz is entirely confined to the veins. Hydrothermal biotite is identified petrographically by its fine grain size and euhedral to shreddy outline as compared to coarser euhedral phenocrysts. Some hydrothermal biotite has a distinct olive cast in contrast to the reddish brown phenocrysts, but shreddy, reddish brown biotite, although mostly disseminated, also occurs in veins. Hydrothermal biotite varies in abundance, averaging about 3 percent (all estimates are volume percent), and does not occur as vein envelopes.

The earliest potassic vein is a barren joint coated with hydrothermal biotite where the joint cuts a biotite or hornblende phenocryst and appears to grade into younger, equally rare, biotite-chalcopyrite veins. The most common potassic vein in the central portion of the El Tiro stock contains the assemblage quartz-biotite-chalcopyrite ± pyrite—in decreasing order of abundance—as a fissure filling and lacks replacement envelopes. These veins vary from 1/64 to 1/16 in. thick, have a random orientation, and are clearly more numerous where disseminated hydrothermal biotite is more abundant. Vein biotite is absent outside of areas averaging less than 0.2 percent Cu as chalcopyrite, regardless of rock type.

The quartz-biotite-chalcopyrite veins in the central portion of the El Tiro stock appear to grade into a thicker and slightly younger vein-type which contains the assemblage quartz-chalcopyrite ± pyrite. This vein, which is also confined to the stock, is the single most abundant copper-bearing vein in El Tiro pit; although it lacks biotite, a close relationship with the biotite-bearing veins is established by the paragenetic position, the presence of chalcopyrite, and the direct relationship between the amounts of chalcopyrite and hydrothermal biotite in the adjacent rock.

The sulfide content of the biotite-potassic assemblage is variable, but averages about 2 percent (volume). The disseminated:vein ratio is 1:1 in the central portion of the stock and appears to decrease to 1:3 near the contact. The pyrite: chalcopyrite ratio varies from 0.5:1 in the central portion of the stock to 2:1 near the contact. Disseminated sulfides are not aligned along joints and appear to have formed by replacement of the rock, often being confined to mafic minerals. Pyrite is subhedral and coarser than chalcopyrite, which is generally irregular in shape. Occasional rounded and embayed sulfide outlines, which might be interpreted as magmatic, are also common in veins. Based on these textures, the sulfides are considered to be of hydrothermal origin, not magmatic as suggested by Mauger (1966).

Hydrothermal biotite is not generally preserved in porphyry outcrops where strong supergene leaching has occurred. However, its presence in a large dike on the southwest crest of El Tiro pit, indicates that it occurs at elevations considerably above the bottom of the pit. Shreddy, disseminated biotite has also been observed in the Daisy stock at the north end of El Tiro pit, and in several porphyry dikes up to one mile south and west of El Tiro pit. The dike occurrences are similar in color to biotite phenocrysts and appear to replace former hornblende phenocrysts. The significance of these occurrences of potassic alteration outside the ore zone in El Tiro pit will be discussed later. Hydrothermal biotite has not been recognized in the monzonite porphyry dikes east of El Tiro pit.

A second potassic assemblage also occurs in the El Tiro stock. It consists of barren joints and quartz-molybdenite ± K-feldspar veins, with pink K-feldspar replacement envelopes and rare small areas of pervasive pink K-feldspar alteration (the term K-feldspar is used for pinkish, hydrothermal orthoclase). The quartz-molybdenite veins have straight, sharp borders, average about 1/4 in. wide, and are clearly fissure fillings. The replacement K-feldspar envelope is generally discontinuous and is never wider than the vein. The presence of molybdenite as thin, continuous seams anywhere within the vein suggests it is slightly younger than the quartz. Disseminated molybdenite either in veins or in the rock is rare. Perhaps 90 percent of these veins strike northeasterly and the larger veins cut the smaller veins.

Veins which contain only pink K-feldspar are rare, discontinuous, and less than 1/2 in. wide, with irregular and gradational walls. The veins are wider where they cut former feldspar phenocrysts, which are more susceptible to replacement than the quartz-orthoclase matrix. They appear to have expanded outward from joints and are of replacement origin. Biotite within the vein envelope is always chloritized. Disseminated chalcopyrite and pyrite are rarely observed in the central portion of the vein.

Alteration K-feldspar has the same general distribution as vein biotite, although K-feldspar is somewhat more widespread and the two minerals never occur together in the same vein. In addition, there is no obvious temporal coincidence between chalcopyrite and K-feldspar as is observed for chalcopyrite and biotite. Although the relationships are not entirely clear, K-feldspar appears to have formed after biotite—possibly overlapping the last stages of chalcopyrite deposition—and does not exceed 2 to 3 percent of the rock.

Vein-related K-feldspar is locally abundant as replacement envelopes along quartz veins in the eastern portion of quartz monzonite porphyry stock adjacent to skarns in the east end of El Tiro pit (referred to as the Imperial stock). These K-feldspar envelopes attack quartz and feldspar phenocrysts with equal intensity. Sulfides are absent in the veins, although they are abundant in the adjacent skarns. Similar quartz–K-feldspar veins with sulfides are present in the Daisy and North Silver Bell quartz monzonite porphyry stocks. Rare, small pods of massive pink K-feldspar, which replace plagioclase and quartz, are present along with epidote in the quartz monzonite porphyry dikes and stocks south and west of El Tiro pit, within and beyond the limits of the pyrite zone. The existence of small grains of disseminated malachite in leached sulfide cavities in the pods suggests the former presence of chalcopyrite. K-feldspar alteration is not observed in the monzonite porphyry dikes.

A weak, pervasive, sericite alteration, which occurs as a replacement of plagioclase phenocrysts, consumes up to 10 percent and averages 4 percent of all rocks in the area. This alteration is not related to rock type, sulfide mineral type, sulfide abundance, or surface weathering and is not part of the phyllic assemblage. The age of this weak sericite alteration is unknown, but its widespread distribution suggests a relationship to potassic and propylitic alteration.

Other minerals perhaps related to potassic alteration in the quartz monzonite porphyry include apatite, chlorite, and epidote. Apatite occurs as blocky grains associated with aggregates of shreddy biotite and sulfide. Chlorite is confined to former mafic sites. Epidote is rarely present adjacent to silicated carbonate rocks. Vein magnetite and bornite are extremely rare and anhydrite and gypsum are absent.

Potassic alteration in the dacite porphyry is most strongly developed adjacent to mineralized quartz monzonite porphyry stocks. The mineralogy is similar to that described above except that average abundances of alteration biotite are roughly twice those in the quartz monzonite porphyry. Approximately one mile northeast of the pit several joint coatings of chlorite-epidote-quartz-leached sulfide have been mapped in dacite porphyry. Chlorite has been recognized only as a replacement of pre-existing mafic minerals in the Silver Bell district, and presumably the vein occurrences represent altered vein biotite at considerable distances outside the pit.

The ratio of disseminated:vein sulfide in the dacite probably averages 2:1 adjacent to the porphyry stocks. Copper as chalcopyrite averages about 0.1 percent Cu, with a pyrite: chalcopyrite ratio of 4:1, which increases away from the porphyry stock. Sulfide textures in the dacite are similar to those in the quartz monzonite porphyry.

In addition to the potassic alteration, the dacite porphyry has been somewhat recrystallized adjacent to the mineralized quartz monzonite porphyry stocks. Recrystallization has resulted in the formation of a microcrystalline matrix of anhedral, blocky quartz and orthoclase grains which resembles silicification in hand specimen. Former quartz phenocrysts have been pseudomorphously recrystallized to a mosaic of interlocking quartz grains. This type of recrystallization, which appears to be confined to potassic-altered zones adjacent to the porphyry stocks, suggests that a hydrothermal fluid and heat were required for the textural modification.

Potassic alteration in the alaskite is very weak and erratically distributed. Within the pit adjacent to the El Tiro stock, traces of hydrothermal vein biotite and K-feldspar after plagioclase were observed in thin section. Erratic occurrences of hydrothermal biotite replacing igneous biotite have also been observed up to 4,000 ft. from the pit. Equally erratic and rare zones of massive pink K-feldspar up to 50 ft. across pervasively replace most pre-existing biotite, plagioclase, and quartz and often contain disseminated epidote. Structural control of the K-feldspar alteration is indicated by its location along the strike of porphyry dikes or well-defined veins. The co-occurrence of K-feldspar and epidote suggests that K-feldspar potassic and propylitic alteration may be time-equivalent assemblages.

Sulfide mineralization associated with potassic alteration in the alaskite is pyritic and does not exceed 1 percent total sulfides. The ratio of pyrite:chalcopyrite generally exceeds 10:1, even adjacent to the El Tiro stock, and sulfides are largely disseminated. The total volume of potassic-related alteration and sulfide mineralization in the alaskite is insignificant and difficult to detect by field mapping.

Propylitic Assemblage. The propylitic assemblage consists of epidote-chlorite ± calcite ± albite ± pyrite and is developed in areas peripheral to potassic alteration. Propylitic alteration is well developed in syenodiorite porphyry dikes east of El Tiro pit. Epidote (2–8%) is mostly confined to sites of former mafic phenocrysts (pyroxene?), along with 1–10 percent chlorite, and minor actinolite and calcite. Chlorite is in part disseminated and appears to be richer in magnesium in the mafic sites. Sericite occurs as a widespread and often pervasive alteration of plagioclase phenocrysts. Similar propylitic alteration is also present in the monzonite porphyry dikes, except that actinolite is absent and epidote is erratic. Pyrite is often absent from the dikes, even though it is present in the adjacent dacite. Propylitic minerals are rare in the quartz monzonite porphyries south and west of El Tiro pit.

The distribution of epidote in the dacite porphyry is

extremely pervasive and is an excellent field guide for mapping propylitic alteration. It forms from 1 to 10 percent of the rock as thin veins, as replacements of limestone clasts near El Tiro pit, and as replacements of plagioclase phenocrysts. The outer limit of epidote is sharp and varies from 500 to 1,500 ft. beyond the outer limit of pyrite. Where thin veins cut the rock, epidote selectively replaces the veinward side of adjacent plagioclase phenocrysts. Chlorite varies from trace to 5 percent, always as a replacement of former biotite phenocrysts. Calcite varies from 0 to 7 percent as a replacement of plagioclase phenocrysts. Pyrite occurs as a thin coating on east-striking joints and as disseminated grains. Within the propylitic zone the ratio of disseminated: joint-controlled pyrite varies from 1:1 near El Tiro pit to 1:20 near the edge of the pyrite zone. The total sulfide content is 2 to 3 percent near the pit and gradually falls to the east. The chemical aspects of propylitic alteration in the dacite porphyry have been studied by Ballantyne (1975).

Recognizable propylitic alteration is very erratic in the alaskite, presumably due to the low mafic and plagioclase content. Rare occurrences of chlorite occur in the pyrite zone south and west of El Tiro pit. Several isolated pods of massive epidote and albite occur along the strike of porphyry dikes outside the pyrite zone about 1 mile west of El Tiro pit. In this general area small occurrences of disseminated and vein epidote with erratic chlorite coincide with a north-striking zone of quartz veins up to 10 ft. thick, in which evidence of sulfide mineralization is absent. The recognition of epidote zoning in the alaskite requires field mapping, as its distribution is too erratic to be determined microscopically.

Phyllic Assemblage. The phyllic assemblage consists of quartz-sericite-pyrite; chalcopyrite is absent. Virtually all occurrences are vein controlled, with a central fissure filling of quartz-pyrite bordered by a replacement envelope of sericite. Areas of pervasive sericite are rare as adjacent replacement envelopes do not generally overlap. Pyrite is coarse grained and forms up to 50 percent of the vein. Pyrite may or may not be present in the adjacent sericite envelopes, although the width of the envelope is often proportional to the abundance of pyrite in the vein. The veins vary up to 1 ft. wide, are widest in the alaskite, and are strongly confined to a northeast strike. Northwest-striking veins are present, but are usually smaller than and cut by northeast-striking veins. Phyllic assemblage veins may grade into earlier quartz-molybdenite veins in which sericite is absent. Phyllic assemblage veins are much less abundant than potassic assemblage veins but contribute over half of the total sulfide in the pit due to their larger size. Within the areas of strongest phyllic assemblage alteration, the total sulfide content by volume averages 5 to 7 percent.

Skarn Assemblage. Skarn refers to the lime-silicate alteration minerals developed in the Paleozoic limestones. The mineralogy of the El Tiro skarn has been briefly studied by Stewart (1912), Buseck (1962), and Merz (1967), and that of the Atlas mine skarn by Agenbroad (1962). Galey (1976) has studied the paragenesis of various vein assemblages in the skarn.

Andradite garnet is the most abundant skarn mineral. Refractive index measurements by Buseck (1962) suggest pure andradite, although a single analysis by Stewart (1912) suggests up to 37 percent grossularite. Megascopically, both brown and green garnets have been recognized by Galey (1976), although the details of their distribution are still unclear. Garnet appears to be more abundant adjacent to porphyry dikes; it is not confined to the contact of the Imperial stock, nor is it always present along porphyry-skarn contacts. Occasional garnet veins in marble attest that its origin is from a hydrothermal fluid and not from isochemical metamorphism.

Diopside, actinolite, tremolite, quartz, and wollastonite are also abundant in the skarn and, although their abundance varies inversely with garnet, they are all spatially coextensive. Lesser amounts of idocrase are present and Agenbroad (1962) has recognized hedenbergite in the Atlas mine. Serpentine occurs most commonly in veins with pyrite cores and discontinuous magnetite borders which occasionally cut the earlier anhydrous silicates. Calcite is present in all skarn assemblages except massive garnet. Marble is absent adjacent to the El Tiro stock, but occurs in contact with and increases uniformly away from the Imperial stock. Marble occurs as highly irregular masses which are converted to skarn by envelopes of garnet and other silicates that expand outward from sulfide-bearing joints. The contacts between blocks of marble and skarn are generally sharp, but are not obvious *loci* of copper mineralization. The various skarn minerals extend at least 1,000 ft. east of the Imperial stock, although their outer limit has not been defined. Endoskarn is so rare as to be considered absent.

Chalcopyrite and pyrite occur as disseminated replacements of earlier Fe-rich skarn silicates; as thin, discontinuous veins—with or without quartz; and as massive sulfide pods with pyrite. The pyrite:chalcopyrite ratio increases to the east from the Imperial stock. Chalcopyrite appears to replace brown garnet, although Buseck (1962) shows several photomicrographs of chalcopyrite being rimmed by magnetite where other silicates are present. Magnetite occurs in small amounts throughout the skarn. Hematite is locally abundant in marble as a hypogene replacement of earlier sulfides. Minor pyrrhotite is also present, although its space-time position is still unknown. Agenbroad (1962) noted that sphalerite is more abundant in areas of mixed garnet and marble than elsewhere in the Atlas mine and this relationship may also hold in El Tiro pit.

Paragenesis

The paragenesis of the various alteration and sulfide minerals has been determined from detailed studies of intersecting veins, mostly in the center of El Tiro pit. This work is summarized in Figure 24.4, along with additional information on the vein geology. The consistent time overlap of most minerals suggests a continuous hydrothermal event during which the chemistry and temperature of the ore fluids were slowly but irreversibly changing. Time overlap of the various minerals results in gradational vein assemblages as discussed earlier; occasionally, early veins have localized minerals of much later assemblages. Figure 24.4 shows that the biotite-potassic assemblage, in which most of the chalcopyrite occurs, is the earliest hydrothermal event. It was followed with

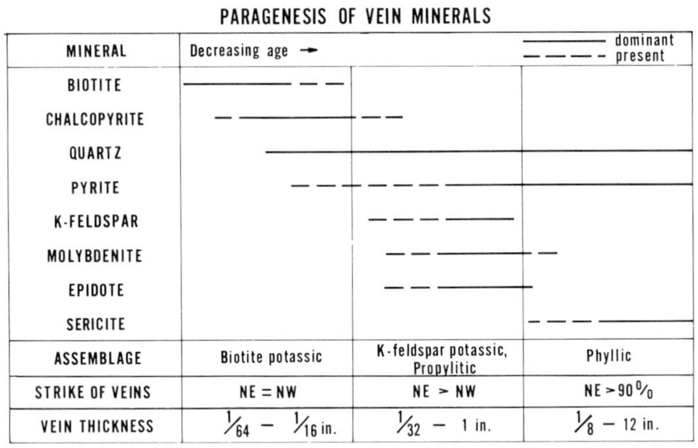

Figure 24.4. Paragenesis of alteration and sulfide minerals, El Tiro area

only minor overlap by the K-feldspar-potassic assemblage, which coincides with an abrupt increase in abundance of quartz-molybdenite veins. Epidote appears to coincide with K-feldspar in time, although these two minerals are not everywhere coextensive so there is some uncertainty in the paragenesis. Epidote and calcite coexist with potassic alteration where potassic and propylitic zones overlap or where potassic alteration overlaps skarn, but these minerals are not considered part of the potassic assemblage. The vein-controlled phyllic assemblage, where the bulk of the pyrite occurs, is clearly the latest of the hydrothermal events and may overlap with the formation of barren quartz veins which are common throughout the pit.

The age of the skarn assemblage with respect to other hydrothermal assemblages is not well established. Textural data suggest that garnet may largely predate chalcopyrite and, thus, may be one of the earliest hydrothermal minerals, possibly equivalent to vein biotite. Quartz veins with K-feldspar replacement envelopes occur in the Imperial stock adjacent to the skarn and extend irregularly into the skarn without envelopes. These veins appear to cut some areas of massive brown garnet. The abundance of pyrite relative to chalcopyrite in serpentine veins and the replacement of chalcopyrite by hematite suggest that serpentine and hematite, although not part of the same assemblage, may be time equivalent with the phyllic assemblage. Additional paragenetic data concerning the skarns are lacking at the present time.

The chemical evolution of the system was accompanied by a structural evolution. Figure 24.4 shows that the size of the veins—both fissure-filling material and replacement envelopes—increases with time. Structural patterns also appear to be time dependent. Although statistical studies have not been made, early biotite-potassic veins appear somewhat randomly oriented, with northwest strikes fully as abundant as northeast strikes. The majority of the later K-feldspar-potassic and phyllic veins strike northeasterly.

Zoning

The total zone of hydrothermal alteration shown on Figure 24.5 covers 4.9 square miles. Coincident with this zone is a slightly smaller zone of pyritic mineralization which covers 3.3 square miles. Central to these zones are several areas containing biotite and K-feldspar veins which coincide with centers of hypogene copper mineralization and contacts of quartz monzonite porphyry stocks. Veins which contain K-feldspar are more widespread than biotite veins and their mineralogy varies with distance from the zoning center. Within and closely adjacent to the El Tiro stock K-feldspar occurs both as veins and disseminated replacements of the porphyry and as replacement envelopes along quartz-molybdenite veins. Elsewhere in the El Tiro area K-feldspar occurs in small, erratically distributed zones which usually contain disseminated chalcopyrite and epidote and no molybdenite. Surrounding the potassic vein zones is a much larger zone of weak and often erratically disseminated biotite and K-feldspar.

The potassic zone is surrounded by a propylitic zone which displays good continuity in the dacite porphyry and extreme discontinuity in the alaskite. The propylitic zone is best defined as the inner and outer limit of epidote, and there is some overlap with irregular occurrences of potassic alteration. This zone is best developed in the dacite porphyry, where it varies from 1,000 to 3,000 ft. wide. The distribution of epidote in the alaskite relative to the center of copper mineralization, although far more erratic, is spatially similar to epidote in the dacite porphyry. In both rocks epidote extends at least 1,000 ft. farther from this center than any visible sulfide and it is clearly more abundant adjacent to areas of altered limestone. Disseminated calcite alteration is generally confined to areas outside the pyrite zone. Within the epidote zone it forms less than 2 percent of the rock, but beyond the epidote zone its abundance abruptly increases to 4 to 7 percent. Its greater abundance to the east of the El Tiro skarns as compared to the North Silver Bell area suggests that the components were partially derived from the replaced limestones in El Tiro pit. Ballantyne (1975) has defined a chlorite-calcite zone roughly 3,000 ft. wide outside the epidote zone in a single petrographic traverse east of the North Silver Bell stock. The existence of this zone of the propylitic assemblage is a distinct possibility, but, as chlorite and calcite occur throughout the Silver Bell Mountains, the outer limit of hydrothermal zoning has not everywhere been defined.

The distribution of phyllic alteration is asymmetric, being largely confined to the alaskite adjacent to the El Tiro and Daisy stocks. It extends roughly 1,000 to 1,500 ft. west of this contact in 4 well-defined vein swarms and east of this contact for a short distance. Similar veining does not occur in the dacite porphyry or Imperial stock east of the center of copper mineralization. Several smaller phyllic zones are erratically scattered throughout the El Tiro area. The overall distribution of phyllic alteration is asymmetric with respect to other alteration zones and it occurs within, not at the outer edge of, the overall potassic zone. It appears to follow highly permeable structures which developed later in the evolution of the system. The pervasive, weak, disseminated sericite is not part of the phyllic assemblage. In addition, the outline of pyrite mineralization is not equivalent to an outline of phyllic alteration, because pyrite is also an integral part

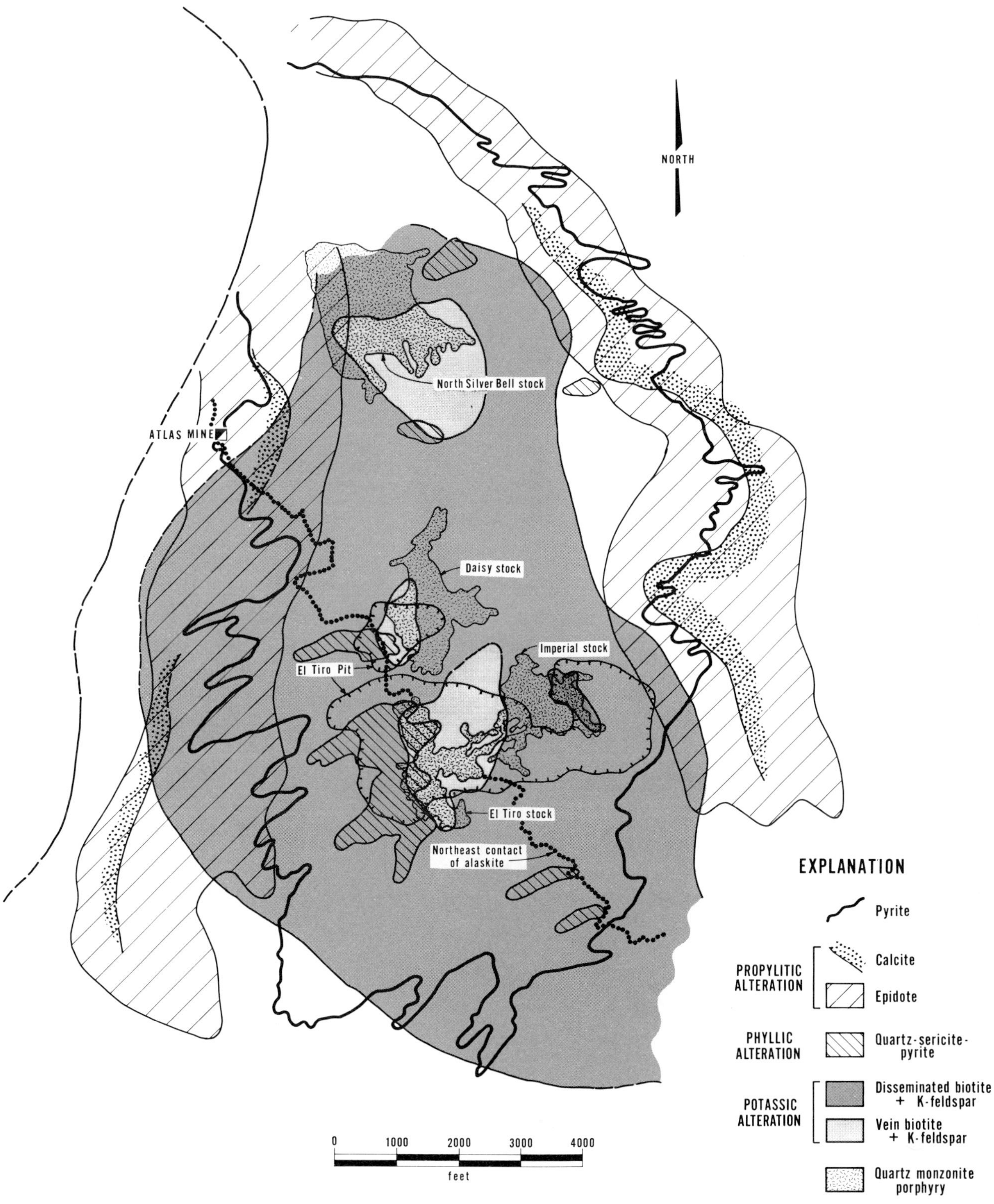

Figure 24.5. Alteration zones in the El Tiro area. Southwest of the alaskite contact potassic and propylitic assemblages are poorly developed and discontinuous, and zone boundaries are drawn on relatively few data points.

of other, earlier assemblages. The overall extent of phyllic alteration at Silver Bell is clearly less than had been previously thought.

Zoning of sulfide mineralization in the El Tiro area follows the general pattern seen in porphyry copper deposits (Lowell and Guilbert, 1970). Within the El Tiro and North Silver Bell stocks the pyrite:chalcopyrite ratio is less than 3:1 and it increases outward to greater than 50:1 in the propylitic zone. Hypogene copper grades in silicate rocks are centered on the El Tiro, Daisy, and North Silver Bell stocks and in dikes near the contact of the Imperial stock and decrease rapidly outward as shown on Figure 24.6. The distribution of molybdenum at the +25 ppm contour is very similar to the distribution of 0.1 percent Cu. Highest Mo values occur as

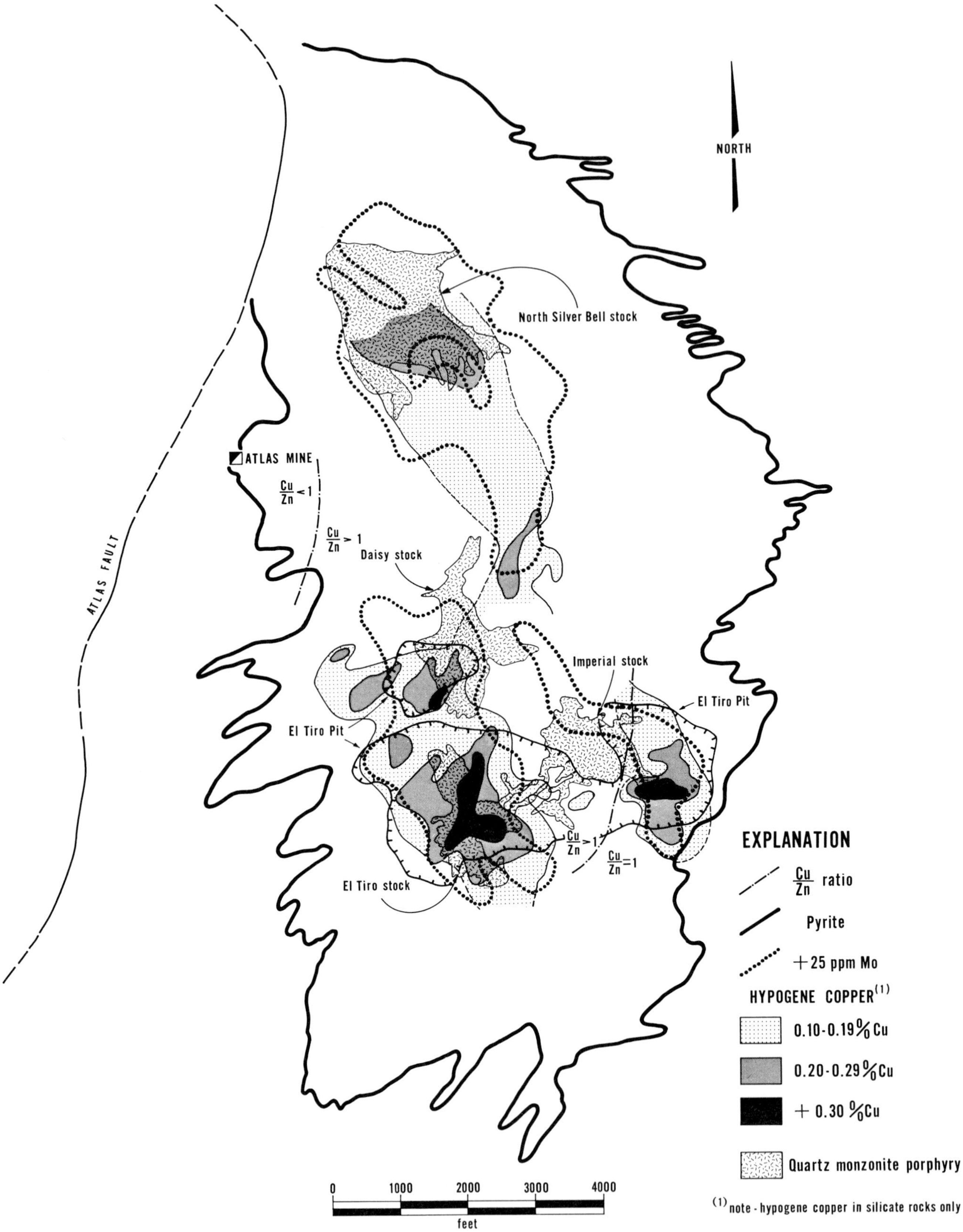

Figure 24.6. Mineralization zones in the El Tiro area

a halo around areas of highest copper and vein biotite and coincide with areas of most abundant vein-related K-feldspar. Zinc is most abundant in the skarns outside the 0.5 percent Cu contour line. The disseminated:vein ratio for sulfides is greatest in the areas of highest-grade chalcopyrite (2:1) and decreases outward with discontinuities at the dacite and the alaskite contacts. Total sulfide contents are generally highest where the phyllic assemblage is superimposed on the potassic assemblage in areas adjacent to, but not coincident with, areas of highest-grade hypogene copper mineralization.

A late assemblage of resinous sphalerite-galena-flourite-barite-calcite-quartz occurs locally throughout the El Tiro area. Its age, Laramide or younger, is uncertain.

On a district scale skarn zones generally occur within the potassic zone. Where intersected by the propylitic zone southeast of El Tiro pit, the limestones are marbleized—a phenomenon which may be related to emplacement of the dacite rather than to hydrothermal alteration. Epidote is mostly absent in the skarn adjacent to El Tiro pit, although it is present in the skarn at the Atlas mine (Agenbroad, 1962). Hydrothermal mineral zoning in the copper-bearing skarn adjacent to and in El Tiro pit has been determined by averaging visually determined mineral abundances in the 250-ft.-thick sulfide zone for 200 diamond drill holes, and the results are shown on Figure 24.7. On the scale of an individual mine bench the patterns are far more irregular, due to overprinting of assemblages of different ages and to fault offsets which juxtapose carbonate rocks of different compositions. Nevertheless, Figure 24.7*a* shows that garnet is generally most abundant adjacent to the Imperial stock. Its occasional distribution in linear patterns not generally parallel to dike trends may reflect fault control. Figure 24.7*b* shows the distribution of residual calcite, which is a reasonable measure of the degree of silication in the carbonate host rocks. The abundance of calcite clearly and very intricately mirrors the shape of the Imperial stock. Figure 24.7*c* shows that hypogene copper is also strongly zoned around the contact of the Imperial stock. In cross section (see Fig. 24.3) higher-grade copper zones are interpreted to dip easterly following the regional dip of the Paleozoic section. The distribution of magnetite is not shown, but it appears to be more abundant in the intermediate and outer portions of the skarn than adjacent to the Imperial stock. The distribution of other silicate alteration minerals and pyrite in the skarn is too erratic to yield uniform zoning patterns over the entire thickness of the sulfide zone.

The data in Figure 24.7 strongly suggest that material added to the carbonate rocks was derived from or moved outward from the Imperial stock. It is interesting that this stock is almost completely barren of sulfide mineralization—generally averaging 0.01 to 0.02 percent Cu—and, with the exception of some quartz-K-feldspar veins along the east contact, is unaltered. Zoning patterns for garnet and copper indicate that fluids moved east and south into the skarns from the Imperial stock. However, on a more district-wide scale, sphalerite zoning appears centered on the El Tiro stock, with sphalerite:chalcopyrite ratios increasing outward. These data permit the interpretation that the source of the materials was the inferred, north-striking structure which passes through the El Tiro stock and that hydrothermal fluids passing through the Imperial stock retained a chemistry dominated by district-scale zoning patterns, rather than by individual intrusive centers.

Highest-grade chalcopyrite mineralization and coincident areas of strong biotite-potassic alteration are unrelated to phyllic alteration. This characteristic is emphasized by the asymmetry of the phyllic zone relative to the centers of copper mineralization, by the widespread (although erratic) occurrence of potassic alteration outside the phyllic zone, and by the paragenesis of the phyllic assemblage, which formed after the deposition of chalcopyrite. The late time of paragenesis of the phyllic alteration has been increasingly recognized in studies of porphyry copper deposits and suggests formation during cooling and decreasing pH of the hydrothermal system; this mechanism is consistent with results of experimental work by Hemley and Jones (1964). The asymmetric distribution of phyllic alteration in the El Tiro area may have resulted from the development of larger, more continuous structures in the alaskite as compared to other rocks as time progressed. Similar asymmetry was noted at Bingham Canyon by Moore and Nash (1974). Zoning diagrams published by Lowell and Guilbert (1970) and theoretical discussions by Rose (1970), implying that the transition between the potassic and phyllic zones was a chemical boundary which controlled ore deposition, need to be modified with respect to time variations of these zones. The boundary between the potassic and phyllic zones did not influence hypogene or deposition in the El Tiro area.

Vertical zoning of alteration or mineralization has not been sufficiently well exposed to reveal well-defined patterns. A 1,550-ft. hole drilled from the bottom of El Tiro pit in the western portion of the porphyry stock revealed decreasing alteration strength at depth, with grades uniformly decreasing from 0.3 percent Cu at the top to 0.06 percent Cu at the bottom. A 2,564-ft. hole drilled in the Imperial skarns within the 0.5 percent Cu contour cut an underlying dacite sill and, under that, more altered limestone; both averaged 0.15 percent Cu. These data suggest that the copper grades decrease with increasing depth and that current exposures in the El Tiro area are relatively deep in the porphyry copper system. Stratigraphic reconstructions place the surface roughly 6,000 ft. above current exposures at the time of mineralization. Drilling has shown that alteration and submarginal mineralization extend at least 2,500 ft. below the surface and suggests that the total vertical extent of mineralization, if it reached the Laramide surface, approached 10,000 ft.

Both the overall zone of hydrothermal alteration and all sulfide and metal zones are elongate in a northerly direction. They are generally parallel to and bisected by a line approximating the position of the concealed structure described earlier which was inferred to have controlled the alignment and elongation of the quartz monzonite porphyry stocks. It is of interest, however, that the aggregate area of all four quartz monzonite porphyry stocks is 0.3 square miles, equivalent to only 6.3 percent of the total alteration zone. Addition of the numerous—but relatively thin—porphyry dikes would not significantly change this figure. Fluid inclusion studies by Ballantyne (1979) in the dacite adjacent to the North Silver Bell stock indicate that a temperature of 278°C was attained 1.5 miles to the northeast. Comparison with the convective cooling model calculated by Cathles (1977)—using a 1.4-km-wide pluton, a depth of 2.3 km, and a permeability of 0.25 millidarcies (reasonable estimates for the North Silver Bell stock)—suggests that temperatures should not have risen above 100°C at a distance of 1.5 miles. Ballantyne has suggested that the unusually large thermal aureole resulted from outward transport of heat by the numerous porphyry dikes in this area. This interpretation may provide an explanation for the well-developed propylitic zone east and west of El

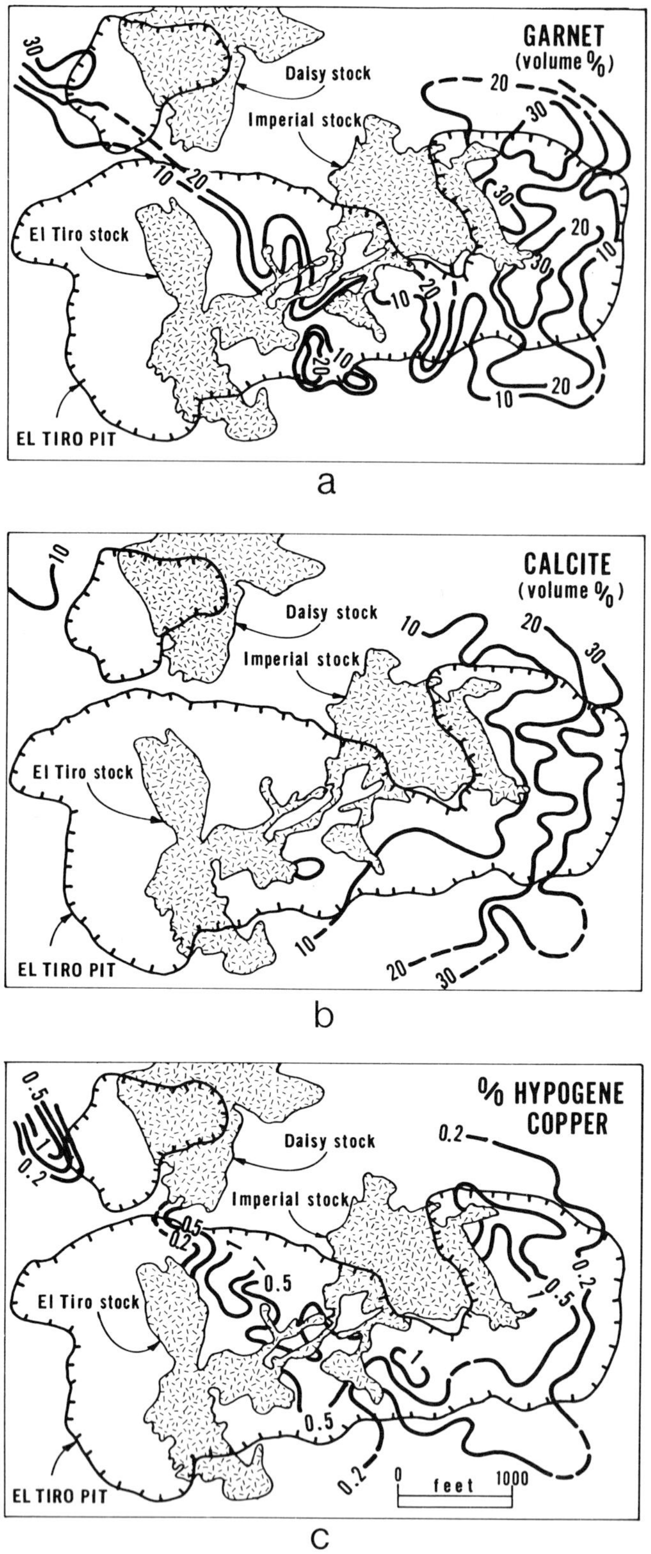

Figure 24.7. Zoning of (*a*) garnet, (*b*) calcite, and (*c*) hypogene copper in skarn in El Tiro pit

Tiro pit which fails to obviously wrap around the southern end of the area; the circulation of the hydrothermal fluid would have been largely in a northeast-southwest direction, parallel to the porphyry dikes.

A possible alternative explanation for the apparently large size of the alteration zones compared to the area of exposed porphyry is that the stocks are apophyses above a single, larger pluton concealed at shallow depth. Although the individual stocks may represent local centers of alteration and mineralization, the zoning pattern for the greater El Tiro area reflects a more district-wide control, illustrated by the large size of the alteration zones as compared to the area of intrusive porphyry. It may also be important that the strongest potassic alteration partly coincides with what may be a low-grade hypogene copper core zone between the El Tiro, Imperial, and Daisy stocks. Finally, the porphyry dikes on Figure 24.2 appear to be fed by a deeper source in that most of them do not connect with the porphyry stocks at the present level of erosion.

The spatial relationship of copper and molybdenum to the El Tiro, Daisy, and North Silver Bell stocks shown on Figure 24.6 is sufficiently close to establish a genetic tie and suggests that the metals were magmatically derived. Had the metals been leached from the adjacent wall rocks by a hot, convecting groundwater cell it is likely that all porphyry stocks would be equally well mineralized. That all porphyry stocks are well mineralized is clearly not the case, as the Imperial stock is virtually barren, averaging overall less than 0.05 percent Cu. In addition, the porphyry stocks south of El Tiro pit are equally unmineralized. Halite-bearing fluid inclusions observed by Nash (1976) indicate that the hydrothermal fluid contained in excess of 25 percent NaCl at one time in its evolution and was probably an efficient complexer of copper.

SUPERGENE ENRICHMENT

The majority of the ore mined in the El Tiro area was derived from a flat-lying, tabular chalcocite blanket which averaged roughly 200 ft. thick at a 0.4 percent Cu cutoff. The top of the chalcocite blanket occurs in sharp contact with the overlying leached capping which, although irregular in detail, is generally conformable in shape to the surface topography. The leached capping is roughly 100 ft. thick and averages about 0.03 percent Cu. The relatively efficient leaching of copper from the capping was undoubtedly due to the overprint of a phyllic assemblage which contained abundant pyrite on a pre-existing potassic assemblage. The mineralogy of the various iron oxide minerals in the capping was studied by Loghry (1972), who confirmed the presence of hematite, goethite, and jarosite. Richard and Courtright (1966) used quantitative studies of the indigenous, maroon to black, hematite-rich limonites as a guide to the presence of chalcocite in the underlying sulfide zone. Copper oxide minerals are generally more common in areas peripheral to the chalcocite blanket; here supergene alteration was insufficient to destroy primary rock-forming minerals, and copper was precipitated on the various feldspars. Traces of chrysocolla, malachite, tenorite, cuprite, native copper, chalcanthite, and sulfides have also been observed in the leached capping over the chalcocite blanket. Chrysocolla is relatively most abundant at the surface, in contrast to cuprite, native copper, and chalcanthite, which are confined to the base of the capping.

The distribution of the chalcocite blanket in the North Silver Bell areas is not discussed, as it is everywhere less than 100 ft. thick, quite discontinuous, and partially oxidized.

Alteration in the capping and in the chalcocite blanket is generally pervasive and strong. All feldspars and mafic minerals have been altered to a variably-birefringent, fine-grained mica, loosely referred to as sericite. Some of this mica may be the "illite" or "hydromica" which Kerr (1951) described as having formed from earlier alteration minerals rather than from igneous minerals. A second, equally common mineral, mostly confined to the feldspars, is brownish, translucent, and poorly crystallized and may be a variety of montmorillonite. Smaller amounts of kaolinite are also present. Although studies of this alteration are incomplete, it appears unrelated to hypogene sulfide assemblages and is not obviously zoned away from specific sulfide veins. In addition, it is confined to areas of higher-grade chalcocite enrichment and the overlying leached capping and weakens with increasing depth in the chalcocite blanket. In some areas the lower limit of the pervasive alteration rises outward from the center of the pit, approximating the shape of a bowl. The overall geometry, close association with the chalcocite blanket, and lack of relationship to hypogene sulfide assemblages or abundances suggest that this pervasive alteration is of supergene origin. In addition to sericite, alunite is most abundant near the top of the leached capping, jarosite is most abundant near the base of the capping, and nontronite is most abundant in the upper part of the chalcocite blanket. These minerals are generally confined to veins and are considered to be entirely of supergene origin.

Chalcocite occurs as a pervasive replacement of disseminated and vein chalcopyrite and, to a lesser extent, vein pyrite. Although detailed microscopic studies are lacking, digenite and covellite are relatively uncommon. The grade of the blanket decreases irregularly from top to bottom and toward the edges. The chalcocite blanket is interpreted to have formed during a period when the rate of leaching of copper sulfides above the water table and replacement of chalcopyrite below the water table by chalcocite was equal to or greater than the rate of erosion.

The distribution of chalcocite at a 0.6 percent Cu cutoff closely coincides with the area of +0.1 percent hypogene Cu as shown on Figure 24.8. Although some of the higher-grade chalcocite follows increased hypogene grades, in detail the distribution of chalcocite appears to reflect control by northeast-striking structures. Note that the shape of the pit only generally follows the shape of the supergene copper contours. Figure 24.9, a typical cross-section through the southern portion of the chalcocite blanket, illustrates the importance of the hypogene phyllic alteration overprint to the development of economic grades of chalcocite. The distribution of grades in the chalcocite blanket is relatively uniform and does not reflect the grade of the underlying hypogene mineralization. Note that the portion of the chalcocite blanket which is ore, shown along the bottom of the graph, is offset west of the center of hypogene copper mineralization. Note also that the sharp drop in the ratio of total:non-sulfide copper coincides with the eastern limit of phyllic alteration. A low ratio means the chalcocite blanket was partly oxidized. Thus, even though mineable grades of copper in the chalcocite blanket extend east of the orebody, the recoverable sulfide component of the chalcocite blanket was reduced below economic grades by oxidation. These relationships establish the importance of the overprint phyllic alteration assemblage, with its relatively high pyrite content, from which sulfuric acid was derived to leach the oxidizing mineralization. The thin, partly oxidized, poorly developed chalcocite blanket below incompletely leached outcrops in the North Silver Bell area also resulted from the relative absence of phyllic alteration.

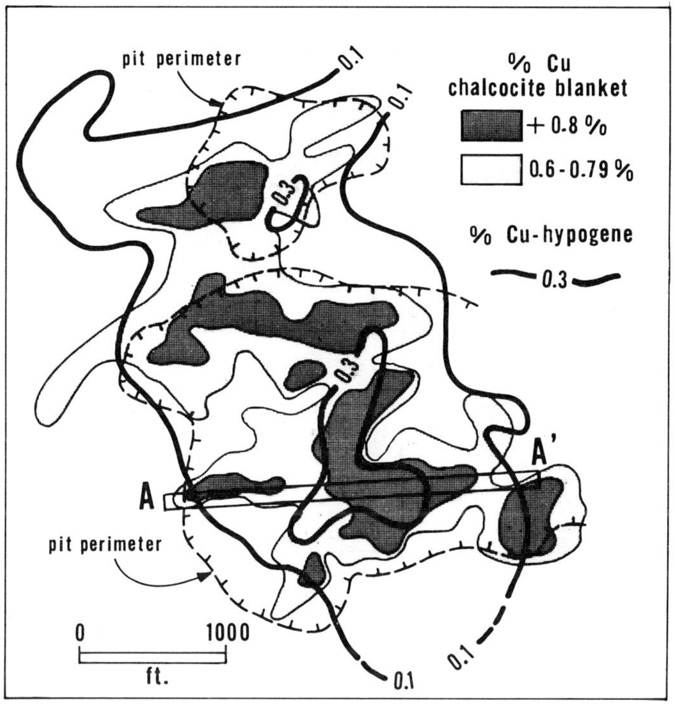

Figure 24.8. Distribution of hypogene and supergene copper in the area of the El Tiro chalcocite blanket

Figure 24.10 shows the distribution of the chalcocite blanket at +50 ft. thickness in the Daisy pit and +100 ft. thickness in El Tiro pit. The close relationship shown between thickness of the blanket and the shape of the pit serves to emphasize that tonnage is equally as important as grade in the definition of an orebody.

Chalcocite enrichment in the Imperial skarns is insignificant because the presence of calcite quickly neutralized the acid generated by the oxidizing sulfides. As a result, copper derived from the oxidation of chalcopyrite was rapidly fixed, usually as malachite. However, the total copper content (at a cutoff of 70.4% Cu) in the oxidized zone averages 1.02 percent Cu, as compared to the sulfide zone, where averages are 0.79 percent Cu. These values suggest that supergene enrichment of copper in some form has occurred in the oxidized zone. The enriched copper may now occur as chrysocolla. Statistical studies of over 100 drill holes show that chrysocolla is most abundant at the surface, where it contains 40 percent of the total non-sulfide copper; it then decreases

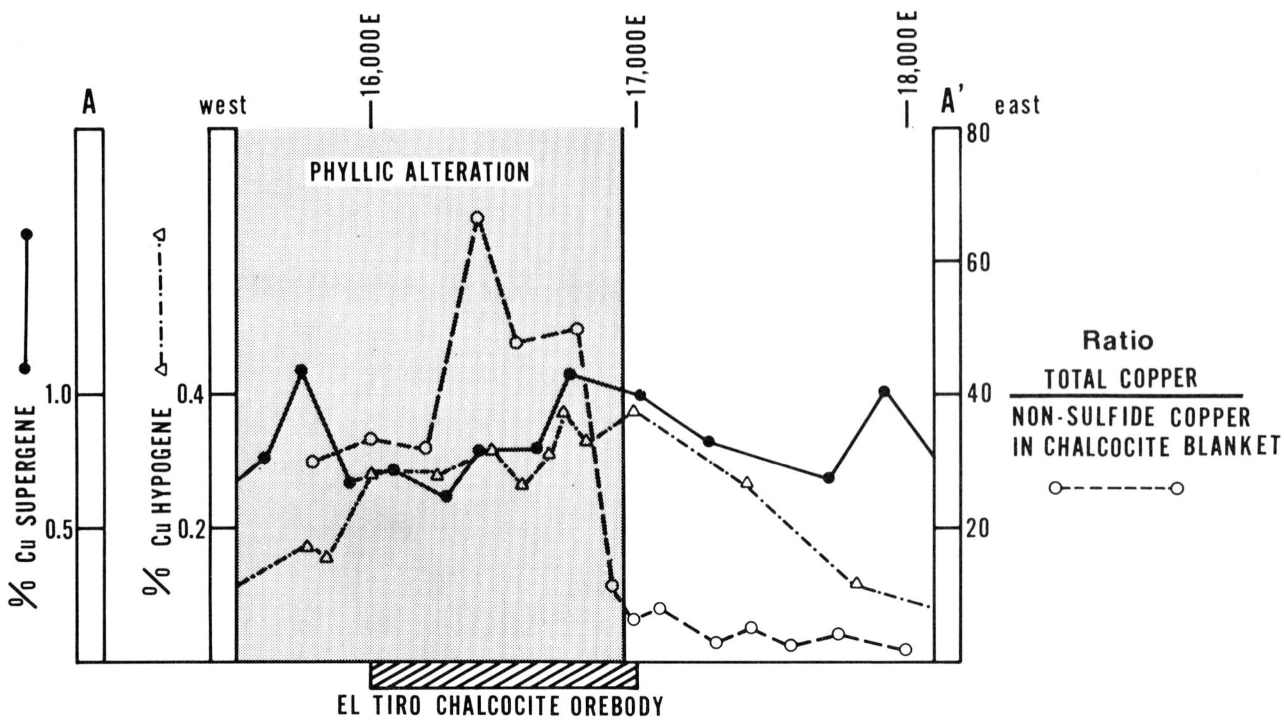

Figure 24.9. Assay cross section through the El Tiro chalcocite blanket (see Fig. 24.8 for location)

progressively to the base of the oxidized zone. This distribution does not correlate well with an increase in abundance of other copper minerals with depth, so the distribution of chrysocolla is not due simply to an in-place breakdown of a pre-existing copper mineral. Supergene enrichment is generally thought to occur only in non-reactive rocks where the pH of groundwater can be kept below 5.3, the hydrolysis point of copper. In the Imperial area supergene sulfide enrichment has been prevented by the relatively alkaline character of the groundwater. However, copper liberated by the breakdown of copper minerals at the surface has apparently moved limited distances near the surface of the oxide zone where it has been fixed as chrysocolla.

The present chalcocite blanket at Silver Bell has been inferred by several writers to have formed during the mid-Tertiary (Livingston et al., 1968; Lowell, 1974) prior to about 25 m.y. These inferences are based on the presence of weakly pyritized clasts of propylitized porphyritic rocks in a conglomerate 5 miles east of Oxide pit which is overlain by an andesite flow dated at 27.9 m.y. Detailed mapping in this area indicates that the clasts are all of local origin and contain no evidence of the former presence or absence of a chalcocite blanket in the Silver Bell district prior to 28 m.y. ago. The clasts do indicate that mineralization was exposed at this time, but proof of enrichment is lacking.

Of particular interest is a small deposit of copper oxide and chalcocite located in a low area 1,500 feet west of Oxide pit (see Fig. 24.1) and referred to as the West Oxide deposit. Host rocks are weakly pyritized alaskite, quartz monzonite porphyry, and post-mineral andesite dikes which may correlate with the 27.9 m.y. flows. Figure 24.11 shows that the thickness of +0.40 percent Cu mineralization is greatest along the post-mineral dikes and thins away from them. The mineralization is dominantly chalcocite northeast of the dikes and oxide copper southwest of the dikes. The evidence plainly suggests that the copper in this area was leached from the strongly altered area northeast of the deposit and was transported in solution downslope, where flow was impeded by the andesite dikes. Clearly, the andesite dikes were emplaced prior to the formation of the chalcocite blanket in the adjacent wall rocks. This blanket is part of a lower-grade, but

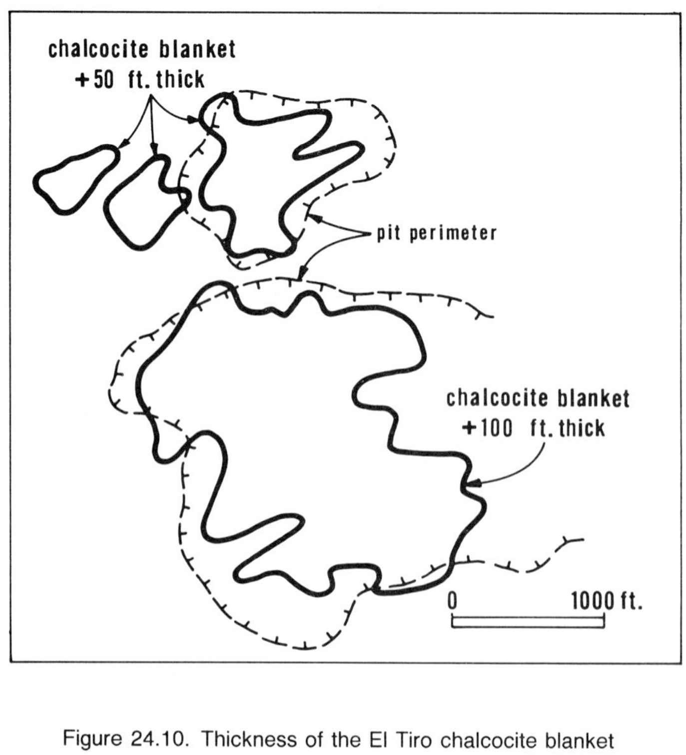

Figure 24.10. Thickness of the El Tiro chalcocite blanket

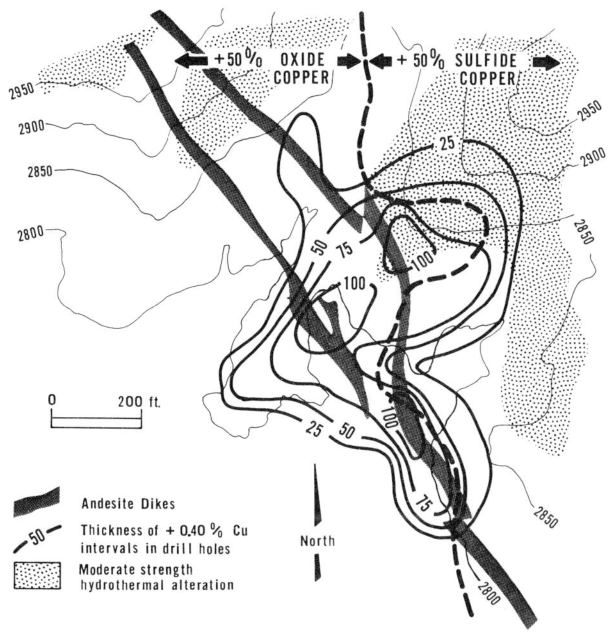

Figure 24.11. Geologic map of the West Oxide deposit

essentially continuous, blanket which extends into Oxide pit. Presumably both the present chalcocite blanket in Oxide pit and the blanket in El Tiro pit formed more recently than the andesite dikes, or within the last 28 m.y.

Ransome (1919) noted that the shapes of the present topography and water table are unrelated to the top of the chalcocite blankets at Ray and Miami, Arizona. He believed that this condition resulted from the development of a chalcocite blanket prior to deposition of the overlying, post-mineral dacite in a terrain where the topography was different from modern topography. The Silver Bell district, on the other hand, provides good examples of the conformable shape of the present topography and the top of the chalcocite blanket. The upper limit of chalcocite probably marks the top of a former water table which has now withdrawn to deeper levels under the influence of a drier climate and/or uplift. The conformable relationship suggests that the formation of the chalcocite blanket is related to the development of the present topographic profile.

Since an absolute date on the supergene enrichment is lacking, an attempt was made to estimate an age based on erosion rates, as follows:

1. The amount of copper added to pre-existing hypogene protore to form the present chalcocite blanket is:

$$\text{grade of chalcocite blanket} - \text{grade of protore} = \begin{matrix}\text{percent copper}\\ \text{added to protore}\end{matrix}$$

$$0.80\%\ \text{Cu} - 0.25\%\ \text{Cu} = .55\%\ \text{Cu}$$

2. The grade of protore which became available to the chalcocite blanket during leaching must be reduced by the grade of copper left in the leached capping as follows:

$$\text{grade of protore} - \text{grade of leached capping} = \begin{matrix}\text{percent copper in}\\ \text{available protore}\end{matrix}$$

$$0.25\%\ \text{Cu} - 0.03\%\ \text{Cu} = 0.22\%\ \text{Cu}$$

3. This allows calculation of the amount of rock leached to form the chalcocite blanket:

$$\left(\frac{\text{percent copper added to protore}}{\text{percent copper in available protore}}\right)\left(\begin{matrix}\text{thickness of}\\ \text{chalcocite blanket}\end{matrix}\right) = \begin{matrix}\text{total rock}\\ \text{leached}\end{matrix}$$

$$\left(\frac{0.55\%\ \text{Cu}}{0.22\%\ \text{Cu}}\right)(200\ \text{ft.}) = 500\ \text{ft.}$$

4. The amount of rock eroded from the deposit during the most recent enrichment cycle is:

$$\text{total rock leached} - \text{remaining leached capping} = \begin{matrix}\text{amount of rock}\\ \text{eroded}\end{matrix}$$

$$500\ \text{ft.} - 100\ \text{ft.} = 400\ \text{ft.}$$

The time required to erode 400 ft. can be roughly estimated from erosion rates given in the literature. Shafiqullah and others (1975) have determined an erosion rate of 0.3 ft./1,000 yr. in the transition zone between the Colorado Plateau and the Basin and Range in Arizona for the mid-Miocene to Recent. This rate is in reasonable agreement with Ruxton and McDougall (1967) who calculate present erosion rates of 0.26 ft./1,000 yr. on an andesitic stratovolcano in northeast Papua for areas of 200 ft. of relief and with Blatt and others (1972) who report erosion rates of 0.20 ft./1,000 yr. for areas underlain by sandstone in South Dakota where rainfall averages 14 in./yr. Applying the lower estimate to Silver Bell, the time required to erode 400 ft. is:

$$\frac{400\ \text{ft.}}{(0.2\ \text{ft.}/1{,}000\ \text{yr.})} = 2\ \text{million years}$$

The uncertainty in the numbers requires comment. The various copper grades and thicknesses are averages, but changes in one value require changes in others that preserve the relationships on a relative basis. The major variable used is the erosion rate; however, the value used was derived from several different environments using different approaches and is believed reasonable. Implicit in the calculation is the assumption that there was no significant loss of copper from the El Tiro blanket by lateral movement of copper-bearing groundwater; this assumption is reasonable, as the blanket underlies a gully, which would have favored inward movement. Also implied is the assumption that erosion of 400 ft. of capping occurred at the same time as leaching and enrichment. Enrichment could have occurred before the erosion of the 400 ft. of capping; however, the extent to which the enrichment cycle is older than the erosion cycle is limited by the thickness of capping through which efficient enrichment can occur. As such thicknesses do not generally exceed 500 to 600 ft., the timing of the enrichment probably coincided rather well with erosion of the 400 ft. of capping in the last 2 million years.

CONCLUSIONS

It has not been the purpose of this chapter to provide a comparative study between the El Tiro orebody and other porphyry copper ore zones. Overall the El Tiro deposit is typical of the classic porphyry copper deposit in the sense that it contains supergene-enriched, disseminated copper mineralization in altered porphyry. It also contains a significant amount of hypogene mineralization in altered carbonate rocks and is, thus, a composite of the intrusion and wall rock types discussed by Titley (1972). In addition, except for the distribution of phyllic alteration, the El Tiro deposit conforms to the generalized zoning patterns found in porphyry copper deposits as summarized by Lowell and Guilbert (1970). Deviations from the generalized model constructed by Lowell and Guilbert, although significant, are no more numerous or severe than in other individual deposits used in their compilation.

Important conclusions of the El Tiro study are listed below:

1. Different silicate rocks had a strong influence on the degree of development of the various hydrothermal assemblages.
2. The zone of sulfide mineralization is elongate NS and probably reflects an as-yet-unidentified structural control.
3. Potassic and propylitic assemblages appear to be time-equivalent.
4. Chalcopyrite has a close space-time association with hydrothermal vein biotite and quartz, but is mostly earlier than alteration K-feldspar and molybdenite.
5. The phyllic zone is later than, and asymmetrically distributed with respect to, potassic alteration and hypogene copper contours.
6. The phyllic-potassic transition did not influence hypogene ore deposition.
7. The strongest supergene enrichment coincides with areas of highest sulfide content, where the phyllic and potassic zones overlap.
8. Pervasive sericite and clay alteration in the leached capping and chalcocite blanket is of supergene origin.
9. Supergene enrichment, which formed the present chalcocite blanket, occurred within the last 2 million years.

It is emphasized that the above conclusions are based largely on mapping and petrographic work and that many research topics remain. One subject for intensive study is the Oxide area. Although similar in many aspects to El Tiro geology, significant differences include the elongate shape of the Oxide ore zone, abundant syenodiorite porphyry as a host rock, higher hypogene copper content, abundant pervasive K-feldspar alteration, and the absence of ore-grade chalcopyrite in the altered carbonate rocks along the north side of the pit. Other research subjects include the extent and type of alteration in dikes east of the pits, the space-time relationships of the skarn with respect to ores in porphyritic rocks, fluid inclusion studies of the ores, sulfide mineralogy, and supergene alteration mineralogy in different rock types.

ACKNOWLEDGMENTS

This chapter is part of a comprehensive study of the Silver Bell region initiated under the direction of W. L. Kurtz. Critical reviews by J. H. Courtright, J. D. Sell, and J. L. Galey have greatly improved the content. Permission to publish was kindly granted by ASARCO Incorporated.

REFERENCES CITED

Agenbroad, L. D., 1962, The geology of the Atlas Mine area, Pima County, Ariz.: Unpub. M.S. Thesis, Univ. of Ariz., Tucson.

Ballantyne, G. H., 1975, Alteration study, North Silver Bell deposit, Pima County, Ariz.: progress report to ASARCO on Ph.D. dissertation research, Univ. of Utah.

———, 1979, Thermal gradients in the North Silver Bell alteration halo: paper given at Society of Economic Geologists Spring Field Conference, Tucson, Ariz.

Banks, N. G., and Dockter, R. D., 1976, Reconnaissance geologic map of the Vaca Hills quadrangle, Arizona: U.S. Geol. Survey Map MF-793.

Blatt, Harvey; Middleton, Gerard; and Murray, Raymond, 1972, Origin of Sedimentary Rocks: New Jersey, Prentice-Hall Inc., 634 p.

Buseck, P. R., 1962, Contact metasomatic deposits at Concepcion del Oro, Mexico; Tem Piute, Nevada; and Silver Bell, Arizona: Unpub. Ph.D. Diss., Columbia University, New York.

Cathles, L. M., 1977, An analysis of the cooling of intrusives by ground-water convection which includes boiling: Econ. Geol., v. 72, p. 804–826.

Cummings, R. B., 1973, Alteration-mineralization zoning study, Silver Bell mine, Pima County, Ariz.: unpublished ASARCO Inc. report.

Davis, S. R., 1974, Geology and geochemistry, North Silver Bell, Pima County, Arizona: unpublished ASARCO Inc. report.

Galey, J. L., 1976, personal communication.

Heidrick, L., 1974, A dynamic model for fracturing and diking in Laramide plutons in Arizona: Geol. Soc. Amer. Abs.. with Prog., Rocky Mtn. Section, v. 6, p. 445–446.

Hemley, J. J., and Jones, W. R., 1964, Chemical aspects of hydrothermal alteration with emphasis on hydrogen metasomatism: Econ. Geol., v. 59, p. 538–569.

Kerr, P. F., 1951, Alteration features at Silver Bell, Arizona: Geol. Soc. America Bull., v. 62, p. 457–480.

Kingsbury, H. M.; Entwistle, L. P.; and Schmitt, Harrison, 1941, Geology and ore deposits of Silver Bell, Arizona: unpublished ASARCO Inc. report.

Livingston, D. E.; Mauger, R. L.; and Damon, P. E., 1968, Geochronology of the emplacement, enrichment, and preservation of Arizona porphyry copper deposits: Econ. Geol., v. 63, p. 30–36.

Loghry, J. D., 1972, Characteristics of favorable cappings from several southwestern porphyry copper deposits: Unpub. M.S. Thesis, Univ. of Ariz., Tucson.

Lowell, J. D., 1974, Regional characteristics of porphyry copper deposits of the Southwest: Econ. Geol., v. 69, p. 601–617.

Lowell, J. D., and Guilbert, J. M., 1970, Lateral and vertical alteration-mineralization zoning in porphyry ore deposits: Econ. Geol., v. 65, p. 373–408.

Mauger, R. L., 1966, A petrographic and geochemical study of Silver Bell and Pima mining districts, Pima County, Ariz.: Unpub. Ph.D. Diss., Univ. of Ariz., Tucson.

McClymonds, N. E., 1959, Paleozoic stratigraphy of the Waterman Mtns., Pima County, Ariz.: in Southern Arizona Guidebook II: Tucson, Ariz. Geol. Soc., p. 67–76.

Merz, J. L., 1967, The geology of the Union Hill area, Silver Bell district, Pima County, Ariz.: Unpub. M.S. Thesis, Univ. of Ariz., Tucson.

Moore, W. J., and Nash, J. T., 1974, Alteration and fluid inclusion studies of the porphyry copper ore body at Bingham, Utah: Econ. Geol., v. 69, p. 631–645.

Nash, J. T., 1976, Fluid inclusion petrology—data from porphyry copper deposits and applications to exploration: U.S. Geol. Survey Prof. Paper 907-D.

Ransome, F. L., 1919, The copper deposits of Ray and Miami, Ariz.: U.S. Geol. Survey Prof. Paper 115.

Richard, K., and Courtright, J. H., 1966, Structure and mineralization at Silver Bell, Arizona, in Titley, S. R., and Hicks, C. L., eds., Geology of the Porphyry Copper Deposits, Southwestern North America: Tucson, Univ. of Ariz. Press, p. 157–163.

Rose, A. W., 1970, Zonal relations of wall rock alteration and sulfide distribution at porphyry copper deposits: Econ. Geol., v. 65, p. 920–936.

Ruxton, B. P., and McDougall, I., 1967, Denudation rates in Northeast Papua from Potassium-Argon dating of lavas: Am. Jour. Sci., v. 265, p. 545–561.

Shafiqullah, M.; Peirce, H. Wesley; and Damon, Paul E., 1975, Rate of structural and geomorphic evolution of the southern margin of the Colorado Plateau in Arizona: Geol. Soc. Amer. Abs.. with Prog., v. 7, p. 373–374.

Stewart, C. A., 1912, The geology and ore deposits of the Silver Bell mining district, Ariz.: AIME Bull., v. 65, p. 455–506.

Titley, S. R., 1972, Intrusion, and wall rock, porphyry copper deposits: Econ. Geol., v. 67, p. 122–123.

Watson, B. N., 1964, Structure and petrology of the eastern portion of the Silver Bell Mtns., Pima County, Ariz.: Unpub. Ph.D. Diss., Univ. of Ariz., Tucson.

———,1968, Updating the geology and ore controls at Silver Bell, Ariz.: manuscript, AIME, Min. Geol. Div., Arizona Section.

25

Geology of the Sacaton Porphyry Copper Deposit

PINAL COUNTY, ARIZONA

Robert B. Cummings

The Sacaton copper deposit is located in Pinal County, Arizona, about 6 miles northwest of Casa Grande and 65 miles northwest of Tucson. The mine is on a gently sloping pediment south of the Sacaton Mountains. In the mine area vegetation is sparse, the climate is semiarid, and the average elevation is 1,450 ft. Early in 1961 Asarco geologists examined a small outcrop of leached capping 1.5 miles south of pre-mineral outcrops in the Sacaton Mountains. This outcrop forms a low hill, about 30 ft. high and 300 ft. in diameter, surrounded by Quaternary alluvium. The hill is underlain by granite and thin monzonite porphyry dikes and exhibits pervasive phyllic alteration. Interpretation of the leached capping suggested that the outcrop contained about 2 percent pyrite by volume with traces of chalcocite.

With the altered outcrop as a positive exploration lead, a drilling program was initiated which eventually outlined two zones of ore-grade copper mineralization. The relative position of the orebodies to the Sacaton Mountains and the discovery outcrop is illustrated in Figures 25.1 and 25.2. Full-scale production from the West orebody commenced in February 1974 and at the end of 1980 averaged approximately 11,500 tons of ore per day. At that time the West orebody was being mined by open-pit methods, and plans for the East orebody called for eventual mining by block-caving methods.

This chapter is based on data obtained from pit mapping at 1 in. = 100 ft. and from diamond drill core logging. Because the East orebody is known only through diamond drilling, most of the discussion and conclusions relate to the West orebody, although generalized comparisons are made between the two orebodies.

GENERAL GEOLOGY

The Sacaton deposit occurs in the desert region of the Basin and Range province of Arizona. At the close of Older Precambrian time the Oracle Granite batholith intruded Pinal Schist. In Younger Precambrian time Apache Group sediments were deposited and igneous activity resulted in the emplacement of the Sacaton Granite northwest of the mine and numerous diabase dikes. During the Paleozoic the Sacaton mine area was probably near the northern limit of the Sonoran Geosyncline. An unknown thickness of Paleozoic sediments was deposited and later eroded along with most of the Apache Group rocks. During the Laramide Orogeny two granitic stocks, the Three Peaks Monzonite and the Sacaton Peak Granite, were emplaced in the vicinity of the mine. The faulting, uplift, and erosion that took place during the Cenozoic resulted in deposition of continental sediments and development of the present topography.

Rock Types

The geology of the Sacaton Mountains is shown in Figure 25.1. Pinal Schist, the oldest rock exposed, occurs almost entirely as quartz-muscovite schist roof pendants in the Precambrian granite. Precambrian granite intrudes the Pinal Schist as a large mass in the northwest portion of the Sacaton Mountains. Smaller exposures are also found in the central portion of the mountains and just south of the Sacaton deposit in the discovery outcrop. The rock is coarse grained, consisting of quartz, orthoclase (some of which occurs as phenocrysts to 1.5 in. long), and minor plagioclase and biotite. Balla (1972) has correlated this granite with the Oracle Granite from the San Manuel area because of petrographic

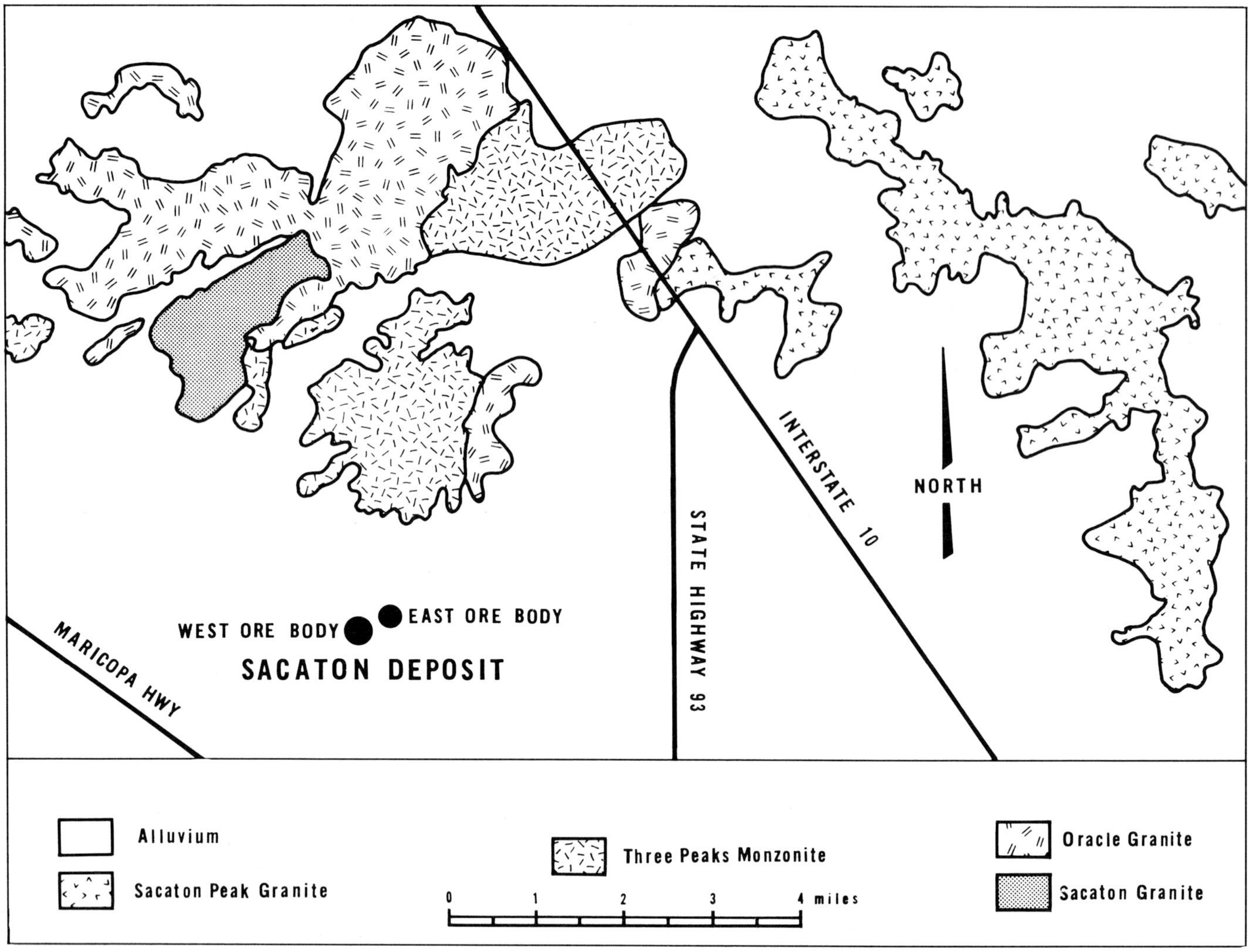

Figure 25.1. Generalized geologic map of the Sacaton Mountains. Modified after Balla (1972).

similarities. His K-Ar date of 1240 m.y. for the rock is younger than the Oracle Granite at San Manuel, but he postulates that this discrepancy is due to an argon loss.

A younger Precambrian granite stock intrudes the Oracle Granite in the southern part of the Sacaton Mountains. Exposures of the granite are elongated roughly parallel to the southern limit of the main mass of Oracle Granite (N60°E). This rock is fine- to medium-grained and contains quartz, orthoclase, muscovite, and minor amounts of plagioclase. Balla (1972) has obtained a K-Ar date of 857 m.y. for the rock and has named it the Sacaton Granite. Numerous northwesterly trending diabase dikes intrude the large mass of Oracle Granite. A whole-rock K-Ar date of 841 m.y. has been obtained on the diabase by Balla (1972).

One small exposure of Paleozoic rocks is found in the Sacaton Mountains about 3.5 miles northeast of the mine. The outcrop consists of quartzite and limestone which have tentatively been identified as Cambrian Bolsa Quartzite and Devonian Martin Limestone (Wilson, 1969). These rocks contain a small corundum deposit and are in probable fault contact with surrounding Laramide intrusive rocks.

Two Laramide granitic stocks comprise most of the eastern two-thirds of the Sacaton Mountains. The Three Peaks Monzonite, oldest of the two rocks, occurs directly north of the mine and intrudes the Oracle and Sacaton granites. Balla (1972, p. 27–28) states: "The Three Peaks stock is a composite, zoned, epizonal pluton which is aligned in a northeasterly direction. The stock consists of four different facies. Beginning at the contact with the Precambrian Oracle Granite, the facies are: a diorite border facies, which is divisible into a fine-grained outer zone and a coarser-grained inner zone; an intermediate monzonite facies; and a central, monzonite, core facies." Exposures of the core facies are the most abundant. This rock is a medium-grained, equigranular, biotite monzonite composed of plagioclase, orthoclase, biotite, quartz, and accessory sphene and magnetite. Balla's average date on biotite from the core facies is 71.3 ± 2 m.y.

The other Laramide stock, the Sacaton Peak Granite, makes up the eastern portion of the Sacaton Mountains. It is similar to the Three Peaks Stock in form (both are composite, zoned stocks) and mineralogy, but distinctly different in texture. Three distinct facies are present. The border facies is a medium-grained biotite quartz monzonite with 15 percent biotite and a gneissic texture. The intermediate facies is a medium-grained, slightly porphyritic, biotite quartz monzonite with prominent quartz phenocrysts and less biotite

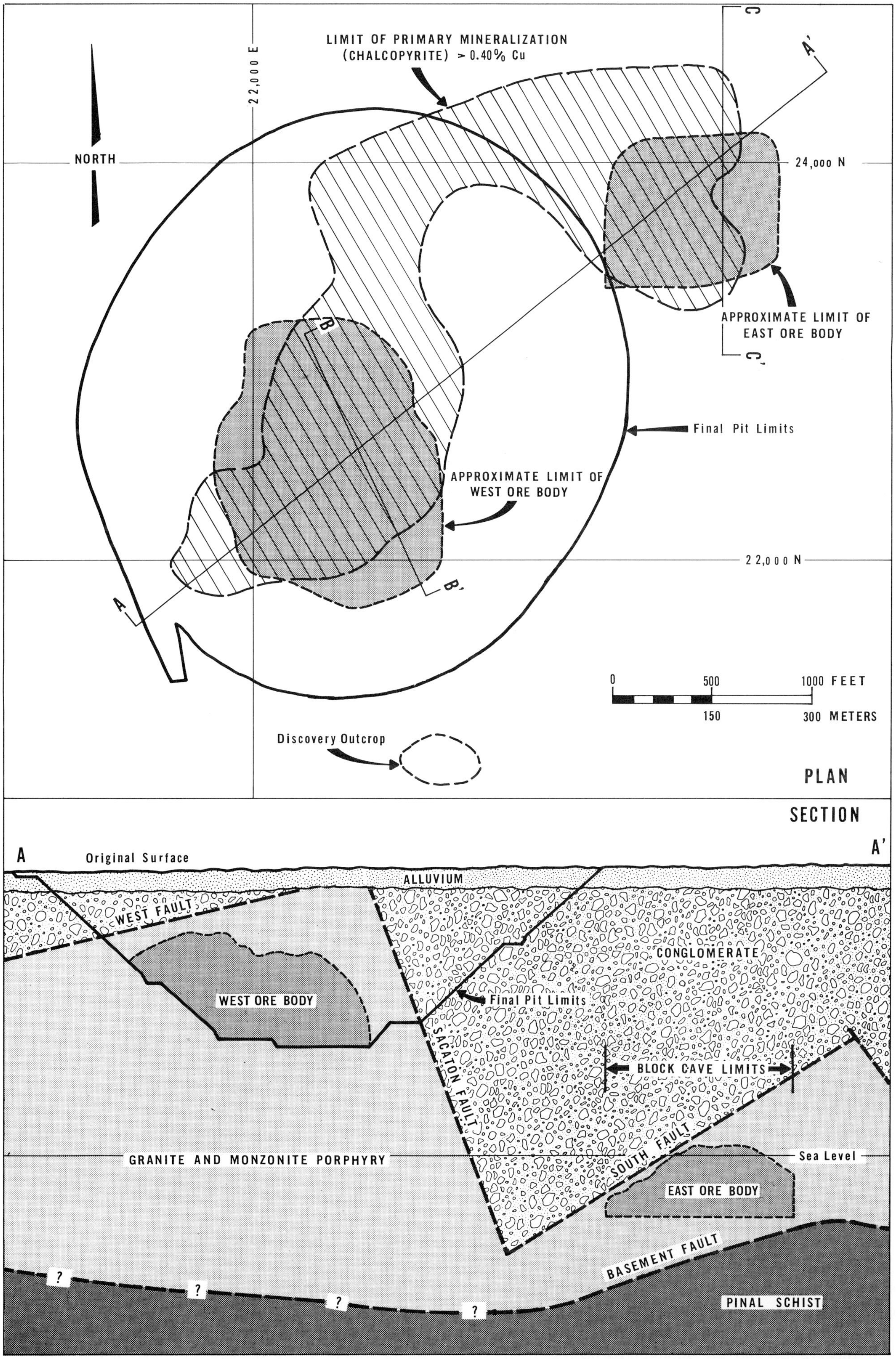

Figure 25.2. Generalized plan and section, showing the limits of the East and West orebodies, Sacaton

than the border facies. The core facies is a medium-to coarse-grained, slightly porphyritic granite with orthoclase phenocrysts up to 1.5 in. in length. The stock is called a granite after the composition of the core, but the overall composition of the stock is that of a quartz monzonite. An isotopic age of 61.2 ± 1.9 m.y. has been found for the intermediate facies (Balla, 1972).

Structure

A major northeasterly trending structural lineament has been recognized passing through the Globe-Miami district toward Ajo. Mayo (1958) named this trend the Jemez Zone. Balla (1972) has postulated that the Jemez Zone was active intermittently from Precambrian to Tertiary time and that this zone controlled the emplacement of the Precambrian Oracle and Ruin granites and the Laramide granitic stocks.

Knowledge of the major structural features in the Sacaton Mine area is derived primarily from drilling information. The Sacaton orebodies and alteration zone are confined to an allochthonous structural block which rests on a low-angle structure referred to as the Basement fault. The allochthon is elongated in a northeasterly direction and measures at least 4 miles in length, up to 1.5 miles in width, and from 1,200 to 2,200 ft. thick. Northwesterly striking normal faults divide the allochthonous rocks into several horst and graben units as shown on Figure 25.2. Autochthonous rocks below the Basement fault are part of the Pinal Schist.

GEOLOGY OF THE OREBODIES

Rock Types

With the exception of the Pinal Schist, found below the Basement fault, all pre-mineral rocks in the vicinity of the orebodies are pervasively altered. In addition, two stages of brecciation are present, often resulting in an intimate mixture of rock types. These features have complicated the delineation and identification of the rocks. Figures 25.3, 25.4*a* and 25.5*a* show the distribution of rock types in the orebodies; Figures 25.4*b* and 25.5*b* show the distribution of sulfides in the West and East orebodies, respectively.

Pinal Schist. A complex of metamorphic rocks which is thought to be Pinal Schist is found below the Basement fault. Rock types include quartz-biotite-chlorite schist, metamorphosed granitic rocks, gneiss, and metavolcanic rocks. These diverse rock types are not found outcropping in Pinal Schist exposures in the area, but, due to the degree of metamorphism, they have been assigned to this unit. Similar rocks have not been identified in the upper plate of the Basement fault.

Oracle Granite. The Oracle Granite varies in composition from granite to quartz monzonite. The rock is coarse-grained, weakly porphyritic, and composed of quartz, orthoclase, plagioclase, and minor biotite. Subhedral phenocrysts of orthoclase up to 1.2 in. long occur locally. A relative increase of plagioclase over orthoclase often accompanies the large orthoclase phenocrysts and results in a quartz monzonite composition. Thin, irregular, and discontinuous aplitic dikes cut the granite and are thought to be related to it. Where intense alteration, brecciation, and granulation occur the only means of identifying the granite is the abundance of coarse-grained, sheared quartz.

The granite is the predominate rock type in the East orebody, where it occurs as a large brecciated mass and as the major constituent of mixed breccias. In the West orebody granite occurs in brecciated masses on both the north and south sides of the pit. It also makes up varying proportions of the mixed breccias in the central portion of the pit.

Diabase. The original composition of the diabase has been masked by hydrothermal alteration, but a good relict diabasic texture is present. The rock now consists of lath-shaped aggregates of sericite and clay after plagioclase in a matrix of fine-grained, shreddy biotite and mafic minerals. A tentative age of Younger Precambrian has been assigned to this rock.

The diabase occurs as irregular dikes intruding granite and as xenoliths in the younger monzonite porphyry. In the West orebody the dikes are generally restricted to the large mass of granite on the north side of the pit. The dikes exposed in the pit strike north to north-northwest, vary greatly in dip, and reach a maximum thickness of 30 ft.

Monzonite Porphyry. Monzonite porphyry intrudes granite and diabase. Although the monzonite porphyry in the mine area cannot be correlated to either of the Laramide stocks in the Sacaton Mountains, it is assumed to be Laramide in age. Variations in the texture and composition of the monzonite porphyry are common. Typically it exhibits phenocryst: groundmass ratios ranging from 40:60 to 60:40. The composition of the medium-grained phenocrysts is typically as follows: 75 percent euhedral plagioclase (0.08 to 0.16 inches in length); 10 to 15 percent euhedral biotite books (0.08 inches in width); 10 percent subhedral quartz (0.08 to 0.12 inches in diameter); and 1 to 3 percent subhedral orthoclase (0.08 to 0.12 inches in diameter). The groundmass is a fine-grained intergrowth of feldspar and quartz but alteration obscures the identification of the feldspars.

Textural and modal variations in the monzonite porphyry include phenocryst:groundmass ratios (from 70:30 to 25:75), accessory hornblende phenocrysts, phenocryst size, phenocryst composition, and megascopic differences in the appearance of the groundmass. The above-mentioned variations in the monzonite porphyry may be gradational over a few tens of feet, but in the mixed breccias variations in texture and composition are common from one fragment to the next. Intense quartz-sericite alteration obscures the quantity of primary quartz which was originally present in the groundmass of the monzonite porphyry. The original composition of the monzonite porphyry may have been quartz monzonite.

Monzonite porphyry intrudes the older rocks in the West orebody and forms mixed breccias; monolithic breccias; large, poorly defined, dike-like masses; and thin, well-defined but discontinuous dikes. Xenoliths of granite are common in the monzonite porphyry. Drilling results and pit mapping indicate that the greatest thickness of monzonite porphyry occurs in the center of and to the west of the West orebody. The monzonite porphyry that intrudes the granite masses on the north and south sides of the pit occurs as dikes. A northeasterly trending mass of monzonite porphyry intrudes the

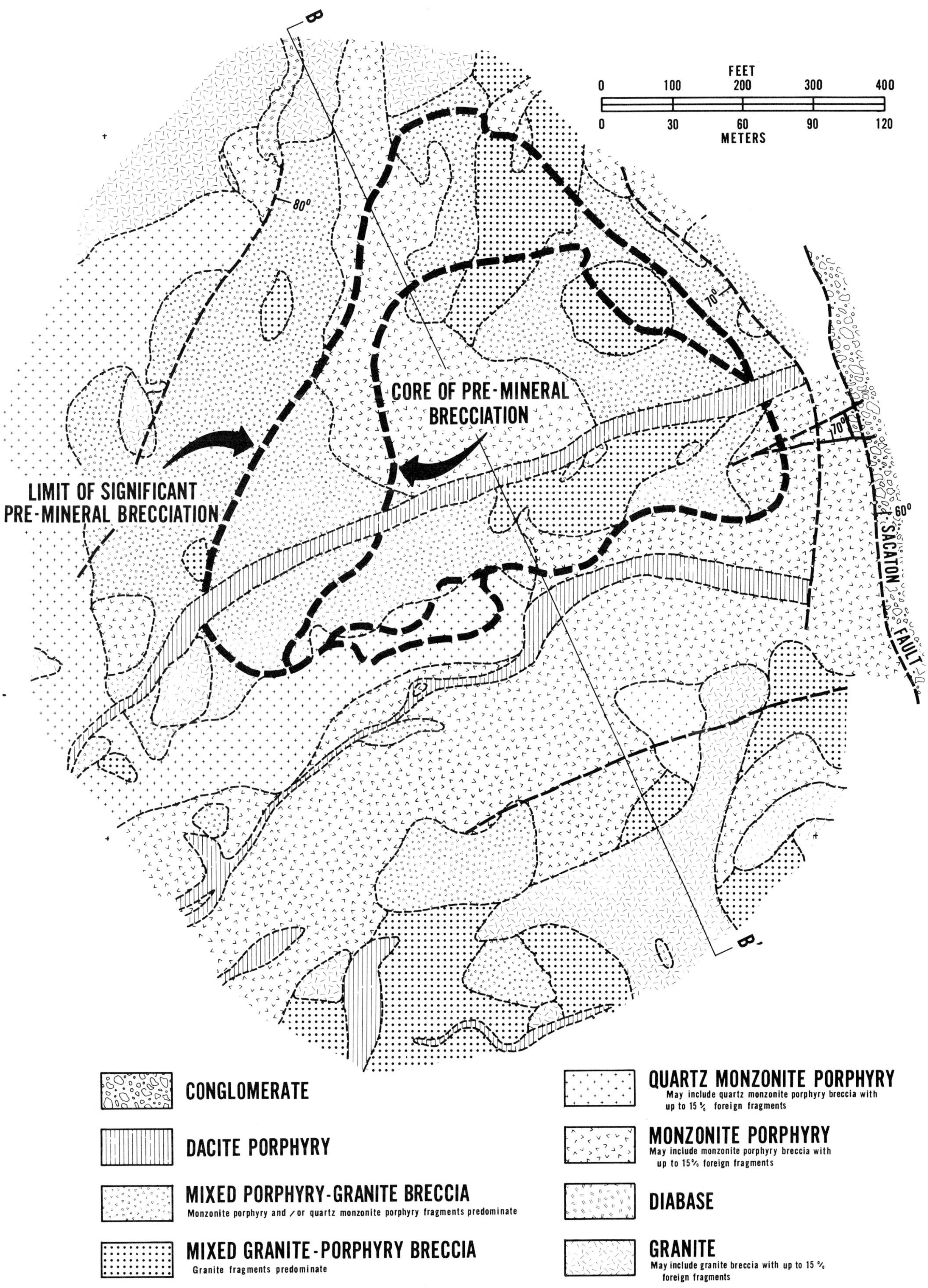

Figure 25.3. Geologic map of the 1,030-ft. bench, West orebody

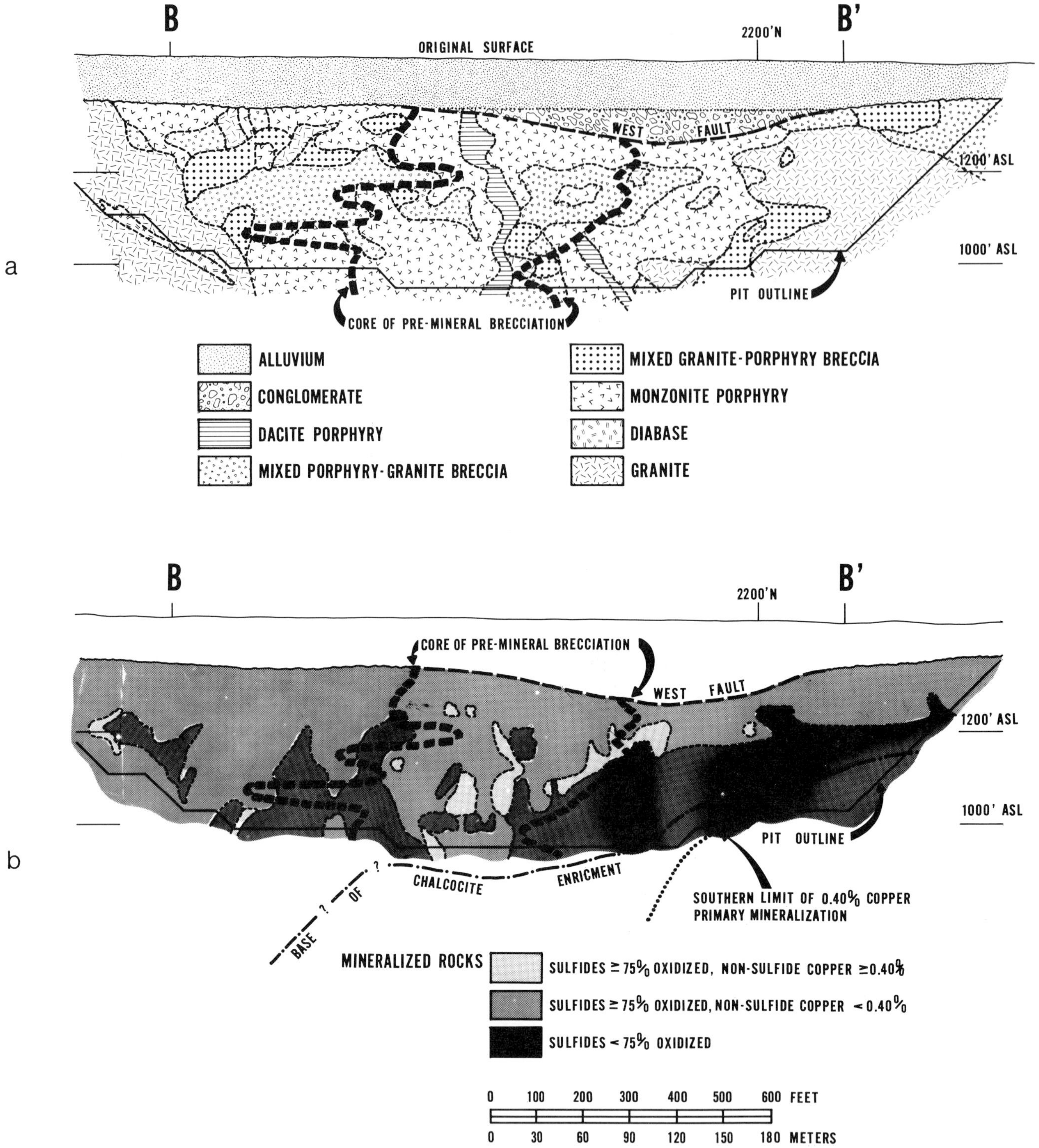

Figure 25.4. Cross section *B-B'* through the West orebody shows (*a*) rock types and (*b*) distribution of sulfides.

granite in the southern portion of the East orebody. Elsewhere it occurs as moderately to steeply dipping dikes and in mixed breccias.

Quartz Monzonite Porphyry. The granite and diabase are intruded by quartz monzonite porphyry, which is thought to be Laramide in age. Texturally and mineralogically this rock is identical to the monzonite porphyry, but is distinguished from it by the presence of 10 percent or more clear quartz phenocrysts. Quartz monzonite porphyry occurs as monolithic and mixed breccias, irregular masses, and dike-like bodies in the west and southwest portions of the West orebody and in the East orebody. Gradational contacts are common between the quartz monzonite porphyry and the monzonite porphyry, and definitive crosscutting relationships have not been found. Because of spatial relationships and similarities in texture and composition, monzonite porphyry and quartz monzonite porphyry are considered to be co-magmatic in origin.

Mixed Breccias. Both the East and West orebodies contain substantial volumes of brecciated rock. The predominant rock types in the breccias are monzonite porphyry, quartz monzonite porphyry, and granite. Differentiation of the mixed breccias is based on the rock type of the dominant breccia fragment. For example, mixed granite-porphyry breccia is mixed breccia in which granite fragments comprise 51 to 84 percent of the total volume of fragments. Mixed porphyry-granite breccia is mixed breccia in which porphyry fragments (monzonite or quartz monzonite) comprise 50 to 84 percent of the total volume of fragments. This differentiation is reflected in the classification of rock types shown in Figures 25.3, 25.4*a* and 25.5*a*. Mixed breccias containing 15 percent or less foreign fragments are not differentiated from corresponding monolithic breccias. For example, a breccia with 10 percent granite fragments and 90 percent monzonite porphyry fragments is designated monzonite porphyry breccia. Contacts between mixed breccias and monolithic breccias are often gradational. In places, however, weakly brecciated monzonite porphyry dikes and masses appear to intrude the mixed brecdias. This relationship suggest that emplacement of the monzonite porphyry post-dates as well as predates the formation of the mixed breccias. Detailed descriptions of the breccias are found in the section on structure.

Mixed breccias are found throughout the West orebody but appear to be concentrated between the granite masses on the north and south sides of the pit. As might be expected, granite-porphyry breccias generally occur in close proximity to masses of granite or granite breccia. Drill hole data suggests that the mixed breccias grade at depth into monzonite porphyry and monzonite porphyry breccia. In the East orebody mixed breccias generally occur in close proximity to monzonite porphyry dikes and masses.

Dacite Porphyry. Dacite porphyry dikes, probably of early Tertiary age, intrude older rocks in both orebodies. The dacite porphyry contains phenocrysts of sodic plagioclase, quartz, and biotite. Phenocrysts make up 15 to 25 percent of the rock and vary in diameter from 0.08 to 0.16 in. The groundmass is an aphanitic granular intergrowth of feldspar, quartz, chlorite, and biotite. Two dacite porphyry dikes, about 250 feet apart, trend N65°E through the central portion of the West orebody (see Fig. 25.3). In the East orebody, a single dacite porphyry dike is found south of the block cave limits. The presence of weak alteration and sulfide mineralization in the dacite porphyry suggests that it was intruded during the later stages of mineralization.

Conglomerate. A Tertiary terrestrial conglomerate has been located in fault contact with the older rocks. The exact age of this unit is not known, but indirect structural evidence suggests it is equivelant in age to the mid-Tertiary Whitetail Conglomerate. The conglomerate at Sacaton contains subangular to sub-rounded clasts comprising 40 to 60 percent of the unit in a silty to gritty, moderately well indurated matrix. Clasts in the conglomerate are mostly Oracle Granite and Pinal Schist, with small amounts of monzonite porphyry. Fragments of leached capping are not uncommon.

Dips in the conglomerate are variable. They average 0 to 20° to the north or northeast on the east side of the pit and 30 to 60° to the north or northeast on the west side of the pit. The conglomerate reaches a maximum thickness of at least 1,750 ft. east of the pit and at least 2,500 ft. to the west of the pit.

Alluvium. An average thickness of 100 ft. of Quaternary alluvium is found over the older rocks in the area of the East and West orebodies. This material is loosely consolidated sand and silt. Occasional fragments of partially decomposed Three Peaks Monzonite are found toward the base of the unit.

Structure

Several periods of deformation have produced a complex structural picture at Sacaton. Each of these periods is characterized by fracturing, faulting, and brecciation.

Fracturing. Rocks occurring in and around the orebodies are well fractured. As a result, much of the rock tends to break into fragments with diameters less than 12 in. Locally, fractures in the leached capping and in the upper portion of the enriched zone are healed by supergene alteration minerals, and the rock breaks into coarser fragments.

Although all possible fracture orientations occur, mapping of fractures indicates that two preferred orientations are present. Mineralized fractures strike from N50°E to E-W (Fig. 25.6) and generally dip greater than 70° in either direction. These fractures are often well healed by supergene sulfides or indigenous limonite and are often unbroken in pit faces. The preferred orientation of barren fractures is N-S to N20°W. Most are close to vertical in dip, but moderate and low-angle dips are also present. Transported limonite often lines these fractures, and many exhibit slickensides which indicate horizontal movement. Displacements on the barren fractures are thought to be minor and are probably the result of adjustment to more significant displacement on faults.

Faulting. A great number of minor faults have been mapped in the West orebody. The faults are often variable in strike and dip and are usually difficult to trace along strike. The prevailing strike direction is N60°E to E-W. Slickensides on some of the faults indicate that horizontal components of displacement are relatively common. Generally, the lack of predictable lithologic contacts to act as markers makes the direction and magnitude of displacement difficult to estimate. Total displacement on most of the faults is thought to be less than 100 ft. Both pre-mineral and post-mineral movement is often present.

Two post-mineral normal faults control the bedrock-conglomerate contact in the vicinity of the West orebody. The Sacaton fault bounds the orebody on the east side. It strikes from N-S to N45°W (the average strike in the pit area is N20°W) and dips about 60° east. Conglomerate in the hanging wall of the fault on the upper benches of the pit is well indurated, but is not crushed or deformed. Chrysocolla often cements the conglomerate in this area. In the footwall of the fault pre-mineral rocks are intensely fractured. On the south side of the pit these rocks are so severely crushed and granulated (for a thickness of up to 40 ft.) that the original rock type cannot be identified. Vertical displacement on the Sacaton fault is at least 1,500 ft. This fault is of major significance because it divides a continuous zone of chalcocite mineralization into two separate orebodies.

The West fault bounds the west side of the West orebody. It strikes N45°W adjacent to the northern portion of the orebody and swings to N20°E adjacent to the southern portion. The dip of the fault varies from 10 to 30° to the west. As with the Sacaton fault, conglomerate occurs in the hanging wall and pre-mineral rocks occur in the footwall. Conglomerate in the hanging wall is well indurated (in the upper benches) but is not crushed or deformed. Pre-mineral footwall rocks contain numerous fractures which parallel the fault, but crushing and granulation are absent. The amount of displacement on the West fault is unknown, but the thickness of conglomerate to the west of the pit suggests that it could be on the order of several thousand feet. Rotational movement is indicated by steep dips in the conglomerate of the hanging wall.

Several minor faults offset the Sacaton and West faults in the area surrounding the West orebody. However, the paucity of these structures here compared to their abundance within the West orebody suggests that movement on the Sacaton and West faults post-dates the bulk of the minor faulting.

The South Fault forms the southern limit of the East orebody. It strikes E-W and dips an average of 45° south. The hanging wall is conglomerate, while pre-mineral rocks occur in the footwall. Maximum vertical displacement is at least 800 ft. Drilling suggests that the South fault is terminated against the Sacaton fault west of the East orebody.

The above-described normal faults and the mineralized rocks containing the Sacaton deposit are terminated at depth on the Basement fault. The fault plane (known only by drilling) takes the shape of a shallow trench, the axis of which trends to the northeast. Along the axis of the trench the fault plane is slightly undulating. It varies in dip from 0 to 20° and is found at depths of 1,800 to 2,200 ft. below the ground

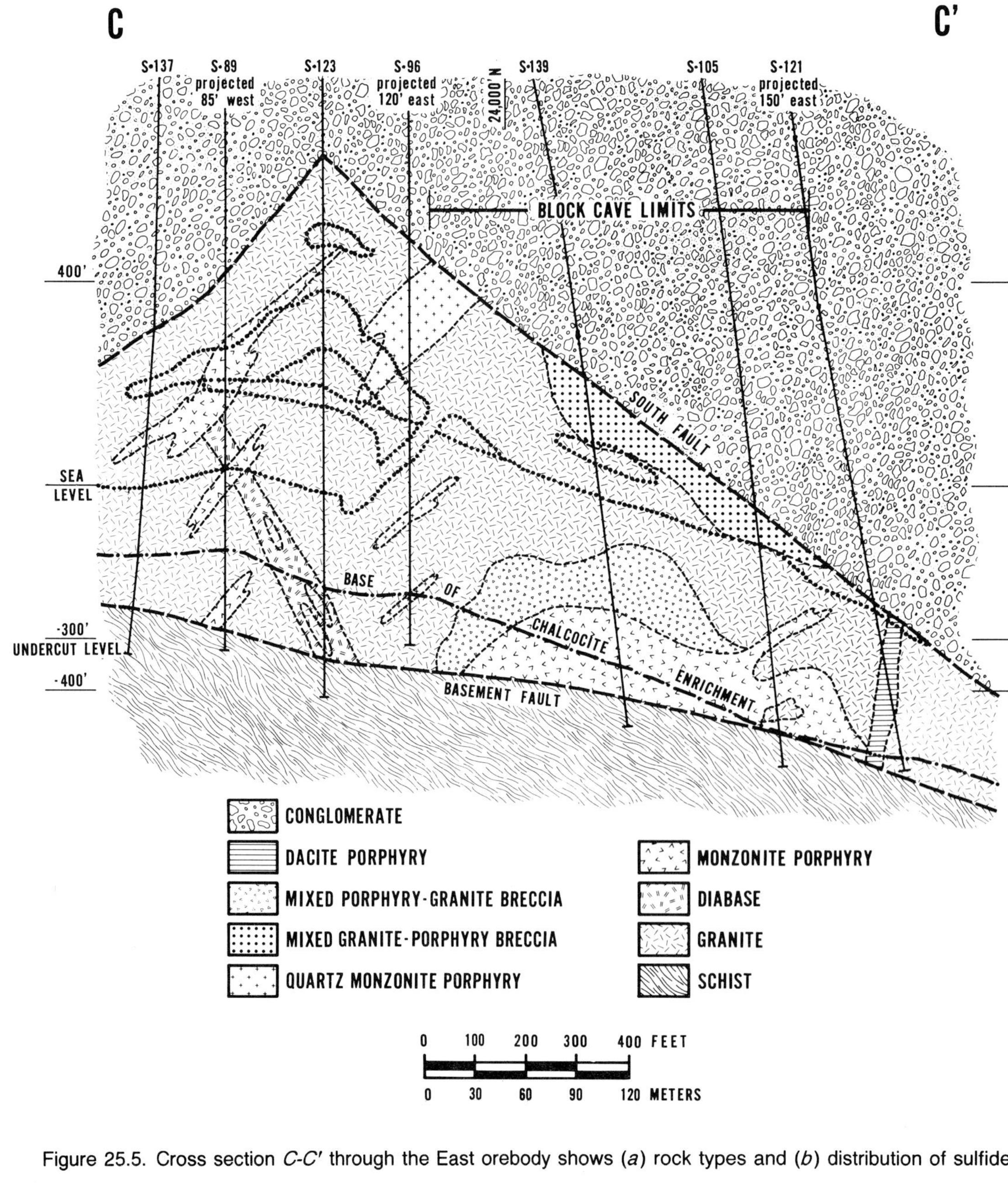

Figure 25.5. Cross section *C-C'* through the East orebody shows (*a*) rock types and (*b*) distribution of sulfides.

surface. The sides of the trench dip from 20 to 40° toward the axis. North of the orebodies drilling suggests that the Basement fault is truncated against a steeply dipping, northeasterly trending structure which brings the Three Peaks Monzonite into fault contact with the rocks of the upper and lower plates.

The plane of the Basement fault is composed of sheared, undulating zones of brecciated upper and lower plate rocks and thin zones of firm but sheared chloritic to hematitic gouge. The average thickness of the fault is about 5 ft. Lower plate rocks of the Pinal Schist complex are often crushed and sheared for distances of up to 40 ft. below the fault. Mineralized upper plate rocks are crushed and brecciated for distances of up to 200 ft. above the fault. The direction of movement of the upper plate of the Basement fault is probably from the southwest. The lack of mineralization in lower plate rocks suggests that movement was on the order of several miles.

Brecciation. Of the two periods of brecciation found at Sacaton, the earliest is pre-mineral. It is related to the intrusion of the monzonite porphyry and is a major ore control in the West orebody. Post-mineral brecciation is superimposed on, and is more extensive than, the earlier brecciation. Both types of brecciation are present in the West orebody, but post-mineral brecciation is the only type occurring in the East orebody.

Pre-mineral brecciation occurs as monolithic breccias and mixed breccias. Diagnostic features of this period of brecciation are subtle and often difficult to recognize because of pervasive hydrothermal alteration, transported iron oxide minerals, and post-mineral brecciation. The breccia consists of tightly packed fragments set in a well-cemented matrix. The diameters of breccia fragments commonly vary from 0.2 in. to 6 ft. The presence of larger fragments or blocks is suspected, but by late 1980 had not been verified. Fragments are usually sub-angular to sub-rounded, but angular and

b

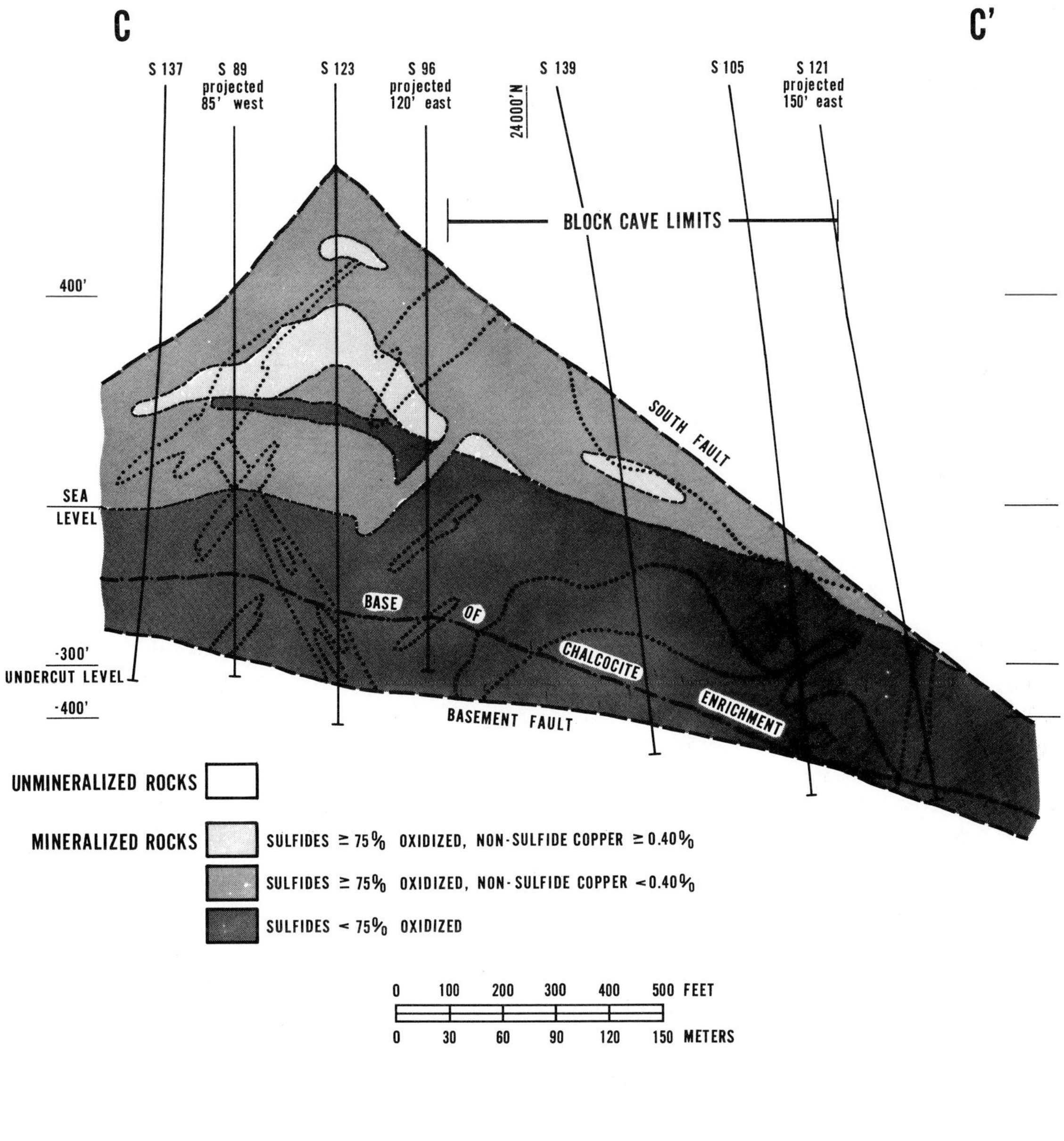

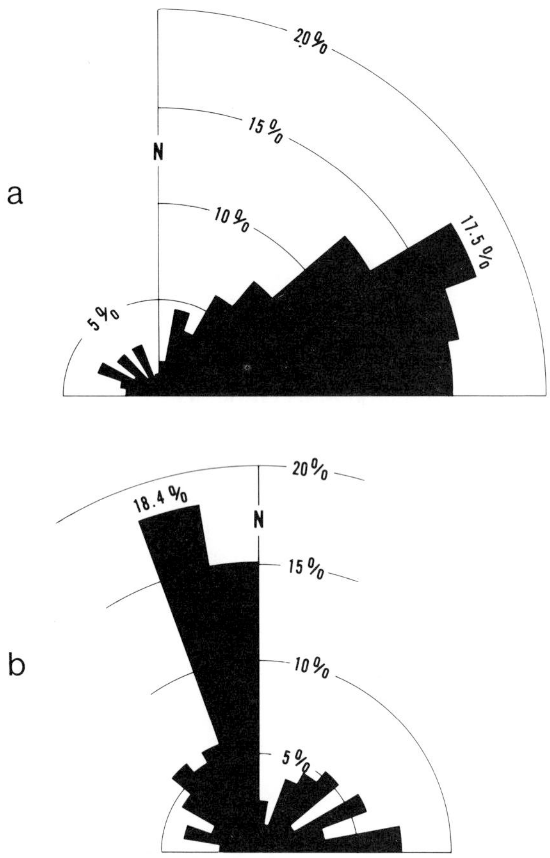

Figure 25.6. Strike frequency diagrams for veins and fractures from the 1,070 bench in the West orebody show the strike frequency for (*a*) 292 veins and mineralized fractures and (*b*) 152 unmineralized fractures. The length of each 10° strike segment is proportional to the percentage of total strike measurements.

rounded forms are also present. The matrix of the breccia consists of small rock fragments and rock flour and usually comprises 5 to 20 percent of the rock. Angular vugs are a diagnostic feature of the pre-mineral breccia. They occur between fragments in the breccia and vary in size from 0.2 to 2.0 in. Breccia vugs commonly occupy 1 to 5 percent of the breccia and are partially to totally filled with one or more of the following: specular hematite, indigenous iron oxide minerals, hypogene sulfides, supergene sulfides, and terminated quartz crystals.

An intimate mixture of rock types occurs as fragments in the pre-mineral breccia. The dominant rock types are monzonite porphyry and granite, with minor quartz monzonite porphyry and rare diabase. The limit of significant pre-mineral brecciation on the 1,030-ft. bench is shown on Figure 25.3. Rock type designations shown on Figures 25.3, 25.4*a* and 25.5*a* do not reflect the intensity of brecciation or differentiate between pre-mineral and post-mineral brecciation. Included in the pre-mineral breccia are the following rock type designations in decreasing order of abundance: monzonite porphyry breccia, mixed porphyry-granite breccia, mixed granite-porphyry breccia, quartz monzonite porphyry breccia, and granite breccia. The relative abundance of granite breccia and granite-porphyry breccia increases outside the limit of significant pre-mineral brecciation. Drilling and pit mapping suggest that the relative abundance of monzonite porphyry in the pre-mineral breccia increases below the 1,030-ft. bench.

The usual measures of brecciation intensity—such as fragment mixing, fragment shape and size, and fragment to matrix ratio—have not identified a center of brecciation or a zonation of brecciation intensity. However, the quantity of vugs in the pre-mineral breccia defines a zonal pattern of brecciation intensity consisting of a strongly brecciated central core, with 3 percent or more breccia vugs, and a border zone of brecciation, with greater than 1 percent but less than 3 percent breccia vugs. The quantity of breccia vugs is thought to be directly related to the intensity of pre-mineral brecciation. Specular hematite is almost always present in the vugs and can be used as a gauge of pre-mineral brecciation intensity.

The breccia core is irregular (see Figs 25.3 and 25.4*a*) and measures roughly 450 ft. by 600 ft., with a slight elongation to the northeast. Although the outline of the core is somewhat variable from bench to bench in the pit, the north and south margins have an overall steep dip to the north. The contact between the core and the border zone is usually gradational. The border zone forms an irregular sheath which almost completely surrounds the core. The limit of significant pre-mineral brecciation as shown in Figure 25.3 corresponds to the outer margin of the border zone or, where the border zone is absent, to the core. Beyond the border zone, the effects of pre-mineral brecciation are lost and post-mineral brecciation predominates.

Post-mineral brecciation has affected the rocks in a number of ways, depending on rock composition, degree and type of alteration, and relative location in the orebodies. Manifestations of this period of brecciation include shattering, crushing and granulation, mixing of rock types, and the presence of linear breccia structures containing crushed sulfides. Shattering occurs as a random network of closely-spaced, through-going fractures. It is ubiquitous in both orebodies, but is more obvious where the dominant rock type is monzonite porphyry or quartz monzonite porphyry. In certain dike-like bodies of monzonite porphyry post-mineral brecciation consists of thoroughly shattered rock. The only significant fragment and matrix development occurs on thin (up to 1 in.) breccia structures. Crushed sulfides occur on some fractures. The absence of significant crushing and clast development may be due, in part, to less intense phyllic and argillic alteration in the groundmass of these monzonite porphyry bodies.

Crushing and granulation are pervasive in the granite. These features occur as discontinuous fissures which cut quartz and orthoclase grains. Where this type of deformation is only weakly developed, igneous textures are easily recognizable and fragment and matrix development is poor. Crushing and granulation in the granite may be equivalent to the intense shattering in the monzonite porphyry. This incipient stage of brecciation is usually restricted to the granite breccias. Granite occurring in the mixed breccias is more intensely deformed.

With increasing post-mineral brecciation the igneous textures of the rocks involved become obscure and fragment and matrix development increases. Matrix commonly makes up to 10 to 30 percent of the rock. It consists of gouge, rock flour, crushed sulfides, and broken mineral grains. Because of intense cataclastic deformation, fragments in well-developed post-mineral breccias are not as well-defined as those in pre-mineral breccias. They commonly range in size from less than 0.2 in. to over 15 ft., and their shape ranges from sub-angular to sub-rounded. Mixing of rock types is common in these breccias. They generally occur as mixed, granite, and monzonite porphyry breccias.

Linear breccia structures are an integral part of the post-mineral brecciation. These structures contain rock and mineral grain fragments (usually comprising 20 to 40 percent of the structure) in a fine-grained matrix. The fragments are rounded to sub-rounded and vary from 0.05 to 2.0 inches in diameter. Frequently the fragments are slightly elongated parallel to the structure walls. The matrix consists of rock flour, gouge, crushed sulfides and small mineral fragments. The bands of varying matrix composition that are common in the structures create a pseudo-flow texture. Crushed, contorted, and sometimes folded sulfide veinlets often occur in the structures. Commonly the breccia structures reach 6 inches in thickness. In the leached capping and chalcocite blanket they are healed by supergene minerals (probably silica and chalcocite). The breccia structures usually strike northeast with steep to moderate dips, but low-angle structures are not uncommon.

Post-mineral brecciation occurs throughout the East and West orebodies. The overall intensity of this brecciation is somewhat variable but seems to be greater on the south side of the West orebody. In the area of the east orebody post-mineral brecciation increases in intensity toward the Basement fault.

Alteration

All pre-mineral rocks in the Sacaton allochthon are altered to some degree. Two distinct hypogene alteration assemblages are present along with a supergene alteration overprint. Typical hypogene alteration zoning patterns have not been identified, but a crude zonation of phyllic alteration is present.

Hypogene Alteration and Zoning. Two hypogene alteration assemblages, potassic and phyllic, have been identified at Sacaton. Propylitic alteration has not been identified. Alteration minerals occurring in rocks of the potassic assemblage include varying quantities of biotite, chlorite, quartz, sericite, and clay, with traces of secondary K-feldspar, calcite, and anhydrite. Secondary biotite and chlorite characterize the potassic assemblage. Since phyllic and supergene alteration are superimposed upon, and largely destroy, potassic alteration, it is uncertain how much of the quartz, sericite, and clay are part of the original potassic suite.

Potassic alteration is often well developed in the monzonite porphyry and quartz monzonite porphyry and is always well developed in the diabase. The granite rarely exhibits weak potassic alteration. In the porphyries fine-grained biotite with a shreddy texture, considered here to be secondary, is found disseminated in the groundmass. The biotite occurs as discrete grains, irregular aggregates, and as fringes around primary biotite phenocrysts. Microscopically, primary biotite is brown while the secondary variety has a greenish cast. Disseminated sulfides are sometimes found with the secondary biotite. Thin biotite veinlets are rarely present. Secondary biotite may make up 40 percent of the groundmass in places where later quartz and sericite alteration is not severe. The original mafic minerals in diabase are almost totally replaced by biotite. In the granite secondary biotite occasionally replaces primary biotite. Intense development of secondary biotite in any of the rocks does not significantly destroy primary igneous textures.

Rocks with potassic alteration may contain chlorite altering from secondary and primary biotite. These rocks always exhibit quartz, sericite, and clay alteration of groundmass and phenocryst feldspars. The chlorite is thought to be part of the potassic assemblage, while most of the quartz, sericite, and clay are probably associated with the later phyllic assemblage. Some quartz veining, along with traces of calcite and anhydrite, are also part of the potassic suite.

The apparent intensity of potassic alteration in the porphyries is variable and is attributed to varying degrees of destruction of secondary biotite by subsequent phyllic alteration. In general the intensity of secondary biotite is greater in monzonite porphyry breecias and dikes than in quartz monzonite porphyry or mixed breccias.

Phyllic alteration is characterized by quartz, sericite, and clay, but quartz and sericite predominate. Secondary silica in the porphyries occurs as a fine-grained replacement of the groundmass (intergrown with sericite and clay). Minor amounts of quartz are also found, with sericite and clay replacing plagioclase phenocrysts in the porphyries and granite. Quartz-sulfide veinlets are associated with the phyllic assemblage and comprise up to 1 percent of the rock by volume.

Sericite is the major alteration product of the phyllic assemblage and constitutes up to 50 percent of the rock. In the porphyries sericite replaces plagioclase phenocrysts, biotite phenocrysts, secondary biotite grains, and the groundmass. It replaces plagioclase, biotite, and orthoclase in granite. Gray alteration selvages bordering quartz-sulfide and sulfide veinlets occur in all the mineralized rocks. The selvages are commonly up to 1 inch thick and are composed of fine-grained intergrowths of sericite and quartz with some clay. Within the selvages igneous textures are often totally destroyed.

Clay minerals make up varying amounts of the phyllic assemblage. Clay generally occurs with sericite in the groundmass of the porphyries as an alteration of feldspar in the porphyries, granite, and diabase. Kaolinite is thought to be the major clay mineral, but others are also present.

Intense phyllic alteration occurs locally in the granite and monzonite porphyry, and, where present, it almost totally obliterates igneous rock textures. Igneous textures are preserved in most of the altered rock, although quartz is the only original mineral remaining. With decreasing alteration, fresh orthoclase is observed in granite and fresh biotite phenocrysts are found in the porphyries. The presence of fresh biotite is interesting because the same rock will exhibit extensive replacement of the groundmass by quartz and sericite and total replacement of plagioclase phenocrysts by sericite and clay.

The phyllic assemblage clearly postdates potassic alteration as evidenced by the alteration of secondary biotite to sericite in phyllic selvages of sulfide veins. Balla (1972) reports a K-Ar age of 64.5 ± 1.4 m.y. for drill core containing sericite and kaolin from the hypogene sulfide zone in the vicinity of the deposit.

The major occurrence for both alteration assemblages is one of pervasive flooding of the rock. Fracture control of alteration minerals occurs rarely in the potassic assemblage but may make up 10 to 20 percent of the alteration minerals in the phyllic assemblage. Occasionally the presence of phyllic selvages seems to be obscured by brecciation and supergene alteration.

The classical hypogene alteration zoning pattern found in some porphyry copper deposits has not yet been recognized at Sacaton, perhaps due to the limited area of available information. Potassic alteration in the Laramide intrusive rocks was originally widespread and probably well developed in both orebodies. Variations in the intensity of potassic alteration appear to be related to the effects of later phyllic alteration and not to a hypogene zoning pattern. The intensity of phyllic alteration does exhibit a crude zonal pattern. A zone of strong phyllic alteration occupies the south and central portion of the West orebody and all of the East orebody. This zone has a northeasterly trend and is continuous between the two orebodies. At right angles to this trend the intensity of phyllic alteration gradually decreases.

Supergene Alteration. Supergene alteration associated with the process of secondary enrichment of sulfides has modified the suite of hypogene alteration minerals. Effects of this supergene overprint are not always assessable because post-enrichment oxidation and leaching often penetrate the chalcocite blanket into the primary sulfide zone.

Erratically distributed silicification of probable supergene origin is found in the oxidized zone and the upper portions of the enriched zone. In areas where supergene silicification is well developed, the rock is very competent and fractures are well healed. Some parts of the chalcocite blanket are well healed enough to prevent oxidation, and pods of supergene sulfide ore up to 100 ft. in diameter are left perched in the leached capping.

An undetermined quantity of the sericite and clay appears to be of supergene origin. The main evidence for this assumption comes from differences in the megascopic appearance of rocks from the oxidized zone and enriched zone compared to rocks from the primary sulfide zone. Igneous textures and phyllic selvages are more readily visible in the primary sulfide zone. It is thought that the selvages and textures are preserved because the rock has not been flooded by supergene solutions.

Minor quantities of supergene alunite occur in the enriched zone as fracture fillings and pods up to 0.1 in. thick.

Mineralization

The West orebody is contained within the limits of the horst formed by the Sacaton and West faults. Within this horst block is a northerly dipping zone of chalcocite enrichment which has been dissected and partially destroyed by post-enrichment oxidation. Ore-grade primary mineralization is present below much of the chalcocite mineralization. Both types of mineralization are mined in the West orebody, which is roughly oval in plan and measures approximately 1,400 ft. by 1,000 ft. with a slight north-south elongation. It varies in thickness from less than 100 ft. at the margins to over 700 ft. in the central portion. Before mining was initiated in 1977 ore reserves were estimated at 33.0 million tons of 0.76 percent copper with a cutoff of 0.30 percent copper. The overall waste:ore ratio was 4.8:1.

The East orebody occurs in the graben on the east side of the Sacaton fault. In late 1980 the bulk of the material to be mined was part of the south-dipping zone of chalcocite enrichment. Primary mineralization did not reach ore grade and plans were to mine it only in order to obtain the overlying chalcocite mineralization. In plan the East orebody measured approximately 750 ft. by 850 ft, and the thickness of ore varied from about 100 ft. to 400 ft. Ore reserves at that time were estimated to be 12 to 14 million tons of +1.0 percent copper.

Hypogene Mineralization. The major hypogene sulfide minerals at Sacaton are pyrite, chalcopyrite, and molybdenite. Traces of bornite and sphalerite have been observed in concentrate samples but have not been identified megascopically. Minor quantities of gold and silver are also present, along with occasional magnetite veins. Quartz occurs as terminated crystals in breccia cavities and as veinlets which usually contain sulfides.

Hypogene sulfides occur as disseminated grains, veins, and vug fillings. Disseminated sulfides are more abundant in granite and strongly brecciated rocks than in the porphyries and weakly brecciated rocks. In the West orebody disseminated grains usually comprise less than 50 percent of the hypogene sulfides, but in the East orebody, where granite breccia is the main rock type, disseminated grains make up over 50 percent of the sulfides. Locally, disseminated sulfides are more abundant in phyllic alteration selvages and in secondary biotite sites. The intensity of mineralization of vugs in the breccia is directly related to the volume of vugs in the rock. In the core of the pre-mineral breccia, sulfides filling these cavities may comprise 30 percent of the total sulfide content.

Four types of sulfide-bearing veins occur at Sacaton. The type which is responsible for the bulk of vein mineralization contains pyrite and varying quantities of chalcopyrite and quartz. Chalcopyrite usually comprises 0 to 40 percent of the veins and quartz is generally less than 10 percent. These structures commonly vary from discontinuous, paper-thin veins to semi-continuous veins up to 0.1 in. thick; rarely they reach a thickness of 6 in. The thicker veins are more continuous along strike. Quartz-pyrite ± chalcopyrite veins up to 1 in. thick are common, but they are relatively unimportant to the total sulfide content of the deposit. Occasional quartz-pyrite ± molybdenite and quartz-molybdenite veins postdate the other vein types.

The total sulfide content for both orebodies is quite variable, ranging from about 1.0 to 4.0 percent by volume. Rock type and pre-mineral brecciation cannot be directly correlated to variations in total sulfide content. North and south of the orebodies the total sulfide content decreases in a fashion similar to the overall alteration intensity. Drilling and pit mapping have defined a zone within which the grade of hypogene mineralization is at least 0.40 percent copper as chalcopyrite. As seen in Figure 25.2, this arcuate shaped zone is continuous between, and underlies most of, both orebodies. Copper grades approaching 0.70 percent are found within the zone in the vicinity of the pre-mineral breccia. Outside the zone the copper grade gradually drops off to less than 0.10 percent copper. The pyrite:chalcopyrite ratio varies from 1:1 to 3:1 within the zone and increases to 10:1 or more outside the zone. Molybdenite occurs in quartz veins and as smears on fractures. The molybdenum content averages approximately 0.010 percent for the West orebody and 0.025 percent for the East orebody.

Supergene Mineralization. Chalcocite and covellite are the only supergene sulfides recognized at Sacaton. Covellite constitutes less than 5 percent of the supergene sulfide content and is generally found near the base of the enriched zone. The paucity of specular hematite below the zone of secondary sulfide enrichment suggests that it is also of supergene origin.

The intensity of secondary enrichment is greatest at the top of the enriched zone and decreases gradually toward the base. In the upper portions of the enriched zone chalcocite completely replaces chalcopyrite and partially replaces pyrite. Toward the base of the zone chalcopyrite is partially replaced and pyrite is rimmed by thin coatings of chalcocite. The enrichment factor (the ratio of supergene copper grade to hypogene copper grade) varies from 3:1 to 5:1 for both orebodies.

The most important control for supergene enrichment is the grade of primary mineralization. The bulk of economic supergene mineralization is underlain by primary sulfides averaging at least 0.40 percent copper. The mode of occurrence of primary sulfides also appears to control the intensity of supergene enrichment. Higher grade chalcocite mineralization in the East orebody is associated with a high percentage of disseminated sulfides. Rock type and structure locally exhibit control over supergene mineralization but predictable patterns have not been recognized.

The chalcocite blanket in the West orebody is irregular in thickness, grade, and continuity. These irregularities are caused by tilting, post-enrichment oxidation, and possibly by fault offsets. In the south and central portion of the orebody the base of the blanket dips gently to the north (see 24.4*b*). Drill hole data suggests that the dip steepens abruptly or that the blanket is downdropped on the order of 200 to 300 ft. on the north side of the breccia core. It is not known whether this drop has been caused by a fault offset or by some unrecognized control that has allowed enrichment to penetrate deeper into the primary zone. On the west side of the orebody the blanket dips to the west. The blanket varies in thickness from less than 50 ft. on the margins to 500 ft. on the north side of the breccia core.

The chalcocite blanket in the East orebody varies in thickness from 200 to 400 ft. On the east side of the orebody the thickness of supergene sulfides is reduced by deep leaching. The top of the blanket on the south side is displaced by the South fault. The base of supergene enrichment dips 20 to 30° to the south.

Leached Capping and Enrichment History

A typical suite of leached capping minerals is found after the oxidation and leaching of primary and secondary sulfides. Hematite, goethite, and jarosite in varying proportions occur as indigenous minerals filling former sulfide sites. Transported iron oxide minerals are common in the leached capping and usually make up a greater volume of the rock than their indigenous equivalents. They commonly occur as fracture fillings and as a flooding of the rock.

The intensity of transported iron oxide has complicated rock type identification and leached capping interpretation. The highest grade supergene mineralization is overlain by leached capping in which the indigenous iron oxides are relatively rich in hematite and exhibit a "live" or pulverulent texture. A relatively high ratio of indigenous iron oxides to transported iron oxides is also indicative of good enrichment.

The thickness of leached capping varies from less than 100 ft. to over 650 ft. in the West orebody, with the thicker intercepts on the north side. Over most of the East orebody the capping varies from about 15 to 225 ft. in thickness; the thin intercepts occur in the southern portion, where the South fault displaces the bulk of the capping. On the east and north margins of the orebody, where greater thicknesses of capping are preserved, intercepts up to 650 ft. are found.

Where thorough leaching has occurred, the capping assays between 0.03 and 0.10 percent copper. Substantial quantities of oxidized copper minerals are found erratically distributed through the capping of both orebodies. In the East orebody the oxide minerals usually occur just above chalcocite mineralization and are thought to have resulted from in-place oxidation of chalcocite along zones of deep oxidation. Copper grades over 1.0 percent are common. In-place oxidation is also found in the West orebody, but generally the oxides occur over a greater horizontal range, and the copper has probably been transported from the point of oxidation. Chrysocolla, brochantite, and malachite are the most common oxidized copper minerals. In upper portions of the capping chrysocolla predominates, while brochantite and malachite predominate in the lower portions. Other oxidized copper minerals present in the capping include atacamite, azurite, antlerite, cuprite, native copper, and neotocite. Metatorbernite and pseudomalachite are rare.

The orebodies at Sacaton have undergone two periods of oxidation and leaching. The first period resulted in the formation of what was probably a uniform high grade chalcocite blanket that was continuous through the East and West orebodies. Although the absolute age of enrichment is not known, clasts of leached capping in hanging wall conglomerate of the Sacaton and West faults indicate that at least some, and probably all, of the original blanket formed prior to movement on these faults.

The second period of oxidation and leaching modified and partially destroyed the original blanket. In the East orebody the effects of this period of post-enrichment oxidation were less severe than in the West orebody. Deep zones of oxidation cut into the chalcocite blanket on the eastern margin of the East orebody, and the bulk of the copper that was oxidized remained *in situ* as oxidized copper minerals. Some of the copper was leached and deposited as chalcocite. The major portion of the area to be mined was unaffected by this process and remained as the economic core of the deposit.

Within the limits of the West orebody the effects of post-enrichment oxidation are diverse and are distributed in an erratic fashion. These effects range from total oxidation of sulfide minerals to partial oxidation, where only 10 or 20 percent of the sulfides are destroyed. Total oxidation of the blanket occurs in zones ranging in width from 650 ft. to less than 3 ft. Complete leaching is common, but in places copper remains as oxides.

The vertical extent of thorough post-enrichment oxidation (where at least 75% of the sulfides have been oxidized) is shown in Figure 25.4*b*. South of the pre-mineral breccia core occasional "fingers" of thorough oxidation penetrate the blanket. Most of the blanket and upper portion of the hypogene zone exhibit a pervasive, partial oxidation of sufides. Copper is generally leached in this area. Within the breccia core thorough post-enrichment oxidation penetrates and destroys a significant portion of the blanket; this oxidation has penetrated to depths of at least 550 ft. below the pre-mine ground surface. Some copper was deposited as oxides, but the bulk was leached. North of the breccia core irregular zones of oxidation cut the blanket; these zones penetrate up to 1,150 ft. below the pre-mine surface.

As a result of the second period of oxidation and leaching, the chalcocite blanket in the West orebody is extremely erratic and discontinuous. Mineable zones of high-grade chalcocite mineralization are often surrounded by completely leached material. This feature requires careful grade control and sorting of the ore during mining.

The fact that post-enrichment oxidation is much more severe in the West orebody than in the East orebody suggests that its intensity is related to movement on the Sacaton fault. Uplift of the West orebody along the fault probably raised the original chalcocite blanket above the existing water table. At that time oxidation and leaching took place in the western blanket and penetrated the margin of the eastern blanket along permeable structural zones. Pre- and post-mineral brecciation acted as local controls for this destructive stage of oxidation and leaching. The abundance of thorough oxidation in the pre-mineral breccia core (see Fig. 25.4*b*) suggests that the permeability of this zone was a major control.

Much copper leached from the original blanket in the West orebody was probably flushed completely out of the mine area by ground water. The possibility also exists that some copper was redeposited as chalcocite. Deep chalcocite mineralization on the north side of the deposit could have resulted from oxidation and redeposition of the central portion of the original blanket.

SUMMARY AND DISCUSSION

In chronological order the major geologic events in the Sacaton mine area include the following:

1. Formation of the Pinal Schist
2. Intrusion of the Precambrian Oracle Granite
3. Intrusion of diabase dikes
4. Intrusion of monzonite porphyry and quartz monzonite porphyry
5. Pre-mineral brecciation
6. Hypogene alteration and sulfide mineralization
7. Intrusion of dacite porphyry dikes
8. Erosion cycle, with formation of original chalcocite blanket
9. Subsidence and deposition of Whitetail(?) conglomerate
10. Normal faulting (West, Sacaton, and South faults) and post-mineral brecciation
11. Post-enrichment oxidation
12. Movement on Basement fault and further post-mineral brecciation
13. Quaternary alluvium

Rather than being discrete events, the intrusions of the porphyries and pre-mineral brecciation were probably overlapping. In addition, post-enrichment oxidation may have taken place in several cycles starting before deposition of the conglomerate and continuing through large scale displacement on the Basement fault.

Although the Sacaton porphyry copper deposit is similar in many respects to other porphyry copper deposits in southwestern North America, significant differences do exist. Any comparison of the area to the "typical" porphyry copper deposit is complicated by the fact that much of the Sacaton deposit and its surrounding alteration zone is known only through drilling. In addition, post-mineral faulting displaces portions of the mineralized system relative to originally adjacent rocks. With these limitations in mind, the model presented by Lowell and Guilbert (1970) can be used to compare Sacaton with the "typical" porphyry copper deposit: the main pre-ore host at Sacaton is Precambrian granite, and the composition, age, and controlling structures of this igneous host rock are similar to the model of Lowell and Guilbert (1970). Drilling suggests the igneous host at Sacaton occurs as a northeasterly elongated stock which measures at least 1,000 by 2,000 ft. The West orebody occurs at the northeastern end of the stock around the zone of pre-mineral brecciation. The 1980 levels of exposure in the West orebody are thought to represent the apex of the stock.

At Sacaton the shape of the deposit, type of deposit boundaries, hypogene plus supergene grade, and hypogene grade are similar to the model of Lowell and Guilbert. On the other hand, roughly equal proportions of ore occur in the pre-ore host and the igneous host at Sacaton, while in most porphyry copper deposits the bulk of the ore is in the igneous host. With total mineable reserves of less than 50 million tons, the Sacaton deposit appeared to be smaller and to contain less tonnage than the typical porphyry copper deposit. However, prior to normal faulting and post-enrichment oxidation, the deposit may well have contained over 200 million tons of ore-grade material. Other differences between Sacaton and the model include the fact that, although potassic alteration is present, secondary K-feldspar is not common.

The potassic assemblage is not recognized as a discrete zone, due to partial destruction by a later pervasive phyllic assemblage, which decreases in intensity away from the center of mineralization. In addition, argillic and propylitic alteration assemblages have not been noted.

Hypogene sulfide minerals at Sacaton are similar to the model except that bornite, sphalerite, and galena are virtually absent, even on the margins of the deposit. Chalcopyrite mineralization is zoned, but is not related to a discrete alteration zone. The lowest pyrite:chalcopyrite ratios occur in both the phyllic and potassic assemblages. As is typical of most porphyry deposits, the total sulfide content is lower in the potassic assemblage than the phyllic assemblage. At Sacaton rocks exhibiting potassic alteration commonly have a total sulfide content of 1.0 to 2.0 percent by volume (1.8 to 3.6% by weight) while rocks with phyllic alteration vary from 1.0 to 4.0 percent by volume (1.8 to 7.2% by weight). The zone of better chalcopyrite mineralization does not appear to be surrounded by a halo of abundant pyrite.

Although mineralized breccia zones are common in porphyry copper deposits, the breccias usually do not make up a significant proportion of the ore in the southwestern United States. At Sacaton a significant proportion of the ore in the West orebody occurs in the pre-mineral breccia.

Supergene enrichment at Sacaton is typical of most porphyry copper deposits. However, the post-enrichment history of the deposit is much more complex than the typical case. Two generations of faulting and tectonic brecciation, followed by destructive oxidation and leaching, modified the chalcocite blankets in both orebodies. The extent and complexity of these activities does not often occur (or evidence of it is not preserved) in porphyry copper deposits.

Pertinent features which must be considered in order to develop a theory of origin for the pre-mineral brecciation are as follows:

1. Pre-mineral brecciation does not occur as a well-defined pipe but as a rather poorly defined zone. Generally the contacts of the zone are gradational. Radial fractures do not occur around the zone.
2. Contacts indicating that the pre-mineral breccias are intrusive have not been found.
3. Certain phases of the monzonite porphyry locally intrude the pre-mineral breccia.
4. The percentage of monzonite porphyry fragments in the pre-mineral breccia increases with depth.
5. Most breccia fragments are sub-angular to sub-rounded and are tightly fitted together.
6. Linear breccia structures described as part of the post-mineral brecciation contain pseudo-flow textures which may have resulted from fluidization. These structures are considered to be post-mineral, due to the presence of crushed sulfides. However, it is possible that the linear breccia structures originated with the pre-mineral breccia as fluidized zones, were later mineralized, and finally re-brecciated during post mineral brecciation.

Pre-mineral brecciation at Sacaton resulted from a complex series of events and probably involved a number of different breccia-forming mechanisms. Subsidence and collapse are thought to be the primary mechanisms of breccia formation. After intrusion of the monzonite porphyry, the overlying granite either collapsed into a void created by exsolution and entrapment of vapors from crystallization of the magma (Norton and Cathles, 1973) or subsided, due to temporary retreat of the magma. In either instance breccias may have developed in the manner envisioned by Gates (1959, p. 812) for breccia pipes in the Shoshone Range, Nevada:

> The pressures of magma and gas open cracks overhead; gas rushes into some of these, tearing fragments from the walls which, in turn, assist in further brecciation by abrasion, attrition, and wedging; magma rushes into others, quickly chills and evolves more gas which brecciates the rocks ahead; still others may be filled with breccia formed by rock bursts.

If the void was formed by magma retreat, caving and rock bursting would have contributed significantly to the filling of the cavity. Several periods of collapse probably occurred along with intermittent intrusive pulses. During the intrusive pulses "mineralization stoping" (Locke, 1926) may have contributed to the brecciation. The result was a zone of thoroughly mixed and brecciated granite and monzonite porphyry which was subsequently altered and mineralized.

Post-mineral brecciation at Sacaton is thought to be tectonic in origin. It is associated with large-scale normal faulting in the area and with movement along the Basement fault.

ACKNOWLEDGMENTS

Credit should be given to former Asarco geologists John E. Kinnison and Arthur G. Blucher for recognizing the significance of the Sacaton discovery outcrop. The exploration program which delineated the Sacaton deposit was directed by Kenyon Richard and J. Harold Courtright.

The writer wishes to acknowledge a number of Asarco geologists for their assistance in the form of stimulating discussions on the geology of Sacaton. These individuals include S. A. Anzalone, G. B. Bailey, J. H. Courtright, S. R. Davis, F. T. Graybeal, H. G. Kreis, W. L. Kurtz, J. D. Sell, G. J. Stathis, and P. G. Vikre. Messrs. Anzalone, Graybeal, and Vikre were particularly helpful in the preparation of this chapter. Donald A. Melhado prepared the illustrations. Permission to publish was granted by ASARCO Incorporated.

REFERENCES CITED

Balla, J. C., 1972, The relationship of Laramide stocks to regional structure in Central Arizona: Unpub. Ph.D. Diss., Univ. Ariz.

Gates, Olcott, 1959, Breccia pipes in the Shoshone Range, Nevada: Econ. Geol., v. 54, p. 790–815.

Locke, Augustus, 1926, The formation of certain ore bodies by mineralization stoping: Econ. Geol., v. 21, p. 431–453.

Lowell, J. D., and Guilbert, J. M., 1970. Lateral and vertical alteration-mineralization zoning in porphyry ore deposits: Econ. Geol., v. 65, p. 373–408.

Mayo, E. B., 1958, Lineament tectonics and some ore districts of the Southwest: AIME Trans. v. 51, no. 211, p. 1169–1175.

Norton, D. L., and Cathles, L. M., 1973, Breccia pipes—products of exsolved vapor from magmas: Econ. Geol., v. 68, p. 540–546.

Wilson, E. D., 1969, Mineral deposits of the Gila River Indian Reservation: Ariz. Bur. Mines Bull., v. 179, 34 p.

26

Geology and Ore Deposits at Mineral Park

MOHAVE COUNTY, ARIZONA

William H. Wilkinson, Jr.; Luis A. Vega; and Spencer R. Titley

The Mineral Park mine is a porphyry copper deposit that contains relatively high molybdenum values. Mineral Park, also known as Ithaca Peak, is located approximately 26 km north of Kingman, Arizona in the Cerbat Mountains. The mine occurs in the central part of the Wallapai mining district. The property was acquired by Duval Corporation in 1958, and production of copper and molybdenum concentrates began in October, 1964. Total production through May, 1979, from the Mineral Park mine was 646,398,730 lbs. of copper; 46,795,013 lbs. of molybdenum; and approximately 5,000,000 oz. of silver. Minable reserves at Mineral Park as of January, 1980, were 49,982,000 tons, averaging 0.20 percent copper and 0.051 percent molybdenum.

STRATIGRAPHY AND PETROGRAPHY IN THE MINERAL PARK AREA

The Cerbat Mountains, where the Mineral Park mine is located, are composed of deformed Precambrian metamorphic and igneous rocks (Thomas, 1949) which are intruded by Laramide quartz monzonite porphyry stocks and rhyolite dikes. The rocks of the Cerbat Complex are represented by an older metamorphic group, the amphibolite; a body of gneiss, and younger intrusive rocks. The distribution of these rock types is shown on the mine-area map in Figure 26.1.

Older Rocks

The oldest exposed rocks in the mine area are Precambrian in age and consist of a sequence of quartz-feldspar gneiss, biotite schist, amphibolite, and quartzite. The occurrence of these rocks in folds and their field relationships suggest that they are part of an old sequence of strata. Exposures are discontinuous and evidence of original stratigraphic facing is lacking. The quartz-feldspar gneiss is strongly resistant to erosion and formed the high peaks of Turquoise Mountain and Gross Peak. Eidel and others (1968) have reported that contacts between the quartz-feldspar gneiss and the Laramide quartz monzonite porphyry were often obscured because of alteration. Where they could not make the distinction between gneiss and quartz monzonite they used the term "hybrid." Exposures created by mining have helped to define quartz-feldspar gneiss–quartz monzonite porphyry contacts (see Fig. 26.1) and have indicated that the rocks originally mapped as hybrid are, in fact, quartz-feldspar gneiss. Table 26.1 gives a typical modal composition for the quartz-feldspar gneiss. Plagioclase in the area is too altered to determine compositions.

Amphibolite schists occur throughout the mine, where they are more abundant than the quartz-feldspar gneiss. The amphibolite forms layers which can be traced for up to 5 km. Amphibolite schists are poorly- to well-foliated and characterized by the presence of hornblende. They are dark colored, fine- to medium-grained, xenoblastic rocks. The overall mineralogy varies somewhat, as shown in Table 26.1, where 3 representative modal analyses are listed. Plagioclase is prominently twinned but unzoned. Hornblende has a neutral to blue-green pleochroism in contrast to the brown pleochroism formed in such schists in the surrounding areas (Thomas, 1953).

Biotite schists are minor in volume and variable in composition. They are fine-grained, strongly-foliated, and contain biotite as a major constituent (40–56%). Quartz varies from 10 to 30 percent by volume and plagioclase varies from 0 to 50 percent. Biotite schist is most abundant just north of the Ithaca Peak stock, but it may be present locally throughout the deposit.

The least abundant rock type in the mine area is a fine-grained quartzite. Outcrops are rare, but Thomas (1953) has reported a layer 12 to 15 m thick near Chloride. The

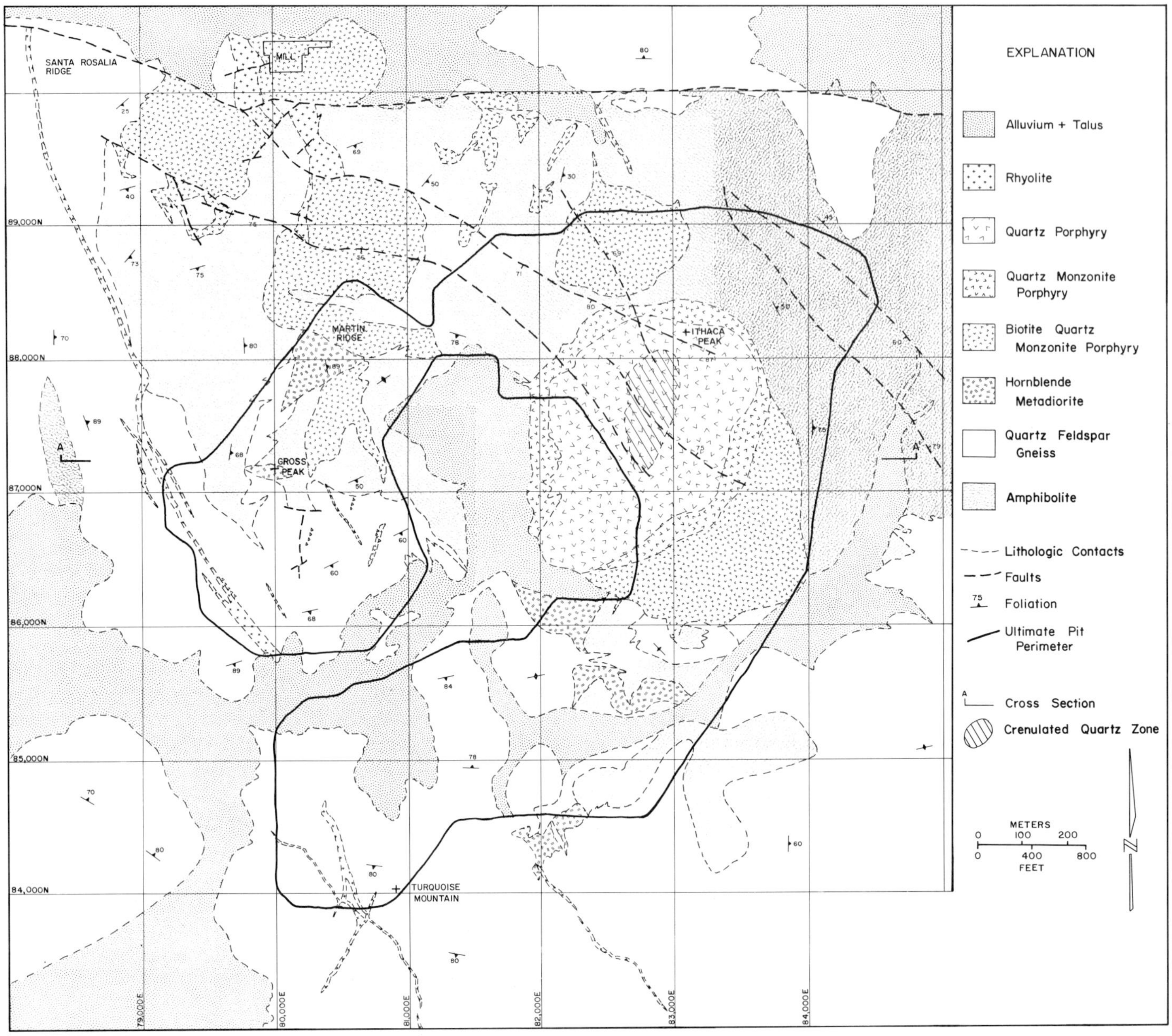

Figure 26.1. Geologic map of the Mineral Park mine area. Most of the rocks of the Wallapi mining district are present in this area.

quartzite has a sugary texture and is garnet-bearing; sparse biotite defines a weak foliation.

Granite Gneisses

The older rocks in the Mineral Park area were intruded by a batholith-sized gneiss complex, varying in composition from biotite quartz monzonite to biotite granite. One of these bodies, the Chloride Granite, has been radiometrically dated (U-Pb) at 1,740 m.y. (Silver, 1967). This age is in agreement with a date (Rb-Sr) derived from similar rocks in the Hualapai Mountains to the south of 1800 ± 470 m.y. (Kessler, 1976). These granite gneisses are the dominant rock types in the Cerbat Mountains, where they form the highest peaks and ridges. The gneisses are medium- to coarse-grained, equigranular rocks in which the development of foliation varies from very strong to indistinct. All of these rock groups are intruded by pegmatites which have been dated (Rb-Sr) from 1,515 to 1,606 m.y. (Wasserburg and Lanphere, 1965).

Diana Granite

The Diana Granite, which locally exhibits weakly developed foliation, is a coarsely porphyritic granite intrusion which has been mapped just west of Chloride. It has been K-Ar dated at 1,350 m.y. (Shafiqullah et al., 1980). The rock is characterized by large (up to 5 cm) orthoclase phenocrysts in a groundmass of orthoclase, microcline, oligoclase, quartz, and biotite (Thomas, 1953). Kessler (1976) has reported data, including Rb-Sr whole rock isochron dates, on 3 plutons of similar lithology in the Northern Hualapai Mountains.

TABLE 26.1
Modal Analyses of Selected Precambrian Rock Samples in the Mineral Park Mine Area

Rock Type	Sample No.	Mineral Composition				
		Quartz	K-feldspar	Plagioclase	Biotite	Hornblende
Quartz Feldspar Gneiss	MP–71	40	45	15	trace	—
Amphibolite Schist	843–1816	23	—	47	5	25
	MP–84	35	—	27	3	35
	905–1012	5	—	40	5	50
Hornblende Metadiorite	843–2734	25	—	50	10	(15)*
	MP–81	25	15	43	5	(12)*
	804–1121	35	20	25	5	(15)*

NOTE: Dash = mineral not present.
*Replaced by secondary biotite.

These plutons are the Hualapai Granite (1,397 ± 69 m.y.), the Holy Moses Granite (1,364 ± 24 m.y.), and an unnamed medium-grained granite (1,337 ± 38 m.y.). This 1,300- to 1,400-m.y.-old intrusive event in the Hualapai and Cerbat mountains is part of the granitic suite recognized by Silver and others (1977) in western North America. These granites and all of the older rocks were intruded by pegmatite dikes dated (Rb-Sr) at 1,100 ± 161 m.y. (Kessler, 1976).

Hornblende Metadiorite

Hornblende metadiorite is the name used at the mine to denote a rock of somewhat variable composition and uncertain age. It is a medium- to coarse-grained, porphyritic-aphanitic, typically non-foliated rock; a weak foliation may be developed adjacent to contacts with other rocks. Near its contacts with amphibolite, fragments of foliated amphibolite schist are often observed.

The distribution of hornblende metadioriate is restricted to the immediate area of the mine and to an area northwest of the mine. The occurrence of hornblende metadiorite only near the Laramide intrusive rocks led Eidel and others (1968, p. 1262) to speculate that the hornblende metadiorite was "metasomatized schist that has been partially remobilized." Several relationships point to an alternate interpretation. The contacts of hornblende metadiorite with other rocks, especially with amphibolite schist, frequently show small-scale interfingering of hornblende metadiorite into the schist along foliation planes; on a larger scale the hornblende metadiorite is commonly discordant to Precambrian foliation. Fragments of foliated amphibolite schist are common in the hornblende metadiorite adjacent to schist contacts. Near these contacts there is often a grain size variation in the hornblende metadiorite from fine-grained near the contacts to increasingly coarser-grained away from the contacts. Together all of these features strongly indicate an intrusive origin for the hornblende metadiorite.

Because the metadiorite is not foliated but intrudes foliated Precambrian rocks, the rock is younger than the last metamorphic event. The hornblende metadiorite is intruded by quartz monzonite porphyry and is, therefore, older than the Laramide porphyry. The petrographic differences between quartz monzonite porphyry and hornblende metadiorite (Table 26.2) further serve to separate these two rock types. The intrusion of the hornblende metadiorite by pegmatites—the documented, widespread 1,300- to 1,400-m.y.-old intrusion event—and the similarity of the hornblende metadiorite to one of Kessler's (1976) 1,300- to 1,400-m.y.-old plutons provide substantial reason to include the hornblende metadiorite as one of the Younger Precambrian plutons.

Laramide Rocks

Biotite quartz monzonite porphyry, biotite quartz diorite porphyry, and rhyolite dikes compose a group of intrusive rocks localized at the Mineral Park mine. A K-Ar age of 71.5 ± 2.6 m.y. (Mauger and Damon, 1965) on vein biotite from Ithaca Peak establishes a Laramide age for early stages of alteration. This date represents a minimum age of intrusion. Rhyolite dikes crosscut the biotite quartz monzonite and quartz diorite porphyries but, in turn, are cut by mineralization and, thus, they may be genetically related to the stock intrusions.

The biotite quartz monzonite porphyry and biotite quartz diorite porphyry are discrete intrusions. Although there is no direct evidence for a connection of these bodies, their "stratigraphic" position in the intrusion-mineralization

TABLE 26.2
Petrographic Differences Between Hornblende Metadiorite and Biotite Quartz Monzonite Porphyry in the Mineral Park Mine Area

Hornblende Metadiorite	Biotite Quartz Monzonite Porphyry
1. Never has aplitic groundmass	1. Often has aplitic groundmass
2. Plagioclase is sharply twinned but *not zoned*	2. Plagioclase is twinned and is *strongly zoned*
3. Contains 5 to 15 percent biotite	3. Contains 2 to 10 percent biotite
4. Biotite is irregular, frayed, clotted	4. Biotite is in books with frayed ends and as isolated grains
5. Hornblende present up to 15 percent, although normally altered to biotite	5. No hornblende
6. Plagioclase is anhedral to subhedral, never euhedral	6. Plagioclase is euhedral to subhedral, often as isolated, euhedral grains

sequences indicates that they represent the same intrusive event. They occur as two main masses, the Ithaca Peak stock and the Gross Peak stock.

Ithaca Peak Stock. The Ithaca Peak stock is a single intrusion of quartz monzonite composition that passively intruded the Precambrian Cerbat Complex (Stringham, 1966). It shows concentric zoning of igneous rock types which range from biotite quartz monzonite porphyry at the contact to quartz porphyry at the center. An intermediate zone called quartz monzonite porphyry is mapped at the mine, but is distinguished from the biotite quartz monzonite porphyry only by the sericitization of biotite. The areal extent of this zone of sericitized biotite diminishes with depth, and the bottom of sericitization coincides with the bottom of chalcocite enrichment. These features suggest that the rock mapped as quartz monzonite porphyry is not a separate rock type, but is instead the product of supergene alteration of the biotite quartz monzonite porphyry.

The biotite quartz monzonite porphyry is a medium-grained, porphyritic-phaneritic to porphyritic-aphanitic rock, with compositions as shown in Table 26.3. The phenocryst phases are euhedral to subhedral; plagioclase is twinned and well zoned with compositions ranging from An_{24} to An_{30}. Rutile, apatite, and zircon are accessory minerals. Two whole rock chemical analyses of the freshest available biotite quartz monzonite porphyry are given in Table 26.4. Although these rocks appear fresh, they contain a high S content, indicating that they are mineralized.

The quartz porphyry is restricted to the central portion of the Ithaca Peak stock, where it forms an elliptical zone with a northeast axis approximately 600 m long and a northwest axis approximately 425 m wide. The quartz porphyry has a quartz monzonite composition, but it is texturally distinct from all other Laramide rocks at Mineral Park. The quartz porphyry is characterized by large (up to 1.5 cm), rounded and embayed quartz "eyes," plagioclase, biotite, and occasional large (up to 4 cm) K-feldspar phenocrysts in an aplitic groundmass. Plagioclase is twinned and well zoned, with compositions ranging from An_{24} to An_{30}.

Near the center of the quartz porphyry is an elliptical core approximately 210 m by 150 m that contains zones of crenulated quartz and large quartz pods, up to 40 m high and 12 m wide. The crenulated quartz veins are sinuous, often tightly folded bands of quartz that cut the matrix of the quartz porphyry but not the phenocrysts. These veins are similar to those described at Henderson (Wallace et al., 1978), though at Mineral Park the veins occur near the center of the quartz porphyry, rather than near the contacts of intrusive phases as at Henderson.

Variations in the original igneous textures of the stock enable recognition of three different textural/lithologic types: (1) seriate-granitic biotite quartz monzonite porphyry, (2) porphyritic-aplitic biotite quartz monzonite porphyry, and (3) porphyritic-aplitic quartz porphyry. The porphyritic-aplitic texture is the most widespread and is developed in two different rock types. This texture is characterized by phenocrysts of quartz, plagioclase, biotite, and K-feldspar in a fine-grained, sugary-textured groundmass that consists of an interlocking mosaic of quartz, orthoclase, and minor biotite.

The distribution of these textural types is shown in Figure 26.2. The seriate-granitic phase forms an incomplete zone 31 to 152 m wide around the southern and eastern margins of the Ithaca Peak stock. The aplitic phases occupy the cen-

TABLE 26.3
Modal Analyses of Selected Laramide Rock Samples From Ithaca Peak and Gross Peak Stocks

Rock Type		Sample No.	Phenocrysts				Groundmass			
			Plagioclase	Biotite	Quartz	K-feldspar	Quartz	K-feldspar	Biotite	Plagioclase
Ithaca Peak	Seriate Biotite Quartz Monzonite Porphyry	MP–63	50	10	5	±2	17	15	—	—
	Aplitic Biotite Quartz Monzonite Porphyry	MP–93	35	4	4	±1	30	25	±2	—
	Aplitic Quartz Porphyry	MP–61–II	20	3	10	±2	23	28	—	13
Gross Peak	Biotite Quartz Monzonite Porphyry	MP–74	45	10	5	—	20	17	3	—
	Biotite Quartz Diorite Porphyry	MP–27	55	3	5	—	25	12	—	—
	Biotite Quartz Monzonite Porphyry Dike	MP–17	40	10	1	—	21	25	3	—

NOTE: Dash = mineral not present.

TABLE 26.4
Whole Rock Chemical Analyses of
Biotite Quartz Monzonite Porphyry From Ithaca Peak Stock

Compound/Element	Sample Number		Average
	MP-78	MP-80	
SiO_2	72.2	71.6	71.9
Al_2O_3	14.7	15.5	15.1
TiO_2	0.036	0.11	0.073
CaO	1.68	2.10	1.89
MnO	0.03	0.01	0.02
MgO	0.71	0.73	0.72
Fe_2O_3	3.35	3.15	3.25
Na_2O	3.37	3.10	3.24
K_2O	3.73	2.89	3.31
S	1.94	1.34	1.64
Less on Ignition	3.0	2.14	2.57
Total	104.75	102.67	103.71
Be (ppm)	3	2	2.5
Cu (ppm)	585	635	610
Mo (ppm)	35	5	20
Pb (ppm)	15	10	12.5
Zn (ppm)	55	85	70
Ni (ppm)	5	5	5
Cr (ppm)	15	15	15
V_2O_5 (ppm)	80	110	95

NOTE: Analyses by Rocky Mountain Geochemical Corp., using atomic absorption.

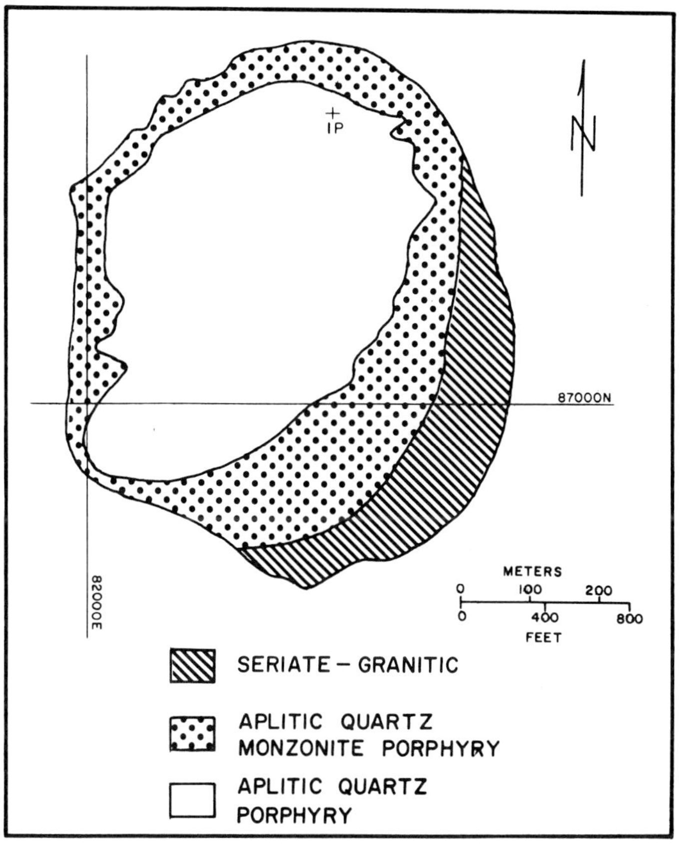

Figure 26.2. Distribution of textural types in the Ithaca Peak *(IP)* stock

tral portions of the stock, with the quartz porphyry in the center. There is textural gradation among the different phases, and the contacts between the two biotite quartz monzonite porphyry phases are not recognizable in exposures at the mine. The contact between biotite quartz monzonite porphyry and quartz porphyry is sub-vertical and gradational over 1 to 2 m. This contact is marked by a gradual disappearance of quartz eyes in the quartz porphyry. Aplites are common near the biotite quartz monzonite porphyry–quartz porphyry contact and in some cases may actually mark the contact. At one location the contact is marked by a fault.

Eidel and others (1968) have recognized this distribution of lithologic types. They have interpreted the zoning to be the result of crystallization of an equigranular rind, with development of the porphyritic texture caused by the fracturing of the pluton and the release of volatiles that produced rapid crystallization in the center of the stock. They have attributed formation of the aplites to injection of some of the rapidly crystallizing liquid along the contacts and into the biotite quartz monzonite porphyry. Similar interpretations for similar textural zoning have been presented by Nielsen (1968) for the Santa Rita stock and by Graybeal (1972) for the Patagonia Batholith.

The contacts of biotite quartz monzonite porphyry and Precambrian rocks are typically very sharp, with no observable thermal effects. Eidel and others (1968) have reported xenoliths of Precambrian schist in the porphyry adjacent to the contacts, but these xenoliths are uncommon at deeper levels of exposure in the mine. Dikes of biotite quartz monzonite porphyry in the Precambrian rocks are common, especially along the northern margin of the Ithaca Peak stock. Dikes of biotite quartz monzonite porphyry have been observed in drill core samples of Precambrian rocks as far as 150 m away from the contact. Bench maps of higher levels indicate that dikes were more common and widespread at higher elevations. Eidel and others (1968) have suggested that the Ithaca Peak stock had an inverted tear-drop shape. Recent drill data indicate that the contacts are irregular and dip sub-vertically.

Gross Peak Stock. The rocks grouped as the Gross Peak stock occur on Martin Ridge, under the mill site, and on Santa Rosalia Ridge (see Fig. 26.1). Most of the discussion in this section concerns the portion of the stock exposed along Martin Ridge, because the quartz monzonite porphyry on Santa Rosalia Ridge and under the mill site are too altered to yield usable samples. Two petrographically distinct rock types, separable only on the basis of microscopic study, make up the Gross Peak stock: biotite quartz monzonite porphyry and biotite quartz diorite porphyry. In thin section the only distinction is in differing amounts of groundmass K-feldspar (see Table 26.3). Plagioclase in both rocks is well zoned, with compositions ranging from An_{25} to An_{35}. The biotite quartz monzonite porphyry from Gross Peak is finer-grained and more biotite-rich than that from the Ithaca Peak stock.

Cross sections indicate the the intrusion on Gross Peak south of 88,000N (Fig. 26.1) is keel-shaped in an east-west direction (Fig. 26.3*A*). It pinches out to the south into 2 large, finger-like projections and, thus, is sill-like from the larger mass to the north. There are no drill data to provide information on the vertical extent of the northern part of the

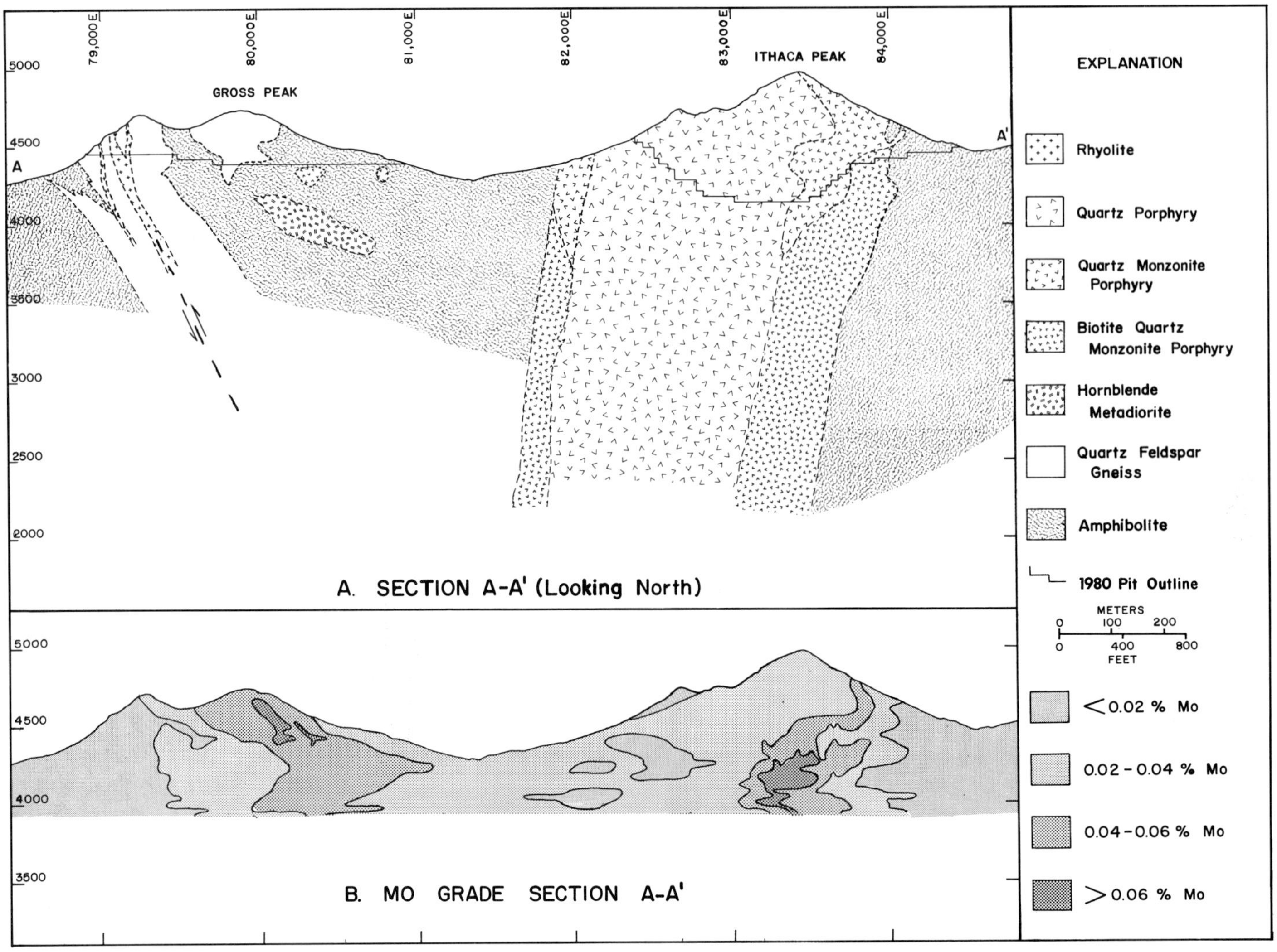

Figure 26.3. Cross sections in the Ithaca Peak–Gross Peak area: *A*, rock distribution at section *A-A'* (looking north); *B*, molybdenum grades at section *A-A'*. Location of section shown in Figure 26.1.

biotite quartz monzonite porphyry. South of 87,000N, several small, north-trending biotite quartz monzonite porphyry dikes were exposed during mining (see Fig. 26.1). These dikes appear to extend to the north into the sill-like mass of the Gross Peak stock. Texturally and compositionally (see Table 26.3) these dikes are identical to the biotite quartz monzonite porphyry to the north.

Rhyolite Dikes. The last intrusive event in the mine area resulted in the emplacement of aphanitic rhyolite dikes. These rocks are white to light pink and only rarely contain small K-feldspar or quartz phenocrysts. The dikes have sharp contacts and typically exhibit flow-banding adjacent to the contacts. The rhyolite dikes cut the biotite quartz monzonite porphyry along Santa Rosalia Ridge and are in turn cut by mineralization. The intrusions at Mineral Park occur at the approximate geographic center of the area containing rhyolite dikes. This coincidence of intrusions and rhyolite dikes and their similarity of ages suggest that they are genetically related.

Breccia Dikes. Several breccia dikes have been noted in bench faces and drill core samples in the Gross Peak area. They are quite erratic in trend, although north-south appears to be a preferred orientation. Commonly they occur along the contacts of biotite quartz monzonite porphyry and rhyolite dikes. The average thickness of the breccia dikes is .5 m, but they range from 1 cm to 6 m.

Angular to sub-rounded fragments occur randomly in a fine-grained matrix that has been strongly altered to secondary biotite, K-feldspar, and quartz. The fragments consist of all the rock types found at the mine except the Laramide porphyries. The breccia dikes are pre-mineral, but their exact relation to the rhyolite and biotite quartz monzonite dikes is problematic. Although the rhyolite cuts the monzonite, only fragments of the rhyolite occur in the breccia dikes. A better understanding of the sequence of events must await an exposure exhibiting definitive relations among the three events.

STRUCTURE OF THE WALLAPAI MINING DISTRICT

The structural evolution of the Cerbat Mountains, where the Wallapai mining district is located, is long and complex. As no Paleozoic rocks remain, structural interpretations are based largely upon discontinuous and incomplete records from the Precambrian rocks. Laramide rocks provide the only record in the gap between Precambrian and mid-Tertiary time. It is not the intent of this study to interpret the regional geologic setting, but an understanding of the structural history of the Wallapai mining district is essential to an understanding of the geologic history at Mineral Park. Because of widespread exposures of Precambrian rocks, and because of the position of the Mineral Park intrusion complex in that terrane, the district affords an excellent opportunity to examine the possible basement influence on control of porphyry mineralization.

The Wallapai mining district is approximately 6.5 km wide and 18 km long and is defined by the known lateral extent of base and precious metal veining (Fig. 26.4). The Ithaca Peak intrusions occur at the geographic center of the district. Orientations of Precambrian foliation vary within the district and define a series of open folds in the older Precambrian rocks. Faulting is expressed as fault-veins and silicified zones, but the lack of marker units precludes determination of offset. Mineralized fractures are important structural elements in the mine area.

Foliation and Folds

Foliation in the Precambrian rocks of the Wallapai mining district is defined by the alignment of biotite in schistose and granitic rocks and by gneissic layering in the granitic gneisses and quartz-feldspar gneiss. Based on foliation trends, the district can be divided into two distinct domains —one in which foliation has a regional northeast trend and one which expresses variable foliation trends. In the first domain there is a strong N40° to 70°E–striking foliation with steep dips. Although there are local variations in attitudes, this trend is present throughout the eastern parts of the Cerbat and Hualapai mountains. This foliation pattern is developed wholly within the batholithic granitic gneisses.

The domain of variable foliation trends is restricted to the western flank of the Cerbat Mountains and involves only the older Precambrian rocks. This domain extends from just north of Chloride at least to the old camp at Cerbat. The foliation within this domain is concordant with lithologic layering and defines a series of steep, rather open synforms and antiforms. Three such series of folds have been identified: (1) the Chloride fold, (2) the Roper Ridge and Turquoise Mountain folds, and (3) the Todd Basin folds (see Fig. 26.4).

The contact between the two structural domains is defined largely by changes in foliation directions and, locally, by lithologies. The structural characteristics at this contact are best observed west of the Keystone Mine (see Fig. 26.4). The number of inclusions of amphibolite in the granitic gneiss increases westward toward the contact. West of the Keystone Mine there is an area of high concentration of amphibolite and schist inclusions in a migmatite zone, and foliation trends are chaotic. Adjacent to the contact, foliation in the amphibolite inclusions in the granitic gneiss still follows the trend of the Roper Ridge fold. To the east, away from the contact, these foliations are gradually rotated until foliation in the amphibolite inclusions parallels foliation in the granitic gneiss.

These characteristics of foliation and the abundance of inclusions of amphibolite in the granitic gneiss suggest that the granitic gneiss intruded an already-folded sequence of meta-sedimentary and meta-volcanic rocks. Folds present are interpreted as remnants of folded terrain that was once more widespread.

The contact between the two domains extends over the distance from Chloride to Cerbat; although the contact is often irregular, its general trend is N30°W. It is noteworthy that both the Ithaca Peak and Alum Wash mineralized centers lie along or near this contact, which is also the locus of major veins and rhyolite dikes in the district. At a point just northwest of Mineral Park, the northernmost major dike makes an abrupt turn to a N25°E trend, and a N10°E strand also diverges from the main group at Todd Basin south of the mine; however, most of these dikes form a series of N30°W-trending swarms that reach a thickness of 30 m (see Fig. 26.4). Thus, although there is no structural break observed on the ground, the contact between the two domains appears to have controlled emplacement of intrusions in the Wallapai mining district.

Faults

Faults are abundant in the district, but the lack of good marker units makes offset and age relationships difficult to interpret. There is evidence that many of the rhyolite dikes were intruded along pre-existing structures. A major fault of probable regional extent occurs west of Gross Peak, where it marks the western edge of mineralization (Fig. 26.1). This fault, named here the Gross Peak fault, is marked by a large rhyolite dike as well as by change in attitudes of foliation in the Precambrian rocks on either side. Eastward, along the trace of the Turquoise Mountain fold limb, the strike of the foliation rotates to east-west around the nose of the fold with dips to the north. The strike of foliation continues across the fault, but dips are rotated from a northerly to a southerly direction at the fault. Cross sections indicate that there is up to 425 m of reverse movement on the Gross Peak fault, with the east side up.

The most obvious faults are those structures which form the major veins of the district. These fault-veins are younger than the rhyolite dikes that they cut. Fault-veins of the district are generally planar to gently curving and form systems of sub-parallel veins. The veins show consistent strikes from N30° to 60°W, with mostly steep dips, although the strikes of veins near Chloride depart from the regional trend and follow the limbs of the Chloride fold. Physical descriptions of these veins are presented by Thomas (1949, 1953) and Dings (1951).

Figure 26.4 shows the distribution of fault veins with an outline envelope drawn around their maximum extent. The long axis of this envelope has a N30°W trend. The majority of the veins occupy the central portion of this envelope; the major groups of veins and the axis of the envelope are centered on the Precambrian contact.

Several large faults are present in the area from Roper Ridge to Ithaca Peak (Fig. 26.4) and near the mill site. Roper Ridge, Santa Rosalia Ridge, and Ithaca Peak (Fig. 26.1) are aligned along a N70°W fault zone. The major bordering faults are shown on Figure 26.1, but between these faults there are numerous smaller faults, together with zones of intense fracturing and silicification. Such silicification has

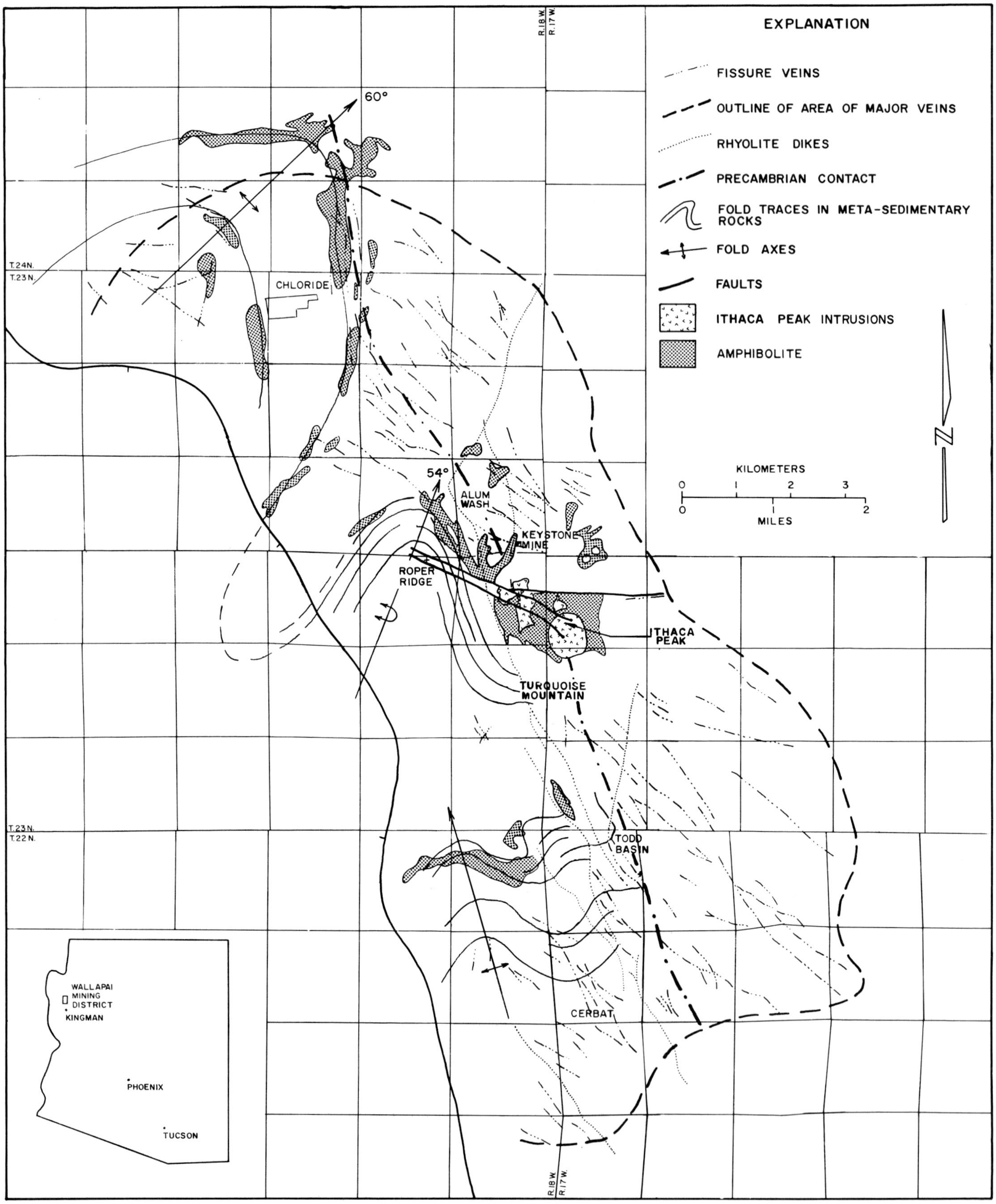

Figure 26.4. Generalized geologic and structural map of the **Wallapai** mining district

created the resistant masses of ridges and peaks at Mineral Park. Near the mill site, an east-striking strand of this zone of faulting is developed and can be traced eastward. The fault zone marks the sharp change from amphibolite schist to quartz-feldspar gneiss north of Ithaca Peak (see Fig. 26.1).

Summary of Major Structural Features

A brief chronological summary of the major structural features of the Wallapai mining district is given below:

1. A screen of folded meta-sedimentary and meta-volcanic rocks occurs along the western flank of the Cerbat Mountains.
2. The folded rocks are intruded by a regionally northeast-foliated granitic gneiss of batholitic proportions.
3. The contact between the folded rocks and the granitic gneisses becomes a major structural element in the district.
4. Intrusion of the Ithaca Peak stocks appears to localize at the intersection of this contact and the Turquoise Mountain fold.
5. The contact is the locus for intrusion of rhyolite dikes and for formation of the major fault-veins of the district.

ALTERATION AND MINERALIZATION IN THE MINERAL PARK DEPOSIT

Hydrothermal alteration associated with the Mineral Park deposit is structurally controlled and has evolved through different stages. Each stage has superimposed its characteristic alteration assemblage on successively earlier stages of alteration. This has resulted in a complex, though systematic, distribution of alteration types for which a paragenetic sequence can be determined. The extensive development of supergene alteration has complicated the alteration picture, but increasing depth in the pit has allowed direct observation of rocks below the base of supergene alteration. This asset, combined with deep drilling, has aided in the separation of hypogene from supergene effects.

Two types of alteration are recognized at Mineral Park: selectively pervasive and veinlet controlled. The characteristics of all the recognized alteration assemblages at Mineral Park are given in Table 26.5 and their paragenetic sequence is shown in Figure 26.5.

Selectively Pervasive Alteration

Selectively pervasive alteration occurs in large rock volumes but affects only certain minerals in the host rock (Titley, 1978). A widely recognized selectively pervasive type of alteration is the replacement of hornblende and primary biotite by secondary biotite. This type is the earliest alteration event recognized at Mineral Park. Secondary biotite is present over an area approximately 1.7 km by 1.45 km (Fig. 26.6); in this area it replaces hornblende in Precambrian amphibolite schist and is present in biotite quartz monzonite porphyry due to recrystallization and to partial pseudomorphic replacement of primary biotite.

Secondary biotite is most easily recognized in the Precambrian amphibolite schists and hornblende metadiorite, where hornblende is partially to totally replaced by aggregates of fine biotite flakes plus quartz and magnetite. At least partial replacement of hornblende was observed in nearly every thin section of the Precambrian rocks examined. Biotite replacement of primary biotite is never total; replacement textures are limited to felty biotite rims around the edges of biotite phenocrysts. The most characteristic feature is the development of a sagenitic rutile texture. A less common manifestation of secondary biotite is the occurrence of scattered, small flakes of biotite in the groundmass of the quartz porphyry and biotite quartz monzonite porphyry. The most abundant secondary biotite observed at Mineral Park, pervasive plus veinlet controlled, occurs at the outer edge of the low-grade copper core. This distribution of secondary biotite is similar to that observed by Carson and Jambor (1974) at Babine Lake, Canada, and by Phillips and others (1974) at the Ray, Arizona, deposit.

A second selectively pervasive alteration assemblage is the rimming and partial to total replacement of plagioclase by K-feldspar. The final result, complete conversion of plagioclase to K-feldspar, was observed in all rock types, but is not as widespread as secondary biotite. K-feldspar may in part be veinlet controlled, but it is pervasive over areas of tens of meters in core samples and in bench faces.

Veinlet-Controlled Alteration

The major portion of alteration effects observed at Mineral Park can be directly attributed to alteration along veins and veinlets. The alteration assemblages may occur either within veinlets or as halos adjacent to veinlets. A paragenetic sequence for these assemblages can be established in terms of evolution through time based on crosscutting relationships (see Table 26.5). Two enigmatic, discordant features—quartz pods and crenulated quartz veins—are not included in the paragenetic sequence because of the lack of crosscutting relationships with other vein types. Sulfides are not associated with these features.

The biotite and K-feldspar veinlets are usually irregular, contain little quartz, and may extend for tens of meters. Biotite and K-feldspar are stable with respect to each other, and biotite, though not obvious in hand specimens, is usually present in K-feldspar veinlets. The K-feldspar veinlets have diffuse contacts with the wall rocks. K-feldspar veining and flooding is essentially co-extensive with, but in part younger than, secondary biotite (see Fig. 26.6).

The coarse-grained quartz-biotite vein assemblage has been observed in two places; in one of these a biotite vein marks the eastern contact of the biotite quartz monzonite porphyry with Precambrian rocks in the Ithaca Peak stock. The vein reaches half a meter in width and consists of intergrown, coarsely crystalline biotite and quartz. There is abundant evidence for the later introduction of quartz into the vein. Sulfides that are present replace biotite and may be related to introduction of the later quartz.

Table 26.5 and Figure 26.5 show two molybdenite-bearing vein sets, one of which is quartz-molybdenite and the other, quartz–K-feldspar–anhydrite–molybdenite. There are sufficient differences in homogenization temperatures, as well as in alteration assemblages, to separate these types in time.

TABLE 26.5
Characteristics of Alteration Vein Assemblages by Rock Type at Mineral Park

	Alteration Type	Biotite Quartz Monzonite Porphyry/Quartz Feldspar Gneiss	Amphibolite Schist	Hornblende Metadiorite
Selectively Pervasive	Biotite	Recrystallization of magmatic biotite with formation of sagenitic rutile Partial replacement of primary biotite along edges Scattered small flakes and clots	Replacement of hornblende by biotite + quartz + magnetite + carbonate Replacement of primary biotite by felty biotite around edges + minor rutile Occasional biotite along fractures and cleavage in plagioclase	Replacement of hornblende by biotite + quartz + magnetite—more complete than in amphibolite Replacement of primary biotite by felty biotite around edges + minor rutile
	K-feldspar	Rimming and partial to total replacement of plagioclase Less abundant than biotite	Some replacement of plagioclase, but may be veinlet-controlled	Rimming and partial replacement of plagioclase Replaces biotite
Veinlet Controlled	Biotite	Veinlets	Replaces hornblende adjacent to veinlets	
	K-feldspar	Diffuse veinlets; replaces wall rock adjacent to veinlets	—	—
	Quartz + K-feldspar + Biotite + Anhydrite + Pyrite + Molybdenite	K-feldspar selvages Sparse carbonate	Biotite replaces hornblende and primary biotite adjacent to veinlets Sparse carbonate	
	Quartz + Molybdenite + Pyrite	No alteration Molybdenite restricted to veinlets	Biotite replaces hornblende Molybdenite restricted to veinlets	Molybdenite restricted to veinlets
	Quartz + Chalcopyrite + Pyrite + Chlorite ± Magnetite + K-feldspar ± Epidote ± Anhydrite	Chlorite in veinlets and replacing biotite adjacent to veinlets Contains minor sphalerite and galena 10% chalcopyrite in mafic sites in halo adjacent to veinlets	Chloritization of biotite adjacent to veinlets Contains minor sphalerite and galena Albite occurs with some of these veinlets 10% chalcopyrite in mafic sites in halo adjacent to veinlets	
	Quartz + Pyrite + Sericite ± Carbonate	Plagioclase and biotite replaced by sericite adjacent to veinlets Wide sericite halos	Chloritization of primary and secondary biotite Carbonate greater than sericite Plagioclase replaced by sericite and carbonate Minor epidote	
	Complex Veins	1. Formation of chlorite + pyrite + epidote + sericite + clay 2. Silicification and white mica adjacent to vein 3. Sericite + clay + sphene replace (1) and (2) (Thomas, 1949)	—	—

NOTE: Vein types are listed in paragenetic order, with oldest at the top and youngest at the bottom. Dash = mineral assemblage not observed.

An identical sequence of early molybdenite + K-feldspar followed by quartz + molybdenite has been described at Butte (Brimhall, 1977).

The chalcopyrite-bearing veins are poorly exposed in the pit, and little is known about them because of supergene replacement of chalcopyrite by chalcocite. The characteristics of chalcopyrite-bearing veins summarized in Table 26.5 were obtained mostly from drill core data supplemented by some observations in the lowest portions of the pit. It is noteworthy that magnetite and chalcopyrite are contemporaneous in these veinlets. The distribution of magnetite in the pit and in drill hole samples falls within the high copper zone similar to distributions at Ray (Phillips et al., 1974). Another important feature of chalcopyrite-bearing veinlets is that the first paragenetic occurrence of chlorite is observed as a phase of this veinlet alteration assemblage. Chlorite occurs as grains in the veinlets or replaces secondary and primary biotite adjacent to the veinlets.

Quartz-pyrite-sericite veinlets represent the last important mineralizing event in the pit and have the greatest degree of development in the more felsic rocks. In the more mafic rocks, sericite is less common; calcite, chlorite, and very minor epidote take its place.

Studies of polished sections indicate that the molybdenite-bearing veinlets contain no observable chalcopyrite except where reopening can be demonstrated. The chalcopyrite veinlets, however, consistently show minor amounts of sphalerite. The quartz-pyrite-sericite veinlets contain pyrite as the dominant sulfide, though very minor amounts of chalcopyrite may be present. Locally, where quartz-pyrite-sericite veinlets cut quartz-molybdenite veinlets, molybdenite is contained in the quartz-pyrite-sericite veinlets, but the amount rapidly diminishes within several centimeters away from the veinlet intersections.

The final major stage of sulfide deposition is represented by the complex quartz-chalcopyrite-pyrite-sphalerite-galena veins, which form the major veins in the Wallapai mining district. These veins cut all other vein types in the pit, but they are of only local importance at the mine. These veins reach widths of 16 m in other parts of the district.

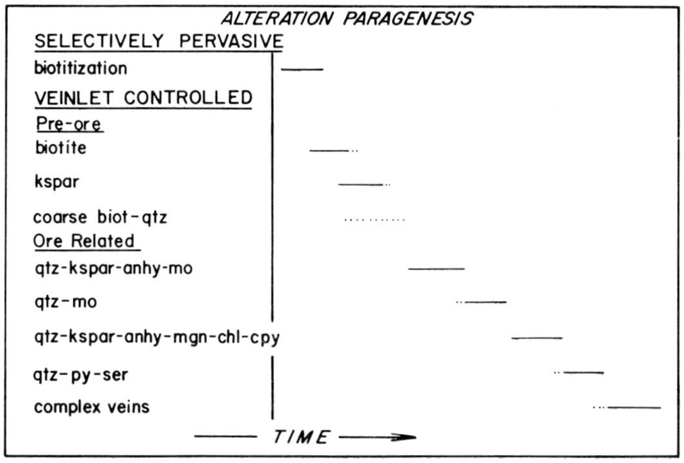

Figure 26.5. Paragenesis of major alteration assemblages at Mineral Park mine. Key: *anhy* = anhydrite, *biot*= biotite, *chl* = chlorite, *cpy* = chalcopyrite, *kspar* = K-feldspar, *mgn* = magnetite, *mo* = molybdenite, *py* = pyrite, *qtz* = quartz, *ser* = sericite.

Distribution of Alteration and Mineralization

Each successively younger alteration assemblage at Mineral Park overlaps and crosscuts earlier alteration assemblages. This relationship is most apparent between early potassic alteration, pervasive and veinlet biotite and K-feldspar alteration, and late quartz-pyrite-sericite alteration. Potassic alteration assemblages recognized in the pit and in drill core samples are extensive (see Fig. 26.6). The quartz-pyrite-sericite assemblage, which completely overprints the volume of potassic alteration, is also abundant throughout the deposit; further, this alteration type extends up to several hundred meters beyond the limits of potassic alteration. At the levels exposed in 1981 no discrete quartz-sericite "shell" (Lowell and Guilbert, 1970) was present.

Diamond drilling and rock chip geochemistry have provided data on which the lateral distribution of molybdenum and copper mineralization may be defined. In Figure 26.7 the 0.01 percent molybdenum contour defines an elliptical zone that is elongated north-northeast. The 0.03 percent molybdenum contour defines a nearly closed elliptical annular zone 200 by 360 m wide around a low-grade core. Grades within the 0.03 percent molybdenum zone are variable, with some areas greater than 0.06 percent molybdenum common. The distribution of molybdenum in the ore zone and in the low-grade core are further emphasized in Figure 26.3*B* (based on blast-hole and drill-hole assays).

The maximum depth of molybdenum mineralization is unknown. Using assay data from 19 drill holes, all greater than 300 m total depth, the lower limits of molybdenum mineralization can be approximated. Based upon the 0.03 percent molybdenum contour as an indication of the bottom of molybdenum mineralization, an approximate lower limit of mineralization occurs at the 870-m elevation (365 m below the lowest pit level in 1980). However, several deep, "root-like" zones extend to at least the 536-m elevation. Grade cross sections to the 1188-m elevation indicate that grade contours are nearly vertical (see Fig. 26.3*B*). Figure 26.8 is a schematic diagram of the best approximation of the vertical extent of molybdenum mineralization at Mineral Park, based on the 0.03 percent molybdenum cutoff. It is emphasized that grades greater than 0.02 percent molybdenum occur locally to an elevation of 158 m below sea level.

The lateral extent of hypogene copper mineralization is not well defined because of supergene effects. The hypogene copper grades presented in Figure 26.6 are based on assay values below the last noted occurrence of chalcocite in drill logs. Within the area of Figure 26.6, copper grades range from 0.05 to 0.15 percent and average 0.069 percent. A low-grade copper core (less than 0.05%) coincides with the low-grade molybdenum core. Primary copper grades decrease with depth, but they bottom at higher elevations than molybdenum grades.

The low-grade cores for both molybdenum and copper mineralization coincide. Coexistence of such low-grade cores have been documented in many porphyry copper deposits (Lowell and Guilbert, 1970). At Mineral Park the low-grade core is not centered on exposed Laramide rocks, but is located partly in quartz porphyry and partly in amphibolite

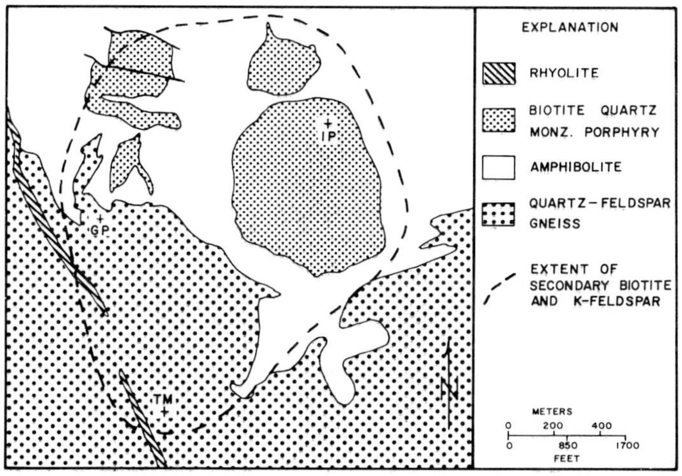

Figure 26.6. Distribution of alteration biotite and K-feldspar at Mineral Park. Key: *GP* = Gross Peak, *IP* = Ithaca Peak, *TM* = Turquoise Mountain.

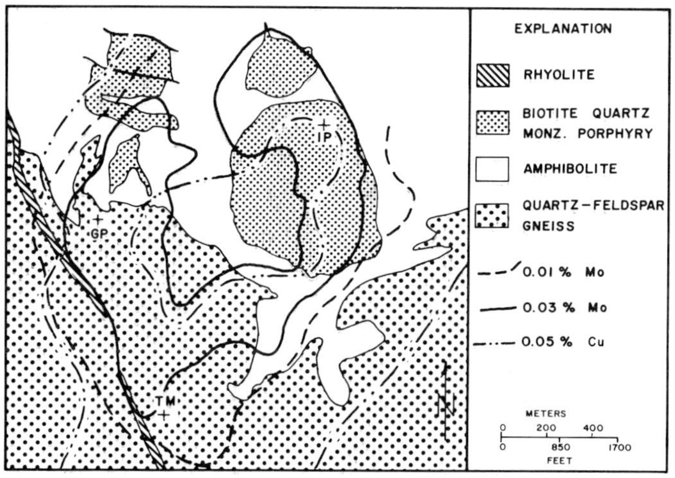

Figure 26.7. Distribution of molybdenum and copper grades at Mineral Park. Key: *GP* = Gross Peak, *IP* = Ithaca Peak, *TM* = Turquoise Mountain.

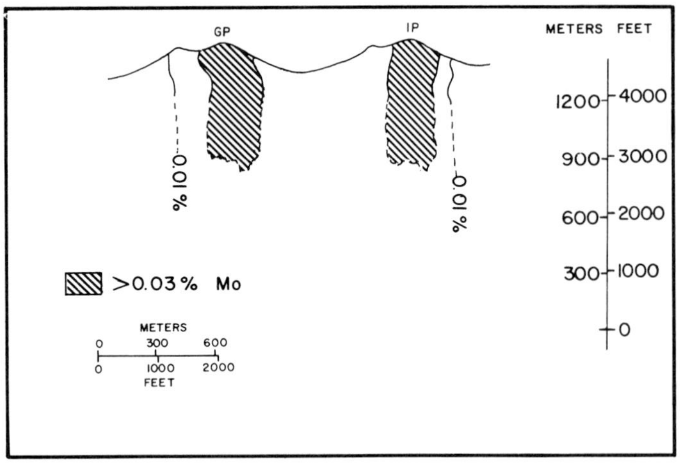

Figure 26.8. Approximate vertical distribution of molybdenum at Mineral Park (looking north). Key: *GP* = Gross Peak, *IP* = Ithaca Peak.

schist (see Fig. 26.7). The quartz porphyry within the core consists of heavily quartz-veined rock and includes the zone of quartz pods and crenulated quartz veins described earlier. Similar quartz-rich cores have been described at OK Tedi, Papua New Guinea (Bamford, 1972) and at Yandera, Papua New Guinea (Titley et al., 1978; Watmuff, 1978).

Copper mineralization has a greater lateral extent than molybdenum (see Fig. 26.7). Diamond drill holes around the eastern and southern margins of the deposit indicate that 0.05 percent copper values extend beyond the 0.01 percent molybdenum contour. Molybdenum values in these same drill holes indicate 0.001 percent molybdenum or less. The district-wide zoning pattern developed from production data on all mines in the Wallapai mining district shows that a central copper-molybdenum zone passes outward into a copper zone, then into a lead-zinc zone, and finally into a peripheral gold-silver zone (Fig. 26.9).

Hypogene copper and molybdenum grades show distinct differences when considered relative to rock type (Table 26.6). Noticeably higher copper grades tend to occur more in the Precambrian mafic rocks than in the more felsic rocks, and molybdenum grades tend to be slightly higher in the more felsic rocks. Molybdenum is almost totally restricted to quartz veins, whereas much of the chalcopyrite is observed in selvages adjacent to veins, where it shows an affinity for mafic mineral sites, especially biotite. This occurrence is consistent with other deposits, such as Ray, where "iron-rich rocks are much better hosts for copper mineralization . . . than are the siliceous rocks . . ." (Phillips et al., 1974, p. 1249).

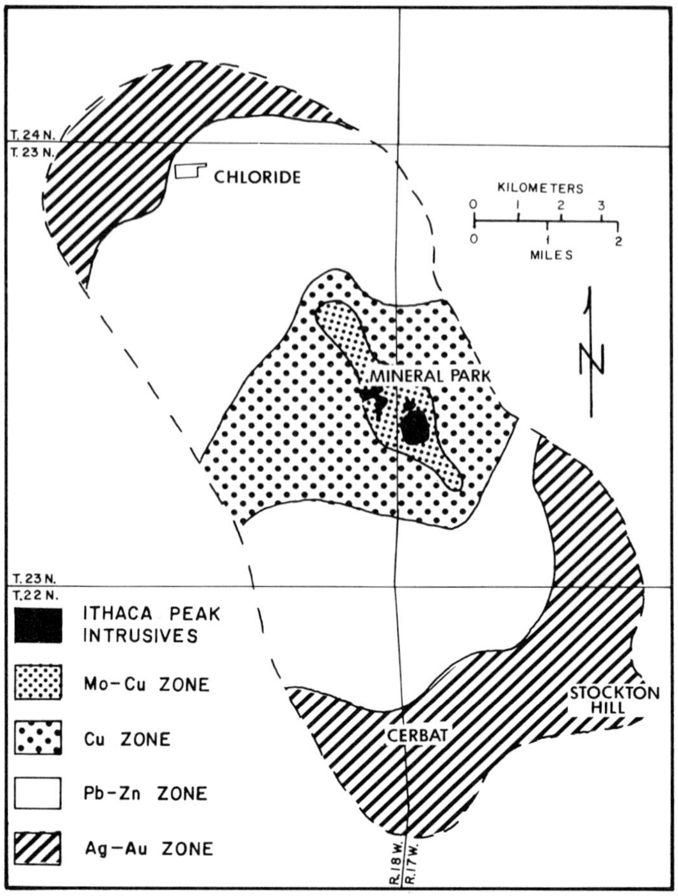

Figure 26.9. Metal zoning of Wallapai mining district, based on production figures for the entire district

TABLE 26.6
Average Grades of Hypogene Copper and Molybdenum by Rock Type at Mineral Park Mine

Rock Type	Cu Grade* (%)	Number of Cu Analyses	Mo Grade* (%)	Number of Mo Analyses
Amphibolite	0.089	376	0.038	390
Hornblende Metadiorite	0.079	245	0.043	245
Quartz Feldspar Gneiss	0.060	713	0.053	714
Biotite Quartz Monzonite Porphyry	0.067	394	0.049	396
Quartz Porphyry	0.065	713	0.039	782

NOTE: Assays by Duval Corporation.
*Grades are for 10-ft. intervals of diamond drill core samples.

FRACTURE ORIENTATIONS AT THE MINERAL PARK MINE

Studies of fracturing by Rehrig and Heidrick (1972) have shown that fracture orientations are more complex at Mineral Park than at the other deposits they have studied. Orientations for all mineralized fractures recorded from the mine are shown in Figure 26.10. No single major trend is apparent. Rehrig and Heidrick (1972) have suggested that this lack of systematic orientations might indicate a radial pattern for fracturing at Mineral Park, but continuing studies of the nature of fracturing at Mineral Park have shown that such a radial pattern is not real.

The results of fracture studies in which vein paragenesis is also considered clearly show a change in mineralized fracture orientations with time from oldest to youngest. The molybdenite veinlets at the mine (Fig. 26.11*A*), which are paragenetically early, are characterized by a dominant east-west strike, which reflects no pre-Laramide structural event

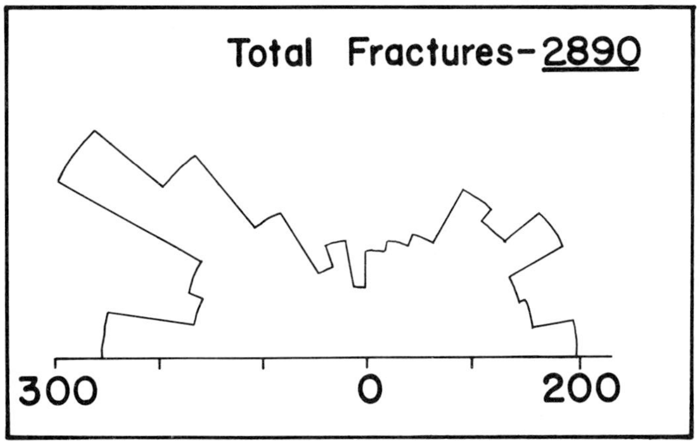

Figure 26.10. Strike diagram of all mineralized fractures at the Mineral Park mine

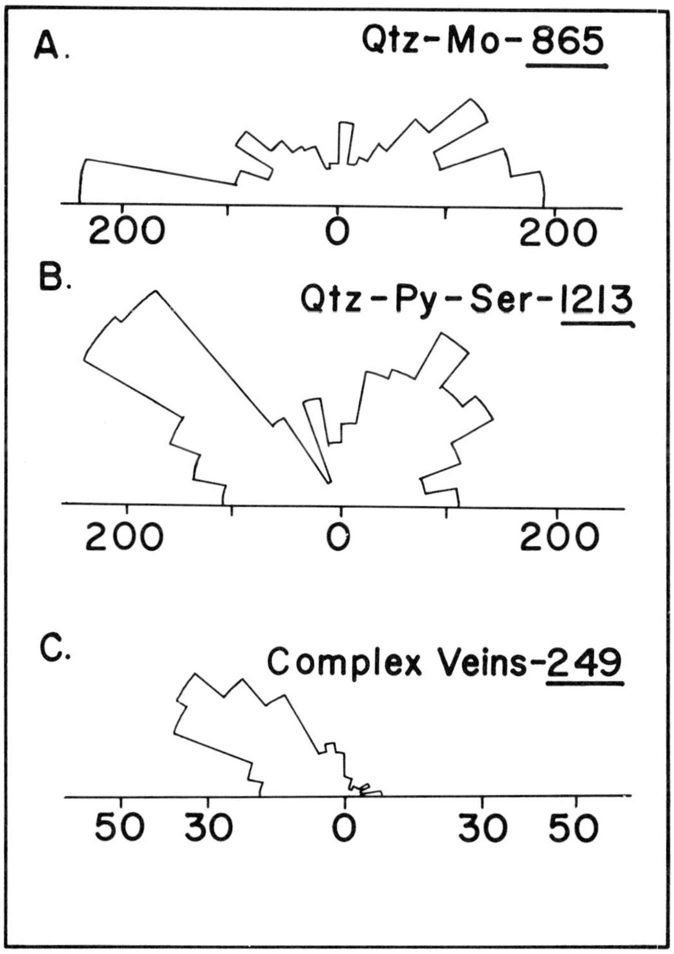

Figure 26.11. Strike diagrams of three types of mineralized fractures at the Mineral Park mine, from oldest to youngest: *A*, quartz-molybdenite *(Qtz-Mo)* veinlets; *B*, quartz-pyrite-sericite *(Qtz-Py-Ser)* veinlets; and *C*, complex sulfide veins.

recognized in the Cerbat Mountains. Two subordinate peaks with strikes of N50 to 60°E and N50 to 60°W are sub-parallel to foliation in the younger Precambrian gneisses and to the Precambrian contact and major fault-veins, respectively. The magnitude of fracturing during the molybdenite stage of mineralization indicated by fracture densities (Titley, 1982) in the ore zone ranges from 0.02 to 0.14 cm^{-1} and it averages 0.05 cm^{-1}.

The quartz-pyrite-sericite veinlets, which cut and are, therefore, younger than the quartz-molybdenite veinlets, show a well-west strike (see Fig. 26.11*B*). Both the northwest and northeast directions are sub-parallel to major structural elements in the Cerbat Mountains. Fracture densities for quartz-pyrite-sericite veinlets in the pit range from 0.05 to 0.33 cm^{-1} (average 0.14 cm^{-1}), which is significantly greater than densities for molybdenum veinlets. Quartz-pyrite-sericite veinlets also extend over a wider area than the quartz-molybdenite veinlets.

The northwest-dominant fracture direction continued during the formation of the paragenetically late complex sulfide veins, and, as Figure 26.11*C* shows, there were no other important fracture directions during the time of their formation. By the time of quartz-pyrite-sericite and complex sulfide vein formation, fractures had evolved from veinlets to major faults, some of which are traceable for over 1.6 km. The fault-vein area extends well beyond the limits of quartz-pyrite-sericite veinlets and defines the 20-km-long Wallapai mining district. The orientation and extent of these fault veins away from the intrusion center at Mineral Park was controlled by the northwest-striking Precambrian boundary in the area.

FLUID INCLUSIONS AT THE MINERAL PARK MINE

Standard fluid inclusion heating and freezing tests were performed on selected vein types in the paragenetic sequence at the Mineral Park mine (Wilkinson, 1980). Reported here are the results of 816 homogenization temperatures and 68 freezing temperatures which were determined from inclusions in quartz intergrown with sulfides in veins representative of the different paragenetic stages. Fluid inclusion analyses were performed after the paragenetic sequence had been established.

An inclusion study by Drake (1972) reported homogenization temperatures from 425 to 450°C in nearly every vein stage; because of mechanical limitations, these temperatures were estimated, rather than measured. The results presented here from the same vein types show that these estimated temperatures were too high.

Two types of fluid inclusions (classifications based on Nash [1976]) were observed at the Mineral Park mine: Type I (liquid-rich inclusions with a vapor bubble and occasional non-halite daughter minerals) and Type III (liquid-rich inclusions with a vapor bubble and a halite daughter mineral).

Type I Inclusions

Type I inclusions are by far the most abundant type observed; they account for 99 percent of the total. They are typically less than 40 μm in average diameter, and most are secondary inclusions occurring along obvious planes. Most of the Type I inclusions consist only of an aqueous liquid and vapor bubble, but occasionally these inclusions contain a birefringent, round or rod-shaped daughter mineral (anhydrite), a reddish opaque phase (hematite), or a triangular-shaped opaque mineral (chalcopyrite?). Multiple daughters are rare. None of the daughter minerals in Type I inclusions changes or dissolves with heating.

Type III Inclusions

Type III fluid inclusions contain an aqueous liquid and a vapor bubble plus a cubic daughter mineral (halite), which disappears upon heating. Only 25 Type III inclusions were recognized and they were observed only in a coarse-grained quartz-biotite vein. Within this vein they occurred only in quartz that was intricately intergrown with biotite; thus, the inclusions are considered co-depositional with the biotite. Several of the Type III inclusions contained rounded, nonbirefringent daughter minerals initially presumed to be sylvite; this presumption was proved incorrect, however, since the minerals did not change size up to homogenization temperatures. A reddish, opaque (hematite) daughter was occasionally present in Type III inclusions, but no chalcopyrite was observed.

Salinities

Salinities for Type I inclusions were calculated from freezing point depressions, as described by Roedder (1972) and Potter and others (1977*a*). In Type III inclusions, NaCl dissolution always occurred before homogenization to the liquid phase, and their salinities were obtained from the temperature of salt dissolution upon heating by using the NaCl solubility data of Potter and others (1977*b*). The distribution of salinities for both types of inclusions is shown in Figure 26.12. Many workers at other deposits have reported two clearly distinct groups of salinities (Roedder, 1971; Nash, 1976; Preece and Beane, in press; Bodnar and Beane, 1980; Reynolds and Beane, 1979). There is no overlap between the two groups present at Mineral Park: Type III inclusions have salinities which group tightly between 31 and 35 weight percent NaCl equivalent, and Type I inclusions have a somewhat wider range of from 1 to 13 weight percent NaCl equivalent. The high salinity fluids are the earliest fluids observed at Mineral Park.

Homogenization Temperatures

Fluid inclusions, abundant in all vein types at the Mineral Park mine, occur mostly as secondary inclusions along planes. An attempt was made initially to distinguish primary from secondary inclusions, but the ambiguities were such that no clearcut distinction could be made. Instead, at least 50 inclusions were analyzed in samples of each vein type in order to establish statistically valid homogenization temperature distributions. Unique peaks of homogenization temperatures were considered characteristic of given vein sets as defined for other deposits by Preece and Beane (in press) and Bodnar and Beane (1980). Histograms of homogenization temperatures for each vein type are presented in paragenetic order in Figure 26.13.

The quartz pods show a unique peak of homogenization temperatures at 350 to 370°C. The quartz pods are spatially restricted to the core of the quartz porphyry, and, since inclusions of this temperature are not seen elsewhere, the fluids forming the quartz pods may have been equally as

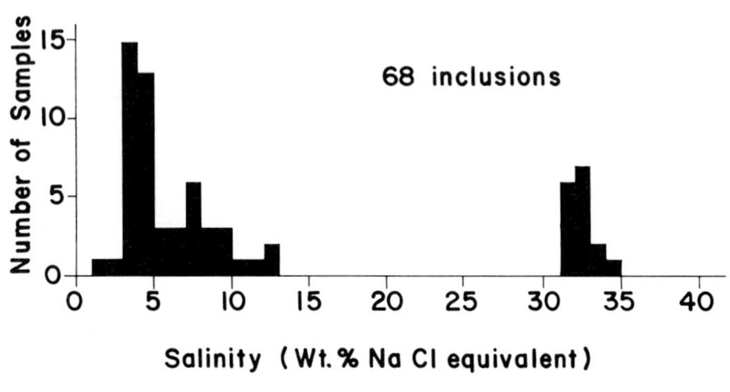

Figure 26.12. Histogram of fluid salinities from all vein types at the Mineral Park mine: *left,* Type I inclusions; *right,* Type III inclusions.

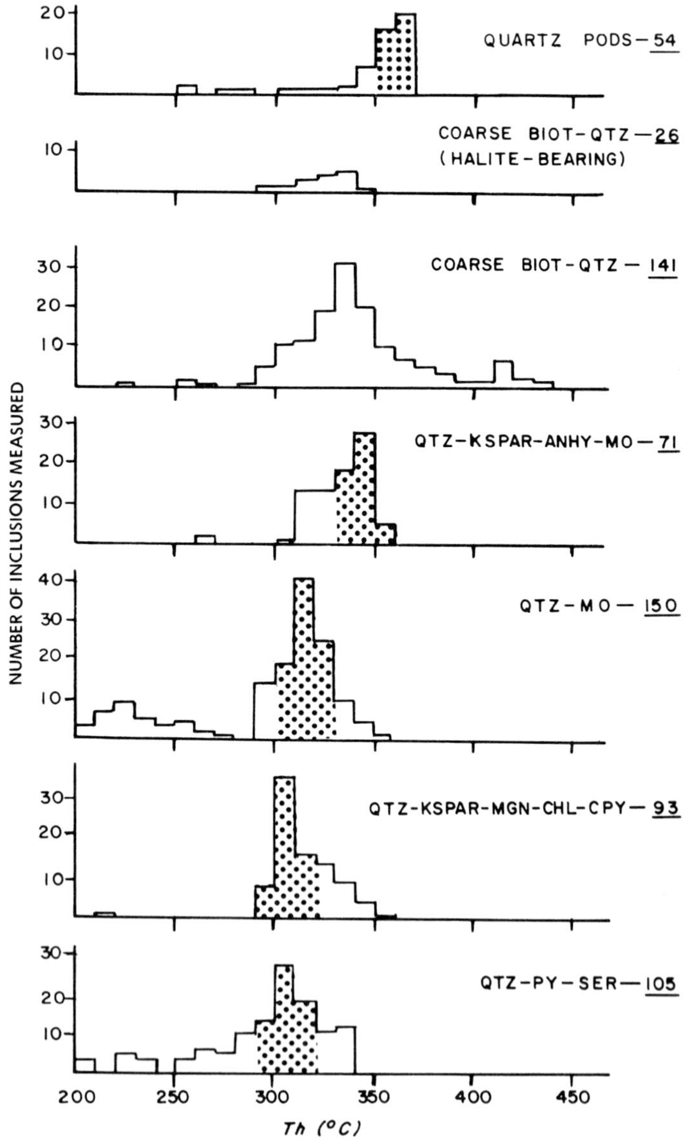

Figure 26.13. Histograms showing distribution of homogenization temperatures for quartz in veinlets (in paragenetic order) at the Mineral Park mine. Numbers of samples tested are shown to the right of each veinlet type. Shaded areas represent unique peaks of temperature. Key: *ANHY* = anhydrite, *BIOT* = biotite, *CHL* = chlorite, *CPY* – chalcopyrite, *KSPAR* = K-feldspar, *MGN* = magnetite, *MO* = molybdenite, *PY* = pyrite, *QTZ* = quartz, *SER* = sericite.

restricted. Their restricted position in the center of the quartz porphyry suggests that the quartz pods preceded other, more widespread vein types. The quartz pods do not record to any extent the fluids from the sulfide-bearing veins. However, occasional sulfides occur along clear quartz veinlets cutting the quartz pods. Homogenization temperatures from these clear quartz veinlets indicate a relationship with fluids of the major sulfide-bearing vein fluids.

The coarse-grained quartz-biotite veins record the most complex fluid evolution of any of the veins examined. Type III inclusions, which were identified as primary, occur only intergrown with biotite and quartz and, thus, can be considered co-depositional with the biotite and quartz. The inclusions in the 410 to 440°C peak of low-salinity fluids occur in quartz not intergrown with biotite; this quartz was introduced later than the biotite. The lower homogenization temperature peak, 300 to 380°C, corresponds to homogenization temperatures of fluids occurring in later sulfide-depositing events. Thus, in the pegmatitic quartz vein there is evidence for an early, moderate-temperature, high-salinity fluid followed by a fluid with a decrease in salinity and increase in homogenization temperature. The same type of sequence has been observed at Sierrita by Preece (1979).

Two unique homogenization temperature peaks occur in molybdenite-bearing veinlets. The 340 to 350°C peak corresponds to quartz–K-feldspar–anhydrite–molybdenite veinlets and the 310 to 330°C peak corresponds to quartz-molybdenite veinlets. The histograms of homogenization temperature peaks for the two vein types are sufficiently different to provisionally define two stages of molybdenum mineralization distinguished from each other by temperature as well as by characteristic alteration assemblages. The quartz-Kspar-chalcopyrite and quartz-pyrite-sericite veinlets have homogenization temperature peaks that are indistinguishable, except that the quartz-chalcopyrite peak is skewed toward higher temperatures and the quartz-pyrite-sericite peak tails off to low temperatures.

All of the vein types observed show evidence for one or two thermal events around 250°C, but these events were well documented in only two samples—quartz phenocrysts and quartz-molybdenite. In all the other samples a brief search was made to insure the presence of such fluid inclusions, but once established, large numbers of homogenization temperatures were not measured; therefore, the number of data in the 200° to 300°C range is small. Because these thermal events were never recognized as unique peaks, the vein assemblages they represent are unknown.

Figure 26.14 is a plot of measured homogenization temperatures versus time for the paragenetic sequence of mineralizing events studied at the Mineral Park mine. There is an early, moderate-temperature, high-salinity event recorded by the pegmatitic quartz. The high-salinity fluids give way abruptly to low-salinity fluids (see Fig. 26.12), the earliest of which shows an increase in homogenization temperature to approximately 420°C. Once the low-salinity fluids predominate, there is a gradual decrease in homogenization temperatures from 420 to 220°C with time. This same sequence of moderate-temperature, high-salinity fluids giving way to higher-temperature, lower-salinity fluids has previously been noted by Preece (1979) at Sierrita.

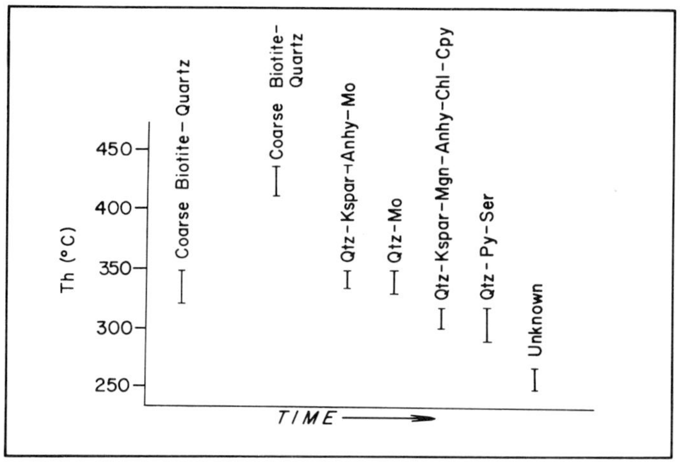

Figure 26.14. Homogenization temperatures vs. time for mineralizing events at Mineral Park

It is important to note that homogenization temperatures during the time of major sulfide deposition varied by only 50°C (from 350 to 300°C). This temperature range represents an almost isothermal temperature regime in which vein alteration assemblages evolve from K-feldspar–biotite stability to K-feldspar–chlorite stability to sericite-chlorite stability, with subsequent deposition of the economic sulfide mineralization at Mineral Park. The nearly isothermal conditions during sulfide deposition and the evolution of alteration assemblages have also been noted by Preece (1979) and by Reynolds (1980) at Santa Rita

In his study of Mineral Park, Drake (1972) has not reported any evidence for boiling; Drake and Ypma (1969) have reported that boiling took place during the chalcopyrite stage, but their evidence was not presented. During the course of this study, no evidence for boiling was observed and no inclusions homogenized to the vapor phase. Since boiling was not indicated at Mineral Park, only minimum pressures can be established for vein formation. Minimum pressure varied considerably during the regime of low-salinity fluids—from approximately 360 to 80 bars. Minimum pressures during sulfide deposition varied from 180 to 80 bars. These pressures correspond to minimum depths of formation of 2 to 3 km. These figures agree well with depths of burial of approximately 3 km, based on restored stratigraphy from the adjacent Colorado Plateau. Because boiling did not occur, a pressure correction is required to obtain trapping temperatures. At a constant pressure (250 bars) and salinity (10 weight % NaCl equivalent), the magnitude of this correction ranges from +10 to +25°C, with the larger value corresponding to lower homogenization temperatures (Potter, 1977).

DISCUSSION

The formation of the Mineral Park deposit reflects the interaction of different geologic events over time: events such as structural setting, intrusion, timing and degree of fracturing, and chemical and structural controls of mineralization acted in concert to produce the deposit being mined.

Structural relationships among rocks in the district provide evidence for interpreting the localization of the Mineral

Park deposit. Because mineralization is of Laramide age and is related to Laramide intrusions, its location reflects the control of the Laramide intrusions. Thomas (1953) has suggested that the emplacement of the Diana Granite at Chloride was controlled by the Chloride Fold, which is of Precambrian age. The nature of the distribution of hornblende metadiorite at the mine suggests that its emplacement was also controlled by a Precambrian fold—the Turquoise Mountain fold. Thus, in Precambrian time, folding served as a structural control for intrusions.

The contact between older and younger Precambrian rocks appears to have exerted an important control over the localization of Laramide intrusions and mineralization. The Ithaca Peak stock and Alum Wash mineralized area are aligned along a northwest trend which is parallel to the strike of the majority of rhyolite dikes in the district. It seems more than coincidental that these northwest trends are also parallel to the recognized Precambrian contact. Furthermore, both mineralized areas occur near intersections of the Precambrian contact and major folds: Alum Wash near the Roper Ridge fold and Ithaca Peak near the Turquoise Mountain fold. These relationships suggest that the emplacement of Laramide intrusions was guided by Precambrian structure and localized at the intersection of folds and the contact between the two Precambrian domains.

A close genetic link between the Mineral Park mine and the veins of the Wallapai mining district is apparent from zoning of different phenomena. Mineral Park occurs at the approximate geographic center of the district. Complex copper-lead-zinc-silver veins are paragenetically late in the mine area. Data presented by Drake (1972) have suggested a thermal link between porphyry copper and vein mineralization. Homogenization temperatures in the complex base-precious metal veins of the district range from 186 to >360°C; the majority of the veins have measured homogenization temperatures from 290 to 350°C. The fluids from these veins have low salinities, ranging from 1 to 4.7 weight percent NaCl equivalent. These fluids are nearly identical to sulfide-depositing fluids recognized in the mine.

Production data acquired from all the veins in the Wallapai mining district have been used to develop zoning maps based on metal ratios. The resulting zoning picture is not as symmetrical as that of Eidel and others (1968), but does show pronounced zoning from a molybdenum-copper zone centered at Mineral Park outward to an intermediate lead-zinc zone and finally to a peripheral gold-silver zone.

The occurrence of Mineral Park at the geographic center of the vein deposits, the metal zoning around the mine, the paragenetic relationships between porphyry copper and vein mineralization, and the similarity of thermosaline properties of the fluids from porphyry copper and vein mineralization strongly indicate a genetic relationship between mineralization at Mineral Park and vein mineralization throughout the district. It is suggested here that the Alum Wash and Mineral Park mineralized areas represent apophyses from a northwest-trending batholith and that the extent of this batholith is outlined by the lateral extent of dikes and veins.

Significant data for interpreting the environment of formation of the ore deposit at Mineral Park are provided by fluid inclusion analyses and by the distribution of mineralization. Fluid inclusion data and reconstructed stratigraphic columns yield a minimum depth of formation of mineralization of approximately 3 km. This is consistent with depths of formation interpreted for many other porphyry copper deposits (Lowell and Guilbert, 1970).

The narrow range of homogenization temperatures (250–440°C) spanning the life of the ancient geothermal system at Mineral Park and the lack of high homogenization temperatures constrain the temperature range and the environment of ore formation. Perhaps the best explanation for the lack of high-temperature fluids at Mineral Park can be found in the numerical simulation studies of Norton and Knight (1977) and Norton (1979). Such studies indicate that high temperatures (>500°C) are characteristic of the immediate pluton environments and occur for only short periods of time. This interpretation is consistent with fluid inclusion results from intrusion-centered deposits such as Bingham (Roedder, 1971; Nash and Cunningham, 1974) and Santa Rita (Reynolds, 1980), where homogenization temperatures greater than 700°C are observed in early veins.

There is a broad vertical region several kilometers high above the cooling pluton—the lithocap region (Norton, 1979)—where temperatures of 200 to 300°C were reached and maintained for long periods of time during the history of the cooling pluton. Norton's results are based on calculations using properties of pure water. The addition of NaCl to the fluid causes a shift—towards higher temperatures—of heat and transport properties of the fluid which would increase temperatures up to the 400°C range above the pluton (Norton, 1979). It is significant that this is the same range (200°C to 400°C) of homogenization temperatures observed at Mineral Park; it is also the same range of homogenization temperatures observed by Bodnar (1978) at Red Mountain in a lithocap environment where the intrusion is unknown.

The lateral extent of both copper and molybdenum mineralization defines an annular zone with a low-grade core. The vertical extent of molybdenum mineralization defines a nearly vertical cylinder which bottoms at approximately the 2,800-ft. elevation; anomalous molybdenum is present to the greatest depths drilled. The distribution of copper and molybdenum with respect to rock types shows that ore-grade mineralization is equally distributed between Laramide- and Precambrian-age rocks, with ore zones cutting across lithologic contacts. There is little suggestion of mineralization zoning relative to exposed Laramide rocks.

The distribution of alteration and mineralization, the narrow range of homogenization temperatures (comparable to predicted results from theoretical modeling), and the lack of high homogenization temperatures suggest that mineralization events at Mineral Park are not related to exposed Laramide rocks. Using Norton's modeling (1979) it can be interpreted that mineralization formed from 1 to 3 km above the causative pluton, but not adjacent to or within the causative pluton. The order of fluid salinities observed at Mineral Park—early high salinity followed by low salinity—is the opposite of that observed by Bodnar (1978) in the lithocap region at Red Mountain.

An important question concerns how deep the buried

source is and whether there might be intrusion-centered mineralization associated with it. Two deep holes were drilled, one to a depth of 1.524 km near the outer edge of the low-grade core, and the other to a depth of 762 m near the center of the low-grade core. Neither encountered evidence for different mineralization zones nor evidence for another intrusive phase. It appears that the causative pluton and possible associated mineralization are very deep.

The controls of mineralization at the Mineral Park deposit consist of a combination of structural and chemical factors. Certain gross structural controls are evident, and it is clear that mineralization was deposited in and adjacent to fractures. The western edge of molybdenum mineralization is controlled to a large degree by the rhyolite-filled Gross Peak fault. The molybdenum grade contours decrease adjacent to the fault and parallel it southward to Turquoise Mountain. The tail in the 0.03 percent molybdenum contour on Turquoise Mountain suggests that mineralizing fluids were trapped against the fault and channeled along it to the south for a short distance. To the east, molybdenum mineralization ceases abruptly at the biotite quartz monzonite porphyry–Precambrian contact. Fracture densities show that the abundance of molybdenite veinlets drops to zero near this contact, although total densities—especially of quartz-pyrite-sericite veinlets—remain high (0.1–0.3 cm^{-1}); the scarcity of quartz-chalcopyrite veinlets prevents a similar analysis for the copper-forming event. Figure 26.7 shows that copper mineralization does extend beyond molybdenum mineralization and, to the west, even crosses the Gross Peak fault. To the east, alteration and mineralization effects die very quickly at or near the Precambrian boundary; there is also a pronounced drop in fracture densities at this boundary, with only quartz-pyrite-sericite veinlets observed east of it.

The distribution of molybdenum grades indicates that the density of molybdenum-bearing fractures must be lower in the low-grade core than in the ore zone. When the shape and position of the annular ore zone is compared to rock types, a significant pattern emerges. The high-grade molybdenum zone (zone of high fracture denisty) occurs largely in quartz monzonite porphyry and quartz-feldspar gneiss, with only minor amounts in the amphibolite schist. The quartz monzonite porphyry and quartz-feldspar gneiss are more susceptible to brittle fracture than is the amphibolite, and they have developed higher fracture densities. The low-grade core can, therefore, be attributed to a combination of poor fracturing characteristics of the amphibolite and the presence of the quartz-rich porphyry. The annulus of mineralization developed in response to different mechanical properties of the various rock types and/or to different stress mechanisms, coupled with changes in the magnitude of strain, which resulted in fracturing.

Chemical controls are less obvious than fracture controls, but they played a major role in sulfide ore deposition. The narrow range of homogenization temperatures measured for different alteration-mineralization events suggests that temperature change was not a major control during sulfide deposition. Ore deposition occurred under nearly isothermal conditions in response to changes in fluid composition manifested by changes in alteration assemblages. The most important chemical control appears to have been changes in the hydrothermal fluid due to water-rock interactions. These chemical changes can be traced through the use of the activity diagram in Figure 26.15. Equilibrium of early fluids with K-feldspar and biotite resulted in the deposition of both minerals in veinlets and left primary K-feldspar and biotite unaffected adjacent to veinlets (see section *A* in Fig. 26.15). Molybdenum deposition occurred near the end of this assemblage. Following molybdenum mineralization, the fluids changed (see section *B,* Fig. 26.15): K-feldspar was still stable, but biotite was altered to chlorite, due to decreasing a_{K^+}/a_{H^+} or to the increasing acidity of the fluid (Beane, 1982). Further increases in acidity then drove the fluid composition into equilibrium with sericite and chlorite (see section *C,* Fig. 26.15), and pyrite became the dominant sulfide mineral. It should be emphasized again that these fluid changes were occurring at essentially isothermal conditions starting at approximately 350°C and ending at 300°C.

Sulfide mineralization decreases with depth, though fracturing persists. The potassic assemblage, K-feldspar–biotite–anhydrite, becomes more abundant with depth and sulfides decrease, copper more rapidly than molybdenum. Molybdenite veinlets from 1.524 km deep yield homogenization temperatures equal to those from the surface (±330°C); however, when temperature corrections are made for the increase in depth, the homogenization temperature rises to approximately 400°C. At such a temperature, sulfides were not a major component of veinlets, and they became so only with the deposition of molybdenite at approximately 350°C. The increase in temperature with depth may have driven hydrothermal fluids into the potassic assemblage stability fields,

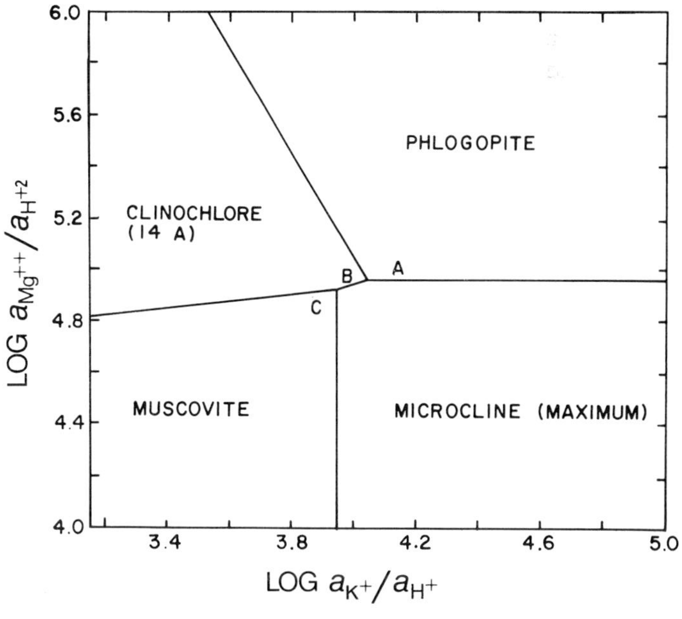

Figure 26.15. Activity diagram showing fluid evolution during mineralization at Mineral Park from the earliest fluids at *A* to the latest fluids at *C*. Diagram is constructed at 300°C and 300 bars pressure. The diagram is balanced on Al^{+3} in the presence of excess SiO_2 and H_2O. The stability field of biotite takes solid solution into account in order to permit stability with K-feldspar, and the chlorite stability field is schematically drawn to depict compatibility with K-feldspar, as suggested for pure phases at 300°C. After Beane (1982).

where sulfides were not abundant. Temperature, then, may have exerted a major control on the vertical distribution of sulfide mineralization.

ACKNOWLEDGMENTS

The authors wish to thank the Duval Corporation for permission to publish this study and for financial support for one author (WHW) during his dissertation (Wilkinson, 1980) research. In particular, the interest and strong support of W. J. Roper, former Resident Manager, and G. P. Boone, Chief Engineer, during the research phase of this study and the continued support of M. R. Miller, Resident Manager, are gratefully acknowledged. Dr. J. I. Sharpe and R. A. Metz, of the Duval Exploration Department, were most helpful with time, logistical support, and critical discussions. Many of the geological data presented in this chapter were collected by many mine geologists at Mineral Park. The help and guidance given by Drs. R. E. Beane, G. A. Davis, J. M. Guilbert, and D. L. Norton of the University of Arizona during the dissertation research are also gratefully acknowledged.

REFERENCES CITED

Bamford, R. W., 1972, The Mount Fubilan (OK Tedi) porphyry copper deposit, Territory of Papua and New Guinea: Econ. Geol., v. 67, p. 1019–1033.

Beane, R. E., 1982, Hydrothermal alteration in silicate rocks, *in* Titley, S. R., ed., Advances in Geology of the Porphyry Copper Deposits, Southwestern North America: Tucson, Univ. Ariz. Press, Chapter 6.

Bodnar, R. J., and Beane, R. E., 1980, Temporal and spatial variations in hydrothermal fluid characteristics during vein filling in pre-ore cover overlying deeply-buried porphyry copper mineralization at Red Mountain, Arizona: Econ. Geol., v. 75, p. 876–893.

Brimhall, G. H. Jr., 1977, Early fracture-controlled disseminated mineralization at Butte, Montana: Econ. Geol., v. 72, p. 37–59.

Carson, D. J. T., and Jambor, J. L., 1974, Mineralogy, zonal relationships, and economic significance of hydrothermal alteration at porphyry copper deposits, Babine Lake area, British Columbia: Can. Min. Metall. Bull., v. 67, p. 110–133.

Dings, M. G., 1951, The Wallapai mining district, Cerbat Mountains, Mohave County, Arizona: U.S. Geol. Survey Bull. 978-E, p. 123–163.

Drake, W. E., 1972, A study of ore-forming fluids at the Mineral Park porphyry copper deposit, Kingman, Arizona: Unpub. Ph.D. Diss., Columbia Univ., 245 p.

Drake, W. E., and Ypma, P. J. M., 1969, Fluid inclusion study of the Mineral Park porphyry copper deposit, Kingman, Arizona: *in* Roedder, E., ed., Proc. of COFFI, 1969, vol. 2, p. 15.

Eidel, J. J.; Frost, J. E.; and Clippinger, D. M., 1968, Copper-molybdenum mineralization at Mineral Park, Mohave County, Arizona, *in* Ridge, J. D., ed., Ore Deposits of the United States 1933–1968: New York, A.I.M.E., p. 1259–1281.

Graybeal, F. T., 1972, The partition of trace elements among coexisting minerals in some Laramide intrusive rocks in Arizona: Unpub. Ph.D. Diss., Univ. Ariz., 220 p.

Kessler, E. J., 1976. Rubidium-strontium geochronology and trace element geochemistry of Precambrian rocks in the northern Hualapai Mountains, Mohave County, Arizona: Unpub. M. S. Thesis, Univ. Ariz., 73 p.

Lowell, J. D., and Guilbert, J. M., 1970, Lateral and vertical alteration-mineralization zoning in porphyry ore deposits: Econ. Geol., v. 65, p. 373–408.

Mauger, R. L., and Damon, P. E., 1965, K-Ar ages of Laramide magmatism and copper mineralization in the Southwest: Atomic Energy Comm. Annual Progress Report No. C00-689-50, p. A-II-1–A-II-8.

Nash, J. T., 1976, Fluid inclusion petrology—data from porphyry copper deposits and applications to exploration: U.S. Geol. Survey Prof. Paper 907-D, 16 p.

Nash, J. T., and Cunningham, C. G., 1974, Fluid inclusion studies of the porphyry copper deposit at Bagdad, Arizona: Jour. Res., U.S. Geol. Survey, v. 2, p. 31–34.

Nielsen, R. L., 1968, Hypogene texture and mineral zoning in a copper-bearing granodiorite porphyry stock, Santa Rita, New Mexico: Econ. Geol., v. 63, p. 37–50.

Norton, Denis, 1979, Transport phenomena in hydrothermal systems: the redistribution of chemical components around cooling magmas: Bull. Mineral., v. 102, p. 471–486.

Norton, Denis, and Knight, Jerry, 1977, Transport phenomena in hydrothermal systems: Cooling plutons: Am. Jour. Sci., v. 277, p. 937–981.

Phillips, C. H.; Gambell, N. A.; and Fountain, D. S., 1974, Hydrothermal alteration, mineralization and zoning in the Ray deposit: Econ. Geol., v. 69, p. 1237–1250.

Potter, R. W. Jr., 1977, Pressure corrections for fluid inclusion homogenization temperatures based on the volumetric properties of the system $NaCl-H_2O$: Jour. Res., U. S. Geol. Survey, v. 5, no. 5, p. 603–607.

Potter, R. W. Jr., Clynne, M. A.; and Brown, D. L., 1977*a,* Freezing point depression of aqueous sodium chloride solutions: Econ. Geol., v. 73, p. 284–285.

Potter, R. W. Jr.; Babcock, R. S.; and Brown, D. L., 1977*b,* A new method for determining the solubility of salts in aqueous solutions at elevated temperatures: Jour. Res., U. S. Geol. Survey, v. 5, no. 3, p. 389–395.

Preece, R. K. III, 1979, Paragenesis, geochemistry, and temperatures of formation of alteration assemblages at the Sierrita deposit, Pima County, Arizona: Unpub. M.S. Thesis, Univ. of Ariz., 106 p.

Preece, R. K. III, and Beane, R. E., in press, Contrasting evolutions of hydrothermal alteration in quartz monzonite and quartz diorite at the Sierrita porphyry copper deposit, Arizona: Econ. Geol., v. 76.

Rehrig, W. A., and Heidrick, T. L., 1972, Regional fracturing in Laramide stocks of Arizona and its relationship to porphyry copper mineralization: Econ. Geol., v. 67, p. 198–213.

Reynolds, T. J., 1980, Variations in hydrothermal fluid characteristics through time at the Santa Rita, New Mexico, porphyry copper deposit: Unpub. M. S. Thesis, Univ. Ariz., 52 p.

Reynolds, T. J., and Beane, R. E., 1979, The evolution of hydrothermal fluid characteristics through time at the Santa Rita, New Mexico, porphyry copper deposit (abs.): Abs. Ann. Mtg. Geol. Soc. America, v. 11, p. 502.

Roedder, E., 1971, Fluid inclusion studies on the porphyry type deposits at Bingham, Utah; Butte, Montana; and Climax, Colorado: Econ. Geol., v. 66, p. 98–120.

———, 1972, Composition of fluid inclusions: U.S. Geol. Survey Prof. Paper 440JJ, 164 p.

Shafiqullah, M.; Damon, P. E.; Lynch, D. J.; Reynolds, S. J.; Rehrig, W. A.; and Raymond, R. H., 1980, K-Ar geochronology and geologic history of southeastern Arizona and adjacent areas: Ariz. Geol. Soc. Digest, v. XII, p. 201-260.

Silver, L. T., 1967, Apparent age relations in the older Precambrian stratigraphy of Arizona (abs.): I.U.G.S. Comm. Geochronology Conf. on Precambrian Stratified Rocks, Edmonton, Canada, p. 87.

Silver, L. T.; Bickford, M. E.; Van Schmus, W. R.; Anderson, J. L.; Anderson, T. H.; and Medaris, L. G., 1977, The 1.4–1.5 B.Y. transcontinental anorogenic plutonic perforation of North America: Geol. Soc. Amer. Abs. with Programs v. 9, no. 7, p. 1176–1177.

Stringham, Bronson, 1966, Igneous rock types and host rocks associated with porphyry copper deposits, *in* Titley, S. R., and Hicks, C. L., eds., Geology of the Porphyry Copper Deposits, Southwestern North America: Tucson, Univ. Ariz. Press, p. 35–40.

Thomas, B. E., 1949, Ore deposits of the Wallapai district, Arizona: Econ. Geol., v. 44, p. 663–705.

———, 1953, Geology of the Chloride quadrangle, Arizona: Geol. Soc. of America Bull., v. 64, p. 391–420.

Titley, S. R., 1978, Geologic history, hypogene features, and processes of secondary sulfide enrichment at the Plesyumi Copper Prospect, New Britain, Papua New Guinea: Econ. Geol., v. 73, p. 768–784.

———, 1982, The style and progress of mineralization and alteration in porphyry copper systems, American Southwest, *in* Titley, S. R., ed., Advances in Geology of the Porphyry Copper Deposits, Southwestern North America: Tucson, Univ. Ariz. Press, Chapter 5.

Titley, S. R.; Fleming, A. W.; and Neale, T. I., 1978, Tectonic evolution of the porphyry copper system at Yandera, Papua New Guinea: Econ. Geol., v. 73, p. 810–828.

Wallace, S. R.; Mackenzie, W. B.; Blair, R. G.; and Muncaster, N. K., 1978, Geology of the Urad and Henderson molybdenite deposits, Clear Creek County, Colorado, with a section on a comparison of these deposits with those at Climax, Colorado: Econ. Geol., v. 73, p. 325–368.

Wasserburg, G. J., and Lanphere, M. A., 1965, Age determinations in the Precambrian of Arizona and Nevada: Geol. Soc. of America Bull, v. 76, p. 735–758.

Watmuff, G., 1978, Geology and alteration-mineralization zoning in the central portion of the Yandera porphyry copper prospect, Papua New Guinea: Econ. Geol., v. 73, p. 829–856.

Wilkinson, W. H. Jr., 1981, The distribution of alteration and mineralization assemblages of the Mineral Park Mine, Mohave County, Arizona: Unpub. Ph.D. Diss., Univ. Ariz., 101 p.

27

Geology of the Copper Canyon Porphyry Copper Deposits

LANDER COUNTY, NEVADA

Ted G. Theodore, David W. Blake, and Edward L. Kretschmer

The Copper Canyon porphyry copper deposits of north-central Nevada, located 19 km southwest of the town of Battle Mountain and about 250 km northeast of Reno, occur in the core of an altered and mineralized area of 9 km^2 in the southeastern part of the Battle Mountain mining district. Mineralized showings along veins were first located in the 1860s at Copper Canyon, and the district was active intermittently until 1961. Recorded production from the district to 1961 includes about 150,000 oz. gold, somewhat more than 2,000,000 oz. silver, 15,000 tons copper, 5,000 tons lead, and about 1,500 tons zinc (Roberts and Arnold, 1965). Most of this metal came from veins and small replacement bodies in the Copper Canyon area. In the early 1960s, emphasis in exploration strategies shifted from a search for relatively low-tonnage, high-grade targets to large-tonnage, low-grade porphyry systems. These exploration efforts culminated in the recognition and development of two porphyry systems in the district that were commercial if mined simultaneously (Sayers et al., 1968)—one at Copper Canyon and one about 10 km to the north-northeast at Copper Basin. Duval Corporation began operating in 1967 from these two systems using open-pit methods. Reserves for milling operations before production are listed in Table 27.1. By 1974, a total of about 102,000 tons of copper contained in concentrates from milling and leaching operations had been shipped from the Copper Canyon and Copper Basin properties. The dollar value of gold produced from the porphyry deposits is second to copper; these deposits are among the smallest porphyry systems that have been exploited by industry in the United States.

TABLE 27.1
Estimated Reserves of Copper Canyon and Copper Basin Deposits, 1967

		Grade		
	Hypogene Ore (tons)	Copper (wt. %)	Gold (oz. per ton)	Silver (oz. per ton)
Copper Canyon	13,875,000	0.79	0.025	0.47
Copper Basin	3,066,000	1.75	0.011	0.26

Many regional and topical investigations contributed toward the authors' understanding of the evolution of the porphyry system at Copper Canyon. Earlier studies in the district by R. J. Roberts, who first unravelled the complex thrust relations there, provided an invaluable geologic framework. Roberts (1964) and Roberts and Arnold (1965) described the geology and the known ore deposits of the district. Theodore and others (1973) reported the K-Ar ages of plutonism and mineralization in the district, and Theodore and Blake (1975, 1978) described in detail the geology and geochemistry of the two major east and west orebodies at Copper Canyon. Blake and others (1978) characterized areal relations between sulfide mineralization and types of silicate alteration. Four other reports (Nash and Theodore, 1971; Theodore and Nash, 1973; Batchelder et al., 1976; Batchelder, 1977) discussed the chemistry, thermometry, and stable-isotope geochemistry of the ore-related fluids in the porphyry system. Theodore et al. (1976) showed the areal distributions and discussed the implications of low, yet measurable amounts of palladium detected near the outer fringes of the porphyry system at Copper Canyon.

GENERAL GEOLOGY OF THE COPPER CANYON DEPOSITS

The Copper Canyon porphyry copper deposits can be found predominantly in fractured and altered sedimentary rocks of late Paleozoic age. The area has been overridden by three successive thrust plates (Fig. 27.1); two moved during

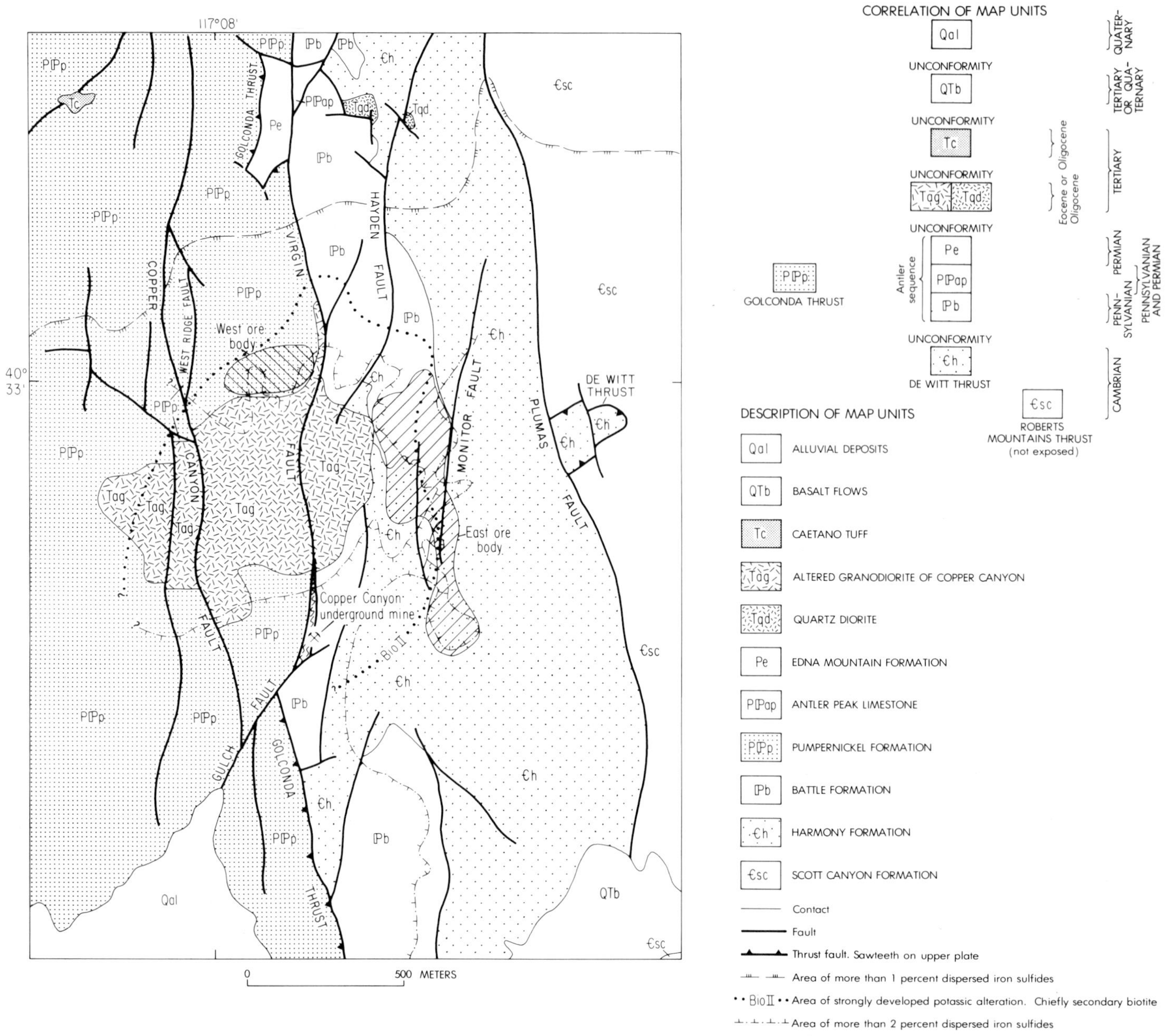

Figure 27.1. Geology of the Copper Canyon area, Lander County, Nevada

middle Paleozoic time and one during the late Paleozoic and (or) early Mesozoic. Between these intervals of major thrusting in north-central Nevada, an autochthonous block of rocks—the Antler sequence (see Correlation of Map Units on Fig. 27.1)—was deposited. This sequence unconformably overlies the two lowermost plates and is itself overridden by the uppermost thrust plate (Table 27.2). Rocks in the thrust plates are floored by (1) the middle Paleozoic Roberts Mountains thrust, (2) the middle Paleozoic Dewitt thrust, and (3) the early Mesozoic Golconda thrust (Roberts, 1964).

The porphyry deposits are related spatially and temporally to a small porphyritic granodiorite emplaced at Copper Canyon during the Eocene or Oligocene Epochs. One deposit formed mainly in rocks belonging to the Antler sequence, and the other mainly in the upper thrust plate or Golconda plate that is structurally above the Antler sequence. According to the classification of Titley (1972), the deposits at Copper Canyon are termed wall rock porphyry copper deposits. As shown in Figure 27.1, the two deposits are within 300 m of a potassically altered granodiorite (Nash and Theodore, 1971; Theodore and Blake, 1975), dated by the K-Ar method as late Eocene or early Oligocene—38 m.y. (Theodore et al., 1973). This middle Tertiary age of porphyry mineralization at Copper Canyon contrasts strikingly with the Mesozoic age of intrusive activity prevalent throughout the northwest half of Nevada (Shawe and Stewart, 1976). Further, these middle Tertiary base metal deposits are notable in that they occur in a region dominated by gold-silver metallization in the Tertiary, as most recently pointed out by Shawe and Stewart (1976) and Silberman and others (1976). The granodiorite of Copper Canyon is one of the shallow-seated bodies of rock emplaced near the northern limit of a diffuse east-west band

TABLE 27.2
Stratigraphic Units Exposed in the Immediate Area of the Ore Deposits at Copper Canyon

Formation	Age	Thickness (meters)	Lithology
Pumpernickel Formation[1]	Pennsylvanian and Permian	150+	Argillite, chert, and limey shale where unmetamorphosed; chief host for the west orebody at Copper Canyon, a copper skarn deposit
	Golconda thrust (early Mesozoic)		
Battle Formation[2]			
Upper Member	Middle Pennsylvanian	60	Quartzite and chert pebble conglomerate
Middle Member		40	Calcareous shale and shaly hornfels
Lower Member		130	Chert pebble conglomerate, calcareous and hematitic where unmetamorphosed; major host for the east orebody
	Major unconformity		
Harmony Formation	Late Cambrian	200+	Sandstone, arkose, feldspathic sandstone where unmetamorphosed; biotite hornfels where metamorphosed; host for the east orebody
	(Base not exposed)		

NOTE: See Roberts (1964) for comprehensive discussion of regional changes in lithology and their tectonic implications.

[1] Lower member of Pumpernickel Formation exposed east of Copper Canyon fault. Entire formation rapidly thickens to the west (Roberts, 1964; Theodore and Blake, 1975).

[2] Basal formation of the Antler sequence.

of Cenozoic intermediate calc-alkalic igneous activity (Stewart et al., 1977) that extended from central Nevada to central Utah 43–34 m.y. ago. Viewed on a somewhat larger scale, however, mineral deposits in this part of Nevada are confined narrowly to northwest- and northeast-trending zones which suggest deep-seated conjugate shear zones that channeled the ore-related intrusions (Roberts, 1966; Shawe and Stewart, 1976). The Battle Mountain mining district anchors the northwest terminus of the Eureka mineral belt (Shawe and Stewart, 1976)—named the Eureka-Battle Mountain mineral belt by Roberts (1966)—along which there is a significant clustering of base and precious metal deposits (see Shawe and Stewart, 1976, for recent modifications of the extent of this belt). The age of metallization along the belt varies markedly and spans at least 95 m.y. The porphyry copper deposit at Ely, Nevada, is Cretaceous in age—110 m.y. (McDowell and Kulp, 1967), and the gold-silver vein deposit at Buckhorn, Nevada, 50 km southeast of Copper Canyon, is late Tertiary—15 m.y. (Wells and Silberman, 1973).

Structural relations in the Copper Canyon area are complex and reflect repeated deformation of the rocks beginning in middle Paleozoic time and continuing until the Tertiary. Deformation during the Paleozoic and Mesozoic Eras primarily involved thrusting, whereas normal faulting was dominant during the Tertiary (Roberts, 1964). The altered granodiorite of Copper Canyon is a generally equidimensional 1,200-m-wide body of rock that lies astride three major tectonic blocks (see Fig. 27.1). It intrudes the Harmony Formation, the Battle Formation, and the Pumpernickel Formation. Although the geologic map of the granodiorite suggests a simple cylindrical configuration, several drill holes indicate that the geometry of the intrusion at depth is very complex (Theodore and Blake, 1975). The granodiorite in a vertical section is shaped somewhat like a doughnut: it contains a thin central part and a thicker rim area. Drill holes collared in the center of the granodiorite have encountered the Harmony Formation at depths in the range of 250 to 375 m. Our detailed geologic mapping suggests that emplacement of the granodiorite was controlled partly by the Virgin fault, and possibly by the Copper Canyon fault, and was helped by some assimilation of the Pumpernickel Formation. The Virgin fault, a geologically and economically significant structure in this area, bounds the Antler sequence on the west. Vertical separations across the Virgin and Copper Canyon fault systems measure about 550 m just north of the granodiorite (Theodore and Blake, 1975). Although most of the displacement along these north-striking faults occurred prior to the emplacement of the granodiorite, displacement along them continued after its emplacement.

The north-striking faults have been offset along both northeast- and northwest-striking faults (see Fig. 27.1). In the general area of the Copper Canyon underground mine, the Gulch fault, a northeast-striking premetallization fault, offsets the Virgin fault with right-lateral separation of 360 m. Just north of the granodiorite, some metallized strands of the Copper Canyon fault have left-lateral separation of 120 m along a northwest-striking postmetallization fault. Northwest-striking faults may therefore be among the youngest structures of the Copper Canyon area.

GEOLOGY OF THE ORE DEPOSITS

West Orebody

The west orebody encloses minable thicknesses of copper-, gold-, and silver-bearing rock containing more than 0.4 weight percent copper equivalent in skarn along the northern margins of the granodiorite of Copper Canyon, predominantly in the Pumpernickel Formation in the upper plate of the Golconda thrust (see Fig. 27.1). Some rocks below the thrust and very close to the granodiorite contain economic concentrations of copper, gold, and silver. The orebody is entirely between the West Ridge and Virgin faults. The uneroded part of the upper thrust plate is only about 60–90 m thick east of the West Ridge fault but thickens rapidly to the west (Roberts, 1964; Theodore and Blake, 1975). Although most of the ore in this plate is in a tectonic block that belongs structurally higher than the block in which the east orebody occurs, the elevation of the west orebody is now about 60 m lower than some of the lowest ore in the east orebody (Theodore and Blake, 1975). The west orebody occupies an irregular ovoid zone about 370 m long in an east-west direction along the northern contact of the granodiorite. On the east it is bounded by a tongue of the granodiorite along the Virgin fault; its base is generally at the Golconda thrust, along which a sill was emplaced—probably as an apophysis from the main intrusive body. This sill underlies most of the orebody. Economic metallization extends about 180 m northward roughly along strike in the metasedimentary rocks, at depths of 12 to 90 m below ground surface; the ore is generally about 45 m thick adjacent to the granodiorite and thins irregularly to about 30 m at the northern margins of the orebody delineated. Near the Virgin fault, the orebody is more or less horizontal. Some rocks are enriched to minable grades and tonnages by secondary concentrations of copper in shattered rocks near the Virgin fault, where it intersects the granodiorite. Just to the east of the Virgin fault, however, the lower and middle units of the Battle Formation between the Virgin and Hayden faults contain relatively low concentrations of hypogene copper sulfides.

Commercial concentrations of copper, gold, and silver in the orebody center more or less on a tabular body of garnet-rich rock or garnetite which has been outlined by drilling (Theodore and Blake, 1978). The garnetite is generally encased sequentially outward by surrounding zones of diopside- and tremolite-bearing rock; the garnetite has been found in the subsurface only between the West Ridge and Virgin faults. Near the granodiorite, however, garnet is conspicuously absent from an irregularly shaped mass of epidote-rich rock that includes about one-third of the orebody. Prior to the beginning of mining operations, garnetite was nowhere exposed. Near the west edge of the orebody, the garnetite is about 11 m thick up against the granodiorite; it thickens irregularly to about 21 to 37 m at distances of 260 to 410 m north of the granodiorite, the greatest distance from the orebody for which we have data from the subsurface.

The orebody occurs within an irregular, sulfide-rich shell that partly surrounds the granodiorite (see Fig. 27.1). Rock within this shell is 2 to 4 volume percent sulfide, and mostly greater than 4 percent around the west orebody (Blake et al., 1978); the granodiorite contains generally less than 2 percent. North of the west orebody, the outer limit of the shell is as yet poorly defined. Chalcopyrite is the major copper mineral in the orebody. Pyrite and pyrrhotite are the dominant iron sulfides in and around the orebody; minor marcasite is present. Pyrrhotite is especially abundant in the garnetite relative to the surrounding rock. At a distance of 410 m from the granodiorite, pyrite plus pyrrhotite constitute about 11 volume percent of the garnetite; the pyrrhotite : pyrite ratio is about 3:1. These iron-sulfide percentages and ratios remain fairly constant through the garnetite to about 90 m from the edge of the granodiorite, where pyrite plus pyrrhotite increase to about 50 percent; the corresponding increase in the pyrrhotite:pyrite ratio is about 9:1. Along this section the rocks achieve ore-grade concentrations of chalcopyrite which are closely coincident with this massive increase of pyrrhotite near the granodiorite. Details at the contact of the granodiorite are sketchy, but from the data available in 1981, economic concentrations of copper, gold, and silver occur only in the metasedimentary wall rock.

East Orebody

The east orebody is a hypogene replacement deposit; most of the copper, gold, and silver metallization occurs in potassic-altered rock in the basal 45 m of the Battle Formation, near the unconformity with the underlying Harmony Formation (Theodore and Blake, 1975). Although some of the ore straddles the narrow parts of the sulfide-rich shell just east of the granodiorite, most ore is within the shell (see Fig. 27.1). Thickness of ore zones ranges from 8 m to more than 60 m, with depth to ore beneath leached capping and waste rock in the 0 to 60 m range. The orebody is irregular in shape; overall north-south dimension is about 1,000 m, the maximum east-west dimension, 400 m. The body lies east of the Virgin fault, mainly between two other sub-parallel faults—the Hayden and the Monitor—that dip to the west. Locally, the orebody tapers sharply, with depth, to widths of about 30 m next to the granodiorite (Blake et al., 1978). Supergene mineralization (chalcocite, chrysocolla, copper carbonates, and copper oxides) and clay alteration are restricted primarily to fault zones and nearby shattered rocks and to the Harmony Formation, particularly in the southeastern part of the orebody.

The overall tonnage of ore in the east orebody was greater than that in the west orebody before mining began. In late 1978, the west orebody was mined out and open-pit mining was started in two gold deposits located about 1,000 m south of the east orebody.

RELATION OF HYPOGENE ALTERATION TO PRIMARY COPPER MINERALIZATION

Skarn

Skarn that contains a spatial zonation of anhydrous and hydrous silicate minerals is the dominant type of hypogene alteration in the general area of the west orebody (Theodore and Blake, 1978). The Pumpernickel Formation here can best be divided into four metamorphic zones: (zone 1) altered argillite, silty sandstone, and chert with biotite as the diagnostic zonal indicator; (zone 2) calc-silicate rock, which can be subdivided further into rock containing locally abundant diopside or tremolite; (zone 3) andradite-diopside-rich garnetite; and (zone 4) epidote-rich rock derived largely from garnetite. The rocks in zone 1 are farthest away from the ore and are probably correlative with the biotite hornfels ascribed to thermal metamorphic effects at many other porphyry copper deposits. The alteration mineralogy of zone 1 reflects a more or less prograde recrystallization contemporaneous with that shown by zones 2 and 3; the mineralogy of zone 4 has developed primarily as a retrograde alteration of garnetite (zone 3). Further, combinations of these mineral assemblages locally can occur in a single hand sample, largely as the result of superposed incomplete metamorphic reactions. Epidote-rich rock, the fourth type of metamorphic rock, is best developed as a replacement of garnetite in an irregular volume of rock near the granodiorite and is largely coincident with ore but less extensive. The fronts of the first three mineral zones in the skarn at Copper Canyon are oriented roughly at right angles to the edge of the granodiorite; implications of this geometry for the overall petrogenesis of the skarn are discussed below. In the immediate area of the west orebody, these mineral assemblages (zones 1–4) were flooded by an even later suite of hydrous silicates—chiefly biotite and sulfides (Fig. 27.1, Bio II).

A flat-lying tabular body of garnetite served as the locus

for most metallization in the west orebody. Copper was deposited during both anhydrous- and hydrous-silicate mineral stages as the skarn evolved at Copper Canyon. Chalcopyrite is the predominant ore mineral, and subeconomic concentrations of chalcopyrite appear to have crystallized first in diopside-pyrrhotite-quartz-K-feldspar assemblages during final stages of diopside growth in the skarn. The bulk of the chalcopyrite was deposited subsequently during hydrous-silicate stages. Ore formed in the anhydrous skarn only after repeated passage through the skarn of copper-bearing fluids, as elsewhere. This type of ore formation caused the paragenetically complex crystallization of secondary hydrous silicates and iron sulfides close to the granodiorite (Theodore and Blake, 1978). Magnetite occurs in very sparse amounts locally near the west orebody.

Rocks altered to skarn mineral assemblages have been found in the Pumpernickel and Battle Formations south of the altered granodiorite of Copper Canyon. The bulk of this skarn occurs in the Pumpernickel Formation in an approximately triangular area bounded by the Copper Canyon, Gulch, and Virgin faults (see Fig. 27.1), extending as far as 400 m south of the granodiorite. Mineral assemblages and parageneses in this skarn are generally the same as those found earlier in the west orebody. Garnetite mostly constitutes andradite-diopside-hematite ±magnetite assemblages containing partly rounded, 0.1- to 1.5-mm-wide andradite crystals that are intensely embayed and corroded by a groundmass consisting of 0.02- to 0.04-mm diopside crystals. Textural relations suggest that during the late anhydrous stage of the skarn crystallization of most diopside followed the growth of andradite—a paragenesis similar to that described earlier for the west orebody (Theodore and Blake, 1978). Pyrrhotite is the most abundant iron sulfide in the skarn; it is concentrated mostly in garnetite along microveinlets and fracture fillings containing minor amounts of chalcopyrite. Some pyrrhotite and chalcopyrite seem to be concentrated near mineral fronts between early diopside-bearing assemblages and late tremolite (actinolite)-biotite-quartz ±epidote ±apatite ±sphene assemblages. There are some notable differences between skarn in the west orebody and skarn south of the granodiorite. South of the granodiorite there is generally less pyrrhotite and more magnetite, less garnetite, and less intense development of post-andradite secondary biotite (Fig. 27.1, Bio II).

Potassic Alteration

The crystallization of minerals principally diagnostic of potassic alteration occurred during two stages of alteration at Copper Canyon. Both of these alteration stages conspicuously contain secondary magnesian biotite as the dominant zonal indicator mineral. As described briefly above, shaly beds of the Pumpernickel Formation were first converted to a biotite hornfels, probably with minimal addition of chemical constituents. This metamorphism occurred penecontemporaneously with the growth of skarn minerals in adjoining beds. Thus early-stage biotite related to skarn development makes up the outermost mineral zone that encloses the tabular flat-lying body of garnetite around the west orebody (Theodore and Blake, 1978). A subsequent stage of potassic alteration, typified by plentiful leafy secondary biotite in veins and as disseminations, centers on the altered granodiorite and forms the hypogene core of the economic mineralization (see Fig. 27.1). The leading edge of the second stage of potassic alteration generally parallels the steeply dipping contacts of the granodiorite and cuts at approximately right angles the silicate mineral zones in the skarn at the west orebody (Theodore and Blake, 1978). Generally, this potassic alteration extends about 300 m out from the granodiorite at the surface.

The granodiorite of Copper Canyon is porphyritic and contains medium- to coarse-grained phenocrysts of plagioclase, quartz, biotite, hornblende, and potassium feldspar set in a fine-grained groundmass that has been altered predominantly to potassic alteration assemblages (Theodore and Blake, 1975). Quartz-potassium feldspar veins are common. Throughout the granodiorite, some 0.01- to 0.02-mm shreds of hydrothermal biotite have recrystallized, both from primary phenocrystic biotite and as replacements of hornblende. Crystals of hornblende locally are replaced by mixtures of secondary biotite, minor chlorite, quartz, and apatite, all crudely pseudomorphous after the original crystals. These secondary, presumably magnesium-rich biotites are pale tan and less pleochroic than relict primary biotites. G. K. Czamanske (written commun., 1974) found by electron microprobe studies of optically similar hydrothermal biotite from the east orebody that the biotite has a mean Mg/Mg+Fe ratio of about 0.78. Primary biotites from three other unaltered Tertiary plutons in the mining district have Mg/Mg+Fe ratios in the 0.49 to 0.56 range; primary biotite from the altered granodiorite of Copper Canyon has a 0.65 to 0.69 ratio (Theodore et al., 1973). In addition, Czamanske determined that TiO_2 is depleted significantly in the hydrothermal biotite relative to the primary biotite of the granodiorite. Newly crystallized quartz and potassium feldspar, including small amounts of white mica, are concentrated in some of the granodiorite dominated by abundant hydrothermal biotite and hydrothermal apatite and sphene. Plagioclase laths, about 4 to 5 mm long, range from calcic oligoclase to andesine. Some are strongly zoned and euhedral, and have cores more calcic than rims, whereas others show oscillatory zoning. Most plagioclase crystals in domains where hydrothermal biotite is extensively developed seem to have remained fairly fresh; they have sharp lamella traces and extinction positions. Sparse white mica has recrystallized preferentially along margins and some crystallographic directions of the plagioclase. Near the northern edge of the granodiorite, sulfides locally make up about 2 volume percent. Pyrite and chalcopyrite are ubiquitous; pyrrhotite, arsenopyrite, sphalerite, molybdenite, and marcasite occur in various associations along veinlets and as disseminations in hydrothermal biotite-rich domains. Pyrrhotite and molybdenite occur more commonly at depth, and paragenetically late chalcocite and covellite are sprinkled throughout. Concentrations of molybdenite in the granodiorite are low—approximately 100 to 200 ppm molybdenum—and most of the molybdenite occurs in quartz-potassium feldspar veinlets in the granodiorite.

Phyllic, Transitional, Propylitic Alteration

Preliminary petrographic studies suggest that rocks between the potassic core and the edge of the iron-sulfide halo include mineral assemblages typical of the other classic alteration zones characteristic of porphyry copper systems. These rocks may be classified broadly as (1) phyllic (sericitic), (2) transitional (including at Copper Canyon minerals typical of the skarn, phyllic, and propylitic zones), and (3) propylitic (Blake et al., 1978). Generally, these three zones, listed in order of occurrence outward from the potassic core, are very weakly developed. Although some rocks altered to and veined by quartz-white mica-pyrite assemblages occur in a narrow irregular phyllic zone just outside the potassic core, similar mineral assemblages occur locally within the potassic core. These occurrences provide compelling evidence from their paragenetic relations that alteration to phyllic assemblages post-dates the potassic alteration at Copper Canyon. In some of the granodiorite a plagioclase destructive type of alteration post-dates the widespread potassic alteration in highly irregular zones that generally are structurally controlled and are near the Virgin fault. Some zones measure about 60 to 90 m in plan and depth. In these zones, plagioclase is strongly replaced by white mica and minor kaolinite to the extent that only euhedral shadows of fine-grained white mica indicate the former presence of plagioclase. In addition, relict primary potassium feldspar phenocrysts locally have been heavily altered to white mica, and some secondary biotite has been converted to white mica and chlorite, whereas secondary potassium feldspar in the groundmass remains unaltered.

Primary copper mineralization is not significant in rocks altered to quartz-white mica-pyrite or phyllic assemblages. There is some notable primary gold mineralization associated with propylitic alteration in two areas. Just north of the east orebody and at the Tomboy mine, 2.0 km south of the east orebody, the Battle Formation in the propylitic zone contains significant concentrations of gold and minimal copper. In these areas of gold mineralization, the pyrite:chalcopyrite ratio is about 15:1, and the total sulfide content, including significant concentrations of sphalerite and galena, is more than 4 percent.

FLUID-INCLUSION PETROLOGY, THERMOMETRY, AND CHEMISTRY

The petrology of the well-developed fluid inclusions prevalent throughout the porphyry copper system at Copper Canyon has been studied intensely (Nash and Theodore, 1971; Theodore and Nash, 1973; Batchelder, 1977; Theodore and Blake, 1978). Briefly, these studies have demonstrated a correspondence among geologic events, related hypogene alteration phenomena, and types of fluid inclusions. Fluid-inclusion studies of skarn from the west orebody suggest that early crystallization of skarn occurred at temperatures of about 500° ±50°C, most likely from moderately saline fluids, generally of about 15 to 20 weight percent NaCl equivalent (Theodore and Blake, 1978). Temperatures were probably about 320° ±40°C during the subsequent crystallization of most of the ores in the skarn and east orebody; the fluids by then were highly saline, possibly about 35-45 weight percent NaCl equivalent (Nash and Theodore, 1971). The evolution of the porphyry system at Copper Canyon through a highly saline hydrothermal stage characterized by halite-bearing and gas-rich inclusions is similar to that of most other porphyry copper deposits (Nash, 1976). Fluid-inclusion relations also suggest that the andradite-bearing assemblages in the skarn at Copper Canyon crystallized under lithostatic or greater than lithostatic conditions, possibly about 380 bars or more, whereas the paragenetically later assemblages (potassic and phyllic) may have formed under hydrostatic conditions of about 150 bars, with the fluid boiling (as indicated by the coexistence of gas-rich and liquid-rich inclusions of the same age). During the final hypogene stages of development of the west orebody, late-stage fluids migrated through the rocks at 160 to 220°C concomitant with the emplacement of minor chlorite-iron oxide-carbonate veinlets (Theodore and Blake, 1978). In the east orebody, temperatures during the late hypogene stages seem to have been somewhat hotter, about 250 to 370°C, and dilute, about 1.2 to 12 weight percent NaCl equivalent (Nash and Theodore, 1971). These late-stage fluids may have deposited some of the gold there.

The areal extent of high-salinity fluid inclusions has been mapped around the deposits at Copper Canyon (Theodore and Nash, 1973; Nash, 1976). The zone within which the high-salinity fluids circulated surrounds the granodiorite unevenly and extends into the Pumpernickel Formation about 300 m from the western contact of the granodiorite and through the Battle, Harmony, and Scott Canyon formations about 2,500 m from the eastern contact. As the zone of high-salinity fluids centers on the east orebody, these fluids thus apparently circulated through a mass of rock smaller than the extent of rock visibly mineralized by more than 1 percent dispersed iron sulfides. Because this zone is smaller than the sulfide halo, mapping of fluid zonations provides an additional method to focus exploration efforts (Nash, 1976). Penetration of the high-salinity fluids into the Pumpernickel Formation may have been retarded partially by the cap-rock effect of a thick sequence of chert in the upper member (Theodore and Blake, 1975). Circulation of these fluids through the Battle, Harmony, and Scott Canyon formations may have been enhanced by abundant pre-mineralization structures and several small granodiorite bodies at depth, east of the altered granodiorite of Copper Canyon. These small intrusive bodies may have acted as additional satellitic heat sources to help drive the circulating fluids. There does not seem to be a strong correspondence between the zone of high-salinity fluid inclusions and a distinct type of silicate alteration (compare Theodore and Nash, 1973, and Blake et al., 1978). West of the altered granodiorite, the high-salinity zone seems to extend only through the phyllic zone, whereas east of the granodiorite, the high-salinity zone extends to the outer edge of the sulfide halo. Moore and Nash (1974) found no detectable difference in the fluid-inclusion populations of the phyllic and potassic alteration zones in the Bingham Canyon, Utah, porphyry copper deposit.

STABLE ISOTOPE STUDIES

Extensive studies of the stable isotopes of oxygen and hydrogen of inclusion fluids and of various hydrothermal minerals from the porphyry system were conducted by Batchelder (1977). The small laccolithic granodiorite associated spatially with the deposits at Copper Canyon is surrounded by widespread visible signs of alteration, as described above. In surficial exposures potassic alteration assemblages are common to 600 m from the granodiorite; hydrothermal biotite is the dominant zonal indicator mineral. Although alteration and metallization at Copper Canyon reflect a relatively dry porphyry system as compared with many other porphyry copper deposits, both the extent of the alteration and the amount of metal deposited seem to require fluids other than those emanating solely from a small magma that crystallizes in an epizonal environment. Fluids in the potassic zones of porphyry deposits are considered generally to be dominated by magmatic water (Taylor, 1974). Batchelder (1977) established the origin of fluids involved in the generation of the porphyry system at Copper Canyon by determination of $\delta^{18}O$ and δD of various minerals.

The $\delta^{18}O$ values of 12 samples of hydrothermal quartz range from +11.3 to +15.1 (Batchelder, 1977). Most of these quartz samples are from sulfide-bearing veins in the east orebody; two are from gold vein deposits peripheral to the core of Cu-Au-Ag metallization centered on the altered granodiorite. Filling temperatures of fluid inclusions are in the 220 to 395°C range; temperatures during crystallization of quartz were inferred from these fluid-inclusion data, then used to calculate the $\delta^{18}O$ of water in equilibrium with quartz. The values of $\delta^{18}O$ of the water calculated to be in equilibrium with quartz are +3.2 to +9.2; most likely water of such a composition reflects isotopic exchange between a light fluid and heavy metasedimentary wall rock (Batchelder, 1977). There is apparently no systematic variation of the calculated isotope composition of these fluids relative to the altered granodiorite of Copper Canyon geographically. Some of the most isotopically heavy fluids in the Copper Canyon area, in fact, are those associated with quartz-pyrite-gold veins at the Tomboy mine, 2.0 km south of the east orebody. The introduction of the bulk of the gold into the west and east orebodies most probably occurred late in their overall paragenetic history (Nash and Theodore, 1971; Theodore and Blake, 1975). The δD values of waters released from fluid inclusions trapped in quartz in the east orebody have values in the –76 to –102 range; values of δD for the inclusion waters released from vein quartz at the two peripheral gold vein deposits studied also fall within this range.

The $\delta^{18}O$ and δD of five samples of biotite were measured by Batchelder (1977): $\delta^{18}O$ values systematically range from +7.8 for an unaltered primary biotite collected from a small pluton 4.8 km west-southwest of Copper Canyon to +3.3 for secondary, very fine grained biotite from the Battle Formation in the east orebody. Determinations of the $\delta^{18}O$ of primary biotites from the altered granodiorite of Copper Canyon yield intermediate values, +7.2 to +6.0. These biotites from the altered granodiorite are seemingly unaltered when viewed under the microscope, but they are set in a fine-grained potassic-altered groundmass. Moreover, δD values show a fairly good correlation of lighter δD values with lighter $\delta^{18}O$ values. δD of the secondary biotite from the east orebody is –139. Temperatures at the time isotope equilibrium was established for these biotites have been calculated from $\delta^{18}O$ values of coexisting quartz and biotite, using the relation qtz-msc = 0.54 qtz-bio (Garlick and Epstein, 1967) and the variability of temperature as a function of muscovite-quartz fractionation determined by Bottinga and Javoy (1973). These temperatures are in fairly good agreement with the filling temperature data (Batchelder, 1977); for example, $\delta^{18}O$ values of coexisting quartz and biotite from the east orebody yield a temperature of 380°C—about the same as the fluid-inclusion data (see Nash and Theodore, 1971, for additional discussion of the thermal history of the east orebody). The isotopic compositions of water in equilibrium with the biotites at these temperatures were then calculated. The calculated isotopic composition of water at 800°C in equilibrium with the unaltered primary biotite obtained from the small pluton west-southwest of Copper Canyon (+10.4 $\delta^{18}O_{H_2O}$, –76 δD_{H_2O}) probably most closely approaches the isotopic makeup of uncontaminated magmatic water evolved from the suite of late Eocene or early Oligocene granodiorites emplaced into the district. The isotopic composition of normal magmatic water has a δD value in the –50 to –85 range and a $\delta^{18}O$ value of about +5.5 to +10.0 (Taylor, 1974). The $\delta^{18}O$ of water calculated to be in equilibrium with three primary biotite samples from the granodiorite is in the +8.6 to +9.8 range; δD of these biotites is in the –91 to –97 range, about 10 per mil lighter than normal magmatic water. It is very likely that the isotopic data from the three biotites obtained from the altered granodiorite of Copper Canyon reflect a subsolidus stage of isotopic exchange established between these biotites and heated water somewhat lighter isotopically than magmatic water. This may be a relatively late event and may have occurred during circulation there of a very high temperature (about 550°C) but low-density fluid of a mixed magmatic and meteoric character.

SUMMARY

A highly simplified overall sequence of geologic events at Copper Canyon might have been (1) recrystallization of andradite-diopside in the skarn and a widespread halo of early potassic assemblages; (2) rise of the granodiorite magma to where it is now exposed; and (3) growth of a second generation of potassic mineral assemblages, partly in the west orebody, but especially concentrated in the east orebody and in the granodiorite. Circulation of heated fluids that were primarily associated with andradite-diopside skarn seems to have focused on rocks west of the Virgin fault. The absence of skarn in the porous, calcareous, and hematitic conglomerate of the Battle Formation that is in contact with the granodiorite at the east orebody strongly suggests that the granodiorite did not provide the fluids involved in generation of the skarn; instead, the skarn probably reflects an intruding magma, precursor to the exposed granodiorite, at depth, initially moving up along the Copper Canyon fault system. Intrusion and alteration may have shifted eastward to the Virgin fault system and continued with a subsequent emplacement of the altered granodiorite of Copper Canyon in its present position. Its emplacement disrupted earlier fluid flow in the immediate wall rocks and contributed significantly toward repeated passage of copper-bearing fluids through the skarn. These fluids caused paragenetically complex mineral assemblages to form in the skarn and eventually led to economic concentrations of copper, gold, and silver in the west orebody. After the granodiorite had reached its present level, the bulk of the ores at Copper Canyon then formed in the east orebody, east of the Virgin fault. Fluids isotopically light relative to normal magmatic ones seem to have equilibrated with quartz and primary and secondary biotite during their crystallization. This relation probably reflects entry during the potassic alteration stage of some meteoric fluids into the core of this porphyry system as it evolved. Access of these meteoric fluids most likely occurred along deeply penetrating pre-metallization structures.

REFERENCES CITED

Batchelder, John, 1977, Light-stable-isotope and fluid-inclusion study of the porphyry copper deposit at Copper Canyon, Nevada: Econ. Geol., v. 72, p. 60–70.

Batchelder, John; Theodore, T. G.; and Blake, D. W., 1976, Stable isotopes and geology of the Copper Canyon porphyry copper deposits, Lander County, Nevada: AIME, SME Trans., v. 260, no. 3, p. 232–236.

Blake, D. W.; Theodore, T. G.; and Kretschmer, E. L., 1978, Alteration and distribution of sulfide mineralization at Copper Canyon, Lander County, Nevada: Ariz. Geol. Soc. Digest XI, p. 67–78.

Bottinga, Y., and Javoy, M., 1973, Comments on oxygen isotope geothermometry, Earth and Planet. Sci. Ltrs., no. 20, p. 250–265.

Garlick, G. D., and Epstein, S., 1967, Oxygen isotope ratios in co-existing minerals of regionally metamorphosed rocks: Geochim. et Cosmochim. Acta, v. 31, p. 181–214.

McDowell, F. W., and Kulp, J. L., 1967, Age of intrusion and ore deposition in the Robinson mining district of Nevada: Econ. Geol., v. 62, p. 905–909.

Moore, W. J., and Nash, J. T., 1974, Alteration and fluid-inclusion studies of the porphyry copper ore body at Bingham, Utah: Econ. Geol., v. 69, p. 631–645.

Nash, J. T., 1976, Fluid-inclusion petrology—data from porphyry copper deposits and applications to exploration: U.S. Geol. Survey Prof. Paper 907-D, p. D1-D16.

Nash, J. T., and Theodore, T. G., 1971, Ore fluids in the porphyry copper deposit at Copper Canyon, Nevada: Econ. Geol., v. 66, p. 385–399.

Roberts, R. J., 1964, Stratigraphy and structure of the Antler Peak quadrangle, Humboldt and Lander Counties, Nevada: U.S. Geol. Survey Prof. Paper 459-A, p. A1–A93.

———, 1966, Metallogenic provinces and mineral belts in Nevada: Nev. Bur. Mines Rept. 13, pt. A, p. 47–72.

Roberts, R. J., and Arnold, D. C., 1965, Ore deposits of the Antler Peak quadrangle, Humboldt and Lander Counties, Nevada: U.S. Geol. Survey Prof. Paper 459-B, p. B1–B94.

Sayers, R. W.; Tippett, M. C.; and Fields, E. D., 1968, Duval's new copper mines show complex geologic history: Min. Eng., v. 20, no. 3, p. 55–62.

Shawe, D. R., and Stewart, J. H. , 1976, Ore deposits as related to tectonics and magmatism, Nevada and Utah: AIME, SME Trans., v. 260, p. 225–232.

Silberman, M. L.; Stewart, J. H.; and McKee, E. H., 1976, Igneous activity, tectonics, and hydrothermal precious-metal mineralization in the Great Basin during Cenozoic time: AIME, SME Trans., v. 260, p. 253–263.

Stewart, J. H.; Moore, W. J.: and Zietz, Isidore, 1977, East-west patterns of Cenozoic igneous rocks, aeromagnetic anomalies, and mineral deposits, Nevada and Utah: Geol. Soc. America Bull., v. 88, p. 67–77.

Taylor, H. P., Jr., 1974, The application of oxygen and hydrogen isotope studies to problems of hydrothermal alteration and ore deposition: Econ. Geol., v. 69, p. 843–883.

Theodore, T. G., and Blake, D. W., 1975, Geology and geochemistry of the Copper Canyon porphyry copper deposit and surrounding area, Lander County, Nevada: U.S. Geol. Survey Prof. Paper 798-B, 86 p.

———, 1978, Geology and geochemistry of the west orebody and associated skarns, Copper Canyon porphyry copper deposits, Lander County, Nevada, *with a section on* Electron microprobe analyses of andradite and diopside *by* N. G. Banks: U-S. Geol. Survey Prof. Paper 798-*C*, 85 p.

Theodore, T. G., and Nash, J. T., 1973, Geochemical and fluid zonation, Copper Canyon, Lander County, Nevada: Econ. Geol., v. 68, p. 565–570.

Theodore, T. G.; Silberman, M. L.; and Blake, D. W., 1973, Geochemistry and K-Ar ages of plutonic rocks in the Battle Mountain mining district, Lander County, Nevada: U.S. Geol. Survey Prof. Paper 798-A, 24 p.

Theodore, T. G.; Venuti, P. E.; Page, N. J; and Carlson, R. R., 1976, Maps showing distribution of palladium and other elements in rocks at Iron Canyon, Lander County, Nevada: U.S. Geol. Survey Map, MF-790, 2 sheets.

Titley, S. R., 1972, Intrusion and wall rock, porphyry copper deposits: Econ. Geol., v. 67, p. 122–123.

Wells, J. D., and Silberman, M. L., 1973, K-Ar age of mineralization at Buckhorn, Eureka County, Nevada: Isochron/West, no. 8, p. 37–38.

About the Contributors

DANIEL M. AIKEN, a graduate of the University of Oregon, has held the position of mine geologist at Duval Corporation's Sierrita and Esperanza mines since 1979. He was previously assigned to Duval Exploration and has also served as pit geologist at Sierrita-Esperanza.

JAMES A. ANDERSON has been executive vice president of exploration and corporate development for Homestake Mining Company in San Francisco since 1975. He earned his doctorate at Harvard in 1965 and has worked as a research geologist with Kennecott Copper and as vice president of U.S. exploration with Occidental Minerals. A member of several professional organizations, in 1978 he was appointed by the Governor to the California State Mining and Geology Board.

KENT D. AVESON joined Conoco in 1974 and was involved with the geological and mine evaluation of the Poston Butte porphyry copper deposit at Florence, Arizona. He joined Union Energy Mining Division of Union Oil Company in 1977 and has been involved in evaluation and feasibility studies of metallic and uranium deposits. While with Union Oil, he has been project engineer and project manager and has worked on the company's oil shale project in Colorado.

NORMAN G. BANKS spent nine years in the detailed study of the Ray porphyry copper deposits and in the mapping of other deposits in south central Arizona. He holds a Ph.D. from the University of California at San Diego and since 1967 has been employed by the U.S. Geological Survey, where he has worked on a variety of projects, including the mapping of porphyry copper mineralization in Washington. He has also worked in volcanology in Hawaii and on Mt. St. Helens.

CHARLES F. BARTER has spent most of his professional life working on the copper deposits of southeastern Arizona. A senior geologist for the ANAMAX Mining Company, he has earned degrees from the University of Illinois and the University of Arizona.

RICHARD E. BEANE, a geochemist with AMAX Exploration, Inc., in Tucson, Arizona, earned his Ph.D. from Northwestern University in 1972. He has taught at the university level, where his research was oriented toward various aspects of the genesis of base metal deposits in the Southwest.

DAVID W. BLAKE has served as mine geologist at Battle Mountain, Nevada, and as regional geologist responsible for precious metal exploration in northern Nevada for the Duval Corporation. He has been with Duval since 1967, and was previously involved in porphyry copper exploration in Arizona and New Mexico with the Bear Creek Mining Company.

MAURICE A. CHAFFEE has participated in a number of geochemical investigations in the western U.S. and northern Mexico. He received his Ph.D. from the University of Arizona in 1964, and, after working in private industry for several years as an exploration and mining geologist, joined the U.S. Geological Survey, Branch of Exploration Research in Denver. His special interest is in the development and improvement of geochemical exploration techniques related to porphyry copper deposits and the arid environment.

DAVID S. COOK has participated in exploration programs in several western states. He has been with Inspiration Consolidated Copper Company since 1974, first as mine geologist at the company's operations at Christmas, and subsequently as superintendent of mine planning and geology at the Christmas division.

HENRY R. CORNWALL joined the U.S. Geological Survey in 1943. His work included eleven years mapping and studying the copper deposits in the Ray area of southern Arizona, ten years mapping and researching gold and silver deposits in Nevada, and eleven years of research in petrology and ore genesis in the Michigan native copper deposits. He retired from U.S.G.S. in 1980.

ROBERT B. CUMMINGS joined ASARCO, Inc. as an exploration geologist in 1967, after earning a B.S. in geological engineering from Michigan Technological University. Since 1973 he has been resident geologist at Asarco's Sacaton mine.

PETER G. DUNN has been involved with porphyry copper exploration since 1965—until 1972 with Bear Creek Mining Company and Kennecott in Arizona and South America and, since 1973, as chief geologist with Quintana Minerals. He earned degrees from Yale and from Stanford University and has worked underground as a mining engineer at Miami Copper and as a geologist with the Bureau of Mineral Resources and with Mount Isa Mines in Australia.

MARCO T. EINAUDI has been a professor of applied earth sciences and geology at Stanford University since 1975. His principle research interests have been the geology and geochemistry of porphyry- and skarn-type mineral deposits. He earned his Ph.D. from Harvard University in 1969 and, before joining the faculty at Stanford, worked for the Anaconda Company in Nevada and Utah, where he concentrated on detailed mine studies and mineral exploration.

PAUL GILMOUR, a consultant in geology since 1968, has worked on a variety of mineral deposits, resource appraisals, and mineral economics studies in North, Central, and South America; the U.K. and western Europe; the Middle East; southern Africa; and Australia. He received his Ph.D. from the University of Edinburgh in 1955 and has worked in several provinces in Canada. He has published articles on petrofabrics, the classification of mineral deposits, ore-reserve estimation, massive pyritic sulfide deposits, and porphyry copper deposits.

FREDERICK T. GRAYBEAL, chief geologist of ASARCO, Inc., was resident geologist at Silver Bell for ASARCO and then spent three years as exploration geologist with West Range Company. He earned his Ph.D. from the University of Arizona in 1972 and taught at the university level before rejoining ASARCO in 1971, where he has also served as exploration geologist and manager of southwest exploration.

TOM L. HEIDRICK, exploration manager of Gulf Mineral Resources, holds an M.S. degree from the University of Colorado. He has taught at Washington State University and the University of Arizona. He has worked in regional geologic studies for the U.S. Geological Survey and was previously employed by Silver King Mines in Nevada and by the Climax Molybdenum Company in Colorado.

LOUIS J. JANSEN, senior geologist in the mine planning division of ASARCO, Inc., spent ten years as mine geologist at the Mission and San Xavier mines near Tucson. He received an M.S. degree in geology from the University of Arizona in 1972 and worked for American Potash at their Searles Lake evaporite deposit before joining ASARCO, where he has also worked in operational geology in New Mexico.

JAMES L. KELLY has been chief geologist at the Twin Buttes mines since exploration and development was started there in 1963 by The Anaconda Company. He graduated from Montana College of Mineral Science and Technology with a B.S. degree in geological engineering in 1941, and has worked in geological exploration for The Anaconda Company in the western U.S., Mexico, Canada, and Chile. He was also chief geologist for Anaconda's uranium operations in New Mexico during the initial stages of exploration and development.

JOHN R. KING, southwest district geologist in charge of metals exploration for the Anaconda Copper Company, has been continuously involved throughout his professional career in exploration for metals throughout the western U.S., eastern Canada, Mexico, and the Philippines. He holds an M.S. degree in geology from Oregon State University and has also worked for ASARCO, Inc.

JOSEPH KOLESSAR, chief geologist at the Tyrone Branch of Phelps Dodge in Tyrone, New Mexico, earned a B.S. degree from the University of Arizona in 1950. Before taking the position at Tyrone, he spent sixteen years as geologist at the Copper Queen Branch of Phelps Dodge in Bisbee.

RANDOLPH A. KOSKI, geologist for the U.S. Geological Survey in the Branch of Pacific-Arctic Geology, Office of Marine Geology, earned his Ph.D. from Stanford University in 1978. He has been involved in studies of massive sulfide and stratiform manganese deposits in the western Cordillera and of sea-floor manganese deposits in the Gulf of Alaska.

EDWARD L. KRETSCHMER spent six years as mine geologist at Duval Corporation's Battle Mountain properties in Nevada. He received a B.S. in geology from the University of Nevada, Reno, in 1974 and, after working for Duval, became a geologist for the Pinson Mining Company.

JACKSON M. LANGTON, manager of the Superior Oil International Minerals Division, received a B.S. in geological engineering and an M.S. in geology from Oklahoma University in 1963. His knowledge of the Dos Pobres deposit is based on his experience as chief geologist of the Phelps Dodge Morenci-Metcalf Branch; in this capacity he had supervision over exploration and development work in Arizona and New Mexico.

PHILIP W. NASON joined CONOCO in 1973 to work on the Poston Butte project and was project geologist through the final phase, which terminated in 1977. He graduated from the University of Massachusetts in 1964 with a degree in geology and carried out post-graduate studies at the Montana School of Mines, while employed by the Anaconda Company. He later joined Casa Grande Copper Company, a subsidiary of the Hanna Mining Company.

DENIS L. NORTON, a professor of geosciences at the University of Arizona, has studied magma-hydrothermal processes and their role in the formation of ore deposits over most of his professional career. His interest in how ore deposits form began in 1960, when he worked as a stope miner at Butte and did graduate work at the Montana School of Mines. After completing graduate studies at the University of California, he pursued the study of ore deposits as a research geochemist with Kennecott Copper Corporation. Since 1973 he has been involved with theoretical analyses that apply transport theory, computer techniques, and field observations to the determination of the geological history of magma-hydrothermal systems.

ALLEN V. SHAW worked as geologist on Conoco's Poston Butte (Florence) project; previously he was an exploration geologist in their Uranium Division. A senior geologist with Conoco Energy Development Company in Dallas, Texas, he earned a B.S. in geology from Tufts University and an M.S. in geology from Michigan State University in 1965.

TED G. THEODORE, a geologist with the Branch of Western Mineral Resources of the U.S. Geological Survey, has carried out extensive research in many aspects of ore genesis, ranging from regional studies to mineral chemistry, and has authored many publications, in both U.S.G.S. media and journals, concerning ore deposits and ore genesis. He completed his Ph.D. at the University of California at Los Angeles and joined the Survey in 1967.

SPENCER R. TITLEY, professor of geosciences at the University of Arizona, has carried out research in metals deposit geology in many regions of the Pacific Basin rim, chiefly in southwestern North America and the southwestern Pacific. He is the author of numerous articles in professional journals and has served on the Editorial Board of *Economic Geology;* he was senior editor of *Geology of the Porphyry Copper Deposits, Southwestern North America.* He earned his Ph.D. from the University of Arizona and was awarded the Medal for Distinguished Achievement in Mineral Engineering by the Colorado School of Mines in 1975.

LUIS A. VEGA has been a geologist at Duval Corporation's Mineral Park property since 1976. He received a B.S. degree from the University of Arizona in 1973 and has worked as an exploration geologist in the western United States.

RICHARD J. WEST joined the Duval Corporation in 1973 as a mining geologist at the Sierrita-Esperanza mine, and in 1975 he was promoted to chief mine geologist. He earned a B.S. degree in geology from MacKay School of Mines and since 1979 has been employed by Pincock, Allen & Holt as an engineering geologist involved in domestic and foreign geotechnical work.

WILLIAM H. WILKINSON, JR., has worked as mine geologist at Duval Corporation's Mineral Park operations and as a geologist in Duval's Exploration Department in Tucson, Arizona. He completed his Ph.D. degree at the University of Arizona in 1981.

SIDNEY A. WILLIAMS has been director of the Geological Laboratory for Phelps Dodge Corporation in Douglas, Arizona, since 1965, where he has been engaged in the application of petrography and geochemistry in base and precious metals exploration. He earned his Ph.D. from the University of Arizona in 1957 and has taught briefly at the university level. He has also worked for Silver King Mines as a mineralogist in precious metals exploration.

Index